THE PILL BOOK, 15th REVISED EDITION: THE ILLUSTRATED GUIDE TO THE MOST PRESCRIBED DRUGS IN THE UNITED STATES

Illustrated with 32 pages of actual-size color photographs

With more than 18.5 million copies in print, *The Pill Book* is the bestselling consumer drug reference ever, offering the most up-to-date, comprehensive information in a newly redesigned format that is even easier to use.

This new 15th edition of *The Pill Book* contains more profiles of commonly prescribed drugs than any other consumer reference. Compiled by a team of eminent pharmacologists, it is based on official, FDA-approved information usually available only to doctors and pharmacists, plus the latest information gathered from computer databases and online resources. It synthesizes the most important facts about each drug in a concise, readable, easy-to-understand entry.

Here are complete profiles on more than 1800 of the most commonly prescribed drugs, including:

- Generic and brand names
- What the drug is for and how it works
- Usual dosages, and what to do if a dose is skipped
- Side effects and possible adverse reactions, highlighted for quick reference
- Interactions with other drugs and foods
- Alcohol-free and sugar-free medications
- The most popular self-injected medications and their safe handling
- Information for seniors, pregnant and breast-feeding women, and others with special needs

This completely revised and updated 15th edition contains dozens of new brand names and more than 20 important new drugs recently approved by the FDA now on sale for the first time.

THE PILL BOOK

15th EDITION

Editor-in-Chief

HAROLD M. SILVERMAN, Pharm. D.

Production

ButterWorks Limited
Kenoza Type, Inc.
Miwako Nishizawa, mouse+tiger design

Consultants

THOMAS SUTHERLAND, R. Ph.
ROBERT KRAUSS, R. Ph.
NEERGARD PHARMACIES, NEW YORK

JUDITH I. BROWN
JENNIFER KITCHIN, MD

Digital Photography and Color Separations

CORAL GRAPHICS
STUDIO 365

Photography

BENN MITCHELL

Original Creators of THE PILL BOOK
HAROLD M. SILVERMAN, Pharm. D.
GILBERT I. SIMON, Sc.D.
LAWRENCE D. CHILNICK
BERT STERN

BANTAM BOOKS
NEW YORK

A Bantam Books Mass Market Original

Published in the United States by Bantam Books, an imprint of The Random House Publishing Group, a division of Random House, Inc., New York.

Previous editions of this book were published by Bantam Books in 1979, 1982, 1986, 1990, 1992, 1994, 1996, 1998, 2000, 2002, 2004, 2006, 2008, and 2010.

ISBN: 978-0-553-59356-3

Printed in the United States of America

www.bantamdell.com

9 8 7 6 5 4 3 2 1

Bantam mass market edition: May 2012

Contents

The purpose of this book is to provide educational information to the public concerning the majority of various types of prescription drugs that are presently used by licensed health care professionals. It is not intended to be complete or exhaustive or in any respect a substitute for personal medical care. *Only a licensed health care professional may prescribe these drugs and their exact dosages.*

While every effort has been made to reproduce products on the cover and insert of this book in an exact fashion, certain variations of size or color may be expected as a result of the printing process. Furthermore, pictures identified as brand-name drugs should not be confused with their generic counterparts. In any event, the reader should not rely solely upon the photographic image to identify any pills depicted herein, but should rely upon the licensed health care professional's prescription as dispensed by the pharmacist.

How to Use This Book

How to Find Your Medication in *The Pill Book*

- *The Pill Book* lists most medications in alphabetic order by generic name because a medication may have many brand names but has only 1 generic name. Most generic medications produce the same therapeutic effects as their brand-name equivalents but are much less expensive. Drugs that are available generically are indicated by the G symbol.
- When a medication has 2 or more active ingredients, it is listed by the most widely known brand name. In some cases, pill profiles are listed by drug type (e.g., Sulfonylurea Antidiabetes Drugs).
- *The Pill Book* includes the names of the top 100 brand-name drugs (cross-referenced to their generic name) in alphabetic order with the pill profiles.
- Most over-the-counter (OTC) medications are not included in *The Pill Book*. For complete information on OTC medications, refer to *The Pill Book Guide to Over-the-Counter Medications.*
- All brand and generic names are listed in the Index. Brand names are indicated by boldface.
- Sugar-free and alcohol-free brand-name drugs are indicated by the S and A symbols in the beginning of each pill profile.

The Pill Book, like pills themselves, should be used with caution. Viewed properly, this book may save you money and, perhaps, your life. It contains life-size pictures of the most prescribed brand-name drugs in the United States. *The Pill Book*'s product identification system is designed to help you check that the medication you are about to take is the one your doctor prescribed. Although many dosage forms are included, not all available forms and strengths of every medication have been shown. While every effort has been made to create accurate photographic reproductions of the products, some variations in size or color may be expected as a result of the printing process. Do not rely solely on the photographic images to identify your pills; check with your pharmacist if you have any product identification questions.

Each pill profile in *The Pill Book* contains the following information:

Generic and Brand Name: The generic name is the common name of the drug approved by the Food and Drug Administration (FDA). It is listed along with the current brand names available for each generic drug. Medications that are available in a generic form are indicated by the G symbol.

Most prescription drugs are sold in more than 1 dosage strength. Also, some drugs, such as oral contraceptives, come in packages containing different numbers of pills. A few manufacturers indicate these variations by adding letters or numbers to the basic drug name; for example, Loestrin 21 1.5/30 and Loestrin 21 1/20. (The numbers here refer to the number of tablets in each monthly packet, 21, and the amount of medication found in the tablets.) Other drugs come in different strengths: This is often indicated by a notation such as "DS" (double strength) or "Forte" (stronger).

The Pill Book lists generic and brand names together only where there are no differences in basic ingredients (e.g., Loestrin). However, the amount of the ingredient may vary from product to product. In most cases, the brand names and generic versions listed for each medication are interchangeable; you can use any version of the drug and expect that it will work for you. *The Pill Book* identifies within the profile those medications for which generic versions are not considered equivalent and which should not be interchanged with a brand-name product or another generic version of the same drug.

Type of Drug: Describes the general pharmacologic class of each drug: "antidepressant," "sedative," "decongestant," "expectorant," and so on.

Prescribed For: All drugs are approved for some symptoms or conditions by federal authorities, but doctors also commonly prescribe drugs for other, as yet unapproved, reasons; in some cases, these are also listed in *The Pill Book*. Check with your doctor if you are not sure why you have been given a certain pill.

General Information: Information on how the drug works, how long it takes for you to feel its effects, or a description of how this drug is similar to or different from other drugs.

Cautions and Warnings: This information alerts you to important and more dangerous reactions. Physical conditions, such as heart disease, that can have serious consequences if the medication is prescribed for you, are in bold type.

Possible Side Effects: Side effects are generally divided into 4 categories—those that are most common, common, less common, and rare—to help you better understand what to expect from your pills. If you are not sure whether you are experiencing a drug side effect, ask your doctor. *The Pill Book* does not include a complete listing of all possible drug side effects. Contact your doctor if you experience anything unusual while taking any medication.

Drug Interactions: Describes what happens when you combine your medication with other drugs and lists which drugs should not be taken at the same time as your medication. Some interactions may be deadly. At every visit, be sure to inform your doctor of any medication you are already taking.

Food Interactions: Provides information on foods to avoid while taking your medication, whether to take your medication with meals or on an empty stomach, and other important facts.

Usual Dose: Tells you the largest and smallest doses usually prescribed and gives dosage instructions for children and seniors, when applicable. You may be given different dosage instructions by your doctor. Do not change the dosage of ANY medication you take without first calling your doctor.

Overdosage: Describes overdose symptoms and what to do if you take too much medication.

Special Information: Includes symptoms to watch for, when to call your doctor, what to do if you forget a dose of your medication, and any special instructions.

Special Populations: *Pregnancy/Breast-feeding:* For women who are or might be pregnant, and what to do if you must take a medication during the time you are nursing your baby. *Seniors:* This section presents the special facts an older adult needs to know about every drug and explains how reactions may differ from those of a younger person.

In an Emergency!

Each year over 1 million people experience some form of drug-related poisoning in the United States. In 2010, more than 500,000 of these poisonings resulted in death or a serious outcome. In fact, drug overdose is a leading cause of fatal poisoning in the United States.

Although each of the pill profiles in *The Pill Book* has specific information on drug overdose, there are a few general rules to remember if you are faced with an accidental poisoning:

1. Make sure the victim is breathing, and call for medical help immediately.
2. Learn the phone number of your local poison control center and post it near the phone. Call the center in an emergency. When you call, be prepared to explain
   - What drug was taken and how much
   - Status of the victim (e.g., conscious, sleeping, vomiting, or having convulsions)
   - The approximate age and weight of the victim
   - Any chronic medical problems of the victim (e.g., diabetes, epilepsy, or high blood pressure), if you know them
   - What medications, if any, the victim takes regularly
3. Remove anything that might interfere with breathing. A person who is not getting enough oxygen will turn blue (the tongue or the skin under the fingernails changes color first). If this happens, lay the victim on his or her back, open the collar, place one hand under the neck, and lift, pull, or push the victim's jaw so that it juts outward. This will open the airway between the mouth and lungs as wide as possible. Begin mouth-to-mouth resuscitation ONLY if the victim is not breathing.
4. If the victim is unconscious or having convulsions, call for medical help immediately. While waiting for the ambulance, lay the victim on his or her stomach and turn the head to one side. Should the victim throw up, this will prevent inhalation of vomit. DO NOT give an unconscious victim anything by mouth. Keep the victim warm.

5. If the victim is conscious, call for medical help and give the victim an 8-oz. glass of water to drink. This will dilute the poison.

Only a small number of poisoning victims require hospitalization. Most may be treated with simple actions or need no treatment at all.

The poison control center may tell you to make the person vomit. The best way to do this is to use ipecac syrup, which is available over-the-counter at any pharmacy. Specific instructions on how much to give infants, children, or adults are printed on the label and will also be given by your poison control center. Remember, DO NOT make the victim vomit unless you have been instructed to do so. Never make the victim vomit if the victim is unconscious, is having a convulsion, or is experiencing a painful, burning feeling in the mouth or throat.

Be Prepared

The best way to deal with a poisoning is to be prepared for it. Do the following now:

1. Write the telephone number of your local poison control center next to your other emergency phone numbers.
2. Decide which hospital you will go to, if necessary, and how you will get there.
3. Buy 1 oz. of ipecac syrup from your pharmacy. The pharmacist will tell you how to use it. Remember, this is a potent drug to be used only if directed and stored out of reach of children.
4. Learn to give mouth-to-mouth resuscitation.

Reduce the Risk of Drug-Related Poisoning

1. Keep all medications in a locked place out of the reach of young children.
2. Do not store medications in containers that previously held food.
3. Do not remove the labels from bottles so that the contents are unknown.
4. To avoid taking the wrong medication, do not take your medicine in the dark or in a dimly lit room.
5. Discard all medications when you no longer need them by flushing them down the toilet.

The Most Commonly Prescribed Drugs in the United States, Generic and Brand Names, with Complete Descriptions of Drugs and Their Effects

Abilify *see **Aripiprazole,** page 121*

Generic Name

Abiraterone (uh-bih-RAT-tir-own)

Brand Names

Zytiga

Type of Drug

Androgen biosynthesis inhibitor.

Prescribed For

Prostate cancer.

General Information

Androgens fuel the growth of prostate cancer, and treatments for the disease generally target androgen production. Abiraterone works by blocking the CYP17 enzyme complex, needed for production of androgens (male hormones) in the testes, adrenal glands, and prostate. It is always prescribed, together with prednisone, for men with metastatic prostate cancer that continues despite treatment with hormones and chemotherapy with docetaxel. Studies have shown it significantly improves the chance of survival by up to about 4 months for those with metastatic prostate cancer that has not responded to other therapies. Abiraterone is broken down by liver enzymes.

Cautions and Warnings

Do not take abiraterone if you are **allergic** or **sensitive** to any of its ingredients.

Abiraterone may cause **liver disease**, as indicated by rising liver enzymes. If liver toxicity develops while you are taking this medicine, your doctor may have you stop taking it. If you resume taking abiraterone, it will be at a lower dose. It should not be used by people with severe liver disease.

This medicine should be used with caution if you have a history of **heart disease**. Its safety in Class III or IV heart failure has not been established. People with a history of heart disease should have their blood pressure and blood-potassium levels checked monthly and must be aware of possible fluid retention (leg, foot, hand, or face swelling; difficulty breathing; chest pain; and reduced urination).

Stressful situations and signs of adrenal gland failure may necessitate a change in your prednisone dose while you are taking abiraterone.

Possible Side Effects

- ▼ Most common: joint swelling or discomfort, arm or leg swelling, muscle discomfort, flushing, diarrhea, urinary infection, and cough.
- ▼ Common: low blood potassium (muscle cramps, possibly altered heart rhythms), high blood pressure, abnormal heart rhythms, frequent urination, nighttime urination, upset stomach, and upper-respiratory infection.
- ▼ Less common: chest pain or chest discomfort and heart failure.
- ▼ Rare: Adrenal insufficiency and other rare side effects may occur. Contact your doctor if you experience anything unusual while taking any medication.

Drug Interactions

- Abiraterone inhibits a principal drug-metabolizing enzyme, which is produced by the liver. Mixing abiraterone with drugs broken down by this enzyme can increase blood levels of such drugs. Abiraterone should not be mixed with antidepressants such as amitriptyline, clomipramine, desipramine, imipramine, and paroxetine; antipsychotics such as haloperidol, risperidone, and thioridazine; beta blockers such as metoprolol, propafenone, and timolol; and other drugs such as aripiprazole, codeine, dextromethorphan, duloxetine, flecainide, mexilletine, ondansetron, tamoxifen, tramadol, and venlafaxine; in some cases your doctor may reduce the dosage of a drug you are taking. Your health care provider or pharmacist can help you identify which drugs are safe to take.
- Avoid mixing abiraterone with atazanavir, clarithromycin, indinavir, itraconazole, ketoconazole, nefazodone, nelfinavir, ritonavir, saquinavir, telithromycin, and voriconazole. These drugs interfere with the production of the liver enzyme that breaks down abiraterone. Consequently, mixing these drugs with abiraterone may raise blood levels of abiraterone.

- Carbamazepine, phenobarbital, phenytoin, rifabutin, rifampin, and rifapentine can lower blood levels of abiraterone by stimulating the production of enzymes that break it down. Avoid mixing these drugs.

Food Interactions

Food increases the amount of abiraterone absorbed into the blood by 10 times. In order to ensure steady dosing, abiraterone must be taken on an empty stomach. Do not eat for at least 2 hours before or 1 hour after you have taken abiraterone.

Usual Dose

Adult: 1000 mg (4 pills) once a day with water on an empty stomach, along with 5 mg of prednisone twice a day; 250 mg once a day with 5 mg prednisone twice a day for people with moderate liver disease.

Child: not recommended.

Overdosage

There is no information on abiraterone overdose. In case of an overdose, take the victim to a hospital emergency room for monitoring and treatment. Heart and liver function should be checked. If you seek treatment, ALWAYS bring the prescription bottle or container.

Special Information

A very small number of people taking this medicine experienced adrenal gland failure. Low blood sugar, dehydration, weight loss, disorientation, weakness, tiredness, low blood pressure, dizziness or fainting especially when rising from a chair or bed, muscle aches, nausea, vomiting, and diarrhea can be signs of this relatively rare event. Patchy (even full body) tanning of the skin can also be a sign of adrenal failure. You may need a larger prednisone dose to accommodate for adrenal failure.

Alert your doctor to any stressful situation you are experiencing or anticipating while taking abiraterone.

If you forget a dose, take it as soon as you remember. If it is almost time for your next dose, skip the dose you forgot and continue with your regular schedule. Do not take a double dose of abiraterone. If you forget a dose of prednisone, take it as soon as you remember, unless it is almost time for your next dose. If that happens, skip the prednisone dose you forgot and continue with your regular schedule. Do not take a double dose. Call your doctor if you forget to take 2 or more abiraterone doses in a row. Your pharmacist can help if you have trouble remembering to take your medicine.

Do not chew or break abiraterone tablets.

It is not known if abiraterone or its breakdown products pass into semen. Use a condom if having sex with a pregnant woman during the time you are taking this medicine and for 1 week after you stop taking it. If the woman is able to become pregnant, use a condom plus one other form of birth control.

Special Populations

Pregnancy/Breast-feeding: Abiraterone is likely to harm a growing fetus. It is not intended for women and should never be used by any woman who is or might become pregnant. Women who must handle abiraterone tablets should wear gloves or other protection to prevent exposure to the drug.

It is not known if this drug passes into breast milk. Nursing mothers who must handle this drug should wear gloves and should consider using infant formula.

Seniors: The majority of people included in studies of this drug were at least 65 years old. No overall differences were seen between seniors and younger adults.

Generic Name

Acamprosate (ah-CAM-pro-sate)

Brand Names

Campral

Type of Drug

Synthetic neurochemical similar to the amino acid homotaurine.

Prescribed For

Alcoholism.

General Information

Acamprosate is used to help alcoholic patients stay alcohol-free after they have stopped drinking. Unlike other drugs used to help people stay away from alcohol, it does not cause people to have a physical reaction to alcohol. Acamprosate restores the balance between two chemical systems in the brain, glutamate and GABA, that are known to become unbalanced in alcoholics, but its exact action is not known. It may reduce alcohol craving. Acamprosate should be part of a program that includes counseling and support, and it should be started as soon as possible after alcohol withdrawal and continued even if the patient starts drinking again. This medication has not been proven to help patients if they are still drinking when they start treatment. Acamprosate has not been studied in patients who abuse other substances together with alcohol. Tolerance or addiction has not developed with acamprosate. It passes out of the body through the kidneys.

Cautions and Warnings

Do not take acamprosate if you are **allergic** or **sensitive** to any of its ingredients or if you have **severe kidney disease**. People with moderate **kidney disease** require a lower dosage of acamprosate.

People taking acamprosate may become depressed or have suicidal thoughts. It should be used with caution in people with a history of **depression** or **suicidal ideation**.

Acamprosate does not eliminate or ease alcohol withdrawal symptoms.

Acamprosate can affect your judgment, thinking, or coordination. Do not drive or operate dangerous machinery if you are taking this medicine.

Possible Side Effects

Almost 2 of every 3 people who take this medicine will experience a drug side effect.

- ▼ Most common: diarrhea.
- ▼ Common: headache, weakness, anxiety, depression, and sleep problems.
- ▼ Less common: pain, accidental injuries, nausea, stomach gas, dizziness, dry mouth, tingling in the hands or feet, itching, sweating, chest pain, loss of appetite, weight gain or loss, impotence, abnormal vision, rash, vomiting, and constipation.
- ▼ Rare: heart or kidney failure, suicidality, psoriasis, hypothyroidism, rheumatoid arthritis, and urinary tract infections. Rare side effects can occur in almost any part of the body. Contact your doctor if you experience anything unusual while taking any medication.

Drug Interactions

- Mixing acamprosate with naltrexone can increase the levels of both drugs in the blood, but no dose adjustments are needed.

Food Interactions

You may take acamprosate with or without food.

Usual Dose

Adult: two 333-mg tablets 3 times a day.
Child: not recommended.

Overdosage

The only symptom associated with acamprosate overdose has been diarrhea. Overdose victims should be taken to a hospital emergency room for observation and treatment. If you seek treatment, ALWAYS bring the prescription bottle or container.

Special Information

Contact your doctor if you are breast-feeding, pregnant, or thinking about becoming pregnant while taking this medicine.

Take care while driving a car or performing complex tasks.

If you forget to take a dose, take it as soon as possible. If you do not remember until it is almost time for your next dose, skip the dose you forgot and continue with your regular schedule. Contact your doctor if you forget to take 2 or more doses in a row. Do not take a double dose.

Acamprosate must be part of an ongoing treatment program. Do not stop taking it on your own, even if you start drinking again.

Special Populations

Pregnancy/Breast-feeding: Acamprosate can damage animal fetuses in doses that are approximately equal to those taken by people on this medicine. Women of childbearing age should use an effective contraceptive while taking this drug. Acamprosate should be taken during pregnancy only if your doctor determines that the potential benefit outweighs the risks.

Acamprosate passes into breast milk. Nursing mothers who must take this drug should use infant formula.

Seniors: Dosage reduction may be needed in seniors because of a general decline in kidney function due to age.

Type of Drug

ACE (Angiotensin-Converting Enzyme) Inhibitors

Brand Names

Generic Ingredients: Benazepril G
Lotensin

Generic Ingredients: Benazepril + Hydrochlorothiazide G
Lotensin HCT

Generic Ingredients: Captopril G
Capoten

Generic Ingredients: Captopril + Hydrochlorothiazide G
Capozide

Generic Ingredients: Enalapril G
Vasotec

Generic Ingredients: Enalapril + Hydrochlorothiazide G
Vaseretic

Generic Ingredients: Fosinopril G
Monopril

Generic Ingredients: Fosinopril + Hydrochlorothiazide G

Generic Ingredients: Lisinopril G
Prinivil Zestril

Generic Ingredients: Lisinopril + Hydrochlorothiazide G
Prinzide Zestoretic

Generic Ingredients: Moexipril G
Univasc

Generic Ingredients: Moexipril + Hydrochlorothiazide G
Uniretic

Generic Ingredients: Perindopril G
Aceon

Generic Ingredients: Quinapril G
Accupril

Generic Ingredients: Quinapril + Hydrochlorothiazide G
Accuretic Quinaretic

Generic Ingredients: Ramipril G
Altace

Generic Ingredients: Trandolapril G
Mavik

Generic Ingredients: Trandolapril + Verapamil
Tarka

Prescribed For

High blood pressure, heart failure, diabetic kidney disease, and post–heart attack management; also used for prevention of heart attacks and strokes, chronic kidney disease, swelling and fluid accumulation, Bartter's syndrome, Raynaud's disease, migraine, and high blood pressure associated with other medical conditions such as scleroderma. ACE inhibitors combined with the diuretic hydrochlorothiazide or the calcium channel blocker verapamil are used to treat high blood pressure.

General Information

ACE inhibitors prevent the conversion of a hormone called angiotensin I to another hormone called angiotensin II, a potent blood-vessel constrictor. Preventing this conversion relaxes blood vessels, thus reducing blood pressure and relieving symptoms of heart failure. These drugs also affect the production of other hormones and enzymes that help regulate blood-vessel dilation. The effects of ACE inhibitors are very similar; these drugs mainly differ in terms of their dosages and how they are eliminated from the body. Some ACE inhibitors need to be converted into an active form in the body before they work while others do not. Also, some ACE inhibitors may have a stronger effect on enzymes in tissues than on those in the blood, but the importance of this difference, or whether one ACE inhibitor is better than another, has not been determined.

Benazepril, captopril, enalapril, lisinopril, moexipril, perindopril, quinapril, and ramipril start working in 1–2 hours and continue to work for about 24 hours. Fosinopril begins working 2–6 hours after you take it.

Many ACE inhibitors contain combinations of antihypertensives. For more information see Hydrochlorothiazide, page 55, and Verapamil, page 225.

Cautions and Warnings

Do not take an ACE inhibitor if you are **allergic** or **sensitive** to another ACE inhibitor or any of its ingredients. Swelling of the face, extremities, or throat has been known to occur with ACE inhibitors, which can be dangerous (see "Special Information"). This effect is 2–4 times more common among **black patients** than other groups. Severe ACE inhibitor sensitivity reactions can also occur in **hemodialysis patients** and in those undergoing **venom immunization**.

ACE inhibitors may increase blood potassium to dangerously high levels, especially when taken with certain drugs (see "Drug Interactions"). Your doctor will monitor your blood-potassium levels while you take this medicine.

ACE inhibitors can damage the liver. Stop taking your medication and call your doctor if your skin or the whites of your eyes become yellow. Patients with **liver disease** may require a lower dosage of some ACE inhibitors.

ACE inhibitors can cause very low blood pressure.

They may affect kidney function. Your doctor should check your urine for protein content during the first few months of treatment. Dosage adjustment may be necessary if you have reduced kidney function.

These medicines can affect white-blood-cell counts, possibly increasing your susceptibility to infection. Your doctor should monitor your blood counts periodically.

These drugs may cause increased sensitivity to the sun. Use sunscreen and wear protective clothing.

ACE inhibitors may be less effective in some **black patients** with high blood pressure, especially when dietary salt intake is high. Nevertheless, they should still be considered useful blood pressure treatments.

Possible Side Effects

Chronic cough is a common side effect of all ACE inhibitors. The cough usually goes away a few days after you stop taking the medication. Benazepril, captopril, enalapril, fosinopril, lisinopril, moexipril, and quinapril are all available in combination with hydrochlorothiazide. For additional information about the side effects of these combinations, see Hydrochlorothiazide, page 55. Rare side effects associated with these drugs can occur in almost any part of the body.

Possible Side Effects *(continued)*

Contact your doctor if you experience anything unusual while taking any medication.

Benazepril

▼ Most common: dizziness, tiredness, headache, and nausea.

▼ Less common: low blood pressure.

Captopril

▼ Most common: rash, itching, and loss of taste.

▼ Less common: dizziness, tiredness, sleep disturbances, headache, tingling in hands or feet, chest pain, heart palpitations, feeling unwell, abdominal pain, nausea, vomiting, diarrhea, constipation, appetite loss, dry mouth, flushing, and difficulty breathing.

Enalapril

▼ Most common: dizziness, fatigue, low blood pressure, and headache.

▼ Less common: chest tightness or pain, fainting, abdominal pain, nausea, vomiting, diarrhea, bronchitis, urinary tract infection, difficulty breathing, weakness, and rash.

Fosinopril

▼ Most common: dizziness and muscle pain.

▼ Less common: chest pain, low blood pressure, fatigue, diarrhea, vomiting, nausea, and altered heart rhythms.

Lisinopril

▼ Most common: dizziness, headache, chest pain, fatigue, and low blood pressure.

▼ Less common: nausea, diarrhea, vomiting, abdominal pain, rash, and muscle weakness.

▼ Rare: Rare side effects can affect your muscles and joints, sex drive, liver, mental status, and respiratory tract.

Moexipril

▼ Most common: dizziness, tiredness, and diarrhea.

▼ Less common: low blood pressure, chest pain, headache, nausea, fainting, abdominal pain, vomiting, difficulty breathing, flushing, muscle aches, swelling in the hands or feet, and rash.

Possible Side Effects *(continued)*

Perindopril

▼ Most common: heart palpitations and protein in urine.

▼ Less common: low blood pressure, sinus irritation, viral infection, fever, upset stomach, pain in hands, and joint stiffness.

Quinapril

▼ Most common: dizziness, tiredness, and low blood pressure.

▼ Less common: nausea, vomiting, chest pain, rash, headache, and diarrhea.

Ramipril

▼ Most common: dizziness and low blood pressure.

▼ Less common: nausea, vomiting, weakness, fatigue, and fainting.

Trandolapril

▼ Most common: dizziness, low blood pressure, upset stomach, fainting, and muscle pain.

▼ Less common: chest pain, heart rhythm changes, and weakness.

For additional information about Tarka, see Verapamil, page 225.

Drug Interactions

- ACE inhibitors may increase blood-potassium levels, especially if taken with dyazide or other potassium-sparing diuretics, aldosterone blockers (e.g., eplerenone), aliskiren, cyclosporine, heparin, or trimethoprim. Left untreated, this can be fatal.
- Mixing any ACE inhibitor with an angiotensin II receptor antagonist (e.g., telmisartan) is not recommended because of the potential for kidney damage.
- All nonsteroidal anti-inflammatory drugs (NSAIDs), including aspirin, can interact with ACE inhibitors. Mixing an NSAID with an ACE inhibitor may carry a higher risk of kidney failure and death, though many people still take this combination. People taking aspirin to prevent a heart attack should use the lowest possible dose.
- When mixed with ACE inhibitors, everolimus increases the risk of swelling of the lips and throat, a potentially life-threatening

condition. Stop taking both drugs if this reaction occurs and call your doctor.

- Severe ACE inhibitor sensitivity reactions can occur in patients taking allopurinol.
- ACE inhibitors increase the effect of lithium by interfering with its passage out of the body via the kidneys; this combination must be used with caution.
- The blood-pressure-lowering effect of ACE inhibitors adds to that of diuretics and beta blockers. Any other drug that causes a rapid drop in blood pressure, including drugs men use for erectile dysfunction, should be used with caution if you are taking an ACE inhibitor.
- ACE inhibitors can decrease the effects of loop diuretics and a dose adjustment may be necessary.
- Mixing an ACE inhibitor with gold salts increases the risk of a nitritoid reaction with symptoms of flushing, low blood pressure, nausea, and vomiting. If these symptoms occur, one medication must be stopped.
- Antacids should be separated by 1–2 hours from each dose of your ACE inhibitor. People taking an acid-reducing pill (a proton-pump inhibitor or H_2 antagonist) may have trouble absorbing ACE inhibitors and may have to use a different medicine for their condition.
- Capsaicin is extremely irritating and may trigger or aggravate the cough associated with ACE inhibitor therapy.
- Phenothiazine sedatives and antivomiting drugs may increase the effects of ACE inhibitors.
- ACE inhibitors increase blood levels of digoxin, which may increase the chance of digoxin-related side effects.
- Mixing ACE inhibitors with a sulfonylurea antidiabetes drug or insulin may increase the risk of low blood sugar in people with diabetes.
- Iron salts reduce blood levels of captopril and should be taken at least 2 hours apart.
- Quinapril decreases the absorption of tetracycline by about ⅓, possibly because of quinapril's high magnesium content.
- Rifampin may reduce the effects of enalapril.
- The combination of perindopril and gentamicin should be used with caution. Mixing these medicines can increase the risk of kidney damage and reduce the effectiveness of perindopril.

Food Interactions

You may take benazepril, enalapril, fosinopril, lisinopril, perindopril, quinapril, ramipril, and trandolapril with food if they upset your stomach.

Captopril and moexipril must be taken on an empty stomach, at least 1 hour before or 2 hours after eating.

Usual Dose

Benazepril

Adult: 5–80 mg once a day or in 2 equally divided doses. People with poor kidney function may need a lower dosage.

Child (age 6 and over): 0.09–0.27 mg per lb. of body weight once a day.

Child (under age 6): not recommended.

Benazepril + Hydrochlorothiazide

Adult: 5/6.25–20/25 mg once or twice a day.

Child: not recommended.

Captopril

Adult: 25–450 mg in 2 or 3 divided doses. Dosage must be tailored to your needs. People with poor kidney function need a lower dosage.

Child (age 7 months to 17 years): 0.4 mg per lb. of body weight up to 450 mg a day in 3 divided doses.

Child (age 2–6 months): 0.01–2.7 mg per lb. of body weight 2–3 times a day.

Child (age 0–1 month): 0.005–0.023 mg per lb. of body weight every 8–12 hours.

Captopril + Hydrochlorothiazide

Adult: 25/15–150/50 mg in divided doses.

Child: not recommended.

Enalapril

Adult (age 16 and over): 2.5–40 mg a day in 1 or 2 doses. People with poor kidney function need a lower dosage.

Child (2 months to 16 years): 0.04 mg per lb. of body weight up to 40 mg once a day or in divided doses.

Enalapril + Hydrochlorothiazide

Adult: 5/12.5–20/50 mg once a day.

Child: not recommended.

Fosinopril

Adult: 10–40 mg once a day. People with liver disease may require lower dosages.

Child (more than 110 lbs.): 5–40 mg once a day.

Fosinopril + Hydrochlorothiazide

Adult: 10/12.5–20/12.5 mg once a day.

Child: not recommended.

Lisinopril

Adult: 5–40 mg once a day. For people with severe kidney disease, the dosage should be 2.5–40 mg once a day.

Child (age 6 and over): 0.03 mg per lb. of body weight once a day up to 40 mg once a day.

Child (age 5 and under): not recommended

Lisinopril + Hydrochlorothiazide

Adult: 10/12.5–40/50 mg once a day.

Child: not recommended.

Moexipril

Adult: 7.5–30 mg once a day or in divided doses. People with poor kidney function should take ½ the usual dose.

Child: not recommended.

Moexipril + Hydrochlorothiazide

Adult: 7.5/12.5–30/50 mg once a day.

Child: not recommended.

Perindopril

Adult: 4–16 mg a day. Seniors (age 65 and over) should take no more than 8 mg a day in 1 or 2 divided doses. People with moderate kidney disease should take 2–8 mg a day, while people with severe kidney disease should not take this drug.

Child: not recommended.

Quinapril

Adult: 5–80 mg a day or in divided doses. People with kidney disease may require a lower dosage.

Child (age 1–17): 5–80 mg once a day.

Quinapril + Hydrochlorothiazide

Adult: 10/12.5–40/50 mg once a day.

Child: not recommended.

Ramipril

Adult: 2.5–20 mg a day. For people with moderate to severe kidney disease, the dosage should be 1.25–5 mg a day.

Child: not recommended.

Trandolapril

Adult: 1–8 mg a day, or 2–8 mg a day for black patients, once a day or in divided doses. A lower starting dose (0.5 mg) may be appropriate when combined with a diuretic and in patients with kidney or liver problems.

Child: not recommended.

Trandolapril + Verapamil

Adult: 1/80–4/240 mg once a day with food.

Child: not recommended.

Overdosage

The principal effect of ACE inhibitor overdose is a rapid drop in blood pressure, as evidenced by dizziness or fainting. Take the overdose victim to a hospital emergency room immediately. If you seek treatment, ALWAYS bring the prescription bottle or container.

Special Information

ACE inhibitor reactions can include swelling of the face, lips, hands, and feet. This swelling can also affect the larynx (throat) and tongue and interfere with breathing. If this happens, go to a hospital at once. Contact your doctor if you develop a sore throat, mouth sores, abnormal heartbeat, sudden difficulty breathing, chest pain, persistent rash, or loss of taste perception.

Some people who start taking an ACE inhibitor after they are already on a diuretic (an agent that increases urination) experience a rapid drop in blood pressure after their first dose or when their dosage is increased. To prevent this from happening, your doctor may tell you to stop taking your diuretic 2 or 3 days before starting the ACE inhibitor or to increase your salt intake during that time. The diuretic may then be restarted gradually.

You may get dizzy if you rise to your feet too quickly from a sitting or lying position when taking one of these medicines.

Avoid strenuous exercise or very hot weather because heavy sweating or dehydration can cause a rapid drop in blood pressure.

Avoid over-the-counter diet pills, decongestants, and other stimulants that can raise blood pressure. Also, do not use potassium supplements or salt substitutes containing potassium without first consulting your doctor.

If you take your medication once a day and forget a dose, take it as soon as you remember. If it is within 8 hours of your next dose, skip the dose you forgot and continue with your regular schedule. If you take benazepril twice a day and miss a dose, take the missed dose right away. If it is within 4 hours of your next dose, take 1 dose immediately and another in 5 or 6 hours, and then go back to your regular schedule. Do not take a double dose.

Special Populations

Pregnancy/Breast-feeding: ACE inhibitors can cause fetal injury or death. Women who are or might become pregnant should not take any ACE inhibitor. If you become pregnant, stop taking the medication and contact your doctor immediately.

ACE inhibitors pass into breast milk. Nursing mothers who must take these medicines should use infant formula.

Seniors: Seniors may be more sensitive to the side effects of these drugs due to age-related changes in kidney and liver function.

Generic Name

Acetaminophen (uh-SEE-tuh-MIN-uh-fen) G

Brand Names

There are many brand-name acetaminophen products and most are available over the counter. Check with your pharmacist about which specific brands are available alcohol- or sugar-free.

Type of Drug

Antipyretic and analgesic.

Prescribed For

Relief of pain and fever for people who cannot or do not want to take aspirin or a nonsteroidal anti-inflammatory drug (NSAID). Acetaminophen may be given to children about to receive a dip-theria, tetanus, and pertussis vaccination to reduce the fever and pain that commonly follow the vaccination.

General Information

Acetaminophen is generally used to relieve pain and fever associated with the common cold, flu, viral infections, or other disorders where pain or fever may occur. It is also used to relieve pain in people who are allergic to aspirin, or those who cannot take aspirin because of potential interactions with other drugs such as oral anticoagulants. It can be used to relieve pain from a variety of sources, including arthritis, headache, muscle ache, menstrual cramping, and tooth and periodontal pain, although it does not reduce inflammation.

Cautions and Warnings

Do not take acetaminophen if you are **allergic** or **sensitive** to any of its ingredients. Do not take acetaminophen for more than 10 days in a row (5 days for children) unless directed by your doctor. Do not take more than is prescribed or recommended on the package.

Use this drug with extreme caution if you have **kidney or liver disease** or **viral infections of the liver**. Large amounts of alcohol increase the liver toxicity of large doses or overdoses of acetaminophen. Avoid **alcohol** if you regularly take acetaminophen. Some people are more sensitive to this effect than others.

Possible Side Effects

This drug is relatively free from side effects when taken in recommended doses. For this reason it has become extremely popular, especially among those who cannot take aspirin.

▼ Rare: large doses or long-term use may cause liver damage, rash, itching, fever, lowered blood sugar, stimulation, yellowing of the skin or whites of the eyes, and/or a change in the composition of your blood. Contact your doctor if you experience anything unusual while taking any medication.

Drug Interactions

- Large doses of barbiturate drugs, phenytoin and similar drugs, and sulfinpyrazone may increase the chances of liver toxicity if taken with acetaminophen.
- Alcoholic beverages increase the chances for liver toxicity and possible liver failure associated with acetaminophen.
- Dosages of warfarin may need to be adjusted if acetaminophen therapy of over 2275 mg a week is started or stopped.

Food Interactions

None known.

Usual Dose

Adult and Child (age 12 and over): 325–650 mg 4–6 times a day, or 1000 mg 3–4 times a day. Avoid taking more than 4 g (twelve 325-mg tablets) a day for long periods of time.

Child (age 11): 480 mg 4–6 times a day.
Child (age 9–10): 400 mg 4–6 times a day.
Child (age 6–8): 320 mg 4–6 times a day.
Child (age 4–5): 240 mg 6 times a day.
Child (age 2–3): 160 mg 6 times a day.
Child (age 1): 120 mg 6 times a day.
Child (age 4–11 months): 80 mg 6 times a day.
Child (under age 4 months): 40 mg 6 times a day.

Overdosage

Acetaminophen is a commonly used ingredient in many over-the-counter (OTC) medications. Always check the list of ingredients when using more than one OTC medication to ensure that the combined dosage is within guidelines and to avoid accidental overdose.

Acute acetaminophen overdose may cause nausea, vomiting, sweating, appetite loss, drowsiness, confusion, abdominal tenderness, low blood pressure, abnormal heart rhythms, yellowing of the skin and whites of the eyes, and liver and kidney failure. Liver damage has occurred with 12 extra-strength tablets or 18 regular-strength tablets, but most people need larger doses—20 extra-strength or 30 regular-strength tablets—to damage their livers. Regular use of large doses for long periods—3000–4000 mg a day for a year—can also cause liver damage, especially if alcohol is involved. In case of overdose, induce vomiting as soon as possible with ipecac syrup—available at any pharmacy—and take the victim to a hospital emergency room. If you seek treatment, ALWAYS bring the acetaminophen bottle or container.

Special Information

Unless abused, acetaminophen is a beneficial, effective, and relatively nontoxic drug. Follow package directions and contact your doctor if acetaminophen does not relieve pain in 10 days for adults or 5 days for children. Contact your doctor if fever gets worse or persists longer than 3 days.

Alcoholic beverages will worsen the liver damage that

acetaminophen can cause. People who take this drug on a regular basis should limit their alcohol intake to less than 3 drinks per day.

If you forget to take a dose, take it as soon as you remember. If it is within an hour of your next dose, skip the dose you forgot and continue with your regular schedule. Do not take a double dose.

Special Populations

Pregnancy/Breast-feeding: Acetaminophen is considered safe during pregnancy when taken in usual doses. Taking continuous high doses of the drug may cause birth defects or interfere with fetal development. Three cases of congenital hip dislocation appear to have been associated with acetaminophen. Check with your doctor before taking this drug if you are or might be pregnant.

Small amounts of acetaminophen may pass into breast milk, but the drug is considered harmless to nursing infants.

Seniors: Seniors may take acetaminophen as directed by a doctor.

Generic Name

Acetazolamide (uh-sete-uh-ZOLE-uh-mide) G

Brand Names

Diamox Sequels

Type of Drug

Carbonic-anhydrase inhibitor.

Prescribed For

Glaucoma, prevention or treatment of mountain sickness, epilepsy, and treatment of drug-induced swelling or swelling due to congestive heart failure.

General Information

By blocking an enzyme in the body called carbonic anhydrase, acetazolamide produces a weak diuretic effect that helps to treat glaucoma by reducing pressure inside the eye. Acetazolamide's antiseizure properties are also produced by its effect on carbonic anhydrase, though exactly how acetazolamide prevents seizure is not well understood.

Cautions and Warnings

Do not take acetazolamide if you are **allergic** or **sensitive** to any of its ingredients or to sulfa drugs. Severe, potentially fatal, allergic reactions have occurred.

Acetazolamide should be taken with caution if you have **low blood sodium or potassium**, **pulmonary obstruction** or **emphysema**, or serious **kidney or liver disease**.

Those with **chronic noncongestive angle-closure glaucoma** should not take acetazolamide as long-term therapy.

People with **diabetes** should be aware that acetazolamide may affect their blood-glucose levels.

Patients on **high-dose aspirin therapy** should take acetazolamide with caution. Weight loss, rapid breathing, lethargy, coma, and death have been reported.

Possible Side Effects

Side effects of short-term therapy are usually minimal.

▼ Most common: nausea or vomiting; tingling feeling in the arms, legs, lips, mouth, or anus; appetite and weight loss; a metallic taste; increased frequency in urination; diarrhea; not feeling well; occasional drowsiness and confusion; and weakness. You may also experience rash, drug crystals in the urine, painful urination, low back pain, urinary difficulty, and low urine volume.

▼ Rare: Rare side effects can affect the liver, mental state, blood sugar, muscles, and senses. Temporary nearsightedness has been reported with the use of this drug. Rarely, severe allergic reactions have occurred in those taking drugs similar to acetazolamide. Contact your doctor if you experience anything unusual while taking any medication.

Drug Interactions

- Avoid drugs (including over-the-counter products) that contain stimulants or anticholinergics, which tend to aggravate glaucoma and cardiac disease.
- Dosages of acetazolamide may need to be adjusted when taken with aspirin.
- Combining diflunisal and acetazolamide can result in an excessive lowering of eye pressure.
- Acetazolamide should not be used with other carbonic-anhydrase inhibitors, such as methazolamide.
- Acetazolamide should be used with caution in those with respiratory disorders who are taking beta blockers.
- Avoid sodium bicarbonate when taking acetazolamide.

- Avoid topiramate when taking acetazolamide due to the increased risk of kidney stone formation.
- The effects of amphetamines may be increased when combined with acetazolamide. These drugs should not be taken together, especially in overdose situations.
- Acetazolamide may increase blood concentrations of cyclosporine, folic acid antagonists, hydantoins (such as phenytoin), and quinidine. Careful monitoring is required when combining these medications.
- Acetazolamide may inhibit the effects of lithium, methenamine, and primidone. Dosage adjustments may be necessary.

Food Interactions

Acetazolamide may be taken with food if it upsets your stomach. Because acetazolamide can increase potassium loss, take this drug with potassium-rich foods such as bananas, citrus fruits, melons, and tomatoes.

Usual Dose

Diuresis in Congestive Heart Failure or Drug-induced Swelling: 250–375 mg or 2.5 mg per lb. of body weight a day.

Epilepsy: 375–1000 mg or 4–15 mg per lb. of body weight a day in divided doses.

Glaucoma: 250–1000 mg a day.

Mountain Sickness: 500–1000 mg a day. If possible begin medication 24–48 hours before ascent.

Overdosage

Symptoms of overdose include drowsiness, loss of appetite, nausea, vomiting, dizziness, tingling in the hands or feet, weakness, tremors, or ringing or buzzing in the ears. In case of overdose, induce vomiting as soon as possible with ipecac syrup—available at any pharmacy—and take the victim to a hospital emergency room. If you seek treatment, ALWAYS bring the prescription bottle or container.

Special Information

Acetazolamide may cause minor drowsiness and confusion, particularly during the first 2 weeks of therapy. Be careful when driving or doing any task that requires concentration.

Contact your doctor if you develop sore throat, fever, unusual bleeding or bruises, tingling in the hands or feet, rash, or unusual pains.

Gradual ascent is recommended to avoid mountain sickness. Taking acetazolamide will not eliminate the need for prompt descent if severe high-altitude sickness symptoms develop.

If you forget a dose, take it as soon as you remember. If it is almost time for your next dose, skip the dose you forgot and continue with your regular schedule. Do not take a double dose.

Special Populations

Pregnancy/Breast-feeding: High doses of this drug may cause birth defects or interfere with fetal development. Acetazolamide should be taken during pregnancy only if your doctor determines that the potential benefit outweighs the risks.

Small amounts of acetazolamide may pass into breast milk. Nursing mothers who must take this drug should use infant formula.

Seniors: Seniors, especially those with impaired kidney function, may require additional monitoring while taking this drug.

Aciphex *see **Proton-Pump Inhibitors,** page 956*

Generic Name

Acitretin (ah-sih-TREH-tin)

Brand Names

Soriatane

Type of Drug

Antipsoriatic.

Prescribed For

Severe psoriasis; also prescribed for a variety of other skin conditions.

General Information

Acitretin is related to vitamin A and prescription drugs such as etretinate and isotretinoin. Acitretin is produced when etretinate is broken down in the body, and its effects are very similar to etretinate. The way that acitretin works is not known. Its full benefit is not likely to be seen until you have taken it for 2 or 3 months. Your doctor is urged to use this medication only in cases of severe psoriasis that have not responded to other treatments because of the risks associated with acitretin.

Cautions and Warnings

Do not take acitretin if you are **allergic** or **sensitive** to any of its ingredients. **Women** who take acitretin must not be **pregnant** during treatment or for 3 years after the completion of treatment. It is not known if acitretin taken by men before conception is also a risk to the fetus.

A small number of people taking this drug have developed liver damage including jaundice (symptoms include yellowing of the skin and whites of the eyes). Acitretin has also been associated with hepatitis. People with kidney failure have much less acitretin in their blood than people with normal kidneys. Caution is advised for people with **liver or kidney damage**.

Cholesterol levels rise in 25–50% of people taking acitretin. Very large increases in triglycerides may be responsible for the few cases of pancreatitis (inflammation of the pancreas) that have been reported. Your doctor should measure your blood-fat levels before you start taking acitretin and monitor them weekly or biweekly until your response to the medication has been determined. People with **diabetes**, who are **obese**, or who have a **history of these conditions** are at increased risk for high cholesterol levels as are people who **drink alcohol excessively**.

Drugs similar to acitretin have been associated with pseudotumor cerebri (increased pressure in the brain). Symptoms of pseudotumor cerebri include visual disturbances, headache, nausea, and vomiting. Report these or any unusual symptoms to your doctor at once.

People taking acitretin who had **spine or bone—including knee or ankle—problems** before starting the drug may find that their problems worsen while on the drug.

People with **diabetes** may find it more difficult to control their blood sugar while on acitretin.

Possible Side Effects

▼ Most common: hair loss or change in texture, peeling skin, and inflammation of the lips.

Possible Side Effects *(continued)*

▼ Common: dry eyes, chills or stiffness, dry skin, fingernail problems, itching, rash, tingling in the hands or feet, increased sensory awareness, loss of some sections of skin, sticky skin, and runny nose.

▼ Less common: drying and thickening of eye tissue; eye irritation; eyebrow or eyelash loss; changes in appetite; swelling; fatigue; hot flashes; flushing; sinus irritation; headache; pain; earache; insomnia; depression; Bell's palsy; crusting of the eyelids; blurred vision; conjunctivitis (pinkeye); double vision; itchy eyes or eyelids; cataracts; swelling inside the eye; unusual sensitivity to bright light; dry mouth; nausea; stomach pain; diarrhea; bleeding gums; joint, back, and muscle pain; and worsening of existing spinal problems.

▼ Rare: Rare side effects can occur in almost any part of the body. Contact your doctor if you experience anything unusual while taking any medication.

Drug Interactions

- People combining acitretin and glyburide (an antidiabetic) may have unusually low blood-sugar levels. Your doctor may have to adjust your diabetic treatment program while you are taking acitretin.
- Combining acitretin with methotrexate increases the risk of liver damage.
- Acitretin reduces the effectiveness of low-progestin contraceptive drugs. If you are taking one of these contraceptives, switch to another type of birth control and use at least 1 other contraceptive method for at least 3 years after treatment is completed. It is not known if acitretin interacts with combined contraceptive drugs.
- Combining alcohol with acitretin produces acitretin's parent compound, etretinate. Etretinate stays in the body much longer than acitretin and may therefore affect the fetus for an even longer period of time than might acitretin. Avoid alcoholic beverages.
- Do not take a vitamin A supplement that has more than the standard minimum daily requirement (1000 mcg). Excess vitamin A plus acitretin exposes you to possible vitamin A toxicity.

- Combining acitretin with tetracyclines may increase the risk of severe pressure on the brain.
- Notify your doctor if you are taking etretinate, isotretinoin, oral or topical tretinoin, or cyclosporine.

Food Interactions

Acitretin is best absorbed when taken with food or meals.

Usual Dose

Adult: 25–50 mg a day with your main meal. Dosage may increase after 4 weeks to 25–75 mg a day. Dosage must be individualized to your specific needs.

Child: not recommended.

Overdosage

Symptoms of acitretin overdose include vomiting, headache, and vertigo. Contact your local hospital emergency room or local poison control center for more information. If you seek treatment, ALWAYS bring the prescription bottle or container.

Special Information

Contact your doctor at once if you become pregnant while taking acitretin or in the 3 years following treatment. The risk of birth defects persists as long as the drug is in your body. In one case, small amounts of etretinate were found in blood plasma and fatty tissue more than 5 years after treatment.

Some people have experienced decreased night vision while taking acitretin. Be careful when driving at night.

Report visual disturbances, headache, nausea, vomiting, or anything unusual to your doctor at once.

Do not drink any alcoholic beverages during acitretin treatment and for at least 2 months after treatment has been completed.

Avoid excess vitamin A (see "Drug Interactions").

Some birth control methods, including low-dose progestin contraceptives and tubal ligation, may fail while taking this drug. Use at least 1 additional form of contraception while taking acitretin to avoid pregnancy.

You may have problems tolerating contact lenses while you are taking acitretin.

Do not donate blood while taking acitretin or for 3 years afterward because your blood might be given to a pregnant woman.

Avoid exposure to excessive sunlight or to sunlamps because of unusual sensitivity caused by acitretin.

If you forget to take a dose of acitretin, take it with food as soon as you remember. If it is almost time for your next dose, skip the one you forgot and continue with your regular schedule. Do not take a double dose.

A worsening of psoriasis may initially occur with treatment, and the full benefit of acitretin may not be seen for 2–3 months.

Special Populations

Pregnancy/Breast-feeding: Acitretin causes birth defects and may damage the fetus. Women who take acitretin must be sure they are not pregnant before starting therapy by using reliable contraception for at least 1 month before starting the drug and taking a pregnancy test within 1 week of starting treatment. Women must use 2 reliable contraceptive methods during treatment and for 3 years following the completion of treatment.

Acitretin may pass into breast milk. Nursing mothers who must take this drug should use infant formula.

Seniors: Seniors have twice as much acitretin in their blood as do younger adults but may take acitretin without special precaution.

Actonel *see **Bisphosphonates,** page 188*

Actos *see **Glitazone Antidiabetes Drugs,** page 529*

Generic Name

Acyclovir (ae-SYE-kloe-vir) G

Brand Names

Zovirax

The information in this profile also applies to the following drugs:

Generic Ingredients: Famciclovir G
Famvir

Generic Ingredients: Ganciclovir G
Cytovene
Zirgan Ophthalmic Gel
Vitrasert

Generic Ingredients: Penciclovir
Denavir Cream

Generic Ingredients: Valacyclovir G
Valtrex

Generic Ingredients: Valganciclovir
Valcyte

Type of Drug

Antiviral.

Prescribed For

Initial treatment and maintenance of genital herpes outbreaks; treatment of herpes zoster (shingles); and treatment of varicella (chickenpox). Ganciclovir is prescribed for herpes and cytomegalovirus (CMV) infections of the eye and CMV infections in other parts of the body, CMV prevention and treatment in people with advanced human immunodeficiency virus (HIV) infection or who have had a kidney and/or heart transplant, and maintenance treatment of CMV retinitis (inflammation of the retina) in people with compromised immune systems. Penciclovir cream is applied topically to cold sores. Cold sores treated with penciclovir cream go away sooner and are less painful than those that are untreated. Penciclovir is converted to its active form inside the viral particle and interferes with DNA production, inhibiting the reproduction process of the herpes virus.

General Information

Acyclovir is the only oral drug that reduces growth rates of the herpes virus and the related viruses, Epstein-Barr, varicella, and CMV; both oral acyclovir and oral ganciclovir work against CMV. Valacyclovir is rapidly reduced to acyclovir. Famciclovir is absorbed into the body and converted to the antiviral penciclovir. Intravenous drugs, including acyclovir injection, may also be used for these viral infections; however, intravenous antiviral drugs are usually reserved for patients with HIV, cancer, or otherwise compromised immune systems.

Acyclovir is selectively absorbed into cells that are infected with the herpes simplex virus, where it is converted into its active form. Acyclovir works by interfering with the reproduction of viral DNA, slowing the growth of existing viruses, but does not affect the DNA of uninfected body cells. It has little effect on recurrent infections. To treat both local and systemic (whole-body) symptoms, acyclovir must be given by intravenous injection or taken by mouth. Local symptoms may be treated with the ointment alone. These drugs may be taken every day to reduce the number and severity of herpes attacks in people who suffer 10 or more attacks a year; it may also be used to treat intermittent attacks as they occur, but treatment must be started as soon as possible to have the greatest effect.

Ganciclovir works by preventing reproduction of CMV. Unlike other antiviral drugs, it works only against this virus and herpes simplex virus. The drug is eliminated through the kidneys. Though most often used for CMV retinitis, ganciclovir has also been used for CMV infections of the urine, blood, throat, and semen. It is also used to prevent CMV infection. Ganciclovir is helpful in controlling CMV infection in heart, kidney, and kidney-pancreas transplant patients. Valganciclovir is not indicated for use in liver transplant patients. Valganciclovir is broken down by the body into ganciclovir; information about ganciclovir in this profile applies to both drugs, unless otherwise noted.

Cautions and Warnings

Do not use these drugs if you are **allergic** or **sensitive** to any of their ingredients. Do not use acyclovir ointment if you have had an allergic reaction to it or to the major component of the ointment base, polyethylene glycol. Do not apply acyclovir ointment inside the vagina because the polyethylene glycol base may cause irritation and swelling of sensitive vaginal tissue. Acyclovir ointment is not intended for use in the eye and should not be used to treat a herpes infection of the eye.

People with **kidney impairment** should have dosages adjusted for all of the antiviral drugs in this profile. Renal failure has occurred in patients using oral acyclovir, in some cases resulting in death.

Maintain adequate hydration while taking oral acyclovir.

Animal testing indicates that acyclovir may affect fertility in men. These effects may be reversible.

Ganciclovir causes anemia, reduced white-blood-cell count, and blood-platelet loss. Regular monitoring of blood and platelet counts is recommended while taking this drug.

Oral ganciclovir is linked to a faster progression of CMV eye infection than the intravenous form of the drug. The risk of rapid progression of eye infection should be balanced against the benefits of taking oral CMV. Ganciclovir eye inserts release their medicine directly on the surface of the eye and are more effective for this purpose.

Ganciclovir and valganciclovir should not be used by people with severe **liver disease** or by those who have had a **liver transplant**. Other drugs in this group can increase liver enzyme production.

Ganciclovir is intended only for people who are **immunocompromised**. It is not intended to treat or prevent CMV infections in **newborns**.

Detachment of the retina has been noted in people taking ganciclovir, as well as in people with CMV who have not taken the drug. The relationship between ganciclovir and this effect is not well known.

Ganciclovir causes increased sensitivity to the sun; use a sunscreen or wear protective clothes when you go outside.

People with **kidney disease** should use ganciclovir with caution and may require treatment at a lower dosage. Famciclovir dosage must be adjusted if you have reduced kidney function.

Studies have shown a trend toward higher blood levels of ganciclovir in white people using the drug than among users from other ethnic groups.

Valganciclovir has been approved for use in **children** following kidney or heart transplants in oral solution form.

Possible Side Effects

Acyclovir

Capsules, Suspension, and Tablets

- ▼ Most common: feeling unwell, headache, diarrhea, nausea, and vomiting.
- ▼ Less common: appetite loss, stomach gas, constipation, fatigue, rash, leg pains, sore throat, a bad taste in the mouth, sleeplessness, and fever.
- ▼ Rare: kidney pain, aching joints, weakness, and tingling in the hands or feet. Contact your doctor if you experience anything unusual while taking any medication.

Ointment

- ▼ Most common: mild burning, irritation, rash, and itching. These effects are more likely to occur when treating an initial herpes attack than a recurrent attack. Women are 4 times more likely to experience burning than men.

Possible Side Effects *(continued)*

Famciclovir

- Most common: headache, nausea, and diarrhea.
- Less common: fever, fatigue, pain, vomiting, constipation, appetite loss, dizziness, tingling in the hands or feet, sleepiness, sore throat, sinus irritation, itching, gas, severe pain during menstruation, and signs of shingles.
- Rare: chills, abdominal pain, back or joint pain, and upset stomach. Contact your doctor if you experience anything unusual while taking any medication.

Ganciclovir and Valganciclovir

- Most common: fever, diarrhea, abdominal pain, reduced white-blood-cell counts, anemia, rash, sweating, nausea, vomiting, and appetite loss.
- Common: infection; chills; stomach gas; low blood-platelet counts (symptoms include bleeding or oozing blood); tingling; burning; numbness or pain in the hands, arms, legs, or feet; itching; pneumonia; weakness; and headache.

Penciclovir

Side effects are generally mild and infrequent. In studies, side effects were similar in type and frequency among people who used penciclovir and those who used an inactive cream.

- Common: headache, redness, and swelling.
- Less common: skin reactions to the cream.
- Rare: loss of skin sensation where the cream has been applied, changes in the sense of taste, and rash. Contact your doctor if you experience anything unusual while taking any medication.

Valacyclovir

- Most common: headache, diarrhea, dizziness, weakness, constipation, abdominal pain, appetite loss, nausea, and vomiting.
- Less common: aching joints, tingling in the hands or feet, stomach gas, fatigue, rash, not feeling well, leg pain, sore throat, a bad taste in the mouth, sleeplessness, and fever.
- Rare: Rare side effects can affect behavior and the nervous system, eyes, gastrointestinal tract, kidneys, and skin. Contact your doctor if you experience anything unusual while taking any medication.

Drug Interactions

- Do not apply acyclovir together with any other ointment or topical medication.
- Combining acyclovir and zidovudine (an HIV drug—also known as AZT) may lead to severe drowsiness and lethargy.
- Cimetidine and probenecid may decrease acyclovir elimination from the body and increase acyclovir levels in the blood, raising the risk of side effects.
- Cimetidine and probenecid slow the rate at which valacyclovir is converted to acyclovir, but this does not change valacyclovir's effectiveness. No adjustments in valacyclovir dosage are necessary.
- Probenecid interferes with famciclovir and ganciclovir release through the kidneys and substantially increases blood levels of ganciclovir.
- Theophylline interferes with the elimination of famciclovir from the body, possibly leading to higher levels of famciclovir in the blood.
- People who took famciclovir and digoxin together experienced increased digoxin in their blood.
- Adriamycin, amphotericin B, flucytosine, pentamidine, trimethoprim-sulfamethoxazole, vincristine, vinblastine, and other cytotoxic drugs may increase the side effects of ganciclovir and should be used together only if absolutely necessary, and only if the potential benefits outweigh the risks.
- People taking imipenem-cilastatin together with ganciclovir have experienced seizures. Avoid this combination.
- Mixing ganciclovir with other drugs that can be damaging to the kidneys may increase the rate and extent of kidney damage.
- Mycophenolate mofetil (MMF) may increase ganciclovir blood levels and MMF in patients with reduced kidney function, increasing the chances of drug side effects.
- Mixing ganciclovir or valganciclovir with the anti-HIV drugs didanosine or AZT may increase didanosine or AZT levels and reduce ganciclovir levels. Because AZT and ganciclovir both cause anemia and low white-blood-cell counts, many people cannot tolerate this combination.

Food Interactions

Acyclovir may be taken with food if it upsets your stomach. High-fat, high-calorie meals can increase the amount of ganciclovir absorbed into the blood. Take ganciclovir with food.

Usual Dose

Acyclovir

Capsules, Suspension, and Tablets

Adult: genital herpes attack—200 mg every 4 hours, 5 times a day for 10 days. Recurrent infections—200 mg every 4 hours, 5 times a day for 5 days. Suppressive therapy for chronic herpes—400 mg twice a day, every day for up to a year. Herpes zoster—800 mg every 4 hours, 5 times a day for 7–10 days.

Child (age 2 and over): Acyclovir has been given to children in daily doses as high as 36 mg per lb. of body weight without any unusual side effects.

Child (under age 2): not recommended.

If you have kidney disease, your doctor should adjust your dose according to the degree of functional loss.

Ointment: Apply every 3 hours, 6 times a day for 7 days. Apply enough medication to cover all visible skin lesions. About ½ in. of ointment should cover about 4 sq. in. of lesions. Your doctor may prescribe a longer course of treatment to prevent the delayed formation of new lesions over the duration of an attack. Begin using ointment at the first sign of an attack.

Famciclovir

Cold Sores

Adult: 1500 mg as a single dose. Initiate therapy at the earliest sign or symptom of a cold sore (tingling, itching, or burning).

Genital Herpes

Adult: 1000 mg twice a day for 1 day; or 250 mg twice a day for up to 1 year for suppression; or 250 mg 3 times a day for 7 days for initial episode. People with reduced kidney function take the same dose but less often, as infrequently as once every 2 days. HIV-infected people should take 500 mg twice a day for 7 days.

Shingles

Adult: 500 mg every 8 hours for 1 week. People with reduced kidney function may require a reduced dose taken as infrequently as once a day.

Ganciclovir

Capsules

Adult and Child (age 13 and over): 3000 mg a day, divided into 3 or 6 equal doses. People with reduced kidney function will need to have their dosage reduced accordingly, possibly to as little as 500 mg 3 times a week.

Child (2 days–12 years): Dosage is calculated for each patient according to a special formula based on kidney function.

Eye Gel

Adult and Child: 1 drop in the affected eye 5 times a day until the ulcer heals and then 1 drop 3 times a day for 7 days.

Penciclovir

Adult and Child (age 12 and over): Apply to affected areas every 2 hours, during waking hours, for 4 days.

Child (under age 12): not recommended.

Valacyclovir

Adult

Cold sores: 2000 mg twice a day for 1 day. Initiate therapy at earliest onset of symptoms (tingling, itching, or burning). Dosage is reduced in people with kidney disease.

Genital herpes: 1000 mg twice a day for 10 days for initial outbreak, preferably within 48 hours; 500 mg twice a day for 3 days for recurrent outbreaks; 500 mg a day for prevention of outbreaks; and 500 mg twice a day in people with HIV or who are immunocompromised.

Shingles: 1000 mg 3 times a day for 7 days.

Child

Chickenpox (age 2–17): 9 mg per lb. of body weight, 3 times a day for 5 days, up to 1000 mg 3 times a day.

Cold Sores (age 12 and over): 2000 mg every 12 hours for 1 day.

Valganciclovir

Adult and Child (age 17 and over): 900 mg twice a day for CMV eye infection to start, then 900 mg once a day, divided into 2 equal doses of 450 mg each; 900 mg once a day to prevent CMV infection in organ-transplant patients. People with reduced kidney function will need to have their dosage reduced accordingly, possibly to as little as 450 mg twice a week.

Child (4 months–16 years): Dosage is calculated for each patient according to a special formula based on kidney function.

Overdosage

Overdose of oral acyclovir may lead to kidney damage due to deposits of acyclovir crystals in the kidneys. Other side effects include agitation, seizures, lethargy, and coma. Little is known about the effects of ganciclovir overdose. As much as 6000 mg of ganciclovir a day has been taken with only temporary lowering of white-blood-cell count. In the case of overdose or accidental ingestion, contact your poison control center. The risk of experiencing toxic side effects from swallowing acyclovir ointment or penciclovir cream is quite small. If you seek treatment, ALWAYS bring the prescription bottle or container.

Special Information

Begin cold sore treatment as early as possible. Early application will help prevent cold sores from appearing and reduce the chance of accompanying pain. Use a finger cot or rubber glove when applying ointment or cream antiviral products to protect against inadvertently spreading the virus. Be sure to apply the medication exactly as directed and to completely cover all lesions. Keep affected areas clean and dry. Loose-fitting clothing will reduce possible irritation of a healing lesion.

Treatment must be started as soon as possible after shingles is diagnosed. The information on the effectiveness of these drugs against shingles was gathered from cases in which treatment was begun within 72 hours of diagnosis.

These drugs are not a cure for genital herpes. Herpes may be transmitted even if you do not have symptoms of active disease. To avoid giving the condition to a sexual partner, do not have intercourse while visible herpes lesions are present. A condom offers some protection against transmission of the herpes virus, but spermicidal products and diaphragms do not. These drugs alone will not prevent herpes transmission.

Initiate therapy at the first sign of symptoms.

Women with genital herpes have an increased risk of cervical cancer. Speak with your doctor about the need for an annual Pap smear.

Contact your doctor if these drugs do not relieve your symptoms, if side effects become severe or intolerable, or if you become pregnant or want to begin breast-feeding. Check with your dentist if you notice swelling or tenderness of the gums.

Avoid exposure to excessive sunlight or sunlamps because of unusual sensitivity caused by oral acyclovir.

Ganciclovir does not cure CMV eye infection, and immunocompromised people taking this drug may find their disease worsening. Regular blood tests are necessary to watch for white-blood-cell or blood-platelet count alterations, and dosage reductions or discontinuation of the drug may be necessary if these counts get too low.

Ganciclovir may cause infertility in men and women. Women of child-bearing age should use effective contraception while taking this drug. Men should use a condom while taking the drug and for at least 90 days afterward to avoid passing the drug to their partners.

Good dental hygiene is important while taking ganciclovir to minimize the risk of infection. If you have dental work done while taking this drug, expect the healing process to take longer.

If you skip several doses or a day or more of acyclovir, the drug will not exert its maximum effect. It is very important to apply penciclovir cream every 2 hours during the day for the drug to work. If you forget to apply a dose of penciclovir, apply it as soon as you remember. If you realize you forgot a dose within 30–45 minutes of your next dose, skip the dose you forgot and continue with your regular schedule. If you forget a dose of famciclovir, take it as soon as you remember. If it is almost time for your next dose, skip the dose you forgot. Do not take a double dose. Contact your doctor if you forget more than 2 doses in a row. It is very important to take ganciclovir exactly as directed. If you forget a dose, take it as soon as you remember and continue with your regular schedule.

Special Populations

Pregnancy/Breast-feeding: These drugs cross into the blood circulation of the fetus. Animal studies have shown that large acyclovir doses—up to 125 times the human dose—cause damage to both mother and fetus. Although there is no information to indicate that acyclovir affects a human fetus, it should be taken during pregnancy only if your doctor determines that the potential benefit outweighs the risks.

Animal studies showed ganciclovir to be toxic to the fetus. There is no reliable information about its effect in pregnant women. Ganciclovir should be taken during pregnancy only if your doctor determines that the potential benefit outweighs the risks. Women who are likely to become pregnant while taking this drug should use reliable contraception.

Acyclovir passes into breast milk in concentrations up to 4 times the concentration in blood, and it has been found in the urine of a nursing infant. Although no side effects have been found in nursing babies, mothers who must take acyclovir should use infant formula.

It is not known if ganciclovir passes into breast milk, but the possible side effects of this drug on a nursing infant indicate that nursing mothers who must take this drug should use infant formula.

Seniors: Shingles attacks in people over age 50 tend to be more severe and respond best to acyclovir treatment if the drug is started within 48–72 hours of the appearance of the first rash. Seniors with reduced kidney function should be given a lower dose of these drugs than younger adults.

Generic Name

Adapalene (uh-DAP-uh-lene)

Brand Names

Differin
Epiduo

Type of Drug

Antiacne.

Prescribed For

Acne.

General Information

Adapalene is similar to a retinoid. Retinoids are compounds related to vitamin A and are used in acne treatment. When adapalene is applied to an acne lesion, it modifies several of the processes involved in skin cell function. It reduces inflammation in the acne lesion and slows the formation of the material that fills the lesion. Very little adapalene is absorbed through the skin.

Cautions and Warnings

Do not use adapalene if you are **allergic** or **sensitive** to any of its ingredients. If you are **sunburned**, wait until your sunburn clears before applying adapalene to your skin. Avoid sun or sunlamp exposure while using adapalene. If you must be in the sun, be sure to apply sunscreen or wear protective clothing over areas where you have applied adapalene. Extreme wind or cold can also be irritating to skin where adapalene has been applied.

Adapalene can irritate the skin if used in combination with products such as medicated or abrasive soaps or cleansers, astringents, or soaps and cosmetics with a strong drying effect. Avoid products containing sulfur, resorcinol, or salicylic acid.

Adapalene can be highly irritating if it gets into your eyes or if it is applied to your lips, the angles of your nose, mucous membranes, cuts, abrasions, or sunburned or damaged skin. Avoid using depilatories or waxing while using adapalene.

Possible Side Effects

- ▼ Most common: redness, irritation, dryness, scaling, itching, and burning are common after applying adapalene to your skin. These effects usually occur during the first 2–4 weeks of adapalene use and subside as treatment continues. Symptoms may be severe enough to cause you to stop using adapalene; contact your doctor if this happens to you.
- ▼ Rare: skin irritation, stinging sunburn, and worsening acne. Contact your doctor if you experience anything unusual while taking any medication.

Drug Interactions

None known.

Usual Dose

Adult and Child (age 12 and over): Wash affected areas with a mild or soapless cleanser and apply a thin layer of adapalene at bedtime.

Child (under age 12): not recommended.

Overdosage

Chronic ingestion of adapalene can cause liver toxicity and other side effects associated with swallowing large amounts of vitamin A. Swallowing adapalene gel is extremely dangerous for pregnant women, who should not take more vitamin A than is contained in their prenatal vitamins. Infants who swallow adapalene should be taken to a hospital emergency room for treatment. If you seek treatment, ALWAYS bring the prescription bottle or container.

Special Information

Stop using adapalene and contact your doctor if you develop a severe skin reaction or any sign of drug allergy or reaction (symptoms include rash, hives, itching, changes in complexion, and breathing difficulties or irregularities).

Adapalene may exacerbate your acne at first, but you should see improvement within 2 weeks.

If you must be in the sun, be sure to apply sunscreen or wear protective clothing over areas to which you have applied adapalene.

Using more than a thin film of adapalene does not produce better results and may be more irritating to the skin.

If you forget to apply a dose of adapalene, apply it as soon as you remember. If it is almost time for your next application of adapalene, skip the dose you forgot and continue with your regular schedule.

Special Populations

Pregnancy/Breast-feeding: Animal studies of adapalene have shown no effects on the fetus. Since the effect of adapalene on pregnant women is not known, the drug should be taken during pregnancy only if your doctor determines that the potential benefit outweighs the risks.

It is not known if adapalene passes into breast milk. Nursing mothers should use infant formula.

Seniors: Seniors may use this drug without special precautions.

Brand Names

Adderall G

Generic Ingredients

Dextroamphetamine Sulfate + Dextroamphetamine Saccharate + Amphetamine Aspartate + Amphetamine Sulfate

Other Brand Names

Adderall XR

The information in this profile also applies to the following drugs:

Generic Ingredients: Dextroamphetamine Sulfate G

Dexedrine
Dextrostat
LiQuadd
ProCentra

Generic Ingredients: Lisdexamfetamine Dimesylate

Vyvanse

Type of Drug

Central-nervous-system (CNS) stimulant.

Prescribed For

Attention-deficit hyperactivity disorder (ADHD) and narcolepsy (uncontrollable desire to sleep).

General Information

Adderall, which is a mixture of two forms of amphetamine, may be prescribed for childhood ADHD, a condition characterized by distractibility, short attention span, hyperactive behavior, emotional instability, and difficulty controlling impulses. They should be used only after a complete evaluation of the child has been done. Frequency and severity of symptoms and their appropriateness for the age of the child determine whether drug therapy is required. Many experts believe that amphetamines offer only a temporary solution because they do not permanently change behavioral patterns. Psychological, educational, and social measures must also be taken to ensure successful treatment in the long term.

Cautions and Warnings

Do not take Adderall if you are **allergic** or **sensitive** to any amphetamine or have **heart disease, a heart defect, high blood pressure, hardening of the arteries, tics or Tourette syndrome, seizures, thyroid disease, glaucoma,** or a history of **agitation** or **drug abuse**.

Amphetamines should be used with extreme caution because they are highly addictive and easily abused.

New or worsening thought patterns, bipolar illness, aggressive or hostile behavior, psychotic behavior, and new manic symptoms can develop during treatment with amphetamines.

Stimulants like amphetamines are not effective and may be dangerous for **children** whose symptoms are related to environmental factors or primary **psychiatric conditions**, including psychosis. A large study suggests that children who take these medicines for ADHD have a higher risk of sudden death. Further research is under way to better define this risk.

Stimulants can cause weight loss and stunted growth in **children** under age 10. Blurred vision and difficulty focusing can occur.

Possible Side Effects

▼ Common: loss of appetite, insomnia, heart palpitations, restlessness, overstimulation, dizziness, increased blood pressure, rapid heartbeat, upper abdominal pain, and weight loss.

Possible Side Effects *(continued)*

- ▼ Less common: euphoria (feeling "high"), hallucinations, aggression, muscle spasms and tremors, headache, dry mouth, unpleasant taste in the mouth, diarrhea, constipation, upset stomach, nausea, vomiting, rash, itching, changes in sex drive, blurred vision, and impotence.
- ▼ Rare: psychotic drug reactions and pathologic skin picking.

Contact your doctor if you experience anything unusual while taking any medication.

Drug Interactions

- Combining an amphetamine and a monoamine oxidase inhibitor (MAOI) antidepressant may cause a severe increase in blood pressure as well as bleeding inside the skull. Wait at least 2 weeks after stopping an MAOI before taking an amphetamine.
- Amphetamines may reduce the effectiveness of high-blood-pressure medicines including adrenergic blockers.
- Gastrointestinal and urinary acidifying agents such as methenamine reduce the effectiveness of amphetamines.
- Gastrointestinal alkalizing agents, such as sodium bicarbonate, and urinary alkalizing agents (acetazolamide, some thiazides) may increase and prolong the effects of amphetamines.
- Antipsychotic medications such as chlorpromazine, haloperidol, and lithium carbonate inhibit the stimulatory effects of amphetamines. Chlorpromazine may be used to treat amphetamine poisoning.
- Amphetamines may enhance the effects of tricyclic antidepressants, norepinephrine, and meperidine.
- Amphetamines may counteract the sedative effect of antihistamines.
- Amphetamines can delay the absorption of ethosuximide, phenobarbital, and phenytoin into the bloodstream.

Food Interactions

These drugs can be taken without regard to food or meals.

Usual Dose

Adderall and Dextroamphetamine

ADHD

Adult and Child (age 6 and over): 5–40 mg a day.

Child (age 3–5): 2–5 mg a day. Dose may be increased weekly until maximum response is achieved.

Child (under age 3): not recommended.

Narcolepsy

Adult and Child (age 12 and over): 5–60 mg a day.

Child (age 6–11): Narcolepsy rarely occurs in children under age 12, but when it does, it can be treated with dextroamphetamine or Adderall. Starting dose is 5 mg a day, increased weekly until maximum response is achieved.

Adderall XR

Adult and Child (age 6 and over): 30 mg a day.

Child (under age 6): Adderall XR has not been studied in children under age 6.

Lisdexamfetamine

Adult and Child (age 6 and over): 30 mg every morning. Daily dose may be increased up to 70 mg.

Overdosage

Symptoms include tremors, muscle spasms, restlessness, exaggerated reflexes, rapid breathing, dry mouth, constipation, hallucinations, confusion, panic, and overaggressive behavior. These may be followed by depression, exhaustion, abnormal heart rhythms, blood-pressure changes, nausea, vomiting, diarrhea, convulsions, and coma. Take the victim to a hospital emergency room immediately. If you seek treatment, ALWAYS bring the prescription bottle or container.

Special Information

Amphetamines should be used very cautiously and only when considered absolutely necessary.

Amphetamines are addictive and commonly abused. If you feel you have developed a tolerance or dependence to Adderall, contact your doctor. Do not increase your dosage without your doctor's approval.

Amphetamines may impair your ability to drive or operate heavy machinery. Use with caution.

To prevent this drug from interfering with sleep, take it at least 6–8 hours before bedtime. Do not crush or chew the sustained-release form.

If you forget your once-daily dose, skip it and go back to your regular schedule the next day. If you take the drug 2–3 times a day and miss a dose, take it as soon as you remember. If it is within 3 hours of your next dose, skip the one you forgot and continue with your regular schedule. Never take a double dose.

Special Populations

Pregnancy/Breast-feeding: Use of amphetamines during the early stages of pregnancy may cause birth defects. Amphetamines also increase the risk of premature delivery and low-birth-weight infants and may cause drug withdrawal symptoms in newborns. Amphetamines should be taken during pregnancy only if your doctor determines that the potential benefit outweighs the risks.

Amphetamines pass into breast milk. Nursing mothers who must take them should use infant formula.

Seniors: Seniors are more sensitive to this drug's effects.

Generic Name

Adefovir (ah-deh-FOE-veer)

Brand Names

Hepsera

The information in this profile also applies to the following drugs:

Generic Ingredients: Entecavir
Baraclude

Generic Ingredients: Lamivudine
Epivir-HBV

Generic Ingredients: Telbivudine
Tyzeka

Generic Ingredients: Tenofovir
Viread

Type of Drug

Hepatitis B antiviral.

Prescribed For

Chronic active hepatitis B in adults.

General Information

Hepatitis B is one of several different types of hepatitis, a viral infection of the liver. These drugs can reduce the amount of hepatitis B virus (HBV) in the bloodstream and slow its spread to healthy liver tissue; however, they cannot cure chronic hepatitis B. People with chronic hepatitis B may develop liver cirrhosis or liver cancer and it is not known if these drugs can prevent these conditions from occurring. Like other viruses and bacteria, HBV can become resistant to the effects of these drugs.

These drugs are eliminated from the body via the kidney. They work against HBV in a way similar to that of certain human immunodeficiency virus (HIV) drugs, interfering with an enzyme called reverse transcriptase, which is an essential component of the viral reproduction process. Almost ½ of each dose is eliminated via the urine within 24 hours of taking it.

Entecavir can reduce the amount of virus in the body, make it harder for new liver cells to be infected by the virus, and improve the general condition of the liver. These drugs work by attacking HBV polymerase, an enzyme essential to the reproduction of HBV inside an infected cell.

Telbivudine does not work against HIV infection and can be taken together with HIV drug therapy.

Lamivudine and tenofovir are antivirals prescribed for HBV and/or HIV. It is important to note that lamivudine products made for HBV contain less medicine than those made for HIV, and these products should not be interchanged. People with mixed HBV/HIV infection should receive the HIV product with more medicine in it. Tenofovir is available in a number of combinations for HIV. People taking tenofovir for HBV should NOT take a combination.

For more information on both lamivudine and tenofovir, see HIV Antivirals, page 555.

These medicines do not cure HBV or stop you from spreading HBV to others, generally through sexual contact or exposure to infected blood. The hepatitis B virus can live outside the body for 1 week.

Cautions and Warnings

Do not take these drugs if you are **allergic** or **sensitive** to any of their ingredients.

Adefovir can be toxic to the kidneys, especially in people who already have some **kidney problems**. Since it is eliminated from the body through the kidneys, people with **kidney disease** are often given lower doses of adefovir.

In some cases, hepatitis can become severely aggravated upon discontinuation of these drugs. Your doctor should check your liver for 12 weeks after the drug is stopped. It is possible that antiviral therapy may have to be restarted.

These drugs have some activity against **HIV**. An HIV blood test is recommended before starting treatment. If you are HIV-positive, these drugs could make the HIV virus resistant to future antiviral drugs.

Severe worsening of **HBV** has occurred in people taking entecavir, mostly **women**, who also had HIV and stopped taking their medication.

People taking these medicines can develop liver disease, liver enlargement, fat degeneration, and lactic acidosis (a potentially fatal metabolic imbalance). This may be a reason for your doctor to stop your treatment with these drugs. This occurs most frequently in **obese women**. Feeling very weak or tired; experiencing unusual muscle pain, difficulty breathing, or stomach pain with nausea and vomiting; feeling cold, especially in your arms and legs; feeling dizzy or lightheaded; and a fast or irregular heartbeat may be signs of lactic acidosis. It is a medical emergency and must be treated in the hospital.

These medicines may cause muscle disease, including persistent aches and pains. If this happens, they should be discontinued to prevent muscle damage. Telbivudine may damage the nervous system, leading to burning or sharp pain, numbness or tingling in the hands or feet that can spread to the arms or legs, extreme sensitivity to touch, poor coordination, weakness or paralysis, and bowel or bladder problems.

Possible Side Effects

Adefovir

In studies, side effects reported in the treated group were similar in frequency to placebo.

- ▼ Most common: weakness, headache, stomach pain, and nausea.
- ▼ Less common: intestinal gas, diarrhea, and upset stomach.

Entecavir

- ▼ Most common: headache, fatigue, dizziness, and nausea.
- ▼ Less common: diarrhea, upset stomach, vomiting, tiredness, hair loss, and sleeplessness.
- ▼ Rare: Rare side effects may affect almost any part of the body. Contact your doctor if you experience anything unusual while taking any medication.

Possible Side Effects *(continued)*

Telbivudine

▼ Most common: upper-respiratory infection, fatigue, not feeling well, muscle tenderness or weakness, abdominal pain, nasal irritation, and sore throat.

▼ Common: influenza or flu-like symptoms, diarrhea or loose stools, and throat pain.

▼ Less common: fever, joint pain, rash, back pain, dizziness, muscle ache, sleeplessness, and upset stomach.

Drug Interactions

These drugs were studied extensively in an attempt to predict possible drug interactions. No major interaction problems have been revealed.

- Taking drugs that can be toxic to the kidneys (such as aminoglycosides, cyclosporine, nonsteroidal anti-inflammatory drugs [NSAIDs], tacrolimus, and vancomycin) together with adefovir can lead to the more rapid appearance of kidney damage.
- Ibuprofen, when taken in dosages of 800 mg 3 times a day, will increase adefovir blood levels by about 20%; however, the importance of this finding is unknown.
- These drugs do not affect liver enzymes and have a low interaction potential.
- Do not take lamivudine and tenofovir together.
- Drugs that affect kidney function may affect blood concentrations of entecavir and telbivudine.
- Other hepatitis B treatments (lamivudine, adefovir, cyclosporine, and pegylated interferon alpha-2a) do not affect either entecavir or telbivudine and are not affected by them.

Food Interactions

Adefovir and telbivudine can be taken without regard to food, but may be taken with food if gastrointestinal (GI) upset occurs. Take entecavir at least 2 hours after a meal and 2 hours before the next meal.

Usual Dose

Adefovir

Adult and Child (age 12 and over): 10 mg once a day. People with kidney disease requiring dialysis may take only 10 mg a week. The exact dosage is based on the severity of kidney disease.

Child (under age 12): not recommended.

Entecavir

Adult and Child (age 16 and over): 0.5–1 mg once a day. People with kidney failure may be treated with as little as 0.05–0.1 mg a day.

Child (under age 16): not recommended.

Lamivudine

Adult (age 18 and over): 100 mg once a day. Daily dose is reduced for people with varying degrees of kidney failure.

Child (age 2–17): 1.3 mg per lb. of body weight a day, up to 100 mg.

Telbivudine

Adult and Child (age 16 and over): 600 mg once a day. People with moderate to severe kidney failure are treated either with a single 600-mg dose every 2, 3, or 4 days depending on the degree of kidney disease or with smaller doses of telbivudine liquid every day.

Child (under age 16): not recommended.

Tenofovir

Adult: 300 mg once a day. Dose reduced for people with kidney disease.

Child: not recommended.

Overdosage

GI symptoms are the most likely outcome of an adefovir overdose. There are no reports of entecavir or telbivudine overdose. People taking single entecavir doses (up to 40 mg) or multiple doses (up to 20 mg per day for up to 14 days) had no unusual side effects. One person accidentally took an overdose with no consequences. People taking up to 1800 mg a day of telbivudine had no increase in side effects. Take the victim to a hospital emergency room. If you seek treatment, ALWAYS bring the prescription bottle or container.

Special Information

Practice safe sex and safe needle use. People taking adefovir may still spread hepatitis B through sexual contact or by sharing needles. Practice safe sex using condoms and dental dams.

Do not share personal items that can have blood or body fluids on them, such as toothbrushes or razor blades.

If you were previously taking lamivudine for hepatitis B and the virus became resistant to it, your doctor will add adefovir to lamivudine to reduce your chances of developing adefovir resistance.

These drugs must be taken continuously to maintain their effectiveness. Try to take your dose at the same time every day. Be sure to keep enough on hand so that you do not run out of medicine. If you take these drugs on a regular schedule and forget a dose, take it as soon as you remember. If it is almost time for your next dose, skip the forgotten dose and continue with your regular schedule. Do not take a double dose of these medicines. Contact your doctor if you forget 2 or more doses in a row. Skipping or forgetting too many doses can make HBV resistant to these drugs.

Your hepatitis B may get worse or become very serious if you stop taking these medications. Do not stop taking them or change your daily dose without talking to your doctor.

Entecavir oral solution is a ready-to-use product and should not be mixed with water or any other liquid product. Each bottle of the oral solution comes with a dosing spoon that is calibrated in 1-mL increments, up to 10 mL. Hold the spoon upright and gradually fill it to the mark next to the prescribed dose. Drink the liquid directly from the dosing spoon. Your pharmacist can help you properly measure your medication dose. Rinse the dosing spoon with water after each daily dose and allow it to air dry.

Contact your doctor at once if you feel very weak or tired, cold (especially in your arms and legs), or dizzy or lightheaded; have unusual muscle pain, difficulty breathing, or stomach pain with nausea and vomiting; or have a fast or irregular heartbeat. These could be signs of lactic acidosis.

Contact your doctor if you experience jaundice (symptoms include yellowing of the skin or whites of the eyes), appetite loss for a few days or more, lower stomach pain, nausea, dark urine, or bowel movements that are light in color. These could be signs of liver toxicity.

Special Populations

Pregnancy/Breast-feeding: Animal studies with adefovir have revealed a tendency for some birth defects when the dosage administered was more than 20 times the average human dose. Entecavir studies revealed slowed development of the skeleton. Animal studies of telbivudine did not reveal any effects on the developing fetus. There is no information on the effect of these drugs during pregnancy. Adefovir should be taken during pregnancy only if your doctor determines that the potential benefit outweighs the risks. A registry has been established to collect information from doctors about pregnant women who take these medicines. You or your doctor may enroll in the registry.

It is not known if adefovir passes into breast milk. Entecavir and telbivudine pass into breast milk. Nursing mothers who must take these drugs should use infant formula.

Seniors: Seniors may be more sensitive to the side effects of these medicines because of the natural loss of kidney function that occurs with age.

Advair Diskus *see **Salmeterol,** page 1029*

Brand Names

Aggrenox

Generic Ingredients

Dipyridamole + Aspirin G

Type of Drug

Antiplatelet.

Prescribed For

Prevention of recurrent stroke or transient ischemic attack (TIA)—"mini-stroke."

General Information

Stroke is often the result of a clot blocking flow in a blood vessel supplying the brain. Aggrenox helps prevent blood clot formation by reducing the "stickiness" of platelets, blood cells that stick together to form the beginnings of all clots. In one study, Aggrenox reduced the risk of stroke by over 30% compared with placebo in people who had recently had a stroke or TIA.

Cautions and Warnings

Do not use this drug if you are **allergic** or **sensitive** to any of its ingredients or any nonsteroidal anti-inflammatory drug (NSAID). People who have **asthma**, **nasal polyps**, or **chronic runny nose**, are likely to be sensitive to aspirin.

The aspirin in Aggrenox can cause Reye's syndrome, a severe reaction (vomiting, lethargy, and belligerence, and possibly worsening to coma) in **children under age 19**.

People with a history of **stomach ulcers** or **stomach problems** should avoid Aggrenox.

People who have **angina** or have had a recent **heart attack** should be very cautious about taking this drug. It may worsen chest pain.

People with **low blood pressure**, **liver disease**, or **kidney failure** should be cautious about taking this drug.

People taking Aggrenox may bleed for longer amounts of time. Those with **bleeding disorders** should avoid Aggrenox.

Possible Side Effects

- ▼ Most common: headache, upset stomach, abdominal pain, nausea, and diarrhea.
- ▼ Common: pain, tiredness, and vomiting.
- ▼ Less common: convulsions, rectal bleeding, blood in the stool, hemorrhoids, back pain, accidental injuries, stomach bleeding, feeling unwell, weakness, fainting, memory loss, arthritis, joint or muscle pain, coughing, and respiratory infection.
- ▼ Rare: Rare side effects can occur in almost any part of the body. Contact your doctor if you experience anything unusual while taking any medication.

Drug Interactions

- Avoid alcohol. People who consume 3 or more alcoholic drinks a day while using any aspirin-containing product are more likely to develop stomach ulcers or bleeding.
- Aspirin may reduce the blood-pressure-lowering effects of angiotensin-converting enzyme (ACE) inhibitor drugs, beta blockers, and diuretics.
- Combining aspirin and acetazolamide or an NSAID can cause kidney problems.
- Aspirin can increase the blood-thinning effects of anticoagulant (blood-thinning) drugs such as warfarin. Avoid this combination.
- Aspirin can increase the effects of oral antidiabetes drugs, possibly leading to low blood sugar.

- Aspirin counteracts the uric-acid-eliminating effects of probenecid and sulfinpyrazone.
- Aspirin can increase the toxic effects of anticonvulsant drugs and methotrexate.
- Dipyridamole increases the level of adenosine in the blood and may increase cardiovascular-related side effects. The adenosine dosage may need to be adjusted when these two drugs are combined.
- Dipyridamole may interfere with cholinesterase inhibitors used to treat myasthenia gravis.

Food Interactions

Aggrenox is best taken on an empty stomach but may be taken with food if it upsets your stomach.

Usual Dose

Adult: 1 capsule (200 mg of sustained-release dipyridamole and 25 mg of aspirin) morning and evening.

Child: not recommended.

Overdosage

Symptoms include a sensation of warmth, flushing, sweating, restlessness, weakness, dizziness, low blood pressure, rapid heartbeat, and ringing in the ears. Take the victim to a hospital emergency room. If you seek treatment, ALWAYS bring the prescription bottle or container.

Special Information

Contact your doctor if you experience blood in your stool, persistent diarrhea, or abdominal or stomach pain.

Avoid alcohol while taking this drug.

In people taking Aggrenox, minor cuts may take longer than normal to stop bleeding.

If you forget a dose, take it as soon as you remember. If it is almost time for your next dose, skip the one you forgot and continue with your regular schedule.

Swallow Aggrenox tablets whole; do not crush or chew them.

Special Populations

Pregnancy/Breast-feeding: Pregnant women should avoid Aggrenox because of its aspirin content. Aspirin can cause bleeding problems in mother and fetus and result in a low-birth-weight infant. Aggrenox should be taken during pregnancy only if your doctor determines that the potential benefit outweighs the risks.

Both ingredients in Aggrenox pass into breast milk. Nursing mothers who must take this drug should use infant formula.

Seniors: Seniors may need a reduced dose of Aggrenox.

Generic Name

Albuterol (al-BUE-tuh-rawl) G

Brand Names

AccuNeb
ProAir HFA
Proventil HFA
Ventolin HFA
VoSpire ER

Combination Products

Generic Ingredients: Albuterol + Ipratropium Bromide

Combivent
DuoNeb

The information in this profile also applies to the following drugs:

Generic Ingredients: Levalbuterol G

Xopenex
Xopenex HFA

Generic Ingredients: Metaproterenol G

Generic Ingredients: Pirbuterol

Maxair

Type of Drug

Bronchodilator.

Prescribed For

Bronchospasm associated with asthma or other obstructive pulmonary diseases, or induced by exercise.

General Information

Albuterol is similar to other bronchodilator drugs, such as metaproterenol and isoetharine, but it has a weaker effect on nerve receptors in the heart and blood vessels; therefore, it is somewhat safer for people with heart conditions. Levalbuterol is a special form of albuterol that carries a lower risk of side effects.

Cautions and Warnings

Do not use albuterol if you are **allergic** or **sensitive** to any of its ingredients. Rare serious reactions including itching, rash, swollen lips, and difficulty breathing have occurred after albuterol use.

Albuterol should be used with caution by people with a history of **angina pectoris** (brief attacks of chest pain), **heart disease**, **irregularities in heartbeat**, **high blood pressure**, **stroke** or **seizure**, **diabetes**, **thyroid disease**, **prostate disease**, or **glaucoma**.

Albuterol may lead to very low blood potassium, which has the potential to affect your heart. This effect usually passes, but your doctor should regularly check your potassium levels.

Excessive use of albuterol inhalants may worsen **asthma** or other **respiratory conditions**, and may increase breathing difficulties rather than relieve them. In the most extreme cases, people have had heart attacks after using excessive amounts of inhalant.

Possible Side Effects

▼ Most common: worsening of asthma, ear infection, upper-respiratory infection, stuffy nose, dizziness, headache, nausea, vomiting, and muscle cramps.

▼ Less common: angina, abnormal heart rhythms, rapid heartbeat and heart palpitations, allergic reaction, fever, tremors, low blood pressure, nervousness, low blood potassium, and high blood sugar. Your blood chemistry can change, making it more acid. Symptoms of this change can include deep and rapid breathing, chest pain, heart palpitations, headache, severe anxiety, visual difficulties, nausea, vomiting, abdominal pain, appetite changes, weight loss, muscle weakness, and bone pains.

Drug Interactions

- Albuterol's effects on the cardiovascular system may be increased by monoamine oxidase inhibitor (MAOI) and tricyclic antidepressants. Do not mix these drugs or use albuterol within 2 weeks after stopping an MAOI or tricyclic antidepressant drug.
- Beta blockers such as propranolol not only block the effects of albuterol but may cause severe bronchospasm in people with asthma.
- Albuterol may reduce the amount of digoxin in the blood of people taking both drugs. Digoxin dose adjustment may be required.
- Albuterol may worsen the potassium-depleting effect of loop or thiazide diuretics.

Food Interactions

Albuterol tablets are more effective when taken on an empty stomach—1 hour before or 2 hours after meals—but can be taken with food if they upset your stomach.

Usual Dose

Albuterol and Pirbuterol Inhalation

Adult and Child (age 4 and over): 1–2 puffs every 4–6 hours. Asthma triggered by exercise may be prevented by inhaling twice 15 minutes before exercising.

Child (under age 4): not recommended.

Albuterol Immediate-Release Tablets

Adult and Child (age 13 and over): starting dose—2 mg 3–4 times a day. Dosage may be cautiously increased to a maximum of 32 mg a day.

Child (age 6–12): starting dose—2 mg 3–4 times a day. Dosage may be cautiously increased to a maximum of 24 mg a day.

Child (under age 6): not recommended.

Albuterol Inhalation Solution

Child (age 4–12): starting dose—0.63 mg or 1.25 mg 3–4 times a day. Deliver over 5–15 minutes by nebulizer.

Child (under age 4): not recommended.

Albuterol Sustained-Release Tablets

Adult and Child (age 13 and over): 4–8 mg every 12 hours. Dosage may be cautiously increased to a maximum of 32 mg a day. People being switched from regular to sustained-release tablets generally take the same dosage per day, in fewer tablets—for example, a 4-mg tablet every 12 hours (1 dose) instead of a 2-mg tablet every 6 hours (2 doses).

Child (age 6–12): 4 mg every 12 hours.

Child (under age 6): not recommended.

Albuterol Syrup

Adult and Child (age 13 and over): 2–4 mg 3–4 times a day. Dosage may be cautiously increased to a maximum of 32 mg a day.

Child (age 6–12): 2 mg 3–4 times a day. Dosage may be cautiously increased to a maximum of 24 mg a day.

Child (age 2–5): starting dose—0.0454 mg per lb. of body weight 3 times a day, not to exceed 2 mg 3 times a day. Dosage may be cautiously increased to a maximum of 12 mg a day.

Levalbuterol Inhalation Solution

Adult and Child (age 12 and over): 0.63 mg 3 times a day every 6–8 hours. Some people may benefit from 1.25 mg at each dose. Deliver over 5–15 minutes by nebulizer.

Child (age 6–11): 0.31 mg 3 times a day every 6–8 hours, by nebulizer.

Overdosage

Overdose of albuterol inhalation usually results in exaggerated side effects, including chest pain and high blood pressure. People who inhale too much albuterol should see a doctor. Overdose of albuterol tablets may lead to changes in heart rate, palpitations, unusual heart rhythm, chest pain, high blood pressure, fever, chills, cold sweats, nausea, vomiting, and dilation of the pupils. Convulsions, sleeplessness, anxiety, and tremors may also develop, and the victim may collapse. If the albuterol overdose was taken within the past ½ hour, give the victim syrup of ipecac to induce vomiting. Do not give ipecac if the victim is unconscious or convulsing. If symptoms have already begun to develop, the victim may need to be taken to a hospital emergency room. Call for instructions, and if you seek treatment, ALWAYS bring the prescription bottle or container.

Special Information

If you are inhaling albuterol, be sure to follow the inhalation instructions that come with the product. The drug should be inhaled during the second ½ of your inward breath, since this will allow it to reach deeper into your lungs. Wait about 1–2 minutes between inhalations. Do not inhale albuterol if you have food or anything else in your mouth.

Do not take more albuterol than your doctor prescribes. Taking more than you need can worsen your symptoms. If your condition worsens after taking your medicine, contact your doctor at once and stop taking it.

Contact your doctor immediately if you develop chest pain, palpitations, rapid heartbeat, muscle tremors, dizziness, headache, facial flushing, or urinary difficulty, or if you continue having breathing difficulties after taking the medicine.

Do not crush or chew the extended-release tablets.

If you forget a dose of albuterol, take it as soon as you remember. If it is almost time for your next dose, skip the one you forgot. Do not take a double dose.

Special Populations

Pregnancy/Breast-feeding: When used during childbirth, albuterol can slow or delay natural labor. It can cause rapid heartbeat and high blood sugar in the mother and rapid heartbeat and low blood sugar in the baby. Albuterol also causes birth defects in animal studies. Albuterol should be taken during pregnancy only if your doctor determines that the potential benefit outweighs the risks.

It is not known if albuterol passes into breast milk. Nursing mothers who must take it should use infant formula.

Seniors: Seniors with cardiovascular disease should use albuterol with caution.

Type of Drug

Aldosterone Blockers (al-DOH-stir-own)

Brand Names

Generic Ingredients: Eplerenone G
Inspra

Generic Ingredients: Spironolactone G
Aldactone

Combination Products
Generic Ingredients: Hydrochlorothiazide + Spironolactone G
Aldactazide

Prescribed For

High blood pressure, cirrhosis, kidney disease, congestive heart failure (CHF), severe heart failure, low blood potassium, and hyperaldosteronism (overproduction of aldosterone). Spironolactone may be prescribed to treat swelling during pregnancy (see "Special Populations").

General Information

Aldosterone blockers limit the access of aldosterone—a hormone that helps to regulate several different body functions—to its receptor. Too much aldosterone results in high sodium levels, which can lead to water retention and potassium loss; it can also affect the size, shape, and function of the heart. Aldosterone blockers are generally combined with other medicines in the management of disease. These drugs are useful in removing excess body fluids in conditions associated with high aldosterone levels.

One in every 10 people with high blood pressure has excess aldosterone in their systems. In people with CHF, aldosterone levels can be 20 times higher than normal, which can worsen their condition, making the use of aldosterone blockers an important part of their treatment. Aldosterone blockers also help the heart return to normal size, shape, and function in people with heart failure. Eplerenone is broken down in the liver, primarily by an enzyme system known as CYP3A4.

Cautions and Warnings

Do not take aldosterone blockers if you are **allergic** or **sensitive** to any of their ingredients.

Spironolactone has been shown to cause tumors in rats when used in high doses. It should only be used for approved medical conditions and only when necessary.

Do not use aldosterone blockers if you have **kidney failure**, **difficulty urinating**, or **high blood potassium**.

People with **liver disease** should be cautious about using aldosterone blockers.

People taking an aldosterone blocker should have their potassium levels checked periodically.

People with **diabetes** who have albumin in their urine should not take aldosterone blockers.

Possible Side Effects

Eplerenone

- ▼ Less common: dizziness, diarrhea, fatigue, flu-like symptoms, coughing, abdominal pain, elevation of blood-cholesterol and/or triglyceride levels, elevation of blood-potassium levels, and albumin in the urine.
- ▼ Rare: enlargement of the breasts in males, irregular menstrual cycles in women, and painful breasts. Contact your doctor if you experience anything unusual while taking any medication.

Spironolactone

- ▼ Less common: drowsiness, lethargy, headache, gastrointestinal upset, cramps and diarrhea, rash, mental confusion, fever, feeling unwell, enlargement of the breasts in males,

Possible Side Effects *(continued)*

impotence, and irregular menstrual cycles or deepening of the voice in women.

Drug Interactions

- Do not combine eplerenone with itraconazole or ketoconazole. These drugs can cause the amount of eplerenone in the blood to increase by up to 500% and may cause fatal increases in blood potassium. Do not use eplerenone with other potent CYP3A4 inhibitors, including clarithromycin, erythromycin, telithromycin, indinavir, nelfinavir, ritonavir, saquinavir, nefazodone, aprepitant, fluconazole, verapamil, diltiazem, and cimetidine due to the risk of high blood potassium (see "Special Information").
- Combining a potassium supplement and an aldosterone blocker can lead to dangerously high blood levels of potassium. Do not use a salt substitute or take any extra potassium unless prescribed by your doctor.
- Combining an aldosterone blocker with an ACE inhibitor or an angiotensin II receptor blocker (ARB) may significantly raise blood potassium. Be sure your doctor monitors your potassium levels if you combine these drugs.
- Spironolactone may interfere with anticoagulant (blood-thinning) drugs and mitotane (an anticancer drug).
- Aspirin can interfere with the diuretic effect of spironolactone but does not alter its effect on high blood pressure or CHF.
- Combining spironolactone with alcohol, barbiturates, or narcotics can lead to dizziness or fainting when rising suddenly from a sitting or lying position.
- Combining spironolactone and a corticosteroid can lead to very low blood potassium.
- Spironolactone may alter your response to drugs used during general anesthesia.
- Lithium generally should not be combined with any diuretic.
- Combining nonsteroidal anti-inflammatory drugs (NSAIDs) with aldosterone blockers can lead to severe elevations of blood potassium and reduce the blood-pressure-lowering effect of the diuretic.
- Spironolactone may raise digoxin blood levels and increase the risk of severe digoxin side effects. Your doctor may have to adjust your digoxin dosage.

- St. John's wort (a CYP3A4 inducer) may decrease eplerenone levels by about 30%.

Food Interactions

Food appears to increase the amount of spironolactone absorbed into the blood. Take this drug with food at the same time every day. Eplerenone can be taken without regard to food or meals. Taking this drug with grapefruit juice increases the amount of drug absorbed into your body.

Usual Dose

Eplerenone

Adult: 25–100 mg a day.

Child: not recommended.

Hydrochlorothiazide + Spironolactone

Adult: 1–8 25-mg tablets a day.

Spironolactone

Adult: Starting dosage is 50–100 mg a day in divided doses for high blood pressure; 25–200 mg a day in divided doses for high fluid levels related to other diseases; 25–100 mg a day for low potassium levels; 100–400 mg a day for hyperaldosteronism.

Child: 0.5–2 mg per lb. of body weight a day in divided doses.

Overdosage

Eplerenone overdose may lead to low blood pressure and high blood potassium. Spironolactone overdose may lead to drowsiness, confusion, rash, nausea, vomiting, dizziness, and diarrhea. Rarely, coma may occur in people with severe liver disease. High blood potassium may also occur, especially in people with kidney disease. Contact your local poison control center or a hospital emergency room for more information. If you seek treatment, ALWAYS bring the prescription bottle or container.

Special Information

Take aldosterone blockers exactly as they are prescribed.

High blood levels of potassium associated with aldosterone blockers may cause weakness, lethargy, drowsiness, muscle pain or cramps, and muscular fatigue. Use caution while doing anything that requires intense concentration, such as driving or operating machinery.

Do not use a salt substitute or take anything else that is a source of extra potassium, including many multivitamin or supplement products.

People with high blood pressure should not self-medicate with over-the-counter cough, cold, or allergy remedies containing stimulants. These drugs can increase the effect of blood pressure medication and have an adverse effect on the heart.

Call your doctor if you are taking spironolactone and develop skin rash or peeling skin, itching, joint aches, and fever. These can be signs of a life-threatening skin disorder.

If you forget a dose, take it as soon as you remember. If it is almost time for your next dose, skip the one you forgot and continue with your regular schedule. Do not take a double dose.

Special Populations

Pregnancy/Breast-feeding: Animal studies with eplerenone showed no effects on a developing fetus. Spironolactone crosses into the fetal circulation. Aldosterone blockers should be taken during pregnancy only if your doctor determines that the potential benefit outweighs the risks.

Aldosterone blockers pass into breast milk. Nursing mothers who must take aldosterone blockers should use infant formula.

Seniors: Seniors may be more sensitive to the effects of these drugs, especially high blood-potassium levels.

Generic Name

Aliskiren (ah-LISS-kih-ren)

Brand Names

Tekturna

Combination Products

Generic Ingredients: Aliskiren + Amlodipine
Tecamlo

Generic Ingredients: Aliskiren + Amlodipine + Hydrochlorothiazide
Amturnide

Generic Ingredients: Aliskiren + Hydrochlorothiazide
Tekturna HCT

Generic Ingredients: Aliskiren + Valsartan
Valturna

Type of Drug

Direct renin inhibitor.

Prescribed For

High blood pressure.

General Information

Renin is produced by the kidney in response to a reduction in blood volume and the amount of blood passing through the kidney. Once in the blood, renin reacts with other hormones to form a very powerful blood vessel constrictor called angiotensin II that directly raises blood pressure. Renin also works with a hormone called aldosterone to raise blood pressure, and it prevents sodium from being eliminated from the body. This increases the amount of water in the system, raising blood volume and increasing blood pressure. Aliskiren inhibits renin and all of its actions, thereby lowering blood pressure. The blood-pressure-lowering effect is usually seen within 2 weeks of starting treatment. When aliskiren treatment is stopped, blood pressure gradually rises to pretreatment levels. Only about 2.5% of any dose is absorbed into the blood and it takes about a week to reach a steady level in the blood. Most of the drug that is absorbed is broken down in the liver. The rest passes out of the body unchanged in the urine. Aliskiren may be used alone or with other hypertensives. For more information see Amlodipine, page 224, Hydrochlorothiazide, page 55, and Valsartan, page 98.

Cautions and Warnings

Do not take aliskiren if you are **allergic** or **sensitive** to any of its ingredients.

These medications may cause injury or death to a developing **fetus**.

Angioedema (a potentially life-threatening swelling of the lips and throat) can occur at any time during aliskiren treatment. If this happens, stop taking the medicine and go to your doctor's office or a hospital emergency room for treatment. This reaction can interfere with your breathing.

Do not take Tekturna HCT if you have **difficulty with urination**.

Hydrochlorothiazide, an ingredient in Tekturna HCT, has been associated with vision problems, specifically temporary nearsightedness and acute angle-closure glaucoma. If glaucoma is left untreated, it can result in permanent vision loss. Contact your doctor if you experience any difficulties with your vision while taking Tekturna HCT.

The safety of aliskiren in people with moderate to severe **kidney disease** or **renal artery disease** is not known.

The combination of aliskiren and an ACE inhibitor, a salt substitute, or a potassium-sparing diuretic can lead to **high blood levels of potassium**, which can affect the heart muscle.

Aliskiren may be less effective in some **black patients with high blood pressure**, especially when dietary salt intake is high. Nevertheless, it should still be considered a useful blood-pressure treatment.

Possible Side Effects

- ▼ Common: nausea, dizziness, and sleeplessness.
- ▼ Less common: diarrhea, abdominal pain, upset stomach, gastroesophageal reflux disease (GERD), cough, rash, high blood levels of uric acid, gout, kidney stones, headache, nose and throat irritation, fatigue, upper-respiratory infection, and back pain.
- ▼ Rare: difficulty breathing; swelling of the hands, face, eyes, or whole body; and seizures. Contact your doctor if you experience anything unusual while taking any medication.

Drug Interactions

- Do not mix these drugs with potassium supplements, potassium-sparing diuretics, amiloride, eplerenone, triamterene, or spironolactone.
- Atorvastatin, cyclosporine, itraconazole, and ketoconazole may substantially increase blood levels of aliskiren. Do not mix these medications.
- Mixing aliskiren with irbesartan can reduce the amount of aliskiren in the blood by 50%. This may reduce the effectiveness of aliskiren.
- Aliskiren should be used cautiously with ACE inhibitors, particularly in patients with diabetes.
- Aliskiren can reduce blood levels of the diuretic furosemide by 30–50%, reducing the diuretic's effect.
- Combining Tekturna HCT and narcotics, barbiturates, or alcohol may lead to dizziness or fainting when rising suddenly from a sitting or lying position.

- Dosage adjustments may be necessary when taking Tekturna HCT with an antidiabetic medication.
- The effects of lithium can be increased when taken with Tekturna HCT; this combination should probably be avoided.
- Nonsteroidal anti-inflammatory drugs (NSAIDs), cholestyramine, and colestipol resins can reduce the effects of Tekturna HCT.
- Combining Tekturna HCT and a corticosteroid can result in very low blood potassium.
- Taking amlodipine and simvastatin may lead to serious side effects. The dose of simvastatin should not exceed 20 mg a day.
- Conivaptan may increase amlodipine levels, increasing side effects. Additional monitoring may be necessary.
- Rifampin and ritonavir may increase levels of valsartan. Dosage adjustments may be necessary.

Food Interactions

Aliskiren may be taken without regard to food or meals. Avoid taking it with high-fat meals because they can drastically reduce the amount of aliskiren absorbed into the blood. Do not use a salt substitute while taking this medication.

Usual Dose

Aliskiren

Adult: 150–300 mg at the same time every day.

Child: not recommended.

Aliskiren + Amlodipine

Adult: one 150/5-mg tablet to start, increasing as needed to one 300/10-mg tablet a day.

Child: not recommended.

Aliskiren + Amlodipine + Hydrochlorothiazide

Adult: one 150/5/12.5-mg tablet a day, increasing as needed to one 300/10/25-mg tablet a day.

Child: not recommended.

Aliskiren + Hydrochlorothiazide

Adult: one 150/12.5-mg tablet to start, increasing as needed to one 300/25-mg tablet a day.

Child: not recommended.

Aliskiren + Valsartan

Adult: One 150/160- or 300/320-mg tablet a day.

Child: not recommended.

Overdosage

The most likely symptom of overdose is low blood pressure (symptoms include dizziness and fainting). If you think you have taken an overdose, contact your doctor or go to a hospital emergency room. If you seek treatment, ALWAYS bring the prescription bottle or container.

Special Information

Contact your doctor at once if you develop swelling of the face, eyes, lips, tongue, or throat; difficulty swallowing or breathing; hoarseness; or other signs of a drug reaction or allergy.

Contact your doctor if you are taking aliskiren and suspect you may be pregnant.

Make sure your doctor knows if you use cyclosporine, a salt substitute, or a potassium-sparing diuretic.

Take your medication at the same time every day; this will help you to take it regularly and not skip doses. If you forget a dose, take it as soon as you remember. If you do not remember until it is almost time for your next dose, skip the dose you forgot and continue with your regular schedule. Do not take a double dose.

Special Populations

Pregnancy/Breast-feeding: Aliskiren can injure or kill a developing fetus. Pregnant women should not take aliskiren. Women who suspect they are pregnant must contact their doctor at once and stop taking aliskiren when pregnancy is confirmed. In those rare cases in which aliskiren is considered life-saving for the mother and there is no substitute for aliskiren, your doctor may advise that you continue on the medicine and then check your baby's development with periodic ultrasound examinations.

It is not known if this drug passes into breast milk. Nursing mothers should use infant formula.

Seniors: Seniors may have higher blood levels of aliskiren and be more susceptible to drug side effects, but starting dose adjustment is not required.

Generic Name

Alitretinoin (al-ih-TRET-in-oin)

Brand Names

Panretin

Type of Drug

Retinoid.

Prescribed For

Skin lesions of Kaposi's sarcoma (KS).

General Information

Alitretinoin binds to and activates retinoid receptors in human cells. Once activated, these receptors help stimulate the body's natural mechanisms for limiting tissue growth—in this case, the growth of KS cells. KS lesions, which are primarily associated with human immunodeficiency virus (HIV), can respond to alitretinoin in as little as 2 weeks, but most people do not start to see results for 4–8 weeks or, in some cases, 14 weeks or more.

Cautions and Warnings

Do not use alitretinoin if you are **allergic** or **sensitive** to any of its ingredients or to retinoids.

Alitretinoin is applied to individual KS lesions. It does not treat systemic KS or prevent new KS lesions from forming.

People requiring **systemic KS treatment** (those who have developed more than 10 new KS lesions within a month) should not use alitretinoin.

People with **swollen lymph glands**, **KS that affects the lungs**, or **other major organ involvement** should not use alitretinoin.

Reduce or discontinue treatment if skin at local application site develops dermal toxicity (severe inflammation and swelling).

Possible Side Effects

- ▼ Most common: rash and burning pain at application site.
- ▼ Common: itching, flaking, peeling, cracking, oozing, swelling, and inflammation at application site.

Drug Interactions

- Do not use insect repellant products that contain DEET, a widely used chemical repellant. Alitretinoin increases DEET toxicity.

Usual Dose

Adult: Apply 2–4 times a day to KS skin lesions. Seniors should use this drug with caution.

Child: not recommended.

Overdosage

Little is known about the effects of accidental ingestion. Contact your local poison control center or a hospital emergency room for information. If you seek treatment, ALWAYS bring the prescription bottle or container.

Special Information

Apply enough alitretinoin gel to cover the entire skin lesion. Allow the gel to dry for 3–5 minutes before covering the area with clothing. Avoid showering, bathing, or swimming for at least 3 hours.

If you use a bandage or dressing, be sure it is not tight and that air can circulate freely over the area.

Avoid applying alitretinoin to unaffected skin because it may be irritated by the drug. Avoid applying near the nose, eyes, or mouth.

Alitretinoin contains alcohol. Always keep it away from any open flame.

Retinoids can cause unusual sensitivity to the sun. Although this has not been seen with alitretinoin, you should avoid prolonged exposure to the sun or use sunscreen while taking this drug.

If you forget a dose, apply it as soon as you remember. If it is almost time for your next dose, apply the forgotten dose and then space the rest of your doses throughout the day. Continue with your regular schedule the next day.

Special Populations

Pregnancy/Breast-feeding: Alitretinoin can harm the fetus when sufficient levels of the drug are present in the mother's bloodstream, but it is not known if these levels are achieved during routine use of alitretinoin. Alitretinoin should be taken during pregnancy only if your doctor determines that the potential benefit outweighs the risks.

It is not known if alitretinoin passes into breast milk. Nursing mothers who must use alitretinoin should use infant formula.

Seniors: There is no information on use of alitretinoin by seniors. Seniors should use it with caution.

Generic Name

Allopurinol (al-oe-PURE-in-nol) G

Brand Names

Zyloprim

The information in this profile also applies to the following drugs:

Generic Ingredients: Febuxostat
Uloric

Type of Drug

Xanthine oxidase inhibitor.

Prescribed For

Gout or gouty arthritis; also prescribed to counter the effects of certain therapies for cancer, ulcers, abnormal heart rhythms in heart bypass patients, seizures, and other conditions that may be associated with too much uric acid in the body.

General Information

Unlike other antigout drugs, which affect the elimination of uric acid from the body, allopurinol and febuxostat act on the system that manufactures uric acid in your body. A high level of uric acid can indicate that you have gout, psoriasis, cancer, or any of a number of other diseases. High levels of uric acid can also be caused by taking certain drugs.

Allopurinol mouthwash helps to prevent mouth, stomach, and intestinal ulcers caused by fluorouracil, an antineoplastic drug. Allopurinol may be given before heart bypass surgery to reduce abnormal rhythms and other surgical complications. It can be used to reduce the relapse rates of duodenal ulcers associated with *Helicobacter pylori* infection and to reduce the vomiting of blood from stomach irritation caused by nonsteroidal anti-inflammatory drugs (NSAIDs). Allopurinol has also been used to control seizures in people for whom standard treatments are not effective.

Cautions and Warnings

Do not take these drugs if you are **allergic** or **sensitive** to any of their ingredients, or if you have ever developed a **severe reaction** to either. Stop taking the medication immediately and contact your doctor if you develop a rash or any other adverse effects while taking allopurinol. Do not start taking allopurinol again if you stopped it because of a severe reaction.

Allopurinol should be used by **children** only if they have high uric-acid levels due to **neoplastic disease** or to **rare metabolic conditions**.

An increase in gout flare-ups or symptoms is common when starting treatment with these drugs. If this happens, your doctor may prescribe colchicines or an NSAID pain reliever for up to 6 months.

Febuxostat is associated with more heart attacks and strokes than allopurinol.

Rare liver irritation and toxicity have occurred with these drugs that improve when drug treatment is discontinued. People taking these drugs should periodically be tested for liver and kidney function. People with severely **compromised kidney function** should take a reduced dose of allopurinol. Febuxostat does not require any alteration in dosage in people with mild or moderate **liver or kidney disease**.

Possible Side Effects

Allopurinol

- ▼ Most common: rash associated with severe, allergic, or sensitivity reaction to allopurinol. If you develop an unusual rash or other sign of drug toxicity, stop taking this medication and contact your doctor.
- ▼ Less common: nausea, vomiting, diarrhea, intermittent stomach pain, gas, upset stomach, headache, insomnia, tingling or numbness in the hands or feet, muscle or joint pain, drowsiness or lack of ability to concentrate, and abnormal liver function tests.
- ▼ Rare: Rare side effects can occur in almost any part of the body. Contact your doctor if you experience anything unusual while taking any medication.

Febuxostat

- ▼ Common: abnormal liver function tests.
- ▼ Less common: rash and nausea.
- ▼ Rare: Rare side effects can occur in almost any part of the body. Contact your doctor if you experience anything unusual while taking any medication.

Drug Interactions

- Large doses of drugs that make your urine more acidic, like megadoses of vitamin C, may increase the risk of kidney stone formation.
- Alcohol, diazoxide, mecamylamine, or pyrazinamide can increase the amount of uric acid in your blood; an increase in your allopurinol dose may be required.
- Do not mix these drugs with azathioprine, cyclophosphamide, mercaptopurine, or other anticancer drugs. They increase the blood levels of the cancer drugs, leading to possible toxicity, bleeding, or infection.
- Allopurinol may prolong the effects of the diabetes drug chloropropamide, and can lead to hypoglycemic reactions in patients with kidney disease.
- Taking allopurinol with probenecid or sulfinpyrazone may cause excessive reduction of uric acid.
- Allopurinol may interact with some anticoagulant (blood thinning) medications, reducing the rate at which the anticoagulant is broken down in the body. Dosage reduction may be necessary.
- People who are susceptible to ampicillin, amoxicillin, bacampicillin, or hetacillin rash are more likely to develop such a reaction while also taking allopurinol.
- Combining a thiazide diuretic or an ACE inhibitor (for high blood pressure or heart failure) with allopurinol increases the risk of a drug-sensitivity reaction.
- Combining vidarabine with allopurinol may increase the risk of neurotoxic effects and anemia, nausea, pain, and itching.
- Large doses of allopurinol—more than 600 mg a day—may increase the effects of and risk of toxic reactions to theophylline by interfering with its clearance from the body.

Food Interactions

Allopurinol is better tolerated if taken with food. Febuxostat may be taken with or without food. Take each dose with a full glass of water. Drink 10–12 glasses of water, juices, soda, or another liquid each day to avoid the formation of uric acid crystals in your urine or kidneys.

Usual Dose

Allopurinol

Adult and Child (age 11 and over): 100–800 mg a day, depending on disease and response.

Child (age 6–10): 300 mg a day.
Child (under age 6): 150 mg a day.

The dose should be reviewed periodically by your doctor to be sure that it is producing the desired therapeutic effect.

Febuxostat

Adult: 40–80 mg once a day.
Child: not recommended.

Overdosage

No overdoses of febuxostat have been reported; the drug was studied in doses up to 300 mg per day for a week. Expected overdose symptoms are exaggerated side effects. Allergic skin reactions to allopurinol can be severe and at times fatal. Overdose victims should be taken to a hospital or emergency room. If you seek treatment, ALWAYS bring the prescription bottle or container.

Special Information

Allopurinol can make you drowsy or make it difficult to concentrate. Take care while driving a car or operating hazardous equipment.

Gout attacks may actually increase during the first few months of taking allopurinol. These attacks should subside.

Contact your doctor at once if you develop rash, hives, itching, chills, fever, nausea, muscle aches, unusual tiredness, fever, yellowing of the skin or whites of the eyes, painful urination, blood in the urine, irritation of the eyes, swelling of the lips or mouth, chest pain, shortness of breath, or symptoms suggestive of a stroke.

Avoid large doses of vitamin C, which can cause the formation of kidney stones during allopurinol treatment. Be sure to drink 10–12 8-oz. glasses of water a day while taking this medication.

If you forget to take a dose of allopurinol, take it as soon as possible. If it is almost time for your next regular dose, double this dose. For example, if your regular dose is 100 mg and you miss a dose, take 200 mg at the next usual dose time.

Special Populations

Pregnancy/Breast-feeding: Animal studies indicate these drugs may cause birth defects or interfere with fetal development. Check with your doctor before taking them if you are or might be pregnant. These drugs should be taken during pregnancy only if your doctor determines that the potential benefit outweighs the risks.

These drugs pass into breast milk. Nursing mothers who must take them should use infant formula.

Seniors: No special precautions are required. Follow your doctor's directions and report any side effects at once.

Type of Drug

Alpha Blockers

Brand Names

Generic Ingredients: Alfuzosin G
Uroxatral

Generic Ingredients: Doxazosin G
Cardura
Cardura XL

Generic Ingredients: Prazosin G
Minipress

Generic Ingredients: Silodosin
Rapaflo

Generic Ingredients: Tamsulosin G
Flomax

Generic Ingredients: Terazosin Hydrochloride G
Hytrin

Prescribed For

High blood pressure (doxazosin, terazosin, and prazosin in combination with a diuretic) and benign prostatic hyperplasia (BPH). Prazosin has also been prescribed for Raynaud's disease. These drugs have also been used to help childhood incontinence, with mixed results.

General Information

These medicines block nerve endings known as alpha-1 receptors. They reduce blood pressure by dilating (widening) and reducing pressure within the blood vessels. The maximum blood-pressure-lowering effect of prazosin and terazosin is seen between 2 and 6 hours after taking a single dose. Terazosin's effect lasts for 24 hours.

In BPH, alpha blockers work by relaxing smooth muscles in the prostate and neck of the bladder. This effect is produced by blockage of alpha-1 receptors in the affected muscles. Despite the fact that these medicines alleviate the urinary symptoms of BPH, their long-term effect on the complications of BPH or the need for urinary surgery is not known. Alpha blockers are broken down in the liver.

Prazosin and terazosin can slightly reduce cholesterol levels and improve the ratio of high-density lipoprotein (HDL)—"good" cholesterol—and low-density lipoprotein (LDL), a positive step for people with a blood-cholesterol problem; however, they are not specifically prescribed as a cholesterol treatment.

Cautions and Warnings

Do not take alpha blockers if you are **allergic** or **sensitive** to any of their ingredients.

Alfuzosin, silodosin, and tamsulosin are only approved for prostate disease and should not be taken by **women**.

Alpha blockers may cause dizziness and fainting, especially after the first few doses. This is known as the "first-dose effect" and may be minimized by limiting the first dose to 1 mg at bedtime. The first-dose effect occurs in about 1% of people and may recur if the drug is stopped for a few days and then restarted.

Do not take alfuzosin or silodosin if you have moderate to severe **liver disease**, since this can drastically increase blood concentrations of the drug.

Alpha blockers should be taken with caution if you have **kidney disease**, since blood concentrations may be increased by 50%. Silodosin may be taken in a reduced dosage if you have **moderate kidney disease**.

Do not take these medicines if you are already taking an alpha blocker for either high blood pressure or prostate problems.

Doxazosin and terazosin may slightly reduce the counts of red and white blood cells.

People taking terazosin may experience a weight gain of about 2 lbs.

Tell your eye surgeon that you are taking an alpha blocker if you are planning **cataract surgery**. These drugs can cause a surgical complication called intraoperative floppy iris syndrome (IFIS).

Doxazosin, tamsulosin, and terazosin may rarely cause priapism (a persistent, painful erection), which should be treated by a doctor.

Possible Side Effects

Alfuzosin

▼ Most common: dizziness, fatigue, upper-respiratory infection, and headache.

Possible Side Effects *(continued)*

- Less common: pain, abdominal pain, upset stomach, constipation, nausea, impotence, bronchitis, sinusitis, sore throat, low blood pressure, dizziness, and fainting.
- Rare: rash; rapid heartbeat; chest pain; leg or ankle swelling; diarrhea; liver damage; runny nose; itching; hives; extreme lip, face, or other swelling; and priapism (a persistent, painful erection). Contact your doctor if you experience anything unusual while taking any medication.

Doxazosin

- Most common: headache, dizziness, and weakness.
- Less common: heart palpitations; abnormal heart rhythms; chest pain; nausea; diarrhea; constipation; abdominal pain or discomfort; gas; breathing difficulties; nosebleed; sore throat; runny nose; muscle or joint pain; visual disturbances; conjunctivitis (pinkeye); ringing in the ears; fainting; depression; decreased sex drive or sexual function; tingling in the hands or feet; nervousness; tiredness; anxiety; sleeplessness; poor muscle coordination; muscle stiffness; poor bladder control; frequent urination; itching; rash; sweating; fluid retention; facial swelling and flushing; and back, neck, shoulder, arm, or leg pain.
- Rare: vomiting, dry mouth, sinus irritation, bronchitis, cold or flu-like symptoms, worsening of asthma, coughing, hair loss, weight gain, and fever. Contact your doctor if you experience anything unusual while taking any medication.

Prazosin

Side effects occur less often with prazosin than with other alpha blockers.

- Most common: dizziness, drowsiness, weakness, nausea, headache, and heart palpitations.
- Less common: low blood pressure, dizziness when rising from a sitting or lying position, rapid heartbeat, vomiting, dry mouth, diarrhea, constipation, abdominal pain or discomfort, breathing difficulties, stuffy nose, nosebleed, joint or muscle pain, blurred vision, conjunctivitis (pinkeye), ringing or buzzing in the ears, depression, nervousness, tingling in the hands or feet, frequent urination, impotence, poor urinary control, priapism (a persistent, painful erection),

Possible Side Effects *(continued)*

itching, sweating, rash, hair loss, fluid retention, and fever. Contact your doctor if you experience anything unusual while taking any medication.

Silodosin

- ▼ Most common: abnormal ejaculation.
- ▼ Less common: dizziness, diarrhea, fainting when getting up from a sitting or lying position, headache, stuffy nose, runny nose, inflammation of the nose and throat, sinus irritation, elevated prostate-specific antigen (PSA) test, abdominal pain, weakness, and sleeplessness.
- ▼ Rare: priapism (a persistent, painful erection), fainting, bruising, severe rash, and liver disease (yellowing of the skin or whites of the eyes and elevated liver enzyme tests). Contact your doctor if you experience anything unusual while taking any medication.

Tamsulosin

- ▼ Most common: dizziness, weakness, and headache.
- ▼ Less common: low blood pressure; rapid heartbeat; abnormal heart rhythms; chest pain; flushing in the face, arms, or legs; fainting; vomiting; dry mouth; diarrhea; constipation; abdominal pain or discomfort; gas; breathing difficulties; stuffy nose; sinus inflammation; cold or flu-like symptoms; cough; bronchitis; worsening of asthma; nosebleed; sore throat; runny nose; shoulder, neck, or back pain; pain in the arms or legs; joint pain; arthritis; muscle pain; blurred vision or other visual disturbances; conjunctivitis (pinkeye); eye pain; nervousness; tingling in the hands or feet; tiredness; anxiety; difficulty sleeping; frequent urination; urinary infection; abnormal ejaculation; itching; rash; sweating; swelling of the face, arms, or legs; and fever.
- ▼ Rare: depression; reduced sex drive or abnormal sexual function, including priapism (a persistent, painful erection); fluid retention; and weight gain. Contact your doctor if you experience anything unusual while taking any medication.

Terazosin

- ▼ Most common: dizziness, weakness, and headache.
- ▼ Rare: depression; reduced sex drive or abnormal sexual function, including priapism (a persistent, painful erection);

Possible Side Effects *(continued)*

fluid retention; and weight gain. Contact your doctor if you experience anything unusual while taking any medication.

Drug Interactions

- Potent inhibitors of CYP3A4 such as clarithromycin, erythromycin, itraconazole, ketoconazole, nefazodone, ritonavir, and telithromycin should not be taken with alfuzosin or silodosin.
- Cyclosporine may raise levels of silodosin. Coadministration is not recommended.
- When taken with other blood-pressure-lowering drugs, including beta blockers, calcium channel blockers, and thiazide diuretics, these drugs reduce blood pressure and can make you dizzy. Terazosin produces a greater blood pressure reduction than the others.
- Mixing sildenafil or another drug for erectile dysfunction with an alpha blocker may lead to a sudden blood pressure drop and some dizziness when rising from a sitting or lying position. This interaction can also increase the risk of dizziness or fainting after the first dose of the alpha blocker (the "first-dose effect").
- Amiodarone increases the effects of alfuzosin, requiring additional monitoring.
- Diltiazem and verapamil may increase levels of alfuzosin, increasing the possibility of side effects. Verapamil also increases blood levels of terazosin.
- Cimetidine increases blood levels of alfuzosin and tamsulosin and should be used with caution.
- The blood-pressure-lowering effect of alfuzosin can be reduced by nonsteroidal anti-inflammatory drugs (NSAIDs), including aspirin.
- People taking any of these drugs for high blood pressure should avoid over-the-counter cough medicines, cold and allergy remedies, and appetite suppressants. These products often contain stimulant ingredients that can increase blood pressure.
- People taking an alpha blocker should avoid alcohol, which increases the risk of low blood pressure.

Food Interactions

Food does not affect the absorption of these drugs. However, it is often recommended to take them after the same meal each day to make it easier to remember to take them.

Usual Dose

Alfuzosin: one 10-mg tablet taken after the same meal every day. Do not crush or chew the tablets.

Doxazosin

Adult: starting dose—1 mg at bedtime; may be increased to a maximum of 8 mg for BPH or 16 mg for high blood pressure, taken once a day.

Child: 1–4 mg a day for pediatric high blood pressure.

Prazosin

Adult: 1 mg 2–3 times a day to start; may be increased to a total daily dose of 20 mg, although 40 mg a day (in divided doses) has been used in some cases.

Child: 0.02–0.22 mg per lb. a day in divided doses for pediatric high blood pressure.

Silodosin: one 8-mg tablet a day with a meal. People with moderate kidney function should take one 4-mg tablet a day.

Tamsulosin: starting dose—0.4 mg ½ hour after the same meal each day. Dosage may be increased to 0.8 mg a day if there has been no response after 2–4 weeks.

Terazosin

Adult: starting dose—1 mg at bedtime. Dosage may be increased in increments of 1–5 mg to a total of 20 mg a day. The usual recommended dose is 10 mg a day for BPH and 5 mg a day for high blood pressure.

Child: 1–20 mg a day for pediatric high blood pressure.

Overdosage

Symptoms may include drowsiness, poor reflexes, and very low blood pressure. Take the victim to a hospital emergency room. If you seek treatment, ALWAYS bring the prescription bottle or container.

Special Information

Take alpha blockers exactly as they are prescribed and do not stop taking them unless directed to do so by your doctor. Avoid over-the-counter drugs that contain stimulants because they may increase your blood pressure.

Alpha blockers may cause dizziness, headache, and drowsiness, especially 2–6 hours after taking your first dose, though these effects may persist after the first few doses. Wait 12–24 hours after taking the first dose before driving, operating machinery, or performing any other task that requires intense concentration. You may take alpha blockers at bedtime to minimize this problem.

Some people undergoing eye surgery who take alpha blockers can experience IFIS. Make sure to tell your eye surgeon if you are taking or have ever been treated with an alpha blocker. There is no benefit to stopping alpha-blocker treatment before cataract surgery.

Prostate cancer and BPH may have similar symptoms. Talk to your doctor about ruling out prostate cancer before beginning treatment for BPH.

Contact your doctor if you develop severe dizziness, heart palpitations, or any bothersome or persistent side effect.

If you are taking an alpha blocker for high blood pressure and stop taking it without gradually reducing the dosage, you may experience a sudden increase in blood pressure, or "rebound effect."

If you forget a dose, take it as soon as you remember. If it is almost time for your next dose, skip the forgotten dose and continue with your regular schedule. Do not take a double dose.

Special Populations

Pregnancy/Breast-feeding: Alfuzosin, silodosin, and tamsulosin should never be used by pregnant women. In animal studies, large dosages of terazosin damaged the fetus and doxazosin has been shown to affect the pregnancy. An alpha blocker should be taken during pregnancy only if your doctor determines that the potential benefit outweighs the risks.

These drugs can pass into breast milk. Nursing mothers who must take an alpha blocker for high blood pressure should use infant formula.

Seniors: Seniors, especially those age 75 and over, and those with heart failure or kidney disease, may be more sensitive to the effects of an alpha blocker.

Generic Name

Alprostadil (al-PROS-tuh-dil) G

Brand Names

Caverject	Edex	Prostin VR
Caverject Impulse	Muse	

Type of Drug

Erectile dysfunction agent.

Prescribed For

Erectile dysfunction; also prescribed for atherosclerosis (hardening of the arteries), gangrene, and pain due to blood vessel disease.

General Information

A male erection happens when blood flows into blood vessels and holding areas inside the penis. Problems occur when blood cannot move into the penis as it normally should. Alprostadil (prostaglandin E1 or PGE1) helps men get and keep an erection by dilating blood vessels that supply the penis and by relaxing muscles to help expand holding areas. Alprostadil also dilates other vessels and reduces platelet stickiness—which slows blood-clotting rates—and relaxes some muscle groups. Alprostadil must be injected into the tissue of the penis or inserted into the urethra.

Cautions and Warnings

Do not take alprostadil if you are **allergic** or **sensitive** to any of its ingredients or to other prostaglandin drugs.

Alprostadil can cause priapism (a persistent, painful erection). People with diseases in which priapism is a possibility—**sickle cell anemia or trait**, **multiple myeloma**, **leukemia**—those with **penile deformities** or **penile implants**, **women**, **children**, or those for whom sexual activity could be dangerous should not use alprostadil.

Penile pain is common after using either form of alprostadil, although it is usually mild or moderate.

Possible Side Effects

Injection

- ▼ Most common: penile pain.
- ▼ Less common: prolonged erection; penile fibrosis (deformity); blood blister or black-and-blue marks at the injection site, usually caused by poor injection technique; penis disorders, including yeast infection, numbness, irritation, sensitivity, itching, redness, and torn skin; penile rash or swelling; headache; dizziness; fainting; respiratory infection; flu-like symptoms; sinus inflammation; runny or stuffy nose; cough; blood-pressure changes; localized pain in places other than injection site; prostate problems; back pain; and general pain.

Possible Side Effects *(continued)*

- ▼ Rare: Rare side effects can affect the penis, kidney and urinary tract, heart and blood, skin, and eyes. Contact your doctor if you experience anything unusual while taking any medication.

Pellets

- ▼ Most common: penile pain.
- ▼ Common: urethral pain, burning or bleeding, and testicular pain.
- ▼ Less common: headache, dizziness, respiratory infection, flu-like symptoms, runny nose, sinus inflammation, low blood pressure, back pain, pelvic pain, and general pain.
- ▼ Rare: Rare side effects can affect the kidney and urinary tract, heart and blood, skin, and eyes. Contact your doctor if you experience anything unusual while taking any medication.

Drug Interactions

- Alprostadil can increase the effect of anticoagulant (blood-thinning) drugs. Your doctor may have to adjust the dose of your anticoagulant.
- The safety of combining alprostadil with other drugs that affect blood vessels is not known. These combinations should be used with caution.

Food Interactions

None known.

Usual Dose

Dosage must be individualized to your need and response.

Overdosage

Alprostadil overdose can lead to an extended and painful erection, as well as other side effects. If this occurs, contact your doctor or go to the nearest emergency room. Overdose victims should seek medical attention. If you seek treatment, ALWAYS bring the prescription container.

Special Information

Patient information leaflets are included with each alprostadil prescription. Read this information before you use your prescription.

You must be trained in proper injection technique by your doctor. Self-injection should be permitted only after your doctor has made sure you know how to do it properly. For more information on how to properly administer this drug, see page 1242.

Alprostadil begins working within 5–10 minutes after taking it. Dosage should be set so that your erection lasts for about 30–60 minutes. Use the lowest dose that works.

You should generally not use alprostadil more than 3 times a week, and wait at least 24 hours between uses.

Do not increase the dosage without consulting your doctor.

Contact your doctor or seek medical assistance if your erection lasts longer than 4 hours.

Special Populations

Pregnancy/Breast-feeding: This product should not be used by women. Men using alprostadil must use a condom if they have intercourse with a pregnant woman. Alprostadil passes into semen and will affect the development of a fetal heart if a condom is not worn.

Seniors: Seniors may use alprostadil without special precaution.

Ambien *see **Zolpidem**, page 1033*

Generic Name

Aminolevulinic Acid

(ah-MEE-noe-lev-u-LIH-nic)

Brand Names

Levulan Kerastick

Type of Drug

Photodynamic therapy (PDT) sensitizer.

Prescribed For

Actinic keratoses.

General Information

Actinic keratoses are skin lesions that develop on sun-exposed areas of the face or hands in older adults with fair skin. Dermatologists consider them precancerous. Aminolevulinic acid solution is applied to the lesions in the doctor's office in preparation for PDT. By enhancing light sensitivity in treated skin, aminolevulinic acid increases the effectiveness of PDT, a form of light therapy that slows the growth of skin cells. PDT is administered 1 day after application of this drug.

Cautions and Warnings

Do not use this drug if you are **allergic** or **sensitive** to any of its ingredients or to porphyrins, or have **porphyria**. Aminolevulinic acid should not be applied around the eyes or inside the nose or mouth.

This drug causes increased sensitivity to the sun and bright indoor lighting. Skin reactions that may occur as a result of this sensitivity cannot be prevented by using sunscreen (see "Special Information").

Possible Side Effects

▼ Most common: scaling, crusting, itching, and changes in skin color. During PDT, which lasts for about 17 minutes, you will experience tingling, stinging, and a prickling or burning sensation in the treated lesions. These effects should begin to go away at the conclusion of PDT, though the lesions and surrounding skin will appear red. Swelling and scaling may also occur. These effects are temporary and should completely resolve within 4 weeks.

▼ Common: skin erosion and welts.

▼ Less common: pain, tenderness, swelling, skin ulcers, small blisters, oozing, loss of sensation in the area of application, scabs, and scratch marks.

Drug Interactions

- Other drugs that enhance your sensitivity to light may increase the effects of aminolevulinic acid. These drugs include griseofulvin, thiazide diuretics, sulfonylureas, phenothiazines, sulfonamides, and tetracycline medications.

Usual Dose

Aminolevulinic acid is applied to lesions in the doctor's office 14–18 hours prior to PDT.

Overdosage

Little is known about the effects of accidental ingestion, which is unlikely to occur because this drug is administered in a doctor's office.

Special Information

Only qualified medical personnel should administer this drug.

After application of the drug, avoid exposing the lesions to sunlight or bright indoor lighting for at least 40 hours. Wear a wide-brimmed hat and protective clothing during this period; sunscreen is not effective. Do not wash treated lesions until PDT has been administered.

If you experience a stinging or burning sensation, you may be able to alleviate these effects by shielding the lesions from light.

Special Populations

Pregnancy/Breast-feeding: The safety of using aminolevulinic acid during pregnancy is not known. Aminolevulinic acid should be used during pregnancy only if your doctor determines that the potential benefit outweighs the risks.

It is not known if aminolevulinic acid passes into breast milk. Nursing mothers who must use it should use infant formula.

Seniors: Seniors may use this drug without special precaution.

Generic Name

Amiodarone (ah-mee-OE-duh-rone) G

Brand Names

Cordarone Pacerone

Type of Drug

Antiarrhythmic.

Prescribed For

Abnormal heart rhythms.

General Information

Amiodarone should be prescribed only in situations in which the abnormal rhythm is so severe as to be life-threatening and it does not respond to other drug treatments. Amiodarone works by decreasing the sensitivity of heart tissue to nervous impulses within the heart. It has not been proven that people taking this drug will live longer than those with similar conditions who do not take it. Amiodarone may exert its effects 2–5 days after you start taking it, but often takes 1–3 weeks to affect your heart.

Amiodarone's antiarrhythmic effects can last for weeks or months after you stop taking it.

Cautions and Warnings

Do not take amiodarone if you are **allergic** or **sensitive** to any of its ingredients or if you have **heart block** or a very **slow heart rate**.

Amiodarone can also cause heart block, a drastic slowing of electrical impulse movement between major areas of the heart, or extreme slowing of the heart rate. Amiodarone heart block occurs about as often as heart block caused by some other antiarrhythmic drugs, but its effects may last longer than those of the other drugs. Amiodarone can also worsen existing **abnormal heart rhythms** in 2–5% of people who take the drug. These effects can be fatal.

Amiodarone can cause potentially fatal drug side effects. At high doses, 10% or more of people taking this drug can develop potentially fatal lung and respiratory effects, beginning with cough and progressive breathing difficulties. Using lower doses is less damaging to the lungs. Liver damage caused by amiodarone is usually mild. In rare cases, amiodarone has been associated with liver failure that resulted in death.

People taking amiodarone may develop optic nerve irritation, leading to partial or complete loss of vision. Most adults who take amiodarone for 6 months or more develop tiny deposits in the corneas of their eyes. These deposits may cause blurred vision or halos in up to 10% of people taking amiodarone. Some people develop dry eyes and sensitivity to bright light.

Nervous system inflammation related to the loss of the nerve's protective covering has occurred after taking amiodarone. Symptoms can include weakness, numbness, tingling, pain and difficulty walking, fainting spells, burning pain in the arms or legs, sudden back pain, or neck pain spreading down the arms or legs.

One in 10 people taking amiodarone can experience unusual sensitivity to the effects of the sun. Use an appropriate sunscreen product and reapply it frequently.

Amiodarone can cause thyroid abnormalities. It may worsen an already sluggish thyroid gland in 2–10% of people taking the drug, and increase thyroid activity in 2% of people taking it. Amiodarone has also been associated with an increase in risk of thyroid tumors.

Antiarrhythmic drugs are less effective and cause abnormal rhythms if **blood potassium** is low.

Possible Side Effects

About 75% of people taking 400 mg or more of amiodarone a day develop some drug side effects. As many as 18% have to stop taking the drug because of a side effect.

▼ Common: fatigue, not feeling well, tremors, unusual involuntary movements, loss of coordination, an unusual walk, muscle weakness, low blood pressure, dizziness, tingling in the hands or feet, reduced sex drive, sleeplessness, headache, nervous system problems, nausea, vomiting, constipation, appetite loss, abdominal pain, dry eyes, unusual sensitivity to bright light, and seeing halos around bright lights. Unusual sun sensitivity is the most common skin reaction to amiodarone, but people taking this drug can develop a blue skin discoloration that may not go away completely when the drug is stopped. Other skin reactions are sun rashes, hair loss, and black-and-blue spots.

▼ Rare: inflammation of the lung or fibrous deposits in the lungs, changes in thyroid function, changes in taste or smell, bloating, unusual salivation, and changes in blood clotting. Amiodarone can cause heart failure, reduced heart rate, and abnormal rhythms. Up to 9% of people taking amiodarone develop abnormalities in liver function. Contact your doctor if you experience anything unusual while taking any medication.

Drug Interactions

Amiodarone affects and is affected by numerous enzyme systems. Many drug interactions are known, but it is likely that many more are yet to be determined.

- Amiodarone increases the effects of metoprolol and other beta blockers, calcium channel blockers such as diltiazem and verapamil, clozapine, cyclosporine, dabigatran, dextromethorphan, digoxin, disopyramide, flecainide, fentanyl, lidocaine, methotrexate, quinidine, theophylline, and warfarin and other anticoagulants. These interactions can take from 2–3 days to several weeks to develop. Some can be life threatening, and for others, drug dosage adjustments may be enough to avoid a serious problem.
- Atorvastatin, azole antifungals, cimetidine, fluoroquinolones, loratadine, macrolide antibiotics, simvastatin, and trazodone increase the effects of amiodarone, which can cause life-threatening abnormal heart rhythms.

- Aprepitant, clarithromycin, diltiazem, erythromycin, fluvoxamine, gestodene, imatinib, mibefradil, mifepristone, nefazodone, norfluoxetine, protease inhibitors (such as indinavir, nelfinavir, ritonavir, and saquinavir), telithromycin, and verapamil can increase blood levels and effects of amiodarone on your heart.
- When amiodarone and phenytoin are taken together, both drugs can be affected. Amiodarone can be antagonized by phenytoin and other hydantoin anticonvulsants, and the effect of phenytoin can be increased by amiodarone.
- Cholestyramine interferes with the absorption of amiodarone into the bloodstream.
- Efavirenz, nevirapine, phenobarbital and other barbiturates, carbamazepine, corticosteroids, modafinil, oxcarbazepine, pioglitazone, rifabutin, rifampin, and St. John's wort increase the formation of enzyme systems that break down amiodarone and may reduce blood levels and drug effectiveness.
- Cimetidine and ritonavir interfere with the breakdown of amiodarone, leading to high drug blood levels and the increased possibility of side effects.
- Azithromycin can interfere with the effectiveness of amiodarone. This interaction may lead to dizziness and cardiac instability.
- Amiodarone can reduce the effectiveness of clopidogrel.

Food Interactions

Amiodarone should be taken on an empty stomach, as food delays its absorption into your bloodstream. If amiodarone upsets your stomach, however, you may take it with food, but then always take it with food to be consistent. Do not eat or drink grapefruit or starfruit products during treatment with amiodarone because they affect how amiodarone is absorbed in the stomach.

Usual Dose

Starting dose—800–1600 mg a day, taken in 1 or 2 doses, usually for 1–3 weeks. Then, 600–800 mg a day for approximately a month. Maintenance dose—400 mg a day. You should take the lowest effective dose to minimize side effects.

Overdosage

The effects of amiodarone overdose include low blood pressure, shock, slow heartbeat, and liver toxicity. Overdose victims should be taken to a hospital emergency room for treatment. If you seek treatment, ALWAYS bring the prescription bottle or container.

Special Information

Side effects are very common with amiodarone; 75% of people taking the drug experience some drug-related problem. Amiodarone stays in the body for months, so side effects may remain even after the drug is stopped.

Contact your doctor if you develop chest pain, breathing difficulties, spitting up blood, nausea, vomiting, abnormal heartbeat, bloating in your feet or legs, tremors, fever, chills, sore throat, unusual bleeding or bruising, changes in skin color, unusual sunburn, or any other unusual side effect. See your doctor for an eye exam if your vision changes at all while taking amiodarone.

Amiodarone can make you dizzy or lightheaded. Take care while driving a car or performing complex tasks.

If you take amiodarone once a day and forget to take a dose, but remember within 12 hours, take it as soon as possible. If you do not remember until later, skip the dose you forgot and continue with your regular schedule. If you take amiodarone twice a day and remember within 6 hours of your regular dose, take it as soon as you remember. Contact your doctor if you forget to take 2 or more doses in a row. Do not take a double dose.

Special Populations

Pregnancy/Breast-feeding: In high doses, amiodarone has been found to be toxic to animal fetuses. Women of childbearing age should use an effective contraceptive while taking amiodarone.

Amiodarone passes into breast milk. Nursing mothers who must take this drug should use infant formula.

Seniors: Dosage reduction may be needed in seniors with poor liver function.

Generic Name

Amlexanox (am-LEX-an-ox) G

Brand Names

Aphthasol

Type of Drug

Skin-ulcer treatment.

Prescribed For

Canker sores in people with normal immune systems.

General Information

Amlexanox slows the production or release of factors involved in the body's inflammatory response. It aids in the healing of mouth ulcers, but the exact way that it accelerates the healing process is not known.

Cautions and Warnings

Do not use amlexanox if you are **allergic** or **sensitive** to any of its ingredients. Stop using this drug if you develop a persistent rash or irritation.

Possible Side Effects

- ▼ Less common: transient local pain, stinging, or burning after application.
- ▼ Rare: mouth irritation, diarrhea, and nausea. Contact your doctor if you experience anything unusual while taking any medication.

Drug Interactions

None known.

Food Interactions

Do not apply amlexanox while you have any food in your mouth.

Usual Dose

Adult: Apply a small amount (¼ in.) to each mouth ulcer 4 times a day, preferably after breakfast, lunch, and dinner, and at bedtime.

Child: not recommended.

Overdosage

Swallowing as much as a whole tube of amlexanox would probably cause only upset stomach, nausea, diarrhea, and vomiting. Contact your local poison control center or hospital emergency room for more information. If you seek treatment, ALWAYS bring the prescription container.

Special Information

Begin using amlexanox as soon as possible after noticing a mouth ulcer and use it until your ulcers heal. Contact your doctor if the pain does not get better or the sores do not heal after 10 days of using amlexanox.

Make sure your teeth, mouth, and hands are clean before applying amlexanox paste. Squeeze ¼ in. of the paste onto your finger and apply it to each mouth ulcer using gentle pressure.

Wash your hands immediately after using amlexanox. If you get the paste into your eyes, wash it out at once using cool water.

If you forget a dose of amlexanox, use it as soon as you remember. If it is almost time for your next dose, skip the dose you forgot and continue with your regular schedule. Do not apply more than the recommended amount at any time.

Special Populations

Pregnancy/Breast-feeding: The effect of amlexanox on pregnancy is not known. Amlexanox should be taken during pregnancy only if your doctor determines that the potential benefit outweighs the risks. Amlexanox passes into the milk of nursing animals, but its effect in humans is not known. Nursing mothers should use this drug with caution.

Seniors: Seniors may use amlexanox without special precaution.

Generic Name

Anagrelide (ah-NAG-rel-ide) G

Brand Names

Agrylin

Type of Drug

Antiplatelet.

Prescribed For

Essential thrombocythemia (ET), to reduce blood-platelet count and the risk of excess blood clotting associated with high blood-platelet levels.

General Information

Blood platelets play an important role in the body. They help to form blood clots that "seal off" minor cuts and wounds and prevent excessive bleeding. When platelet counts are too high, as in ET, unwanted clots may form almost anywhere in the body. These clots may obstruct blood vessels, leading to leg cramps, heart attack, stroke, or other medical problems. Exactly how anagrelide reduces blood-platelet count is not known, but it may interfere with the formation of new platelets. Anagrelide is not approved for general use by children under age 16, but it has been used without apparent harm by 8 children between the ages of 8 and 17, who took it in doses of up to 4 mg a day.

Cautions and Warnings

Do not take anagrelide if you are **allergic** or **sensitive** to any of its ingredients.

This drug should be used with caution by people who have **heart disease**. Use of anagrelide may cause heart palpitations, rapid heart rate, and congestive heart failure.

Unusually low blood-platelet counts can develop in people treated with anagrelide. Platelet counts should be periodically checked while you are taking this drug; they usually rise soon after the drug is stopped.

People with **liver or kidney disease** should use this drug with caution. Anagrelide can cause liver or kidney toxicity and worsen diseases of those organs.

Interstitial lung diseases have been reported with use of anagrelide, including difficulty breathing and inflammation of lung tissue, with the time of onset being 1 week to several years. In most cases, symptoms improved after the drug was discontinued.

Possible Side Effects

- ▼ Most common: heart palpitations, diarrhea, abdominal pain, nausea, gas, headache, weakness, swelling, pain, dizziness, and difficulty breathing.
- ▼ Common: chest pain, rapid heartbeat, vomiting, upset stomach, appetite loss, rash or itching, tingling in the hands or feet, back pain, and not feeling well.
- ▼ Less common: fever, flu-like symptoms, chills, neck pain, sensitivity to bright light, abnormal heart rhythms, bleeding, heart disease, stroke, angina, heart failure, dizziness when rising from a sitting or lying position, flushing, migraine, fainting, depression, confusion, tiredness, high blood pressure, nervousness, memory loss, itching, skin disease, hair loss, stomach bleeding, blood in the stool, stomach irritation, anemia, thrombocytopenia (low blood-platelet count), black-and-blue marks, swollen lymph glands, painful urination, blood in the urine, muscle and joint ache,

Possible Side Effects *(continued)*

leg cramps, runny nose, nosebleeds, lung disease, sinus inflammation, pneumonia, bronchitis, asthma, double vision or other visual difficulties, ringing or buzzing in the ears, liver inflammation, and dehydration.

Drug Interactions

- Sucralfate may interfere with the absorption of anagrelide. Do not combine these drugs.
- Anagrelide may increase the blood-thinning effect of aspirin.
- Amiodarone, cimetidine, ciprofloxacin, fluoroquinolone antibiotics, fluvoxamine, interferon, methoxsalen, and mibefradil may increase blood levels of anagrelide by interfering with its breakdown.
- Anagrelide may interfere with the breakdown of amitriptyline, amrinone, caffeine, cilostazol, clomipramine, clozapine, cyclobenzaprine, enoximone, estradiol, fluvoxamine, haloperidol, imipramine, mexiletine, milrinone, naproxen, olanzapine, olprinone, ondansetron, phenacetin, acetaminophen, propranolol, riluzole, ropivacaine, theophylline, tizanidine, verapamil, warfarin, zileuton, and zolmitriptan in the body.

Food Interactions

Anagrelide can be taken without regard to food or meals.

Usual Dose

Adult: 0.5 mg 4 times a day or 1 mg twice a day, to start, with a maximum daily dose of 10 mg and no more than 2.5 mg in a single dose. After at least a week, the lowest effective dose should be sought.

Child: Limited information is available for the use of anagrelide in children. Children ranging in age from 7–17 have been given starting dosages similar to adults with similar side effects.

Overdosage

Little is known about the effects of anagrelide overdose, but symptoms are likely to include a sudden drop in blood-platelet count and heart or central-nervous-system side effects that could result in abnormal bleeding. Overdose victims should be taken to a hospital emergency room at once. If you seek treatment, ALWAYS bring the prescription bottle or container.

Special Information

Blood-platelet counts should be checked every 2 days when beginning anagrelide for 1 week. Until a maintenance dose has been established, platelet counts should then be taken once a week.

Women who might become pregnant should use a reliable form of birth control while taking anagrelide.

If you forget a dose, take it as soon as possible. If it is almost time for your next dose, skip the dose you forgot and continue with your regular schedule. Contact your doctor if you forget 2 or more doses in a row. Do not take a double dose.

Special Populations

Pregnancy/Breast-feeding: At high doses, anagrelide caused birth defects in animal studies. Anagrelide should be taken during pregnancy only if your doctor determines that the potential benefit outweighs the risks.

It is not known if this drug passes into breast milk. Nursing mothers who must take anagrelide should use infant formula.

Seniors: Seniors may take anagrelide without special precaution.

Generic Name

Anakinra (an-ah-KIN-rah)

Brand Names

Kineret

The information in this profile also applies to the following drugs:

Generic Ingredients: Abatacept
Orencia

Type of Drug

Immune system modulator.

Prescribed For

Moderate to severe rheumatoid arthritis (RA) in adults. Abatacept is also used for juvenile arthritis.

General Information

Anakinra blocks the biological activity of a substance called interleukin-1, which is produced in response to inflammation. Anakinra may be prescribed together with methotrexate, azathioprine, leflunomide, sulfasalazine, or other drugs for the treatment of rheumatoid arthritis. It must be injected under the skin every day.

Abatacept is a T-cell costimulation modulator and may be prescribed with other RA drugs, except the tumor necrosis factor (TNF) antagonist medicines. It may be prescribed with methotrexate for children age 6 and older with arthritis.

Cautions and Warnings

Do not use these drugs if you are **allergic** or **sensitive** to any of their ingredients.

Serious infections, including **tuberculosis**, are possible in people using these medicines because of their ability to suppress the immune response. This may be more common in people with other conditions that predispose them to conditions such as asthma or advanced or uncontrolled diabetes. People with previous tuberculosis may experience a reactivation of the dormant infection. Stop using these drugs if a serious infection develops.

The safety and effectiveness of using these drugs in people with **suppressed immune systems** has not been established.

People with **chronic obstructive pulmonary disease** (COPD) may be more likely to develop respiratory side effects with these medicines.

Levels of some white blood cells may be reduced in rare cases, leading to persistent fever or pale skin color. Contact your doctor if any of these symptoms develop.

Anakinra is cleared through the kidneys. People with severe **kidney disease** may accumulate anakinra in their blood.

People with a history of **hepatitis B** may experience a reactivation of their hepatitis while taking these medicines.

People taking these medicines should not receive any **live virus vaccines**, because the body may not be able to respond as expected to the vaccine. **Children** receiving abatacept should be fully immunized before starting their treatments.

Possible Side Effects

Abatacept

- ▼ Most common: headache, upper-respiratory infections, stuffy nose, and nausea. In children: upper-respiratory infection and stuffy nose.
- ▼ Less common: dizziness, cough, back pain, upset stomach, and urinary infection. In children: headache, nausea, cough, fever, and abdominal pain.

Possible Side Effects *(continued)*

▼ Rare: rash and arm or leg pain. Contact your doctor if you experience anything unusual while taking any medication.

Anakinra

▼ Most common: infections and injection-site reactions.

▼ Common: reduced white-blood-cell counts, headache, nausea, and diarrhea.

▼ Less common: sinusitis, flu-like symptoms, and abdominal pain.

▼ Rare: Rare side effects can occur in almost any part of the body. Contact your doctor if you experience anything unusual while taking any medication.

Drug Interactions

- Do not mix these drugs in the same syringe as another drug.
- Anakinra and abatacept should not be used in combination with etanercept or any other TNF-blocking agent because of the increased risk of infection.
- Abatacept for injection under the skin does not affect blood sugar, but intravenous (IV) abatacept contains a sugar that can give high blood-sugar readings on the day you get an IV dose.

Food Interactions

None known.

Usual Dose

Abatacept

Adult: 500–1000-mg IV infusion given every 2 weeks after the first infusion for 1 month, then every 4 weeks or 125 mg weekly at home, self-injected under the skin using the silicone-free syringe in the manufacturer's package. Inject the entire contents of the syringe.

Child (age 6–17): 4.5 mg per lb. of body weight up to 1000 mg per dose.

Child (under age 6): not recommended.

Anakinra

Adult: 100 mg a day, at the same time each day, injected under the skin via pre-filled syringe. Inject the entire contents of the syringe.

Child: 0.45–0.9 mg per lb. of body weight a day up to 100 mg injected under the skin. Special anakinra syringes are not available in sizes suitable for children, so the syringes must be prepared by a qualified pharmacist to avoid the risk of overdose.

Overdosage

In animal studies, doses up to 35 times the maximum human dose of anakinra and up to 5 times the maximum human dose of abatacept have been used with no evidence of serious toxicities. Contact your doctor or local poison control center for more information. If you seek treatment, ALWAYS bring the prescription bottle or container.

Special Information

Do not use a syringe if the contents are discolored or contain particles. Keep anakinra refrigerated.

Tell your doctor about all the medicines you take, including nonprescription drugs, herbal supplements, and vitamins.

Make sure your doctor knows if you have the flu or any infection, even a small cut or open sore; tuberculosis or an infection that keeps coming back; hepatitis or any other liver inflammation (which can be reactivated by these medicines); lung disease (especially COPD); or diabetes or any other reason to check your blood sugar.

Tell your doctor if you are pregnant or breast-feeding, going to have surgery, or have recently been vaccinated or are scheduled for a vaccination. You should not receive any live virus vaccine while taking these drugs or for 3 months after you stop taking them.

Call your doctor if you develop a cough that does not go away, weight loss, fever, or night sweats. These can be signs of tuberculosis or another serious infection.

Hives; swollen face, eyelids, lips, or tongue; or difficulty breathing can be a sign of an allergic reaction.

Reactions may develop at the site where the medicine is injected. Injection sites should be rotated among the thigh, abdomen, and upper arm to avoid excessive bruising or other skin damage.

If you forget a dose of anakinra or abatacept, take it as soon as you remember. If it is almost time for your next dose, skip the dose you forgot and continue with your regular schedule.

For more information on how to properly administer this drug, see page 1242.

Special Populations

Pregnancy/Breast-feeding: Animal studies at doses 29 times the human dose of abatacept and 100 times that of anakinra indicate no harm to the fetus. However, there is no conclusive information on the use of these drugs by pregnant women. These drugs should be taken during pregnancy only if your doctor determines that the potential benefit outweighs the risks.

It is not known if these drugs pass into breast milk. Nursing mothers who must take them should use infant formula.

Seniors: The risk of anakinra side effects is greater in seniors because of the natural decline in kidney function. Caution should be exercised with these drugs because of the greater risk of infection and malignancy in seniors.

Generic Name

Anastrozole (ah-NAS-troe-zole) G

Brand Names

Arimidex

The information in this profile also applies to the following drugs:

Generic Ingredients: Letrozole G
Femara

Type of Drug

Aromatase inhibitor.

Prescribed For

Breast cancer in postmenopausal women. Anastrozole may also be prescribed for breast cancer prevention and male infertility. Letrozole may be prescribed for delayed puberty in males.

General Information

Anastrozole is used for breast cancer that has advanced or spread despite treatment with tamoxifen, as an initial treatment for estrogen-receptor-positive breast cancer, or for breast cancer in which the hormone receptor status is unknown. Anastrozole reduces the amount of estradiol, an estrogenic hormone, in the blood. It does this by interfering with the action of the aromatase enzyme, an element involved in the manufacture of estradiol. Most of anastrozole is broken down in the liver.

Cautions and Warnings

Do not take anastrozole if you are **allergic** or **sensitive** to any of its ingredients. Severe reactions, including lip swelling and choking, have rarely occurred.

These drugs should not be used in women who are or may become **pregnant** as they are harmful to a developing fetus.

Anastrozole should be used with caution in women who have pre-existing **heart disease** in which blood flow to the heart is limited.

These medications increase blood-cholesterol levels.

Women with **estrogen-receptor-negative disease** and those who did not respond at all to tamoxifen are not likely to respond to anastrozole.

Deterioration of bone density may occur in women taking anastrozole or letrozole.

People with severe **liver disease** may need reduced dosages of letrozole.

Possible Side Effects

Anastrozole

- ▼ Most common: weakness, nausea, headache, flushing, generalized pain, and back pain.
- ▼ Less common: muscle and joint pain; cough; diarrhea; constipation; abdominal pain; appetite loss; bone pain; sore throat; dizziness; rash; dry mouth; swelling in the arms, legs, or feet; pelvic pain; unexpected vaginal bleeding; depression; chest pain; and tingling in the hands or feet.
- ▼ Rare: Rare side effects can occur in almost any part of the body. Contact your doctor if you experience anything unusual while taking any medication.

Letrozole

Almost 90% of women taking letrozole for 2 years experience at least 1 drug side effect.

- ▼ Most common: flushing/hot flashes, arthritis, joint pain, back pain, arm or leg pain, night sweats, and weight gain.
- ▼ Common: nausea, diarrhea, vomiting, weight loss, fatigue, weakness, not feeling well, vaginal dryness, difficulty breathing, rash, chest pain, sleeplessness, infections, leg or ankle swelling, muscle pain, broken bones, heart

Possible Side Effects *(continued)*

or kidney disease, urinary infection, high blood pressure, and swollen lymph glands (after mastectomy).

- ▼ Less common: vaginal bleeding, vaginal irritation, headache, dizziness or lightheadedness, osteoporosis, constipation, itching, appetite loss, new cancers, stroke. Stray blood clots can break off and block blood flow to areas of the body, including the lungs, brain, gastrointestinal tract, kidney, or leg.
- ▼ Rare: blurred vision; liver irritation; endometrial disorders, including endometrial cancer; heart attack; and angina. Contact your doctor if you experience anything unusual while taking any medication.

Drug Interactions

- Usual doses of anastrozole do not affect other medications; however, high doses of anastrozole can reduce the ability of the liver to break down certain drugs.
- Tamoxifen reduces blood levels of anastrozole without increasing treatment benefit. These drugs should not be taken together.
- Estrogen-containing therapies should not be used with anastrozole.

Food Interactions

These drugs can be taken without regard to food or meals.

Usual Dose

Anastrozole

Adult: 1 mg once a day.

Letrozole

Adult: 2.5 mg once a day.

Overdosage

Symptoms of overdose can be exaggerated side effects. Overdose victims should be taken to a hospital emergency room. If you seek treatment, ALWAYS bring the prescription bottle or container.

Special Information

Contact your doctor if your side effects become severe or intolerable.

Use a condom, diaphragm, or other non-hormonal contraceptive while taking anastrozole or letrozole.

You may need to have routine bone density tests while taking these medications.

Letrozole may cause fatigue or dizziness. Use extra caution while doing anything that requires concentration, such as driving a car or operating hazardous machinery.

If you forget a dose of anastrozole or letrozole, take it as soon as you remember if it is within 12 hours of the missed dose. If it is over 12 hours, skip the missed dose and continue with your regular schedule. Contact your doctor if you forget more than 2 doses in a row.

Special Populations

Pregnancy/Breast-feeding: These drugs are intended only for postmenopausal women. Animal studies have shown that exposure to them can harm the fetus. Women who think they may become pregnant while taking these drugs should use a condom, diaphragm, or other non-hormonal contraceptive.

Seniors: Seniors may take this drug without special precaution.

AndroGel *see **Testosterone,** page 1114*

Type of Drug

Angiotensin II Blockers

(AN-jee-oe-TEN-sin)

Brand Names

Generic Ingredients: Azilsartan Medoxomil
Edarbi

Generic Ingredients: Azilsartan Medoxomil + Chlorthalidone
Edarbychlor

Generic Ingredients: Candesartan Cilexetil
Atacand

Generic Ingredients: Candesartan Cilexetil + Hydrochlorothiazide
Atacand HCT

Generic Ingredients: Eprosartan Mesylate G
Teveten

Generic Ingredients: Eprosartan Mesylate + Hydrochlorothiazide
Teveten HCT

Generic Ingredients: Irbesartan
Avapro

Generic Ingredients: Irbesartan + Hydrochlorothiazide
Avalide

Generic Ingredients: Losartan Potassium G
Cozaar

Generic Ingredients: Losartan Potassium + Hydrochlorothiazide G
Hyzaar

Generic Ingredients: Olmesartan Medoxomil
Benicar

Generic Ingredients: Olmesartan Medoxomil + Hydrochlorothiazide
Benicar HCT

Generic Ingredients: Olmesartan Medoxomil + Amlodipine + Hydrochlorothiazide
Tribenzor

Generic Ingredients: Telmisartan
Micardis

Generic Ingredients: Telmisartan + Amlodipine
Twynsta

Generic Ingredients: Telmisartan + Hydrochlorothiazide
Micardis HCT

Generic Ingredients: Valsartan
Diovan

Generic Ingredients: Valsartan + Hydrochlorothiazide
Diovan HCT

Generic Ingredients: Valsartan + Amlodipine
Exforge

Prescribed For

High blood pressure; kidney damage in type 2 diabetes (irbesartan and losartan); high blood pressure with enlarged left ventricle (losartan); prevention of heart attack or stroke (telmisartan); heart failure (candesartan and valsartan); and treatment following heart attack (valsartan). May also be used for prevention of migraine (candesartan and olmesartan).

General Information

These drugs work by blocking the effects of angiotensin II (AII), a hormone found in blood vessels and other tissue. AII plays an important role in regulating blood pressure. Unlike angiotensin-converting enzyme (ACE) inhibitors—another group of blood-pressure-lowering medication—AII blockers do not cause chronic cough. AII blockers can be used alone or with a thiazide diuretic such as hydrochlorothiazide, as in Hyzaar, Avalide, and Diovan HCT, for example. Although these are single tablets, your doctor may prescribe an AII blocker and a diuretic as separate pills. Combining an AII blocker and a diuretic may reduce blood pressure twice as much as an AII blocker alone.

AII blockers may be useful in treating heart failure and may slow the progression of kidney disease in people with diabetes and high blood pressure.

Many AII blockers contain combinations of antihypertensives. For more information see Amlodipine, page 224, and Hydrochlorothiazide, page 55.

Cautions and Warnings

Do not take an AII blocker if you are **allergic** or **sensitive** to any of its ingredients. You may be sensitive to one AII blocker and tolerant of another.

Do not take AII blockers if you are or think you might be **pregnant**.

Patients with **heart failure** given an AII blocker generally experience a drop in blood pressure. If this happens, a temporary dosage reduction may be needed. People who are **dehydrated** or who have **low blood sodium**, such as those being treated with diuretics or on dialysis, may also experience a sudden drop in blood pressure (symptoms include dizziness and fainting). Once your body has adjusted to a diuretic-AII blocker combination, this problem should subside.

Some people who take an AII blocker develop kidney function changes similar to those associated with ACE inhibitor drugs.

Telmisartan is noticeably less effective in **black patients**. Other AII blockers may also be somewhat less effective in black patients, although the addition of a diuretic such as hydrochlorothiazide is usually beneficial.

People with serious **liver disease** or **cirrhosis** should receive a lower starting dosage of losartan and telmisartan. People with liver disease or cirrhosis should be cautious about taking candesartan and valsartan, although no initial dosage adjustment is required.

Possible Side Effects

AII blockers are generally very well tolerated. In clinical studies, the risk of side effects was about the same for an AII blocker as for a placebo (sugar pill).

Azilsartan

- ▼ Less common: diarrhea.
- ▼ Rare: Rare side effects can occur in almost any part of the body. Contact your doctor if you experience anything unusual while taking any medication.

Candesartan

- ▼ Common: respiratory infection, dizziness, and back pain.
- ▼ Less common: headache, fatigue, diarrhea, nausea and vomiting, abdominal pain, joint pain, sinus problems, sore throat, runny nose, cough, bronchitis, chest pain, and swollen arms or legs.
- ▼ Rare: Rare side effects can occur in almost any part of the body. Contact your doctor if you experience anything unusual while taking any medication.

Eprosartan

- ▼ Common: respiratory infection.
- ▼ Less common: urinary tract infection, dizziness, headache, diarrhea, upset stomach, muscle pain or cramps, cough, sore throat, runny nose, and swelling.
- ▼ Rare: Rare side effects can occur in almost any part of the body. Contact your doctor if you experience anything unusual while taking any medication.

Irbesartan

- ▼ Common: diarrhea, upset stomach or heartburn, and fatigue.
- ▼ Less common: dizziness, headache, anxiety, nervousness, muscle aches, nausea and vomiting, abdominal pain, cough, sinus problems, sore throat, runny nose, flu-like

Possible Side Effects *(continued)*

symptoms, swelling, chest pain, rash, rapid heartbeat, and urinary infection.

▼ Rare: Rare side effects can occur in almost any part of the body. Contact your doctor if you experience anything unusual while taking any medication.

Losartan

▼ Common: respiratory infection.

▼ Less common: dizziness, sleeplessness, diarrhea, upset stomach, heartburn, pain, muscle cramps, muscle aches, cough, stuffy nose, rash, sore throat, fatigue, swelling, and sinus problems.

▼ Rare: Rare side effects can occur in almost any part of the body. Contact your doctor if you experience anything unusual while taking any medication.

Olmesartan

▼ Common: dizziness.

▼ Less common: headache, diarrhea, back pain, bronchitis, flu-like symptoms, sore throat, stuffy nose, sinus problems, and respiratory infection.

▼ Rare: Rare side effects can occur in almost any part of the body. Contact your doctor if you experience anything unusual while taking any medication.

Telmisartan

▼ Common: respiratory infection.

▼ Less common: dizziness, headache, fatigue, anxiety or nervousness, diarrhea, upset stomach, heartburn, nausea, abdominal pain, back pain, muscle aches, cough, sinus irritation, sore throat, flu-like symptoms, chest pain, urinary infection, swelling in the arms or legs, and high blood pressure.

▼ Rare: Rare side effects can occur in almost any part of the body. Contact your doctor if you experience anything unusual while taking any medication.

Valsartan

▼ Common: headache and dizziness.

▼ Less common: fatigue, diarrhea, nausea, abdominal pain, joint pain, respiratory infection, cough, sore throat, sinus problems, runny nose, virus infection, and swelling.

Possible Side Effects *(continued)*

▼ Rare: Rare side effects can occur in almost any part of the body. Contact your doctor if you experience anything unusual while taking any medication.

Drug Interactions

- Alcohol and narcotic and barbiturate drugs may increase the blood-pressure-lowering effects, such as dizziness or fainting, of AII blockers.
- Combining an AII blocker and another blood-pressure-lowering drug, especially a diuretic, reduces blood pressure more efficiently than either drug used alone. People taking a diuretic who start an AII blocker may initially experience a rapid blood pressure drop and should start with a lower AII-blocker dosage.
- Combining nonsteroidal anti-inflammatory drugs (NSAIDs) and an AII blocker may result in decreased effectiveness of the AII blocker and potential kidney damage. These medications should be combined cautiously.
- Taking an AII blocker with potassium-sparing diuretics or potassium supplements may lead to excess levels of blood potassium and require additional monitoring.
- Candesartan, telmisartan, and valsartan may increase levels of lithium leading to toxicity. Lithium doses may need adjusting.
- Fluconazole may increase the effects of losartan.
- Rifampin may reduce the effectiveness of losartan.
- Combining telmisartan and digoxin can increase digoxin blood levels by up to 50%, leading to possible drug side effects. This combination should be used with caution.
- Cyclosporine, rifampin, and ritonavir may increase levels of valsartan.

Food Interactions

For optimal effectiveness, take valsartan at least 1 hour before or 2 hours after meals. Other AII blockers can be taken with or without food.

Usual Dose

Azilsartan

Adult: 80 mg once a day.

Child: not recommended.

Candesartan

Adult and Child (age 17 and over): 8–32 mg once a day. Usual starting dose is 4 or 16 mg a day.

Child (age 6–16): over 110 lbs.: 4–32 mg a day; under 110 lbs.: 2–16 mg a day.

Child (age 1–5): 0.02–0.2 mg per lb. a day.

Child (under age 1): not recommended.

Eprosartan

Adult: 400–800 mg a day in 1 or 2 doses. Usual starting dose is 600 mg.

Child: not recommended.

Irbesartan

Adult and Child (age 13 and over): 150 mg once a day to start, increasing to 300 mg once a day if necessary. A lower dosage (75 mg) may be prescribed for people who are dehydrated or salt-depleted.

Child (age 6–12): 75–150 mg a day.

Child (under age 6): not recommended.

Losartan

Adult: 25–50 mg once a day to start, increasing gradually up to 100 mg in 1 or 2 doses a day.

Child (age 6 and over): 0.35 mg per lb. of body weight a day to start and then adjusted as necessary. Dosage not to exceed 100 mg per day.

Child (under age 6): not recommended.

Olmesartan

Adult and Child (age 17 and over): 20–40 mg a day. Usual starting dose is 20 mg a day.

Child (age 6–16): 44–76 lbs.: 10–20 mg once a day; over 76 lbs.: 20–40 mg once a day.

Child (under age 6): not recommended.

Telmisartan

Adult: 20–80 mg a day. Usual starting dose is 40 mg a day.

Child: not recommended.

Valsartan

Adult: 40–320 mg a day. Usual starting dose is 80–160 mg a day.

Child (age 6 and over): 0.75 mg per lb. of body weight a day to start and then adjusted as necessary. Dosage not to exceed 160 mg per day.

Child (under age 6): not recommended.

Overdosage

Little is known about AII-blocker overdose, although it could be fatal. The most likely overdose symptoms are very low blood pressure, dizziness, and rapid heartbeat. Overdose victims should be taken to a hospital emergency room. If you seek treatment, ALWAYS bring the prescription bottle or container.

Special Information

Avoid strenuous exercise and very hot weather because heavy sweating or dehydration can cause a rapid blood pressure drop.

People on dialysis who take telmisartan may become dizzy or faint when rising quickly from a sitting or lying position at the beginning of treatment.

Avoid over-the-counter diet pills, decongestants, and stimulants because they may contain ingredients that can raise blood pressure. People taking losartan should avoid using potassium supplements.

Contact your doctor if you develop any of the following symptoms: dry mouth, thirst, weakness, tiredness, drowsiness, restlessness, confusion, seizures, muscle pains or cramps, muscular fatigue, dizziness or fainting, drastically reduced urine output, rapid heartbeat, and nausea or vomiting.

If you take an AII blocker once a day and forget a dose, take it as soon as you remember. If it is within 8 hours of your next dose, skip the one you forgot and continue with your regular schedule. If you take an AII blocker twice a day and forget a dose, take it as soon as you remember. If it is within 4 hours of your next dose, take 1 dose right away and another in 5 or 6 hours, then go back to your regular schedule. Never take a double dose.

Special Populations

Pregnancy/Breast-feeding: AII blockers should not be taken during pregnancy because they can cause fetal injury or death. If necessary, you should take another drug for high blood pressure if you are or might be pregnant.

It is not known if AII blockers pass into breast milk, although they do in animal studies. Nursing mothers who must take an AII blocker should use infant formula.

Seniors: Seniors may take AII blockers without special precautions.

Type of Drug

Antiemetics ($5HT_3$ Type)

Brand Names

Generic Ingredients: Alosetron
Lotronex

Generic Ingredients: Dolasetron
Anzemet

Generic Ingredients: Granisetron G
Granisol
Sancuso

Generic Ingredients: Ondansetron G
Zofran
Zofran ODT

Prescribed For

Nausea and vomiting caused by chemotherapy and other cancer treatments and general anesthesia. Alosetron is prescribed only for women with severe irritable bowel syndrome (IBS) whose main symptom is diarrhea. Ondansetron is also prescribed for bulimia, excessive vomiting during pregnancy, post-surgical shivering, and itching.

General Information

These drugs prevent nausea and vomiting by interfering with a form of the neurohormone serotonin (5HT) known as $5HT_3$. They block its effects in the part of the brain that controls vomiting and in the vagus nerve in the stomach and intestines. These drugs are very effective and often work in cases in which older antiemetics have failed. Alosetron works against IBS by blocking the action of serotonin in the intestines. This reduces the cramping, abdominal discomfort, urgency, and diarrhea caused by IBS. Blood concentrations of alosetron are 30–50% higher in women than in men.

Cautions and Warnings

Do not use antiemetics if you are **allergic** or **sensitive** to any of their ingredients.

Serious and possibly fatal colitis and serious complications of constipation leading to hospitalization, blood transfusions, and surgery have developed in people taking alosetron. People with a history of **gastrointestinal (GI) difficulties** including chronic or severe constipation, colitis, intestinal obstruction, or diverticulitis should not take this drug.

People with **heart rhythm problems**, especially those taking diuretics and antiarrhythmic drugs, should be cautious about taking dolasetron. Due to its effect on heart rhythm, dolasetron injection should not be prescribed to prevent chemotherapy-related nausea and vomiting in children or adults; the tablet should be used instead.

People with **liver problems** need lower doses of alosetron and may consider using other drugs in this group.

These drugs should only be used when the risk of nausea and vomiting is relatively high or if vomiting must be avoided following surgery.

Possible Side Effects

Alosetron

- ▼ Most common: constipation.
- ▼ Common: nausea and abdominal or GI discomfort or pain.
- ▼ Rare: Rare side effects can occur in any part of the body. Contact your doctor if you experience anything unusual while taking any medication.

Dolasetron

- ▼ Common: headache, low blood pressure, slowed heart rate, and dizziness.
- ▼ Less common: high blood pressure, abdominal pain, diarrhea, rapid heartbeat, fever or chills, and tiredness.
- ▼ Rare: blood in the urine; chest pain; kidney problems; painful or difficult urination; pain; severe stomach pain with nausea or vomiting; rash; hives; itching; swollen face, feet, or lower legs; and breathing difficulties. Contact your doctor if you experience anything unusual while taking any medication.

Granisetron

- ▼ Most common: headache, constipation, and weakness.
- ▼ Common: abdominal pain, diarrhea, nausea, vomiting, appetite loss, chills, and anemia.
- ▼ Less common: dizziness, fever, anxiety, sleeplessness, hair loss, and low blood-platelet count.
- ▼ Rare: drug-sensitivity reactions, chest pain, and fainting. Contact your doctor if you experience anything unusual while taking any medication.

Possible Side Effects *(continued)*

Ondansetron

▼ Most common: headache, feeling unwell, and constipation.

▼ Less common: anxiety, agitation, dizziness, fever, lightheadedness, diarrhea, gynecological problems, itching, abnormal heart rhythms, and low blood pressure.

Drug Interactions

- Dolasetron and ondansetron should be used with caution with antiarrhythmic agents (such as amiodarone, bretylium, disopyramide, dofetilide, quinidine, and sotalol), arsenic trioxide, chlorpromazine, cisapride, droperidol, mefloquine, mesoridazine, moxifloxacin, pentamidine, pimozide, tacrolimus, thioridazine, and ziprasidone. The potential for serious heart arrhythmias is increased when these medications are combined.
- Alosetron should be taken with caution with drugs that decrease gastrointestinal movement such as anticholinergics.
- Alosetron may reduce the amount of hydralazine and isoniazid in the blood.
- Fluvoxamine, cimetidine, ciprofloxacin and the quinolone antibiotics should not be taken with alosetron because they interfere with the enzyme system (CYP1A2) that breaks it down. Other weaker CYP1A2 inhibitors are amiodarone, interferon, methsoxalen, and mibefradil.
- Ketoconazole may increase blood concentrations of alosetron by 30%. Other CYP3A4 inhibitors such as clarithromycin, itraconazole, protease inhibitors, telithromycin, and voriconazole should be used with caution.
- Blood levels of dolasetron may be increased when combined with cimetidine or atenolol.
- Combining rifamycins and dolasetron or ondansetron may reduce the level of antiemetic in the blood.
- Apomorphine should not be combined with ondansetron.
- Phenytoin and carbamazepine lower blood levels of ondansetron.
- Blood levels of cisplatin and cyclophosphamide may be reduced when either of these drugs is taken with ondansetron.

Food Interactions

These drugs may be taken without regard to food or meals.

Usual Dose

Alosetron

Adult: 0.5 mg twice a day to start. Dosage may be increased to 1 mg twice a day if the lower dose is not working. Alosetron should be discontinued if adequate results are not seen after 4 weeks at 1 mg twice a day.

Dolasetron

Adult and Child (age 17 and over): a single dose of 100 mg.

Child (age 2–16): 0.8 mg per lb. of body weight, up to 100 mg.

Granisetron

Adult and Child (age 17 and over): 2 mg once a day or 1 mg twice a day.

Child (age 2–16): not recommended.

Ondansetron

Adult and Child (age 12 and over): 8 mg twice a day; 8 mg 3 times a day may be prescribed for adults over age 17 for nausea and vomiting associated with radiation therapy. People with liver failure should take no more than 8 mg a day. A single 24-mg dose 30 minutes before starting chemotherapy may be recommended.

Child (age 4–11): 4 mg 3 times a day.

Child (under age 4): not recommended.

Overdosage

Symptoms may include severe constipation, temporary blindness, high blood pressure, fainting, and mild headache. Contact your local poison control center or a hospital emergency room for more information. If you seek treatment, ALWAYS bring the prescription bottle or container.

Special Information

Contact your doctor if you develop chest tightness, wheezing, breathing difficulties, chest pain, or any bothersome or persistent side effect.

Contact your doctor at once and immediately stop taking alosetron if you develop constipation or symptoms of ischemic colitis, including abdominal pain, cramps, nausea, vomiting, and bloody diarrhea.

Maintain good dental hygiene while taking these drugs. Chronic dry mouth can increase the risk of tooth decay and gum disease.

If you forget a dose, take it as soon as you remember. If it is almost time for your next dose, skip the dose you forgot and continue with your regular schedule. Missing more than 1 dose may increase the risk of vomiting.

To use Zofran ODT, make sure your hands are dry. Peel back the foil on a blister and gently remove the tablet. Do not push the tablet through the foil. Immediately place the tablet on top of the tongue, where it will dissolve in seconds, then swallow with saliva.

Special Populations

Pregnancy/Breast-feeding: There are no adequate studies of the effects of these drugs in pregnant women. An antiemetic should be taken during pregnancy only if your doctor determines that the potential benefit outweighs the risks.

These drugs may pass into breast milk. Nursing mothers who must take any of these drugs should consider using infant formula.

Seniors: Seniors may take these drugs without special precaution, although elderly women taking alosetron may be at increased risk of serious constipation.

Type of Drug

Antihistamine Eye Drops

Brand Names

Generic Ingredients: Alcaftadine
Lastacaft

Generic Ingredients: Azelastine G
Optivar

Generic Ingredients: Bepotastine
Bepreve

Generic Ingredients: Emedastine
Emadine

Generic Ingredients: Epinastine G
Elestat

Generic Ingredients: Olopatadine
Pataday Patanol

Prescribed For

Eye itching due to allergy.

General Information

These drugs clear conjunctivitis (pinkeye) by preventing the release of chemicals from mast cells in the eye that cause allergic symptoms. They also work to minimize the response of nerve endings to any of these allergy-causing chemicals that might be present.

Cautions and Warnings

Do not use antihistamine eye drops if you are **allergic** or **sensitive** to any of their ingredients.

Do not use these drugs to treat redness caused by contact lens irritation. If you wear contact lenses, take them out before you put these drops into your eye.

Possible Side Effects

Side effects are generally mild and subside as your body gets used to the medicine.

Alcaftadine

▼ Less common: eye irritation, burning or stinging, eye redness and itching, runny nose, headache, and flu-like symptoms.

Azelastine

▼ Most common: burning or stinging sensation in the eyes, headache, and bitter taste in the mouth.

▼ Less common: asthma, conjunctivitis (pinkeye), difficulty breathing, eye pain, fatigue, flu-like symptoms, sore throat, itching, runny nose, and temporary blurred vision.

Bepotastine

▼ Common: bitter taste in the mouth after use.

▼ Less common: eye irritation, headache, and sore nose and throat.

Emedastine and Olopatadine

▼ Common: headache.

▼ Less common: mild burning or stinging of the eye, eye fatigue, itching of the eye, weakness, abnormal dreams, bad taste in the mouth, blurred vision, staining of the cornea, dry eyes, red eye, eye discomfort, sensation of something in the eye, inflammation of the cornea, sinus irritation, rash, runny nose, and tearing.

Epinastine

▼ Most common: burning sensation in the eye and itching.

Possible Side Effects *(continued)*

▼ Less common: headache, runny nose, sinus irritation, cough, and sore throat.

Drug Interactions

None known.

Usual Dose

Alcaftadine

Adult and Child (age 3 and over): 1 drop once a day in the affected eye.

Azelastine

Adult and Child (age 3 and over): 1 drop twice a day in the affected eye.

Bepotastine

Adult and Child (age 2 and over): 1 drop twice a day in the affected eye.

Child (under age 2): not recommended.

Emedastine

Adult and Child (age 3 and over): 1 drop in the affected eye up to 4 times a day.

Epinastine and Olopatadine

Adult and Child (age 3 and over): 1–2 drops twice a day at 6–8 hour intervals in the affected eye.

Overdosage

Little is known about overdose of antihistamine eye drops, but it is unlikely to lead to drug side effects. Accidental ingestion of these drugs is not likely to be severe because each bottle contains small amounts of active drug. Contact your local poison control center or hospital emergency room for more information. If you seek treatment, ALWAYS bring the prescription bottle or container.

Special Information

Do not wear contact lenses if your affected eye is red. If you wear soft contact lenses and your eye is not red, wait at least 15 minutes after using these medicines before putting in your lenses, this will prevent the preservatives in the eye drops from being absorbed into the lenses.

To avoid infection, do not touch the dropper tip to your finger, eyelid, or any other surface. Wait at least 5 minutes before using another eye drop or eye ointment.

If you forget a dose, administer it as soon as you remember. If it is almost time for your next dose, skip the one you forgot and continue with your regular schedule. Do not take a double dose.

Special Populations

Pregnancy/Breast-feeding: These drugs can cause birth defects at extremely high oral doses in laboratory animals but there is no information on their effect in women. These drugs should be taken during pregnancy only if your doctor determines that the potential benefit outweighs the risks.

Emedastine may pass into breast milk. It is not known if alcaftadine, azelastine, bepotastine, epinastine, or olopatadine pass into breast milk. Nursing mothers who must use antihistamine eye drops should use infant formula.

Seniors: Seniors may use these drugs without special precaution.

Type of Drug

Antihistamine-Decongestant Combination Products

Brand Names

There are many brand-name antihistamine-decongestant combination products, most of which are available over the counter. Check with your pharmacist about which specific brands are available as generics or as alcohol- or sugar-free.

Generic Ingredients

Acrivastine + Pseudoephedrine
Brompheniramine + Phenylephrine
Brompheniramine + Pseudoephedrine
Carbinoxamine + Phenylephrine
Carbinoxamine + Pseudoephedrine
Cetirizine + Pseudoephedrine
Chlorpheniramine Maleate + Phenylephrine Hydrochloride
Chlorpheniramine Maleate + Phenyltoloxamine + Phenylephrine Hydrochloride

Chlorpheniramine Maleate + Pseudoephedrine
Chlorpheniramine Polistirex + Pseudoephedrine Polistirex
Chlorpheniramine Tannate + Pyrilamine Tannate + Phenylephrine Tannate
Chlorpheniramine Tannate + Phenylephrine Tannate
Desloratadine + Pseudoephedrine
Dexbrompheniramine + Pseudoephedrine
Dexchlorpheniramine Maleate + Pseudoephedrine Hydrochloride
Diphenhydramine Hydrochloride + Phenylephrine Hydrochloride
Diphenhydramine Tannate + Phenylephrine Tannate
Fexofenadine + Pseudoephedrine
Loratadine + Pseudoephedrine
Promethazine + Phenylephrine Hydrochloride
Pyrilamine + Pseudoephedrine + Phenyltoloxamine + Pheniramine
Pyrilamine Tannate + Phenylephrine Tannate
Triprolidine Hydrochloride + Pseudoephedrine Hydrochloride

Prescribed For

Sneezing, watery eyes, runny nose, itchy or scratchy throat, nasal congestion, and other symptoms of the common cold, allergies, and upper-respiratory conditions.

General Information

The basic formula for each of these antihistamine-decongestant combinations is the same: An antihistamine is used to relieve allergy symptoms and a decongestant is used to treat the symptoms of either a cold or allergy.

Most of these products are taken several times a day, while others are long-acting and are taken once or twice a day. Since nothing can cure a cold or allergy, the best you can hope to achieve from a cold and allergy remedy is relief from symptoms.

Cautions and Warnings

Do not use antihistamines if you are **allergic** or **sensitive** to any of their ingredients.

Antihistamines in these products may cause drowsiness. Decongestants may cause anxiety and nervousness and may interfere with sleep.

People with **narrow-angle glaucoma**, very **high blood pressure**, severe **coronary artery disease**, **prostate disease**, certain

stomach ulcers, **bladder obstruction**, and those having **asthma attacks** or **difficulty urinating** should not use these products.

A recent FDA panel recommended that pediatric use of antihistamines and decongestants should be banned for **children under age 6**.

Possible Side Effects

- ▼ Most common: restlessness, nervousness, sleeplessness, drowsiness, sedation, excitation, dizziness, poor coordination, and upset stomach.
- ▼ Less common: low blood pressure; heart palpitations, rapid heartbeat, and abnormal heart rhythms; chest pain; anemia; fatigue; confusion; tremors; headache; irritability; euphoria (feeling "high"); tingling or heaviness in the hands; tingling in the feet or legs; blurred or double vision; convulsions; hysterical reaction; ringing or buzzing in the ears; fainting; increase or decrease in appetite; nausea; vomiting; diarrhea or constipation; frequent urination; difficulty urinating; early menstrual periods; loss of sex drive; breathing difficulties; wheezing with chest tightness; stuffy nose; itching; rash; unusual sensitivity to the sun; chills; excessive perspiration; and dry mouth, nose, or throat.

Drug Interactions

- Combining these products with alcoholic beverages, antianxiety drugs, sedatives, or narcotic pain relievers may lead to excessive drowsiness or difficulty concentrating.
- Avoid these products if you are taking a monoamine oxidase inhibitor (MAOI) antidepressant or if you have stopped taking an MAOI in the past 14 days. The MAOI may cause a very rapid rise in blood pressure or increase side effects such as dry mouth and nose, blurred vision, and abnormal heart rhythms.
- The decongestant component of these products may interfere with the normal effects of blood-pressure-lowering medications and can aggravate diabetes, heart disease, hyperthyroid disease, high blood pressure, prostate disease, stomach ulcer, and urinary blockage.
- If your doctor has prescribed one of these products, do not self-medicate with an additional over-the-counter drug for

the relief of cold symptoms. This combination may aggravate high blood pressure, heart disease, diabetes, or thyroid disease.

Food Interactions

These drugs are best taken on an empty stomach but may be taken with food if they upset your stomach.

Usual Dose

Dosages vary. Generally, these products are taken every 4–12 hours.

Overdosage

Symptoms of overdose are drowsiness, chills, dry mouth, fever, nausea, nervousness, irritability, rapid or irregular heartbeat, chest pain, and urinary difficulties. Most cases should be treated by inducing vomiting as soon as possible with ipecac syrup—available at any pharmacy. Then contact your local poison control center for more information or take the victim to a hospital emergency room. If you seek treatment, ALWAYS bring the medicine's bottle or container.

Special Information

Use extra caution while doing anything that requires concentration, such as driving a car or operating hazardous machinery.

Contact your doctor if your side effects are severe or become intolerable.

If you forget to take a dose of your medication, take it as soon as you remember. If it is almost time for your next dose, skip the dose you forgot and continue with your regular schedule. Do not take a double dose.

Special Populations

Pregnancy/Breast-feeding: Animal studies suggest that some older antihistamines cause birth defects, but the antihistamines in these products have not been proven harmful. If you are or might be pregnant, do not take any of these products without your doctor's knowledge.

Small amounts of antihistamine or decongestant pass into breast milk. Nursing mothers who must use these products should use infant formula.

Seniors: Seniors are more sensitive to the side effects of these medications.

Generic Name

Apraclonidine (ah-prah-KLON-ih-dene) G

Brand Names

Iopidine

Type of Drug

Sympathomimetic.

Prescribed For

Post-surgical increases in eye pressure and additional short-term treatment in people who are using other glaucoma medicines.

General Information

Apraclonidine reduces both elevated and normal fluid pressure inside the eye and selectively blocks certain nerve endings without acting as a local anesthetic. The exact way it works is not known, but apraclonidine, like other drugs that reduce eye pressure, may work by decreasing the production of eye fluid. The drug starts to work within 1 hour after it is put into the eye and reaches its maximum effect in 3–5 hours.

Cautions and Warnings

Do not use apraclonidine if you are **allergic** or **sensitive** to any of its ingredients or to clonidine. This drug can cause an allergic-like reaction, including red eye, swelling of the lid and white of the eye, itching, burning, and the feeling of something in your eye. If this happens, stop using the drug and contact your doctor.

Taking this drug with a **monoamine oxidase inhibitor (MAOI) antidepressant** may result in severe side effects—do not combine them.

Using this medicine with other eye-pressure-lowering drugs may not provide additional benefit—other drugs work in the same way and a further effect may not be possible.

The ability of apraclonidine to lower eye pressure decreases over time. Most people continuously benefit for less than 1 month.

People with **kidney, liver, heart, or vascular disease** should be monitored by their doctors while taking this medicine.

Apraclonidine has been associated with **depression**. People with depression or a history of depression should be monitored by their doctors while taking this medication.

Possible Side Effects

- ▼ Most common: eye redness, dry eye, discharge from the eye, tearing, eye discomfort, lid swelling, feeling of something in your eye, itching, dry nose, changes in taste, dizziness, drowsiness, dry mouth, headache, and weakness.
- ▼ Less common: blanching of the eye; lid crusting; abnormal vision; eye pain; runny nose; sore throat; worsening asthma; constipation and nausea; abnormal heart rhythms; chest pain; difficulty sleeping; depression; body pain; nervousness; distorted sense of smell; decreased coordination; pain, numbness, or tingling in the hands or feet; and rash.

Drug Interactions

- Apraclonidine can reduce pulse and blood pressure. If you are also taking drugs to treat high blood pressure or other cardiovascular drugs, check your pulse and blood pressure.
- MAOI antidepressants can slow the breakdown of apraclonidine and increase the risk of drug side effects. This combination should be avoided. You should also wait 14 days after stopping an MAOI before starting apraclonidine.

Usual Dose

Adult: 1–2 drops in the affected eye 3 times a day.

Overdosage

Exaggerated side effects, especially those that affect the nervous system, are symptoms of overdose. Contact your local poison control center for more information. If you seek treatment, ALWAYS bring the prescription bottle or container.

Special Information

Apraclonidine can cause dizziness and tiredness. Be careful doing anything that requires concentration, coordination, or alertness while taking this medication.

To prevent infection, do not touch the dropper tip to your finger or eyelid. Wait 5 minutes before using any other eye drop or ointment.

Remove contact lenses before applying apraclonidine and wait 15 minutes before reinserting them.

If you forget a dose of apraclonidine, take it as soon as you remember. If it is almost time for your next dose, take 1 dose as soon as you remember and then go back to your regular schedule. Do not take a double dose.

Special Populations

Pregnancy/Breast-feeding: In animal studies, apraclonidine was toxic to embryos when given by mouth. Apraclonidine should be taken during pregnancy only if your doctor determines that the potential benefit outweighs the risks.

It is not known if this drug passes into breast milk. Nursing mothers who must take this medication should use infant formula.

Seniors: Seniors may use this medicine without special precaution.

Generic Name

Aprepitant (ah-PRE-pih-tant)

Brand Names

Emend

Type of Drug

Antinauseant and antiemetic (an agent that prevents or relieves nausea and vomiting).

Prescribed For

Acute and delayed nausea and vomiting associated with chemotherapy and prevention of nausea and vomiting following anesthesia.

General Information

Aprepitant works against nausea and vomiting by selectively inhibiting the substance P/neurokinin 1 (NK 1) receptor. This is a unique approach to nausea therapy and it complements other nausea therapies, such as corticosteroids and 5HT receptor antagonists that should be used together with aprepitant. Aprepitant is broken down in the liver.

Cautions and Warnings

Do not take aprepitant if you are **allergic** or **sensitive** to any of its ingredients. Severe allergic reactions to this drug can develop.

Aprepitant should be used with caution if you have severe **liver disease**. People with mild to moderate liver disease can tolerate the drug.

Aprepitant is not intended for normal nausea and vomiting in those not undergoing chemotherapy treatment or for chronic continuous therapy. It should not be used for the chronic management of nausea and vomiting.

Possible Side Effects

▼ Most common: fatigue, nausea, appetite loss, hiccups, and constipation and diarrhea.

▼ Common: dizziness, dehydration, heartburn, headache, and vomiting.

▼ Less common: abdominal pain, fever, upset stomach, stomach pains, ringing or buzzing in the ears, mucous membrane swelling, and sleeplessness.

▼ Rare: Rare side effects can occur in almost any part of the body. Contact your doctor if you experience anything unusual while taking any medication.

Drug Interactions

- Aprepitant may slow the breakdown of astemizole, cisapride, pimozide, or terfenadine, leading to serious drug side effects. Do not combine these medicines with aprepitant.
- Clarithromycin, diltiazem, itraconazole, ketoconazole, nefazodone, nelfinavir, and ritonavir may raise blood levels of aprepitant, increasing the chances for drug side effects and toxicity. These drugs should be combined with caution.
- Carbamazepine, phenytoin, and rifampin may reduce the effectiveness of aprepitant.
- Blood levels of aprepitant and paroxetine are both reduced by about 25% when they are combined.
- Blood levels of the hormones ethinyl estradiol and norethindrone—used in many hormonal contraceptive products—can be reduced, compromising the effectiveness of these products. Use a non-hormonal contraceptive method while taking aprepitant and for 1 month after you stop.
- Aprepitant may decrease blood levels of tolbutamide when given concurrently, reducing its effectiveness.
- The breakdown of warfarin may be increased by aprepitant, reducing the blood thinner's effectiveness. If you take warfarin and have to use aprepitant, your doctor should closely monitor your warfarin in the 2-week period (especially days 7–10) after the beginning of each aprepitant cycle.

- Aprepitant can increase the amount of corticosteroid drug that is absorbed into your blood. Oral dexamethasone and methylprednisolone doses should be decreased by ½ when combined with aprepitant.
- Aprepitant increases blood levels of midazolam, increasing the chances for drug side effects. Levels of other benzodiazepine sedatives (such as alprazolam and triazolam) may rise as well.
- Aprepitant is often given with cancer chemotherapy drugs that are broken down by the same enzymes. This combination might be expected to raise the amount of chemotherapeutic in the blood, but this was not a problem in clinical studies of the drug. Drugs that may have this effect, and should be used with caution, include docetaxel, paclitaxel, etoposide, irinotecan, ifosfamide, imatinib, vinorelbine, vinblastine, and vincristine.

Food Interactions

This drug can be taken without regard to food or meals.

Usual Dose

Adult: 125 mg 1 hour before starting chemotherapy, followed by 80 mg on the 2 days following chemotherapy. Aprepitant should be used in combination with a corticosteroid (such as dexamethasone) and a $5HT_3$ receptor antagonist (such as ondansetron).

Child: not recommended.

Overdosage

There is limited information about aprepitant overdose, but drowsiness and headache may occur. Overdose victims should be taken to a hospital emergency room. If you seek treatment, ALWAYS bring the prescription bottle or container.

Special Information

Contact your doctor if you develop itching, rash, hives, or difficulty breathing. These can be signs of a drug reaction.

Aprepitant is given in a 3-day cycle. Take the first dose 1 hour before chemotherapy. Take the next 2 doses on the morning of the 2 days following your chemotherapy treatment.

Special Populations

Pregnancy/Breast-feeding: While animal studies of aprepitant revealed no adverse effects on a developing fetus, there is no information on how this drug will affect pregnant women. Aprepitant should be taken during pregnancy only if your doctor determines that the potential benefit outweighs the risks.

Aprepitant passes into milk in animal studies. Nursing mothers who must take it should use infant formula.

Seniors: Seniors may be more sensitive to the effects of aprepitant, but dosage adjustments are not needed.

Apri *see **Contraceptives,** page 316*

Aricept *see **Cholinesterase Inhibitors,** page 286*

Generic Name

Aripiprazole (ah-rih-PIP-rah-zole)

Brand Names

Abilify Abilify Discmelt

Type of Drug

Antipsychotic.

Prescribed For

Schizophrenia and bipolar disorder, major depressive disorder, and irritability in autism spectrum disorders. It may also be prescribed for cocaine addiction, restless legs syndrome, and Tourette syndrome.

General Information

Aripiprazole is an antipsychotic that works on serotonin and dopamine receptors in the brain. Unlike other antipsychotics that only decrease dopamine, it may both increase and decrease dopamine, targeting specific areas of the brain where the neurotransmitter is too plentiful or too reduced. However, the exact way it works is not known.

The effectiveness of aripiprazole was established by studying hospitalized schizophrenics for 4–6 weeks, and later studies also proved its effectiveness for 6 months or beyond.

Children age 6–17 with an autism spectrum disorder may take this medication as part of a total treatment program including psychological, educational, and social intervention.

Cautions and Warnings

Do not take aripiprazole if you are **allergic** or **sensitive** to any of its ingredients. Severe allergic reactions to this drug can develop.

Aripiprazole has been associated with increased mortality in seniors with **dementia** or **Alzheimer's disease**. The specific causes of death related to atypical antipsychotic drugs were either due to a heart-related event or infection, mostly pneumonia.

Antipsychotics have been associated with a higher risk of suicidal thinking and behavior in **children**, **adolescents**, and **young adults**. Use in this population must be carefully balanced with need.

People with **major depressive disorder** may experience a worsening of depression. Families and caregivers should be alert for signs of worsening depression or the emergence of suicidal thinking or behavior. Suicide is a danger with all antipsychotic medications. To reduce the possibility of overdose, people taking this drug should have no more than a 30-day supply of medication at any one time.

A serious set of side effects known as neuroleptic malignant syndrome (NMS) may occur while taking aripiprazole. Symptoms include high fever, convulsions, difficult or fast breathing, rapid heartbeat, rapid or irregular pulse or blood pressure, increased sweating, muscle rigidity, and mental changes. NMS can be fatal and requires immediate medical attention. This condition has been associated with most antipsychotic medicines.

Tardive dyskinesia (a group of severe side effects associated with antipsychotic and other drugs) may occur while taking aripiprazole and is often considered a reason to stop taking this drug. Symptoms include lip smacking or puckering, puffing of the cheeks, rapid or wormlike tongue movements, uncontrolled chewing motions, and uncontrolled arm or leg movements. Symptoms can increase with the length and dosage of antipsychotic drug therapy and may become permanent. Report any of these side effects to your doctor.

People taking this medicine have developed **high blood sugar** and **diabetes**. People with a diagnosis of high blood-sugar levels or diabetes should have their blood-sugar levels checked regularly while taking aripiprazole. People with a family history of diabetes or other diabetes risk factors should be tested periodically during treatment. Others should be monitored for symptoms of diabetes (increased thirst, increased food consumption, increased urination, and fatigue).

People with **liver or kidney disease** may have higher blood levels of aripiprazole than healthy people, but this is not a reason to adjust the drug dose.

Levels of some white blood cells can drop drastically in people taking aripiprazole, making it harder to fight infection. Your doctor will monitor your blood count.

Aripiprazole can cause dizziness or fainting when rising from a sitting or lying position, especially when people start taking the drug. People with a history of **heart disease** or **stroke** are more likely to experience dizziness or fainting when rising from a sitting or lying position while taking aripiprazole, especially upon initiation of the drug.

Seizures occur in a small number of people taking aripiprazole. It should be taken with care if you have had or are at increased risk of seizures.

Avoid exposure to **extreme heat**. Antipsychotics can upset your body's temperature-regulating mechanism, making you more prone to heatstroke.

Swallowing problems and inhaling food can be a problem with all antipsychotics, including aripiprazole.

Possible Side Effects

In studies of aripiprazole, reported side effects were similar in people taking aripiprazole and those taking an inactive placebo (sugar pill).

- ▼ Most common: headache, nausea, vomiting, constipation, weight gain, anxiety, lightheadedness, tiredness, sleeplessness, and an uncontrollable feeling of restlessness.
- ▼ Common: weakness and rash.
- ▼ Less common: fever, tremors, runny nose, cough, blurred vision, abnormal heart rhythms, and weight gain.
- ▼ Rare: Rare side effects can occur in almost any part of the body. Contact your doctor if you experience anything unusual while taking any medication.

Drug Interactions

- Aripiprazole should not be combined with alcohol or other central-nervous-system depressants; motor skills may be impaired.
- Carbamazepine reduces blood levels of aripiprazole. If carbamazepine is added to aripiprazole treatment, the dose of aripiprazole should be doubled. Aripiprazole dosage should be reduced to normal levels when carbamazepine is stopped.
- Aripiprazole has the potential to increase the effects of certain drugs used to treat high blood pressure.
- Clarithromycin, fluoxetine, itraconazole, ketoconazole, paroxetine, and quinidine increase blood levels of aripiprazole. If any of these drugs are combined with aripiprazole, the dosage of aripiprazole should be reduced by ½ until the other drug is stopped. In addition, aripiprazole may increase levels of fluoxetine and decrease levels of paroxetine.

Food Interactions

This drug can be taken without regard to food or meals.

Usual Dose

Adult: 10–15 mg once a day. Maximum dose is 30 mg.

Child (age 6–17): 2 mg a day to start, increased gradually to 10–15 mg a day if needed.

Overdosage

Symptoms of overdose include tiredness and vomiting. Take the victim to a hospital emergency room. If you seek treatment, ALWAYS bring the prescription bottle or container.

Special Information

Aripiprazole may cause drowsiness. Use caution when doing anything that requires intense concentration, such as driving or operating machinery.

Avoid alcoholic beverages while taking aripiprazole.

If you get dizzy while taking aripiprazole, avoid sudden changes in posture and avoid climbing stairs.

Do not open the blister pack until you are ready to take aripiprazole. Do not push the tablet through the foil but instead peel the foil back. Handle the tablet with clean, dry hands.

If you forget to take a dose of aripiprazole, take it as soon as you remember and continue with your regular dose on the next day. Tell your doctor or pharmacist if you forget more than 1 dose of aripiprazole. Do not take a double dose of this medication unless advised to do so by your doctor.

Be sure to tell your doctor about any other medicines you are taking, including over-the-counter remedies.

Special Populations

Pregnancy/Breast-feeding: Newborns whose mothers were taking any antipsychotic medicine during pregnancy are more likely to experience agitation, abnormally increased or decreased muscle tone, tremor, sleepiness, severe difficulty breathing, and difficulty in feeding. In some newborns, the symptoms subside within hours or days and do not require specific treatment; other newborns may require longer hospital stays. If you are or might be pregnant, do not stop taking this medication without talking to your doctor, because suddenly stopping antipsychotic medications can cause significant treatment complications.

Aripiprazole passes into breast milk. Nursing mothers who must take it should use infant formula.

Seniors: Seniors eliminate 20% less aripiprazole than younger adults, but there is no need for dosage adjustments.

Generic Names

Aspirin, Buffered Aspirin (AS-prin) G

Brand Names

There are many brand-name aspirin products, most of which are available over the counter. Check with your pharmacist about which specific brands are available buffered or with antacids.

Type of Drug

Analgesic and anti-inflammatory agent.

Prescribed For

Mild to moderate pain, fever, arthritis, and inflammation of bones, joints, or other body tissues. People who have had a stroke or transient ischemic attack (TIA)—oxygen shortage to the brain—may have aspirin prescribed to reduce the risk of having another such attack. Aspirin may also be prescribed as an anticoagulant (blood thinning) drug in people with unstable angina and to protect against heart attack. Aspirin has a definite beneficial effect if it is taken as soon as possible after having a heart attack.

General Information

Aspirin may be the closest thing we have to a wonder drug. It has been used for more than a century for pain and fever relief and is now used for its effect on the blood as well.

Aspirin is the standard against which all other drugs are compared for relieving pain and for reducing inflammation. Chemically, aspirin is a member of the group of drugs called salicylates. Other salicylates include sodium salicylate, sodium thiosalicylate, choline salicylate, and magnesium salicylate (trilisate). These drugs are no more effective than regular aspirin, although 2 of them—choline salicylate and magnesium salicylate—may be a little less irritating to the stomach. They are all more expensive than aspirin.

Aspirin reduces fever by causing the blood vessels in the skin to open, allowing heat to leave the body more rapidly. Its effects on pain and inflammation are thought to be related to its ability to prevent the manufacture of complex body hormones called prostaglandins. Of all the salicylates, aspirin has the greatest effect on prostaglandin production.

Many people find that they can take buffered aspirin but not regular aspirin. The addition of antacids to aspirin can be important to people who must take large doses of aspirin for chronic arthritis or other conditions. In many cases, aspirin is the only effective drug and can be tolerated only with the antacids present.

Cautions and Warnings

Do not take aspirin if you are **allergic** or **sensitive** to any of its ingredients, or to nonsteroidal anti-inflammatory drugs (NSAIDs) such as indomethacin, sulindac, ibuprofen, fenoprofen, naproxen, tolmetin, and meclofenamate sodium or to products containing tartrazine (a commonly used orange dye and food coloring). People with **asthma**, a history of **hives**, or **nasal polyps** are more likely to be allergic to aspirin.

Reye's syndrome is a life-threatening condition characterized by vomiting and stupor or dullness and may develop in children with **fever** that is treated with aspirin or other salicylates. Up to 30% of people who develop Reye's syndrome can die, and permanent brain damage is possible in those who survive. Because of this, authorities advise against giving **children** under age 19 aspirin or another salicylate, especially those with **viral infections with or without fever**; acetaminophen should be given instead.

People with severe **liver or kidney disease** or **gout** should avoid aspirin.

People on a **restricted salt diet** should avoid sodium-containing buffered aspirin because of its high salt content.

Alcoholic beverages may worsen the stomach irritation caused by aspirin. Alcohol increases the risk of aspirin-related ulcers.

Stop taking aspirin if you develop dizziness, hearing loss, or ringing or buzzing in the ears.

Aspirin interferes with normal blood clotting and should therefore be avoided for 1 week before surgery. Ask for your surgeon or dentist's recommendation before taking aspirin for pain after surgery.

Aspirin should not be taken by people with **hemophilia**, **other bleeding disorders**, or **bleeding ulcers**, or those who are in a state of **bleeding**.

Possible Side Effects

- ▼ Most common: nausea, upset stomach, heartburn, loss of appetite, and small amounts of blood in the stool.
- ▼ Less common: hives, rashes, liver damage, fever, thirst, and visual difficulties. Aspirin may contribute to the formation of stomach ulcers and bleeding. People who are allergic to aspirin and those with a history of nasal polyps, asthma, or rhinitis may experience difficulty breathing and a stuffy nose.

Drug Interactions

- People taking anticoagulant (blood thinning) drugs should avoid aspirin because it increases the effect of the anticoagulant.
- Taking aspirin and acetazolamide may lead to high blood levels of acetazolamide and possible toxicity.
- Aspirin may increase the possibility of stomach ulcer when taken together with alcoholic beverages.
- Aspirin may counteract the blood-pressure-lowering effect of ACE inhibitors and beta blockers. Aspirin may also counteract the effects of some diuretics in people with liver or kidney disease.
- Aspirin may increase blood levels of methotrexate, leading to increased chances of drug toxicity.

- Aspirin may increase blood levels of phenytoin and valproic acid, leading to increased chances of drug toxicity.
- Do not take aspirin with an NSAID. There is no benefit to the combination, and the chance of side effects—especially stomach irritation—is vastly increased.
- Large aspirin doses (2000 mg a day or more) can lower blood sugar. This can be a problem in people with diabetes who take insulin or oral antidiabetes drugs to control their condition.
- Aspirin will counteract the uric-acid-eliminating effect of probenecid and sulfinpyrazone.

Food Interactions

Because aspirin can cause upset stomach and bleeding, take each dose with food, milk, or a glass of water.

Usual Dose

Adult

Aches, Pains, and Fever: 324–1000 mg every 4–6 hours; not to exceed 4000 mg per day.

Arthritis and Rheumatic Conditions: 3000 mg a day in divided doses to start; dose can be increased as needed until blood-salicylate levels reach 150–300 mcg/mL.

Heart Attack Prevention, Stroke, or TIA: 50–325 mg a day.

Child (under age 19): not recommended because of the risk of Reye's syndrome (see "Cautions and Warnings").

Overdosage

Aspirin may be lethal for adults in overdoses of 30 regular-strength tablets—325 mg each—or 20 maximum-strength tablets—500 mg. Aspirin may be lethal for children in overdoses of 12 regular-strength tablets or 8 maximum-strength tablets.

Aspirin is a commonly used ingredient in many over-the-counter (OTC) medications. Always check the list of ingredients when using more than one OTC medication to ensure that the combined dosage is within guidelines and to avoid accidental overdose.

Symptoms of mild overdose are rapid and deep breathing, nausea, vomiting, dizziness, ringing or buzzing in the ears, flushing, sweating, thirst, headache, drowsiness, diarrhea, and rapid heartbeat.

Severe overdose may cause fever, excitement, confusion, convulsions, liver or kidney failure, coma, and bleeding.

The initial treatment of aspirin overdose involves inducing

vomiting to remove any drug remaining in the stomach. Further treatment depends on how the situation develops and what must be done to maintain the patient. Do not induce vomiting until you have spoken with your doctor or poison control center. If in doubt, go to a hospital emergency room. If you seek treatment, ALWAYS bring the aspirin bottle or container.

Special Information

Contact your doctor if you develop continuous stomach pain or ringing or buzzing in the ears.

Do not use an aspirin product if it has a strong odor of vinegar. This is an indication that the product has started to break down in the bottle.

Do not crush or chew a sustained-release preparation of aspirin.

Check with your doctor if pain lasts more than 10 days, if pain worsens, or redness or swelling develop. Also, report a fever that persists for longer than 3 days.

If you are taking aspirin regularly, report to your doctor if you notice a ringing or buzzing in the ears or experience severe or continuing headache. You should also report gastrointestinal symptoms that become bothersome, such as stomach pain, heartburn, nausea, and vomiting. These may be signs of an ulcer.

If you forget to take a dose of aspirin, take it as soon as you remember. If it is almost time for your next dose, skip the dose you forgot and continue with your regular schedule. Do not take a double dose.

Special Populations

Pregnancy/Breast-feeding: Check with your doctor before taking any aspirin-containing product during pregnancy. Aspirin may cause bleeding problems in the fetus during the last 2 weeks of pregnancy. Taking aspirin during the last 3 months of pregnancy may extend the length of pregnancy, prolong labor, and lead to a low-birth-weight infant. It can also cause bleeding in the mother before, during, or after delivery. Anemia may also result from taking aspirin during pregnancy.

Aspirin passes into breast milk, but has not caused any problems in nursing babies. Nursing mothers should speak to their doctors before using aspirin.

Seniors: Aspirin, especially in larger doses that a senior may take for arthritis and rheumatic conditions, may be irritating to the stomach. Seniors with liver disease should not use aspirin.

Generic Name

Atomoxetine (ah-tom-OX-eh-teen)

Brand Names

Strattera

Type of Drug

Selective norepinephrine reuptake inhibitor.

Prescribed For

Attention-deficit hyperactivity disorder (ADHD).

General Information

Atomoxetine is used for attention-deficit hyperactivity disorder. This drug may be used by children, teenagers, and adults. Unlike most other medicines used for ADHD, it is not a stimulant.

Cautions and Warnings

Do not take atomoxetine if you are **allergic** or **sensitive** to any of its ingredients.

Suicidal thoughts and actions have occurred in **children** and **teens** taking atomoxetine. Warning signs to look for include agitation, irritability, and unusual behavior changes, especially during the first few months of drug therapy or when drug dosage is increased or decreased.

Separate atomoxetine from any **monoamine oxidase inhibitor (MAOI) antidepressant** by at least 2 weeks. Serious, sometimes fatal, symptoms, including body-temperature elevations, rigidity, muscle stiffness, or rapid changes of vital signs or mental status (including extreme agitation, progressing to delirium and coma), may occur.

Atomoxetine is not recommended for people with **narrow-angle glaucoma**. Atomoxetine should also not be taken by those with a **pheochromocytoma** (adrenal gland tumor), or those with a history of pheochromocytoma.

In rare cases, atomoxetine may cause severe liver injury. Atomoxetine should be discontinued in patients with jaundice or evidence of liver dysfunction. People with **liver disease** may require a lower dosage of atomoxetine.

Children or adolescents with **structural heart abnormalities** or other **serious heart problems** should not take atomoxetine.

Adults with these conditions should take this medication with caution or not at all due to the risk of sudden death.

Atomoxetine can increase blood pressure and heart rate. People with **high blood pressure**, **rapid heartbeat**, or **cardiovascular or cerebrovascular disease** should use it with caution. Atomoxetine may bring on or exacerbate symptoms of **Raynaud's disease** (a condition involving blood circulation at the extremities). People taking atomoxetine may feel dizzy or faint when rising quickly from a sitting or lying position.

Children taking atomoxetine grow more slowly and gain less weight than other children their age for the first 9–12 months they are taking the medicine. After that, they start growing more quickly and generally catch up with their peers after 3 years.

People with **bipolar disorder** who take atomoxetine may be at risk for experiencing a manic reaction and should be carefully monitored.

Atomoxetine may cause an increase in aggression or hostility, which should be reported to a doctor immediately. Atomoxetine may also bring on manic behavior, hallucinations, or delusional thinking. Children and adolescents beginning treatment with atomoxetine should be carefully monitored for changes in behavior.

Atomoxetine may cause hesitation or difficulty in urinating.

Rare cases of priapism (a persistent, painful erection) have been reported in adults and children taking atomoxetine. Suspected cases warrant immediate medical attention.

Possible Side Effects

Children and Adolescents

In clinical studies, drug side effects were similar to those reported by people taking an inactive placebo (sugar pill).

- ▼ Most common: headache, upper abdominal pain, vomiting, and coughing.
- ▼ Common: dizziness, tiredness, and irritability.
- ▼ Less common: constipation, upset stomach, runny nose, urinary difficulties, appetite loss, weight loss, crying, tiredness, reduced sense of touch, tingling in the hands or feet, mood swings, and skin rash.

Adults

- ▼ Most common: dry mouth, headache, nausea, and sleeplessness.

Possible Side Effects *(continued)*

- ▼ Common: hesitation or difficulty urinating, constipation, upset stomach, tiredness or fatigue, sinus infection, appetite loss, dizziness, sleeping problems, painful menstruation, erectile dysfunction, and reduced sex drive or other sexual concerns.
- ▼ Less common: abdominal gas, fever and chills, weight loss, abnormal dreams, sinus headache, tingling in the hands or feet, muscle ache, impotence, delayed onset of menstruation, irregular or other menstrual issues, prostate irritation, skin rash, increased sweating, and hot flashes.
- ▼ Rare: chest pain and heart palpitations. Contact your doctor if you experience anything unusual while taking any medication.

Drug Interactions

- Atomoxetine should not be used 2 weeks before or after taking an MAOI antidepressant (see "Cautions and Warnings").
- Atomoxetine should be used with caution with the following drugs: antiarrhythmic agents (such as amiodarone, bretylium, disopyramide, dofetilide, quinidine, and sotalol), arsenic trioxide, chlorpromazine, cisapride, dolasetron, droperidol, gatifloxacin, halofantrine, levomethadyl, mefloquine, mesoridazine, moxifloxacin, pentamidine, pimozide, probucol, sparfloxacin, thioridazine, and ziprasidone. Serious heart rhythm disorders are possible.
- Atomoxetine increases the effects of albuterol, causing high blood pressure and rapid heartbeat. Dosage adjustments may be required.
- Fluoxetine, paroxetine, and quinidine substantially increase the amount of atomoxetine in the blood. Atomoxetine dosage adjustments may be necessary.
- Atomoxetine raises blood pressure and should be given with caution to people who are already taking medicines that raise blood pressure. It may counter the effects of some drugs used to treat high blood pressure.
- Atomoxetine may reduce the efficacy of iobenguane. Atomoxetine should be discontinued for approximately 24 hours prior to administration of iobenguane.

Food Interactions

Atomoxetine can be taken without regard to food or meals.

Usual Dose

Adult and Child (155 lbs. and over): 40–80 mg a day in a single or divided dose. Maximum dose is 100 mg a day. Divided doses should be taken in the morning and late afternoon or early evening.

Child (age 6 and over and less than 155 lbs.): starting dose—0.23 mg per lb. of body weight. Dose can be gradually increased up to 0.55 mg per lb. as a single dose in the morning or 2 doses, one in the morning and the second in the late afternoon or early evening.

People with moderate liver disease should take ½ of the regular dose and those with severe liver disease should take ¼ of the regular dose.

Overdosage

Little is known about the effects of atomoxetine overdose. Contact your local poison control center or a hospital emergency room for information. If you seek treatment, ALWAYS bring the prescription bottle or container.

Special Information

Contact your doctor if your skin or eyes develop a yellowish tinge or if you develop thirst, heart palpitations, constipation, urinary problems, fatigue, appetite loss, or a light-colored stool. These can be signs of liver disease.

Patients taking atomoxetine and their caregivers should be alerted to new signs of agitation, aggression, anxiety, depression, hostility, mood swings, impulsive behavior, insomnia, irritability, mania, panic attacks, or any other unusual changes in behavior or talk of suicide. Contact your doctor immediately.

If you forget a dose of atomoxetine, take it as soon as you remember. If it is almost time for your next dose, skip the one you forgot and continue with your regular schedule. Do not take a double dose.

Use caution while driving or operating machinery when you start taking atomoxetine until you can determine how it will affect your abilities.

Special Populations

Pregnancy/Breast-feeding: Animal studies show that atomoxetine may affect a developing fetus. Atomoxetine should be taken during pregnancy only if your doctor determines that the potential benefit outweighs the risk.

Atomoxetine may pass into breast milk. Nursing mothers who must take this drug should use infant formula.

Seniors: Atomoxetine has not been studied in older adults.

Generic Name

Atovaquone (ah-TOE-vuh-quone)

Brand Names

Generic Ingredients: Atovaquone

Mepron [$]

Combination Products

Generic Ingredients: Atovaquone + Proguanil

Malarone Malarone Pediatric

Type of Drug

Anti-infective.

Prescribed For

Prevention and treatment of mild to moderate *Pneumocystis carinii* pneumonia (PCP); prevention and treatment of malaria caused by *Plasmodium falciparum*.

General Information

Atovaquone is an anti-infective with specific activity against PCP, an infection commonly associated with HIV. It is used in people who cannot take the combination of trimethoprim and sulfamethoxazole. In studies comparing atovaquone with trimethoprim-sulfamethoxazole (TMP-SMZ), approximately 60% of people with PCP improved on each drug. However, more people died of PCP and other infections while being treated with atovaquone. Of those who died, most had less atovaquone in their bloodstream than those who lived. In studies comparing oral atovaquone with intravenous pentamidine for treating PCP in people with HIV, both drugs were equally effective, at 14%. Again, there was a direct correlation between the amount of atovaquone in the blood and survival. The drug stays in the body for several days and is eliminated through the liver.

Atovaquone + proguanil is effective against *P. falciparum*, an organism that causes malaria and that may be resistant to other antimalaria drugs such as chloroquine, halofantrine, mefloquine, and amodiaquine.

Cautions and Warnings

Do not take atovaquone if you are **allergic** or **sensitive** to any of its ingredients.

This drug has not been studied for severe PCP or in those who are failing on TMP-SMZ.

Atovaquone only works against PCP. People with PCP who have **bacterial, viral, fungal, or other infections of the lung** may continue to worsen despite atovaquone therapy. If this happens, it may be a sign that another kind of infecting organism is the cause. Additional medicine will be necessary.

Atovaquone absorption is strongly influenced by food. People with **gastrointestinal disorders** or those who are unable to take atovaquone with food may not be able to absorb enough medicine for it to be effective. Intravenous treatments with other PCP anti-infectives may be necessary.

Atovaquone may not work as well in people with **liver disease.** Your doctor should carefully monitor your progress.

Possible Side Effects

Because atovaquone was evaluated in people with advanced HIV, it is difficult to discern side effects of the drug use from those caused by the disease. Overall, only 4–9% of people studied stopped taking the drug because of side effects, a much smaller percentage than occurs with other PCP treatments.

- ▼ Most common: rash, nausea, diarrhea, headache, vomiting, fever, sleeplessness, weakness, itching, oral fungal infections, abdominal pain, upset stomach, appetite loss, constipation, cough, dizziness, pain, increased sweating, anxiety, sinus inflammation, and runny nose.
- ▼ Less common: changes in sense of taste, low blood sugar, and low blood pressure.

Drug Interactions

- Atovaquone may increase blood levels of warfarin, oral antidiabetes drugs, digoxin, and other drugs that bind strongly to blood proteins.

- Rifampin and rifabutin may reduce blood levels of atovaquone, possibly diminishing its effectiveness. Use of these agents with atovaquone is not recommended.
- Metoclopramide reduces the availability of atovaquone in the body. Other antiemetic drugs should be used whenever possible.
- Tetracycline reduces blood levels of atovaquone and may reduce its effectiveness. If both drugs are needed to treat different infections, your doctor should carefully monitor your progress.
- Taking atovaquone with TMP-SMZ has resulted in reduced blood levels of TMP-SMZ. This should not reduce TMP-SMZ's effectiveness.
- Taking atovaquone with zidovudine (AZT) drastically reduces the rate at which zidovudine is eliminated from the body. For most people, this is not a problem.

Food Interactions

Take atovaquone with food or meals to improve drug absorption. A high-fat meal can increase the amount absorbed by 300%.

Usual Dose

Atovaquone

Adult

Prevention: 1500 mg once a day with food.

Treatment: 750 mg twice a day for 3 weeks, taken with food.

Child (age 13–17)

Prevention: 1500 mg once a day with food.

Treatment: 750 mg twice a day for 3 weeks, taken with food.

Child (under age 13): not recommended.

Atovaquone + Proguanil

Adult

Prevention: 250/100 mg (1 tablet) once a day beginning 1–2 days before traveling to an area known for malaria. Continue taking this dose throughout the trip and for 7 days after returning home.

Treatment: 1000/400 mg (4 tablets) once a day for 3 days.

Child

Prevention: 11–18 lb.: 31.3/12.5 mg (½ pediatric tablet) once a day; 19–24 lb.: 46.9/18.8 mg (¾ pediatric tablet) once a day; 25–44 lb.: 62.5/25 mg (1 pediatric tablet) once a day;

45–66 lb.: 125/50 mg (2 pediatric tablets) once a day; 67–88 lb.: 187.5/75 mg (3 pediatric tablets) once a day; at least 89 lb.: 150/100 mg (1 adult tablet) once a day. Begin taking the medicine 1–2 days before traveling to an area known for malaria and continue taking it throughout the trip and for 7 days after returning home. Not recommended for children under 11 lb.

Treatment: 11–18 lb.: 125/50 mg (2 pediatric tablets) once a day; 19–24 lb.: 187.5/75 mg (3 pediatric tablets) once a day; 25–44 lb.: 150/100 mg (1 adult tablet) once a day; 45–66 lb.: 500/200 mg (2 adult tablets) once a day; 67–88 lb.: 750/300 mg (3 adult tablets) once a day; at least 89 lb.: 1000/400 mg (4 adult tablets) once a day. Take the medicine for 3 consecutive days. Not recommended for children under 11 lb.

Overdosage

Atovaquone overdose may change red blood cells, making them unable to carry oxygen through the body, resulting in a bluish tint to the skin. Rash has also been reported. Contact your local poison control center or hospital emergency room for more information. If you seek treatment, ALWAYS bring the prescription bottle or container.

Special Information

Taking atovaquone regularly and with food is essential to the drug's effectiveness. If you cannot eat 2 meals a day, your doctor may have to prescribe another PCP treatment.

If you forget a dose, take it as soon as you remember. If it is almost time for your next dose, space your remaining doses equally throughout the rest of the day so that you can still take a total daily dose of 1500 mg, or 2 tsp.

Special Populations

Pregnancy/Breast-feeding: In animal studies, atovaquone affected fetal development. This drug should be taken during pregnancy only if your doctor determines that the potential benefit outweighs the risks.

Atovaquone is likely to pass into breast milk because of its affinity for body fat. Nursing mothers who must take this drug should use infant formula.

Seniors: Atovaquone has not been tested systematically in people over age 65. Seniors, especially those with kidney, heart, or liver disease, may be more sensitive to its side effects.

Avalide *see **Angiotensin II Blockers,** page 97*

Avapro *see **Angiotensin II Blockers,** page 97*

Avelox *see **Fluoroquinolone Anti-infectives,** page 512*

Avodart *see **Finasteride,** page 494*

Generic Name

Azithromycin (uh-ZIH-throe-MYE-sin) G

Brand Names

AzaSite Eye Drops
Zithromax
Zmax

Type of Drug

Macrolide antibiotic.

Prescribed For

Upper- and lower-respiratory-tract infections, skin infections, sexually transmitted diseases (STDs), middle ear infections, streptococcal infections of the throat and tonsils, bacterial sinusitis, and bacterial conjunctivitis (pinkeye).

General Information

Azithromycin is an azalide antibiotic, a subgroup of the macrolides. Macrolide drugs are either bactericidal (bacteria-killing) or bacteriostatic (inhibiting bacterial growth) depending on the organism in question and amount of antibiotic present.

Cautions and Warnings

Do not take azithromycin if you are **allergic** or **sensitive** to any of its ingredients or any macrolide antibiotic. Serious allergic reactions have rarely occurred in patients taking azithromycin.

Azithromycin is excreted primarily through the liver. People with **liver disease or damage** should not take this medication because of possible severe reactions, including liver failure and death. Azithromycin should be stopped if you develop signs of liver damage (see "Special Information").

Colitis (bowel inflammation), ranging from mild to life-threatening, has been associated with all antibiotics (see "Possible Side Effects").

People with severe **kidney disease** may be more susceptible to gastrointestinal (GI) side effects. Use with caution.

People taking azithromycin have developed new or worsened **myasthenia gravis**. Symptoms include muscle weakness or paralysis, difficulty standing, drooping head, difficulty swallowing, gagging or choking, and vision problems.

Azithromycin is considered appropriate only for the treatment of more mild forms of **pneumonia** in nonhospitalized patients. People with other underlying conditions, those who are **immunocompromised**, and those who contract pneumonia in a hospital or other institutional setting probably should be treated with other antibiotics.

Possible Side Effects

Most side effects are mild and go away once you stop taking azithromycin.

- ▼ Most common: diarrhea, nausea, vomiting, and abdominal pain. Colitis (symptoms include severe abdominal cramps and severe, persistent, and possibly bloody diarrhea) may develop.
- ▼ Less common: heart palpitations; chest pain; vaginal irritation; stomach upset; gas; dizziness; headache; tiredness; unusual sun sensitivity; rash; itching; swelling; fungal infection of the mouth or vagina; dark, tarry stools; kidney inflammation; and vertigo.
- ▼ Rare: angioedema (a potentially life-threatening swelling of the lips and throat) and jaundice (yellowing of the skin and whites of the eyes). Contact your doctor if you experience anything unusual while taking any medication.

Drug Interactions

- Nilotinib and pimozide should not be taken with azithromycin. Potentially fatal cardiac abnormalities may develop.

- Potentially life-threatening heart rhythm abnormalities (arrhythmias) may develop if azithromycin is taken with antiarrhythmic drugs or with fluoroquinolone antibiotics. Azithromycin should not be taken with levofloxacin or sparfloxacin and should be used with caution with moxifloxacin. Other drugs that may cause arrhythmias when used with azithromycin include arsenic trioxide, chlorpromazine, cisapride, dolasetron, droperidol, gatifloxacin, halofantrine, levomethadyl, lithium, maprotiline, mefloquine, mesoridazine, methadone, paliperidone, perflutren, pentamidine, probucol, propafenone, tacrolimus, tetrabenazine, thioridazine, and ziprasidone.
- All macrolide antibiotics increase blood levels of cyclosporine, which may cause kidney or nerve damage.
- Mixing azithromycin with rifabutin may reduce white-blood-cell levels. Use with caution.
- Do not mix azithromycin with dronedarone as it may increase the blood levels and side effects of this medication.
- Antacid products containing aluminum magnesium may delay the absorption of azithromycin into the blood. Separate your antacid dose from azithromycin by at least 1 hour. Zmax may taken without regard to antacids.
- Taking azithromycin with a benzodiazepine sedative, carbamazepine, digoxin, dihydroergotamine, ergotamine, hexobarbital, phenytoin, theophylline, or warfarin may increase these medications' blood levels. Blood monitoring and dosage adjustments may be necessary.
- Combining azithromycin and nelfinavir may increase azithromycin side effects.

Food Interactions

Tablets and oral suspension (except Zmax) can be taken with or without food, although food may help prevent GI side effects. Zmax should be taken on an empty stomach, 1 hour before or 2 hours after meals.

Usual Dose

Azithromycin

Respiratory Tract Infections, Skin Infections, STDs, and Bacterial Sinusitis

Adult and Child (age 16 and over): 500 mg as a single dose for 3 days, or 500 mg as a single dose on day 1, then 250 mg once a day on days 2–5 of treatment. STDs are treated with a single dose of 1000–2000 mg.

Mycobacterium avium **Infection; Adult and Child (age 16 and over)**

Prevention: 1200 mg once a week with or without approved dosage regimen of rifabutin.

Treatment: 600 mg/day in combination with ethambutol at the recommended daily dose of 6.8 mg per lb. of body weight.

Middle Ear Infections, Bacterial Sinusitis,* and Pneumonia; Child (age 6 months and over)

1-Day Regimen: 13.6 mg per lb. of body weight a day for 1 day.

3-Day Regimen: 4.5 mg per lb. of body weight a day for 3 days.

5-Day Regimen: 4.5 mg per lb. of body weight a day for day 1, and 2.27 mg per lb. of body weight a day for days 2–5.

**3-day regimen preferred for bacterial sinusitis.*

Tonsillitis and Sore Throat

Child (age 2 and over): 5.5 mg per lb. of body weight a day for 5 days.

Eye Drops

Adult and Child (age 1 and over): 1 drop in affected eye twice a day for 2 days, then 1 drop once a day for 5 days.

Zmax

Adult and Child (age 16 and over): 2000 mg once a day for 1 day.

Child (6 months–15 years): 27.3 mg per lb. of body weight once a day for 1 day. Children weighing more than 75 lb. should be given the adult dose (2000 mg).

Overdosage

Overdose may cause severe side effects, especially nausea, vomiting, stomach cramps, and diarrhea. Contact your local poison control center or hospital emergency room for more information. If you seek treatment, ALWAYS bring the prescription bottle or container.

Special Information

Contact your doctor if you develop nausea, vomiting, diarrhea, stomach cramps or severe abdominal pain, muscle weakness or paralysis, difficulty standing, drooping head, difficulty swallowing, gagging or choking, or vision problems. Stop taking this drug and immediately contact your doctor if you experience signs of a drug reaction, including breathing difficulties, chest pain, hives, rash, itching, mouth sores, or unusual sensitivity to light. Yellowing of the skin or whites of the eyes, severe itching, appetite loss, fatigue, and nausea can be signs of a severe liver reaction to azithromycin.

It is crucial that you follow your doctor's directions on how to take the drug and how many days to take it—even if you feel well sooner. This drug's effectiveness may be severely reduced otherwise. Taking azithromycin at the same time each day may help you remember your medication.

If you forget a dose of azithromycin, take it as soon as you remember. If it is almost time for your next dose, skip the dose you forgot and go back to your regular schedule.

Special Populations

Pregnancy/Breast-feeding: It is not known if azithromycin taken during pregnancy will harm a fetus. Azithromycin should be taken during pregnancy only if your doctor determines that the potential benefit outweighs the risks.

It is not known if azithromycin passes into breast milk, but other macrolide antibiotics do. Animal studies suggest azithromycin is unlikely to harm an infant, but nursing mothers who must take this drug should consider using infant formula.

Seniors: Seniors with liver disease should use caution. Seniors who have pneumonia or are especially sickly or debilitated probably should be treated with other medications.

Type of Drug

Azole Antifungals

Brand Names

Generic Ingredients: Fluconazole G
Diflucan

Generic Ingredients: Itraconazole G
Sporanox

Generic Ingredients: Ketoconazole G
Extina
Ketozole
Nizoral
Nizoral Shampoo
Xolegel

Generic Ingredients: Posaconazole
Noxafil

Generic Ingredients: Voriconazole G
Vfend

Prescribed For

Fungal infections of the blood, mouth, throat, vagina, skin, toenails, urinary tract, or respiratory or central nervous system.

Fluconazole, itraconazole, posaconazole, and voriconazole can be used to treat or prevent opportunistic fungal infections that afflict many people with HIV or cancer whose immune systems have been compromised.

General Information

Azole antifungals are used to treat a variety of fungal infections, including *Candida, Aspergillus, Cryptococcus, Blastomycosis, Fusarium, Histoplasmosis,* and *Scedosporium.* They work by inhibiting important enzyme systems in the organisms they attack. These drugs are broken down in the liver.

Cautions and Warnings

Do not take azole antifungals if you are **allergic** or **sensitive** to any of their ingredients. People who are allergic to one azole antifungal may also be allergic to the others, but cross-reactions are not common and serious allergic reaction is rare.

Itraconazole should not be used in people who have evidence of **heart failure** or a history of heart failure.

Azole antifungals can affect heart rhythm and should be used with caution if you have a history of **abnormal heart rhythms**. Intravenous doses of these drugs can reduce your heart's pumping efficiency. People with heart failure or those who may develop it should use these drugs with caution.

Rarely, azole antifungals can cause liver damage. These drugs should be used with caution in people with **liver disease**. Fluconazole, itraconazole, and ketoconazole have been associated with serious liver toxicity. People taking these drugs should have their liver function monitored.

Azole antifungals should be used with caution in people with **kidney disease**.

Voriconazole tablets contain lactose. They should not be taken by patients with rare hereditary problems of **galactose intolerance, Lapp-lactase deficiency**, or **glucose-galactose malabsorption**.

Rash may be an important sign of drug toxicity, especially in people with HIV or others with compromised immune function. Report any rashes, especially ones that do not heal readily, to your doctor.

Temporary or permanent hearing loss can occur rarely with these drugs, especially if they are combined with **quinidine**.

These drugs can have very serious effects if combined with other medicines. See "Drug Interactions" for specific information.

Possible Side Effects

Side effects are generally more common among people with HIV.

Fluconazole

- ▼ Most common: nausea, headache, rash, vomiting, abdominal pain, and diarrhea.
- ▼ Less common: liver toxicity, as measured by increases in specific lab tests. These changes in lab values are more common in people with HIV or cancer, who are more likely to be taking several drugs.
- ▼ Rare: seizures and exfoliative skin disorders. People with HIV or cancer who take fluconazole for fungal infections may develop severe liver or skin problems. Contact your doctor if you experience anything unusual while taking any medication.

Itraconazole

- ▼ Most common: nausea, vomiting, and rash.
- ▼ Less common: diarrhea, abdominal pain, appetite loss, swelling in the legs or feet, fatigue, fever, feeling unwell, itching, headache, dizziness, reduced sex drive, tiredness, high blood pressure, liver or kidney function abnormalities, low blood potassium, and impotence.
- ▼ Rare: gas, sleeplessness, depression, ringing or buzzing in the ears, bronchitis, chest pain, coughing, and swollen or painful breasts in men or women. Contact your doctor if you experience anything unusual while taking any medication.

Ketoconazole

- ▼ Common: nausea, vomiting, upset stomach, abdominal pain or discomfort, itching, and swollen breasts in men.

Possible Side Effects *(continued)*

- ▼ Less common: headache, dizziness, sleepiness, fever and chills, diarrhea, impotence, blood abnormalities.
- ▼ Rare: severe allergic reactions. Contact your doctor if you experience anything unusual while taking any medication.

Posaconazole

- ▼ Most common: fever, headache, chills, swelling in the legs, appetite loss, dizziness, fluid accumulation, weakness, blood-pressure changes, anemia, low white-blood-cell counts with or without fever, vaginal bleeding, diarrhea, nausea, vomiting, abdominal pain, constipation, upset stomach, mucous membrane irritation, rapid heartbeat, bacteria in the blood, herpes infection, cytomegalovirus infection, infection, sore throat, low blood potassium, low blood magnesium, high blood sugar, muscle and joint pain, back pain, low blood-platelet levels, black-and-blue marks, sleeplessness, cough, difficulty breathing, nosebleeds, and rash and itching.
- ▼ Common: upper-respiratory infection, low blood calcium, and anxiety.
- ▼ Less common: tiredness, weakness, blurred vision, taste changes, and heart rhythm changes.

Voriconazole

- ▼ Most common: visual disturbances.
- ▼ Common: fever, rash, nausea, blood infections, swelling in the arms or legs, and respiratory disorder.

Drug Interactions

- Do not mix astemizole, cisapride, pimozide, quinidine, or terfenadine with posaconazole or voriconazole. Posaconazole should also not be combined with halofantrine. Ketoconazole should not be taken with astemizole, cisapride, or terfenadine, and itraconazole should not be mixed with cisapride, dofetilide, pimozide, or quinidine. Severe, possibly fatal cardiac side effects, including heart attack or abnormal heart rhythms, may occur. Similarly, combining fluconazole with terfenadine or cisapride may cause cardiac events. Do not mix these medicines.

- Antacids interfere with the absorption of ketoconazole and itraconazole. Take antacids more than 2 hours after taking these drugs.
- St. John's wort reduces blood levels of voriconazole and can interfere with its effectiveness. Long-acting barbiturates can also interfere with the effectiveness of voriconazole. Do not mix these drugs.
- Fluconazole and ketoconazole may interfere with contraceptive drugs. Consider using an alternative form of birth control.
- Fluconazole, itraconazole, ketoconazole, and voriconazole may increase the amount of the sulfonylurea-type antidiabetes drugs (e.g., tolbutamide, glyburide, and glipizide) in the blood, causing low blood sugar.
- Fluconazole, itraconazole, ketoconazole, posaconazole, and voriconazole increase blood levels of certain benzodiazepines such as triazolam and midazolam. Ketoconazole should not be combined with oral triazolam and itraconazole should not be combined with oral midazolam or triazolam. Other azole/benzodiazepine combinations should be monitored, and dose reductions may be necessary.
- Fluconazole, itraconazole, ketoconazole, and voriconazole increase blood levels of the anticoagulant warfarin. Dosage adjustments and blood monitoring may be necessary.
- Ergot alkaloids such as ergotamine and dihydroergotamine should not be used with posaconazole or voriconazole and should be used with caution with itraconazole.
- Fluconazole, itraconazole, ketoconazole, posaconazole, and voriconazole increase blood levels of HMG-CoA reductase inhibitors, also known as statin drugs. Reduced dosages of these drugs are necessary when combined with an azole antifungal.
- When azoles are combined with the immunosuppressant medications cyclosporine, sirolimus, and tacrolimus, increased blood concentrations of these medications may result. Dosages may need to be adjusted.
- Fluconazole, itraconazole, ketoconazole, and voriconazole increase blood levels of protease inhibitors such as indinavir, ritonavir, and saquinavir. Itraconazole and voriconazole levels may be affected by these drugs as well. Voriconazole and ritonavir should not be taken together.

- The effects of corticosteroids, such as dexamethasone and prednisolone, may be enhanced by fluconazole, itraconazole, ketoconazole, and voriconazole.
- Carbamazepine blood levels may be increased by fluconazole, itraconazole, ketoconazole, and voriconazole, increasing the risk for side effects. Carbamazepine should not be combined with voriconazole.
- Itraconazole, posaconazole, and voriconazole may cause elevated levels of calcium channel blockers. Dosage adjustments may be necessary.
- Vinca alkaloid use should be avoided when taking azoles. The risk of vinca alkaloid toxicity (symptoms include muscle aches and constipation) is increased when these medications are combined.
- Ketoconazole may also increase blood levels of HIV drugs, including didanosine (ddI).
- Use caution when combining fluconazole with alfentanil, buspirone, haloperidol, losartan, nisoldipine, phenytoin, rifabutin, rifampin, theophylline, tolterodine, tricyclic antidepressants, zidovudine, and zolpidem. Dosage adjustments may be necessary.
- Hydrochlorothiazide may increase blood levels of fluconazole up to 40%.
- Ketoconazole interacts with buspirone, didanosine, donepezil, histamine$_2$ antagonists, isoniazid, nisoldipine, quinidine, sucralfate, proton-pump inhibitors, rifampin, theophyllines, and zolpidem. Dosage adjustments may be required.
- Use caution when combining itraconazole with alfentanil, aripiprazole, buspirone, budesonide, busulfan, cilostazol, clarithromycin, digoxin, disopyramide, docetaxel, eletriptan, erythromycin, halofantrine, haloperidol, nevirapine, phenobarbital, phenytoin, rifabutin, and trimetrexate. Dosage adjustments may be necessary.
- Use of cimetidine, phenytoin, or rifabutin with posaconazole should be avoided if possible. Frequent monitoring and dosage adjustments may be needed to avoid side effects.
- Caution should be used when combining voriconazole and cimetidine, methadone, phenytoin, or proton-pump inhibitors such as omeprazole.
- Voriconazole may increase blood levels of rifabutin significantly, while voriconazole levels may be significantly

decreased. Voriconazole should not be combined with rifabutin or rifampin.

- Combining voriconazole with a non-nucleoside reverse transcriptase inhibitor (NNRTI) for HIV can either increase or decrease blood levels of voriconazole and increase blood levels of the NNRTI. Drug side effects may occur.
- Voriconazole should not be combined with efavirenz.

Food Interactions

Take itraconazole and voriconazole at least 1 hour before or 2 hours after a meal. Take ketoconazole with food or meals. Posaconazole must be taken with food or a nutritional supplement. Another treatment should be considered if this requirement cannot be met.

Usual Dose

Fluconazole

Adult and Child (age 14 and over): 50–400 mg once a day.

Child (under age 14): 1.3–5.5 mg per lb. of body weight once a day; no more than 600 mg a day.

Itraconazole

Itraconazole capsules and liquid are not interchangeable because of differences in how they are absorbed. If you must switch from one to the other, your doctor will have to recalibrate your dosage.

Adult and Child (age 16 and over): 200–400 mg a day.

Child (age 3–15): 100 mg a day has been prescribed, but the long-term effects of itraconazole in children are not known.

Ketoconazole

Oral

Adult: usual dose—200–400 mg once a day. Dosages of up to 1200 mg a day have been used. Treatment may continue for several months, depending on the type of infection being treated.

Child (age 2 and over): 1.5–3 mg per lb. of body weight once a day.

Child (under age 2): not recommended.

Topical: Apply to affected and immediately surrounding areas 1–2 times a day for 2–6 weeks, depending on the type of infection being treated.

Posaconazole

Adult and Child (age 13 and over): 200–800 mg a day.

Child (under age 13): not recommended.

Voriconazole

Adult and Child (age 12 and over): 100–300 mg every 12 hours.

Child (under age 12): not recommended.

Overdosage

Overdose is likely to result in exaggerated drug side effects. Doses of posaconazole up to 1600 mg a day have been taken without any adverse reactions. Take the victim to a hospital emergency room. If you seek treatment, ALWAYS bring the prescription bottle or container.

Special Information

When taking these medications, regular doctor visits are necessary to monitor liver function and general progress. Contact your doctor if you develop severe diarrhea; vomiting; reddening, loosening, blistering, or peeling of the skin; darkening of the urine; jaundice (yellowing of the skin or whites of the eyes); loss of appetite; or abdominal pain, especially on the right side.

When taking itraconazole, tell your doctor if you find it hard to do mild exercise, experience difficulty breathing, or have swelling in your legs or ankles. These can be signs of heart failure. Report other symptoms that are bothersome or persistent.

If you forget a dose of 1 of these medicines, take it as soon as you remember. If it is almost time for your next dose, skip the dose you forgot and continue with your regular schedule. Do not take a double dose.

Special Populations

Pregnancy/Breast-feeding: Animal studies with these medicines show effects on the fetus, some of which have been seen in humans, although in most a direct link has not been established. Taking large (400–800 mg) daily doses of fluconazole for most of the first 3 months of pregnancy has been linked to a specific set of serious birth defects. This effect has not been seen with the lower (150 mg) single dose used for yeast infections. An azole antifungal should be taken during pregnancy only if your doctor determines that the potential benefit outweighs the risks. These drugs pass into breast milk. Nursing mothers who must take these drugs should use infant formula.

Seniors: Seniors may require a reduced dosage of fluconazole due to age-related loss of kidney function. No dosage adjustments are necessary with other azole antifungals. Several cases of hearing loss have been reported in seniors taking itraconazole with or without quinidine.

Generic Name

Baclofen (BAK-loe-fen) G

Brand Names

Gablofen   Lioresal

Type of Drug

Skeletal muscle relaxant.

Prescribed For

Muscle spasms associated with multiple sclerosis (MS), spinal cord injury or disease, or other nervous system conditions; may also be used to treat trigeminal neuralgia (tic douloureux), Tourette syndrome, cerebral palsy, hiccups, and acid reflux, and to prevent migraine.

General Information

Baclofen may work by interfering with nervous system reflexes at the spinal cord, although it may also have some effect outside the spinal cord. Baclofen is chemically similar to a natural nerve transmitter known as GABA; baclofen's effect on muscle spasm may be related to its effect on GABA nerve receptors.

Cautions and Warnings

Do not take baclofen if you are **allergic** or **sensitive** to any of its ingredients.

It should not be taken for muscle spasm resulting from **stroke** or **Parkinson's disease** because its benefit in these situations has not been proven and it is generally poorly tolerated. The condition of people with **epilepsy** or **psychotic disorders** may worsen while taking baclofen.

Baclofen should not be taken by people for whom stiff or rigid muscles are helpful in maintaining upright posture or increasing functionality.

About 4% of **women with MS** who take baclofen for less than 1 year develop ovarian cysts that usually disappear on their own.

This is within the normal range for all women (1–5%) for developing ovarian cysts.

Baclofen is excreted primarily through the kidneys, so patients with **kidney disease** or **impaired kidney function** should use baclofen with caution.

Abruptly stopping baclofen can lead to hallucinations and seizure. Dosage should always be gradually reduced, except in cases of severe side effects.

Possible Side Effects

Baclofen may affect lab tests for liver function and can raise blood-sugar levels.

- ▼ Most common: drowsiness, low blood pressure, weakness, dizziness, lightheadedness, nausea, constipation, headache, confusion, frequent urination, and sleeplessness.
- ▼ Less common: fatigue or lethargy, euphoria, excitement, depression, hallucinations, tingling in the hands or feet, muscle pain, ringing or buzzing in the ears, coordination difficulties, tremors, rigidity, loss of muscle tone, unusual eye movement and other muscle-control problems, double vision, pinpoint or wide-open pupils, breathing difficulties, heart palpitations, dry mouth, appetite loss, changes in sense of taste, abdominal pain, diarrhea, bedwetting, difficulty urinating, painful urination, impotence, rash, itching, swelling of the ankles, excessive sweating, weight gain, and stuffy nose.
- ▼ Rare: slurred speech, blurred vision, seizure, fainting, chest pain, blood in the urine, and testing positive for blood in the stool. Contact your doctor if you experience anything unusual while taking any medication.

Drug Interactions

- Avoid alcoholic beverages and other nervous system depressants such as antihistamines, sedatives, or narcotic pain relievers while taking baclofen.

Food Interactions

This drug can be taken without regard to food or meals.

Usual Dose

Adult and Child (age 12 and over): 5 mg 3 times a day for 3 days, gradually increased every 3 days until the desired effect is achieved, usually at 40–80 mg a day. People with kidney disease require lower doses.

Child (under age 12): not recommended.

Overdosage

Symptoms of baclofen overdose include vomiting, loss of muscle tone, twitching, convulsions, pinpoint or wide-open pupils, drowsiness, blurred or double vision, breathing difficulties, seizure, and coma. Overdose victims should be taken to a hospital emergency room for treatment. If you seek treatment, ALWAYS bring the prescription bottle or container.

Special Information

Baclofen is a nervous system depressant. Take care when driving or doing anything that requires concentration and physical coordination.

Contact your doctor if you develop persistent symptoms such as a frequent urge to urinate, painful urination, constipation, nausea, headache, sleeplessness, or confusion.

Do not stop taking baclofen on your own. Abruptly stopping this drug may lead to hallucinations or seizure.

Your pharmacist may prepare a baclofen liquid. This mixture should be kept in the refrigerator and must be thrown away after 1 month.

If you forget a dose of baclofen and remember within 1 hour of your scheduled time, take it immediately. If you do not remember until more than 1 hour later or if you forget it completely, skip the dose you forgot and continue with your regular schedule. Do not take a double dose.

Special Populations

Pregnancy/Breast-feeding: Baclofen increases the chances of certain birth defects in lab animals. Baclofen should be taken during pregnancy only if your doctor determines that the potential benefit outweighs the risks.

Baclofen taken by mouth passes into breast milk. Nursing mothers who must take this drug should use infant formula or receive the drug by injection directly into the spinal cord, because baclofen administered by injection does not pass into breast milk.

Seniors: Seniors may be more sensitive to nervous system side effects, including hallucinations, depression, drowsiness, and confusion.

Generic Name

Becaplermin (beh-CAP-ler-min)

Brand Names

Regranex

Type of Drug

Human growth factor.

Prescribed For

Diabetic foot and leg wounds.

General Information

Becaplermin is a type of human growth factor produced in a laboratory. Although it is not a substitute for good wound care, becaplermin can stimulate wound tissue to heal faster. Studies of the drug have produced mixed results. In some studies, people using becaplermin were 1½–2 times more likely to have complete healing of their wounds. In another study, the results with becaplermin were the same as those with good wound care alone.

Cautions and Warnings

Do not use becaplermin if you are **allergic** or **sensitive** to any of its ingredients.

Becaplermin should not be used to speed the healing of wounds that are healing by themselves.

Becaplermin should not be applied to **skin cancer** or **tumors** or exposed bones, joints, tendons, or ligaments because its effect on these body structures is not known.

The cancer death rate is 5 times higher in people who have used 3 or more tubes of becaplermin than people who have never used the drug. However, the risk of new cancer is not increased.

Becaplermin should not be used for wounds that do not extend to subcutaneous tissue or are caused by poor circulation.

Possible Side Effects

People treated with becaplermin plus wound care had a slightly larger risk of developing a rash than those who received wound care alone.

Drug Interactions

None known.

Usual Dose

Adult and Child (age 16 and over): The amount of gel used depends on the size of the wound and will be determined by your doctor. Apply a thin, continuous layer ($\frac{1}{16}$ in.) to the wound and cover with a saline-moistened bandage; leave in place for 12 hours. Then, remove the becaplermin bandage, rinse the wound, and cover it with a new saline-soaked bandage for the rest of the day. Continue this process until the wound has healed completely.

Child (under age 16): not recommended.

Overdosage

Little is known about the effects of accidental ingestion. Contact your local poison control center or a hospital emergency room for information. If you seek treatment, ALWAYS bring the prescription container.

Special Information

Contact your doctor if your wound worsens or is irritated by becaplermin.

Wash your hands before applying becaplermin.

Do not allow the tip of the becaplermin tube to touch any surface, including the wound being treated.

Your doctor should reassess your treatment if the wound is not 30% smaller in 10 weeks and completely healed in 20 weeks.

Applying more becaplermin than recommended will not make your wound heal better or faster.

If you forget a dose, apply it as soon as you remember. If it is almost time for your next dose, skip the missed dose and continue with your regular schedule.

Special Populations

Pregnancy/Breast-feeding: The safety of using becaplermin during pregnancy is not known. Becaplermin should be used during pregnancy only if your doctor determines that the potential benefit outweighs the risks.

It is not known if becaplermin passes into breast milk. Nursing mothers who must use this drug should use infant formula.

Seniors: Seniors may use this drug without special precaution.

Generic Name

Belimumab (beh-LIM-u-mab)

Brand Names

Benlysta

Type of Drug

B lymphocyte stimulator (BLyS) inhibitor.

Prescribed For

Lupus erythematosus.

General Information

Belimumab is the first new treatment for lupus since the approval of corticosteroid medicines for lupus in 1955. It is intended for people with active, autoantibody-positive lupus who are also receiving other lupus treatments. Belimumab is a man-made monoclonal antibody that is given as an hour-long intravenous (IV) infusion by your health care provider. It interferes with the activity of BLyS, a protein needed for the survival of B-cells, which play a key role in the body's immune system but which also can produce autoantibodies that attack and destroy healthy tissues in the body. In lupus, rheumatoid arthritis, and certain other autoimmune diseases, elevated levels of BLyS are thought to contribute to the production of these autoantibodies.

Cautions and Warnings

Do not use belimumab if you are **allergic** or **sensitive** to any of its ingredients or have had a previous reaction to belimumab. Serious sensitivity reactions can develop while you are taking this drug. Your doctor may give you an antihistamine and corticosteroid before the IV to prevent a serious reaction from developing. Your doctor will be prepared to manage a serious reaction if one occurs.

During clinical studies, a small percentage of people died while undergoing treatment, with more deaths among people taking belimumab than those taking placebo. The causes of death varied without a detectable pattern.

Belimumab suppresses the immune system and can make you more likely to develop a serious infection. Use special caution if you have or are being treated for a chronic infection. Your doctor will check your blood for infection during belimumab treatment. Tell your doctor if you develop a fever or other sign of infection.

Depression and suicidal thoughts can develop while you are taking belimumab.

Belimumab has not been tested in **severe active lupus of the kidney or nervous system**.

Black patients participating in drug studies did not respond as well to belimumab as others studied. African-Americans should use this drug with caution.

Possible Side Effects

- ▼ Most common: drug-sensitivity reactions (low blood pressure, hives, itching, rash, rapid swelling of the lips and throat, or difficulty breathing), nausea, and diarrhea.
- ▼ Common: fever, common cold symptoms, bronchitis, sleeplessness, arm and leg pain, migraines, sore throat, and depression.
- ▼ Less common: bladder infection, stomach virus, and low white-blood-cell count.
- ▼ Rare: A very small number of people develop antibodies to belimumab. Contact your doctor if you experience anything unusual while taking any medication.

Drug Interactions

- Live virus vaccines should be avoided starting 30 days before you start taking belimumab and while you are taking it, due to the increased infection risk.
- Corticosteroids and ACE inhibitors lower blood levels of belimumab, but the decrease is not clinically important.

Food Interactions

This drug can be taken without regard to food or meals.

Usual Dose

Adult: 4.5 mg per lb. of body weight every 2 weeks for 3 doses, then every 4 weeks. Belimumab is given by IV infusion over at least 1 hour in your doctor's office or another health care setting.

Child: not recommended.

Overdosage

There is no experience with belimumab overdose. Because it is administered by a health professional, the chances of overdose are small and the means of treatment are at hand during administration.

Special Information

Call your doctor if you develop a fever, chills, swollen glands, or other sign of possible blood infection or if you experience a sign of a drug reaction, including wheezing, difficulty breathing, tongue or lip swelling, or rash.

Special Populations

Pregnancy/Breast-feeding: Belimumab enters the developing fetus but its effect on pregnant women is not known. It has caused fetal death in animal studies. Belimumab should be taken during pregnancy only if your doctor determines that the potential benefit outweighs the risks. You or your doctor can enroll in a registry that has been created to gather information on pregnant women who decide to take belimumab.

Belimumab may pass into breast milk, but it is not known if it can affect a nursing infant. Nursing mothers who must take it should use infant formula.

Seniors: Seniors should use this medicine with caution because little is known about the effect of this drug in older adults.

Benicar *see **Angiotensin II Blockers,** page 97*

Type of Drug

Benzodiazepine Antianxiety/ Seizure Drugs

Brand Names

Generic Ingredients: Alprazolam G
Niravam Xanax Xanax XR

Generic Ingredients: Chlordiazepoxide G
Librium

Generic Ingredients: Clobazam
Onfi

Generic Ingredients: Clonazepam G
Klonopin

Generic Ingredients: Clorazepate G
Gen-Xene
Tranxene
Tranxene T-Tab

Generic Ingredients: Diazepam G
Diastat
Diazepam Intensol
Valium

Generic Ingredients: Lorazepam G
Ativan
Lorazepam Intensol

Generic Ingredients: Oxazepam G

Prescribed For

Anxiety, tension, fatigue, agitation (particularly due to alcohol withdrawal), muscle spasm, and seizures; some are also prescribed for irritable bowel syndrome and panic attacks.

General Information

Benzodiazepines directly affect the brain. They can relax you and make you more tranquil or sleepy, or they can slow nervous system transmissions in such a way as to act as an anticonvulsant. This is especially valuable in managing disorders in which seizures are a major symptom. Many doctors prefer benzodiazepines to other drugs that can be used to similar effect because they tend to be safer, have fewer side effects, and are usually as effective, if not more so.

Cautions and Warnings

Do not take a benzodiazepine if you know you are **allergic** or **sensitive** to any of its ingredients or to another benzodiazepine drug.

Benzodiazepines can aggravate narrow-angle **glaucoma**, but you may take them if you have open-angle glaucoma and are receiving therapy for it.

Other conditions in which benzodiazepines should be avoided are severe **depression**, severe **lung disease**, **sleep apnea** (intermittent cessation of breathing during sleep), **myasthenia gravis** (a neuromuscular disease), **severe liver disease**, **drunkenness**, and **kidney disease**. In all of these conditions, the depressive effects of benzodiazepines may be enhanced, which could be detrimental to your overall condition. Reduced doses of these medicines are required by people with **mild to moderate liver disease**.

Benzodiazepines should not be taken by **psychotic patients**. They are not effective for them and can trigger unusual excitement, stimulation, and rage.

Benzodiazepines taken for epilepsy can increase the risk of **suicidal thoughts or actions**. Call your doctor in the event of worsening depression, suicidal thoughts or actions, or any unusual mood or behavior changes.

These drugs are generally not intended for more than 3–4 months of continuous use. Your condition should be reassessed before continuing your medication beyond that time.

Benzodiazepines can be addictive. They should be used with caution in people with a history of **drug dependence**. Drug withdrawal may develop if you stop taking it after only 4 weeks of regular use but is more likely after longer use. It may start with anxiety and progress to tingling in the hands or feet, sensitivity to bright light, sleep disturbances, cramps, tremors, muscle tension or twitching, poor concentration, flu-like symptoms, fatigue, appetite loss, sweating, and changes in mental state. Your dosage should always be reduced gradually to prevent drug withdrawal symptoms.

Severe withdrawal symptoms may include convulsions, psychosis, hallucinations, tremors, anxiety, behavioral changes, and seizures. People with a history of any **seizure disorder** should be especially cautious when discontinuing benzodiazepines. They may also need to increase the dosage of their anticonvulsant medication if taking either diazepam or clonazepam.

Possible Side Effects

▼ Most common: mild drowsiness during the first few days of therapy. Weakness and confusion may occur, especially in seniors and in those who are sickly. If these effects persist, contact your doctor.

▼ Less common: depression, weakness, lethargy, disorientation, aggression, irritability, fever, headache, cough, bronchitis, pneumonia and other respiratory infections, joint pain, inactivity, slurred speech, stupor, dizziness, tremors, constipation, dry mouth, appetite changes, nausea, vomiting, swallowing difficulty, drooling, inability to control urination, sexual difficulties, irregular menstrual cycle, changes in heart rhythm, low blood pressure, fluid retention, blurred or double vision, itching, rash, hiccups,

Possible Side Effects *(continued)*

hyperactivity, nervousness, hysteria, psychosis, inability to fall asleep, and occasional liver dysfunction. If you have any of these symptoms, stop taking the drug and contact your doctor at once.

▼ Rare: Rare side effects can affect your heart, stomach and intestines, urinary tract, blood, muscles, and joints. Contact your doctor if you experience anything unusual while taking any medication.

Drug Interactions

- Benzodiazepines are central-nervous-system depressants. Avoid alcohol, other sedatives, narcotics, barbiturates, monoamine oxidase inhibitor (MAOI) and other antidepressants, and antihistamines. Taking diazepam with these drugs may lead to excessive depression, drowsiness, or difficulty breathing.
- Alcohol increases clobazam blood levels by 50%.
- Smoking may reduce these drugs' effectiveness by increasing the rate at which they are broken down by the body.
- Effects of benzodiazepines may be prolonged when taken with cimetidine, contraceptive drugs, disulfiram, fluoxetine, isoniazid, ketoconazole, metoprolol, probenecid, propranolol, rifampin, and valproic acid.
- Lower clobazam doses are needed if you mix it with lansoprazole, omeprazole, pantoprazole, rabeprazole, chloramphenicol, cimetidine, felbamate, fluoxetine, fluvoxamine, indomethacin, ketoconazole, modafinil, oxcarbazepine, probenecid, ticlopidine, and topiramate.
- Lower doses of beta blockers, antidepressants, $5HT_3$ antiemetics, antipsychotic medicines, atomoxetine, chlorpheniramine, narcotic pain relievers, and tamoxifen are required by those using clobazam.
- Theophylline may reduce the sedative effects of diazepam.
- If you take antacids, separate them from your benzodiazepine dose by at least 1 hour to prevent them from interfering with the passage of diazepam into the bloodstream.
- These drugs may increase blood levels of digoxin and the chances for digoxin toxicity.
- Levodopa + carbidopa's effects may be decreased if it is taken with a benzodiazepine.

- Combining a benzodiazepine and phenytoin may increase phenytoin blood concentrations and the risk of phenytoin toxicity.

Food Interactions

These drugs are best taken on an empty stomach, but may be taken with food if they upset your stomach.

Usual Dose

Alprazolam

Anxiety Disorder

Adult: 0.25–0.5 mg 3 times a day. Dosage must be tailored to your individual needs with a maximum dose of 4 mg a day.

Child: not recommended.

Panic Disorder

Adult: 1–10 mg a day.

Child: not recommended.

Chlordiazepoxide

Adult: 5–100 mg a day. This range is due to individual response related to age, weight, disease severity, and other characteristics.

Child (age 6 and over): may be given if deemed appropriate by a doctor. Starting dose—5 mg 2–4 times a day. Maintenance dose—up to 30 mg a day for some children, but must be individualized to obtain maximum benefit.

Child (under age 6): not recommended.

Clobazam

Clobazam is broken down by different enzyme systems produced in the liver. One of them, called CYP2C19, can be deficient in some people and they should start out at 5 mg a day regardless of body weight and increase slowly to ½ the recommended dose for others.

Adult and Child (weighing 65 lbs. and over): 10–40 mg a day divided into 2 doses.

Child (weighing under 65 lbs.): 5–20 mg a day divided into 2 doses. Doses larger than 5 mg a day should be split into 2 doses.

Child (under 2 years old): not recommended.

Senior: The lowest effective dose should be used.

Clonazepam

Clonazepam is available in either tablets or orally disintegrating tablets called wafers. Wafers should not be opened until immediately before the dose is to be taken. Do not push the wafer through the foil. Use dry hands to remove the wafer. The wafer will disintegrate quickly in saliva.

Seizures

Adult and Child (age 11 and over): starting dose—0.5 mg 3 times a day. The dose is increased by 0.5–1 mg every 3 days until seizures are controlled or side effects develop. The maximum daily dose is 20 mg.

Child (under age 11): starting dose—0.004–0.013 mg per lb. of body weight a day in 2 or 3 divided doses. The dose is increased by 0.25–0.5 mg every 3 days until a maintenance dose of 0.05–0.09 mg per lb. of body weight is reached.

Panic Attacks

Adult: starting dose—0.25 mg twice a day. The dose is increased to 1 mg a day after 3 days. Most people do not require a higher dose. The maximum daily dose is 4 mg.

Other uses for clonazepam involve doses from 0.5–16 mg a day, depending on the condition and its severity.

Clorazepate

Immediate-Release

Adult and Child (age 9 and over): 15–60 mg a day. The average dose is 30 mg in divided quantities, but dosage must be adjusted to individual response for maximum effect. Maximum recommended daily dose is 90 mg. For treatment of anxiety, clorazepate may be taken as a single dose at bedtime.

Child (under age 9): not recommended.

Sustained-Release

Adult: The sustained-release form of clorazepate may be given as a single dose, either 11.25 or 22.5 mg, once every 24 hours. Sustained-release tablets are not recommended for the initial dosage.

Child: not recommended.

Diazepam

Solution or Tablets

Adult: 2–40 mg a day. Dosage must be adjusted to individual response for maximum effect. In seniors, less of the drug is usually required to control tension and anxiety.

Child (6 months and over): 1–2.5 mg 3 or 4 times a day; more may be needed to control anxiety and tension.

Child (under 6 months): not recommended.

Rectal Gel

Adult and Child (age 12 and over): 0.09 mg per lb. of body weight. Approximate dosage: 5 mg if 31–60 lbs., 10 mg if 61–110 lbs., 15 mg if 111–165 lbs., or 20 mg if 166–244 lbs.

Child (age 6–11): 0.14 mg per lb. of body weight. Approximate dosage: 5 mg if 22–40 lbs., 10 mg if 41–82 lbs., 15 mg if 83–121 lbs., or 20 mg if 122–163 lbs.

Child (age 2–5): 0.23 mg per lb. of body weight. Approximate dosage: 5 mg if 13–24 lbs., 10 mg if 25–49 lbs., 15 mg if 50–73 lbs., or 20 mg if 74–97 lbs.

An extra 2.5 mg of the rectal gel may be given if a more precise dosage is needed or as a partial replacement for people who do not retain the full dosage after it is first inserted rectally.

Lorazepam

Adult and Child (age 12 and over): 2–3 mg a day divided into 2 or 3 doses for anxiety disorder. Daily dosage may range from 1–10 mg. For bedtime anxiety that interferes with sleep, 2–4 mg may be given.

Child (under age 12): not recommended.

Senior or Sickly People: 1–2 mg a day divided into 2 or 3 doses. Dose may be increased as needed.

Oxazepam

Adult and Child (age 13 and over): 10–30 mg 3 or 4 times a day.

Child (age 6–12): 0.45 mg per lb. of body weight a day, divided into 3 or 4 doses.

Child (under age 6): not recommended.

Overdosage

Symptoms of overdose include confusion, sleepiness, poor coordination, lack of response to pain, loss of reflexes, shallow breathing, low blood pressure, and coma. The victim should be taken to a hospital emergency room. If you seek treatment, ALWAYS bring the prescription bottle or container.

Special Information

Benzodiazepines can cause tiredness, drowsiness, inability to concentrate, or similar symptoms. Be careful if you are driving, operating machinery, or performing other activities that require concentration.

People taking benzodiazepines for more than 3 or 4 months at a time may develop drug withdrawal reactions if the medication is stopped suddenly (see "Cautions and Warnings"). Do not stop taking benzodiazepines, or increase or decrease the dosage, without first consulting your doctor.

The effectiveness of hormonal contraceptives can be reduced by antiepileptic medicines, including clobazam, which increases the risk of unintended pregnancy. Additional non-hormonal contraceptive methods are recommended while you are taking these drugs.

If you forget a dose, take it as soon as you remember. If it is almost time for your next dose, skip the one you forgot and continue with your regular schedule. Do not take a double dose.

Special Populations

Pregnancy/Breast-feeding: Benzodiazepines may cause birth defects if taken during the first 3 months of pregnancy. Avoid taking any benzodiazepine if you are or might be pregnant.

A registry has been established to gather information on pregnant women and their use of antiepileptic medicine such as clobazam.

These drugs can pass into breast milk. Nursing mothers who must take benzodiazepines should use infant formula.

Seniors: Seniors, especially those with liver or kidney disease, are more sensitive to the effects of diazepam and generally require smaller doses to achieve the same effect.

Generic Name

Benzyl Alcohol (BEN-zill AL-ka-hol)

Brand Names

Ulesfia Lotion

Type of Drug

Pediculicide.

Prescribed For

Head lice infestation.

General Information

Benzyl alcohol lotion should be used as part of an overall program for head lice treatment, including washing or dry-cleaning all recently worn clothes and personal care items (clothes, hats, towels, and bedding) and using a special fine-tooth comb to remove dead lice and nits. It acts by interfering with the louse's breathing system, effectively smothering it. By 2 weeks after treatment, ¾ of people using this product are free of live lice.

Cautions and Warnings

Do not use benzyl alcohol if you are **allergic** or **sensitive** to any of its ingredients. This product is highly irritating, and may cause skin irritation and allergic reactions.

Preemies and babies less than 1 month old may be at risk for an unusual group of symptoms called "gasping syndrome." This product should not be used in children younger than 6 months old.

Possible Side Effects

Side effects increase noticeably as the drug dose increases.

- ▼ Most common: itching and swelling.
- ▼ Common: pus discharge on the skin and eye irritation.
- ▼ Less common: skin irritation with or without loss of sensation and pain.
- ▼ Rare: dry skin; skin abrasions; tingling, redness, itching, peeling, and burning of the skin; and dandruff rash. Contact your doctor if you experience anything unusual while taking any medication.

Drug Interactions

None known.

Usual Dose

Adult and Child (age 6 months and over): Apply enough benzyl alcohol lotion to completely saturate the dry scalp and hair; leave on for 10 minutes, then thoroughly rinse off with water. The recommended amount of lotion per treatment depends on hair length:

0–2 inches:	½–¾ bottle
2–4 inches:	¾–1 bottle
4–8 inches:	1–1½ bottles
8–16 inches:	1½–3 bottles
16–22 inches:	3–4 bottles
Over 22 inches:	4–6 bottles

Repeat this treatment again in 7 days.

Overdosage

Overapplication may cause extra skin irritation and reaction. If this product is accidentally swallowed, take the victim to a hospital emergency room. If you seek treatment, ALWAYS bring the bottle or container.

Special Information

This product is to be only applied to the hair and skin. It should not be applied to the mouth, eyes, or vaginal area.

Remember to administer a second benzyl alcohol treatment 7 days after the first. This is important to kill any lice remaining from the first treatment.

Tell your doctor if you have any skin conditions or especially sensitive skin.

Special Populations

Pregnancy/Breast-feeding: There is no indication that enough benzyl alcohol is absorbed through the skin to affect a developing fetus; however, benzyl alcohol should be used during pregnancy only if your doctor determines that the potential benefit outweighs the risks.

It is not known if benzyl alcohol enters breast milk. Nursing mothers who must use it should use infant formula for a short time because of possible effects on a nursing infant.

Seniors: Benzyl alcohol lotion has not been tested in people older than 60 years. Seniors may be more sensitive to it.

Generic Name

Beta Blockers

Brand Names

Generic Ingredients: Acebutolol G
Sectral

Generic Ingredients: Atenolol G
Tenormin

Generic Ingredients: Betaxolol G
Betoptic Eye Drops
Betoptic S Eye Drops

Generic Ingredients: Bisoprolol G
Zebeta

Generic Ingredients: Carteolol G
Ocupress Eye Drops

Generic Ingredients: Levobunolol G
Betagan Eye Drops

Generic Ingredients: Metipranolol G
Optipranolol Eye Drops

Generic Ingredients: Metoprolol G
Lopressor
Toprol-XL

Generic Ingredients: Nadolol G
Corgard

Generic Ingredients: Nebivolol
Bystolic

Generic Ingredients: Penbutolol
Levatol

Generic Ingredients: Pindolol G
Visken

Generic Ingredients: Propranolol G
Inderal
Inderal LA
Innopran XL

Generic Ingredients: Sotalol G
Betapace
Betapace AF
Sorine

Generic Ingredients: Timolol G
Istalol Eye Drops
Timoptic Eye Drops
Timoptic Ocudose Eye Drops
Timoptic-XE Eye Drops

Combination Products
Generic Ingredients: Atenolol + Chlorthalidone G
Tenoretic

Generic Ingredients: Bisoprolol + Hydrochlorothiazide G
Ziac

Generic Ingredients: Metoprolol + Hydrochlorothiazide
Lopressor-HCT

Generic Ingredients: Nadolol + Bendroflumethiazide G
Corzide

Generic Ingredients: Propranolol + Hydrochlorothiazide G
Inderide
Inderide LA

Generic Ingredients: Timolol + Brimonidine
Combigan

Type of Drug

Beta-adrenergic blocking agent.

Prescribed For

Beta-adrenergic blocking drugs, or beta blockers, are prescribed alone or in combination for a variety of different uses, including high blood pressure—often in combination with other blood pressure medicines—abnormal heart rhythms, angina pectoris, heart failure, and prevention of second heart attack and migraine. They can also be used to treat alcohol withdrawal, stage fright, and other anxieties as well as to manage some of the side effects of antipsychotic medications. Beta-blocker eye drops are used to treat glaucoma.

General Information

Beta blockers interfere with the action of a specific part of the central nervous system. Beta receptors are found all over the body and affect many body functions; these drugs interfere with the action of adrenaline and other chemicals on these receptors. There are 2 types of beta receptors, $beta_1$ and $beta_2$. Each of these medicines has particular characteristics that make it suitable for different conditions or individuals. Though some beta blockers are approved for only 1 use because of limitations in how they were studied, all beta blockers share the same characteristics with some differences between them.

Atenolol primarily blocks the $beta_1$ receptor. Nebivolol blocks both receptors when taken at high doses by people whose liver breaks down the drug more slowly than average. Pindolol is a mild heart stimulant, which can be advantageous for some patients. Sotalol is approved only for serious, proven abnormal rhythms that occur in the ventricles (lower chambers) of the heart. Sotalol has both potent beta-blocker and antiarrhythmic activity.

When used to treat high blood pressure, beta blockers may be used either alone or concurrently with other antihypertensive drugs, particularly with a thiazide-type diuretic.

Some beta blockers are available in sustained-release formulations, which maintain a steady blood level of the drug for about 24 hours and permit the medicine to be taken only once a day.

Beta-blocker eye drops reduce ocular pressure (pressure inside the eye) by slowing the production of eye fluids and by slightly increasing the rate at which these fluids flow through and leave the eye. Small amounts of these drugs are absorbed into the general blood circulation after they are instilled in the eye and may affect areas of the body other than the eye.

Cautions and Warnings

Do not take these drugs if you are **allergic** or **sensitive** to any of their ingredients or to other beta blockers. People with a severe allergy to any substance may be more sensitive to that allergen while taking a beta blocker. People with a history of **severe anaphylactic reaction** to allergens may be unresponsive to usual doses of epinephrine while taking beta blockers.

People with **angina** who take these medicines for high blood pressure risk aggravating their angina if they suddenly stop taking the drug. If you are stopping this medicine, your doctor will gradually reduce your drug dosage—including beta-blocker eye drops—over 1–2 weeks.

These drugs reduce the amount of blood pumped by the heart with each beat. This reduction in blood flow may aggravate the condition of people with **poor circulation** or **circulatory disease**.

Beta blockers should be avoided by those with **slow heartbeat**, moderate to severe **heart block** (a condition affecting the heart's conduction system), **congestive heart failure** (unless it is due to a quickened heart rate that can be treated with a beta blocker), or **acute heart failure**. Beta blockers have become a cornerstone of heart-failure treatment when prescribed in low doses and closely managed by your doctor. Carvedilol, an alpha-beta blocker was the first drug with beta-blocking properties to be approved for heart-failure treatment.

These drugs should be used with caution if you have **liver or kidney disease**, because your ability to eliminate these drugs from your body may be impaired. Dose adjustments may be needed. Sotalol dose must be modified in people with kidney disease.

If you are undergoing **major surgery**, your doctor may want you to stop taking these drugs at least 2 days before surgery because of possible interaction with general anesthetics.

Beta blockers should be used with caution if you have an untreated **pheochromocytoma** (adrenal gland tumor).

Beta blockers should be used with caution by those with **chronic bronchitis**, **emphysema**, or other non-diseases that cause bronchospasm, because they worsen these conditions.

All beta-blocker medicines, including eye drops, can raise blood sugar and mask the physical signs of **hypoglycemia**. People with **diabetes** who must take insulin or oral medications to lower blood sugar and those subject to hypoglycemia must use beta blockers with caution and may need their dosage adjusted for this effect.

A portion of each dose of beta-blocker eye drop is absorbed into your blood. If you cannot tolerate oral beta blockers, you may also be intolerant of the eye drops.

Beta blockers may worsen **psoriasis**.

Ironically, sotalol taken on its own can cause abnormal heart rhythms. A cardiologist must supervise the use of both sotalol and solatol AF by monitoring your heart with an electrocardiogram (ECG) in a clinic or hospital for 3 days after your maintenance dose has been reached.

If you have a history of **symptomatic atrial fibrillation/flutter (AFIB/AFL)** and are receiving solatol treatment, you should discuss with your doctor a switch to the AF formulation of solatol, as there are critical differences in terms of dosage and safety information. You should not substitute solatol with solatol AF because of these distinct differences.

Possible Side Effects

Beta-blocker side effects are relatively infrequent and generally mild; normally they develop early in the course of treatment and are rarely a reason to stop taking the medication. People are more likely to stop their beta blocker because of inconvenient side effects such as dulling of the sex drive rather than because of medically important effects.

Acebutolol

- ▼ Most common: fatigue.
- ▼ Common: dizziness and headache.
- ▼ Less common: chest pain, swelling in the legs or arms, depression, sleeplessness, abnormal dreams, rashes, constipation, diarrhea, upset stomach, stomach gas, nausea, frequent urination, back pain, joint and muscle pain, difficulty breathing, stuffy nose, and vision changes.
- ▼ Rare: cough, low blood pressure, slow heartbeat, anxiety, impotence, changes in response to touch stimulation, itching, vomiting, abdominal pain, painful urination, nighttime urination, liver changes, sore throat, wheezing, eye irritation

Possible Side Effects *(continued)*

or pain, dry eye, and lupus erythematosus (a chronic autoimmune disease). Contact your doctor if you experience anything unusual while taking any medication.

Atenolol

- Most common: impotence.
- Less common: unusual tiredness or weakness, slow heartbeat, heart failure (symptoms include swelling of the legs, ankles, or feet), dizziness, bronchospasm, depression, confusion, anxiety, nervousness, sleeplessness, disorientation, short-term memory loss, emotional instability, cold hands and feet, constipation, diarrhea, nausea, vomiting, upset stomach, increased sweating, urinary difficulties, cramps, blurred vision, hair loss, stuffy nose, chest pain, back or joint pain, colitis, drug allergy (symptoms include rash, itching, difficulty breathing, and swelling of the mouth, face, lips, or tongue), and liver toxicity.
- Rare: lupus erythematosus (a chronic autoimmune disease). Contact your doctor if you experience anything unusual while taking any medication.

Beta-Blocker Eye Drops (Betaxolol, Carteolol, Levobunolol, Metipranolol, and Timolol)

- Common: eye discomfort.
- Less common: blurred vision; inflammation of the cornea; sensation of something in the eye; sensitivity to light; tearing; eye pain, dryness, or itching; redness, inflammation, discharge, cloudy vision; and crusting of the lashes.
- Rare: unusual tiredness or weakness, slow heartbeat, low blood sugar, lupus erythematosus (a chronic autoimmune disease), heart failure, dizziness, breathing difficulties, bronchospasm, depression, rash, and hair loss. Contact your doctor if you experience anything unusual while taking any medication.

Bisoprolol

- Most common: impotence.
- Less common: unusual tiredness or weakness, slow heartbeat, heart failure, dizziness, bronchospasm, depression, confusion, anxiety, nervousness, sleeplessness, disorientation, short-term memory loss, emotional instability, cold

Possible Side Effects *(continued)*

hands and feet, constipation, diarrhea, nausea, vomiting, upset stomach, increased sweating, urinary difficulties, cramps, blurred vision, hair loss, stuffy nose, aggravation of lupus erythematosus (a chronic autoimmune disease), chest pain, back or joint pain, colitis, drug allergy (symptoms include rash, itching, difficulty breathing, and swelling of the mouth, face, lips, or tongue), and liver toxicity.

Metoprolol and Nadolol

▼ Less common: impotence, unusual tiredness or weakness, slow heartbeat, heart failure, dizziness, bronchospasm, depression, confusion, anxiety, nervousness, sleeplessness, disorientation, short-term memory loss, emotional instability, cold hands and feet, constipation, diarrhea, nausea, vomiting, upset stomach, increased sweating, urinary difficulties, cramps, blurred vision, hives, hair loss, stuffy nose, aggravation of lupus erythematosus (a chronic autoimmune disease), chest pain, back or joint pain, colitis, drug allergy (symptoms include rash, itching, difficulty breathing, and swelling of the mouth, face, lips, or tongue), and liver toxicity.

Nebivolol

▼ Common: headache.

▼ Less common: fatigue, dizziness, diarrhea, nausea, sleeplessness, chest pain, slow heartbeat, difficulty breathing, rash, and swelling in the legs and arms.

▼ Rare: weakness, abdominal pain, high blood levels of cholesterol and uric acid, and tingling in the hands or feet. Contact your doctor if you experience anything unusual while taking any medication.

Penbutolol

▼ Common: headache.

▼ Less common: fatigue, dizziness, diarrhea, nausea, upset stomach, sleeplessness, chest pain, slow heartbeat, weakness, chest pain, arm or leg pain, respiratory infections, cough, difficulty breathing, and excess sweating.

▼ Rare: sexual impotence. Contact your doctor if you experience anything unusual while taking any medication.

Possible Side Effects *(continued)*

Pindolol and Propranolol

- ▼ Most common: impotence.
- ▼ Less common: unusual tiredness or weakness, slow heartbeat, heart failure, dizziness, bronchospasm, depression, confusion, anxiety, nervousness, sleeplessness, disorientation, short-term memory loss, emotional instability, cold hands and feet, constipation, diarrhea, nausea, vomiting, upset stomach, increased sweating, urinary difficulties, cramps, blurred vision, hair loss, stuffy nose, aggravation of lupus erythematosus (a chronic autoimmune disease), chest pain, back or joint pain, colitis, drug allergy (symptoms include rash, itching, difficulty breathing, and swelling of the mouth, face, lips, or tongue), and liver toxicity.

Sotalol

- ▼ Most common: difficulty breathing, slow heartbeat, chest pain, and heart palpitations.
- ▼ Common: swollen arms or legs, abnormal cardiogram, low blood pressure, abnormal heart rhythms, and fainting.
- ▼ Less common: infection, fever, localized pain, fatigue, dizziness, lightheadedness, weakness, nausea, and vomiting.
- ▼ Rare: leg pain due to blood vessel spasm; heart disease; flushing; high blood pressure; headache; difficulty sleeping; excess sweating; anxiety; diarrhea; upset stomach; abdominal pain; colon problems; stomach gas; lung problems; loss of sex drive; urinary problems; pain in the arms, legs, or back; rash; bleeding; and visual problems. Contact your doctor if you experience anything unusual while taking any medication.

Drug Interactions

- Atenolol may interact with surgical anesthetics to increase the risk of heart problems during surgery. Some anesthesiologists recommend gradually stopping the drug by 2 days before surgery.
- Beta blockers raise blood sugar. Your insulin dose may have to be altered and your response to oral antidiabetic drugs may change.
- Beta blockers increase the blood-pressure-lowering effects of other blood-pressure-reducing agents, including clonidine,

guanabenz, and reserpine, and calcium channel blockers such as nifedipine.

- Aspirin-containing drugs, indomethacin, and sulfinpyrazone may interfere with the blood-pressure-lowering effect of beta blockers.
- Cocaine reduces the effectiveness of all beta blockers.
- Beta blockers may worsen the cold hands and feet associated with taking ergot alkaloids, used to treat migraine. Gangrene is a possibility in people taking both an ergot and atenolol.
- Beta blockers will counteract thyroid-hormone replacements. Your dose may have to be adjusted for this effect.
- Calcium channel blockers, contraceptive drugs, diphenhydramine, flecainide, haloperidol, hydralazine, phenothiazine sedatives, propafenone, and quinolone antibacterials may increase the amount of beta blocker in the bloodstream, increasing the beta-blocking effect.
- Beta blockers should not be taken within 2 weeks of taking a monoamine oxidase inhibitor (MAOI) antidepressant.
- Cimetidine increases the amount of atenolol, metoprolol, and propranolol absorbed into the bloodstream from oral tablets.
- Beta blockers may interfere with the effectiveness of some antiasthma drugs, including aminophylline and theophylline, and especially ephedrine and isoproterenol. They have opposite effects on the same receptors.
- Mixing a beta blocker with digitalis drugs, disopyramide, phenytoin, or quinidine may result in excessive slowing of the heart, possibly causing heart block (disruption of the electrical impulses that control heart rate).
- Smoking increases the rate at which these and many other drugs are broken down by liver enzymes. Your dose may need to be reduced if you stop smoking.
- Aluminum salts, ampicillin, barbiturates, calcium salts, cholestyramine, colestipol, and rifampin may reduce the effectiveness of the beta blockers.
- Beta blockers may increase the effects of gabapentin, lidocaine, or prazosin, leading to undesirable reactions or toxicity.
- Mixing a beta blocker and prazosin may increase the lightheadedness associated with prazosin.
- Beta blockers may block the effects of epinephrine.
- Bupropion, duloxetine, fluoxetine, paroxetine, propafenone, quinidine, and terbinafine can substantially increase the

amount of beta blockers in the blood by interfering with their breakdown by liver enzymes. Amiodarone, cimetidine, and sertraline also have this interaction, but the effect is smaller. Avoid these combinations.

- Other drugs that can increase beta-blocker levels but to a lesser extent are antihistamines, celecoxib, chlorpheniramine, chlorpromazine, citalopram, clemastine, clomipramine, diphenhydramine, doxepin, doxorubicin, escitalopram, halofantrine, haloperidol, histamine, hydroxyzine, levomepromazine, methadone, metoclopramide, mibefradil, midodrine, moclobemide, perphenazine, ranitidine, ritonavir, ticlopidine, and tripelennamine.
- Dexamethasone, rifampin, and sildenafil reduce blood levels of the beta blockers, but the combined effect on blood pressure is moderate.

Food Interactions

Sustained-release metoprolol (Toprol-XL) may be taken with food if it upsets your stomach. Because food increases the amount of short-acting metoprolol (Lopressor) absorbed into the blood, take the short-acting form without food.

It is best to take propranolol without food or on an empty stomach, but it may be taken with food if it upsets your stomach. However you take propranolol, it is important to be consistent about taking it with or without food in order to maintain consistent effects.

Other beta blockers can be taken without regard to food or meals.

Usual Dose

Acebutolol

High Blood Pressure

Adult: starting dose—100 mg a day, taken all at once or in 2 divided doses. The daily dose may be gradually increased. Maintenance dose—400–800 mg a day.

Child: not recommended.

Senior: Older adults may respond to lower doses and should be treated more cautiously, beginning with 100 mg a day, increasing gradually to a maximum of 400 mg a day.

Abnormal Heart Rhythms

Adult: starting dose—200 mg a day. Maintenance dose—200–600 mg a day in 2 divided doses.

Child: not recommended.

Senior: Older adults may respond to lower doses and should be treated more cautiously, beginning with 100 mg a day, increasing gradually to a maximum of 400 mg a day.

Atenolol

Adult: 50 mg a day. Some people may require doses of 100–200 mg a day. Dosages over 100 mg a day are not likely to produce additional benefit to those being treated for hypertension. People with kidney disease may need only 50 mg every other day.

Child: not recommended.

Senior: Older adults should be treated more cautiously and may need a lower dose.

Beta-Blocker Eye Drops

Adult: 1–2 drops in the affected eye twice a day.

Bisoprolol

Adult: starting dose—5 mg once a day. The daily dose may be gradually increased up to 20 mg. Maintenance dose—5–10 mg once a day. People with kidney or liver disease may need only 2.5 mg a day to start.

Child: not recommended.

Senior: Lower doses may be needed to achieve the same effect.

Metoprolol

Adult

Metoprolol: 100–450 mg a day: dosage must be tailored to your specific needs.

Metoprolol + Hydrochlorothiazide: 1 tablet a day. This is available in a number of dosage strengths for individualized treatment options.

Child: not recommended.

Nadolol

Adult: 40–80 mg a day.

Child: not recommended.

Senior: Lower doses may be needed to achieve the same effect.

Nadolol + Bendroflumethiazide

Adult: starting dose—2.5–20 mg a day, either in 1 dose or divided into 2 doses. Maintenance dose—2.5–5 mg a day.

Child: not recommended.

Senior: Lower doses may be needed to achieve the same effect.

Nebivolol

Adult: 5 mg a day to start, increasing gradually to 40 mg a day as needed.

Child: not recommended.

Senior: Dose adjustment is not necessary.

Penbutolol

Adult: 20 mg once a day. Larger doses are well tolerated but do not produce a better effect. The full effect is seen in 2–4 weeks. A 10-mg daily dose takes 4–6 weeks to work. People with liver disease may require lower doses.

Child: not recommended.

Senior: Dose adjustment may be required.

Pindolol

Adult: 5–60 mg a day.

Child: not recommended.

Senior: Lower doses may be needed to achieve the same effect.

Propranolol

Adult: 30–700 mg a day. Take once a day at bedtime to minimize side effects.

Child: not recommended.

Senior: Lower doses may be needed to achieve the same effect.

Sotalol

Sotalol treatment is started and adjusted in a hospital where you can be closely monitored until you are stabilized. The dosage of this medicine must be customized for each person.

Adult: 80 mg twice a day to start, increased gradually to 160–320 mg a day. Some people may need up to 640 mg a day but side effects are more common with increased dose. Dose must be reduced for people with kidney disease.

Senior: A lower dose may be required to achieve the same result due to reduced kidney function.

Child: Dosage is customized to each child's requirement and is based on height and weight. Sotalol has not been well studied in children with kidney disease. It will take much more time to reach a satisfactory dosage in this group.

Sotalol AF

Sotalol AF treatment is started and adjusted in a hospital where you can be closely monitored until you are stabilized Solatol AF has distinct differences in dosage from sotalol and must be individualized for each patient.

Adult: 80 mg twice a day to start. Maximum dose of 160 mg twice a day. Dose must be reduced for people with kidney disease.

Senior: A lower dose may required to achieve the same result due to reduced kidney function.

Child: Dosage is customized to each child's requirement and is based on height and weight. Sotalol AF has not been well studied in children with kidney disease. It will take much more time to reach a satisfactory dosage in this group.

Overdosage

Overdose symptoms include changes in heartbeat—unusually slow, unusually fast, or irregular—severe dizziness or fainting, breathing difficulties, bluish-colored fingernails or palms, and seizures.

Very low blood pressure, heart failure, and shock may also result from a beta-blocker overdose. The victim should be taken to a hospital emergency room. If you seek treatment, ALWAYS bring the prescription bottle or container.

If the overdose occurs in the eye, flush the eye immediately with water or saline.

Special Information

These drugs are meant to be taken continuously. When ending treatment, beta-blocker dosage should be reduced gradually over a period of about 2 weeks. Do not stop taking your medicine unless directed to do so by your doctor. Abrupt withdrawal may cause chest pain, breathing difficulties, increased sweating, and unusually fast or irregular heartbeat. This is especially true of sotalol, which must be taken on a regular schedule without interruption.

Contact your doctor at once if you develop back or joint pain, breathing difficulties, cold hands or feet, depression, rash, or changes in heartbeat. These drugs may produce an undesirable lowering of blood pressure, leading to dizziness or fainting; contact your doctor if this happens. Also contact your doctor if you experience persistent or bothersome anxiety, diarrhea, constipation, impotence, headache, itching, nausea or vomiting, nightmares or vivid dreams, upset stomach, insomnia, stuffy nose, frequent urination, unusual tiredness, or weakness.

Consult your doctor or pharmacist before taking other

medications and supplement products with your beta blocker, including over-the-counter medications.

Beta blockers can cause drowsiness, lightheadedness, dizziness, or blurred vision. Be careful when driving or performing complex tasks.

It is best to take your beta blocker at the same time each day. If you forget a dose, take it as soon as you remember. If you take nebivolol and do not remember until your next dose, continue with your regular schedule. If you take your beta blocker once a day and it is within 8 hours of your next dose, skip the dose you forgot and continue with your regular schedule. If you take it twice a day and it is within 4 hours of your next dose, skip the one you forgot and continue with your regular schedule. Never take a double dose of your beta blocker.

Do not crush or chew the sustained-release form of any beta-blocker drug.

Do not use beta-blocker eye drops with contact lenses in your eye. Do not touch the dropper to any surface.

Special Populations

Pregnancy/Breast-feeding: These medicines cross the placenta. Infants born to women who took a beta blocker while pregnant had lower birth weights, low blood pressure, and slower heart rates. Beta blockers reduce blood flow to the placenta, raising the risk of fetal death and premature and immature births. Also, beta blockers produced low blood sugar and slowed the heart rate of the developing fetus. The newborn continues to experience beta-blocker effects for 3–5 days after birth and must be closely monitored in a neonatal unit. These drugs should be taken during pregnancy only if your doctor determines that the potential benefit outweighs the risks.

Some beta blockers can pass into breast milk, especially if you are taking a large dose. Nursing mothers should use infant formula.

Seniors: Seniors taking a beta blocker may be more likely to suffer from cold hands and feet, reduced body temperature, chest pain, general feelings of ill health, sudden breathing difficulties, increased sweating, or changes in heartbeat. They should use the lowest effective dose, as this group is more likely to have decreased heart, kidney, and liver function and to be taking additional medications. Dosage adjustment of nebivolol is not necessary in seniors.

Generic Name

Betaine (BEE-tane)

Brand Names

Cystadane

Type of Drug

Homocysteine antagonist.

Prescribed For

Homocysteinuria.

General Information

Homocysteinuria is a group of 3 disorders of the metabolism characterized by too much homocysteine in the blood and urine. People with this problem tend to have skeletal problems, problems with the lens of the eye, and blood-clotting problems that can cause chest pain or heart attack. Virtually all people treated with betaine experience a decrease of homocysteine in their blood. When used together with other homocysteinuria treatments, including folate and vitamins B_{12} and B_6, betaine's effect has been additive to those treatments. Betaine starts working in several days and has been used for several years with no loss of effect. Most patients treated with betaine have been children. The effects of homocysteinuria can be devastating in children and include developmental problems, lethargy, seizures, and eye problems.

Cautions and Warnings

None known.

Possible Side Effects

Side effects, which are uncommon, include nausea, upset stomach, diarrhea, choking if the powder is inhaled, and bad odors. Reported psychological changes from betaine are questionable.

Drug Interactions

None known. Betaine has been used successfully together with folate and vitamins B_{12} and B_6.

Food Interactions

Betaine should be taken with food.

Usual Dose

Adult and Child: 3 g twice a day. Dosage for children under age 3 may be started at about 45 mg per lb. of body weight a day and then increased in weekly 45-mg steps. Dosage should be increased in all patients until homocysteine is either undetectable in the blood or present in small amounts; doses up to 20 g a day have been required. Carefully measure all doses with the scoop provided. Each level scoopful is equal to 1 g of betaine.

Overdosage

Little is known about the effects of betaine overdose. People have been safely and successfully treated at doses up to 20 g a day. Contact your poison control center or a hospital emergency room for more information. If you seek treatment, ALWAYS bring the prescription bottle or container.

Special Information

Shake the bottle lightly before removing the cap to loosen the powder. Protect the powder from moisture.

Mix each dose with 4–6 oz. of water until it dissolves completely, then drink it at once.

Do not use the product if the final solution is either not clear or colored, or if the powder does not completely dissolve.

If you forget a dose, take it as soon as you remember. If it is almost time for your next dose, skip the dose you forgot and continue with your regular schedule. Tell your doctor about any missed doses.

Special Populations

Pregnancy/Breast-feeding: The safety of using betaine during pregnancy is unknown. Betaine should be used during pregnancy only if your doctor determines that the potential benefit outweighs the risks.

It is not known if betaine passes into breast milk. Nursing mothers who must take this drug should use infant formula.

Seniors: Seniors may use this drug without special precaution.

Generic Name

Bicalutamide (bye-kal-UTE-uh-mide) G

Brand Names

Casodex

The information in this profile also applies to the following drugs:

Generic Ingredients: Flutamide G

Generic Ingredients: Nilutamide
Nilandron

Type of Drug

Antiandrogen.

Prescribed For

Prostate cancer. Flutamide may also be prescribed for acne and hirsutism (excessive hair growth in women).

General Information

Antiandrogens are prescribed together with another hormone product for prostate cancer. Bicalutamide competes with testosterone and other natural androgens (male hormones) by binding to the same places in body tissue where androgens normally bind. Prostate cancer is androgen-sensitive and responds to treatments that counteract the effects of androgen or remove the sources of androgen. These drugs are always prescribed together with a luteinizing hormone-releasing hormone drug.

Cautions and Warnings

Do not take these drugs if you are **allergic** or **sensitive** to them or any of their ingredients.

People taking these medications may develop severe liver failure. People with **liver disease** may be at greater risk for serious side effects and should use this medicine with caution. People with severe liver impairment should not take flutamide or nilutamide.

Male breast cancer is a risk with these medicines. Almost 40% of men taking bicalutamide as single therapy for **prostate cancer** develop breast pain and enlargement. Bicalutamide may also reduce sperm count.

These drugs can increase blood sugar. The increase can be enough to push people with prediabetes into active disease. People with **diabetes** must carefully monitor their blood sugar.

Two of every 100 people taking nilutamide develop interstitial pneumonitis (symptoms include cough, chest pain, fever, and breathing difficulties). People with **lung disease** and **Asians** may be at greater risk. Report any breathing difficulties or worsening of pre-existing breathing difficulties to your doctor immediately.

Flutamide may cause jaundice and severe blood conditions, including hemolytic anemia. People with certain **blood disorders** and **people who smoke** are at greater risk for these side effects. Isolated cases of aplastic anemia (a potentially fatal blood disorder) have been reported in people taking nilutamide, but the relationship between the drug and the disease is not established.

Possible Side Effects

Bicalutamide

- ▼ Most common: hot flashes, general pain, headache, weakness, back pain, nausea, constipation, sleeplessness, breathing difficulties, and swollen breasts.
- ▼ Common: diarrhea and pelvic pain.
- ▼ Less common: vomiting, abdominal pain, chest pain, flu-like symptoms, high blood pressure, swelling in the ankles or lower legs, high blood sugar, weight loss, dizziness, tingling in the hands or feet, sweating, rash, nighttime urination, blood in the urine, urinary or other infection, loss of libido, impotence, breast pain, painful urination, anemia, and bone pain.
- ▼ Rare: Rare side effects can occur in almost any part of the body. Contact your doctor if you experience anything unusual while taking any medication.

Flutamide

- ▼ Most common: diarrhea, cystitis, and bleeding from the rectum.
- ▼ Common: rectal irritation, blood in the urine, hot flashes, loss of libido, impotence, nausea, rash, and swollen breasts.
- ▼ Less common: drowsiness, confusion, depression, anxiety, nervousness, appetite loss, stomach problems, anemia, low white-blood-cell and blood-platelet counts, arm or leg swelling, urinary and muscle problems, and high blood pressure.
- ▼ Rare: hepatitis, jaundice, and breathing difficulties. Contact your doctor if you experience anything unusual while taking any medication.

Nilutamide

Side effects are more pronounced when taken together with leuprolide.

- ▼ Most common: hot flashes and difficulty adapting to the dark.

Possible Side Effects *(continued)*

- ▼ Common: high blood pressure, nausea, constipation, dizziness, visual changes, urinary infection, and elevated liver enzymes.
- ▼ Less common: not feeling well, angina, heart failure, diarrhea, gastrointestinal disorders and bleeding, alcohol intolerance, leg swelling, weight loss, arthritis, dry mouth, nervousness, tingling in the hands or feet, stuffy nose, itching, and abnormal kidney function.
- ▼ Rare: lung irritation.

Drug Interactions

- Bicalutamide and flutamide increase the effect of oral anticoagulant (blood thinning) drugs such as warfarin. Dosage adjustment may be necessary.
- Bicalutamide increases blood levels of midazolam and may increase the effects of other drugs that work in a similar way.
- Nilutamide may increase the risk of the potentially serious side effects of phenytoin, theophylline, or vitamin K antagonists.

Food Interactions

None known.

Usual Dose

Bicalutamide

Adult: 50 mg once a day, morning or night.

Child: not recommended.

Flutamide

Adult: 500–1500 mg a day, once a day or in 2 doses. Daily doses of 125, 250, or 375 mg may be given for acne or hirsutism.

Child: not recommended.

Nilutamide

Adult: 300 mg a day, reduced to 150 mg a day after 30 days.

Child: not recommended.

Overdosage

Symptoms of overdose may include nausea, vomiting, tiredness, headache, dizziness, slow breathing, weakness, tearing, appetite loss, swollen and tender breasts, and liver inflammation. Overdose victims should be taken to a hospital emergency room. If you seek treatment, ALWAYS bring the prescription bottle or container.

Special Information

Report anything unusual to your doctor, especially pain or tenderness in the upper-right abdomen, yellowing of the skin or whites of the eyes, severe itching, dark urine, persistent appetite loss, and unexplained flu-like symptoms. These may be signs of severe liver toxicity. Also report any breathing difficulties, cough, chest pain, or fever.

Women who are prescribed this medicine for acne or hirsutism should use non-hormonal contraception during treatment and for at least 1 month after treatment is stopped to avoid becoming pregnant.

Flutamide can turn your urine amber or yellow-green and cause unusual sun sensitivity. Use sunscreen and wear long-sleeve protective clothing while you are taking flutamide.

Up to ½ of people taking nilutamide can take from a few seconds to a few minutes to adapt to darkness. This can be a problem especially when driving at night or through tunnels. Wearing tinted glasses minimizes this effect.

Up to 5% of people taking nilutamide may experience intolerance to alcohol. Symptoms include flushing, tiredness, and lightheadedness. If you experience this reaction, you should avoid alcohol.

Take these medicines at the same time each day for best results. If you forget a dose of bicalutamide, take it as soon as you remember. If it is almost time for your next dose, skip the dose you forgot and continue with your regular schedule. Contact your doctor if you forget to take more than 1 dose. Do not stop taking these medicines unless directed to do so by your doctor.

Special Populations

Pregnancy/Breast-feeding: These drugs can harm a growing fetus and must never be taken by a pregnant woman. Make sure your doctor knows if you are or are planning to become pregnant.

It is not known if these drugs pass into breast milk. Nursing mothers who must take them should use infant formula.

Seniors: Seniors may take this drug without special precaution.

Brand Names

BiDil

Generic Ingredients

Isosorbide Dinitrate + Hydralazine Hydrochloride

Type of Drug

Vasodilator combination.

Prescribed For

Heart failure in black patients, in combination with other heart-failure treatments.

General Information

BiDil is a combination of two drugs that dilate (open) both arteries and veins. It is the first drug product to be specifically approved for people in a single racial group for any indication. The 2 ingredients in BiDil have been available generically for years and are prescribed for a variety of uses. Isosorbide dinitrate is prescribed for angina, heart failure, and spasms of the esophagus. Hydralazine hydrochloride is prescribed to treat high blood pressure and heart failure. When people with heart failure take this drug combination, it makes it easier for the heart to pump blood throughout the body by widening arteries and veins.

Cautions and Warnings

Do not take BiDil if you are **allergic** or **sensitive** to any of its ingredients.

Do not use erectile dysfunction drugs with BiDil.

This drug may be inappropriate for you if you have had a recent **heart attack** or have **cardiomyopathy** (loss of blood-pumping ability due to damaged heart muscle) or **low blood pressure**, especially postural low blood pressure (symptoms include dizziness or fainting when rising from a sitting or lying position).

Long-term administration of more than 200 mg a day of hydralazine may produce symptoms of lupus erythematosus (a chronic autoimmune disease), including muscle and joint pain, skin reactions, fever, kidney inflammation, and anemia, although they usually disappear when the drug is discontinued. Report any fever, chest pain, feelings of ill health, or other unexplained symptoms to your doctor. The risk of developing lupus increases with higher dosages; approximately 5–10% of people taking 200 mg a day of hydralazine develop lupus. The daily dosage of hydralazine when you take BiDil can be as high as 225 mg.

Hydralazine may cause a very rapid heartbeat, potentially leading to angina or a heart attack.

Taking pyridoxine (vitamin B_6) may relieve tingling or numbness in the hands or feet caused by hydralazine.

Possible Side Effects

- ▼ Most common: headache, nausea, dizziness, weakness, and chest pain.
- ▼ Common: low blood pressure.
- ▼ Less common: blurred vision, dry mouth, sinus irritation, rapid heartbeat, heart palpitations, high blood sugar, runny nose, numbness or tingling in the hands or feet, vomiting, and high blood-fat levels.
- ▼ Rare: flushing; tearing, itching, or redness of the eyes; tremors; muscle cramps; depression; disorientation; anxiety; itching; rash; fever; chills; occasional hepatitis (symptoms include yellowing of the skin or whites of the eyes); constipation; urinary difficulties; and adverse effects on normal blood composition. Rare side effects can occur in almost any part of the body. Contact your doctor if you experience anything unusual while taking any medication.

Drug Interactions

- Do not take sildenafil, vardenafil, or tadalafil with BiDil. The combination can result in a rapid and potentially fatal drop in blood pressure.
- Taking this drug with a monoamine oxidase inhibitor (MAOI) antidepressant may increase the blood-pressure-lowering effect of the hydralazine component of BiDil. This combination should be used with caution.
- Do not self-medicate with over-the-counter appetite suppressants or cough, cold, and allergy remedies, as many contain ingredients that may aggravate heart disease.
- Taking this drug with large amounts of alcohol may rapidly lower blood pressure, resulting in weakness, dizziness, and fainting.

Food Interactions

Take this drug on an empty stomach. It is unknown how food affects BiDil.

Usual Dose

Adult: 1 or 2 tablets 3 times a day, 1 hour before or 2 hours after eating.

Overdosage

There have been no reports of BiDil overdose. Symptoms of BiDil overdose would be related to the specific effects of each active ingredient and can include reduced oxygen supply to heart muscle, leading to a heart attack, abnormal heart rhythms, and profound shock. Fainting, coma, and death may follow unless the victim is treated. Overdose victims must be taken to a hospital emergency room at once. If you seek treatment, ALWAYS bring the prescription bottle or container.

Special Information

Avoid alcohol.

Contact your doctor if you develop a persistent headache, dizziness, facial flushing, blurred vision, or dry mouth.

It is important to make sure you drink plenty of fluids every day and pay attention to hot weather and exercise situations in which you might lose unusual amounts of fluids and salts. Fluid loss may lead to low blood pressure, dizziness, and possibly fainting.

If you forget to take a dose of BiDil, take it as soon as you remember. If it is almost time for your next dose, skip the dose you forgot and continue with your regular schedule. Never take a double dose.

Special Populations

Pregnancy/Breast-feeding: Isosorbide dinitrate crosses into the fetal circulation, and hydralazine can cause low blood pressure in pregnant women and their babies. BiDil should be taken during pregnancy only if your doctor determines that the potential benefit outweighs the risks.

It is not known if BiDil passes into breast milk. Nursing mothers who must take it should use infant formula.

Seniors: Specifics about how seniors react to this drug are not known. The lowest effective dose of BiDil should always be used, especially in people with reduced kidney and/or liver function.

Type of Drug

Bisphosphonates (bis-FOS-fun-ates)

Brand Names

Generic Ingredients: Alendronate G
Fosamax

Generic Ingredients: Alendronate + Vitamin D
Fosamax Plus D

Generic Ingredients: Etidronate G
Didronel

Generic Ingredients: Ibandronate
Boniva
Boniva Injection

Generic Ingredients: Pamidronate G
Aredia

Generic Ingredients: Risedronate G
Actonel
Atelvia

Generic Ingredients: Tiludronate
Skelid

Generic Ingredients: Zoledronic Acid
Reclast
Zometa

Prescribed For

Prevention and treatment of osteoporosis (a condition characterized by loss of bone mass due to calcium depletion) in postmenopausal women, older men, and people taking high doses of corticosteroids; Paget's disease of bone; growth of bone into soft tissues after bone surgery; high blood calcium associated with cancer; bone cancer spread; and multiple myeloma (advanced cancer in multiple tissues).

General Information

Bisphosphonates have been used for many years to treat a variety of conditions associated with low bone mass caused by calcium depletion. They work on cells called osteoclasts that normally break down bone tissue, making bones stronger by preventing loss of bone mass. In osteoporosis, bones become weak and brittle, increasing the risk of spine, hip, and other bone fractures, which are a major cause of death and disability in older people. Although alendronate and etidronate have been studied in children, little benefit has been shown and bisphosphonates generally are considered safe and effective only for adults. Information taken from large studies, including the 150,000+ patient Women's Health Initiative indicates that postmenopausal women who take bisphosphonates for a year or more can substantially reduce their risk of breast cancer.

Cautions and Warnings

Do not use bisphosphonates if you are **allergic** or **sensitive** to any of their ingredients.

Do not use bisphosphonates if you have severe **kidney disease**.

Avoid oral bisphosphonates if you have active **stomach or intestinal disease** such as difficulty swallowing, ulcers, or stomach irritation. Notify your doctor if you experience any gastrointestinal (GI) problems while taking oral bisphosphonates. Contact your doctor if your stomach problems persist or get worse; he or she may stop this treatment.

Do not use oral bisphosphonates if you cannot stand or sit upright for 30 minutes (see "Special Information").

Do not use etidronate if you have very soft bones due to severe **vitamin D deficiency** as your risk of broken bones is increased.

People taking bisphosphonates for osteoporosis can experience an uncommon thigh bone fracture in which the bone breaks just below the hip bone.

Jawbone decay (osteonecrosis) may occur in people taking bisphosphonate drugs and having dental work, especially those with **cancer**, taking **corticosteroids**, or with **poor oral hygiene**. Symptoms include bone infection and slow healing. Dental surgery can worsen the decay if performed after the process has begun. Nevertheless, you should contact a dental surgeon to provide specific care if osteonecrosis develops.

Long-term bisphosphonate treatment may raise the risk of cancer of the esophagus.

These drugs may rarely increase the risk of abnormal heart rhythms.

Bisphosphonates can cause low blood calcium and should not be used by people with **low blood calcium**.

Bisphosphonates can cause severe and sometimes incapacitating bone, joint, and/or muscle pain. If muscle or bone pain persists or gets worse while you are taking a bisphosphonate, contact your doctor, who may consider stopping your medicine.

Possible Side Effects

Side effects are generally mild and similar to those reported by people taking a placebo (sugar pill). Rare side effects may occur in almost any part of the body. Contact your doctor if you experience anything unusual while taking any medication.

Possible Side Effects *(continued)*

Alendronate

- ▼ Most common: bone pain and abdominal pain and discomfort.
- ▼ Less common: upset stomach, constipation, diarrhea, nausea, difficulty swallowing, muscle pain, headache, acid reflux, vomiting, gas, and stomach ulcers.
- ▼ Rare: changes in taste.

Etidronate

- ▼ Most common: headache, stomach pain, leg cramps, arthritis pain, nausea, and diarrhea.
- ▼ Less common: hair loss, broken bones, irritation of the esophagus, swelling and changes in the appearance and texture of the tongue, allergic reactions (swelling of the lips and throat, rash, and itching), softening of the bones, amnesia, confusion, depression, hallucinations, and tingling in the hands and feet.
- ▼ Rare: decreases in red- and/or white-blood-cell counts.

Ibandronate (Injection)

- ▼ Most common: fever, back pain, abdominal pain, high blood pressure, upset stomach, nausea, headache, diarrhea, and flu-like symptoms.
- ▼ Less common: constipation, dizziness, rash, fatigue, sleeplessness, urinary infection, muscle aches, leg pain, bronchitis, upper-respiratory infection, and high cholesterol.

Ibandronate (Oral)

- ▼ Most common: fever, high blood pressure, abdominal pain, back pain, and upset stomach.
- ▼ Common: constipation, ulcers, nausea, headache, high cholesterol, and urinary infections.
- ▼ Less common: dizziness, rash, sleeplessness, depression, cold symptoms, fatigue, diarrhea, bronchitis, upper-respiratory infection, and leg pain.

Pamidronate

- ▼ Most common: fever; injection-site reaction; nausea; appetite loss; low calcium, magnesium, potassium, and/or phosphate; and fatigue.

Possible Side Effects *(continued)*

- Less common: sleepiness, heart rhythm changes, loss of thyroid hormone function, fainting, constipation, anemia, lung congestion, and runny nose.

Risedronate

- Most common: fever, headache, diarrhea, abdominal pain, rash, and back pain.
- Common: upset stomach, nausea, flu-like symptoms, swelling in the hands and feet, chest pain, dizziness, constipation, bronchitis, sinus irritation, and high blood pressure.
- Less common: depression, insomnia, vomiting, bone pain, muscle pain, weakness, eye irritation, and respiratory infection.
- Rare: urinary infection, arthritis, sore throat, accidental injury.

Tiludronate

- Most common: pain, diarrhea, and nausea.
- Common: headache, upset stomach, respiratory infection, runny nose, and sinus irritation.
- Less common: vomiting, dizziness, accidental injury, flu-like symptoms, tingling in the hands or feet, chest pain, fever, coughing, sore throat, gas, cataracts, eye redness, glaucoma, rash, skin disorders, tooth problems, joint problems, swelling in the hands or feet, high parathyroid hormone levels, infection, and vitamin D deficiency.

Zoledronic Acid

- Most common: fever, constipation, nausea, fatigue, and headache.
- Common: anemia, difficulty breathing, bone pain, weakness, muscle pain, coughing, sleeplessness, diarrhea, appetite loss, and dizziness.
- Less common: leg or ankle swelling; agitation; anxiety; confusion; depression; nerve pain; low blood pressure; loss of sensation in hands or feet; hair loss; back pain; vomiting; muscle spasms; urinary infection; low potassium, magnesium, or phosphate; and upper-respiratory infection.
- Rare: dehydration and injection-site reaction.

Drug Interactions

- Bisphosphonates may increase the GI-irritating effects of aspirin, ibuprofen, and other nonsteroidal anti-inflammatory drugs (NSAIDs).
- Bisphosphonates reduce the ability of teriparatide to build new bone.
- Aminoglycoside antibiotics may add to the blood-calcium-lowering effect of bisphosphonates, reducing calcium to an undesirable level.
- Antacids and calcium- and iron-containing supplements can interfere with the absorption of oral bisphosphonates. Separate doses of an oral bisphosphonate from these drugs by at least 30 minutes.
- Etidronate may affect the action of warfarin.
- Risendronate should not be mixed with H_2 agonists such as cimetidine or proton pump inhibitors such as omeprazole because these agents decrease the amount of risedronate absorbed into your body.
- Ranitidine may increase the amount of alendronate and ibandronate in the blood, but the degree of increase is not likely to be clinically important.
- Aspirin can interfere with the absorption of tiludronate.
- Indomethacin can increase the amount of tiludronate absorbed into the blood by 2–4 times.
- Loop diuretics may increase the blood-calcium-lowering effect of zoledronic acid, leading to excessive decreases in calcium levels.
- Mixing zoledronic acid with thalidomide increases the risk of kidney damage.
- Using zoledronic acid with drugs that are primarily eliminated from your body through the kidneys may increase blood levels of those drugs and may lead to kidney damage.

Food Interactions

Take these medicines with plain water on an empty stomach (such as when you first wake up in the morning). Food and drink—even mineral water, orange juice, or coffee—interfere with the absorption of these drugs. Take alendronate or risedronate at least 30 minutes and ibandronate at least 1 hour before eating, drinking, or taking other medications. Wait 2 hours after taking etidronate and 4 hours after taking tiludronate before consuming any food, drink (other than plain water), or other medications.

Usual Dose

Alendronate

Adult: 5–40 mg a day or 35–70 mg once a week.

Child: 5–10 mg a day.

Alendronate + Vitamin D

Adult: 70 mg/2800 International Unit (IU) or 70 mg/5600 IU once a week.

Child: not recommended.

Etidronate

Adult and Child: 2.3–9 mg per lb. of body weight a day.

Ibandronate

Adult

Injection: 3 mg by injection once every 3 months.

Oral: 2.5 mg once a day or one 150-mg tablet once a month.

Child: not recommended.

Pamidronate

Adult: 90 mg by intravenous (IV) infusion given as a single dose over 2–24 hours or in divided doses over 3 consecutive days, depending on the disease being treated.

Risedronate

Adult: 5–30 mg a day, 35 mg once a week, or 150 mg once a month.

Child: 2.5–5 mg a day.

Tiludronate

Adult: 400 mg a day.

Child: not recommended.

Zoledronic Acid

Adult

Reclast: 5 mg by IV infusion for at least 15 minutes once every 1 or 2 years for osteoporosis; usually only a single dose is given for Paget's disease of the bone.

Zometa: 4 mg by IV infusion for high blood-calcium levels associated with cancer, bone cancer spread, and multiple myeloma, which may be repeated in 1 week or every 3–4 weeks depending on the condition treated. Dosage is reduced for people with mild to moderate kidney damage.

Child: 0.02 mg per lb. of body weight by IV injection

Overdosage

Little is known about the effects of bisphosphonate overdose. Very low blood calcium is the most serious symptom and requires emergency treatment. Kidney damage and reduced levels of magnesium and phosphate in the blood are also possible. Other symptoms may include upset stomach, heartburn, ulcer, and irritation of the esophagus. Milk or antacids may reverse these effects. Do not let the victim lie down or vomit. Overdose victims should be taken to a hospital emergency room. If you seek treatment, ALWAYS bring the prescription bottle or container.

Special Information

Food interferes with the effectiveness of these drugs. Carefully follow the directions in "Food Interactions" above.

Do not suck on any of these tablets or allow them to dissolve in your mouth because they can cause mouth sores.

To reduce the risk of stomach and throat irritation, do not lie down for at least 30 minutes after taking alendronate or risedronate. Do not lie down for 60 minutes after taking ibandronate.

Separate doses of calcium, iron, and vitamin D supplements from your bisphosphonate by at least 2 hours.

If you forget a dose, take it as soon as you remember. If it is almost time for your next dose, skip the dose you forgot and continue with your regular schedule. If you forget a morning dose and take it later in the day, you must still follow the instructions in "Food Interactions" about avoiding food.

Special Populations

Pregnancy/Breast-feeding: Bisphosphonates cause abnormal bone development in animal fetuses and are toxic to pregnant animals. Pregnant women should not use them.

It is not known if bisphosphonates pass into breast milk. Because these drugs affect bone formation, nursing mothers who must take a bisphosphonate should use infant formula.

Seniors: Kidney function should be monitored in seniors taking these drugs.

Boniva *see **Bisphosphonates,** page 188*

Generic Name

Bosentan (boh-SEN-tan)

Brand Names

Tracleer

The information in this profile also applies to the following drugs:

Generic Ingredients: Ambrisentan
Letairis

Type of Drug

Endothelin receptor antagonist.

Prescribed For

Pulmonary arterial hypertension.

General Information

These drugs lower blood pressure by working on the endothelin system. Endothelin is a hormone that plays an important role in maintaining blood pressure. It is normally found in blood vessels, but endothelin levels are very high in the blood and lungs of people with pulmonary arterial hypertension (high blood pressure in the arteries that carry oxygen to the lungs). People with this condition have high blood pressure and difficulty breathing and get very tired even when walking or doing other moderate exercise. Pulmonary arterial hypertension can be fatal.

Cautions and Warnings

Do not take these drugs if you are **allergic** or **sensitive** to any of their ingredients.

Bosentan can cause liver injury. People taking it should have their liver enzymes checked monthly. Enzyme increases can be a sign of liver injury and may be a reason to stop taking bosentan. People with moderate to severe **liver damage** should avoid these drugs.

These drugs should not be taken during **pregnancy** as they are likely to cause birth defects (see "Special Populations").

These medications can drastically reduce sperm count, making it very difficult to father a child. In a small study, ¼ of men taking bosentan experienced a 50% drop in sperm count. Sperm count returned to normal when the drug was stopped.

These medicines cause water retention and swelling and may require the addition of a diuretic or discontinuation of therapy.

These drugs lead to a reduction in red blood cells, resulting in anemia. Larger doses of these drugs cause a greater loss of red blood cells.

Possible Side Effects

Ambrisentan

Most side effects are mild. Only stuffy nose increases with increased dosage.

▼ Most common: swelling in the arms or legs, stuffy nose, sinusitis, flushing, heart palpitations, abdominal pain, constipation, difficulty breathing, and headache.

Bosentan

▼ Most common: headache and sore throat and nose.

▼ Common: flushing, abnormal liver function, leg swelling, low blood pressure, and heart palpitations.

▼ Less common: upset stomach, swelling, itching, anemia, tiredness, difficulty swallowing or breathing, and swelling of the lips, tongue, face, or throat.

Drug Interactions

- It is possible that bosentan may cause failure of hormonal contraceptives.
- Cyclosporine, used to prevent transplant rejection, increases blood levels of bosentan and ambrisentan. Do not combine these drugs.
- Mixing glyburide, an antidiabetes drug, with bosentan increases the risk of elevated liver enzyme levels while decreasing the effectiveness of both medications. Do not combine these drugs.
- When clarithromycin is combined with bosentan, the risk of liver injury is increased. Close monitoring of liver enzyme levels is required when these drugs are taken together.
- Ketoconazole significantly increases blood levels of bosentan by slowing its breakdown in the liver, possibly leading to

increased side effects. When these drugs are taken together, careful monitoring is required.

- When bosentan is taken with sildenafil, bosentan blood levels may increase while sildenafil levels are decreased. Dosage adjustments may be needed.
- Combining either of these drugs with rifampin may cause an initial increase in the amount of bosentan or ambrisentan in the blood. Caution is advised.
- Ritonavir may increase bosentan concentrations, requiring dosage adjustments.
- Combining bosentan with a statin-type cholesterol-lowering drug such as simvastatin, lovastatin, or atorvastatin reduces the amount of statin drug in the blood. Dose increases may be needed.
- Although not studied in humans, animal testing shows increased bosentan levels when used with tacrolimus. Caution is advised when combining these drugs.
- Bosentan can reduce the amount of warfarin in the blood by about ⅓. Changes in warfarin dosage may be needed.

Food Interactions

These drugs may be taken without regard to food or meals.

Usual Dose

Ambrisentan

Adult: 5–10 mg once a day. Do not crush, split, or chew these tablets.

Child: not recommended.

Bosentan

Adult: 62.5 mg twice a day for 4 weeks, then 125 mg twice a day.

Child: not recommended.

Overdosage

Massive overdose may result in severe lowering of blood pressure, requiring emergency attention. The most common effects associated with overdose are headache, low blood pressure, increased heart rate, and nausea and vomiting. Overdose victims should be taken to a hospital emergency room for treatment. If you seek treatment, ALWAYS bring the prescription bottle or container.

Special Information

Do not stop taking these drugs without gradually reducing the dosage as instructed by your doctor.

If you forget to take a dose, take it as soon as you remember. If it is almost time for your next dose, skip the dose you forgot and continue with your regular schedule. Do not take a double dose.

Contact your doctor at once if you develop severe itching, yellowing of the skin or whites of the eyes, tiredness, swelling in the arms or legs, nausea, vomiting, fever, or abdominal pain.

Doctors must enroll in special restricted distribution programs before they can prescribe these medicines, because of the risks of liver injury and birth defects associated with them. These medicines are not available in regular pharmacies but are mailed to you from a central pharmacy only after the testing and other program requirements have been met by your doctor.

Special Populations

Pregnancy/Breast-feeding: These medicines are very likely to cause major birth defects and should not be taken by pregnant women. Women must be sure they are not pregnant before beginning these treatments.

Women should also use non-hormonal contraceptives while on these drugs. Hormone-based contraceptives such as birth control pills, injections, and implants may not work in women taking bosentan or ambrisentan.

It is not known if either of these medicines passes into breast milk. Nursing mothers should use infant formula.

Seniors: The greater chance of kidney, liver, and cardiac function side effects in seniors may affect drug dosage. Seniors may also experience more swelling in the arms or legs.

Type of Drug

Bowel Anti-inflammatory Drugs (5-ASA Type)

Brand Names

Generic Ingredients: Balsalazide G
Colazal

Generic Ingredients: Mesalamine G

Apriso
Asacol HD
Canasa
Lialda
Pentasa
Rowasa

Generic Ingredients: Olsalazine

Dipentum

Prescribed For

Ulcerative colitis and prevention of recurrence of ulcerative colitis; rectal products prescribed for distal ulcerative colitis, proctitis, and proctosigmoiditis.

General Information

Chemical cousins of aspirin, these bowel anti-inflammatory drugs (5-ASA type) are used to treat symptoms of bowel inflammation. No one knows exactly how they work, but they are believed to have a local effect on the bowel. The tablet forms are made to delay drug release until they reach the colon. Little of the drug is absorbed into the blood; 70–90% remains in the colon.

Cautions and Warnings

Do not take bowel anti-inflammatories if you are **allergic** or **sensitive** to any of their ingredients or to aspirin. Although people who are sensitive or allergic to sulfasalazine have generally been able to tolerate mesalamine—which is an active agent in sulfasalazine—they should be cautious.

People with **asthma** should use these medications with caution.

Bowel anti-inflammatories may worsen **colitis** or cause cramping, sudden abdominal pain, bloody diarrhea, fever, headache, or rash. Stop taking the drug at once and contact your doctor if any of these symptoms develop.

Mesalamine has caused myocarditis and pericarditis (inflammation of the membranes lining the heart). People who have **conditions that predispose them to myocarditis or pericarditis** should use mesalamine with caution.

People with **pyloric stenosis** (narrowing of the opening between the stomach and the intestines) may experience prolonged gastric retention of mesalamine.

Some people taking mesalamine have developed kidney problems. People who have or have had **kidney disease** should be cautious about using these drugs. All people taking mesalamine should have kidney function tests before and during drug therapy.

Possible Side Effects

Bowel anti-inflammatories are generally well tolerated. Tablets and capsules have the most side effects, suppositories the fewest.

Capsules

- ▼ Less common: abdominal pain, cramps, or discomfort; diarrhea; nausea; headache; respiratory infection; rash; and skin spots.
- ▼ Rare: worsening of colitis, constipation, gas, vomiting, dizziness, fever, sleeplessness, belching, upset stomach, sweating, feeling unwell, tiredness, itching, acne, achy joints, leg or joint pain, muscle aches, conjunctivitis (pinkeye), swelling, and hair loss. Other rare side effects can occur in almost any part of the body. Contact your doctor if you experience anything unusual while taking any medication.

Rectal Suspension

- ▼ Common: abdominal pain, cramps, or discomfort; gas; nausea; headache; and flu-like symptoms.
- ▼ Less common: bloating; diarrhea; hemorrhoids; pain on enema insertion; rectal pain, soreness, or burning; dizziness; fever; feeling unwell; tiredness; cold symptoms; sore throat; itching; rash; skin spots; back pain; leg pain; and joint pain.
- ▼ Rare: constipation, muscle weakness, sleeplessness, swelling, hair loss, and urinary burning or infection. Contact your doctor if you experience anything unusual while taking any medication.

Suppositories

- ▼ Common: headache.
- ▼ Less common: abdominal pain, cramps, or discomfort; diarrhea or frequent stools; worsening of colitis; flatulence or gas; nausea; rectal pain, soreness, or burning; dizziness; dry mouth; fever; sore throat; cold symptoms; acne; rash; skin spots; and swelling.

Tablets

- ▼ Most common: headache; abdominal pain, cramps, or discomfort; diarrhea; belching; nausea; sore throat; and generalized pain.

Possible Side Effects *(continued)*

▼ Common: constipation, upset stomach, vomiting, muscle weakness, dizziness, fever, runny nose, rash, skin spots, achy joints, back pain, and stiff muscles.

▼ Less common: worsening of colitis, gas, chills, sweating, feeling unwell, tiredness, acne, itching, arthritis, chest pain, conjunctivitis (pinkeye), painful menstruation, swelling, depression, feeling lightheaded, appetite loss, sleeplessness, and flu-like symptoms.

▼ Rare: sleeplessness, hair loss, leg or joint pain, and urinary burning or infection. Other rare side effects can occur in almost any part of the body. Contact your doctor if you experience anything unusual while taking any medication.

Drug Interactions

- Mesalamine should be used with caution with drugs that can cause kidney damage, such as nonsteroidal anti-inflammatory drugs (NSAIDs) due to increased risk for effects on the kidneys.
- When mesalamine is combined with azathioprine or mercaptopurine, the potential for blood disorders may be increased. Blood monitoring is necessary and dosages may need adjusting.
- The anticoagulant effects of warfarin may be reduced by mesalamine and olsalazine.

Food Interactions

Take the tablet and capsule with food.

Usual Dose

Balsalazide

Adult: 2250 mg 3 times a day for 8 weeks. Treatment may be required for up to 12 weeks.

Child (age 5–17): 750–2250 mg 3 times a day for 8 weeks.

Child (under age 5): not recommended.

Mesalamine

Adult

Tablets and Capsules: 1500–4000 mg a day for up to 6 months.

Once-Daily Tablets or Capsules: 2–4 pills once a day with a meal.

Suppositories: one 1000-mg suppository at bedtime for 3–6 weeks. Retain the suppository for 1–3 hours for maximum benefit.

Rectal Suspension: 1 bottle of suspension taken as an enema at bedtime every night for 3–6 weeks. The enema liquid should be retained for about 8 hours.

Child: not recommended.

Olsalazine

Adult: 1000 mg a day in 2 divided doses.

Child: not recommended.

Overdosage

Symptoms of overdose are likely to include ringing or buzzing in the ears, fainting or dizziness, headache, lethargy, confusion, drowsiness, sweating, rapid breathing, vomiting, and diarrhea. In case of overdose, contact your local poison control center or hospital emergency room. You may be told to induce vomiting with ipecac syrup—available at any pharmacy—before taking the victim to the emergency room. If you seek treatment, ALWAYS bring the prescription bottle or container.

Special Information

The tablets and capsules must be swallowed whole. Contact your doctor if they are visible in your stool. When using suppositories, handle them as little as possible to prevent melting.

Contact your doctor if you develop chest pain, breathing or urinary difficulties, fever, unusual bleeding or bruising, worsening of colitis, or any bothersome or persistent side effects.

If you forget to administer a dose, do so as soon as you remember. If you take a tablet or capsule and it is within 4 hours of your next dose, skip the dose you forgot and continue with your regular schedule. If you take the suppositories or rectal solution and you do not remember until it is almost time for the next dose, skip the one you forgot and continue with your regular schedule. Do not take a double dose.

Special Populations

Pregnancy/Breast-feeding: Bowel anti-inflammatories can pass into the fetal circulation. A bowel anti-inflammatory should be taken during pregnancy only if your doctor determines that the potential benefit outweighs the risks.

Small amounts of these drugs can pass into breast milk. Nursing mothers who must take these drugs should consider using infant formula.

Seniors: Seniors may use these drugs without special precaution.

Generic Name

Brimonidine (brim-ON-ih-dene) G

Brand Names

Alphagan P

Type of Drug

Alpha agonist.

Prescribed For

Glaucoma and ocular hypertension (high pressure inside the eye).

General Information

Brimonidine stimulates alpha-2 receptors in the eye and lowers pressure there. The maximum effect occurs 2 hours after the drops are administered. Brimonidine reduces the amount of aqueous humor (liquid) produced inside the eye and increases the rate at which fluid flows out of the eyeball. That portion of brimonidine that finds its way into the bloodstream is broken down by the liver.

Cautions and Warnings

Do not use brimonidine if you are **allergic** or **sensitive** to any of its ingredients.

People with **kidney or liver disease** should use this drug with caution. People with **cardiovascular disease** should exercise caution with this medication because it can affect blood pressure. It should be used with caution in people with **depression**, **cerebral or coronary insufficiency**, and **Raynaud's disease**.

Brimonidine may cause fatigue, drowsiness, and dizziness or fainting when rising from a sitting or lying position.

Brimonidine's effectiveness may decrease over time. Your doctor should check your eye pressure periodically to make sure the drug is still working.

Possible Side Effects

- ▼ Most common: dry mouth; redness, burning, and stinging of the eye; headache; blurred vision; sensation of something in the eye; drowsiness; and eye allergy and itching.
- ▼ Common: staining or erosion of the cornea, unusual sensitivity to bright light, eyelid redness or swelling, eye pain or ache, dry eye, respiratory symptoms, dizziness, eye

Possible Side Effects *(continued)*

irritation, upset stomach, weakness, abnormal vision, and muscle pain.

▼ Less common: crusty deposit on the eyelid, eye bleeding, abnormal taste sensation, sleeplessness, eye discharge, high blood pressure, anxiety, depression, heart palpitations, dry nose, and fainting.

Drug Interactions

- Do not combine brimonidine with monoamine oxidase inhibitor (MAOI) antidepressants.
- Brimonidine may enhance the effects of alcohol, barbiturates, sedatives, anesthetics, beta-blocking drugs, blood-pressure-lowering drugs, and cardiac glycosides.
- Tricyclic antidepressants can increase the breakdown of brimonidine.

Usual Dose

Adult and Child (age 2 and over): 1 drop in the affected eye every 8 hours, 3 times a day.

Child (under age 2): not recommended.

Overdosage

Little is known about the effects of accidental ingestion. Victims should be taken to a hospital emergency room for treatment. If you seek treatment, ALWAYS bring the prescription bottle or container.

Special Information

If you wear soft contact lenses, wait at least 15 minutes between the time you put the drops in your eye and when you put your lenses in.

To prevent possible infection, do not allow the dropper to touch your fingers, eyelids, or any surface. Wait at least 5 minutes before using any other eye drops.

Brimonidine may make you drowsy. Be careful while driving or doing anything else that requires concentration while you are taking this drug.

It is important that brimonidine be used according to your doctor's directions. If you forget to administer a dose of brimonidine, do so as soon as you remember. If it is almost time for your next dose, skip the dose you forgot and continue with your regular schedule. Do not take a double dose.

Special Populations

Pregnancy/Breast-feeding: A small amount of brimonidine may pass into the circulation of the fetus. Brimonidine should be used during pregnancy only if your doctor determines that the potential benefit outweighs the risks.

It is not known if brimonidine passes into breast milk. Nursing mothers who must use this drug should use infant formula.

Seniors: Seniors may use brimonidine without special precaution.

Generic Name

Bupropion (bue-PROE-pee-on) G

Brand Names

Generic Ingredients: Bupropion Hydrobromide
Aplenzin

Generic Ingredients: Bupropion Hydrochloride
Budeprion SR
Budeprion XL
Buproban
Wellbutrin
Wellbutrin SR
Wellbutrin XL
Zyban

Type of Drug

Antidepressant and smoking deterrent.

Prescribed For

Depression, seasonal affective disorder (Wellbutrin XL), and nicotine addiction (Zyban).

General Information

Bupropion is used for major depression and seasonal affective disorder and may work as a smoking deterrent by acting on key hormone systems in the brain. It works primarily on dopamine and noradrenaline, unlike the selective serotonin reuptake inhibitor (SSRI) antidepressants, which primarily work on serotonin. Bupropion may not act until you have taken it for 2–4 weeks. The drug clears your system about 2 weeks after you stop taking it.

Cautions and Warnings

Do not take bupropion if you are **allergic** or **sensitive** to any of its ingredients.

Antidepressants have been associated with an increased risk of suicide, especially in **children** and **teenagers**. Suicide is always a risk in depressed people, who should only be allowed to have minimal quantities of medication in their possession. Clinical worsening of a depressed person's condition may also occur early in therapy with antidepressants. People taking bupropion for smoking cessation should also be vigilant for symptoms of agitation, hostility, depressed mood, changes in thinking or behavior that are not typical, and talking about suicide or suicidal behavior. Caregivers should also be alert.

People with **seizure disorders**, people who have had a seizure in the past, and people with **bulimia** or **anorexia nervosa** should not take bupropion because they are at a higher risk of having a seizure. About 4 in 1000 people taking bupropion in dosages up to 450 mg a day develop a seizure. The risk of developing a seizure increases by about 10 times with dosages between 450 and 600 mg a day. About ½ of the people who developed a seizure on bupropion had a risk factor such as a history of head injury, a previous seizure, or a nervous system tumor, or they were taking another drug associated with increased seizure risk.

People who have abruptly stopped drinking alcohol or taking sedatives should not be prescribed bupropion.

People with unstable **heart disease** or those who have had a recent **heart attack** should take this drug with caution because of possible side effects.

Many people taking bupropion experience some restlessness, agitation, anxiety, and sleeplessness, especially soon after they start taking the drug. Some even require sleeping pills to counter this effect, and others find the stimulation so severe that they have to stop taking bupropion.

Bupropion may trigger a manic episode in those with **depression** or **bipolar disorder**.

People taking bupropion may experience hallucinations, delusions, or psychotic episodes. Dosage reduction or drug withdrawal is usually necessary to manage these reactions.

One-quarter of those who take bupropion lose their appetite and 5 or more lbs. of body weight. People who have lost weight due to their depression should be cautious about taking bupropion.

People switching from bupropion to a **monoamine oxidase inhibitor (MAOI) antidepressant**, or vice versa, should allow at least 2 weeks to pass between stopping 1 drug and starting the other.

People with **kidney or liver disease** require less bupropion at the beginning of treatment. Dosage should be increased cautiously.

An antidepressant other than bupropion should be seriously considered for people with a history of **drug abuse** because of the mild stimulation bupropion causes. These people may require larger-than-usual dosages, but they are still susceptible to seizures at these higher dosages.

Possible Side Effects

About 10% of people stop taking bupropion due to side effects.

▼ Most common: dry mouth; dizziness; rapid heartbeat; headache, including migraine; excessive sweating; nausea; vomiting; constipation; appetite loss; weight changes; sedation; agitation; sleeplessness; and tremors.

▼ Less common: upset stomach; diarrhea; increased appetite; menstrual complaints; impotence; urinary difficulties; slowness of movement; salivation; muscle spasms; warmth; uncontrolled muscle movement; compulsion to move around or change positions; abnormal heart rhythms; blood-pressure changes; heart palpitations; fainting; itching; redness and rash; confusion; hostility; loss of concentration; reduced sex drive; anxiety; delusions; euphoria (feeling "high"); fatigue; joint pain; fever or chills; respiratory infection; and visual, taste, and hearing disturbances.

Drug Interactions

- Phenelzine (an MAOI) increases the risk of bupropion side effects. Allow at least 2 weeks to pass between stopping an MAOI and starting bupropion. Serious side effects can occur.
- Do not mix bupropion with other drugs that increase the risk of seizures, including antidepressants, antipsychotics, systemic steroids, and theophylline.
- Use of bupropion and linezolid should be avoided. The risk of serious high blood pressure may be increased with this combination.
- Bupropion should be administered with caution with certain antidepressants (such as desipramine, fluoxetine, imipramine, nortriptyline, paroxetine, and sertraline), antipsychotics (such as haloperidol, risperidone, and thioridazine),

beta blockers (such as metoprolol), type 1C antiarrhythmics (such as flecainide or propafenone), iloperidone, and tamoxifen. When people are taking bupropion, dosages of these medications should be initiated at the lower end of the dose range.

- Careful monitoring should occur when bupropion is administered with guanfacine. The risk of bupropion toxicity is increased with this combination.
- Carbamazepine, efavirenz, phenobarbital, phenytoin, rifamycins, and ritonavir may reduce blood concentrations of bupropion.
- People taking both bupropion and carbidopa + levodopa or amantadine experience increased side effects. People taking these drugs should have their bupropion dosage increased gradually.
- Cyclosporine concentrations may be reduced when bupropion is added. Monitoring of cyclosporine levels should occur whenever bupropion is started or stopped.
- Combining bupropion with a nicotine-replacement drug can cause high blood pressure.
- Combining bupropion with cimetidine, clopidogrel, or ticlopidine can increase the risk of bupropion side effects.
- Do not combine Wellbutrin and Zyban, as they contain the same active ingredient.
- The risk of seizures may be increased when bupropion is combined with tiagabine.
- Taking bupropion with an anticoagulant such as warfarin may increase the blood-clotting effects of warfarin.
- People taking bupropion should avoid alcohol.

Food Interactions

Bupropion may be taken with food if it upsets your stomach.

Usual Dose

Bupropion Hydrobromide

Depression

Adult: 174–522 mg a day; normal daily dosage is 348 mg.
Child: not recommended.

Bupropion Hydrochloride

Depression

Adult: 200–450 mg a day; normal daily dosage is 300 mg.
Child: not recommended.

Smoking Cessation

Adult: 150 mg twice a day. Begin treatment while you are still smoking.

Child: not recommended.

Overdosage

Symptoms of overdose are likely to include severe side effects, such as seizures—present in ⅓ of overdoses—hallucinations, loss of consciousness, and abnormal heart rhythms. Overdose victims should be taken to a hospital emergency room at once. If you seek treatment, ALWAYS bring the prescription bottle or container.

Special Information

Do not stop taking bupropion without your doctor's knowledge. Suddenly stopping the drug may cause withdrawal reactions and side effects.

Contact your doctor if you experience agitation or excitement, restlessness, confusion, difficulty sleeping, anxiety, panic attacks, sleeplessness, irritability, hostility, aggressiveness, acting impulsively, a manic reaction, deepening depression, suicidal thinking, fast or abnormal heart rhythm, severe headache, seizure, rash, fainting, or any unusual or persistent side effect.

Bupropion may make you tired, dizzy, or lightheaded. Be careful when driving or doing any task that requires concentration.

Alcohol, sedatives, and other nervous system depressants increase the depressant effects of this drug. Alcohol also increases the risk of a seizure.

If you forget a dose, take it as soon as you remember. If it is almost time for your next dose and you take it several times a day, take 1 dose as soon as you remember and another in 3 or 4 hours, then go back to your regular schedule. Do not take a double dose.

Special Populations

Pregnancy/Breast-feeding: The safety of using bupropion during pregnancy is not known. Bupropion should be taken during pregnancy only if your doctor determines that the potential benefit outweighs the risks. Pregnant women trying to quit smoking should use nondrug methods until their pregnancy is completed.

Bupropion passes into breast milk. Nursing mothers who must use bupropion should use infant formula.

Seniors: Seniors with reduced kidney or liver function may require a reduced dosage.

Buspirone (bue-SPYE-rone) G

Brand Names

BuSpar

Type of Drug

Minor sedative and antianxiety drug.

Prescribed For

Anxiety and generalized anxiety disorders; also prescribed for the aches, pains, fatigue, and cramps of premenstrual syndrome (PMS).

General Information

Buspirone has a potent antianxiety effect. It is approved by the U.S. Food and Drug Administration for short-term relief of anxiety, but it may apparently be used safely for more than 4 weeks. The exact way in which buspirone works is not known, but it seems to lack the addiction dangers associated with other antianxiety drugs, including benzodiazepines. It neither severely depresses the nervous system nor acts as an anticonvulsant or muscle relaxant, as other antianxiety drugs do. Minor improvement will be apparent after only 7–10 days of drug treatment, but the maximum effect does not occur for 3 or 4 weeks.

Cautions and Warnings

Do not take buspirone if you are **allergic** or **sensitive** to any of its ingredients.

Buspirone should be used cautiously by people with **liver or kidney disease** and not at all by those with severe disease.

Buspirone does not have any antipsychotic effect and should not be taken for symptoms of **psychosis**.

Although buspirone has not shown a potential for drug abuse, you should be aware of this possibility.

Buspirone should not be used with **monoamine oxidase inhibitor (MAOI) antidepressants**.

Possible Side Effects

- ▼ Most common: dizziness, drowsiness, nausea, and headache.
- ▼ Common: fatigue, nervousness, lightheadedness, excitement, dry mouth, and insomnia.
- ▼ Less common: heart palpitations, muscle aches and pains, tremors, rash, sweating, clamminess, rapid heartbeat,

Possible Side Effects *(continued)*

difficulty concentrating, anger or hostility, depression, loss of interest, diarrhea, constipation, vomiting, and blurred vision.

▼ Rare: Rare side effects can occur in almost any part of the body. Contact your doctor if you experience anything unusual while taking any medication.

Drug Interactions

- Combining buspirone with an MAOI antidepressant may produce severe hypertension and may be dangerous. These medications should not be combined.
- The effects of combining buspirone with other drugs that work in the central nervous system (CNS) are not known. Do not take other sedatives or antianxiety or psychoactive drugs with buspirone unless prescribed by a doctor familiar with your complete medical history.
- When buspirone is combined with cimetidine, buspirone concentrations may be elevated.
- Erythromycin, itraconazole, ketoconazole, clarithromycin, diltiazem, verapamil, fluvoxamine, and ritonavir may increase blood levels of buspirone. When used in combination, your buspirone dosage may need to be adjusted.
- Buspirone may increase the side effects of haloperidol and diazepam.
- Studies show that buspirone is not affected by alcohol, but this combination should still be used with caution because buspirone causes drowsiness and dizziness.
- The combination of buspirone and trazodone may cause liver inflammation.
- Nefazodone may increase buspirone side effects. A lower buspirone dose may be necessary.
- Combining rifampin, rifabutin, phenytoin, phenobarbitol, carbamazepine, or dexamethasone with buspirone may decrease buspirone's effectiveness.

Food Interactions

This drug may be taken either with or without food, but for the most consistent results, always take your dose at the same time of day in the same way—that is, with or without food. Avoid drinking large amounts of grapefruit juice with this drug.

Usual Dose

Adult: starting dose—7.5 mg twice a day. Dosage may be increased gradually to 60 mg a day.

Overdosage

Symptoms of overdose are nausea, vomiting, dizziness, drowsiness, pinpoint pupils, and upset stomach. The overdose victim should be taken to a hospital emergency room. If you seek treatment, ALWAYS bring the prescription bottle or container.

Special Information

Buspirone may cause CNS depression, drowsiness, and dizziness. Be careful while driving or operating hazardous equipment. Avoid other CNS drugs and alcoholic beverages because they will enhance buspirone's effects.

Contact your doctor if you become restless, develop uncontrolled or repeated movements of the head, face, or neck, or have any intolerable side effects.

If you forget a dose, take it as soon as you remember. If it is almost time for your next dose, skip the dose you forgot and go back to your regular schedule. Do not take a double dose.

Special Populations

Pregnancy/Breast-feeding: Though buspirone has not been found to cause birth defects, be sure to inform your doctor if you are or might be pregnant while taking this drug. Buspirone should be taken during pregnancy only if your doctor determines that the potential benefit outweighs the risks.

It is not known how much buspirone passes into breast milk. Nursing mothers who must take this drug should use infant formula.

Seniors: Several hundred seniors participated in drug evaluation studies without any unusual problems. However, the effect of this drug in seniors is not well known, and special problems may surface, particularly in those with kidney or liver disease.

Generic Name

Butenafine (bue-TEN-uh-fene)

Brand Names

Mentax Mentax-TC

The information in this profile also applies to the following drugs:

Generic Ingredients: Terbinafine

Desenex Max
Lamisil AT
Lamisil
Terbinex

Type of Drug

Antifungal.

Prescribed For

Fungal infections of the skin, fingernails or toenails; athlete's foot; jock itch; and ringworm.

General Information

Butenafine works by blocking the natural synthesis of a chemical—ergosterol—essential to the cell membrane (outer skin) of the fungus cell. Butenafine may actually kill the fungus if enough of it is present. Some butenafine is absorbed into the bloodstream.

Terbinafine is a general-purpose antifungal that also works against *Candida* and other fungal infections of the skin. Terbinafine is unique because it accumulates in the skin and continues to kill the fungus even after you stop using it. Most other antifungals do not kill the fungus; they only stop it from growing.

Cautions and Warnings

Do not use butenafine or terbinafine if you are **allergic** or **sensitive** to any of its ingredients.

Terbinafine is not recommended for those with **kidney or liver disease.**

Terbinafine may precipitate symptoms of **systemic lupus erythematosus** (a chronic autoimmune disease). People with pre-existing lupus should not use terbinafine.

Terbinafine should be used only for specific fungal infections and only as prescribed. Rarely, people taking terbinafine have experienced severe eyesight changes or a severe drop in white-blood-cell count, leading to serious infection and fever. Serious skin reactions to terbinafine have been reported; if skin rash occurs, contact your doctor immediately.

Possible Side Effects

Butenafine

▼ Common: rash, burning, stinging, worsening of the infection, swelling, irritation, and itching.

Possible Side Effects *(continued)*

Terbinafine

Topical

- ▼ Most common: itching and irritation of the skin immediately after application.
- ▼ Less common: burning, irritation, and dryness of the skin.

Oral

- ▼ Most common: headache.
- ▼ Common: diarrhea and rash (including psoriasis-type rashes or worsening psoriasis and pinhead-sized pustules).
- ▼ Less common: upset stomach, abdominal pain, nausea, gas, itching, liver irritation, taste changes, and temporary eyesight changes.
- ▼ Rare: aching joints and muscles, yellowing of the skin or whites of the eyes, loss of appetite, severe reactions of the liver or skin, low white-blood-cell count, and allergic reactions. Contact your doctor if you experience anything unusual while taking any medication.

Drug Interactions

- When you apply these medicines to your skin, do not mix them with any other topical medication, unless directed to do so by your doctor.
- Cimetidine and fluconazole increase the amount of terbinafine in the blood.
- Do not combine terbinafine and rifampin.
- Terbinafine may reduce the effect of cyclosporine.
- When terbinafine is combined with certain antiarrythmic medications or beta blockers, terbinafine levels may be increased, requiring additional monitoring and dosage adjustments.
- Terbinafine may increase the effect of caffeine.
- Terbinafine may raise blood levels of dextromethorphan, certain monoamine oxidase inhibitor (MAOI) drugs, selective serotonin reuptake inhibitors (SSRI), and tricyclic antidepressants.
- Warfarin levels may increase or decrease when taken with terbinafine.

Food Interactions

Take terbinafine tablets 1 hour before or 2 hours after eating.

Usual Dose

Butenafine

Adult and Child (age 12 and over): Apply enough to cover the affected area and surrounding skin once a day for 2–4 weeks, or twice a day for 1 week. Wash your hands after each application.

Child (under age 12): not recommended.

Terbinafine

Cream

Adult and Child (age 12 and over): Apply to affected areas morning and night for 1–4 weeks. Wash your hands after each application.

Child (under age 12): Consult your doctor.

Spray

Adult and Child (age 12 and over): once or twice a day for 1 week.

Child (under age 12): Consult your doctor.

Tablets

Adult: 250 mg a day for 6–12 weeks, depending on the condition being treated.

Child: 125–250 mg a day for 6 weeks, depending on body weight.

Overdosage

Terbinafine overdose may lead to nausea, vomiting, abdominal pain, dizziness, rash, frequent urination, and headache. Little is known about the effect of swallowing butenafine. Overdose victims should be taken to a hospital emergency room. If you seek treatment, ALWAYS bring the prescription bottle or container.

Special Information

These drugs may irritate sensitive skin. Contact your doctor if this happens—another medication may be more appropriate. Also contact your doctor if you experience redness, itching, burning, blistering, swelling, or oozing.

Athlete's foot is relatively common and may be caused by a number of different kinds of fungi. Do not use these drugs without your doctor's knowledge.

These topical medications are to be applied only to your skin. They should not be applied to other areas, including the eyes, nose, mouth, or vagina.

Do not bandage the area where the medication has been applied unless otherwise directed by your doctor.

If you apply the cream after bathing, be sure that your feet are completely dry, especially the areas between your toes. Do not wear socks made from wool or synthetic material or shoes that do not have adequate ventilation.

As is often the case when using an anti-infective, your symptoms may begin to improve before you have completed the full course of treatment. Be sure to use all of the medication as directed. If you are taking butenafine for jock itch or ringworm, wear loose-fitting clothing and keep the area cool and dry.

Contact your doctor if the condition does not improve after 4 weeks of using the cream.

If you forget to administer a dose, do so as soon as you remember. If it is almost time for your next dose, skip the one you forgot and continue with your regular schedule.

Special Populations

Pregnancy/Breast-feeding: Butenafine should be taken during pregnancy only if your doctor determines that the potential benefit outweighs the risks. The effect of taking terbinafine during pregnancy is not known. Women who are pregnant should not use terbinafine because the treatment of toenail or fingernail fungal infections can be postponed until after pregnancy.

Terbinafine passes into breast milk. Nursing mothers who must use this drug should use infant formula. It is not known if butenafine passes into breast milk. Nursing mothers who must use this drug should use infant formula.

Seniors: Seniors may use this medication without special precaution.

Bystolic *see **Beta Blockers,** page 166*

Generic Name

C1 Esterase Inhibitors (ESS-tuh-raze)

Brand Names

Berinert
Cinryze

Type of Drug

Serine protease inhibitor.

Prescribed For

Type I and II hereditary angioedema.

General Information

Hereditary angioedema (HAE) is a very rare and potentially life-threatening genetic disease accounting for 0.4% of all cases of angioedema. HAE symptoms include edema (swelling) in various body parts, including the hands, feet, genitals, face, and airway or throat. Swelling in the intestinal wall can cause severe abdominal pain, nausea, and vomiting. There are 3 types of HAE. Type I HAE is defined by low blood levels of a protein in the body called C1 inhibitor. Type II HAE is characterized by the presence of normal or high blood levels of a dysfunctional form of C1 inhibitor. Type III HAE is an estrogen-dependent inherited form of angioedema occurring mainly in women; C1 inhibitor proteins function normally and are present in normal amounts in type III HAE.

Cinryze is used to prevent HAE attacks, while Berinert is used to treat them. Both of these C1 esterase inhibitors are given by intravenous (IV) injection. Anyone trained in the proper administration of IV medicines may give this drug, including patients who can self-administer it during an HAE attack.

Cautions and Warnings

Do not use C1 esterase inhibitors if you are **allergic** or **sensitive** to any of their ingredients. Symptoms of an allergic reaction include hives, itching, chest tightness, wheezing, low blood pressure, dizziness, or fainting during or after injecting this medicine. Call your doctor if you experience any of these symptoms.

Laryngeal edema (throat closing) is the most dangerous of all HAE symptoms. If you must treat yourself for a laryngeal attack, contact your doctor immediately afterward.

Blood clotting may occur after C1 esterase inhibitor is injected, especially if used at larger than recommended doses. Call your doctor if you experience any of the following signs of a blood clot: new swelling; pain in the arms, legs or abdomen; chest pain; difficulty breathing; loss of feeling or ability to control movements; loss of consciousness; or vision or speech changes.

This product is made from human blood plasma and may contain infectious viruses and other agents.

Possible Side Effects

- ▼ Common: headache, nausea, and abdominal pain.
- ▼ Less common: taste changes, vomiting, muscle spasms, and pain.
- ▼ Rare: viral infections, injection-site pain and redness, chills, and fever. Contact your doctor if you experience anything unusual while taking any medication.

Drug Interactions

None known.

Usual Dose

Berinert

Adult and Child (age 12 and over): 9 units per lb. of body weight by IV injection at a rate of 4 mL per minute.

Child (under age 12): not recommended.

Cinryze

Adult and Child (age 12 and over): 1000 units by IV injection at a rate of 1 mL per minute for 10 minutes every 3–4 days.

Child (under age 12): not recommended.

Overdosage

Blood clotting has occurred in newborns and young children given high doses of this drug during or after heart surgery. In case of an overdose, take the victim to a hospital emergency room for monitoring and treatment. If you seek treatment, ALWAYS bring the prescription bottle or container.

Special Information

Because this product is injected directly into a vein, it is important to have epinephrine available at all times in case of a hypersensitivity reaction (see "Cautions and Warnings").

Talk to your doctor when planning a trip. Make sure to take a sufficient supply of C1 esterase inhibitor with you and prepare for proper medication storage (refrigeration) at your destination.

Patients and caregivers who give this medicine must be trained to recognize HAE symptoms and when and how to mix each medication dose and prepare it for IV administration. Follow your doctor's instructions and record the lot number of each vial of medicine you use for future reference.

Special Populations

Pregnancy/Breast-feeding: The effect of this drug on a growing fetus is not known. Make sure your doctor knows if you are pregnant or intend to become pregnant while using this medication. Pregnant women have taken up to 3500 units during pregnancy to treat an HAE attack with no ill effects, but this drug should be taken during pregnancy only if your doctor determines that the potential benefit outweighs the risks.

It is not known if this drug passes into breast milk. Nursing mothers who must take this medicine should use infant formula.

Seniors: Too few seniors have taken this drug to determine if they respond differently than younger adults.

Generic Name

Calcitonin (kal-sih-TOE-nin) G

Brand Names

Fortical
Miacalcin

Type of Drug

Polypeptide hormone.

Prescribed For

Osteoporosis (condition characterized by loss of bone mass due to depletion of minerals, especially calcium) in postmenopausal women.

General Information

Calcitonin helps to strengthen bone by adding more calcium to it and slowing the natural process by which bone is broken down. The calcitonin used in this drug is essentially identical to human calcitonin except that it is more potent. It is a synthetic version of the natural calcitonin found in salmon. Calcitonin can increase bone density and reduce the risk of fractures of the vertebrae (bones that comprise the spinal column), which are associated with back pain and loss of height. Calcitonin has been available for years as an injection, but the development of the nasal spray makes the drug easier to use.

Cautions and Warnings

Do not use calcitonin if you are **allergic** or **sensitive** to any of its ingredients. Serious allergic reactions are possible with this medication.

Changes in the tissues lining your nose are possible with long-term use of this product. An initial nasal examination and then periodic examinations are recommended.

Possible Side Effects

- ▼ Most common: stuffy nose, runny nose, and other nasal symptoms; and back pain.
- ▼ Less common: joint pain, nosebleed, and headache.

Drug Interactions

None known.

Usual Dose

Adult: 1 spray (200 IU) a day.

Child: not recommended.

Overdosage

Little is known about the effects of calcitonin overdose or accidental ingestion. Nausea and vomiting have been reported after high doses. Contact your local poison control center for more information. Overdose victims should be taken to a hospital emergency room. If you seek treatment, ALWAYS bring the prescription bottle or container.

Special Information

Alternate nostrils daily when using the nasal spray.

Before you take your first dose, you must activate the pump. Hold the bottle upright and press the two white arms toward the bottle 6 times until a faint spray is emitted. Once this occurs, the pump is activated and ready for use. It is not necessary to reactivate the pump every day.

Store new, unassembled bottles in the refrigerator. Keep the bottle in use at room temperature and discard after 30 days.

If you forget to administer a dose of the nasal spray, do so as soon as you remember. If it is almost time for the next dose, skip the dose you forgot and continue with your regular schedule. Contact your doctor if you forget 2 or more doses.

Contact your doctor if you develop severe nose irritation or any unusual or intolerable symptom. Follow your doctor's recommendations regarding calcium and vitamin D supplements. This drug is not intended to replace the need for dietary calcium.

Special Populations

Pregnancy/Breast-feeding: Calcitonin does not cross into the fetal circulation, though animal studies have associated the injectable form of the drug with low birth weight. Calcitonin should be used during pregnancy only if your doctor determines that the potential benefit outweighs the risks.

It is not known if calcitonin passes into breast milk, though animal studies have shown that it reduces the amount of milk produced. Nursing mothers who must use calcitonin should use infant formula.

Seniors: Seniors may use this product without special precaution.

Generic Name

Calcitriol (kal-SIH-tree-ohl)

Brand Names

Vectical Ointment

Type of Drug

Vitamin D analogue.

Prescribed For

Mild to moderate plaque psoriasis.

General Information

Calcitriol is a form of vitamin D that has been prescribed for kidney disease and osteoporosis for many years. When applied to psoriasis lesions, it helps them to improve, but the exact way it produces this effect is not known. Up to ¼ of people using calcitriol showed improvement. Calcitriol ointment should be used only for mild to moderate psoriasis. It is not approved for more serious forms of psoriasis.

Cautions and Warnings

Do not use calcitriol if you are **allergic** or **sensitive** to any of its ingredients.

Calcitriol is a potent form of vitamin D and, as such, can affect your calcium and bones. Your doctor will test your blood calcium and may temporarily stop this drug if the level is too high. It is not yet known if people with pre-existing calcium disorders should avoid this product.

Calcitriol ointment intensifies the effects of natural and artificial sunlight on your skin, increasing the risk of skin cancer.

Possible Side Effects

- ▼ Most common: raised blood-calcium levels (usually within 10% of normal).
- ▼ Common: abnormal laboratory tests.
- ▼ Less common: urine abnormality, skin discomfort, itching, psoriasis, and calcium in the urine.
- ▼ Rare: kidney stones, skin blistering, rash, redness and itching, and burning sensation with discomfort. Contact your doctor if you experience anything unusual while taking any medication.

Drug Interactions

- This drug should be used with caution by people taking medicines that can affect blood-calcium levels, including thiazide diuretics, calcium and vitamin D supplements, and osteoporosis medicines.

Usual Dose

Adult: Apply to psoriasis plaques morning and night. Do not use more than 2 large tubes per week.

Child: not recommended.

Overdosage

Applying excess quantities of this product can cause drug side effects, especially high blood calcium. Do not use more than 2 large tubes per week. Overdose victims should be taken to a hospital emergency room. If you seek treatment, ALWAYS bring the prescription bottle or container.

Special Information

Calcitriol ointment intensifies the effects of natural and artificial sunlight on your skin, increasing the risk of skin cancer. Wear protective clothing and avoid direct sun exposure to areas where you have applied it. Do not use a sunlamp or tanning booth while using this product.

Do not apply this ointment to sensitive areas such as your lips, face, eyes, or vagina.

Special Populations

Pregnancy/Breast-feeding: Oral calcitriol is toxic to the developing fetus. Some calcitriol will be absorbed into the bloodstream from this ointment, but the exact amount cannot be predicted. Calcitriol should be used during pregnancy only if your doctor determines that the potential benefit outweighs the risks.

It is not known if calcitriol passes into breast milk. Nursing mothers who must use calcitriol should use infant formula.

Seniors: Seniors may use this product without special precaution.

Type of Drug

Calcium Channel Blockers

Generic Ingredients: Amlodipine G
Norvasc

Generic Ingredients: Diltiazem G
Cardizem
Cardizem CD
Cardizem LA
Cartia XT
Dilacor XR
Dilt-CD
Dilt-XR
Diltia XT
Diltzac
Matzim LA
Taztia XT
Tiazac

Generic Ingredients: Felodipine G

Generic Ingredients: Isradipine G
DynaCirc CR

Generic Ingredients: Nicardipine G
Cardene
Cardene SR

Generic Ingredients: Nifedipine G
Adalat CC
Afeditab CR
Nifediac CC
Nifedical XL
Procardia
Procardia XL

Generic Ingredients: Nimodipine G

Generic Ingredients: Nisoldipine G
Sular

Generic Ingredients: Verapamil G
Calan
Calan SR
Covera-HS
Isoptin SR
Verelan
Verelan PM

Combination Products
Generic Ingredients: Amlodipine + Benazepril G
Lotrel

Generic Ingredients: Amlodipine + Valsartan
Exforge

Generic Ingredients: Verapamil + Trandolapril G
Tarka

Prescribed For

High blood pressure, angina pectoris (brief attacks of chest pain), Prinzmetal's angina, and heart rhythm disorders; may also be prescribed for migraine headache prevention, high blood pressure in children, muscle cramps that do not respond to other therapy, tardive dyskinesia, Raynaud's disease, and gallbladder and kidney stone attacks.

Nimodipine is prescribed only for functional losses after a hemorrhagic (bleeding) stroke and for the prevention of migraine and cluster headaches.

General Information

Currently there are 2 chemical classes of calcium channel blockers available in the United States. The vast majority of these (including nifedipine) belong to the *dihydropyridine* class, widely prescribed for high blood pressure and angina. Verapamil is a *phenylalkylamine* and is often prescribed for angina because it is more selective for heart muscle. Verapamil helps stop spasms of blood vessels in the heart, making it easier to supply oxygen-rich blood to heart muscle. The choice of one calcium channel blocker over another is often based on individual experience. These drugs block the passage of calcium, an essential factor in muscle contraction, into the heart and smooth muscles. Such blockage of calcium interferes with the contraction of these muscles, which in turn dilates (widens) the veins and vessels that supply blood to them. This dilating effect reduces blood pressure, the amount of oxygen used by the heart muscle, and the risk of blood vessel spasm.

These medicines only affect the movement of calcium into muscle cells; they have no effect on calcium levels in the blood.

Lotrel combines the calcium channel blocker amlodipine with the angiotensin-converting enzyme (ACE) inhibitor benazepril. Both drugs are often prescribed individually for hypertension. Lotrel is not intended as a first treatment for hypertension. You should take Lotrel only after you have tried an ACE inhibitor or calcium channel blocker alone and your doctor feels you need an additional drug to control your blood pressure. (See Benazepril, page 7, for more information.)

Other products that combine a calcium channel blocker with another medicine, often for high blood pressure, are prescribed. (See Trandolapril, page 8, and Valsartan, page 98, for more information.)

Cautions and Warnings

Do not take these medicines if you are **allergic** or **sensitive** to any of their ingredients. Sensitivity to one chemical group does not mean you will be sensitive to a member of another chemical group.

The combination products Exforge and Lotrel should not be used during **pregnancy** as injury or death to the fetus can occur.

Patients taking a beta-blocking drug who begin taking these drugs may develop an increase in episodes of **angina**. Angina may also intensify when these drugs are first started, when they are increased, or if they are stopped abruptly.

Diltiazem can slow your heart and interfere with normal electrical conduction. Diltiazem should not be taken by those with the heart conduction disorders **sick sinus syndrome** or second- or third-degree **atrioventricular (AV) block** unless a functioning pacemaker is in place.

Diltiazem should not be taken if you are having a **heart attack** or if you have **lung congestion**. People with **congestive heart failure** or **compromised ventricular function** should take calcium channel blockers with caution, especially in combination with a beta blocker. Congestive heart failure has, on rare occasions, developed in people taking nifedipine.

You should not use nicardipine if you have had a **stroke** or

bleeding in the brain or if you have advanced **narrowing of the arteries**—particularly of the aorta.

Calcium channel blockers may cause low blood pressure, particularly if taken with beta blockers.

Felodipine, isradipine, and nifedipine may cause mild to moderate swelling of the hands and feet.

People with **hypertrophic cardiomyopathy** (progressive weakening and destruction of heart muscle) who are taking up to 720 mg a day of verapamil are at risk of developing severe cardiac side effects. Most of these effects respond to dose reduction, and people generally may continue on verapamil at lower dosages.

Verapamil may slow the transmission of nerve impulses to the muscles of people with **Duchenne's muscular dystrophy**, possibly leading to the failure of respiratory muscles.

People with **kidney disease** or severe **liver disease** may require dosage adjustments. Diltiazem can cause liver damage.

Possible Side Effects

Amlodipine

- ▼ Most common: headache, dizziness or lightheadedness, anxiety, nausea, swelling in the arms or legs, heart palpitations, and flushing.
- ▼ Less common: sleepiness, muscle weakness, cramps or abdominal discomfort, itching, rash, sexual difficulties, wheezing or shortness of breath, muscle cramps, pain, and inflammation.
- ▼ Rare: Rare side effects can occur in almost any part of the body. Contact your doctor if you experience anything unusual while taking any medication.

Diltiazem

- ▼ Common: dizziness; lightheadedness; weakness; headache; and fluid accumulation in the hands, legs, or feet.
- ▼ Less common: low blood pressure; fainting; increase or decrease in heart rate; abnormal heart rhythm; heart failure; nervousness; fatigue; nausea; rash; tingling in the hands or feet; hallucinations; temporary memory loss; difficulty sleeping; diarrhea; vomiting; constipation; upset stomach; itching; unusual sensitivity to sunlight; painful or stiff joints; liver inflammation; and increased urination, especially at night.

Possible Side Effects *(continued)*

Felodipine

- ▼ Most common: swelling in the ankles, feet, or legs; dizziness; lightheadedness; muscle weakness or cramps; facial flushing; and headache.
- ▼ Less common: respiratory infections, cough, tingling in the hands or feet, upset stomach, abdominal pain, chest pain, nausea, constipation, diarrhea, heart palpitations, sore throat, runny nose, back pain, and rash.
- ▼ Rare: Rare side effects can affect the heart, stomach, blood, and joints. It can affect your mood, sex drive, and urinary tract. Contact your doctor if you experience anything unusual while taking any medication.

Isradipine

Isradipine side effects are generally mild and self-limiting.

- ▼ Most common: headache.
- ▼ Less common: low blood pressure; chest pain; abdominal pain; rapid heartbeat; dizziness; diarrhea; a feeling of warmth; nausea; lightheadedness; fatigue and lethargy; itching; rash; flushing; changes in certain blood-cell components; and swelling of the legs, ankles, or feet.

Nicardipine

- ▼ Most common: dizziness or lightheadedness; fluid accumulation in the hands, legs, or feet; headache; weakness or fatigue; heart palpitations; angina; and facial flushing.
- ▼ Less common: low blood pressure; abnormal heart rhythms; fainting; increase or decrease in heart rate; heart failure; nausea; rash; nervousness; tingling in the hands or feet; hallucinations; temporary memory loss; difficulty sleeping; weakness; diarrhea; vomiting; constipation; upset stomach; itching; unusual sensitivity to the sun; painful or stiff joints; liver inflammation; increased urination, especially at night; infection; allergic reactions; sore throat; and hyperactivity.

Nifedipine

Nifedipine side effects are generally mild and rarely cause people to stop taking the drug.

- ▼ Most common: swelling of the ankles, feet, and legs; dizziness or lightheadedness; flushing; a feeling of warmth; and headache.

Possible Side Effects *(continued)*

- ▼ Less common: nausea; weakness, shakiness, or jitteriness; giddiness; muscle cramps, inflammation, and pain; nervousness; mood changes; heart palpitations; heart failure; heart attack; breathing difficulties; coughing; fluid in the lungs; wheezing; stuffy nose; fever and chills; and sore throat.
- ▼ Rare: Rare side effects can occur in the heart, stomach or intestines, urinary tract, and joints and muscles and can affect mental and sexual function, hearing, and balance. Contact your doctor if you experience anything unusual while taking any medication.

Nimodipine

- ▼ Most common: diarrhea, low blood pressure, rash, and headache.
- ▼ Less common: swelling of the arms or legs, high blood pressure, heart failure, rapid heartbeat, changes in the electrocardiogram, depression, memory loss, psychosis, paranoid feelings, hallucinations, nausea, itching, acne, anemia, bleeding or bruising, abnormal blood clotting, flushing, breathing difficulties, stomach bleeding, and muscle cramps.
- ▼ Rare: dizziness, heart attack, liver inflammation or jaundice, vomiting, intestinal blockage, and sexual difficulties. Contact your doctor if you experience anything unusual while taking any medication.

Nisoldipine

- ▼ Most common: headache and swelling in the arms or legs.
- ▼ Common: sore throat, sinus irritation, heart palpitations, and dizziness.
- ▼ Less common: chest pain, nausea, and rash.

Verapamil

Verapamil generally causes fewer side effects than other calcium channel blockers.

Some people taking verapamil have experienced a heart attack and abnormal heart rhythms, but these effects have not been directly linked to verapamil.

- ▼ Most common: rash; low blood pressure; slowed heartbeat; heart failure or lung congestion marked by coughing,

Possible Side Effects *(continued)*

wheezing, or breathing difficulties; tiredness or weakness; swelling of the ankles, feet, or legs; upper-respiratory infection; flu-like symptoms; headache; dizziness; lightheadedness; constipation; and nausea.

▼ Rare: chest pain, rapid or irregular heartbeat, unusual production of breast milk, bleeding or tender gums, fainting, flushing, and feeling warm. Other rare side effects can occur in almost any part of the body. Contact your doctor if you experience anything unusual while taking any medication.

Drug Interactions

- Diltiazem should not be given with macrolide antibiotics such as erythromycin and telithromycin.
- Diltiazem should not be taken concurrently with tolvaptan.
- Mixing dantrolene and verapamil may lead to high blood-calcium levels and heart muscle depression. If you are taking dantrolene, a calcium channel blocker *other* than verapamil should be prescribed for you.
- Carbamazepine, dexamethasone, phenobarbital, phenytoin, rifabutin, rifampin, and St. John's wort should not be combined with nifedipine.
- Flecainide, a drug for abnormal heart rhythms, should not be combined with nifedipine. Flecainide and verapamil should be used together cautiously.
- The combination of nisoldipine and phenytoin should be avoided.
- Verapamil should not be taken with dofetilide or tolvaptan.
- When quinidine and verapamil are taken together, quinidine levels are increased. They should be taken together only when no other alternative exists. The combination of quinidine and verapamil should be avoided in patients with hypertrophic cardiomyopathy.
- Verapamil and beta blockers taken together may cause excessively low blood pressure. Verapamil use should be avoided in people who have any degree of ventricular dysfunction who are taking beta blockers.
- Disopyramide should not be taken within 48 hours of taking verapamil.
- Severe low blood pressure has been reported during fentanyl anesthesia with the combination of a calcium channel

blocker and a beta blocker. Blood-pressure monitoring is necessary during administration.

- Mixing two calcium channel blockers can substantially reduce blood pressure.
- Taking any drug for erectile dysfunction while you are on a calcium channel blocker can lead to an unexpected drop in blood pressure. These medicines should be mixed with caution.
- When amlodipine or verapamil are combined with simvastatin, the risk of muscle disease is increased. Doses of simvastatin should not exceed 20 mg a day.
- Cimetidine increases blood concentrations of diltiazem, isradipine, nicardipine, nifedipine, nimodipine, and verapamil.
- Very slow heart rate has been reported with the combination of diltiazem or verapamil and clonidine.
- Efavirenz and rifampin lower blood levels of diltiazem.
- Taking diltiazem or verapamil with dronedarone causes the effects of both drugs to be increased. Diltiazem or verapamil doses should be initiated at a lower range.
- Moricizine reduces diltiazem levels while diltiazem increases moricizine levels. Monitoring is required when either drug is started, stopped, or adjusted in dosage.
- Protease inhibitors such as ritonavir increase levels of diltiazem.
- The combination of diltiazem or verapamil with anesthetics such as enflurane and halothane may increase the cardiac depressing effects of the anesthetics. Careful monitoring and dosage adjustment are required.
- Diltiazem may also increase the sedative effects of benzodiazepines such as midazolam and triazolam.
- Although diltiazem and beta blockers such as propranolol are generally well tolerated, a dose reduction in the beta blocker may be necessary and monitoring is required.
- Diltiazem may increase the effects of buspirone, carbamazepine, cilostazol, colchicine, corticosteriods, cyclosporine, digoxin, everolimus, quinidine, ranolazine, sirolimus, statin drugs, tacrolimus, and theophylline. Additional monitoring and dosage adjustments may be necessary.
- The potential for serious cardiac arrhythmias exists when isradipine or nicardipine is combined with antiarrhythmic agents (such as amiodarone, bretylium, disopyramide, dofetilide, quinidine, and sotalol), arsenic trioxide, chlorpromazine,

cisapride, dolasetron, droperidol, mefloquine, mesoridazine, moxifloxacin, pentamidine, pimozide, tacrolimus, thioridazine, and ziprasidone.

- Protease inhibitors such as amprenavir, indinavir, nelfinavir, and ritonavir may increase the effects of nicardipine and nifedipine.
- Nicardipine increases the effects of cyclosporine and digoxin.
- When nifedipine is combined with an ACE inhibitor such as benazepril, very low blood pressure and slow heart rate may result. Regular blood-pressure monitoring is necessary.
- Taking doxazosin with nifedipine increases the effects of nifedipine and decreases the effects of doxazosin. Regular blood-pressure monitoring is necessary and nifedipine dosages may need adjusting.
- Azole antifungal medications such as ketoconazole, itraconazole, and voriconazole may increase the effects of nifedipine, nisoldipine, and verapamil, possibly requiring a dosage reduction.
- The combination of nifedipine and a beta blocker such as propranolol may increase the risk of congestive heart failure, severe low blood pressure, and exacerbation of angina in people with cardiovascular disease.
- Nifedipine and delavirdine should be combined cautiously with regular blood-pressure monitoring.
- Cisapride, fluoxetine, *Ginko biloba*, ginseng, imatinib, diuretics such as furosemide and chlorothiazide, certain antibiotics such as erythromycin and telithromycin, methyldopa, nefazodone, prazosin, quinidine, quinupristin, dalfopristin, and valproic acid increase the blood-pressure-lowering effects of nifedipine. Dosage adjustments of nifedipine may be necessary.
- Melatonin and nafcillin decrease the effects of nifedipine. Blood-pressure monitoring should take place whenever these medications are started or stopped in people taking nifedipine.
- Nifedipine may cause hypoglycemia (low blood-sugar levels) in those taking acarbose for diabetes management. Blood-glucose levels should be carefully monitored when these medications are taken concurrently.
- Nifedipine decreases the blood-clotting effects of clopidogrel.
- Nifedipine increases blood levels of digoxin, metformin, tacrolimus, and warfarin. Dosage adjustments of these medications may be necessary when given with nifedipine.

- Quinidine reduces the amount of nisoldipine in the blood, but maximum levels remain unaffected.
- Verapamil should be used with caution with other drugs that treat high blood pressure, such as ACE inhibitors, diuretics, and vasodilators.
- Verapamil interacts with certain drugs used in chemotherapy treatment for cancer. Verapamil blood levels may be reduced by cyclophosphamide, procarbazine, prednisone, vincristine, and the vindesine, adriamycin, and cisplatin drug regimens. Verapamil can increase doxorubicin and paclitaxel concentrations.
- Verapamil's effectiveness and side effects may be reversed by taking calcium supplements or antacids.
- Verapamil may reduce the amount of lithium in your body, leading to a possible loss of mania control, lithium toxicity, and psychotic symptoms.
- Barbiturates, phenytoin and similar antiseizure medicines, rifampin, St. John's wort, and sulfinpyrazone may interfere with verapamil's effects.
- Verapamil increases the effects of alcohol, aspirin, buspirone, carbamazepine, colchicine, cyclosporine, digoxin, eletriptan, eplerenone, everolimus, imipramine, midazolam, muscle relaxants such as pancuronium, prazosin, ranolazine, risperidone, and theophyllines. Blood levels of these drugs should be monitored while taking verapamil and the dosages adjusted as necessary.
- Combining a diuretic and Lotrel lowers blood pressure, possibly excessively.
- Use alcohol cautiously with Lotrel.

Food Interactions

Calcium channel blockers are best taken on an empty stomach, 1 hour before or 2 hours after a meal.

Avoid drinking grapefruit juice if you are taking a calcium channel blocker and be sure to stop drinking or eating grapefruit at least 3 days before you start taking the medicine. Avoid fatty foods when taking nisoldipine.

Usual Dose

Amlodipine

Adult: 5–10 mg once a day. Do not stop taking amlodipine abruptly. The dosage should be gradually reduced over a period of time. Seniors, especially those with liver disease may be more sensitive to the effects of amlodipine.

Child: not recommended.

Amlodipine + Benazepril

Adult: Daily doses range from 2.5 mg of amlodipine and 10 mg of benazepril to 10 mg of amlodipine and 40 mg of benazepril. Dosage depends on your need for each of the 2 ingredients. Small or frail people or those with liver failure should follow dosage recommendations for seniors.

Child: not recommended.

Senior: Start with 2.5 mg of amlodipine and 10 mg of benazepril a day and increase gradually. You may need to take amlodipine and benazepril in separate pills until your daily needs are established.

Diltiazem

Immediate-Release: 120–360 mg a day in 3–4 doses.

Sustained-Release/Extended-Release: 120–540 mg once a day.

Felodipine: 2.5–10 mg a day. No patient should take more than 20 mg a day. Do not stop taking felodipine abruptly. The dosage should be reduced gradually over a period of time to the lowest effective dose.

Isradipine: 5–20 mg a day in 2 doses. Do not stop taking the drug abruptly. The dosage should be reduced gradually over a period of time to the lowest effective dose.

Nicardipine

Immediate-Release: 20–40 mg 3 times a day. People with kidney disease should take 20 mg 3 times a day. People with liver disease should take 20 mg twice a day. Seniors should start with 20 mg 2–3 times a day and increase dosage gradually.

Sustained-Release: 30–60 mg twice a day. People with kidney disease should take 30 mg twice a day.

Nifedipine

Immediate-Release: 10–30 mg 3 times a day. Do not take more than 180 mg a day.

Sustained-Release: 30–60 mg once a day. Do not take more than 120 mg a day.

Nimodipine

Stroke: 60 mg every 4 hours, beginning within 96 hours after the stroke and continuing for 21 days.

Migraine Headache: 40 mg 3 times a day.

Nisoldipine

Adult: starting dose—17 mg a day. Maintenance dose—17–34 mg. Seniors and those with liver disease should start with 8.5 mg a day.

Child: not recommended.

Verapamil: Dosages range between 120–540 mg a day, depending on your condition and dose requirement.

Verapamil + Trandolapril: 1 tablet a day. This sustained-release combination is available in a variety of strengths.

Overdosage

Overdose of these drugs can cause very low blood pressure, slow heartbeat, nausea, weakness, dizziness, drowsiness, confusion, and slurred speech. If you think someone has taken a calcium-channel-blocker overdose, take the victim to a hospital emergency room right away. If you seek treatment, ALWAYS bring the prescription bottle or container.

Special Information

Contact your doctor if you develop constipation, nausea, very low blood pressure, swelling in the arms or legs, worsening angina, swelling in the hands or feet, breathing difficulties, increased heart pain, or dizziness or lightheadedness, or if other side effects are particularly bothersome or persistent. Swelling of the hands or feet may develop within 2 or 3 weeks of starting your medication. The chances of this happening depend on age and dosage. It occurs in fewer than 10% of people under age 50 taking a small dose and in more than 30% of those over age 60 taking a larger one.

Do not open, crush, or chew any sustained-release or long-acting calcium-channel-blocker product. You may notice what looks like a tablet in your stool. This is not a cause for alarm, because some drug products are made in a way that normally releases the medicine without actually destroying the tablet.

If you are taking one of these medications for high blood pressure, be sure to continue taking your medication and follow any instructions for diet restriction or other treatments. Do not suddenly stop taking them. The dose should be gradually reduced to prevent angina from developing.

Some capsules contain liquid medication. When the drug is needed in the blood immediately, or the patient is unable to swallow, the capsules may be punctured and their content squeezed under the tongue; the medication is rapidly absorbed into the blood when taken in this manner. Nifedipine capsules are particularly useful when extremely high blood pressure must be lowered as quickly as possible. Some researchers assert that biting the capsule and swallowing the contents is an even faster way of absorbing the drug.

It is important to maintain good dental hygiene while taking nifedipine and to use extra care when using your toothbrush or dental floss. The drug may make you more susceptible to some infections.

If you forget a dose of calcium channel blocker and you take it 3 or more times a day, take it as soon as you remember. If it is almost time for your next dose, take the dose you forgot and space the rest evenly throughout the remainder of the day. If you take your medicine once or twice a day and forget a dose, take it as soon as you remember. If it is almost time for your next dose, skip the dose you forgot and continue with your regular schedule. Do not take a double dose.

Special Populations

Pregnancy/Breast-feeding: Calcium channel blockers can cross into the fetal blood circulation, and some have been used to treat severe high blood pressure associated with pregnancy without causing any damage to the fetus. Others have been shown to interfere with the development of the fetus and may cause fetal damage or death. Lotrel should not be taken by pregnant women. If you are taking Lotrel and become pregnant, see your doctor at once about changing drugs. Women of childbearing age who must take Lotrel must use an effective contraceptive method. Women who are or might be pregnant should not take a calcium channel blocker without their doctor's knowledge and approval. These medicines should be taken during pregnancy only if your doctor determines that the potential benefit outweighs the risks.

Some calcium channel blockers can pass into breast milk. Nursing mothers who must take one should use infant formula.

Seniors: Seniors can be more sensitive to the effects of these medicines because of normal reductions in liver and kidney function and may require less medicine to achieve the same benefit as younger adults.

Generic Name

Capecitabine (cape-SE-tah-been)

Brand Names

Xeloda

Type of Drug

Antimetabolite.

Prescribed For

Breast cancer and colorectal cancer.

General Information

Capecitabine is prescribed for stages of breast and colorectal cancer in place of 5-FU, an injected drug that has been the basis for many chemotherapy programs. Capecitabine is converted in the body to 5-FU. Unlike many anticancer medications, capecitabine can be taken by mouth and has relatively few serious side effects.

Cautions and Warnings

Do not take capecitabine if you are **allergic** or **sensitive** to any of its ingredients or to 5-FU.

People taking **warfarin** or certain other **blood-thinning medications** are at risk of potentially fatal bleeding when capecitabine is added to their therapy. People taking these medications together should be closely monitored for changes in their response to the blood thinner.

Capecitabine is largely eliminated through the kidneys. People with severe **kidney disease** should not take it. Dose adjustments are required for those with moderate kidney disease.

People with **liver disease** should be carefully monitored by their doctors because capecitabine's effect on the liver is not known.

Capecitabine may reduce fertility.

Capecitabine use is associated with heart and blood-vessel disease. These reactions may be more common in those with a history of **coronary artery disease**.

Capecitabine may cause severe diarrhea. Contact your doctor if you experience symptoms (see "Special Information").

Jaundice has occurred in patients taking capecitabine, requiring an interruption of medication until symptoms resolved.

Possible Side Effects

▼ Most common: diarrhea, constipation, nausea, vomiting, mouth sores, abdominal pain, hand-and-foot syndrome (see "Special Information"), inflammation of the skin, tingling or pain in the hands or feet, fatigue, loss of appetite, low blood-cell counts, eye irritation, and fever.

▼ Common: upset stomach, nail problems, headache, dizziness, sleeplessness, dehydration, swelling, muscle aches, and pain in the arms or legs.

▼ Less common and rare side effects can affect the stomach and intestines; skin; nervous system; tear ducts; lungs and respiratory system; heart and blood vessels; blood, urinary, and reproductive tracts; liver; and other organs. Contact your doctor if you experience anything unusual while taking any medication.

Drug Interactions

- Combining capecitabine with warfarin can cause excessive bleeding.
- Combining antacids and capecitabine can increase the amount of drug absorbed by about 20%. Separate doses of antacids and capecitabine by 2 hours.
- Leucovorin (a drug used in cancer treatment) increases the side effects of 5-FU. This combination has caused death in several seniors.
- When combining capecitabine with phenytoin, doses of phenytoin may need to be reduced due to an increase in side effects.

Food Interactions

Capecitabine should be taken within 30 minutes of a meal to avoid stomach problems.

Usual Dose

Adult: 3000–5600 mg a day, depending on height and weight, in 2 doses. Capecitabine is used in 3-week cycles: 2 weeks on the drug, followed by 1 week off. Dosage may be reduced by 50% in people who experience severe side effects.

Child: not recommended.

Overdosage

Symptoms include nausea, vomiting, diarrhea, bleeding and reduced blood-cell counts, and stomach irritation. Overdose victims should be taken to a hospital emergency room. If you seek treatment, ALWAYS bring the prescription bottle or container.

Special Information

Stop taking capecitabine and contact your doctor if you have 4–6 more bowel movements a day than normal, vomit 2–5 times in 1 day, or become very nauseous. Depending on the severity of your symptoms, your doctor may reduce your dosage.

Capecitabine has caused hand-and-foot syndrome. Symptoms of this condition include numbness, tingling, pain, swelling, redness, skin loss, and blistering of the hands or feet. Stop taking the drug and contact your doctor if you experience any of these symptoms.

People who develop stomatitis (symptoms include swelling, pain, or sores in the area of the mouth or tongue) should stop taking the drug and contact their doctor at once.

Contact your doctor, but do not stop taking the drug, if you develop a fever of 100.5°F or higher or other signs of infection.

If you forget a dose, take it as soon as you remember. If it is almost time for your next dose, take 1 dose right away and space the remaining daily dosage evenly throughout the day. Go back to your regular schedule the next morning. Contact your doctor if you miss more than 2 doses in a row.

Special Populations

Pregnancy/Breast-feeding: Capecitabine can harm the fetus. Effective contraception is absolutely necessary while taking this drug. Capecitabine should be taken during pregnancy only if your doctor determines that the potential benefit outweighs the risks.

It is not known if capecitabine passes into breast milk. Nursing mothers who must take this drug should use infant formula.

Seniors: Seniors may be more sensitive to side effects, especially diarrhea and other stomach problems.

Generic Name

Capsaicin (cap-SAY-sin)

Brand Names

Qutenza Skin Patch 8%

Type of Drug

TRPV1 nerve channel stimulator.

Prescribed For

Pain due to shingles.

General Information

Capsaicin is a synthetic version of capsicum, the active component of chili peppers. It temporarily relieves pain by stimulating and then reducing the number of pain-specific nerve endings where it is applied. It depletes or interferes with substance P, a chemical involved in transmitting pain impulses to the brain. In order for capsaicin to work, your pain must originate in nerves near the surface of the skin, as is the case with shingles. Another treatment may be required in several months due to regrowth of pain receptors into the affected area. Low-dose (0.075%) capsaicin products are used for relieving pain associated with osteoarthritis, rheumatoid arthritis, and diabetic nerve damage. Capsaicin lotions, creams, and gels are sold over the counter to relieve muscle, joint, or nerve pain. Capsaicin is also the active ingredient in pepper spray products used for self-defense.

Cautions and Warnings

Do not take capsaicin if you are **allergic** or **sensitive** to any of its ingredients or if you have ever had a reaction to any other capsaicin product or to hot peppers.

Capsaicin should not be applied to broken or irritated skin.

You may cough or sneeze because of capsaicin irritation during the patch placement process.

Capsaicin can temporarily raise your blood pressure. Make sure your doctor knows if you have **high blood pressure**.

Possible Side Effects

- ▼ Most common: skin redness and pain during application.
- ▼ Common: itching and rash after application of the patch and nausea.
- ▼ Less common: nose and throat irritation, bronchitis, sinusitis, vomiting, and elevated blood pressure.
- ▼ Rare: skin peeling, loss of feeling in treated skin, coughing, and abnormal skin odor.

Drug Interactions

- Do not apply any other capsaicin product to the area where the patch was applied. This can result in pain and damage to the skin.

Food Interactions

This drug can be taken without regard to food or meals. Handling hot peppers during food preparation may temporarily irritate treated areas.

Usual Dose

Adult: 1–4 patches applied to painful areas by a health care professional for 1 hour. The area may be retreated no sooner than 3 months after the previous treatment.

Child: not recommended.

Overdosage

Accidental overdose may occur only during product application. If this happens, the affected area will be cleaned and cooled. Capsaicin is highly irritating and should not be applied near the eyes, nose, or other sensitive tissue.

Special Information

Skin treated with a capsaicin patch can be sensitive to hot showers or baths, sunlight, and vigorous exercise for a few days after treatment.

If capsaicin comes into contact with skin that is not meant to be treated, apply a cleansing gel to the affected area for 1 minute, wipe off with clean gauze, then wash with soap and water.

You may need additional pain relievers during or after capsaicin treatment until it starts working.

Special Populations

Pregnancy/Breast-feeding: Lab studies have not shown that capsaicin applied to the skin damages a developing fetus; however, there is no information on the effect of this product during pregnancy. Capsaicin should be used during pregnancy only if your doctor determines that the potential benefit outweighs the risks.

Capsaicin may pass into breast milk. To minimize the potential for damage to nursing infants, mothers should not nurse on treatment days. Capsaicin is removed from the bloodstream within 3–6 hours after treatment.

Seniors: Seniors may use this product without special restriction.

Generic Name

Carbamazepine (car-bam-A-zuh-pene) G

Brand Names

Atretol
Carbatrol

Epitol
Equetro
Tegretol
Tegretol-XR
Teril

The information in this profile also applies to the following drugs:

Generic Ingredients: Oxcarbazepine
Trileptal

Type of Drug

Anticonvulsant.

Prescribed For

Seizure disorders and trigeminal neuralgia (all but Equetro) and bipolar disorder (Equetro); also used to treat borderline personality disorder, psychotic disorders, withdrawal from alcohol, restless leg syndrome, and diabetes insipidus. Oxcarbazepine is prescribed for partial seizures in adults and children over age 2.

General Information

Carbamazepine was first approved for relief of the severe pain of trigeminal neuralgia. Over the years, it has gained wide use in seizure control, especially in people whose seizures are uncontrolled with phenytoin, phenobarbital, or primidone, or who have suffered severe side effects from these drugs. Carbamazepine is not a simple pain reliever and should not be taken for everyday aches and pains. It is associated with potentially fatal side effects.

Oxcarbazepine is similar in structure to carbamazepine but it is broken down differently in the body, resulting in several clinical advantages over carbamazepine. Both work by blocking calcium channels in the brain.

Cautions and Warnings

Carbamazepine and oxcarbazepine should not be used if you are **allergic** or **sensitive** to any of their ingredients or to any tricyclic antidepressant.

Rarely, severe, possibly fatal skin reactions can develop in a few people taking these medications. Tell your doctor at once if you experience any type of skin reaction while taking carbamazepine or oxcarbazepine. **Asians** are 10 times more likely to develop these reactions than non-Asians.

Carbamazepine may cause severe, possibly life-threatening blood reactions. People who have had **blood reactions to other drugs** are at particular risk for another reaction with carbamazepine. Your doctor should take a complete blood count before you start taking this drug and repeat these blood tests weekly during the first 3 months of treatment, and then every month for the next 2–3 years. Unexplained fever or infection may be a sign of a blood reaction.

People taking this drug are more likely to have suicidal thoughts or actually attempt suicide.

Carbamazepine should not be used if you have had **bone marrow depression**.

Monoamine oxidase inhibitor (MAOI) antidepressants should be discontinued 2 weeks before starting carbamazepine.

Carbamazepine should be used with caution in those with **kidney, heart**, **or liver disease** and avoided in those with **hepatic porphyria**, an enzyme deficiency of the liver.

Carbamazepine may aggravate **glaucoma** and should be used with caution by people with this condition.

Carbamazepine may activate underlying **psychosis** and, in **older adults**, **confusion** or **agitation**.

A small number of allergic reactions involving multiple organs have occurred just after starting oxcarbazepine in adults and children. Many of these people were hospitalized and some had life-threatening circumstances. Typical signs and symptoms of this reaction are fever and rash associated with swollen lymph glands, hepatitis, abnormal liver and blood tests, itching, kidney inflammation, inability to urinate, joint pain, and weakness.

People taking oxcarbazepine occasionally develop very low blood-sodium levels (symptoms include nausea, feeling sick, headache, tiredness, confusion, and reduced pain sensitivity) during the first 3 months of treatment. Your doctor will check your blood periodically and may stop the drug or lower the dose to eliminate this problem.

Oxcarbazepine has been associated with adverse reactions related to the central nervous system. These reactions include difficulty with concentration, speech or language problems, sleepiness or fatigue, and coordination abnormalities, including poor muscle coordination and difficulty walking.

Oxcarbazepine should be gradually withdrawn to reduce seizure risk.

Those with **kidney disease** should begin with lower doses of oxcarbazepine.

These drugs are not for the relief of minor aches or pains.

Possible Side Effects

Carbamazepine

- ▼ Most common: dizziness, drowsiness, unsteadiness, nausea, vomiting, headache, infection, pain, and dry mouth.
- ▼ Less common: blurred or double vision, depression, manic depressive reaction, anxiety, memory disturbances, weakness, itching, rash, diarrhea, upset stomach, and constipation.
- ▼ Rare: Rare side effects can affect your breathing, speech, emotions, liver function, urinary function, and many other parts of the body. Contact your doctor if you experience anything unusual while taking any medication.

Oxcarbazepine

- ▼ Most common: nausea, vomiting, abdominal pain, upset stomach, fatigue, headache, dizziness, tiredness, tremor, and double vision or abnormal vision.
- ▼ Common: poor muscle coordination, unusual eye movements, abnormal walking, memory loss, worsened convulsions, and fainting.
- ▼ Less common: emotional upset, reduced sensitivity to stimulation, nervousness, taste changes, earache, fever, allergy, weakness, swollen legs, weight gain, low blood pressure, speech or language problems, confusion, abnormal thinking, acne, flushing, rash, appetite loss, dry mouth, rectal bleeding, toothache, diarrhea, constipation, stomach irritation, thirst, runny nose, coughing, bronchitis, sore throat, nosebleed, and back pain.
- ▼ Rare: Rare side effects can occur in almost any part of the body. Contact your doctor if you experience anything unusual while taking any medication.

Drug Interactions

- Carbamazepine blood levels may be increased by azoles (such as ketoconazole), acetazolamide, cimetidine, dalfopristin, danazol, delavirdine, diltiazem, fluoxetine, fluvoxamine, haloperidol, isoniazid, loratadine, levetiracetam, macrolide antibiotics, MAOIs, nefazodone, niacinamide, nicotinamide, protease inhibitors, quetiapine, quinine, quinupristin, terfenadine, tricyclic antidepressants, valproate, verapamil, or zileuton, leading to possible carbamazepine toxicity.

- These medications may reduce the effectiveness of contraceptive drugs and cause breakthrough bleeding.
- Antimalarials (such as chloroquine and mefloquine), cisplatin, doxorubicin, felbamate, phenobarbital and other barbiturates, phenytoin, primidone, rifampin, succinimides (such as methsuximide), and theophylline may decrease the absorption of carbamazepine.
- Levels of phenobarbital, a breakdown product of primidone, may be increased by combining primidone and carbamazepine.
- Carbamazepine may reduce the effects of acetaminophen, anticoagulants (blood thinners, such as warfarin), certain antidepressants, benzodiazepines (such as diazepam and lorazepam), bupropion, buspirone, calcium channel blockers (such as felodipine), cyclosporine, doxycycline, glucocorticoids (such as dexamethasone and hydrocortisone), lamotrigine, levothyroxine, methadone, mirtazapine, certain muscle relaxants, oxcarbazepine, praziquantel, statin drugs, succinimides, tiagabine, topiramate, tramadol, trazodone, and zonisamide.
- Combining carbamazepine and other antiseizure drugs, including felbamate, hydantoins, succinimides, and valproic acid, may cause unpredictable results. Combination treatments to control seizures must be customized to each person.
- Combining carbamazepine and lithium may increase nervous system side effects such as muscular twitching or impaired consciousness.
- Carbamazepine suspension should not be combined with other liquid medicines or diluents.
- Carbamazepine, phenobarbital, phenytoin, and valproic acid reduce the amount of oxcarbazepine in the blood.
- Oxcarbazepine may increase the amount of phenobarbital and phenytoin in the blood.
- Verapamil and felodipine reduce oxcarbazepine levels in the blood.
- Oxcarbazepine reduces blood levels of lamotrigine.

Food Interactions

Take carbamazepine with food if it causes stomach upset. Avoid taking carbamazepine with grapefruit products. Oxcarbazepine can be taken without regard to food or meals.

Usual Dose

Carbamazepine

Adult and Child (age 13 and over): 400–1200 mg a day, depending on the condition. The maximum dose is 1200 mg a day for adults and children over age 15 and 1000 mg a day for children age 13–15. Rarely, dosages of 1600 mg a day have been used in adults. Usual maintenance dose is 400–800 mg a day in divided doses for trigeminal neuralgia and 800–1200 mg a day for epilepsy.

Child (age 6–12): 200–1000 mg a day. Dosage should be adjusted to the minimum effective level, usually 400–800 mg a day. Do not exceed 1000 mg a day.

Child (under age 6): 5–9 mg per lb. of body weight a day to start. Dosage may increase until optimal therapeutic response is reached, not to exceed 16 mg per lb. of body weight a day in divided doses.

Dosage varies according to form. Liquid carbamazepine must be taken 3 times a day, regular carbamazepine tablets twice a day, and sustained-release tablets once a day. Never change your dosage schedule without first checking with your doctor.

Oxcarbazepine

Adult and Child (age 17 and over): 600–2400 mg a day. People with poor kidney function should start at ½ the dosage and increase slowly until the desired response is reached.

Child (age 4–16): 3.75–4.5 mg per lb. of body weight up to 600 mg a day to start. Increase gradually to 900–1800 mg a day, according to body weight.

Overdosage

Carbamazepine is a potentially lethal drug. Overdose symptoms appear in 1–3 hours. These include irregularity in or difficulty breathing, rapid heartbeat, changes in blood pressure, shock, loss of consciousness or coma, convulsions, muscle twitching, restlessness, uncontrolled body movements, drooping eyelids, psychotic mood changes, nausea, vomiting, and reduced urination. Induce vomiting right away with ipecac syrup (available at any pharmacy). Then take the victim to a hospital emergency room.

All oxcarbazepine overdose patients have recovered with treatment. Symptoms are likely to be exaggerated drug side effects. Overdose victims should be taken to a hospital emergency room.

If you seek treatment, ALWAYS bring the prescription bottle or container.

Special Information

These drugs may cause dizziness and drowsiness. Take care while driving or doing any task that requires concentration.

Contact your doctor at once if you experience rash, yellowing of the skin or whites of the eyes, unusual bleeding or bruising, abdominal pain, pale stools, dark urine, impotence, mood changes, nervous system symptoms, swelling, fever, chills, sore throat, or mouth sores. These may be signs of potentially fatal drug reactions.

These drugs may reduce the effectiveness of hormonal contraceptives. Use a non-hormonal contraceptive method while taking them.

Like all anticonvulsant medicines, these medicines must be gradually stopped to avoid experiencing sudden seizures.

Alcohol can enhance the depressive effects of these drugs.

If you forget a dose of carbamazepine, skip it and go back to your regular schedule. If you miss more than 1 dose in a day, contact your doctor. Do not stop taking this drug without first consulting your doctor.

If you forget to take a dose of oxcarbazepine, take it as soon as you remember. If it is almost time for your next dose, skip the dose you forgot and continue with your regular schedule. Do not take a double dose of oxcarbazepine. Contact your doctor if you forget 2 or more doses in a row.

Special Populations

Pregnancy/Breast-feeding: These drugs caused birth defects in animal studies. Seizure disorder itself also increases the risk of birth defects. Carbamazepine and oxcarbazepine should be taken during pregnancy only if your doctor determines that the potential benefit outweighs the risks.

These drugs pass into breast milk. Nursing mothers who must take carbamazepine or oxcarbazepine should use infant formula.

Seniors: Seniors taking these drugs are more likely to develop heart problems, confusion, or agitation.

Type of Drug

Carbonic-Anhydrase Inhibitors, Eye Drops (kar-BON-ik an-HYE-drase)

Brand Names

Generic Ingredients: Brinzolamide
Azopt

Generic Ingredients: Dorzolamide G
Trusopt

Combination Products
Generic Ingredients: Dorzolamide + Timolol G
Cosopt

Prescribed For

Glaucoma.

General Information

These drugs are similar to acetazolamide, a carbonic-anhydrase inhibitor taken by mouth. Carbonic anhydrase is an enzyme found in many parts of the body, including the eyes. By blocking the effects of this enzyme, dorzolamide and brinzolamide slow the production of fluid inside the eye, reducing pressure. This effect is useful in treating open-angle glaucoma because the disease is characterized by elevated eye pressure. Dorzolamide and brinzolamide are sulfonamides, or sulfa drugs, and although they are administered topically, they affect the entire body.

Cautions and Warnings

Do not use these drugs if you are **allergic** or **sensitive** to any of their ingredients or to other sulfa drugs. Small amounts of these drugs enter the bloodstream. Rarely, people using them experience side effects or allergies associated with sulfa drugs.

These drugs have not been studied in people with very **poor kidney or liver function**. Because these drugs are eliminated via the kidneys, people with impaired kidney function should use an alternative glaucoma medication.

Swelling of the cornea, the eye's outer layer, has developed in some people using dorzolamide eye drops.

These drugs have not been studied in people with **acute angle-closure glaucoma**.

See Timolol, page 167, for more information on the combination product Cosopt.

Possible Side Effects

Brinzolamide

- ▼ Common: blurred vision and a bitter, sour, or unusual taste in the mouth.
- ▼ Less common: eyelid inflammation; conjunctivitis (pinkeye); rash; dry eye; sensation of something in the eye; headache; eye redness, itching, discharge, or pain; and runny nose.
- ▼ Rare: allergic reactions, hair loss, chest pain, diarrhea, nausea, sore throat, tearing, itchy rash, double vision, dizziness, dry mouth, breathing difficulties, upset stomach, tired eyes, kidney pain, cornea problems, and formation of a crust or sticky sensation around the eyelid. Brinzolamide can cause the same types of side effects as other sulfa drugs, but this is very unlikely. Contact your doctor if you experience anything unusual while taking any medication.

Dorzolamide

- ▼ Most common: eye burning, stinging, or discomfort and a bitter taste in the mouth immediately after administering the eye drops.
- ▼ Less common: allergic reactions, conjunctivitis (pinkeye), blurred vision, tearing, dry eye, and increased sensitivity to bright light.
- ▼ Rare: headache, nausea, weakness, tiredness, rash, and kidney stones. Dorzolamide can cause the same types of side effects as other sulfa drugs, but this is very unlikely. Contact your doctor if you experience anything unusual while taking any medication.

Drug Interactions

- If you are using more than 1 eye-drop product, separate doses of these drugs by at least 10 minutes.
- These medications should not be used with oral carbonic-anhydrase inhibitors.

Usual Dose

Brinzolamide

Adult: 1 drop in the affected eye 3 times a day.

Child: not recommended.

Dorzolamide

Adult and Child: 1 drop in the affected eye 3 times a day.

Overdosage

Accidental ingestion of a bottle of dorzolamide or brinzolamide may affect blood levels of potassium and other electrolytes. The victim should be taken to a hospital emergency room. If you seek treatment, ALWAYS bring the prescription bottle or container.

Special Information

Contact your doctor and stop using your eye drops if you develop any unusual eye reaction or condition, including swollen eyelids and conjunctivitis (pinkeye).

Vision may be temporarily blurred when using the eye drops. Use caution when driving or operating machinery.

If you wear soft contact lenses, take them out before using the eye drops and put them back in 15 minutes after a dose.

To prevent infection, do not allow the eyedropper tip to touch your fingers, eyelids, or any surface. Wait at least 10 minutes before using any other eye drops.

If you forget to administer a dose, do so as soon as you remember. If it is almost time for your next dose, skip the one you forgot and continue with your regular schedule. Do not take a double dose.

Special Populations

Pregnancy/Breast-feeding: Very high dosages of dorzolamide or brinzolamide caused birth defects in animal studies. Although the risks of using these drugs during pregnancy are small in humans, dorzolamide or brinzolamide should be taken during pregnancy only if your doctor determines that the potential benefit outweighs the risks.

It is not known if these drugs pass into breast milk. Nursing mothers who must use either drug should use infant formula.

Seniors: Seniors may use this medication without special precaution.

Generic Name

Carvedilol (car-VAY-dih-lol) G

Brand Names

Coreg Coreg CR

Type of Drug

Alpha-beta-adrenergic blocker.

Prescribed For

Heart failure, high blood pressure, and reduced left ventricular function following heart attack; also used for angina and cardiomyopathy.

General Information

Carvedilol was the first beta blocker approved for heart failure. It is also the only beta blocker approved for severe heart failure.

Carvedilol blocks both the alpha- and beta-adrenergic portions of the central nervous system. This dual action reduces the amount of blood pumped with each heartbeat and also decreases the risk of tachycardia (very rapid heartbeat). Carvedilol's beta-blocking effects begin within an hour of taking the first dose; maximum blood pressure lowering occurs after 1 or 2 weeks. The drug also causes blood vessels to dilate (widen), allowing the heart to pump blood more efficiently.

Cautions and Warnings

Do not take carvedilol if you are **allergic** or **sensitive** to any of its ingredients, or if you have **atrioventricular (AV) block**, **sick sinus syndrome**, or **severe bradycardia** (slow heart rate) without the use of a pacemaker.

Carvedilol should not be taken by patients with **bronchial disease**, such as **chronic bronchitis**, **emphysema**, or **asthma**.

Carvedilol therapy should not be stopped suddenly due to the risk of worsening the heart condition.

In studies, carvedilol caused mild and reversible liver injury in about 1 of every 100 people who took it. Those with severe **liver disease** should not take this medication. Contact your doctor at once if you develop signs of liver damage (symptoms include severe itching, dark-colored urine, flu-like symptoms, appetite loss, and yellowing of the skin or whites of the eyes).

People with **peripheral vascular disease** should use carvedilol with caution, as their symptoms can worsen.

Check with your doctor about continuing carvedilol if you are to receive **general anesthesia**; heart function that is depressed by anesthetics can worsen if carvedilol is used at the same time.

Make sure your doctor knows if you have **diabetes**. Carvedilol can mask signs of **low blood sugar** and may increase the effects of insulin or oral antidiabetes drugs, making it more difficult to recover from the effects of low blood sugar.

People taking carvedilol may experience excessive low blood pressure or slow heart rate.

Those with **congestive heart failure** or **angina** may experience an initial worsening of their condition while taking carvedilol.

Those with **kidney disease** should have their kidneys monitored during initiation of carvedilol and should stop taking it or have their dosage reduced if kidney function declines. Rarely, carvedilol has caused reduced kidney function, which returns to its original state after discontinuation of the drug.

Carvedilol can mask symptoms of an **overactive thyroid gland**. Abruptly stopping carvedilol can trigger an attack of hyperthyroidism.

People with **pheochromocytoma** (adrenal gland tumor) should take carvedilol with caution.

If you are scheduled for cataract surgery, make sure your ophthalmologist knows you are taking carvedilol. A condition called intraoperative floppy iris syndrome has been reported during cataract surgery with those taking carvedilol.

Possible Side Effects

Most side effects are considered mild or moderate.

- ▼ Most common: dizziness, fatigue, headache, sleepiness or sleeplessness, diarrhea, nausea, vomiting, weight gain, abdominal pain, slow heartbeat, dizziness when rising from a sitting or lying position, swelling of the hands or feet, sore throat, breathing difficulties, tiredness, back pain, urinary infection, and viral infection.
- ▼ Less common: extra heartbeats; palpitations; blood-pressure changes; fainting; reduced blood supply to the arms and legs (symptoms include aches, cramps, pain, or tiredness on walking, or pain in the foot, thigh, hip, or buttocks); tingling in the hands or feet; reduced sensation; depression; nervousness; constipation; gas; liver irritation; cough; impotence and reduced sex drive in men; itching; rash; visual difficulties; ringing or buzzing in the ears; high blood-cholesterol levels, sugar, or uric acid; anemia; weakness; hot flashes; leg cramps; dry mouth; not feeling well; sweating; and muscle ache.

Possible Side Effects *(continued)*

▼ Rare: Rare side effects can affect the heart, mental status, the respiratory tract, the urinary tract, and the kidney. It can also cause hair loss, weight gain, high blood-triglyceride levels, low blood-platelet counts, and sugar in the urine. Contact your doctor if you experience anything unusual while taking any medication.

Drug Interactions

- Carvedilol increases the effects of insulin and oral antidiabetes drugs. People taking this combination must monitor their blood-sugar levels regularly. Contact your doctor if there is any change from your normal pattern.
- Carvedilol increases the effects of verapamil, diltiazem, and similar calcium-channel-blocker drugs.
- Carvedilol may increase the effects of catecholamine-depleting agents such as monoamine oxidase inhibitor (MAOI) antidepressants and reserpine.
- Carvedilol increases the blood-pressure-lowering effect of clonidine. People taking this combination may need less clonidine to control their pressure.
- Carvedilol increases the amount of digoxin in the blood by about 15%. Your digoxin dosage may need to be adjusted.
- Cyclosporine levels may be elevated when it is taken with carvedilol. Dosage adjustments may be necessary.
- Cimetidine increases the amount of carvedilol absorbed into the blood by about 30%, but the importance of this interaction is not clear.
- Rifampin reduces the amount of carvedilol in the blood by about 70%. Dosage adjustment is necessary.
- The breakdown of carvedilol by liver enzymes can be interfered with by amiodarone, fenofibrate, fluconazole, fluvastatin, fluvoxamine, isoniazid, lovastatin, phenylbutazone, probenecid, sertraline, sulfamethoxazole, sulfaphenazole, teniposide, voriconazole, and zafirlukast. This interaction can result in elevated carvedilol blood concentrations and possible unwanted effects.
- Diphenhydramine, hydroxychloroquine, propafenone, quinidine, and selective serotonin reuptake inhibitor (SSRI) antidepressants may increase concentrations of carvedilol.

Monitoring is necessary when giving hydroxychloroquine and carvedilol simultaneously.

- Salicylates (such as aspirin) may inhibit the actions of carvedilol. Blood pressure should be monitored during coadministration.
- Do not consume alcohol (including medicines that contain alcohol) within 2 hours of taking carvedilol.

Food Interactions

Take carvedilol with food to reduce the risk of dizziness or fainting.

Usual Dose

Heart Failure

Adult: 3.125 mg twice a day for 2 weeks. Dose may be doubled every 2 weeks to the highest level tolerated. Maximum daily dosage is 25 mg twice a day in people weighing less than 187 lbs., and 50 mg twice a day in people who weigh more.

High Blood Pressure and Cardiomyopathy

Adult: 6.25 mg twice a day to start, increased after 7–14 days to 12.5 mg twice a day, then again to 25 mg twice a day if needed.

Child: children weighing 137.5 lbs. or less: 0.09–0.18 mg per lb. twice a day; children weighing over 137.5 lbs.: 12.5–25 mg twice a day.

Ventricular Dysfunction Following Heart Attack

Adult: 6.25 mg twice a day, increased after 3–10 days—based on tolerability—to 12.5 mg twice a day, then again to the target dose of 25 mg twice a day.

Studies of carvedilol in children age 2 months to 17 years with heart failure have not shown consistent improvement in heart function.

Overdosage

Overdose may lead to very low blood pressure (symptoms include dizziness and fainting); slow heartbeat and other cardiac symptoms, including shock and heart attack; breathing difficulties; bronchial spasm; vomiting; periods of unconsciousness; and seizures. Overdose victims must be taken to a hospital emergency room. If you seek treatment, ALWAYS bring the prescription bottle or container.

Special Information

Carvedilol should be taken continuously. Do not stop taking it without your doctor's knowledge, because abrupt withdrawal may cause chest pain, breathing difficulties, increased sweating, and unusually fast or irregular heartbeat. The dose should be gradually reduced over a period of about 2 weeks.

Contact your doctor if you develop any allergic reaction to this drug, including hives or swelling of the face, lips, tongue, and/or throat that can make it hard to breathe or swallow. These reactions are rare but can be deadly.

People taking carvedilol may become dizzy or faint when rising quickly from a sitting or lying position. If this happens to you, sit or lie down until you feel better. Carvedilol can also cause drowsiness, lightheadedness, or blurred vision. Be careful when driving or doing any task that requires concentration.

Contact-lens wearers are more likely to experience dry eyes with carvedilol.

Swallow extended-release tablets whole; do not crush or break them.

It is best to take carvedilol at the same time each day. If you forget a dose, take it as soon as you remember. If it is within 4 hours of your next dose, skip the dose you forgot and continue with your regular schedule. Do not take a double dose.

Special Populations

Pregnancy/Breast-feeding: Animal studies indicate that carvedilol passes into the fetal bloodstream and may interfere with pregnancy. Carvedilol should be taken during pregnancy only if your doctor determines that the potential benefit outweighs the risks.

It is not known if carvedilol passes into human breast milk, though it passes into rat breast milk. Beta-blocker drugs such as carvedilol may affect babies' hearts. Nursing mothers who must take this drug should use infant formula.

Seniors: Seniors are more likely to develop dizziness and may require reduced dosages.

Celebrex *see **Celecoxib,** below*

Celecoxib (sel-eh-KOX-ib)

Brand Names

Celebrex

Type of Drug

Cyclooxygenase-2 (COX-2) inhibitor nonsteroidal anti-inflammatory drug (NSAID).

Prescribed For

Osteoarthritis, rheumatoid arthritis, juvenile rheumatoid arthritis, acute pain, menstrual pain, and arthritis of the spine (ankylosing spondylitis).

General Information

Traditional NSAIDs work primarily by blocking the effects of COX-2, a body enzyme that plays an important role in regulating pain and inflammation. But these NSAIDs also have an unwanted effect: They interfere with cyclooxygenase-1 (COX-1), a related enzyme that helps to maintain the stomach's protective lining. NSAIDs that block the effects of this enzyme may produce side effects such as stomach irritation, gas, and stomach ulcers.

Celecoxib is different from other NSAID pain relievers in that it inhibits primarily the COX-2 enzyme and does not affect COX-1. All other NSAIDS act on both COX-1 and COX-2, although the degree to which they act on each enzyme varies. All NSAIDs work in a similar manner, and 200–400 mg of celecoxib and 500 mg of naproxen are about equally effective. However, celecoxib is less likely to cause the gastrointestinal (GI) side effects often associated with other NSAIDs. Another advantage of celecoxib is that it does not cause thinning of the blood or affect blood platelets as can happen with older NSAIDs. Celecoxib is broken down in the liver.

Black patients absorb about 40% more celecoxib than Caucasians; its importance is unclear. Celecoxib is the first drug proven effective in reducing the number of intestinal polyps in people with the rare genetic disorder familial adenomatous polyposis.

Cautions and Warnings

Do not take celecoxib if you are **allergic** or **sensitive** to any of its ingredients or to sulfa drugs. NSAIDs should not be taken by people with **asthma** or by those who have had an **allergic reaction to aspirin or another NSAID**. They can develop a group of symptoms (runny nose with or without nasal polyps and a severe bronchial spasm) known as the aspirin triad.

COX-2 inhibitors, including celecoxib, have been associated with high blood pressure, heart attacks, and stroke. People with **cardiovascular disease** or risk factors for cardiovascular disease may be at higher risk for cardiac events while taking this medication. Celecoxib may also cause water retention and swelling and should be used with caution in those with **congestive heart failure** or **fluid retention** or in those taking medications to treat **high blood pressure**. Blood-pressure monitoring should occur regularly while taking celecoxib. It should not be used to treat pain associated with **heart-bypass surgery**. Two other COX-2 inhibitors were taken off the market because of safety concerns. Rofecoxib was removed because safety issues were noted after people had taken it for 18 months or more. Valdecoxib was taken off the market because of the lack of safety data, severe skin rashes, and concerns raised in people taking the drug after having had heart surgery.

NSAIDs can cause GI bleeding and ulcers and stomach perforation. This can occur at any time, with or without warning, in people who take NSAIDs regularly. Celecoxib should be used with caution by people who have had **stomach ulcers** or **GI bleeding**. Minor upper-GI problems, such as upset stomach, are common and may occur at any time during NSAID therapy. People who develop bleeding or ulcers and continue NSAID treatment should be aware of the risk of developing more serious side effects. Risk of GI bleeding and ulcers is increased with longer duration of therapy as well as treatment with oral corticosteroids and anticoagulants, smoking, alcoholism, older age, and general poor health.

Children taking celecoxib may be more likely to vomit blood, suffer acute kidney failure, or develop rashes.

Celecoxib has not been studied in people with severe **kidney disease**. They should not use this drug unless their doctors closely monitor their kidney function.

Celecoxib can cause liver irritation and should be used with caution by people with **hepatitis** or **cirrhosis**. People with moderate **liver disease** can have twice as much celecoxib in their blood and require a reduced dosage. The effect of celecoxib in people with severe **liver failure** is not known.

Serious life-threatening skin reactions are possible while taking this medication. Stop taking celecoxib and contact your doctor at the first sign of a rash or other skin reaction.

Possible Side Effects

Side effects are similar to those of traditional NSAIDs. Stomach and intestinal side effects are about ½ as common.

Possible Side Effects *(continued)*

- ▼ Most common: headache.
- ▼ Common: diarrhea, upset stomach, sinus irritation, and respiratory infection.
- ▼ Less common: abdominal pain, gas, nausea, back pain, swelling in the legs or arms, accidental injuries, sleeplessness, dizziness, sore throat, runny nose, and rash.
- ▼ Rare: Rare side effects can occur in almost any part of the body. Contact your doctor if you experience anything unusual while taking any medication.

Drug Interactions

- Celecoxib may interact with certain agents to cause serious heart rhythm disturbances. These agents include antiarrhythmic agents (such as amiodarone, bretylium, disopyramide, dofetilide, quinidine, and sotalol), arsenic trioxide, chlorpromazine, cisapride, dolasetron, droperidol, mefloquine, mesoridazine, moxifloxacin, pentamidine, pimozide, tacrolimus, thioridazine, and ziprasidone.
- Alcohol may increase the risk of serious GI-related side effects. Avoid alcohol.
- Combining celecoxib with an aluminum and magnesium antacid slightly reduces the amount of drug absorbed. Separate doses of these antacids and celecoxib by 1–2 hours.
- Azole antifungals such as fluconazole and voriconazole and corticosteroids such as prednisone increase blood concentrations of celecoxib.
- Amiodarone, metronidazole, ritonavir, and zafirlukast may increase levels of celecoxib.
- Celecoxib may increase concentrations of carvedilol, mexiletine, and tramadol.
- Although celecoxib may be combined with low dosages of aspirin, taking these drugs together increases the risk of stomach or intestinal ulcers or other complications. The ulcer risk associated with this combination is less than that posed by single-drug therapy with a traditional NSAID.
- You should not use celecoxib with a traditional NSAID, as the potential for GI-related side effects is increased.
- Celecoxib can reduce the blood-pressure-lowering effect of angiotensin-converting enzyme (ACE) inhibitors and

angiotensin II receptor antagonists. These combinations can also increase the risk of kidney damage after chronic celecoxib use.

- Celecoxib may elevate lithium blood levels.
- Celecoxib can reduce the effect of furosemide and thiazide-type diuretics. The risk of kidney disease is increased with these combinations.
- Celecoxib should be used cautiously with warfarin. Concurrent use of these drugs may cause an increased risk of bleeding complications.

Food Interactions

Celecoxib can be taken without regard to food or meals. For optimal effectiveness, avoid taking this drug with high-fat meals.

Usual Dose

Adult: 100–200 mg twice a day.

Child (age 2–17): juvenile rheumatoid arthritis—22–55 lbs.: 50 mg twice a day; over 55 lbs.: 100 mg twice a day.

Child (under age 2): not recommended.

Overdosage

Overdosage symptoms include lethargy, drowsiness, nausea, vomiting, and stomach pain. Stomach or intestinal bleeding or severe allergic reactions can occur. High blood pressure, kidney failure, breathing difficulties, and coma are rare.

The victim should be taken to a hospital emergency room. If you seek treatment, ALWAYS bring the prescription bottle or container.

Special Information

Contact your doctor if you develop rash, itching, unexplained weight gain, nausea, fatigue, jaundice (yellowing of the skin or whites of the eyes), flu-like symptoms, lethargy, swelling, black stools, severe stomach pain, persistent headache, or any bothersome or persistent side effect.

If you forget a dose and remember within 1 or 2 hours of your scheduled time, take it right away. If you do not remember until later, skip the forgotten dose and continue with your regular schedule.

Special Populations

Pregnancy/Breast-feeding: Celecoxib has caused birth defects in animal studies. Any NSAID may affect fetal heart development during the second ½ of pregnancy. Pregnant women should not take celecoxib without their doctor's approval. Celecoxib should be taken during pregnancy only if your doctor determines that the potential benefit outweighs the risks.

NSAIDs may pass into breast milk. There is a possibility that a nursing mother taking celecoxib could affect her baby's heart or cardiovascular system. Nursing mothers who must take this drug should use infant formula.

Seniors: Generally, seniors can take this drug without special precaution. Those who weigh less than 110 lbs. should begin with the lowest possible dosage.

Type of Drug

Cephalosporin Antibiotics

(CEF-uh-loe-SPOR-in)

Brand Names

Generic Ingredients: Cefaclor G
Raniclor

Generic Ingredients: Cefadroxil G

Generic Ingredients: Cefdinir G
Omnicef

Generic Ingredients: Cefditoren Pivoxil
Spectracef

Generic Ingredients: Cefixime G
Suprax

Generic Ingredients: Cefpodoxime Proxetil G

Generic Ingredients: Cefprozil G

Generic Ingredients: Ceftibuten
Cedax

Generic Ingredients: Cefuroxime Axetil G
Ceftin

Generic Ingredients: Cephalexin G
Keflex

Prescribed For

Bacterial infections.

General Information

These antibiotics are related to cephalosporin C, which is similar to penicillin and is isolated from the *Cephalosporium acremonium* fungus. Of the more than 20 different antibiotic drugs derived from cephalosporin C, only those that are taken by mouth are included in *The Pill Book*. Most common infections can be treated with these antibiotics, but they are not interchangeable. Your doctor must select the appropriate antibiotic for a particular infection.

Cautions and Warnings

Do not take cephalosporin antibiotics if you are **allergic** or **sensitive** to any of their ingredients. Up to 15% of people allergic to penicillin may also be allergic to cephalosporins. The most common cephalosporin allergic reaction is a hive-like rash condition with redness over large areas of the body. Other sensitivity reactions include general rash, fever, and joint aches or pain. Such reactions generally begin after a few days of taking the antibiotic and resolve within a few days after the antibiotic is stopped.

A serious, potentially life-threatening skin reaction called Stevens-Johnson syndrome has occurred in some people taking a cephalosporin. Symptoms include fever, sore throat, fatigue, peeling skin, and blisters. Contact your doctor if you develop any type of skin reaction.

Prolonged or repeated use of a cephalosporin may lead to a secondary infection not susceptible to the antibiotic.

Occasionally, people taking a cephalosporin develop colitis. Contact your doctor if you develop severe diarrhea while taking one of these drugs.

People with **poor kidney function** may require less medicine to treat their infections. Rarely, people taking a cephalosporin have had a seizure, especially those with kidney disease whose dose was not reduced.

Cefaclor may cause serum sickness (symptoms include fever, joint pain, and rash). Symptoms generally resolve after discontinuation of therapy.

Rarely, severe anemia occurs in people taking cephalosporin antibiotics. Report any signs of anemia (such as pale skin color, weakness, tiredness, difficulty breathing, and abnormal heart rhythms) to your doctor.

Cefprozil oral suspension contains phenylalanine and cannot be taken by people with **phenylketonuria**.

Possible Side Effects

Most side effects are mild.

- ▼ Most common: diarrhea, headache, abdominal pain, constipation, gas, upset stomach, nausea, vomiting, itching, and rash.
- ▼ Less common: dizziness, tiredness, weakness, tingling in the hands or feet, confusion, appetite loss, changes in taste perception, and genital and anal itching. Colitis may develop.

Drug Interactions

- Antacids can reduce the amounts of cefaclor, cefdinir, cefditoren, and cefpodoxime in the blood. Do not take antacids within 2 hours of these antibiotics.
- Cimetidine, famotidine, ranitidine, or nizatidine can reduce the effectiveness of cefpodoxime and cefuroxime.
- Iron and iron-fortified foods may interfere with the absorption of cefdinir. Separate your iron dose from the antibiotic by at least 2 hours. Iron-fortified infant formula does not have this effect.
- Probenecid may increase blood levels of some cephalosporins.
- Potent (loop-type) diuretics can lead to kidney damage if mixed with a cephalosporin antibiotic.

Food Interactions

Generally, cephalosporins may be taken with food or milk if they upset your stomach. Ceftibuten oral suspension should be taken at least 2 hours before or 1 hour after a meal. Cefditoren should be taken with a meal. Food increases the absorption of cefpodoxime and cefuroxime.

Usual Dose

Cefaclor

Adult: 250 mg every 8 hours, or 375–500 mg every 12 hours.
Child: 9 mg per lb. of body weight a day in 2–3 equal doses.

Cefadroxil

Adult: 1–2 g a day in 1–2 doses.
Child: 13 mg per lb. of body weight a day in 1–2 doses.

Cefdinir

Adult and Child (age 13 and over): 600 mg a day in 1–2 doses.

Child (age 6 months–12 years): 6.5 mg per lb. of body weight a day in 1–2 doses.

Cefditoren

Adult and Child (age 12 and over): 200–400 mg twice a day for 10–14 days.

Child (under age 12): not recommended.

Cefixime

Adult and Child (age 12 and over): 400 mg a day in 1–2 doses.

Child (age 6 months–11 years): 3.5 mg per lb. of body weight a day in 1–2 doses.

Cefpodoxime

Adult and Child (age 12 and over): 200–800 mg a day in 1–2 doses.

Child (age 2 months–11 years): 4.5 mg per lb. of body weight a day in 1–2 doses. Maximum daily dose for middle-ear infections and sinus infections is 400 mg; 200 mg for sore throat or tonsillitis.

Cefprozil

Adult and Child (age 13 and over): 500–1000 mg a day.

Child (age 2–12 years): 7–13 mg per lb. of body weight a day in 1–2 doses.

Ceftibuten

Adult and Child (age 12 and over): 400 mg once a day for 10 days.

Child (age 6 months–11 years): 4 mg per lb. of body weight, up to 400 mg, once a day.

Cefuroxime

Adult and Child (age 13 and over): 500–1000 mg a day in 1–2 doses.

Child (age 3 months–12 years): tablets (must be able to swallow tablets whole)—250 mg every 12 hours; liquid—9–13 mg per lb. of body weight every 12 hours.

Cephalexin

Adult: 1000–4000 mg a day in divided doses, usually 250 mg every 6 hours or 500 mg every 12 hours.

Child: 11–23 mg per lb. of body weight a day in divided doses. The dose may be increased to 46 mg per lb. of body weight for middle-ear infections.

Overdosage

Common symptoms of overdose are nausea, vomiting, and upset stomach. These can often be treated with milk or an antacid. Cephalosporin overdoses are generally not serious; contact a hospital emergency room or local poison control center for more information. If you seek treatment, ALWAYS bring the prescription bottle or container.

Special Information

Contact your doctor if you develop severe abdominal cramps or diarrhea. Stop taking this drug and immediately contact your doctor if you experience fever, chest tightness, breathing difficulties, redness, muscle aches, or swelling.

You must take the full course of treatment prescribed—even if you feel better in 2 or 3 days—to obtain the maximum benefit from any antibiotic.

Proper diagnosis is key to the effectiveness of an antibiotic: Do not take any antibiotic without consulting your doctor.

You should be aware that all cephalosporins may cause false results for certain urine tests for sugar. Cefuroxime may cause false results for blood sugar. Diabetics taking cefuroxime should not change their diet or diabetes medication without consulting their doctor.

If you miss a dose that you take once a day, take it as soon as you remember. If it is almost time for your next dose, take the dose you forgot right away and your next one 10–12 hours later. Then go back to your regular schedule. If you take the medication twice a day, take the dose you forgot right away and the next dose 5–6 hours later. Then go back to your regular schedule. If you take the medication 3 or more times a day, take the dose you missed right away and your next dose 2–4 hours later. Then go back to your regular schedule.

Most cephalosporin liquids must be kept in the refrigerator to maintain their strength. Only cefixime liquid does not require refrigeration. All of the liquid cephalosporins have a very limited shelf life. Do not keep any of these liquids beyond the 10 days–2 weeks specified on the label. Follow your pharmacist's storage instructions.

Special Populations

Pregnancy/Breast-feeding: These drugs are considered relatively safe during pregnancy, though small amounts pass into the fetus. Little information is available about the newer members of the group. Also, cephalosporins pass more quickly out of the bodies of pregnant women. A cephalosporin antibiotic should be taken during pregnancy only if your doctor determines that the potential benefit outweighs the risks.

Small amounts of most cephalosporin antibiotics pass into breast milk. Nursing mothers who must take a cephalosporin should use infant formula.

Seniors: Seniors may require a lower dosage if they have reduced kidney function.

Generic Name

Cetirizine (seh-TERE-ih-zene) G

Brand Names

Zyrtec

The information in this profile also applies to the following drugs:

Generic Ingredients: Azelastine
Astelin Astepro

Generic Ingredients: Fexofenadine G
Allegra

Generic Ingredients: Levocetirizine G
Xyzal

Type of Drug

Antihistamine.

Prescribed For

Azelastine: runny nose, sneezing, nasal itching, and post-nasal drip. Cetirizine: stuffy and runny nose, itchy eyes, and scratchy throat caused by seasonal and year-round allergy, and for other symptoms of allergy such as rash, itching, and hives; also prescribed for chronic itching and for asthma. Fexofenadine: sneezing, stuffy and runny nose; scratchy throat and mouth; and itchy, watery, and red eyes caused by seasonal allergies. Levocetirizine: hives, runny nose, sneezing, itching of the nose or throat, and/or itchy, watery eyes due to hay fever or other upper-respiratory allergies; also used for asthma, year-round allergy, and for other symptoms of allergy such as rash, itching, and hives; also prescribed for chronic itching.

General Information

Antihistamines generally work by blocking the release of histamine (a chemical released by body tissue during an allergic reaction) from the cell at the H_1 histamine receptor site, drying up secretions of the nose, throat, and eyes. Cetirizine causes less sedation than older antihistamines and appears to be just as effective. Levocetirizine is the active portion of the cetirizine molecule and is as effective as cetirizine with a similar side effect profile.

Cautions and Warnings

Do not take these medications if you are **allergic** or **sensitive** to any of their ingredients.

People with **kidney disease** should receive reduced dosages of cetirizine and levocetirizine. Do not take these drugs if kidney disease is severe. **Children** with kidney disease should not receive levocetirizine.

Possible Side Effects

- ▼ Common: headache, drowsiness, fatigue, dry mouth, bitter taste in the mouth, dizziness, runny nose, and sore throat.
- ▼ Less common: nosebleeds, stuffy nose, sneezing, cough, nausea, upset stomach, changes in bowel habits, nervousness, and fever (children).
- ▼ Rare: fainting and weight gain. Contact your doctor if you experience anything unusual while taking any medication.

Drug Interactions

- Cimetidine may increase the level of azelastine in the blood.
- Cetirizine is less likely than other antihistamines to interact with drugs.
- Aluminum- and magnesium-containing antacids may inhibit the effects of fexofenadine by nearly ½.
- Azole antifungals such as itraconazole, ketoconazole, and voriconazole may increase the effects of fexofenadine.
- When erythromycin and fexofenadine are taken together, fexofenadine levels may be increased.
- Rifampin decreases blood levels of fexofenadine.
- Serious heart rhythm problems are possible if fexofenadine is taken with antiarrhythmic agents (such as amiodarone, bretylium, disopyramide, dofetilide, quinidine, and sotalol), arsenic trioxide, chlorpromazine, cisapride,

dolasetron, droperidol, mefloquine, mesoridazine, moxifloxacin, pentamidine, pimozide, tacrolimus, thioridazine, and ziprasidone.

- Ritonavir increases the amount of levocetirizine and slows its breakdown in the body. This may result in increased levocetirizine side effects.
- Theophylline may cause small increases in levocetirizine levels if given together.

Food Interactions

These medications can be taken without regard to food or meals.

Usual Dose

Azelastine Nasal Spray

Adult and Child (age 12 and over): 1–2 sprays in each nostril twice a day.

Child (age 5–11): 1 spray in each nostril twice a day.

Cetirizine

Adult and Child (age 6 and over): 5–10 mg once a day depending on symptoms. Reduce dosage in people with kidney disease.

Child (age 2–5): 2.5–5 mg a day.

Child (age 6–23 months): 2.5 mg a day.

Fexofenadine

Adult (age 12 and over): 60 mg twice a day or 180 mg once a day. People with kidney disease should take 60 mg a day.

Child (age 2–11): 30 mg twice a day.

Child (age 6–23 months): 15 mg twice a day.

Levocetirizine

Adult and Child (age 12 and over): 5 mg every evening.

Child (age 6–11): 2.5 mg (½ tablet) every evening. Dosage for children should not exceed 2.5 mg a day.

Child (age 6 months–5 years): 1.25 mg (¼ tsp.) oral solution every evening. Dosage should not exceed 1.25 mg a day.

Overdosage

Drug overdose is likely to cause severe side effects. Overdose victims should be given ipecac syrup—available at any pharmacy—to make them vomit and be taken to a hospital emergency room. If you seek treatment, ALWAYS bring the prescription bottle or container.

Special Information

Use extra caution while doing anything that requires concentration, such as driving a car or operating hazardous machinery.

Report sore throat, unusual bleeding, bruising, tiredness, weakness, or any other unusual side effect to your doctor.

Do not combine these drugs with alcohol or other nervous system depressants.

Do not put azelastine nasal solution into your eyes.

If you forget to take a dose of antihistamine, take it as soon as you remember. If it is almost time for your next dose, skip the one you forgot and continue with your regular schedule. Do not take a double dose.

Special Populations

Pregnancy/Breast-feeding: Oral antihistamines are generally considered safe for use during pregnancy. But do not take any antihistamine without your doctor's knowledge if you are or might be pregnant—especially during the last 3 months of pregnancy, because newborns may have severe reactions to antihistamines.

Small amounts of antihistamine pass into breast milk. Nursing mothers who must take cetirizine should use infant formula.

Seniors: Antihistamines are more likely to cause dizziness, sleepiness, and confusion in seniors. Dosage reduction may be recommended depending on kidney function.

Generic Name

Cevimeline (seh-VIM-ih-lene)

Brand Names

Evoxac

Type of Drug

Cholinergic.

Prescribed For

Dry mouth in people with Sjögren's syndrome.

General Information

Sjögren's syndrome is a group of symptoms related to a lack of bodily secretions. People with this condition have very dry eyes and mucous membranes, facial lesions, and neck swelling. It often occurs in menopausal women and is often associated with rheumatoid arthritis, poor blood circulation in the legs, and tooth decay. Cevimeline increases secretions in the mouth by binding to specific nervous system receptors and causing the release of more saliva.

Cautions and Warnings

Do not take cevimeline if you are **allergic** or **sensitive** to any of its ingredients.

This drug may make breathing more difficult and worsen **lung conditions** such as asthma, chronic bronchitis, or chronic obstructive pulmonary disease (COPD). Those with uncontrolled asthma should not take this medication.

Eye conditions such as **glaucoma** or **inflammation of the iris** may be worsened by cevimeline.

Cevimeline may affect the heart, and some people with severe **heart disease**, including those with a history of severe angina or heart attack, may not be able to compensate for this effect.

Cevimeline may worsen **gallstones** and **kidney stones** and should be avoided by people with a history of these conditions.

Cevimeline may cause blurred vision, especially at night.

Possible Side Effects

- ▼ Most common: excessive sweating, headache, nausea, sinus irritation, respiratory infection, runny nose, and diarrhea.
- ▼ Common: upset stomach, abdominal pain, urinary infection, coughing, and sore throat.
- ▼ Less common: vomiting, back pain, injury, rash, conjunctivitis (pinkeye), dizziness, bronchitis, severe joint pain, fatigue, bone pain, sleeplessness, hot flashes, excess salivation, chills, and anxiety.
- ▼ Rare: frequent urination, weakness, and flushing. Other rare side effects can occur in almost any part of the body. Contact your doctor if you experience anything unusual while taking any medication.

Drug Interactions

- Combining cevimeline with a beta blocker can lead to heart rhythm disturbances.

- Cevimeline may interfere with the effects of anticholinergics, found in some medications for abdominal or stomach spasms or cramps.
- Cholinergics such as bethanechol, donepezil, physostigmine, pilocarpine, and pyridostigmine can add to the effects of cevimeline.
- Some drugs may interfere with the breakdown of cevimeline in the liver, increasing the chance of drug side effects. These include amiodarone, celecoxib, chlorpheniramine, cimetidine, ciprofloxacin, clarithromycin, clomipramine, cocaine, diltiazem, erythromycin, fluconazole, fluoxetine, halofantrine, indinavir, itraconazole, ketoconazole, methadone, mibefradil, nelfinavir, paroxetine, quinidine, ranitidine, ritonavir, saquinavir, and terbinafine.

Food Interactions

Grapefruit juice may interfere with the breakdown of cevimeline in the liver, increasing the chance of drug side effects. Food interferes with the absorption of cevimeline into the bloodstream. Take this drug on an empty stomach.

Usual Dose

Adult: 30 mg 3 times a day.
Child: not recommended.

Overdosage

Overdose symptoms can include exaggerated drug side effects, including headache, visual impairment, excess tearing and/or sweating, difficulty breathing, stomach or intestinal spasms, nausea, vomiting, diarrhea, changes in heart rhythm, blood-pressure changes, shock, mental confusion, and tremors. Overdose victims should be taken to a hospital emergency room. If you seek treatment, ALWAYS bring the prescription bottle or container.

Special Information

Cevimeline may cause blurred vision, possibly interfering with driving or performing tasks that require reliable vision, especially at night or in low light.

If you sweat excessively while taking cevimeline, be sure to drink a lot of water. Excessive sweating can lead to dehydration.

If you miss a dose, take it as soon as you remember. If it is almost time for your next dose, skip the missed dose and continue with your regular schedule. Do not take a double dose.

Special Populations

Pregnancy/Breast-feeding: Cevimeline's effect on the developing fetus is not known. Cevimeline should be used during pregnancy only if your doctor determines that the potential benefit outweighs the risks.

It is not known if cevimeline passes into breast milk. Nursing mothers who must take this drug should use infant formula.

Seniors: Older adults should be cautious about using this drug because of its possible effects on the kidney, liver, and heart, and on other diseases or medications.

Chantix *see **Varenicline,** page 1201*

Generic Name

Chlorpheniramine Maleate

(KLOR-fen-ERE-uh-mene MAL-ee-ate) G

Brand Names

There are many brand-name antihistamine products, the most common of which is listed here. Most are available over the counter.

Chlor-Trimeton

The information in this profile also applies to the following drugs:

Generic Ingredients: Cyproheptadine Hydrochloride G

Generic Ingredients: Dexchlorpheniramine Maleate G

Generic Ingredients: Tripelennamine G

Type of Drug

Antihistamine.

Prescribed For

Stuffy and runny nose, itchy eyes, and scratchy throat caused by seasonal allergy, and other symptoms of allergy such as rash, itching, and hives.

General Information

Antihistamines generally work by blocking the release of histamine (a chemical released by body tissue during an allergic reaction) from body cells at the H_1 histamine receptor site, drying up secretions of the nose, throat, and eyes.

Cautions and Warnings

Do not use this drug if you are **allergic** or **sensitive** to any of its ingredients.

Chlorpheniramine should not be used by people who have **deep-breathing problems** such as asthma, emphysema, or chronic bronchitis.

Antihistamines should not be given to **premature or newborn infants**. Because antihistamines pass into breast milk, nursing mothers should also not use antihistamines.

Use chlorpheniramine with care if you have a history of **thyroid disease**, **heart disease**, **high blood pressure**, or **diabetes**. This drug should be avoided or used with extreme care if you have **narrow-angle glaucoma**, **stomach ulcer** or other **stomach problems**, **enlarged prostate**, or **problems passing urine**.

Possible Side Effects

▼ Less common: rash or itching; sensitivity to bright light; increased sweating; chills; lowered blood pressure; headache; rapid heartbeat; sleeplessness; dizziness; disturbed coordination; confusion; restlessness; nervousness; irritability; euphoria (feeling "high"); tingling in the hands or feet; blurred or double vision; ringing in the ears; upset stomach; appetite loss; nausea; vomiting; constipation; diarrhea; urinary difficulties; chest tightness; wheezing; stuffy nose; and dryness of the mouth, nose, or throat. Young children may also develop nervousness, irritability, tension, and anxiety.

Drug Interactions

- Chlorpheniramine should not be taken with a monoamine oxidase inhibitor (MAOI) antidepressant or tricyclic antidepressants, because the combination may cause severe side effects.
- The effects of sedatives, benzodiazepines such as diazepam, and sleeping medications are increased when any of these

drugs is combined with chlorpheniramine. It is extremely important for your doctor to know if you are taking any other medication with chlorpheniramine so that the dosage of that medication can be properly adjusted.

- Anticholinergenics may cause an increase in side effects of chlorpheniramine.
- Be extremely cautious when drinking alcoholic beverages while taking this drug, which enhances the intoxicating and sedating effects of alcohol.

Food Interactions

You may take this drug with food if it upsets your stomach.

Usual Dose

Chlorpheniramine

Adult and Child (age 12 and over): 4 mg every 4–6 hours; do not take more than 24 mg a day.

Child (age 6–11): tablets or syrup: 2 mg every 4–6 hours; do not take more than 12 mg a day; oral suspension: 2.5–5 mL every 12 hours.

Child (age 2–5): tablets or syrup: consult your physician; oral suspension: 1.25 mL every 12 hours.

Child (under age 2): consult your physician.

Chlorpheniramine, Sustained-Release

Adult: 8–12 mg at bedtime, or every 8–12 hours during the day; do not take more than 24 mg a day.

Child (age 12–17): 8 mg during the day or at bedtime.

Child (under age 12): not recommended.

Cyproheptadine

Adult and Child (age 15 and over): 4–20 mg a day; do not exceed 32 mg a day.

Child (age 7–14): 4 mg 2–3 times a day; do not exceed 16 mg a day.

Child (age 2–6): 2 mg 2–3 times a day; do not exceed 12 mg a day.

Dexchlorpheniramine

Adult and Child (age 12 and over): 2 mg every 4–6 hours.

Child (age 6–11): 1 mg every 4–6 hours.

Child (age 2–5): 0.5 mg every 4–6 hours.

Dexchlorpheniramine, Sustained-Release

Adult and Child (age 12 and over): 4–6 mg every 8–10 hours and at bedtime.

Child (age 6–11): 4 mg once a day and at bedtime.
Child (under age 6): not recommended.

Tripelennamine

Adult and Child (age 12 and over): 25–50 mg every 4–6 hours; do not take more than 600 mg a day. Adults may take up to three 100-mg, sustained-release tablets a day, although this much is not usually needed.

Child (under age 12): 2 mg per lb. of body weight a day in divided doses; no more than 300 mg a day should be given.

Overdosage

Symptoms of overdose include depression or stimulation, especially in children; dry mouth; fixed or dilated pupils; flushing of the skin; upset stomach; unsteadiness; and convulsions. Overdose victims should be made to vomit as soon as possible with ipecac syrup—available at any pharmacy—to remove excess drug from the stomach. Take the victim to a hospital emergency room immediately if the victim is unconscious or if you cannot induce vomiting. If you seek treatment, ALWAYS bring the prescription bottle or container.

Special Information

Antihistamines may cause tiredness or loss of concentration. Be extremely cautious when driving or doing anything that requires close attention.

If you forget a dose, take it as soon as you remember. If it is almost time for your next dose, skip the one you forgot and continue with your regular schedule. Do not take a double dose.

Special Populations

Pregnancy/Breast-feeding: Animal studies have shown that some antihistamines may cause birth defects. Do not take any antihistamine without your doctor's knowledge if you are or might be pregnant—especially during the last 3 months of pregnancy, because newborns may have severe reactions to antihistamines.

Small amounts of some antihistamines pass into breast milk. Nursing mothers who must take them should use infant formula.

Seniors: Seniors are more sensitive to antihistamine side effects. Dosage reduction may be needed.

Generic Name

Chlorpromazine (klor-PROE-muh-zene) G

Brand Names

Only available in generic form.

The information in this profile also applies to the following drugs:

Generic Ingredients: Fluphenazine Hydrochloride G

Generic Ingredients: Pimozide
Orap

Generic Ingredients: Thioridazine Hydrochloride G

Generic Ingredients: Thiothixene G
Navane

Generic Ingredients: Trifluoperazine Hydrochloride G

Type of Drug

Antipsychotic.

Prescribed For

Psychotic disorders; manic symptoms related to manic-depressive disorder; agitation or aggressiveness in children with attention-deficit hyperactivity disorder (ADHD) or behavioral problems; nausea, vomiting, and hiccups; acute intermittent porphyria; and apprehension before surgery or other procedures. Pimozide is prescribed for Tourette syndrome.

General Information

Chlorpromazine and similar antipsychotics act upon a portion of the brain called the hypothalamus. Antipsychotic medications affect parts of the hypothalamus that control metabolism, body temperature, alertness, muscle tone, hormone balance, and vomiting. These medications are available in suppositories and as a liquid for those who have trouble swallowing tablets.

Cautions and Warnings

Do not take these medications if you are **allergic** or **sensitive** to any of their ingredients or to any antipsychotic drug.

Antipsychotic medications should not be used to treat **dementia-related psychosis in the elderly**.

Tardive dyskinesia, a syndrome consisting of potentially

irreversible, involuntary, jerky movements, may develop in people taking antipsychotic drugs. Generally, longer duration of treatment is related to increased risk of developing tardive dyskinesia and the likelihood that it will be irreversible.

Antipsychotic drugs have also been associated with a potentially fatal condition sometimes referred to as neuroleptic malignant syndrome (NMS). Symptoms of NMS include high fever, muscle rigidity, altered mental states, irregular or fast heartbeat, irregularities in blood pressure, and excessive sweating.

Levels of some white blood cells can drop drastically in people taking one of these medicines, making it harder to fight infection. Your doctor will monitor your blood count.

These medications may depress the cough reflex. People have accidentally choked to death because the cough reflex failed to protect them.

Because of their effect in reducing vomiting, antipsychotics may obscure symptoms of disease or toxicity due to overdose of another drug. Children who show signs or symptoms of **Reye's syndrome** should not be given these medications for this reason.

These medications should be used under your doctor's strict supervision if you have **heart**, **liver**, **or kidney disease**, **low blood pressure**, a **seizure disorder** or a history of **seizures**, or **depression**.

Avoid exposure to extreme heat, because these drugs may upset your body's temperature-control mechanism. Do not allow the liquid forms of these drugs to come in contact with your skin because they are highly irritating.

Possible Side Effects

▼ Most common: drowsiness, especially during the first or second week of therapy. If drowsiness becomes troublesome, contact your doctor.

▼ Less common: changes in blood components, including anemias; raised or lowered blood pressure; abnormal heart rate; heart attack; sensitivity to light; and faintness or dizziness.

▼ Rare: Rare side effects can occur in almost any part of the body. Contact your doctor if you experience anything unusual while taking any medication.

Jaundice (symptoms include yellowing of the skin or whites of the eyes) may appear; when it does, it is usually within the

Possible Side Effects *(continued)*

first 2–4 weeks of treatment. Normally the jaundice goes away when the drug is discontinued, but there have been cases when it has not.

Antipsychotics may produce extrapyramidal side effects, including spasm of the neck muscles, rolling back of the eyes, convulsions, difficulty swallowing, and symptoms associated with Parkinson's disease. These side effects seem very serious but usually disappear after the drug has been withdrawn; however, symptoms affecting the face, tongue, or jaw may persist for as long as several years, especially in older adults with a history of brain damage.

These medications may cause an unusual increase in psychotic symptoms or may cause paranoid reactions, tiredness, lethargy, restlessness, hyperactivity, confusion at night, bizarre dreams, sleeplessness, depression, decreased sex drive, increased appetite, or euphoria (feeling "high").

Drug Interactions

- Do not mix these drugs with medications to treat heart rhythm, such as amiodarone, bretylium, disopyramide, dofetilide, quinidine, and sotalol; arsenic trioxide; cisapride; dolasetron; droperidol; mefloquine; mesoridazine; moxifloxacin; pentamidine; tacrolimus; and ziprasidone. These combinations can affect your heart rhythm.
- Other drugs that should not be combined with pimozide due to the risk of dangerous heart rhythm disorders include aprepitant, cimetidine, dalfopristin, delavirdine, efavirenz, fluoroquinolones (such as gatifloxacin, moxifloxacin, and sparfloxacin), halofantrine, haloperidol, levomethadyl, macrolide antibiotics (such as azithromycin, clarithromycin, dirithromycin, and erythromycin) nefazodone, nilotinib, probucol, protease inhibitors (such as indinavir, nelfinavir, ritonavir, and saquinavir), quinupristin, certain selective serotonin reuptake inhibitor (SSRI) antidepressants (citalopram, fluvoxamine, paroxetine, and sertraline), tricyclic antidepressants such as amitriptyline, and zileuton.
- Taking lithium together with an antipsychotic drug may lead to disorientation, loss of consciousness, or uncontrolled muscle movements. Patients should be closely monitored with this combination.

- Be cautious about taking these medications with over-the-counter cough, cold, or allergy medications, barbiturates, alcohol, sleeping pills, narcotics or other sedatives, or any other drug that may produce a depressive effect.
- Anticholinergic drugs may reduce the effectiveness of these medications and increase the chance of side effects.
- Chlorpromazine, thiothixene, and trifluoperazine may counter the blood-pressure-lowering effect of guanethidine.
- Chlorpromazine may reduce the effectiveness of oral anti-coagulant (blood thinning) medications.
- Combining propranolol and chlorpromazine, thioridazine, or trifluoperazine may lead to unusually low blood pressure. Thioridazine should not be taken with propranolol, fluvox-amine, or pindolol.
- Combining tricyclic antidepressants with chlorpromazine can lead to antidepressant side effects.
- Taking chlorpromazine or trifluoperazine with a thiazide diuretic may cause excessively low blood pressure.
- Thiothixene should not be combined with tramadol.
- Carbamazepine may significantly reduce the effectiveness of thiothixene.

Food Interactions

Take liquid chlorpromazine with fruit juice or other liquids. You may also take it with food if it upsets your stomach.

Usual Dose

Chlorpromazine

Adult and Child (age 13 and over): 10–50 mg 3–4 times a day, individualized according to your disease and response. Dosages of up to 800 mg a day have been used for some disorders.

Child (age 6 months–12 years): 0.25 mg per lb. of body weight every 4–6 hours. Dosages above 500 mg a day have not shown to be effective.

Child (under 6 months): not recommended.

Fluphenazine

Adult: 2.5–10 mg a day to start. Dose is individualized according to your response up to 20–40 mg a day.

Seniors: 1–2.5 mg per day to start; increased to lowest effective dose depending on response.

Child: not recommended.

Pimozide

Adult: 1–2 mg a day in divided doses to start. Dose is increased according to your response, usually up to 10 mg a day.

Child: 0.02 mg per lb. of body weight every day, divided into several doses to start, increased according to response to a maximum of 0.9 mg per lb. or 10 mg per day.

Thioridazine

Adult: 50–100 mg 3 times a day, increasing gradually to a maximum of 800 mg a day.

Child: 0.02 mg per lb. of body weight to start, increased according to response to a maximum of 1.35 mg per lb.

Thiothixene

Adult and Child (age 12 and over): 2 mg 3 times a day, increasing gradually to a maximum of 15 mg a day. Some people may require 5 mg twice a day to start. Dose is increased according to your response, usually to 10–30 mg a day, although 60 mg a day may be required.

Child (under age 12): not recommended.

Trifluoperazine

Adult and Child (age 12 and over): 1–5 mg twice a day, increasing gradually, usually to 15–20 mg a day. Reduced doses should be used for seniors and smaller people.

Child (age 6–11): 1 mg 1–2 times a day to start, increasing gradually until symptoms are controlled. Final daily dose is usually no more than 15 mg.

Overdosage

Overdose symptoms include depression, extreme weakness, tiredness, lowered blood pressure, agitation, restlessness, uncontrolled muscle spasms, convulsions, fever, dry mouth, abnormal heart rhythms, and coma. The victim should be taken to a hospital emergency room immediately. If you seek treatment, ALWAYS bring the prescription bottle or container.

Special Information

Contact your doctor at once if you develop sore throat, fever, rash, weakness, visual problems, tremors, muscle movements or twitching, yellowing of the skin or whites of the eyes, or darkening of the urine.

Do not stop taking these medications without your doctor's knowledge. It may take several weeks before this drug takes effect.

These drugs may cause drowsiness. Use caution when driving or operating hazardous equipment. Avoid alcoholic beverages.

Antipsychotics may cause unusual sensitivity to the sun and may turn your urine reddish brown to pink.

If dizziness occurs, avoid rising quickly from a sitting or lying position and avoid climbing stairs. Use caution in hot weather, because these drugs may make you more prone to heatstroke.

If you are using sustained-release capsules, do not chew or break them. Liquid forms of these medications must be protected from light. Do not take them out of their opaque bottles.

If you take an antipsychotic medication more than once a day and forget to take a dose, take it right away if you remember within an hour. If you do not remember within an hour, skip the dose you forgot and continue with your regular schedule. If you take 1 dose a day and forget a dose, skip the dose you forgot and continue your regular schedule the next day. Never take a double dose.

Special Populations

Pregnancy/Breast-feeding: Infants born to women taking this drug have experienced side effects, including jaundice and nervous system effects. Newborns whose mothers are taking any antipsychotic medicine are more likely to experience agitation, abnormally increased or decreased muscle tone, tremor, sleepiness, severe difficulty breathing, and difficulty in feeding. In some newborns, the symptoms subside within hours or days and do not require specific treatment; other newborns may require longer hospital stays. Check with your doctor about taking chlorpromazine if you are or might be pregnant. Do not stop taking this medication without talking to your doctor, because suddenly stopping antipsychotic medications can cause significant treatment complications. These drugs should be taken during pregnancy only if your doctor determines that the potential benefit outweighs the risks.

These drugs may pass into breast milk. Nursing mothers who must take an antipsychotic medication should use infant formula.

Seniors: Seniors with dementia-related psychosis are at a greater risk of dying while taking these and other antipsychotic medicines. Seniors are generally more sensitive to the effects of these drugs and usually achieve desired results with lower dosages. Some experts feel that seniors should receive ¼–½ the usual adult dose.

Generic Name

Chlorzoxazone (klor-ZOX-uh-zone) G

Brand Names

Lorzone
Parafon Forte DSC
Remular-S

Type of Drug

Skeletal muscle relaxant.

Prescribed For

Pain and spasm of muscular conditions, including strain, sprain, bruising, and lower back problems.

General Information

Chlorzoxazone works primarily on the spinal cord level and on the brain, acting as a mild sedative. This results in fewer spasms, less pain, and greater mobility. Chlorzoxazone provides only temporary relief and is not a substitute for other types of therapy, such as rest, surgery, and physical therapy.

Cautions and Warnings

Do not take chlorzoxazone if you are **allergic** or **sensitive** to any of its ingredients, or if you have a condition known as **porphyria**.

People with **poor liver function** should take this drug with caution because serious liver toxicity has rarely occurred in people using chlorzoxazone.

Chlorzoxazone may interact with other drugs that cause nervous system depression (see "Drug Interactions").

Because it is possible to become dependent on this drug, people with a history of **substance abuse** should take chlorzoxazone with caution.

Possible Side Effects

- ▼ Most common: dizziness, drowsiness, lightheadedness, malaise, and overstimulation.
- ▼ Less common: headache, stomach cramps or pain, diarrhea, constipation, heartburn, nausea, and vomiting.
- ▼ Rare: internal bleeding, liver problems, severe allergic-type skin reactions, and breathing problems. Contact your doctor if you experience anything unusual while taking any medication.

Drug Interactions

- The depressive effects of chlorzoxazone may be enhanced by taking it with alcohol, sedatives, sleeping pills, or other nervous system depressants. Avoid these combinations.

Food Interactions

Take this drug with food if it upsets your stomach. The tablets may be crushed and mixed with food.

Usual Dose

Adult: 250–750 mg 3–4 times a day.

Overdosage

Early signs of chlorzoxazone overdose may include nausea, vomiting, diarrhea, drowsiness, dizziness, lightheadedness, and headache. Victims may also feel sluggish or sickly and lose the ability to move their muscles. Breathing may become slow or irregular, and blood pressure may drop. Contact a doctor immediately or go to a hospital emergency room for treatment. If you seek treatment, ALWAYS bring the prescription bottle or container.

Special Information

Chlorzoxazone may make you drowsy or reduce your ability to concentrate. Be extremely careful while driving or operating hazardous equipment. Avoid alcoholic beverages.

Chlorzoxazone may turn your urine orange to purple-red; this is not dangerous.

Contact your doctor if you develop drowsiness, weakness, an allergic reaction, skin rash or itching, breathing difficulties, black or tarry stools, vomiting of material that resembles coffee grounds, liver problems, or any other severe or bothersome side effect.

If you miss a dose of chlorzoxazone by more than an hour, skip the dose you forgot and continue with your regular schedule. Do not take a double dose.

Special Populations

Pregnancy/Breast-feeding: The safety of chlorzoxazone in pregnant women has not been established. Chlorzoxazone should be taken during pregnancy only if your doctor determines that the potential benefit outweighs the risks.

It is not known if chlorzoxazone passes into breast milk. Nursing mothers should use infant formula.

Seniors: Seniors, especially those with severe liver disease, are more sensitive to the effects of chlorzoxazone.

Generic Name

Cholestyramine (kol-es-TYE-rah-meen) G

Brand Names

LoCHOLEST
LoCHOLEST Light
Prevalite
Questran
Questran Light

The information in this profile also applies to the following drugs:

Generic Ingredients: Colesevelam Hydrochloride
WelChol

Generic Ingredients: Colestipol Hydrochloride G
Colestid

Type of Drug

Cholesterol-lowering agent. Antidiabetic (colesevelam only).

Prescribed For

High blood-cholesterol levels, high blood-sugar levels, generalized itching associated with bile duct obstruction, diarrhea, colitis, digitalis overdose, hyperthyroidism, or hyperoxaluria (a condition that may lead to kidney stones).

General Information

These drugs are called "bile acid sequestrants" because they lower blood-cholesterol levels by absorbing bile acids in the bowel. Because the body uses cholesterol to make the bile acids—needed to digest fat—fat digestion can only continue by making more bile acid from blood cholesterol. This results in lower blood-cholesterol levels 4–7 days after starting one of these medicines.

The bile acid sequestrants work entirely within the bowel and are never absorbed into the bloodstream. The cholesterol-lowering effect of these drugs may be increased when they are taken with a statin, fibrate, or nicotinic acid.

Cautions and Warnings

Do not use these medicines if you are **allergic** or **sensitive** to any of their ingredients or if your **bile duct is blocked**.

If you are being treated for **hypothyroidism**, **diabetes**, **kidney or blood vessel disorder**, **obstructive liver disease**, or **alcoholism**, consult your doctor before taking cholestyramine.

These agents can reduce absorption of vitamins A, D, E, K, and folic acid. You may need to take additional vitamin supplements.

Colesevelam should not be used if your **blood triglyceride level is over 500**, if you have had an **inflamed pancreas** because of very high triglyceride levels, or if you have a **blocked colon**.

Colesevelam should be used with caution if you have **difficulty swallowing** or **digestive problems**, or you have undergone surgery on your stomach or intestines.

Cholestyramine may cause or worsen **constipation** and **hemorrhoids**. Most constipation is mild, but it may become severe and result in bowel impaction. Some people may need to stop the medication or take less of it.

Possible Side Effects

- ▼ Most common: constipation, bloating, and flatulence.
- ▼ Less common: abdominal pain, bleeding disorders or black-and-blue marks due to interference with the absorption of vitamin K, belching, gas, nausea, vomiting, diarrhea, heartburn, appetite loss, blood in stool, and changes in the appearance of stool due to a high fat level.
- ▼ Rare: Rare side effects can affect your mouth, stomach and intestines, muscles and joints, mental status, urinary tract, breathing, or eyes (night blindness). Contact your doctor if you experience anything unusual while taking any medication.

Drug Interactions

- Cholestyramine interferes with the absorption of virtually all oral drugs, including contraceptive drugs, corticosteroids, digitalis, doxepin, furosemide, gemfibrozil, glipizide, hydrocortisone, imipramine, nonsteroidal anti-inflammatory drugs (NSAIDs), mycophenolate, penicillin, phenobarbital, phosphate supplements, propranolol, statins, tetracycline, thiazide diuretics, thyroid drugs, ursodiol, valproic acid, sustained-release verapamil, warfarin and other anticoagulant (blood thinning) drugs, and vitamins A, D, E, and K. Take other medications at least 1 hour before or 4–6 hours after taking cholestyramine.

Food Interactions

Take this medication with food. The powder may be mixed with soda, water, juice, cereal, or pulpy fruits, such as applesauce or crushed pineapple.

Usual Dose

Cholestyramine

Adult: 4–16 g (1–4 packets or 1–4 level scoopfuls) taken 1–6 times a day.

Child: 108 mg per lb. of body weight up to a total of 8 g a day in divided doses.

Colesevelam

Adult: 6 tablets once a day or in 2 divided doses; or 3.75-g packet once a day or 1.875-g packet twice a day.

Child (age 10 and over): 3.75-g packet once a day or 1.875-g packet twice a day.

Child (under age 10): not recommended.

Colestipol

Adult: 2–16 tablets once a day or in divided doses; or 5–30 g (1–6 packets) once a day or in divided doses.

Child: not recommended.

Overdosage

The most severe effect of overdose is obstruction of the gastrointestinal tract. Take the overdose victim to a hospital emergency room. If you seek treatment, ALWAYS bring the prescription bottle or container.

Special Information

Do not swallow the granules or powder in their dry form; doing so may result in the inhalation of powder into your lungs or a clogged esophagus. Prepare each packet of powder by mixing it with soup, cereal, or pulpy fruit or by adding the powder to a 6-oz. glass of water or another noncarbonated beverage. If some of the drug sticks to the sides of the glass, rinse it with liquid and drink the remainder. Do not sip the drink containing your medication or hold it in your mouth without swallowing, as this may lead to undesirable changes in the color or feel of your teeth.

Colestipol and colesevelam tablets should be swallowed whole.

Constipation, gas, nausea, and heartburn may occur and then disappear with continued use of this medication. If constipation is a problem, your doctor may recommend drinking more fluids and taking a fiber supplement. Contact your doctor if these side effects persist or if you develop unusual problems such as bleeding from the gums or rectum.

If you miss a dose, skip it and continue with your regular schedule. Do not take a double dose.

Special Populations

Pregnancy/Breast-feeding: Although these drugs do not affect the fetus directly, it may prevent the absorption of vitamins A, D, and E and other nutrients essential to the fetus' proper development—even when you take a prenatal vitamin supplement. These drugs should be taken during pregnancy only if your doctor determines that the potential benefit outweighs the risks.

These drugs are not absorbed into the body. However, reduced absorption of vitamins A, D, and E and other nutrients may make your milk less nutritious. Nursing mothers who must take these drugs should use infant formula.

Seniors: Seniors are more likely to experience side effects, especially those relating to the bowel.

Type of Drug

Cholinesterase Inhibitors

(KO-lin-ESS-tuh-rase)

Brand Names

Generic Ingredients: Donepezil G

Aricept　　Aricept ODT

Generic Ingredients: Galantamine G

Razadyne　　Razadyne ER

Generic Ingredients: Rivastigmine G

Exelon　　Exelon Transdermal System

Prescribed For

Alzheimer's disease. Also used for vascular dementia, dementia associated with Parkinson's disease, post-stroke aphasia (problems with language), and improvement of memory in multiple sclerosis patients.

General Information

Cholinesterase inhibitors work by increasing the function of certain receptors in the brain that are stimulated by the hormone acetylcholine. They do this by interfering with cholinesterase, the enzyme that breaks down acetylcholine. People with Alzheimer's disease (a degenerative condition of the central nervous system) develop a shortage of this brain chemical early in the disease.

There is no evidence that cholinesterase inhibitors reverse the degenerative effects of Alzheimer's, but they may slow the rate at which the disease worsens.

Cautions and Warnings

Do not take cholinesterase inhibitors if you are **allergic** or **sensitive** to any of their ingredients.

Cholinesterase inhibitors must be discontinued before **surgery** because they increase the effects of anesthetic drugs.

People with **heart disease** should use cholinesterase inhibitors with caution because they may slow heart rate and cause fainting. Two studies of people with mild symptoms of Alzheimer's disease taking **galantamine** revealed a higher rate of death from heart attack, stroke, or sudden death.

Cholinesterase inhibitors may be expected to cause increased stomach acid production and increased activity of the gastrointestinal tract. Possible complications include **ulcers** or **bleeding**. Nausea, vomiting, and weight loss are common side effects. **Alcohol** and **nonsteroidal anti-inflammatory drugs (NSAIDs)** such as aspirin or ibuprofen may worsen this effect.

Using cholinesterase inhibitors may also lead to urinary blockage, increase the risk of generalized seizures, and worsen **asthma** or other **pulmonary diseases**. Use with caution if you have these conditions.

People with severe **liver or kidney dysfunction** should not take galantamine.

Possible Side Effects

People taking cholinesterase inhibitors generally experience side effects at about the same rate as those taking a placebo (sugar pill).

- ▼ Most common: headache, general pain, accidents, nausea, diarrhea, sleeplessness, and dizziness.
- ▼ Common: tiredness, vomiting, appetite loss, and muscle cramps.
- ▼ Less common: arthritis, depression, abnormal dreams, fainting, black-and-blue marks, and weight loss.
- ▼ Rare: Rare side effects can occur in almost any part of the body. Contact your doctor if you experience anything unusual while taking any medication.

Drug Interactions

- Cholinesterase inhibitors interfere with anticholinergic drugs (often prescribed for stomach disorders).
- Cholinesterase inhibitors can be expected to increase the effects of cevimeline, surgical anesthetic drugs, and drugs that irritate the stomach and intestines, such as aspirin, ibuprofen, and other NSAIDs.
- The breakdown of cholinesterase inhibitors (except rivastigmine) in the liver can be slowed by amiodarone, celecoxib, chlorpheniramine, cimetidine, ciprofloxacin, clarithromycin, clomipramine, cocaine, delavirdine, diltiazem, doxorubicin, erythromycin, fluconazole, fluoxetine, fluvoxamine, halofantrine, haloperidol, indinavir, itraconazole, ketoconazole, levopromazine, methadone, mibefradil, mifepristone, nefazodone, nelfinavir, norfloxacin, paroxetine, quinidine, ranitidine, ritonavir, saquinavir, terbinafine, and grapefruit juice.
- The breakdown of cholinesterase inhibitors (except rivastigmine) in the liver can be increased by barbiturates, carbamazepine, corticosteroids, efavirenz, nevirapine, pioglitazone, phenytoin, and rifampin.

Food Interactions

Donepezil and galantamine can be taken without regard to food or meals.

Rivastigmine should be taken with morning and evening meals.

The rivastigmine transdermal patch can be used without regard to food or meals.

Usual Dose

Donepezil

Adult: 5 or 10 mg once a day.

Galantamine

Adult: 8–24 mg a day in 1–2 doses.

Rivastigmine

Adult: 3–12 mg a day divided into 2 doses.

Rivastigmine Transdermal Patch

Adult: Apply one 4.6-mg patch a day to start. Dose may be increased to one 9.5-mg patch a day.

Overdosage

Cholinesterase inhibitor overdose can be very serious. Symptoms include severe nausea, vomiting, salivation, sweating, slow heart rate, low blood pressure, slow breathing rate, convulsions, muscle weakness, and collapse. Take the overdose victim to a hospital emergency room at once. If you seek treatment, ALWAYS bring the prescription bottle or container.

Special Information

Donepezil should be taken just before bedtime.

Follow the special package directions for rivastigmine solution.

Do not remove the rivastigmine patch from its packaging until just before you are ready to apply it. Apply the patch to clean, dry, and hairless skin on the upper or lower back, upper arm, or chest that is also free of any powder, oil, moisturizer, or lotion that could keep the patch from sticking to your skin properly; skin should also be free of cuts, rashes, and irritations. Avoid places where the patch can be rubbed off by tight clothing. When changing your patch, apply your new patch to a different spot of skin (for example, on the right side of your body one day, then on the left side the next day). Do not use the same spot more than once every 14 days. Wear only one patch at a time and change it every 24 hours. If the patch falls off, apply a new patch for the rest of the day, then replace the patch the next day at the same time as usual.

Tobacco or nicotine use increases the rate at which rivastigmine is cleared from the body.

If you forget a dose and take your medication once a day, take it as soon as you remember. If it is almost time for your next dose, skip the dose you forgot and continue with the regular schedule. If you take your medication 2 or more times a day, take your dose as soon as you remember. If it is almost time for your next dose, skip the dose you forgot and continue with your regular schedule. Do not take a double dose.

Special Populations

Pregnancy/Breast-feeding: One animal study of a cholinesterase inhibitor indicated a small risk of birth defects. A cholinesterase inhibitor should be taken during pregnancy only if your doctor determines that the potential benefit outweighs the risks.

It is not known if cholinesterase inhibitors pass into breast milk. Nursing mothers who must take this drug should use infant formula.

Seniors: Seniors with moderate kidney function loss should not take galantamine. Dosage adjustments are not needed for donepezil or rivastigmine.

Cialis *see **Erectile Dysfunction Drugs,** page 453*

Generic Name

Ciclopirox (sye-kloe-PEER-ox) G

Brand Names

Loprox

Penlac

Type of Drug

Antifungal.

Prescribed For

Fungus and yeast infections of the nails and skin, including athlete's foot, candida, and dandruff.

General Information

Ciclopirox slows the growth of a variety of fungus organisms and yeasts and kills many others. The drug penetrates the skin, hair, hair follicles, and sweat glands. Ciclopirox nail lacquer is used for toenail and fingernail fungus infections. Ciclopirox shampoo is used for dandruff.

Cautions and Warnings

Do not use this product if you are **allergic** or **sensitive** to any of its ingredients.

Possible Side Effects

▼ Common: burning, itching, stinging, or oozing at the application site.

Drug Interactions

None known.

Usual Dose

Cream/Lotion

Adult and Child (age 10 and over): Massage into cleansed affected skin and surrounding area twice a day.

Nail Lacquer

Adult: Apply to infected nails once a day. Use in conjunction with monthly visits to a health care professional.

Shampoo

Adult and Child (age 17 and over): Wet hair and apply 1–2 tsp. to the scalp. Lather and leave on hair and scalp for 3 minutes, then rinse. Avoid contact with eyes. Repeat twice a week for 4 weeks.

Child (under age 16): not recommended.

Overdosage

Accidental ingestion may cause nausea and upset stomach. Contact your local poison control center or hospital for more information. If you seek treatment, ALWAYS bring the prescription bottle or container.

Special Information

This product can be expected to relieve symptoms within the first week of use. Follow your doctor's directions for the complete 2–4-week course of treatment with the cream or lotion to gain maximum benefit. The nail lacquer may be used for up to 48 weeks. Stopping the medication too soon can lead to a relapse.

When using ciclopirox nail lacquer, do not apply it to any skin other than that which surrounds the infected nails, because of possible irritation. Do not apply nail polish or any other nail lacquer to infected nails while you are using this product.

Avoid using ciclopirox nail lacquer near an open flame because the product is flammable.

Do not cover cream or lotion with a bandage.

Contact your doctor if the affected area burns, stings, or becomes red after you use this product, or if your symptoms do not clear up after 4 weeks of treatment; by then it is unlikely that this product will be effective.

If you forget a dose of ciclopirox, apply it as soon as you remember. Do not apply more than the amount prescribed to make up for the missed dose.

Special Populations

Pregnancy/Breast-feeding: Ciclopirox may pass to the fetus in very small amounts. In animal studies, high doses of ciclopirox given by mouth did not harm the fetus. Ciclopirox should be taken during pregnancy only if your doctor determines that the potential benefit outweighs the risks.

It is unknown if ciclopirox passes into breast milk. Nursing mothers who must use this drug should use infant formula.

Seniors: Seniors may use this drug without special precaution.

Generic Name

Cilostazol (sil-oe-STAY-zol) G

Brand Names

Pletal

Type of Drug

Antiplatelet.

Prescribed For

Intermittent claudication.

General Information

In intermittent claudication, leg muscles go into spasm due to reduced blood flow. This occurs when plaque buildup narrows blood vessels leading to the calf or other leg muscles. People with this condition often develop leg pain after walking only a short distance. Cilostazol prevents blood platelets from "clumping together" to begin the process of forming a blood clot, which can further obstruct arteries and worsen intermittent claudication. This drug is broken down in the liver.

Cautions and Warnings

Do not take this drug if you are **allergic** or **sensitive** to any of its ingredients.

People with **congestive heart failure** should not take cilostazol. Some studies indicate that long-term use of this drug may cause cardiovascular problems.

People with **hemostatic disorders**, including **thrombocytopenia (low blood-platelet count)** or **active pathologic bleeding** should not take cilostazol.

Cilostazol should be used with caution in people with moderate to severe **liver or kidney disease**.

Possible Side Effects

The risk of side effects increases with dosage.

- ▼ Most common: headache, infection, abdominal pain, abnormal stool, and diarrhea.
- ▼ Common: heart palpitations, rapid heartbeat, dizziness, upset stomach, nausea, sore throat, runny nose, back pain, and swelling in the arms or legs.

Possible Side Effects *(continued)*

- ▼ Less common: gas, cough, fainting, and muscle aches.
- ▼ Rare: Rare side effects can occur in almost any part of the body. Contact your doctor if you experience anything unusual while taking any medication.

Drug Interactions

- Avoid mixing cilostazol with fluconazole, fluoxetine, fluvoxamine, itraconazole, ketoconazole, miconazole, nefazodone, or sertraline because this interaction may slow the breakdown of cilostazol, prolonging its effects. Cilostazol dosage is reduced by ½ when it is combined with any of these drugs.
- Aspirin can increase the anticoagulant (blood thinning) effect of cilostazol, but this combination has not caused serious bleeding problems. There is no information on the effect of combining cilostazol and other antiplatelet or anticoagulant drugs. Cilostazol dosage is reduced by ½ when it is combined with any of these drugs.
- Diltiazem increases cilostazol blood levels by about 50%. Cilostazol dosage is reduced by ½ when it is combined with diltiazem.
- Erythromycin and similar antibiotics increase cilostazol blood levels. Take ½ the regular dose of cilostazol when combining it with any of these drugs.
- Combining cilostazol and omeprazole increases the effects of cilostazol. Cilostazol dosage is reduced by ½ when it is combined with omeprazole.
- Smoking reduces the effectiveness of cilostazol by causing the liver to break it down faster.

Food Interactions

Take this drug on an empty stomach at least 30 minutes before or 2 hours after meals. Do not drink grapefruit juice at any time while taking cilostazol because it can interfere with the breakdown of the drug.

Usual Dose

Adult: 100 mg twice a day; 50 mg twice a day when combined with other drugs that may increase the effect of cilostazol (see "Drug Interactions").

Child: not recommended.

Overdosage

Symptoms of overdose are likely to be the most common side effects. Overdose victims should be taken to a hospital emergency room. If you seek treatment, ALWAYS bring the prescription bottle or container.

Special Information

Several weeks of cilostazol treatment may be necessary before you notice any improvement in symptoms. Maximum benefit usually occurs after 12 weeks.

If you forget a dose, take it as soon as you remember. If it is almost time for your next dose, skip the forgotten dose and continue with your regular schedule. Do not take a double dose.

Special Populations

Pregnancy/Breast-feeding: Animal studies suggest that cilostazol may harm the fetus, but there is no information on the effect of cilostazol in pregnant women. Cilostazol should be taken during pregnancy only if your doctor determines that the potential benefit outweighs the risks.

Cilostazol may pass into breast milk. Nursing mothers who must take this drug should use infant formula.

Seniors: Seniors can take this drug without special precaution.

Ciprodex Ear Drops *see **Fluoroquinolone Anti-infectives,** page 512*

Generic Name

Clemastine (KLEH-mas-tene) G

Brand Names

Allerhist-1
Contac 12 Hour Allergy
Dailyhist-1
Dayhist-1
Dayhist Allergy
Tavist Allergy

Combination Products

Generic Ingredients: Acetaminophen + Clemastine + Pseudoephedrine
Tavist Allergy/Sinus/Headache

Type of Drug

Antihistamine.

Prescribed For

Sneezing, stuffy and runny nose, itchy eyes, and scratchy throat caused by seasonal allergies and for other symptoms of allergies such as rash, itching, and hives.

General Information

Antihistamines generally work by blocking the release of naturally occurring histamine (a chemical released by body tissue during an allergic reaction) from cells at the H_1 histamine receptor site, drying up secretions of the nose, throat, and eyes. Clemastine is less sedating than most antihistamines, but not less sedating than astemizole, cetirizine, or loratadine.

Cautions and Warnings

Clemastine should not be taken if you are **allergic** or **sensitive** to any of its ingredients.

People with **asthma** or other **deep-breathing problems**, **heart disease**, **high blood pressure**, **diabetes**, **enlarged prostate**, **difficulty urinating**, a history of **seizures**, **glaucoma**, **stomach ulcers** or other **stomach problems**, and **hyperthyroidism** should use clemastine with caution because its side effects can aggravate these problems.

Possible Side Effects

- ▼ Most common: drowsiness; dizziness; headache; weakness; nervousness; stomach upset; loss of appetite; nausea; vomiting; cough; stuffy nose; diarrhea; constipation; sore throat; nosebleeds; and dry mouth, nose, or throat.
- ▼ Less common: allergic reaction (symptoms include rash, itching, hives, and breathing difficulties), sleeplessness, menstrual irregularities, muscle aches, sweating, tingling in the hands or feet, frequent urination, visual disturbances, and ringing or buzzing in the ears.

Drug Interactions

- Combining clemastine with alcohol, sedatives, sleeping pills, or other nervous system depressants may increase the depressant effects of clemastine. Do not combine these drugs.

- The effects of oral anticoagulant (blood thinning) drugs may be decreased by clemastine. Do not take this combination without your doctor's knowledge.
- Monoamine oxidase inhibitor (MAOI) antidepressants may increase the drying and other effects of clemastine. This combination can also worsen urinary difficulties.
- When taking antihistamines on a regular basis, notify your doctor if you are taking large amounts of aspirin. Effects of too much aspirin may be masked by the antihistamine.

Food Interactions

Clemastine is best taken on an empty stomach at least 1 hour before or 2 hours after eating; it may be taken with food if it upsets your stomach.

Usual Dose

Adult and Child (age 12 and over): 1.34 mg twice a day, up to 8.04 mg, of the syrup; or 2.68 mg of the tablets in 24 hours.

Child (age 6–12): 0.67 mg twice a day, up to 4.02 mg, of the syrup.

Overdosage

Overdose is likely to cause severe side effects. Overdose victims should be given ipecac syrup—available at any pharmacy—to induce vomiting and should then be taken to a hospital emergency room. If you seek treatment, ALWAYS bring the prescription bottle or container.

Special Information

Clemastine may make it difficult for you to concentrate or perform complex tasks such as driving a car. Be sure to report any unusual side effects to your doctor.

Antihistamines may occasionally produce excitability, particularly in children.

If you forget to take a dose of clemastine, take it as soon as you remember. If it is almost time for your next dose, skip the one you forgot and continue with your regular schedule. Do not take a double dose.

Special Populations

Pregnancy/Breast-feeding: Do not take any antihistamines without your doctor's knowledge if you are or might be pregnant—especially during the last 3 months of pregnancy, because newborns may have severe reactions to antihistamines.

Small amounts of clemastine pass into breast milk. Nursing mothers who must take clemastine should use infant formula.

Seniors: Seniors may be more likely to experience side effects.

Generic Name

Clindamycin (klin-duh-MYE-sin) G

Brand Names

Cleocin
Cleocin T
Clinda-Derm
Clindagel
Clindesse
Clindets
Evoclin

Combination Products

Generic Ingredients: Clindamycin + Benzoyl Peroxide

Acanya
Benzclin
Duac

Generic Ingredients: Clindamycin + Tretinoin

Veltin
Ziana

Type of Drug

Antibiotic.

Prescribed For

Serious bacterial infections. The vaginal cream is used to treat bacterial vaginosis. Topical clindamycin is used to treat acne and rosacea.

General Information

Clindamycin is one of the few oral drugs that is effective against anaerobic bacteria, which grow only in the absence of oxygen and are often found in infected wounds, lung abscesses, abdominal infections, and infections of the female genital tract. It also works against bacteria usually treated with penicillin or erythromycin, including serious respiratory-tract infections. Clindamycin may be useful for treating certain skin or soft tissue infections. It kills the bacteria that frequently cause acne.

Clindamycin is not used to treat vaginal fungus or yeast infections.

Cautions and Warnings

Do not take clindamycin if you are **allergic** or **sensitive** to any of its ingredients or to lincomycin, another antibiotic.

Clindamycin can cause a severe intestinal irritation called colitis, which can be fatal. Signs of colitis are diarrhea, blood in the stool, and abdominal cramps. Any form of this drug, including products applied to the skin and the vaginal cream, can provoke colitis. Because of this, clindamycin should be reserved for serious infections or those that cannot be treated with other drugs.

People with **asthma** or a history of **allergies** should use clindamycin capsules with caution.

Clindamycin should be used with caution if you have **gastrointestinal disease** or **kidney or severe liver disease**.

Possible Side Effects

Capsules

▼ Most common: diarrhea, stomach pain, nausea, vomiting, and pain when swallowing.

▼ Less common: itching, rash, signs of serious drug sensitivity such as difficulties breathing and yellowing of the skin or the whites of the eyes, colitis (see "Cautions and Warnings"), effects on blood components, and vaginal irritation.

▼ Rare: scaling of the skin and joint pain. Contact your doctor if you experience anything unusual while taking any medication.

Topical Lotion

▼ Most common: dry skin, redness, burning, peeling, oily skin, and itching.

▼ Less common: abdominal pain, upset stomach, and headache.

▼ Rare: diarrhea and colitis (see "Cautions and Warnings"). Contact your doctor if you experience anything unusual while taking any medication.

For further information on the side effects of Veltin or Ziana, see Tretinoin, page 1175.

Vaginal Cream and Suppositories

▼ Most common: vaginal yeast infections; vaginal itching or irritation; thick, white vaginal discharge; and pain during intercourse.

Possible Side Effects *(continued)*

▼ Less common: yeast infections in the body, nausea, vomiting, diarrhea, constipation, abdominal pain, dizziness, headache, vertigo, and colitis (see "Cautions and Warnings").

Drug Interactions

- Do not combine clindamycin and erythromycin.
- The absorption of clindamycin capsules into the bloodstream is delayed by Kaolin-Pectin suspension (prescribed for diarrhea). Separate these drugs by at least 2 hours.
- Clindamycin should be used with caution by people also using neuromuscular agents.
- Clindamycin may reduce levels of cyclosporine; dosages of cyclosporine may need to be increased to be effective.
- If clindamycin is combined with paclitaxel, side effects of paclitaxel may be increased.

For more information on Veltin or Ziana, see Tretinoin, page 1175.

Food Interactions

Take the oral medication with a full glass of water or with food to prevent irritation of the stomach and intestine.

Usual Dose

Capsules

Adult and Child (age 16 and over): 150–450 mg every 6 hours.

Child (under age 16): 4–9 mg per lb. of body weight a day in 3–4 doses.

Foam: Wash the skin and pat dry before application. Dispense enough to cover the affected area(s) onto a cool surface (the foam will melt on contact with warm skin). Use fingertips to pick up foam and massage small amounts into the affected area(s) until the foam disappears. Use once a day.

Suppositories: Insert 1 suppository a day for 3 consecutive days.

Topical Lotion: Wash the skin and pat dry before application. Apply enough to cover the affected area(s) with a thin coat twice a day.

Vaginal Cream: Insert 1 applicator's worth at bedtime for 3–7 consecutive days.

Overdosage

Clindamycin overdose may lead to severe diarrhea and other drug side effects. Do not treat this diarrhea on your own. Discontinue use of this drug and contact your local poison control center or hospital emergency room for information. If you seek treatment, ALWAYS bring the prescription bottle or container.

Special Information

Prolonged or unsupervised use of clindamycin may lead to secondary infections from other organisms, such as fungi. Take this drug for the full course of therapy as indicated by your physician.

Contact your doctor immediately if you develop severe diarrhea, abdominal pain, breathing difficulties, or jaundice (yellowing of the skin or whites of the eyes).

Women using the vaginal cream should not have vaginal intercourse or use other vaginal products such as tampons or douches until treatment is complete.

The vaginal creams or suppositories may reduce the efficacy of latex condoms or diaphragms. Use an alternative method of birth control for 72 hours (3 days) after the last dose.

The topical lotion is for external use only. Avoid contact with your eyes or mucous membranes.

If you miss a dose of oral clindamycin, take it as soon as you remember. If it is almost time for your next dose of clindamycin, double that dose and go back to your regular dosage schedule.

Special Populations

Pregnancy/Breast-feeding: This drug crosses into fetal blood circulation. Clindamycin should be taken during pregnancy only if your doctor determines that the potential benefit outweighs the risks.

Clindamycin passes into breast milk but is considered safe for nursing infants.

Seniors: Seniors with other illnesses may be unable to tolerate diarrhea and other clindamycin side effects.

Generic Name

Clonidine (KLAH-nih-dene) G

Brand Names

Catapres Catapres-TTS-1

Catapres-TTS-2 Nexiclon XR
Catapres-TTS-3

Type of Drug

Alpha receptor stimulant.

Prescribed For

High blood pressure, including hypertensive emergency (diastolic blood pressure over 120). The extended-release formulation is used for attention-deficit hyperactivity disorder (ADHD). Clonidine is also used for excess sweating, childhood growth delay, Tourette syndrome, restless leg syndrome, schizophrenic psychosis, ulcerative colitis, painful or difficult menstruation, hot flashes related to menopause, diagnosis of pheochromocytoma (adrenal-gland tumor), kidney poisoning associated with cyclosporine, diabetic diarrhea, smoking cessation, methadone and opiate detoxification, withdrawal from alcohol and benzodiazepines such as Valium, nerve pain following herpes attack, and allergic reactions in the presence of asthma triggered by external sources.

General Information

Clonidine stimulates nerve endings in the brain called alpha-adrenergic receptors. It reduces blood pressure by dilating (widening) blood vessels. Clonidine works quickly, decreasing blood pressure within 1 hour. The other uses of clonidine relate to its stimulation of alpha receptors in the body.

Cautions and Warnings

Do not take clonidine if you are **allergic** or **sensitive** to any of its ingredients.

People who have had a **stroke** or recent **heart attack** or who have **cardiac insufficiency** or **chronic kidney failure** should avoid taking clonidine.

Some people develop a tolerance of their clonidine dosage. If this happens, your blood pressure may increase and your doctor may prescribe a higher dose.

Never stop taking clonidine without your doctor's knowledge. If you abruptly stop taking clonidine, you may experience an unusual increase in blood pressure accompanied by agitation, headache, nervousness, and severe reactions, possibly death. Restarting clonidine therapy or taking another antihypertensive can reverse these effects.

Clonidine may cause degeneration of the retina. See your eye doctor for regular checkups if you are taking this drug.

If you require **surgery**, your doctor will continue your clonidine therapy until about 4 hours before surgery and resume it as soon as possible afterward.

People who develop skin sensitivity (symptoms include rash, itching, and swelling) to the transdermal patch form of clonidine may experience the same reactions with oral clonidine.

Possible Side Effects

Tablets

- Most common: dry mouth, drowsiness, dizziness, constipation, and sedation.
- Common: headache and fatigue. These effects tend to diminish within 4–6 weeks.
- Less common: appetite loss, swelling or pain in the glands of the throat, nausea, vomiting, weight gain, blood-sugar elevation, breast pain or enlargement, worsening of congestive heart failure, heart palpitations, rapid heartbeat, painful blood-vessel spasm, abnormal heart rhythms, electrocardiogram changes, feeling unwell, changes in dream patterns, nightmares, difficulty sleeping, hallucinations, delirium, anxiety, depression, nervousness, restlessness, rash, hives, thinning or loss of scalp hair, difficult or painful urination, nighttime urination, retaining urine, decrease or loss of sex drive, weakness, muscle or joint pain, leg cramps, increased alcohol sensitivity, dryness and burning of the eyes, dry nose, loss of color, and fever.

Transdermal Patch

- Most common: dry mouth and drowsiness.
- Less common: constipation; nausea; changes in sense of taste; dry throat; fatigue; headache; lethargy; changes in sleep patterns; nervousness; dizziness; impotence; sexual difficulties; and mild skin reactions, including itching, swelling, contact dermatitis, discoloration, burning, peeling, throbbing, white patches, and generalized rash. Rashes of the face and tongue have also occurred but cannot be specifically tied to transdermal clonidine.

Drug Interactions

- Avoid combining clonidine and tizanidine. Very low blood pressure may result.
- Combining clonidine and a beta-adrenergic blocker may increase the severity of a drug-withdrawal reaction and rebound high blood pressure. This reaction may be very serious.
- Combining clonidine with a calcium channel blocker such as diltiazem or verapamil may lead to very low blood pressure and atrioventricular (AV) block (abnormality in heartbeat patterns). A similar reaction is possible when combining clonidine and digitalis. This reaction may be very serious.
- Avoid alcohol, barbiturates, and sedatives because they increase the depressive effects of clonidine.
- Tricyclic antidepressants, mirtazapine, and prazosin may counteract the effects of clonidine.
- Clonidine increases the effects of cyclosporine. Clonidine dosages may need adjusting.

Food Interactions

The tablets are best taken on an empty stomach but may be taken with food if they upset your stomach.

Usual Dose

Immediate-Release Tablets

Adult and Child (age 12 and over): high blood pressure—0.02–0.06 mg a day in divided doses to a maximum of 2.4 mg a day. Seniors should start with a lower dose and increase more slowly.

Child (under age 12): not recommended.

Extended-Release Tablets

Child (age 6 and over): ADHD–maximum dose of 0.4 mg a day. Dosages over 0.1 mg a day should be divided into 2 doses taken morning and evening.

Transdermal Patch

Adult and Child (age 12 and over): 100 mcg delivered daily from a patch applied once every 7 days. Up to two 300-mcg patches may be needed to control blood pressure. Transdermal dosage exceeding 600 mcg a day has not been shown to increase effectiveness.

Child (under age 12): not recommended.

Overdosage

Symptoms of overdose are slow heartbeat, central-nervous-system depression, very slow breathing, low body temperature, pinpoint pupils, seizures, lethargy, agitation, irritability, nausea, vomiting, abnormal heart rhythms, mild increases in blood pressure followed by a rapid drop in blood pressure, dizziness, weakness, loss of reflexes, and vomiting. Victims should be taken to a hospital emergency room immediately. If you seek treatment, ALWAYS bring the prescription bottle or container.

Special Information

Clonidine causes drowsiness in about ⅓ of people who take it. Be extremely careful while driving or performing any task that requires concentration. This effect is prominent during the first few weeks of clonidine therapy and then tends to decrease.

Do not take over-the-counter cough and cold medications unless directed by your doctor.

Contact your doctor if you become depressed or have vivid dreams or nightmares while taking clonidine, or if you develop swelling in your feet or legs, paleness or coldness in your fingertips or toes, or any persistent or bothersome side effect.

Apply the transdermal patch to a hairless area of skin such as the upper arm or torso. Use a different skin site each time. If the patch becomes loose, apply the supplied adhesive directly over it. If the patch falls off before 7 days are up, apply a new one. Do not remove the patch while bathing.

If you forget a dose of oral clonidine, take it as soon as possible and then go back to your regular schedule. If you miss 2 or more consecutive doses, consult your doctor; missed doses may cause blood pressure increases and severe adverse effects. Do not take a double dose.

Special Populations

Pregnancy/Breast-feeding: Clonidine passes into the fetal bloodstream. Animal studies show that clonidine may damage the fetus in doses as low as ⅓ the maximum dose. Clonidine should be taken during pregnancy only if your doctor determines that the potential benefit outweighs the risks.

Clonidine passes into breast milk. Nursing mothers who must take this drug should use infant formula.

Seniors: Seniors are more susceptible to the effects of this drug and should begin with lower doses.

Generic Name

Clotrimazole (kloe-TRIM-uh-zole) G

Brand Names

Desenex
FungiCure
Gyne-Lotrimin
Lotrimin AF
Mycelex

The information in this profile also applies to the following drugs:

Generic Ingredients: Betamethasone Dipropionate + Clotrimazole G
Lotrisone

Generic Ingredients: Econazole G

Generic Ingredients: Sertaconazole
Ertaczo

Type of Drug

Antifungal. Lotrisone is an antifungal and corticosteroid combination product.

Prescribed For

Fungal infections of the mouth, skin, and vaginal tract.

General Information

Clotrimazole is useful against a variety of fungal organisms that other drugs do not affect. The exact way in which clotrimazole works is unknown. Econazole and Lotrisone are prescribed for severe skin infections such as athlete's foot, jock itch, and ringworm. Sertaconazole is used for athlete's foot in people age 12 and older with compromised immune systems.

Cautions and Warnings

Do not use this product if you are **allergic** or **sensitive** to any of its ingredients.

If these products cause local itching or irritation, stop using them.

Do not use these products in your eyes.

Do not use Lotrisone to treat diaper rash.

Lotrisone may increase glucose levels in the blood or urine, especially in people with severe **diabetes**.

Proper diagnosis is essential for effective treatment. Do not use these products without first consulting your doctor.

Possible Side Effects

Side effects are infrequent and usually mild.

Cream and Solution

▼ Most common: redness, burning, stinging, blistering, peeling, itching, and swelling of local areas.

Lozenge

▼ Most common: stomach cramps or pain, diarrhea, nausea, and vomiting.

Vaginal Tablet

▼ Most common: mild burning, rash, mild cramps, and frequent urination. Your sexual partner may also experience some burning or itching.

Drug Interactions

None known.

Food Interactions

The oral form of clotrimazole is best taken on an empty stomach, at least 1 hour before or 2 hours after meals. However, you may take it with food as long as you allow the lozenge to dissolve fully in your mouth.

Usual Dose

Cream and Solution

Adult: Apply to clean, dry, affected areas morning and night for 1–4 weeks depending on the condition being treated.

Child: Clotrimazole and econazole may be used on children age 2 and over in the same dosage as adults. Lotrisone is not recommended for children under age 17. Sertaconazole is not recommended for children under age 12.

Lozenge

Adult and Child (over age 3): 1 lozenge 5 times a day for 2 weeks or more.

Vaginal Cream

Adult: 1 applicator's worth at bedtime for 3–7 consecutive days.

Vaginal Tablet

Adult: 1 tablet inserted into the vagina at bedtime for 3 days, or 2 tablets a day for 3–7 consecutive days.

Overdosage

Little is known about the effects of clotrimazole overdose or accidental ingestion. Contact your local poison control center for more information. If you seek treatment, ALWAYS bring the prescription bottle or container.

Special Information

If treating a vaginal infection, you should refrain from sexual activity. Contact your doctor if burning or itching develops or if the condition does not improve within 7 days.

If you are using the vaginal cream, you may want to wear a sanitary napkin to avoid staining your clothing. Do not use a tampon during treatment.

Dissolve the lozenge slowly in the mouth. This may take up to 30 minutes.

When using these products for skin infections, do not cover the area with any kind of bandage unless directed to do so by your doctor. Wear loose-fitting clothing (preferably cotton), especially after application to the genital area. For athlete's foot, wear well-fitting, ventilated shoes, and change your socks at least once a day.

Although prolonged treatment with Lotrisone is not recommended, it is important to take this drug for the entire period prescribed by your doctor, even if you are no longer experiencing symptoms.

People with ringworm should wash their clothes separately from other household members' clothes.

Clotrimazole is not effective on scalp or nails.

These products must be used or taken on consecutive days. If you forget a dose of oral clotrimazole, take it as soon as you remember. Do not double your dose.

Special Populations

Pregnancy/Breast-feeding: Women who are or might be pregnant should talk to their doctor about these medications' risks and benefits. Women who are in the first 3 months of pregnancy should use clotrimazole and Lotrisone only if directed to do so by their doctors. Econazole should be strictly avoided during the first 3 months of pregnancy and used only if absolutely necessary in the last 6 months. If you are pregnant, your doctor may want you to insert vaginal tablets by hand rather than use a vaginal applicator.

It is unknown whether the drug passes into breast milk. Use with caution or use infant formula.

Seniors: Seniors may use this medication without special precaution.

Brand Name

Coartem (ko-AR-tem)

Generic Ingredients

Artemether + Lumefantrine

Type of Drug

Antimalarial.

Prescribed For

Uncomplicated malaria in people resistant to other therapies.

General Information

Coartem is the first artemesinin antimalarial to be made available in the United States. The artemesinins are derived from the leaves of the *Artemisia annua* plant used to treat malaria. Coartem should not be used to prevent malaria or to treat serious malaria and it may be effective when other antimalarial drugs fail. Of the 350–500 million new malaria cases each year, 90% occur in sub-Saharan Africa, but it is also found in parts of Asia and Latin America. Americans who travel to these or other high-risk areas can develop malaria if bitten by an infected mosquito.

Cautions and Warnings

Do not take this drug if you are **allergic** or **sensitive** to any of its ingredients.

This drug should used with caution if you have an **abnormal electrocardiogram (ECG), a family history of heart disease or sudden death, low blood levels of potassium or magnesium**, or if you take **other drugs that also affect the heart**.

Many drugs can interact with Coartem to affect your heart. Be sure all your doctors, especially your primary care physician and cardiologist, know you are taking it.

People with severe **liver or kidney disease** should use this drug with caution.

Possible Side Effects

Adult:

- ▼ Most common: headache, appetite loss, dizziness, weakness, tiredness, fever and chills, joint and muscle pain, nausea, vomiting, abdominal pain, sleeping problems, and heart palpitations.
- ▼ Common: diarrhea and liver and bile disorders.
- ▼ Less common: not feeling well, malaria recurrence, and nose and throat inflammation.
- ▼ Rare: Other side effects can affect almost any part of the body. Contact your doctor if you experience anything unusual while taking any medication.

Child:

- ▼ Most common: fever, cough, vomiting, appetite loss, headache, and malaria reinfection.
- ▼ Common: chills, weakness, tiredness, abdominal pain, diarrhea, nausea, runny nose, liver or spleen enlargement, and anemia.
- ▼ Less common: dizziness, bone or joint pain, rash, and changes in lab tests for liver injury.
- ▼ Rare: Other side effects can affect almost any part of the body. Contact your doctor if you experience anything unusual while taking any medication.

Drug Interactions

- Halofantrine, another antimalarial, and Coartem tablets should not be taken within 1 month of each other because they both affect the heart.
- Quinidine and quinine should be used with caution after Coartem treatment because of their effect on the heart.
- The following drugs slow the enzyme system in the liver that breaks Coartem down, which can result in higher blood levels of the medicine and an exaggerated effect on your heart: amiodarone, aprepitant, chloramphenicol, clarithromycin, delavirdine, diltiazem, erythromycin, fluconazole, fluoxetine, fluvoxamine, gestodene, imatinib, indinavir, itraconazole, ketoconazole, mibefradil, miconazole, mifepristone, nefazodone, nelfinavir, norfloxacin, norfluoxetine, ritonavir, saquinavir, sertraline, telithromycin, verapamil, and voriconazole.
- The following drugs can increase the breakdown of Coartem, reducing its effectiveness: barbiturates, carbamazepine,

corticosteroids, efavirenz, mefloquine, modafinil, nevirapine, oxcarbazepine, phenobarbital, phenytoin, pioglitazone, rifabutin, rifampin, and St. John's wort.

- The following drugs may interact with Coartem to produce drug side effects, including a possible effect on your heart; report anything unusual to your doctor if you are taking any of these drugs while you are taking Coartem: alprenolol, amitriptyline, amphetamine, aripiprazole, atomoxetine, carvedilol, chlorpheniramine, chlorpromazine, clomipramine, codeine, debrisoquine, desipramine, dextromethorphan, donepezil, duloxetine, encainide, flecainide, haloperidol, imipramine, lidocaine, methoxyamphetamine, metoclopramide, metoprolol, mexiletine, nebivolol, nortriptyline, ondansetron, oxycodone, paroxetine, perhexiline, perphenazine, phenacetin, phenformin, promethazine, propafenone, propranolol, risperidone, sparteine, tamoxifen, thioridazine, timolol, tramadol, venlafaxine, and zuclopenthixol.
- Coartem can reduce the effectiveness of all contraceptive drugs. Use an additional birth control method during the entire month in which you take these pills.

Food Interactions

This drug must be taken with a fatty meal or fatty food to obtain maximum drug absorption into the bloodstream. If you have trouble swallowing the pills, Coartem tablets may be crushed and mixed with 1 or 2 tsp. of water just before they are taken. The mixture should be followed by food or drink other than water.

Do not drink or eat any grapefruit or starfruit products while on this treatment. They can slow the breakdown of this drug by the liver and increase its effect on your heart.

Usual Dose

Six doses of Coartem over 3 days—day 1: the first dose then a second dose 8 hours later; days 2 and 3: one dose morning and evening. The number of Coartem pills you take each time is based on body weight.

Adult and Child (age 2 months and over)

71 lbs. and over: 4 tablets per dose.
55–70 lbs.: 3 tablets per dose.
33–54 lbs.: 2 tablets per dose.
11–32 lbs.: 1 tablet per dose.
Under 11 lbs.: not recommended.

Overdosage

There is no information on Coartem overdose, though likely symptoms include effects on the heart and blood. Overdose victims should be taken to a hospital emergency room. If you seek treatment, ALWAYS bring the prescription bottle or container.

Special Information

Malaria patients often cannot tolerate food. If you vomit within 2 hours after taking a dose, take a repeat dose right away. If the second dose is vomited, contact your doctor at once. An alternative malaria medicine may be prescribed.

The entire Coartem treatment program takes 3 days; you must try to take it exactly as prescribed. If you forget a dose, take it as soon as you remember. If you forget more than one dose of Coartem, contact your doctor at once. An alternative malaria medicine may be prescribed.

If you experience a serious allergic reaction to Coartem, stop taking it immediately and contact your doctor. Allergic symptoms include serious skin rash; swelling; hives; fast heartbeat; difficulty swallowing, breathing, or speaking; swelling of the lips, tongue, or face; and tightness of the throat.

Special Populations

Pregnancy/Breast-feeding: Coartem has been used by more than 1500 pregnant women with no increase in injuries to the developing fetus or general pregnancy problems. However, studies of Coartem in pregnant animals have shown variable results. Coartem should be taken during pregnancy only if your doctor determines that the potential benefit outweighs the risks.

The ingredients in Coartem may pass into breast milk. Nursing mothers who must take it should use infant formula because of the possible risk of drug side effects to the nursing infant.

Seniors: Seniors are more likely to be taking other medicines and to have reduced kidney and liver function and heart disease. These factors must be considered before taking Coartem.

Generic Name

Colchicine (KOLE-chih-seen)

Brand Names

Colcrys

Type of Drug

Antigout medication.

Prescribed For

Mediterranean fever and prevention and treatment of gouty arthritis; also prescribed for chronic progressive multiple sclerosis; cirrhosis of the liver; biliary cirrhosis; Behçet's disease; pseudogout (a condition caused by calcium deposits); amyloidosis; very low blood-platelet count (also known as idiopathic thrombocytopenic purpura [ITP]); skin reactions, including scleroderma, psoriasis, Sweet syndrome, and other conditions; and nerve disability associated with chronic progressive multiple sclerosis.

General Information

Although no one knows exactly how colchicine works, it appears to help people with gout by reducing the inflammatory response to uric acid crystals that form inside joints and by interfering with the body's mechanism for making uric acid. Unlike drugs that affect uric-acid levels, colchicine does not block the progression of gout to chronic gouty arthritis; it will, however, relieve the pain of acute attacks and lessen the frequency and severity of attacks. It has no effect on other kinds of pain.

Cautions and Warnings

Do not use colchicine if you are **allergic** or **sensitive** to any of its ingredients or if you suffer from any serious **blood**, **kidney**, **liver**, **stomach**, **or cardiac condition**. Dose adjustments may be required depending on the seriousness of your condition.

Colchicine can cause muscle weakness, damage, and pain. These symptoms are frequently related to high levels of colchicine in the blood caused by poor kidney function or a drug interaction (see "Drug Interactions") and improve on their own 1 week to several months after the drug is stopped. This reaction can be mistaken for other conditions.

Colchicine can cause a sudden drop in red- and white-blood-cell and blood-platelet counts. Periodic blood counts should be done if you are taking colchicine for long periods of time.

Colchicine interferes with the absorption of vitamin B_{12} by affecting the lining of the gastrointestinal (GI) tract.

Colchicine may affect the process of sperm generation in men.

The safety and effectiveness for use by **children** have not been established.

Possible Side Effects

Side effects generally subside when the colchicine dose is reduced.

- ▼ Most common: nausea, vomiting, diarrhea, and abdominal pain.
- ▼ Common: severe diarrhea, kidney and blood-vessel damage, blood in the urine, and reduced urination.
- ▼ Less common: hair loss, rash, appetite loss, and muscle and nerve weakness.
- ▼ Rare: Usually with long-term colchicine therapy—reduced blood-cell and platelet counts, nerve inflammation, severe blood-clotting problems, unusual bleeding or bruising, tingling in the hands or feet, red or purple spots under the skin, lactose intolerance, stomach cramps and pain, and other reactions. Colchicine may interfere with sperm formation. Contact your doctor if you experience anything unusual while taking any medication.

Drug Interactions

- Mixing colchicine with atazanavir, clarithromycin, darunavir, indinavir, itraconazole, ketoconazole, nefazodone, nelfinavir, ritonavir, saquinavir, or telithromycin drastically increases the amount of colchicine in the blood. Do not mix these drugs, especially if you have kidney and/or liver disease.
- Cyclosporine, dipyridamole, quinidine, ranolazine, and verapamil can slow colchicine's release from your body via the kidneys, increasing blood levels of the drug. Do not mix these drugs, especially if you have kidney and/or liver disease.
- Amiodarone, aprepitant, chloramphenicol, cimetidine, ciprofloxacin, delavirdine, diltiazem, erythromycin, fluconazole, fluvoxamine, fosamprenavir, gestodene, imatinib, mibefradil, mifepristone, norfloxacin, norfluoxetine, and voriconazole can also raise colchicine blood levels, but less than the drugs listed above. These drugs should be avoided if you are taking colchicine because of increased side effect and toxicity risk.
- Barbiturates, carbamazepine, corticosteroid drugs, efavirenz, glitazone antidiabetes drugs, modafinil, nevirapine, oxcarbazepine, phenobarbital, phenytoin, rifabutin, rifampin, and St. John's wort can speed the breakdown of colchicine in

the liver, reducing its effectiveness. Dose adjustments may be required.

- Atorvastatin, benzafibrate, fenofibrate, fenofibric acid, fluvastatin, gemfibrozil, pravastatin, and simvastatin increase the risk of muscle damage with colchicine. Take this combination with care and report any changes to your doctor.
- Mixing colchicine with digoxin increases the risk of muscle pain and damage.
- Colchicine interferes with the absorption of vitamin B_{12}.
- Colchicine may increase sensitivity to central-nervous-system depressants, such as sedatives and alcohol.
- The following drugs may reduce colchicine's effectiveness: anticancer drugs, bumetanide, diazoxide, thiazide diuretics, ethacrynic acid, furosemide, mecamylamine, pyrazinamide, and triamterene.
- Taking phenylbutazone with colchicine increases the risk of side effects.

Food Interactions

Avoid eating grapefruit or drinking grapefruit juice while taking colchicine, as they can increase the chance of serious side effects.

Usual Dose

Acute Gout Attack: 1.2 mg (2 tablets) at first sign of a gout flare, followed by 0.6 mg (1 tablet) 1 hour later. This initial dose may be followed by another 0.6 mg every 1–2 hours until pain is relieved or nausea, vomiting, or diarrhea occurs. The maximum recommended dose is 1.8 mg over a 1-hour period. The total dose needed to control pain and inflammation during an attack varies from 4–8 mg, with a 3-day interval between courses to minimize drug toxicity.

Amyloidosis: 0.5 mg 1–2 times a day.

Behçet's Disease: 0.5–1.5 mg a day.

Biliary Cirrhosis: 0.6 mg twice a day.

Cirrhosis of the Liver: 1 mg a day for 5 days each week.

Familial Mediterranean Fever

Adult and Child (age 13 and over): 1.2–2.4 mg a day in 1 or 2 divided doses. Dosage must be tailored to your individual needs with a maximum dose of 4 mg a day.

Child (age 7–12): 0.9–1.8 mg a day.

Child (age 4–6): 0.3–1.8 mg a day.
Child (under age 4): not recommended.

Gout Prevention: 0.5–1.2 mg a day. In mild cases, 0.5 mg or 0.6 mg may be taken 3–4 days a week.

ITP: 1.2–1.8 mg a day for 2 weeks or more.

Pseudogout: 0.6 mg twice a day.

Scleroderma: 1 mg a day.

Sweet Syndrome: 0.5 mg 1–3 times a day.

Other Skin Disorders: up to 1.8 mg a day, depending on the specific condition.

Overdosage

The lethal dose is estimated at 65 mg, although people have died after taking as little as 7 mg over 4 days, while others have lived after taking 60 mg or more. Usually 1 day passes between the overdose and first symptoms. Overdose symptoms start with nausea, vomiting, stomach pain, diarrhea—which may be severe and bloody—and burning sensations in the throat or stomach or on the skin. Serious and life-threatening complications begin within 1–3 days after the overdose. The overdose victim should go to a hospital emergency room. If you seek treatment, ALWAYS bring the prescription bottle or container.

Special Information

Contact your doctor if you develop rash, sore throat, fever, unusual bleeding or bruising, tiredness, muscle pain or weakness, tingling or numbness in the fingers or toes, or if your lips, tongue, or palms become pale or turn gray. Vomiting, abdominal pain, diarrhea, nausea, kidney damage, and blood in the urine may occur with colchicine, especially at maximum doses. This can worsen existing GI or other conditions. Stop taking the medication and contact your doctor if you develop one of these symptoms.

Stop taking maximum doses of colchicine as soon as gout pain is relieved, and reduce your dose to a maintenance level if your doctor has prescribed it for gout prevention.

Take this medication every day. If you forget a dose of colchicine, take it as soon as possible. If it is almost time for your next dose, skip the dose you forgot and continue with your regular schedule. Do not take a double dose.

Special Populations

Pregnancy/Breast-feeding: Colchicine passes into the blood circulation of the developing fetus. Animal studies indicate it can harm the fetus, but there is no conclusive information on the safety of this drug in humans. Colchicine should be taken during pregnancy only if your doctor determines that the potential benefit outweighs the risks.

Colchicine passes into breast milk and a nursing infant receives less than 10% of the mother's dose in its milk. No problems in nursing infants are known, but nursing mothers who must take colchicine should consider using infant formula.

Seniors: Seniors, especially those with kidney, liver, GI, or heart disease, are more likely to develop drug side effects and should use colchicine with caution, beginning at the low end of the dosing range.

Combivent *see* ***Ipratropium,*** *page 644*

Concerta *see* ***Methylphenidate,*** *page 742*

Type of Drug

Contraceptives

Brand Names

Generic Ingredients: Low-Dose Estrogen + Low-Dose Progestin + Low Androgen Activity (Single-Phase Combination) G

Aviane
Lutera
Lybrel
Orsythia

Generic Ingredients: Low-Dose Estrogen + High-Dose Progestin + Intermediate Androgen Activity (Single-Phase Combination)

Junel Fe 1/20
Loestrin 21 1/20
Loestrin 24 Fe
Loestrin Fe 1/20
Microgestin Fe 1/20

Generic Ingredients: Low-Dose Estrogen + Intermediate-Dose Progestin + Intermediate Androgen Activity (Single-Phase Combination) G

Altavera
Cryselle
Levlen
Lo/Ovral
LoSeasonique
Nordette-28
Seasonique

Generic Ingredients: Low-Dose Estrogen + High-Dose Progestin + Low Androgen Activity (Single-Phase Combination) G

Junel Fe 1.5/30
Kariva
Mircette
Zovia 1/35E

Generic Ingredients: Low-Dose Estrogen + High-Dose Progestin + High Androgen Activity (Single-Phase Combination)

Loestrin 21 1.5/30
Loestrin Fe 1.5/30

Generic Ingredients: Intermediate-Dose Estrogen + Low-Dose Progestin + Low Androgen Activity (Single-Phase Combination) G

Ortho-Cyclen

Generic Ingredients: Intermediate-Dose Estrogen + Intermediate-Dose Progestin + Intermediate Androgen Activity (Single-Phase Combination) G

Norinyl 1 + 50

Generic Ingredients: Intermediate-Dose Estrogen + High-Dose Progestin + Low Androgen Activity (Single-Phase Combination) G

Desogen
Ortho-Cept
Zovia 1/50E

Generic Ingredients: Intermediate-Dose Progestin + Low-Dose Estrogen + No Androgen Activity (Single-Phase Combination)

Beyaz
Yaz

Generic Ingredients: Intermediate-Dose Progestin + Intermediate-Dose Estrogen + No Androgen Activity (Single-Phase Combination)

Yasmin

Generic Ingredients: Intermediate-Dose Progestin + High-Dose Estrogen + Intermediate Androgen Activity (Single-Phase Combination) G

Norinyl 1 + 35
Nortrel 1/35
Ortho-Novum 1/35
Ovcon-50

Generic Ingredients: High-Dose Estrogen + Low-Dose Progestin + Low Androgen Activity (Single-Phase Combination)

Balziva-28
Brevicon
Briellyn
Modicon
Neocon 0.5/35
Nortrel 0.5/35
Ovcon-35

Generic Ingredients: Low-Dose Progestin + High-Dose Estrogen + Low Androgen Activity (3-Phase Combination) G

Tri-Norinyl

Generic Ingredients: High-Dose Estrogen + Intermediate-Dose Progestin + Low Androgen Activity (2-Phase Combination)

Necon 10/11
Ortho-Novum 10/11

Generic Ingredients: Low-Dose Estrogen + Low-Dose Progestin + Low Androgen Activity (3-Phase Combination)

Ortho Tri-Cyclen Lo

Generic Ingredients: Low-Dose Estrogen + High-Dose Progestin + Intermediate Androgen Activity (3-Phase Combination) G

Estrostep Fe
Tilia Fe
Tri-Legest Fe

Generic Ingredients: Low-Dose Estrogen + High-Dose Progestin + Low Androgen Activity (3-Phase Combination)

Cyclessa

Generic Ingredients: Intermediate-Dose Estrogen + Low-Dose Progestin + Low Androgen Activity (3-Phase Combination) G

Aranelle
Ortho Tri-Cyclen
Tri-Levlen
TriNessa
Trivora
Velivet

Generic Ingredients: High-Dose Estrogen + Intermediate-Dose Progestin + Low Androgen Activity (3-Phase Combination) G
Ortho-Novum 7/7/7

Generic Ingredients: High-Dose Estrogen + High-Dose Progestin + Intermediate-Dose Estrogen + Intermediate-Dose Progestin (4-Phase Combination)
Natazia

Generic Ingredients: High-Dose Progestin (Mini-Pill) G
Nor-QD Ortho Micronor

Generic Ingredients: Low-Dose Estrogen + Low-Dose Progestin (Patch)
Ortho Evra

Generic Ingredients: Low-Dose Estrogen + Low-Dose Progestin (Vaginal Ring)
NuvaRing

Generic Ingredients: Etonogestrel (Implant)
Implanon

Generic Ingredients: Progestin (Implant)

Generic Ingredients: Levonorgestrel (Intrauterine Insert)
Mirena

Generic Ingredients: Progesterone Agonist/Antagonist (Emergency Contraceptive)
Ella

Prescribed For

Prevention of pregnancy, endometriosis, excessive menstruation, and cyclic withdrawal bleeding. Several of these products can be prescribed for moderate acne in women age 15 and over. The Mirena intrauterine insert may be prescribed to treat heavy menstrual bleeding. Products containing drosperinone (a progestin) may help women with premenstrual syndrome (PMS).

General Information

Contraceptive drugs are synthetic hormones containing either progestin or a progestin-estrogen combination. The overall effects of any contraceptive are influenced by the interaction of all active ingredients, including those with androgenic and antiestrogenic activity. These drugs are similar to natural female hormones, which cannot be used as contraceptives because very large dosages would be required. Synthetic hormones are more potent and are effective at smaller dosages. Contraceptive drugs work by preventing sperm from reaching the unfertilized egg, preventing the implantation of a fertilized egg in the uterus, or preventing ovulation (the release of an unfertilized egg from the ovaries). They prevent acne by balancing hormone levels.

Hormonal contraceptives can be 97–99% effective at preventing pregnancy. These products vary in their effectiveness and in the amount and type of estrogen or progestin used. The side effects of these drugs tend to increase with the amount of hormone they contain. Although low hormone dosages are preferred, contraceptives with the smallest amounts of estrogen may be less effective in some women than others.

Single-phase products provide constant levels of estrogen and progestin throughout the entire month-long pill cycle. In 2-phase combinations, the amount of estrogen remains at a steady low level throughout the cycle, while progestin levels increase and then decrease. This variation in progestin allows normal changes to take place in the uterus. Three-phase products are meant to simulate the normal hormone cycle and reduce breakthrough bleeding. Throughout the cycle, estrogen levels remain the same while those of progestin change to create a 3-part wave pattern. The amount of estrogen in 3-phase products is considered low. Breakthrough bleeding may occur with the older combination products from day 8 through 16 of the cycle. Natazia, a "4-phase" contraceptive, contains 5 different pills that must be taken in a specific order: a high dose of estradiol (the first time this estrogen has been used in a contraceptive product); a moderate dose of estradiol plus a moderate dose of dienogest (a progestin new to the United States that has been used in Europe for menopausal symptoms); a moderate estradiol plus high dienogest; a low-dose estradiol; and inactive placebo pills.

The mini-pill, a progestin-only product, may cause irregular menstrual cycles and may be less effective than estrogen-progestin combinations. Mini-pills may be recommended to older women or women who should avoid estrogens (see "Cautions and Warnings").

The contraceptive patch releases small amounts of progestin and estrogen continuously over 3 weeks. The medication is absorbed into the blood vessels just below the skin. The patch works in the same way as contraceptive pills do.

The vaginal ring releases small amounts of etonorgestrel, a progestin, and estradiol, an estrogen, in the vaginal canal over 3 weeks. The combination prevents pregnancy in the same way as combination pills do but may be less effective than contraceptive pills because some people find them harder to use.

Most contraceptive drugs are designed to simulate a normal menstrual cycle. By not taking the hormones 1 week out of the month, you continue to have your regular period. In fact, these products are often used to stabilize a woman's period. Seasonique comes in a 91-pill packet and is taken once a day for 3 months. This means you will only have your period once every 3 months. Another, Lybrel, is designed to be taken every day, eliminating monthly menstruation. Drosperinone, the progestin found in Beyaz, Yasmin, and Yaz, has been found to relieve PMS symptoms in addition to acting as an effective contraceptive hormone. Beyaz also contains a folic acid supplement.

Levonorgestrel, a progestin, is used in implants that provide effective contraception for up to 5 years after surgical implantation under the skin of the upper arm or inside the uterus. Levonorgestrel implants should be replaced at least once every 5 years. Etonorgestrel implants are effective for 3 years. Implants can be removed at any time, reversing the contraceptive effect. The progestin intrauterine inserts provide effective contraception for about 1 year. The implant and intrauterine systems contain the same hormone found in the mini-pill and are associated with many of the same side effects and precautions as oral contraceptives.

Emergency contraceptives (sometimes referred to as the "morning-after pill") contain high doses of estrogen and progestin. Ella works against progesterone needed to establish a pregnancy. They are intended for use only after contraceptive failure or unprotected intercourse. They should never be taken to end an existing pregnancy.

Contraceptive drugs in any form are associated with risks. These risks are greatest in women over age 35 who smoke and have high blood pressure.

Cautions and Warnings

Do not take contraceptives if you are **allergic** or **sensitive** to them or any of their ingredients.

These drugs are intended only for women who have periods. They should not be taken by girls who have not yet menstruated and menopausal women. **Smokers** in their mid-30s or older who use contraceptive drugs are 5 times more likely to have a heart attack than nonsmokers taking contraceptives and 10–12 times more likely to have a heart attack than nonsmokers who do not use the pill. Death due to circulatory disease also increases substantially in smokers taking contraceptive drugs, especially in women at least 35 years old. The risk of stroke is also increased in this group. **Heavy smokers** (more than 15 cigarettes a day) should not use hormonal contraceptives.

You should not use contraceptive drugs if you are or might be **pregnant** or have a history of **jaundice during a previous pregnancy or hormonal contraceptive use**. You must wait at least 4 weeks after completing a pregnancy to start taking any contraceptive drug. The risk of blood clots is highest during those 4 weeks.

You should not use contraceptive drugs if you have a history of **blood clots** in veins or arteries, **heart valve disease with associated blood clots, stroke, heart attack**, or any **blood-coagulation disorder**, or if you are to undergo surgery involving a long period of immobility. Products with drosperinone (a progestin), more estrogen, or those that provide higher sustained blood levels of estrogen, such as the contraceptive patch, are more likely to be associated with an increased risk of life-threatening blood clots. The risk of developing serious blood clots is greater with the Ortho Evra contraceptive patch than with similar traditional contraceptive pills.

You should not use contraceptive drugs if you have known or suspected **cancer** of the breast, sex organs, or liver. The risk of breast cancer may be slightly higher among current and recent users of combination contraceptive drugs. This risk appears to decline after contraceptive use is stopped and is gone by 10 years after stopping combination contraceptive products. Breast cancers found in contraceptive users tend to be less advanced than those in noncontraceptive users.

You should not use contraceptives if you have serious **liver disease, migraine**, uncontrolled **high blood pressure, varicose veins**, or **diabetes with vascular disease**.

Contraceptive drugs may cause eye lesions. Call your doctor at once if you develop visual difficulties of any kind.

Women taking the combination product Seasonique will have their period only once every 3 months and those taking Lybrel will not have a regular monthly period. It is absolutely essential for you to verify you are not pregnant if you think you may be pregnant for any reason.

The risks of contraceptive drugs increase if you are **physically immobile** or have **asthma**; **cardiac insufficiency**; **epilepsy**; **kidney problems**; **benign breast disease**; **diabetes**; **endometriosis**; **gallbladder disease or gallstones**; **liver problems**, including **jaundice**; **high blood cholesterol**; **estrogen or progestin intolerance**; **depression**; or **tuberculosis**.

There is an increased risk of heart attack in women who have used contraceptive drugs for more than 5 years, or who are **between age 40 and 49** and have other coronary risk factors such as **smoking**, **obesity**, **high blood pressure**, **diabetes**, and **high blood cholesterol**. This risk remains even after the medication is stopped.

Contraceptive drugs may mask the onset of **menopause**.

Progestin-only products are associated with an increased risk of blood-clotting problems.

The progestin in Beyaz, Yasmin, and Yaz raises blood-potassium levels. Women with **kidney**, **liver**, **or adrenal gland disease** should use either product with caution.

Intrauterine inserts have been associated with an increased risk of pelvic inflammatory disease. The highest risk usually occurs within the first 20 days after insertion. Do not use intrauterine inserts if you have had an **ectopic pregnancy**.

Toxic shock syndrome has been associated with tampons, some barrier contraceptives, and the vaginal ring, although there is no proof that the product was the cause of the infection.

Possible Side Effects

▼ Common: Common side effects often result from using a product that is poorly suited to your body chemistry. Determining the right amount and type of hormone often minimizes these effects. If you are taking too much estrogen, you may experience nausea, bloating, high blood pressure, migraine and other headaches, excess cervical

Possible Side Effects *(continued)*

mucous, skin discoloration, colon polyps, water retention and swelling, and breast fullness or tenderness. Too little estrogen may cause early or mid-cycle breakthrough bleeding, spotting, or reduced periodic flow. Too much progestin is associated with weight gain and increased appetite, tiredness or fatigue, low periodic flow, acne, depression, breast regression, and androgen-related side effects (acne, oily scalp, hair loss, or excess hair growth). Too little progestin may cause late breakthrough bleeding, excessive periodic bleeding, or missed periods.

▼ Less common: abdominal cramps, infertility after discontinuance of the drug, breast tenderness, weight change, headache, rash, vaginal itching and burning, general vaginal infection, nervousness, dizziness, depression, cataracts, changes in sex drive, hair loss, and increased sensitivity to the sun.

▼ Rare: Women who use contraceptive drugs are more likely to develop several serious conditions, including blood clots in the deep veins, stroke, heart attack, liver cancer, gallbladder disease, and high blood pressure. Women who smoke cigarettes are at much higher risk for some of these adverse effects. Contact your doctor if you experience anything unusual while taking any medication.

Drug Interactions

- Ampicillin, barbiturates, bexarotene, bosentan, carbamazepine, chloramphenicol, efavirenz, felbamate, fluconazole, griseofulvin, ketoconazole, nelfinavir, neomycin, nitrofurantoin, oxcarbazepine, penicillin drugs, phenylbutazone, phenytoin, protease inhibitor drugs for HIV, rifampin, rifamycin, rifapentine, sedatives, statin drugs (atorvastatin and rosuvastatin), St. John's wort, sulfa drugs, and tetracycline products can make contraceptives less effective by making them leave the body faster. Use backup birth control while taking these medications together.
- Contraceptive drugs may elevate blood levels of benzodiazepine sedatives and sleeping pills (midazolam, lorazepam, oxazepam, and temazepam), caffeine, corticosteroids, cyclosporine, imatinib, metoprolol, selegiline, theophylline

drugs, tizanidine, tricyclic antidepressants, and triptan-type migraine drugs, increasing the risk of side effects. Discuss mixing these medicines with your doctor. Dosage reductions may be needed.

- Contraceptive drugs may increase the toxic liver effects of acetaminophen and reduce the drug's effectiveness. Contraceptive drugs may increase or decrease the effect of anticoagulant (blood thinning) drugs. Discuss the risks of this combination with your doctor.
- Mycophenolate interferes with only those contraceptives that contain levonorgestrel (Aviane, Lutera, Lybrel, Mirena, and Seasonique). Backup contraception is recommended.
- Exenatide may reduce the effectiveness of contraceptive pills. Take them at least 1 hour before an injection of exenatide.
- Contraceptive drugs may reduce the effectiveness of clofibrate for elevated blood triglycerides, sulfonylurea drugs for diabetes, ursodiol for gallbladder disease, and pain relievers, including salicylates (aspirin).
- Acetaminophen may increase blood levels of ethinyl estradiol, a common contraceptive drug ingredient, increasing side effects and reducing contraceptive effectiveness.
- Beyaz, Yasmin, and Yaz raise blood-potassium levels. They should not be used if you are taking spironolactone or another potassium-sparing diuretic, potassium supplements, angiotensin-converting enzyme (ACE) inhibitors, angiotensin receptor antagonists, aldosterone antagonists, heparin, nonsteroidal anti-inflammatory drugs (NSAIDs), or other medications on a long-term basis that may further increase potassium levels.
- Contraceptive drugs may interfere with the effects of insulin for diabetes.
- Acitretin interferes with the contraceptive effect of progestin-only mini-pills. It is not known if it also interferes with combination contraceptive drugs.

Food Interactions

Avoid grapefruit products while you are taking a contraceptive drug because they can raise blood levels of some hormone ingredients.

Usual Dose

Single-Phase, 2-Phase, and 3-Phase Combinations: The first day of bleeding is day 1 of the menstrual cycle. Beginning on the first day of the cycle, take 1 pill a day for 20–21 days according to the number of pills supplied by the manufacturer. If menstrual flow has not begun 7 days after taking the last pill, begin the next month's cycle of pills. Some manufacturers recommend starting the pills on a Sunday to make it easy to remember to take them. In this case, start taking your pills on the first Sunday after your period begins. If menstruation begins on a Sunday, take the first pill that day.

Natazia: Take 1 pill every day in the exact order they appear in the manufacturer's blister pack. Do not skip any days in between cycles, whether or not you actually have your period.

Seasonique: Take 1 light blue-green tablet containing levonorgestrel and ethinyl estradiol a day for 84 consecutive days, followed by 7 days of ethinyl estradiol tablets. Do not stop if spotting or breakthrough bleeding occurs. Report prolonged bleeding to your doctor.

Progestin-Only Mini-Pill: Take 1 pill every day.

Contraceptive Patch: Apply a new patch to the thigh, abdomen, or arm. Remove the patch after 3 weeks and then reapply a new patch after 1 week. Be sure to always apply a new patch on the same day of the week. If you are switching from birth control pills, apply the first patch on the same day you would start a new cycle of pills.

Vaginal Ring: Keep the vaginal ring in the vaginal canal for 3 weeks. Remove it and put a new one in 1 week later. If you did not use a hormonal contraceptive in the previous month, insert the ring between day 1 and day 5 of your cycle.

If you are switching from a combination birth control pill, insert the ring at any time during the week after you took your last pill but before you would have started your next cycle of pills. No additional contraception is necessary.

If you are switching from a mini-pill, insert the ring on the day after you take your last mini-pill.

If you are switching from a progestin implant or an intrauterine device (IUD), insert the ring on the same day your implant or IUD is removed.

If you are switching from a progestin injection, insert the ring on the same day you would have received your next injection.

If you are switching from a progestin-only mini-pill, implant, injection, or IUD, use another form of contraception for the first 7 days after you insert the ring.

Emergency Contraception: Emergency contraceptive kits have only a few pills. They should be taken with a full meal. Take ½ the pills (1 or 2 depending on the brand you use) within 72 hours of unprotected sex; however, they are most effective when taken within the first 24 hours. Take the rest of the pills 12 hours after the first dose. Emergency contraceptives reduce the risk of pregnancy by 75%.

The pregnancy test in the kit can be used to determine if you became pregnant earlier in your cycle or during a previous cycle. If the test is positive, consult your doctor before taking emergency contraception. If you vomit within 1 hour of taking either dose, contact your doctor.

The dose of the emergency contraceptive Ella is one 30-mg tablet. It can be taken up to 5 days after intercourse or suspected contraceptive failure without regard to food or meals.

Overdosage

An overdose may cause nausea and withdrawal bleeding in adult women. Overdose victims should be taken to a hospital emergency room. If you seek treatment, ALWAYS bring the prescription package.

Special Information

Use backup birth control to prevent pregnancy in the first 3 weeks after you begin taking contraceptive drugs.

You must take birth control pills every day, even if you do not have sexual intercourse very often. Women who start to take Natazia must use a backup non-hormonal contraceptive until they have taken the pills for 9 days in a row. One or 2 out of 100 women taking Natazia may become pregnant during the first year of treatment.

Contraceptive drugs do not protect against sexually transmitted diseases, including HIV/AIDS.

Take your pill at the same time each day to establish a routine and ensure maximum contraceptive protection.

Contact your doctor immediately if you experience severe abdominal pain; severe or sudden headache; pain in the chest, groin, or leg, especially the calf; sudden slurring of speech; changes in vision; weakness, numbness, or pain in the arms or legs; coughing up of blood; loss of coordination; or shortness of breath. These symptoms may require emergency treatment.

Other problems that may require medical attention are bulging eyes; changes in vaginal bleeding; fainting; frequent or painful urination; a gradual increase in blood pressure; breast lumps or secretions; depression; yellowing of the skin or whites of the eyes; rash; redness or irritation; upper abdominal swelling, pain, or tenderness; an unusual or dark-colored mole; thick, white vaginal discharge; or vaginal itching or tenderness.

See your doctor for a checkup every 6–12 months.

Some manufacturers include 7 inert or iron pills in their packaging to be taken on days when the drug is not taken. This makes it easier for women to stay on schedule with their pills. The 7 pills bridge the gap between contraceptive cycles and allow women to take 1 pill every day without stopping.

Good dental hygiene is essential while taking contraceptive drugs. See your dentist regularly and brush and floss carefully, because contraceptive drugs may increase the risk of an oral infection.

Contraceptive drugs may increase your sensitivity to the sun.

Wearing contact lenses may be uncomfortable while taking contraceptive drugs because the pills can cause minor changes in the shape of your eyes.

All contraceptive prescriptions come with "Patient Information." Read it thoroughly, as it gives detailed information about the drug and its use.

What if I Forget My Pill?

For single- or 2-phase combinations: If you forget to take a pill for 1 day, take 2 pills the following day. If you miss 2 consecutive days, take 2 pills for the next 2 days. Then return to your schedule of 1 pill a day. If you miss 3 consecutive days, do not take any pills for the next 7 days and use another form of contraception; then start a brand new cycle.

Natazia: You should not skip pills or delay your regular pill by more than 12 hours. Your chances of becoming pregnant go up with every forgotten pill and as you get closer to the end of your cycle. If you forget a pill and it is within 12 hours of your regular time, take the forgotten pill and continue with your regular schedule. On days 1–17 of your cycle, if you delay a pill more than 12 hours after your usual time, take the pill immediately and take your next pill at the regular time. Use a backup contraceptive for the next 9 days. You may have to take 2 pills on the same day. If you forget a pill during days 18–24 and it is more than 12 hours after your regular time, stop taking the pills and throw the pack away. Instead, open a new pack and start from day 1. Continue using your new pack as usual and use a backup contraceptive for 9 days. If you forget a pill during days 25–28, take your missed pill right away and continue with your regular schedule. No backup contraceptive is needed.

If you forget 2 pills in a row during days 1–17, skip the forgotten pills and continue with your regular schedule. Use a backup contraceptive for 9 days. If you forget 2 pills during days 17–25, do not take anything from your current pack and throw it away. Instead, start a new pack from day 1 and use a backup contraceptive for 9 days. If you forget 2 pills on days 25–28, throw your current pack away, start a new pack from day 1, and continue with your regular schedule. Backup contraception is not needed.

Spotting or light bleeding is normal when you first start taking Natazia. Missing pills can also lead to spotting. If you forget to take 1 or more pills or if you vomit or have diarrhea within 4 hours after taking a dose of Natazia, take another pill of the same color from your extra blister pack.

If you have unprotected sex during a hormone-free interval or in the first week of pill taking AND have missed 2 or more pills in that first week, talk to your doctor about emergency contraception pills.

Seasonique: The risk of ovulation and pregnancy increases with each forgotten light blue-green pill. If you miss 1 light blue-green pill, take it as soon as you remember and take the next pill at your regular time. This may mean you will take 2 pills on the same day. You don't need to use a backup birth control method if you forget only 1 pill. If you forget 2 light blue-green pills in a row, take 2 pills on the day you remember and take 2 pills the next day. Then go back to taking 1 pill a day until you finish your pack. If you miss 2 or more light blue-green pills in a row, you must use non-hormonal backup contraception until you have taken a light blue-green pill for 7 days in a row. If you miss 1 or more yellow tablets, you are still protected against pregnancy provided you begin taking light blue-green pills again on the proper day.

For 3-phase combinations: If you forget to take a pill for 1 day, take 2 pills the following day. If you miss 2 consecutive days, take 2 pills for the next 2 days. Then return to your schedule of 1 pill a day. If you forget to take a pill for 3 days in a row, stop taking the drug and use a non-hormonal backup contraceptive until your period starts. ALWAYS use a backup contraceptive method for the remainder of your cycle if you forget even 1 pill of a 3-phase combination.

If you forget to apply the contraceptive patch on the same day of the week once every 4 weeks, you risk a loss of effectiveness on the days after you should have applied it. If the patch comes off or is partially detached in mid-cycle, you must start a new 3-week cycle at once by removing the old patch and applying a new one.

If the vaginal ring is accidentally expelled during the 3 weeks it is normally retained, rinse it off with water and replace it within 3 hours. Do not use hot water. If the ring is not reusable, insert a new ring and continue with your regular schedule. If you do not replace the ring within 3 hours, its effectiveness may be reduced. If you are in week 3 of the cycle, throw the ring away; you may insert a new one immediately, which will begin a new 3-week cycle and cause you to skip a period. Or you may wait a week, during which time you will have periodic bleeding, and insert a new ring no later than 7 days after the vaginal ring was expelled. This option should be chosen if you had used the ring for 7 days in a row before it was expelled.

If, when it is expelled, you are in week 1 or 2 of your cycle and the ring is out for more than 3 hours, reinsert it and use an additional form of contraceptive until the ring has been worn for 7 consecutive days. A vaginal ring may break and then slip out or cause discomfort. Throw the ring away if this happens.

Missing a pill reduces your protection. If you keep forgetting to take your pills, you must use another birth control method.

Special Populations

Pregnancy/Breast-feeding: Contraceptive hormones cause birth defects and may interfere with fetal development. They are not safe for use during pregnancy, although no birth defects have been reported after 1 or 2 days of inadvertent use of birth control pills. If you think you are pregnant, use a non-hormonal form of contraception and stop taking your birth control pills.

Contraceptive hormones pass into breast milk. Combination contraceptive products may reduce the amount of milk produced. Nursing mothers who must use any of these drugs should use infant formula.

Seniors: These products are not intended for women who have completed menopause.

Coreg *see **Carvedilol,** page 250*

Type of Drug

Corticosteroids, Eye Products

(kor-tih-koe-STER-oids)

Brand Names

Generic Ingredients: Dexamethasone G
Maxidex

Generic Ingredients: Dexamethasone + Ciprofloxacin
Ciprodex

Generic Ingredients: Dexamethasone + Tobramycin G
Tobradex
Tobradex ST

Generic Ingredients: Dexamethasone + Neomycin Sulfate + Polymyxin B Sulfate G
Dexasporin
Maxitrol

Generic Ingredients: Difluprednate
Durezol

Generic Ingredients: Fluorometholone G
Flarex
FML
FML Forte

Generic Ingredients: Loteprednol Etabonate
Alrex
Lotemax

Generic Ingredients: Loteprednol Etabonate + Tobramycin
Zylet

Generic Ingredients: Prednisolone Acetate G

Omnipred
Pred Forte
Pred Mild

Generic Ingredients: Prednisolone Acetate + Gentamicin Sulfate

Pred G

Generic Ingredients: Prednisolone Acetate + Sulfacetamide Sodium

Blephamide
Blephamide S.O.P.

Generic Ingredients: Prednisolone Acetate + Neomycin Sulfate + Polymyxin B Sulfate

Poly-Pred

Generic Ingredients: Prednisolone Sodium Phosphate G

Generic Ingredients: Prednisolone Sodium Phosphate + Sulfacetamide Sodium G

Vasocidin

Generic Ingredients: Rimexolone

Vexol

Generic Ingredients: Tobramycin G

Aktob
Tobrex

Prescribed For

Allergic and inflammatory eye conditions and to speed healing and relieve pain after eye surgery or injury.

General Information

Corticosteroid eye products are prescribed for general relief of inflammation due to allergy and other causes. They are also used after eye surgery or serious eye injury to aid the healing process by reducing the natural inflammatory process. Very severe eye conditions that do not respond to these products may require treatment with corticosteroid drugs taken by mouth. Fluorometholone and prednisolone (up to 0.125%) are preferred for long-term treatment because they are least likely to raise the fluid pressure inside the eye. Corticosteroid eye products have not been widely studied in children, though fluorometholone has been proven safe for use in children age 2 and over.

Cautions and Warnings

Do not use a corticosteroid eye product if you are **allergic** or **sensitive** to corticosteroids.

These products should not be used if you have a **fungal, herpes, tuberculosis, or viral infection of the eye**. They should be used with caution if you have **cataracts**, **glaucoma**, or **diabetes**. Do not use any of these products without your doctor's knowledge.

Long-term use of these products can lead to eye damage, including glaucoma, infection, and nerve damage.

Do not use any of these products in **children** without consulting a doctor.

Possible Side Effects

▼ Rare: watery eyes; glaucoma; optic nerve damage; gradual blurring, reduction, or loss of vision; eye pain or infections; drooping eyelid; eye burning, stinging, or redness; nausea; and vomiting. Contact your doctor if you experience anything unusual while taking any medication.

Drug Interactions

- Corticosteroids applied to the eye may interfere with the effect of antiglaucoma drugs.
- The risk of raising fluid pressure inside the eye is increased when corticosteroid eye products are taken with anticholinergic drugs, especially atropine, over a long period of time.

Food Interactions

None known.

Usual Dose

Eye Drops: 1–2 drops several times a day. When used after surgery, the eye drops are continued for 2 to 3 weeks according to your doctor's instructions.

Eye Ointment: Place a thin strip of ointment into the affected eye several times a day.

Overdosage

Swallowing a container of corticosteroid eye drops or ointment usually does not produce serious effects. Contact your local poison control center or a hospital emergency room for more information. If you seek treatment, ALWAYS bring the prescription container.

Special Information

If you forget to administer a dose, do so as soon as you remember. If it is almost time for your next dose, skip the one you forgot and continue with your regular schedule.

To prevent infection, keep the eyedropper from touching your fingers, eyelids, or any surface. Wait at least 5 minutes before using any other eye drops.

If the brand you are taking contains benzalkonium chloride, wait at least 15 minutes before inserting contact lenses. In some cases, you may be instructed not to wear contact lenses for the duration of treatment.

Special Populations

Pregnancy/Breast-feeding: Using large amounts of corticosteroid eye drops during pregnancy may affect the adrenal gland of the fetus. A corticosteroid eye product should be taken during pregnancy only if your doctor determines that the potential benefit outweighs the risks.

Oral corticosteroids pass into breast milk, but it is not known if this is also true of corticosteroid eye drops. Nursing mothers who must use one of these medications should use infant formula.

Seniors: Seniors may use these products without special precaution.

Type of Drug

Corticosteroids, Inhalers

(kor-tih-koe-STER-oids)

Brand Names

Generic Ingredients: Beclomethasone Dipropionate

QVAR 40 QVAR 80

Generic Ingredients: Budesonide G

Pulmicort Pulmicort Flexhaler

Generic Ingredients: Budesonide + Formoterol

Symbicort

Generic Ingredients: Ciclesonide

Alvesco

Generic Ingredients: Flunisolide

AeroBid Aerospan HFA

Generic Ingredients: Fluticasone Propionate
Flovent Diskus   Flovent HFA

Generic Ingredients: Fluticasone Propionate + Salmeterol Xinafoate
Advair Diskus   Advair HFA

Generic Ingredients: Mometasone Furoate
Asmanex Twisthaler

Generic Ingredients: Triamcinolone Acetonide
Azmacort

Prescribed For

Chronic asthma and bronchial disease.

General Information

Corticosteroid inhalers relieve the symptoms associated with asthma and bronchial disease by reducing inflammation of bronchial mucous membranes, making it easier to breathe. Corticosteroid inhalers produce the same treatment effect as oral corticosteroids, with some important differences. Because inhalers deliver the drug directly to the lungs, smaller dosages can be used. They also have fewer side effects because little of the drug reaches the bloodstream. Corticosteroid inhalers can prevent asthma attacks if used regularly but do not relieve them once they start.

Cautions and Warnings

Do not use a corticosteroid inhaler if you are **allergic** or **sensitive** to any of its ingredients.

In people with **asthma**, death from adrenal gland failure has occurred during and after switching from an oral corticosteroid to an inhaler. Adrenal function is impaired for several months after the switch. Corticosteroid inhalers should not be used as the primary treatment of **severe asthma**. They are recommended only for people who take prednisone or another oral corticosteroid, or for people who do not respond to other asthma drugs. These drugs cannot relieve asthma attacks once they start.

Those who use any corticosteroid product, including inhalers, are more likely to have reduced immune system function. This reduces the body's ability to fight infection from any source, including **chickenpox**, **shingles**, and **measles**. Adults who have not had these viral infections should take care to avoid becoming infected while using any corticosteroid product. Do not receive a **live virus vaccine** while taking corticosteroids of any kind, as they interfere with the body's reaction to the vaccine.

People with **lung disease** who use a corticosteroid inhaler may develop lung infections or pneumonia more easily than others.

Combining an oral corticosteroid with a corticosteroid inhaler may cause pituitary gland suppression.

During a period of **severe stress**, you may have to switch to an oral corticosteroid if the inhaler does not control your asthma. During periods of stress or a severe asthma attack, people who have stopped using an inhaler should ask their doctors about taking an oral corticosteroid.

Corticosteroid inhalers may be associated with immediate or delayed drug reactions, including breathing difficulties, rash, and bronchospasm.

Inhaled corticosteroids can rarely cause your bones to lose calcium, which can lead to broken bones and degeneration of the large bones in the hip from calcium loss (aseptic necrosis of the femoral and humoral heads).

Use corticosteroids with caution if you have respiratory **tuberculosis**, **herpes** of the eye, a **bacterial**, **fungal**, **or parasitic infection**, or any other untreated **systemic infection**.

Children using an inhaled corticosteroid for asthma control may grow at a slower pace than children who do not. Whether this is due to the asthma or the corticosteroid is unknown.

The combination products Advair and Symbicort both contain beta-2 agonists. In some asthma patients, beta-2 agonists may increase the risk of asthma-related death. See Salmeterol, page 1029, for more information on these drugs.

Possible Side Effects

- ▼ Most common: dry mouth, hoarseness, rash, bronchospasm, respiratory infections, fungal infection of the mouth, runny nose, headache, upset stomach, and palpitations.
- ▼ Rare: depression, cough, wheezing, infection, and facial swelling. Cough and wheezing are probably caused by an ingredient in the inhaler other than the corticosteroid itself. Contact your doctor if you experience anything unusual while taking any medication.

Drug Interactions

- Women on long-term corticosteroid therapy should not take mifepristone for termination of pregnancy.
- Budesonide should not be taken with quinolones such as levofloxacin. The risk of tendon rupture is increased with this combination.
- Budesonide should not be combined with aldesleukin.
- The combination of fluticasone and ritonavir is not recommended.
- Barbiturates, carbamazepine, and rifamycins (such as rifampin) may decrease the effects of budesonide.
- Hormonal contraceptives may increase the effects of budesonide. Dosage reductions may be necessary.
- Dosages of both phenytoin and budesonide may need to be increased if they are taken together.
- Budesonide may increase the blood-thinning effects of warfarin, adding to the risk of serious bleeding.
- Budesonide may decrease the effects of aspirin.
- Azole antifungals (such as itraconazole and ketoconazole), delavirdine, and protease inhibitors (such as ritonavir) may increase the effects of ciclesonide.
- Ketoconazole may increase blood levels of fluticasone and mometasone. These combinations should be monitored.
- Using an inhaled corticosteroid and an oral corticosteroid together may increase the effect of both drugs. Use with caution.
- See Formoterol, page 1029, for further drug interactions for the combination product Symbicort.
- See Salmeterol, page 1029, for further drug interactions for the combination product Advair.

Food Interactions

Large amounts of grapefruit and starfruit products can slow the breakdown of budesonide and fluticasone. Avoid these foods if you use one of these drugs regularly.

Usual Dose

Beclomethasone

Adult and Child (age 12 and over): starting dose—40–160 mcg twice a day; maximum dose is 320 mcg twice a day.

Child (age 5–11): starting dose—40 mcg twice a day; maximum dose is 80 mcg twice a day.

Child (under age 5): not recommended.

Budesonide

Adult: starting dose—360 mcg twice a day. Do not exceed 720 mcg twice a day.

Child (age 6 and over): 180 mcg twice a day. Do not exceed 360 mcg twice a day.

Child (under age 6): not recommended.

Budesonide Nebulizer

Child (age 1–8): 0.5 mg once a day or twice a day in divided doses via jet nebulizer connected to an air compressor.

Child (under age 1): Consult your doctor.

Budesonide and Formoterol Inhalation

Adult and Child (age 12 and over): 2 inhalations morning and evening.

Child (under age 12): not recommended.

Ciclesonide

Adult and Child (age 12 and over): starting dose—80 mcg twice a day. Maximum dose is 320 mcg twice a day.

Child (under age 12): not recommended.

Flunisolide

AeroBid

Adult and Child (age 16 and over): 2 inhalations (500 mcg) morning and evening. Do not exceed 8 inhalations a day.

Child (age 6–15): 2 inhalations (500 mcg) morning and evening. Higher doses in this group have not been studied.

Child (under age 6): not recommended.

Aerospan HFA

Adult and Child (age 12 and over): 160–320 mcg morning and evening.

Child (age 6–11): 80–160 mcg morning and evening.

Child (under age 6): not recommended.

Fluticasone Inhalation

Adult and Child (age 12 and over): 88–880 mcg twice a day.

Child (4–11): 88–440 mcg twice a day.

Child (under age 4): not recommended.

Fluticasone Diskus

Adult and Child (age 12 and over): 100–500 mcg twice a day.

Child (age 4–11): 50–100 mcg twice a day.

Child (under age 4): not recommended.

Fluticasone and Salmeterol

Advair Diskus

Adult and Child (age 12 and over): one 500/50 dose inhalation morning and evening.

Child (age 4–11): one 100/50 dose inhalation morning and evening.

Child (under age 4): not recommended.

Advair HFA

Adult and Child (age 12 and over): 2 inhalations morning and evening.

Child (under age 12): not recommended.

Mometasone

Adult and Child (age 12 and over): 220–880 mcg once a day in the evening.

Child (age 4–11): 110 mcg once a day in the evening.

Child (under age 4): not recommended.

Triamcinolone

Adult and Child (age 6 and over): 2 inhalations (220 mcg) once a day.

Child (age 2–5): 2 inhalations (110 mcg) once a day.

Child (under age 2): not recommended.

Overdosage

Serious adverse effects are unlikely. Excessive use of large amounts of an inhaled corticosteroid may cause overdose symptoms and require gradually stopping the drug. Contact your local poison control center or a hospital emergency room for more information. If you seek treatment, ALWAYS bring the prescription container.

Special Information

People using both a corticosteroid inhaler and a bronchodilator, such as albuterol, should use the bronchodilator first, wait a few minutes, and then use the corticosteroid inhaler. This allows more corticosteroid to be absorbed.

These drugs are for preventive therapy only and will not affect an asthma attack. Inhaled corticosteroids must be taken regularly, as directed. Wait at least 1 minute between inhalations.

To properly take this medication, thoroughly shake the inhaler if it is one that must be shaken. Take a drink of water to moisten your throat. Place the inhaler 2 finger-widths away from your mouth and tilt your head back slightly. While activating the inhaler, take a slow, deep breath for 3–5 seconds, then hold your breath for about 10 seconds, and finally breathe out slowly. Allow at least 1 minute between puffs. Rinse your mouth after each use to reduce dry mouth and hoarseness.

If you forget to administer a dose, do so as soon as you remember. If it is almost time for your next dose, skip the dose you forgot and continue with your regular schedule. Do not take a double dose. Tell your doctor or pharmacist if you forget to take more than 1 dose.

Special Populations

Pregnancy/Breast-feeding: Corticosteroids may cause birth defects or interfere with fetal development. An inhaled corticosteroid product should be taken during pregnancy only if your doctor determines that the potential benefit outweighs the risks.

It is not known if inhaled corticosteroids pass into breast milk, though oral corticosteroids do. Nursing mothers who must take an inhaled corticosteroid should use infant formula.

Seniors: Seniors may use corticosteroid inhalers without special precaution. Tell your doctor if you have bone or bowel disease, colitis, diabetes, glaucoma, fungal or herpes infections, high blood pressure, high blood cholesterol, an underactive thyroid, or heart, kidney, or liver disease.

Type of Drug

Corticosteroids, Nasal

(kor-tih-koe-STER-oids)

Brand Names

Generic Ingredients: Beclomethasone Dipropionate
Beconase AQ

Generic Ingredients: Budesonide
Rhinocort Aqua

Generic Ingredients: Ciclesonide
Omnaris

Generic Ingredients: Flunisolide G

Generic Ingredients: Fluticasone Furoate
Veramyst

Generic Ingredients: Fluticasone Propionate G
Flonase

Generic Ingredients: Mometasone Furoate
Nasonex

Generic Ingredients: Triamcinolone Acetonide G
Nasacort AQ

Prescribed For

Rhinitis (nasal inflammation) associated with seasonal or chronic allergy and other causes; also used to prevent recurrence of nasal polyps.

General Information

Nasal corticosteroids are used to treat severe symptoms of seasonal allergy that have not responded to other drugs such as decongestants. They work by reducing inflammation of the mucous membranes that line the nasal passages, making it easier to breathe. These drugs may take several days to produce an effect. Some nasal corticosteroids are approved for both allergic and nonallergic rhinitis.

Cautions and Warnings

Do not use a nasal corticosteroid if you are **allergic** or **sensitive** to corticosteroids. Rarely, serious and life-threatening drug-sensitivity reactions, including choking, throat swelling leading to suffocation, and skin reactions, have occurred.

Very rarely, deaths caused by failure of the adrenal gland have occurred in people taking adrenal corticosteroid tablets or syrup who were switched to a nasal corticosteroid. This is a rare complication and usually results from stopping the liquid or tablets suddenly instead of gradually.

Temporary or permanent loss of the sense of smell and taste has been reported with flunisolide use.

Combining prednisone or another oral corticosteroid with a nasal corticosteroid may cause **pituitary gland suppression**, although nasal corticosteroids alone rarely cause this problem.

Use nasal corticosteroids with caution if you have **tuberculosis**, **chickenpox**, **measles**, **shingles**, or any serious **fungal, bacterial, or viral infection**. These illnesses can be more serious if your immune system has been affected by a corticosteroid drug.

Do not receive a **live virus vaccine** while taking corticosteroids of any kind, as they interfere with the body's reaction to the vaccine.

Rarely, nasal *Candida* infections develop in people using a nasal corticosteroid. These infections may require treatment with an antifungal drug, as well as the discontinuance of the nasal corticosteroid.

During a period of severe **stress**, you may have to switch to an oral corticosteroid drug if the nasal form does not control your symptoms.

You should not use a nasal corticosteroid if you have recently experienced a nasal **wound** or **surgery** or have chronic **nose-bleeds** or nasal **ulcers**.

Rare cases of cataracts, glaucoma, and increased eye pressure have occurred in people using a nasal corticosteroid. You should use these medications with caution if you have a history of **cataracts** or **glaucoma**.

Children using nasal corticosteroids may experience reduction in growth velocity.

Possible Side Effects

- ▼ Most common: mild irritation of the nose, nasal passages, and throat; burning; stinging; dryness; and headache.
- ▼ Less common: lightheadedness, nausea, nosebleed or bloody mucous, unusual nasal congestion, bronchial asthma, sneezing attacks, runny nose, sore throat, and loss of the sense of taste.
- ▼ Rare: ulcers of the nasal passages, watery eyes, vomiting, hypersensitivity reactions (symptoms include itching, rash, swelling, bronchospasms, and breathing difficulties), nasal infection, wheezing, perforation of the wall between the nostrils, and increased eye pressure. Contact your doctor if you experience anything unusual while taking any medication.

Drug Interactions

- Do not use fluticasone propionate with ritonavir.
- Azole antifungals (such as itraconazole and ketoconazole), delavirdine, and protease inhibitors (such as ritonavir) may increase the effects of ciclesonide. Use caution when combining ketoconazole with any nasal corticosteroid.
- Ephedrine, phenobarbital, and rifampin may decrease the effect of nasal corticosteroids.

Usual Dose

Beclomethasone

Adult and Child (age 6 and over): 1–2 sprays (42–84 mcg) in each nostril twice a day. The maximum daily dose should not exceed 2 sprays twice a day, or 336 mcg.

Child (under age 6): not recommended.

Budesonide

Adult and Child (age 6 and over): starting dose—1 spray in each nostril (64 mcg) once a day. The maximum recommended daily dose is 4 sprays in each nostril once a day, or 256 mcg.

Child (under age 6): not recommended.

Ciclesonide

Adult and Child (age 6 and over): 2 sprays (50 mcg/spray) in each nostril once a day.

Child (under age 6): not recommended.

Flunisolide

Adult and Child (age 15 and over): 2 sprays (58 mcg) in each nostril twice a day to start; may be increased up to 8 sprays a day in each nostril.

Child (age 6–14): 1 spray (29 mcg) in each nostril 3 times a day, or 2 sprays in each nostril twice a day.

Child (under age 6): not recommended.

Fluticasone Furoate

Adult and Child (age 12 and over): 2 sprays in each nostril (110 mcg) once a day to start. Dose may be reduced to 1 spray in each nostril after symptoms are controlled.

Child (age 2–11): 1 spray in each nostril (55 mcg) once a day. Dose may be increased to 2 sprays in each nostril once a day if necessary.

Child (under age 2): not recommended.

Fluticasone Propionate

Adult and Child (age 4 and over): 2 sprays in each nostril (200 mcg) once a day or divided in 2 doses to start. Dose may be reduced by ½ in a few days.

Child (under age 4): not recommended.

Mometasone

Adult and Child (age 12 and over): 2 sprays in each nostril (200 mcg) once a day; may be increased to 4 sprays a day in each nostril for people age 18 and older.

Child (age 2–11): 1 spray in each nostril (110 mcg) once a day.
Child (under age 2): not recommended.

Triamcinolone

Adult and Child (age 13 and over): 2 sprays in each nostril (220 mcg) once a day; may be decreased to 1 spray a day in each nostril when symptoms are under control.

Child (age 6–12): 1 spray in each nostril once a day (110 mcg); may be increased to 2 sprays a day in each nostril, if needed, and then reduced to 1 spray in each nostril per day once symptoms are controlled.

Child (age 2–5): 1 spray in each nostril once a day.

Child (under age 2): not recommended.

Overdosage

Serious adverse effects are unlikely after accidental ingestion. Rarely, excessive use of large amounts of nasal corticosteroids may cause overdose symptoms such as irregular menses, acne, facial puffiness, and weight gain. These symptoms require gradual, not immediate, discontinuation of the drug. Contact your local poison control center or a hospital emergency room for more information. If you seek treatment, ALWAYS bring the prescription container.

Special Information

It may be necessary to clear your nasal passages with a nasal decongestant before using a nasal corticosteroid to allow it to reach the mucous membranes.

Some of these drugs take 10–14 days to start working. Beclomethasone, budesonide, and triamcinolone work faster, in 3–7 days; ciclesonide starts working within 1 or 2 days and shows additional benefits after several weeks of use; in some cases, triamcinolone and budesonide provide relief in 12 hours. Flunisolide may take up to 2 weeks. Do not use any of these drugs continuously for more than 3 weeks unless you have experienced a definite benefit.

If you are using more than one spray at a time, wait at least 1 minute between sprays. Be careful to avoid getting any of the spray in your eyes.

Nasal corticosteroids may cause irritation and drying of mucous membranes in the nose. Contact your doctor if this effect persists or if symptoms get worse.

Contact your doctor if you are exposed to measles or chicken-pox while using any of these medicines.

People using a nasal corticosteroid to prevent the return of nasal polyps after surgery may experience nosebleeds because the drug can slow healing of the wound.

If you forget to administer a dose, do so as soon as you remember. If it is almost time for your next dose, skip the dose you forgot and continue with your regular schedule. Do not take a double dose.

Special Populations

Pregnancy/Breast-feeding: Taking large amounts of corticosteroids during pregnancy may slow fetal growth. Although the small amount of drug absorbed into the blood after nasal application is unlikely to have any effect, consult your doctor before taking any corticosteroid if you are or might be pregnant.

It is not known if nasal corticosteroids pass into breast milk, though oral corticosteroids do. Nursing mothers should use infant formula.

Seniors: Seniors may use nasal corticosteroids without special precaution. Tell your doctor if you have bone or bowel disease, colitis, diabetes, glaucoma, fungal or herpes infections, high blood pressure, high blood cholesterol, an underactive thyroid, or heart, kidney, or liver disease.

Type of Drug

Corticosteroids, Oral

(kor-tih-koe-STER-oids)

Brand Names

Generic Ingredients: Betamethasone
Celestone

Generic Ingredients: Budesonide G
Entocort EC

Generic Ingredients: Cortisone Acetate G

Generic Ingredients: Dexamethasone G
Baycadron
DexPak 6 Day
DexPak 10 Day
DexPak 13 Day

Generic Ingredients: Fludrocortisone G

Generic Ingredients: Hydrocortisone G
Cortef

Generic Ingredients: Methylprednisolone G
Medrol

Generic Ingredients: Prednisolone G
Millipred
Millipred DP
Pediapred
Prelone

Generic Ingredients: Prednisone G

Prescribed For

A wide variety of disorders from rash to cancer, including adrenal disease, adrenal hormone replacement, bursitis, arthritis, severe skin diseases such as psoriasis and other rashes, severe or disabling allergies, asthma, drug or serum sickness, attacks of multiple sclerosis (MS), severe respiratory diseases such as pneumonitis, blood disorders, gastrointestinal (GI) disease such as ulcerative colitis and Crohn's disease, and inflammation of the nerves, heart, or other organs. Dexamethasone is also used to treat mountain sickness, vomiting, bronchial disease in premature babies, excessive hairiness, and hearing loss associated with bacterial meningitis. Fludrocortisone is used to treat Addison's disease and for symptomatic orthostatic hypotension. Prednisone is used to improve strength and function of some muscular dystrophy patients. Methylprednisolone is used to decrease mortality in some patients suffering from severe alcoholism and chronic active hepatitis.

General Information

Produced by the adrenal gland, natural corticosteroids are hormones that affect almost every body system. The major differences among corticosteroid drugs are potency and variation in secondary effects. Doctor preference and past experience with a corticosteroid usually determine which drug to prescribe for a specific disease.

Cautions and Warnings

Do not use an oral corticosteroid if you are **allergic** or **sensitive** to any of its ingredients.

Corticosteroids may mask symptoms of an **infection**. Because these drugs compromise the immune system, new infections may occur during corticosteroid treatment; when this happens, a relatively minor infection that would respond to ordinary treatment can turn serious. Corticosteroids may impair immune response to **hepatitis B**, prolonging recovery. They may reactivate dormant **amebiasis** (a parasitic infection). Corticosteroids should not be taken if you have a **fungal blood infection**, because they can allow the infection to spread more easily. They should be used with caution by people with **herpes eye infection**, **tuberculosis**, or any other **bacterial**, **fungal**, **or viral infections**.

Long-term use of any corticosteroid may increase the risk of developing cataracts, glaucoma, or eye infections, especially viral or fungal.

When stopping a corticosteroid, dosage must be reduced gradually under a doctor's supervision—otherwise you may experience adrenal gland failure.

If you are taking large corticosteroid doses, you should not receive any **live virus vaccine**, because corticosteroids interfere with the body's reaction to the vaccine.

Hydrocortisone and cortisone may lead to high blood pressure. Other corticosteroids are less likely to affect blood pressure.

Corticosteroids should be used with caution if you have severe **kidney disease**.

High-dose or long-term corticosteroid therapy may aggravate or worsen **stomach ulcers**. This may occur when total dosage reaches 1000 mg of prednisone, 150 mg of betamethasone or dexamethasone, 5000 mg of cortisone, 4000 mg of hydrocortisone, 1000 mg of prednisolone, or 800 mg of methylprednisolone.

People who have recently stopped taking a corticosteroid and are going through a period of **stress** may need small doses of a rapid-acting corticosteroid, such as hydrocortisone, to get them through this period. Contact your doctor if you think you might be experiencing this kind of stress reaction.

Use corticosteroids with caution if you have had a recent **heart attack** or have **ulcerative colitis**, **heart failure**, **high blood pressure**, **blood-clotting tendencies**, **thrombophlebitis**, **osteoporosis**, **antibiotic-resistant infections**, **Cushing's disease**, **myasthenia gravis**, **metastatic cancer**, **diabetes**, **underactive thyroid disease**, **cirrhosis of the liver**, or **seizure disorders**.

Corticosteroid psychosis (symptoms include euphoria or feeling "high," delirium, sleeplessness, mood swings, personality changes, and severe depression) may develop in people taking dosages greater than 40 mg a day of prednisone. These symptoms may also develop with other corticosteroids taken in equivalent doses (see "Usual Dose" for relative equivalencies). Symptoms of corticosteroid psychosis usually develop within 15–30 days of beginning treatment. These symptoms may also be linked to other factors—women and those with a family history of psychosis are more at risk.

Corticosteroids can cause loss of calcium, which may result in bone fractures and aseptic necrosis of the femoral and humoral heads (a condition in which the large bones in the hip degenerate from loss of calcium).

Prednisone may aggravate **emotional instability**.

Children using oral corticosteroids may experience reduction in growth velocity.

Corticosteroids do not cure **MS** or slow its progression, though they may speed recovery from attacks of the disease.

Corticosteroid products often contain **tartrazine dyes** and **sulfite preservatives**. Many people are allergic to these chemicals.

Possible Side Effects

- ▼ Most common: headache, respiratory infections, acne, and bruising.
- ▼ Common: water retention (swollen ankles), back pain, heart failure, upset stomach (possibly leading to stomach or duodenal ulcer), potassium loss, dizziness, fatigue, insomnia, weight gain, increased appetite, nausea, stomach gas, abdominal pain, general pain, muscle weakness, loss of muscle mass, slowed healing of wounds, increased sweating, allergic rash, itching, convulsions, excess hair growth, and worsening of a pre-existing psychiatric condition.
- ▼ Less common: irregular menstruation; slowed growth in children, particularly after lengthy periods of corticosteroid treatment; adrenal or pituitary gland suppression; diabetes; drug sensitivity or allergic reactions; blood clots; moon face; feeling unwell; euphoria; mood swings; personality changes; and severe depression.
- ▼ Rare: Rare side effects can appear in any part of the body. Contact your doctor if you experience anything unusual while taking any medication.

Drug Interactions

- Women on long-term betamethasone therapy should not take mifepristone for termination of pregnancy.
- Tell your doctor if you are taking any oral anticoagulant (blood thinning) drug. If you begin taking a corticosteroid, your anticoagulant dosage may need to be adjusted.
- Azole antifungals (such as itraconazole and ketoconazole), hormonal contraceptives, and macrolide antibiotics (such as clarithromycin) may increase the effects of betamethasone. A reduced dosage may be necessary. Ketoconazole may increase blood levels of other corticosteroids. This combination should be used cautiously.
- Corticosteroids may decrease the effects of aspirin and other salicylates.
- Barbiturates, carbamazepine, cholestyramine, hydantoins (such as phenytoin), and rifamycins (such as rifampin) may decrease the effects of betamethasone. Dosage adjustments may be necessary.
- Both betamethasone and cyclosporine levels are increased when these medications are taken together. This combination should be used cautiously.
- The risk of GI side effects is increased when betamethasone is taken with nonsteroidal anti-inflammatory drugs (NSAIDs).
- Levels of blood potassium may become dangerously low if betamethasone is taken with other drugs that lower potassium, such as diuretics.
- The risk of tendon rupture is increased when betamethasone is taken with quinolones (such as ciprofloxacin).
- Betamethasone may decrease the effects of aldesleukin, oral antidiabetes medications, and isoniazid. Dosages may need to be increased when these drugs are taken with betamethasone.
- Risk of dangerous heart rhythm disorders is increased when betamethasone is taken with digoxin.
- Limit your intake of alcohol while on oral corticosteroids.

Food Interactions

Take corticosteroids with food or a small amount of antacid to avoid stomach upset. If stomach upset continues, notify your doctor. Grapefruit juice doubles the amount of some oral corticosteroids absorbed into the blood.

Usual Dose

Once-daily doses should be taken in the morning. Dosages vary greatly and depend on age, the disease being treated and its severity, and response to treatment.

Betamethasone: 0.6–7.2 mg a day.

Budesonide: 9 mg a day.

Cortisone: 25–300 mg a day.

Dexamethasone: 0.75–9 mg a day. Daily dosage sometimes exceeds 9 mg. A temporary dosage increase may be necessary if you are experiencing emotional stress. In alternate-day therapy, twice the usual daily dose is taken every other day.

Fludrocortisone: 0.1 mg 3 times a week to 0.2 mg a day, with cortisone or hydrocortisone pills.

Hydrocortisone: 20–240 mg a day.

Methylprednisolone: starting dose—4–48 mg or more a day. Maintenance dose varies. A temporary dosage increase may be necessary if you are experiencing emotional stress. In alternate-day therapy, twice the usual daily dose is taken every other day.

Prednisolone and Prednisone: 5–60 mg a day. Daily dose sometimes exceeds 60 mg. A temporary dose increase may be necessary if you are experiencing emotional stress. In alternate-day therapy, twice the usual daily dose is taken every other day.

Equivalent Doses: Using 5 mg of prednisone as the basis for comparison, equivalent doses of other corticosteroids are 0.6 mg–0.75 mg of betamethasone, 25 mg of cortisone, 0.75 mg of dexamethasone, 20 mg of hydrocortisone, 4 mg of methylprednisolone, and 5 mg of prednisolone.

Overdosage

Symptoms of overdose are anxiety, depression or stimulation, joint or muscle pain, blurred vision, stomach bleeding, increased blood sugar, high blood pressure, and water retention. The victim should be taken to a hospital emergency room immediately. If you seek treatment, ALWAYS bring the prescription bottle or container.

Special Information

Do not stop taking this medication without your doctor's knowledge. Suddenly stopping any corticosteroid drug may have severe consequences; the dosage must be gradually reduced by your doctor.

Contact your doctor if you develop unusual weight gain, black or tarry stools, swelling of the feet or legs, muscle weakness, vomiting of blood, menstrual irregularity, prolonged sore throat, fever, cold or infection, appetite loss, nausea and vomiting, diarrhea, weight loss, weakness, dizziness, or low blood sugar.

If you take several doses a day and forget a dose, take the dose you forgot as soon as possible. If it is almost time for your next dose, skip the one you forgot and double the next dose. If you take 1 dose a day and forget a dose, skip the dose you forgot and continue with your regular schedule. Do not take a double dose.

If you take a corticosteroid every other day and forget a dose, take it immediately if you remember it in the morning of your regularly scheduled day. If it is much later in the day, skip the dose you forgot and take it the following morning, then go back to your regular schedule. Do not take a double dose.

Special Populations

Pregnancy/Breast-feeding: Studies have shown that long-term corticosteroid therapy at high dosages may cause birth defects, as may chronic corticosteroid use during the first 3 months of pregnancy. An oral corticosteroid should be taken during pregnancy only if your doctor determines that the potential benefit outweighs the risks.

Corticosteroids taken by mouth may pass into breast milk. Most nursing mothers who must take a corticosteroid should use infant formula, though low dosages of some of these drugs may be taken for short periods while breast-feeding. Consult your doctor.

Seniors: Seniors are more likely to develop high blood pressure while taking an oral corticosteroid. Older women are more susceptible to osteoporosis (a condition characterized by loss of bone mass due to depletion of minerals, especially calcium) associated with high dosages of oral corticosteroids. Lower dosages are just as effective in seniors and cause fewer side effects.

Type of Drug

Corticosteroids, Topical

(kor-tih-koe-STER-oids)

Brand Names

CLASS 1—Super-potent topical products

Generic Ingredients: Betamethasone Dipropionate gel, ointment 0.05% G

Diprolene ointment

Generic Ingredients: Clobetasol Propionate cream, foam, gel, lotion, shampoo, ointment 0.05% G

Clobex
Cormax
Embeline
Embeline E
Olux
Olux E
Temovate
Temovate E

Generic Ingredients: Diflorasone Diacetate 0.05% G

Generic Ingredients: Fluocinonide cream 0.1% G
Vanos

Generic Ingredients: Flurandrenolide tape 4 mcg/cm^2
Cordran Tape

Generic Ingredients: Halobetasol Propionate cream/ ointment 0.05% G
Ultravate

CLASS 2—High-potency topical products
Generic Ingredients: Amcinonide ointment 0.1% G

Generic Ingredients: Betamethasone Dipropionate ointment 0.05% G
Diprolene AF

Generic Ingredients: Betamethasone Dipropionate (0.064%) + Calcipotriene (0.005%) ointment
Taclonex

Generic Ingredients: Desoximetasone cream, ointment 0.25% and 0.05%; gel 0.05% G
Topicort
Topicort LP

Generic Ingredients: Diflorasone Diacetate cream, ointment 0.05% G
ApexiCon
ApexiCon E

Generic Ingredients: Fluocinonide cream, gel, ointment, solution 0.05% G

Generic Ingredients: Halcinonide cream, ointment, solution 0.1%
Halog

Generic Ingredients: Mometasone Furoate ointment 0.1% G
Elocon

Generic Ingredients: Triamcinolone Acetonide ointment 0.5% G

CLASS 3—Upper mid-strength topical products
Generic Ingredients: Amcinonide lotion 0.1% G

Generic Ingredients: Betamethasone Dipropionate cream 0.05% G
Diprolene

Generic Ingredients: Betamethasone Valerate ointment and foam 0.1% G
Luxiq Foam

Generic Ingredients: Fluticasone Propionate cream 0.05% G
Cutivate

Generic Ingredients: Triamcinolone Acetonide cream 0.5% G
Triacet Trianex

CLASS 4—Mid-strength topical products
Generic Ingredients: Amcinonide cream 0.1% G

Generic Ingredients: Betamethasone Dipropionate lotion 0.05% G

Generic Ingredients: Desoximetasone cream 0.05% G
Topicort

Generic Ingredients: Fluocinolone Acetonide 0.025% G
Synalar

Generic Ingredients: Flurandrenolide ointment 0.05% G
Cordran

Generic Ingredients: Fluticasone Propionate lotion 0.05% G
Cutivate

Generic Ingredients: Hydrocortisone Valerate ointment 0.2% G
Westcort

Generic Ingredients: Mometasone Furoate 0.1% G
Elocon

Generic Ingredients: Prednicarbate ointment 0.1% G
Dermatop

Generic Ingredients: Triamcinolone Acetonide 0.1% G
Triderm

CLASS 5—Lower mid-strength topical products

Generic Ingredients: Betamethasone Valerate cream, lotion 0.1% G
Beta-Val
Valnac
Dermabet

Generic Ingredients: Clocortolone Pivalate cream 0.1%
Cloderm

Generic Ingredients: Desonide ointment 0.05% G
Desonil
DesOwen

Generic Ingredients: Fluocinolone Acetonide cream 0.025% G
Synalar

Generic Ingredients: Flurandrenolide cream, lotion 0.05% G
Cordran Lotion
Cordran SP

Generic Ingredients: Fluticasone Propionate ointment 0.005% G
Cutivate

Generic Ingredients: Hydrocortisone Butyrate cream, ointment, solution 0.1% G
Locoid

Generic Ingredients: Hydrocortisone Probutate 0.1%
Pandel

Generic Ingredients: Hydrocortisone Valerate cream 0.2% G
Westcort

Generic Ingredients: Prednicarbate cream 0.1% G

CLASS 6—Mild topical products

Generic Ingredients: Alclometasone Dipropionate cream, ointment 0.05% G
Aclovate

Generic Ingredients: Desonide cream, lotion 0.05% G
DesOwen

Generic Ingredients: Fluocinolone Acetonide cream, shampoo, solution 0.01% G
Capex Shampoo

Generic Ingredients: Flurandrenolide cream 0.025% G
Cordran

Generic Ingredients: Triamcinolone Acetonide cream 0.1% G
Triderm

Generic Ingredients: Triamcinolone Acetonide cream 0.025% G

CLASS 7—Least potent topical products
Generic Ingredients: Hydrocortisone 1% and 2.5% G

Ala-Cort
Ala-Scalp
Anti-Itch Maximum Strength
Auqanil HC
Aveno Anti-Itch Maximum Strength
Beta HC
Caldecort
Cortaid Advanced 12 Hour
Cortaid Intensive Therapy
Cortaid Maximum Strength
Corticool
Cortizone-10
Cortizone-10 Plus
Demarest Dricort
First Hydrocortisone
Gynecort 10
HydroSkin
Instacort 5
Instacort 10
Itch-X
Kericort 10
Med-Derm
Monistat Soothing Care
Noble Formula HC
Preparation H
Recort Plus
Rederm
Sarnal HC
Scalpicin Maximum Strength
Texacort
TheraCort

Generic Ingredients: Hydrocortisone Acetate cream, ointment 0.5% and 1% G

Cortaid Maximum Strength
Demarest Dricort
Gynecort 10
Lanacort 10
Medi-First
Tucks Anti-Itch

Prescribed For

Inflammation, itching, eczema, dermatitis and allergic reactions, vitiligo (patchy loss of skin color), blistering skin diseases, lupus and other connective tissue diseases, psoriasis, and many other specialized skin problems; may also be used in limited quantities to treat severe diaper rash.

General Information

Topical corticosteroids do not cure the underlying cause of skin problems, but they can relieve symptoms of rash, itching, or inflammation by interfering with the body mechanisms that produce them. You should never use a topical corticosteroid without your doctor's knowledge, because it could mask a symptom important in diagnosing your condition. Also, improper use of a topical corticosteroid could lead to unwanted and sometimes permanent side effects, such as stretch marks and thin fragile skin. Ointments are also less likely to cause allergic reactions because they contain fewer inactive ingredients.

Generic products in this group can vary in potency and produce different results from their brand-name counterparts, even though they contain the identical quantity of active ingredient. Topical steroids are rated from 1 (most potent) to 7 (least potent). Generally, products within a potency class are interchangeable. Ask your doctor or pharmacist which products are interchangeable. The lowest potency products are available without a prescription. Ointments tend to be more potent than creams, lotions, and solutions, and different product concentrations affect their classification.

Super-potent topical corticosteroids (class 1) should not be used on the face and neck, under the arms, or in the groin area. These products are generally reserved for situations in which less potent products have not worked. They should be used sparingly with caution, and should only be applied to the areas that are affected with the rash. Using a product in this category for longer than 2 weeks at a time increases the risk of permanent skin damage.

High-potency topical corticosteroids (classes 2 and 3) are best for the trunk, arms, and legs, but should not be used on the face and neck, under the arms, or in the groin area. Using a product in this category for longer than 2 weeks at a time increases the risk of permanent skin damage.

Intermediate-potency topical corticosteroids (classes 4 and 5) can be used in children for up to 1–2 weeks at a time. This type of medication is best for the trunk and extremities, and is more effective on thin skin than on thicker skin.

Low-potency topical corticosteroids (classes 6 and 7) can be used on any part of the body and can be used in children. They are the best choice for the face, neck, underarms, groin, and other occluded areas such as skin folds.

Cautions and Warnings

Do not use a topical corticosteroid if you are **allergic** or **sensitive** to corticosteroids or to any ingredients of the aerosol, cream, gel, lotion, ointment, or solution.

Do not use a topical corticosteroid as the sole treatment for **bacterial skin infections** such as impetigo, **viral skin diseases** such as herpes, **fungal skin infections** such as athlete's foot, or known **tuberculosis** of the skin. These drugs should not be used in the ear if the eardrum is perforated. Do not use a topical corticosteroid on **ulcerated skin** or to treat **acne**.

Skin problems can become less responsive if a product is applied continuously over a long period of time. This can result in a flare-up of the problem when the medication is stopped. Using a less potent product may avoid this problem.

Rectal corticosteroid products should not be used if you have any serious **bowel condition**, including bowel perforation, obstruction, abscess, and systemic fungal infection.

The rectal foam is not expelled after it has been applied and may result in higher drug blood levels than those associated with rectal enema products. The risk of systemic (whole-body) side effects is greater when more of the drug enters the blood. If there is no improvement after 2 or 3 weeks of using a rectal corticosteroid, contact your doctor.

Using a topical corticosteroid around the eyes for prolonged periods may cause cataracts, glaucoma, and/or permanent thinning and fragility of the skin around the eyes where the corticosteroid is being applied.

Children may be more susceptible to serious systemic side effects from topical corticosteroids, including growth retardation, Cushing's syndrome, and suppression of natural corticosteroid production, requiring a tapering of the medication, especially if the medications are applied to large areas over long periods. Superpotent topical corticosteroids are not recommended for children.

Possible Side Effects

Side effects are more likely with extended use of high-potency topical corticosteroid products and when the treated area is covered with a bandage that completely prevents skin contact with water and air.

Significant amounts of corticosteroids may be absorbed into the bloodstream if large amounts are used for long periods. This can result in systemic effects and may cause serious problems, particularly in people with liver disease. Systemic side effects include lightheadedness, hives, growth suppression, and adrenal suppression.

▼ Most common: burning; itching; irritation; "steroid" acne; skin thinning, tightening, or discoloration; stretch marks; dry cracked skin; spider veins; skin color changes; bruising; and secondary infection.

Drug Interactions

None known.

Usual Dose

Adult

Cream, Ointment, Solution, Foam, and Aerosol: Apply a thin film to the skin 2–3 times a day. High- and super-potent products should be applied no more than twice a day and should be used for short-term treatment, usually 2–3 weeks at a time. Some may need to be applied only once a day.

Rectal Enema: 100 mg nightly for 21 days.

Rectal Foam: 1 applicator's worth, 1–2 times a day for 2–3 weeks.

Child: Dosages for children should be limited to the lowest possible potency.

Overdosage

Serious adverse effects are unlikely after accidental ingestion. Excessive use of large amounts of topical corticosteroids may cause overdose symptoms and require gradual discontinuation of the drug. Contact your local poison control center or a hospital emergency room for more information. If you seek treatment, ALWAYS bring the prescription bottle or container.

Special Information

To prevent secondary infection, clean the skin before applying the drug. Apply a very thin film and rub in gently—effectiveness depends on contact area, not the thickness of the layer applied.

Do not wash, rub, or put clothing on the area until the medication has dried.

Topical corticosteroids have an additive effect: with continuous use, 1 or 2 applications a day may be as effective as 3 or more. Once the drug begins to take effect, your doctor may recommend reducing the dose to the minimum level needed to control the condition.

Flurandrenolide tape comes with specific directions for use; follow them carefully.

If your doctor instructs you to apply plastic wrap or any other occlusive dressing, follow directions carefully. These dressings can increase the penetration of the drug into your skin by as much as 10 times, which may be a crucial element in the medication's effectiveness. Occlusive dressings should not be used with any of the super-potent topical products.

If you are using one of these products for diaper rash, do not use tight-fitting diapers or plastic pants, which can cause too much drug to be absorbed into the blood.

Your doctor may prescribe a specific form of the product with good reason. Do not change forms without your doctor's knowledge; a different form may not be as effective.

If you forget to administer a dose, do so as soon as you remember. If it is almost time for your next dose, skip the one you forgot and continue with your regular schedule. Do not administer a double dose.

Special Populations

Pregnancy/Breast-feeding: Large amounts of corticosteroids applied to the skin for long periods of time may increase the risk of birth defects. A topical corticosteroid should be used during pregnancy only if your doctor determines that the potential benefit outweighs the risks. Do not use any over-the-counter hydrocortisone product for more than a few days without your doctor's knowledge.

Nursing mothers who must use a topical corticosteroid should consider using infant formula. If you apply a corticosteroid to the nipple area, be sure to completely clean the area prior to nursing. Nursing mothers should never use the highest potency corticosteroids (classes 1, 2, or 3) because of the risk of absorbing large amounts of drug into the system that could find its way into breast milk. Nursing mothers should discuss topical corticosteroid use with their doctor before applying any product.

Seniors: Seniors are more susceptible to high blood pressure and osteoporosis (a condition characterized by loss of bone mass due to depletion of minerals, especially calcium) associated with large dosages. These effects are unlikely with topical corticosteroids unless a high-potency medication is used over a large area for an extended period.

Brand Names

Cortisporin Otic

Generic Ingredients

Hydrocortisone + Neomycin Sulfate +
Polymyxin B Sulfate [G]

Other Brand Names

AK-Spore H.C.
Antibiotic Otic
Cortatrigen Ear Drops
Drotic
Ear-Eze
LazerSporin-C
Octicair Otic
Otic-Care
Otocort
Pediotic
UAD Otic

Type of Drug

Antibiotic and corticosteroid combination.

Prescribed For

Superficial ear infection, ear inflammation or itching, and other outer-ear problems.

General Information

Cortisporin Otic contains a corticosteroid to reduce inflammation and 2 antibiotics to treat local ear infections. This combination can be quite useful for local ear problems because of its dual method of action and its relatively broad applicability.

Cautions and Warnings

Do not use Cortisporin Otic if you are **allergic** or **sensitive** to any of its ingredients.

Cortisporin Otic is designed for use in the ear. It can be very damaging if placed into the eye.

Cortisporin should not be used if you have **herpes simplex**, **vaccinia**, or **chickenpox**. It also should not be used by patients sensitive to **sulfite**.

Cortisporin Otic should not be used if you have a **perforated eardrum**.

Possible Side Effects

▼ Local irritation, such as itching or burning, may occur as a drug-sensitivity or allergic reaction.

Drug Interactions

None known.

Usual Dose

3–4 drops in the affected ear 3–4 times a day. Treatment should not last beyond 10 days.

Overdosage

The amount of drug contained in each bottle is too small to cause serious problems. Contact a hospital emergency room or your local poison control center for more information. If you seek treatment, ALWAYS bring the prescription bottle or container.

Special Information

Use only when prescribed by a physician. Overuse of this or similar products can result in the growth of new organisms, such as fungi. If new infections or problems appear, stop using the drug and contact your doctor.

Before administering drops, wash your hands then hold the closed bottle in your hand for a few minutes to warm it to body temperature. Shake well for 10 seconds. For best results, drops should not be self-administered, but given by another person. The person receiving the drops should lie on his or her side with the affected ear facing upward. Fill the dropper and instill the required number of drops directly in the ear canal.

If the drops are being given to an infant, hold the earlobe down and back to allow the drops to run in. If the drops are being given to an older child or adult, hold the earlobe up and back to allow them to run in. Do not put the dropper into the ear or allow it to touch any part of the ear or bottle. Keep the ear tilted for about 5 minutes after the drops have been put in or insert a soft cotton plug, whichever is recommended by your doctor.

If you forget to administer a dose of Cortisporin Otic, do so as soon as you remember. If it is almost time for your next dose, skip the dose you forgot and continue with your regular schedule. Do not apply a double dose.

Special Populations

Pregnancy/Breast-feeding: There are no studies of Cortisporin Otic in pregnant women but it does contain a corticosteroid, which when used over long periods of time in other formulations may increase the risk of birth defects. Cortisporin Otic should be used during pregnancy only if your doctor determines that the potential benefit outweighs the risks.

Nursing mothers who must take this drug should use infant formula.

Seniors: Seniors may use this product without special precaution.

Coumadin *see **Warfarin,** page 1224*

Cozaar *see **Angiotensin II Blockers,** page 97*

Crestor *see **Statin Cholesterol-Lowering Agents,** page 1065*

Generic Name

Cromolyn (KROE-muh-lin) G

Brand Names

Crolom
Gastrocrom
Intal
Opticrom

The information in this profile also applies to the following drugs:

Generic Ingredients: Nedocromil
Alocril

Type of Drug

Allergy preventive and antiasthmatic.

Prescribed For

Prevention of severe allergic reactions, including asthma, runny nose, and mastocytosis; also prescribed for food allergies, eczema, dermatitis, chronic itching, and hay fever. It may be used to treat and prevent chronic inflammatory bowel disease. The eye drops are used to treat conjunctivitis (pinkeye) and other eye irritations.

General Information

Unlike antihistamines, which work against histamine that has been released into the system, cromolyn sodium prevents allergy, asthma, and other conditions by stabilizing mast cells, a key component in any allergic reaction because they release histamine. Cromolyn prevents the release of histamine and other chemicals from mast cells. The drug works only in the areas to which it is applied; only 7–8% of an inhaled dose and 1% of a swallowed capsule is absorbed into the blood. Even the oral capsules, which one would normally expect to be absorbed into the blood, treat only gastrointestinal-tract allergies. Cromolyn products must be used on a regular basis to be effective in reducing the frequency and intensity of allergic reactions.

Cautions and Warnings

Do not take cromolyn if you are **allergic** or **sensitive** to any of its ingredients. Rarely, people have experienced severe allergic attacks after taking cromolyn.

Cromolyn should never be used to treat an acute allergy attack. It is intended only to prevent or reduce the number of allergic attacks and their intensity. Once the proper dosage level has been established for you, reducing that level may result in a recurrence of attacks.

People with **kidney or liver disease** require reduced dosage.

Cough or bronchial spasm may occasionally occur after the inhalation of a cromolyn dose. Severe bronchospasm is rare.

Cromolyn aerosol should be used with caution in people with **abnormal heart rhythm** or **diseased coronary blood vessels** because of a possible reaction to the propellants used in the product.

Possible Side Effects

- ▼ Most common: rash and itching. Headache and diarrhea (for capsules). Watery, itchy, dry, or puffy eyes; and styes (for eye drops). Most capsule and eye-drop side effects are minor and may be attributable to the underlying condition; a variety have been reported but cannot be tied conclusively to the drug.
- ▼ Less common: local irritation, including nasal stinging, sneezing, tearing, cough, and stuffy nose; urinary difficulty or frequency; dizziness; headache; joint swelling; muscle pain; a bad taste in the mouth; sore throat; nosebleeds; abdominal pain; and nausea.
- ▼ Rare: severe drug reactions consisting of coughing, difficulty in swallowing, hives, itching, breathing difficulties, and swelling of the eyelids, lips, or face. Contact your doctor if you experience anything unusual while taking any medication.

Drug Interactions

None known.

Food Interactions

Inhaled or swallowed cromolyn products should not be mixed with any food, juice, or milk. The nasal and eye products can be taken without regard to food or meals.

Usual Dose

Aerosol

Adult and Child (age 5 and over): up to 2 sprays 4 times a day, spaced equally throughout the day. To prevent exercise asthma, 2 puffs may be inhaled up to 1 hour before exercise.

Eye drops

Adult and Child (age 4 and over): 1–2 drops in each eye 4–6 times a day at regular intervals.

Inhaled Capsules or Solution

Adult and Child (age 2 and over): starting dose—20 mg 4 times a day. Children under age 5 may inhale cromolyn powder if their allergies are severe. The solution must be given with a power-operated nebulizer and face mask. Handheld nebulizers are not adequate. To prevent exercise asthma, 20 mg may be inhaled up to 1 hour before exercise.

Nasal Solution

Adult and Child (age 6 and over): 1 spray in each nostril 3–6 times a day at regular intervals. First blow your nose and then inhale the spray.

Oral Capsules

Adult and Child (age 13 and over): 2 dissolved capsules (200 mg) 4 times a day taken 30 minutes before meals and at bedtime.

Child (age 2–12): 1 dissolved capsule (100 mg) 4 times a day 30 minutes before meals and at bedtime. Dosage may be increased to about 13–18 mg per lb. of body weight in 4 equal doses.

Child (under age 2): about 10 mg per lb. of body weight a day divided into 4 equal doses. This product is recommended for infants and young children only if absolutely necessary.

Overdosage

No action is necessary other than medical observation. Contact your local poison control center or a hospital emergency room for more information. If you seek treatment, ALWAYS bring the prescription bottle or container.

Special Information

Cromolyn is taken to prevent or minimize severe allergic reactions. It is imperative that you take cromolyn products on a regular basis to provide equal protection throughout the day.

If you are taking cromolyn to prevent seasonal allergies, it is essential that you start taking the medication before you come into contact with the cause of the allergy and that you continue treatment while you are exposed to it.

Cromolyn oral capsules should be opened and their contents mixed with about 4 oz. of hot water. Stir until the powder completely dissolves and the solution is completely clear, then fill the rest of the glass with cold water. Drink the entire contents of the glass. Do not mix the solution with food, juice, or milk.

Do not wear soft contact lenses while using cromolyn eye drops. The lenses may be reinserted a few hours after you stop taking the drug. To prevent contamination, do not touch the applicator tip to any surface, including your eyes or fingers.

Contact your doctor if you develop wheezing, coughing, a severe drug reaction (see "Possible Side Effects"), rash, or any bothersome or persistent side effect.

Contact your doctor if your symptoms do not improve or if they worsen.

If you forget to administer a dose, do so as soon as you remember, and space the remaining daily dosage evenly throughout the day. Do not take a double dose.

Special Populations

Pregnancy/Breast-feeding: In animal studies, very large dosages of cromolyn administered by vein have affected the fetus, though no birth defects were reported. Cromolyn should be used during pregnancy only if your doctor determines that the potential benefit outweighs the risks.

It is not known if cromolyn passes into breast milk. Nursing mothers who must use cromolyn should use infant formula.

Seniors: Older adults with reduced kidney or liver function may require lower dosages.

Generic Name

Cyclobenzaprine (sye-cloe-BEN-zuh-prene) G

Brand Names

Amrix Flexeril

Type of Drug

Skeletal muscle relaxant.

Prescribed For

Serious muscle spasm and acute muscle pain; also used to treat fibrositis (muscular rheumatism).

General Information

Cyclobenzaprine is used to treat severe muscle spasms; it is prescribed as part of a coordinated program of rest, physical therapy, and other measures.

Cautions and Warnings

Do not take cyclobenzaprine if you are **allergic** or **sensitive** to any of its ingredients.

This drug should not be taken for several weeks following a **heart attack** or by people with **abnormal heart rhythms**, **heart failure**, **heart block** (disruption of the electrical impulses that control heart rate), or **hyperthyroidism** (overactive thyroid gland).

People with severe **liver disease** should not use cyclobenzaprine and those with moderate liver disease should use it with caution.

Cyclobenzaprine should be used with caution by people with **urinary retention**, **glaucoma**, or **increased eye pressure**.

This drug may increase the chances of cavities or gum disease.

Cyclobenzaprine is intended only for short-term use of 2–3 weeks.

Cyclobenzaprine is chemically similar to tricyclic antidepressants and may produce some of the more serious side effects associated with those drugs. Abruptly stopping cyclobenzaprine may cause nausea, headache, and feelings of ill health; this is not a sign of addiction.

Possible Side Effects

- ▼ Most common: dry mouth, drowsiness, and dizziness.
- ▼ Less common: muscle weakness, fatigue, nausea, constipation, upset stomach, unpleasant taste, blurred vision, headache, nervousness, and confusion.

Possible Side Effects *(continued)*

▼ Rare: Rare side effects can occur in almost any part of the body. Contact your doctor if you experience anything unusual while taking any medication.

Drug Interactions

- The combination of cyclobenzaprine and a monoamine oxidase inhibitor (MAOI) antidepressant may produce very high fever, convulsions, and possibly death. Do not take these drugs within 14 days of each other.
- The effects of alcohol, sedatives, or other nervous system depressants may be increased by cyclobenzaprine.
- Cyclobenzaprine may increase some side effects of atropine, ipratropium, and other anticholinergic drugs.
- Cyclobenzaprine may increase the effects of haloperidol, loxapine, pimozide, anticoagulant (blood thinning) drugs, anticonvulsants, thyroid hormones, antithyroid drugs, phenothiazines, thioxanthenes, and nasal decongestants such as naphazoline, oxymetazoline, phenylephrine, and xylometazoline.
- Barbiturates and carbamazepine may counteract the effects of cyclobenzaprine.
- Fluoxetine, ranitidine, cimetidine, methylphenidate, estramustine, estrogens, and contraceptive drugs may increase the effects and side effects of cyclobenzaprine.
- Cyclobenzaprine may counteract the effects of clonidine, guanadrel, and guanethidine.

Food Interactions

None known.

Usual Dose

Amrix

Adult: 15–30 mg once a day.

Flexeril

Adult: 5–10 mg 3 times a day.

Overdosage

Cyclobenzaprine overdose may cause confusion, loss of concentration, hallucinations, agitation, overactive reflexes, fever, vomiting, rigid muscles, and other side effects of the drug. It may also cause drowsiness, low body temperature, rapid or irregular heartbeat and other kinds of abnormal heart rhythms, heart failure, dilated pupils, convulsions, very low blood pressure, stupor, coma, and sweating. Overdose victims must be taken to a hospital emergency room. If you seek treatment, ALWAYS bring the prescription bottle or container.

Special Information

Cyclobenzaprine causes drowsiness, dizziness, or blurred vision in more than 40% of people who take it, which may interfere with the ability to perform complex tasks such as driving or operating equipment. Avoid alcohol, sedatives, and other nervous system depressants because they can enhance the sedative effects of cyclobenzaprine.

Contact your doctor if you develop rash; hives; itching; urinary difficulties; clumsiness; confusion; depression; convulsions; difficulty breathing; irregular heart rate; chest pain; fever; yellowing of the skin or whites of the eyes; swelling of the face, lips, or tongue; or any other persistent or bothersome side effect.

If you forget a dose of cyclobenzaprine, take it as soon as you remember. If you take cyclobenzaprine once a day and it is almost time for your next dose, skip the one you forgot and continue with your regular schedule. If you take cyclobenzaprine twice a day and it is almost time for your next dose, take 1 dose as soon as you remember, another in 5 or 6 hours, and then go back to your regular schedule. If you take cyclobenzaprine 3 times a day and it is almost time for your next dose, take 1 dose as soon as you remember, another in 3 or 4 hours, and then go back to your regular schedule. Never take a double dose.

Special Populations

Pregnancy/Breast-feeding: The safety of cyclobenzaprine in pregnant women has not been established. Cyclobenzaprine should be used during pregnancy only if your doctor determines that the potential benefit outweighs the risks.

It is not known if cyclobenzaprine passes into breast milk, but antidepressants with a similar chemical structure do pass into breast milk. Nursing mothers who must take this drug should use infant formula.

Seniors: Seniors are more likely to be sensitive to the effects of cyclobenzaprine. Use of Amrix in particular is not recommended in the elderly.

Generic Name

Cyclosporine (sye-kloe-SPOR-in) G

Brand Names

Gengraf
Neoral
Restasis Ophthalmic Emulsion
Sandimmune

Type of Drug

Immunosuppressant.

Prescribed For

Kidney, heart, or liver transplantation; also used for bone marrow, heart-lung, and pancreas transplants. Cyclosporine is also prescribed for severe psoriasis and rheumatoid arthritis, aplastic anemia, atopic dermatitis, Behçet's disease, cirrhosis of the liver, ulcerative colitis, dermatomyositis, patchy hair loss, eye symptoms of Graves' disease, kidney inflammation, leukemia, multiple sclerosis, psoriasis-related arthritis, myasthenia gravis, pemphigus, sarcoidosis of the lung, and pyoderma gangrenosum. Cyclosporine eye emulsion is prescribed for dry eyes.

General Information

Cyclosporine is primarily used to prevent rejection of transplanted organs. It works by blocking the activity of T-cells, which protect the body against invading microorganisms or foreign substances. Cyclosporine also prevents the production of a substance known as interleukin-II that activates T-cells. Cyclosporine eye emulsion treats dry eye caused by inflammation of the cornea and tissue that covers the white part of the eye. It reduces inflammation and allows tears to form and flow.

Cautions and Warnings

Cyclosporine should be prescribed only by doctors experienced in immunosuppressive therapy and the care of organ-transplant patients. Sandimmune is always used with corticosteroid drugs like prednisone and should never be used with other immunosuppressive medicines. When combined with other immune suppressants, Neoral and Gengraf must be used with great care because oversuppression of the immune system may lead to lymphoma or another malignancy as well as extreme susceptibility to infection.

Do not substitute Neoral or Gengraf for Sandimmune; they are not equivalent to each other. Sandimmune is poorly absorbed into the bloodstream and usually requires a larger dose than the other forms of cyclosporine. People taking this drug by mouth for a long period of time should have their blood checked for cyclosporine levels so that the dosage may be adjusted if necessary.

Cyclosporine may increase the risk of skin cancer in people with psoriasis who are undergoing other treatments at the same time, including radiation therapy, ultraviolet light therapy, and certain psoriasis medications (see "Drug Interactions").

Cyclosporine causes kidney toxicosis (kidney poisoning, which is different from transplant rejection) in 25–35% of people taking it to prevent organ rejection. Mild symptoms usually start after about 2 or 3 months of treatment. Your doctor will carefully monitor your kidney function while you take cyclosporine, and reducing the dosage may control this effect. In one study, clonidine skin patches used before and after surgery decreased toxic risks to the kidney.

Liver toxicosis is seen in about 5% of transplant patients taking cyclosporine. It usually appears in the first month and may be controlled by reducing dosage.

Convulsions may develop, especially in people also taking high dosages of **corticosteroids**. Other nervous system side effects are listed below (see "Possible Side Effects").

Cyclosporine may cause high blood pressure, and this effect may last after cyclosporine treatment has been stopped. You may require blood-pressure-lowering medication but should avoid using medicines that increase your blood-potassium levels (see "Drug Interactions").

Live vaccines should not be given to people taking cyclosporine, because cyclosporine blocks the body's response to the vaccine, making it ineffective. This effect lasts several months to years after stopping cyclosporine. Do not take any vaccine without informing your doctor that you are taking cyclosporine or have taken it in the past.

Do not use cyclosporine eye drops if you have an **eye infection**.

Small amounts of cyclosporine eye emulsion may be absorbed into the bloodstream, but the risk of body-wide side effects is small.

Possible Side Effects

▼ Most common: kidney damage, tremor, high blood pressure, increased hair growth, infection, and enlargement of the gums.

Possible Side Effects *(continued)*

▼ Less common: abdominal pain, acne, appetite loss, drug allergy (symptoms include rash, itching, hives, and breathing difficulties), high blood sugar, low blood-magnesium levels, high blood-potassium levels, brittle hair or fingernails, convulsions, confusion, conjunctivitis (pinkeye), cramps, diarrhea, dizziness, fluid retention and swelling, flushing, gas, hair loss, headache, hearing loss, hiccups, muscle pain, nausea or vomiting, reduced counts of red and white blood cells and platelets, sinus inflammation, sleeplessness, swollen and painful male breasts, ringing or buzzing in the ears, tingling in the hands or feet, upset stomach, and increased urinary frequency.

▼ Rare: blood in the urine, heart attack, itching, anxiety, depression, lethargy, weakness, mouth sores, difficulty swallowing, intestinal bleeding, constipation, pancreas inflammation, night sweats, chest pain, joint pain, visual disturbances, and weight loss. Contact your doctor if you experience anything unusual while taking any medication.

Eye Drops

▼ Most common: burning sensation.

▼ Less common: red eye, discharge from the eye, overflow of tears, eye pain, a sensation of something in the eye, itching, stinging, and blurred vision and other visual disturbances.

Drug Interactions

- Do not mix bosentan and cyclosporine, as blood levels of bosentan may be increased, raising the chance of side effects, whereas cyclosporine blood levels may be reduced, increasing the risk of organ rejection.
- Do not use cyclosporine with berberine or colchicine, as these combinations dramatically increase the risk of kidney damage.
- Cyclosporine raises blood levels of aliskiren and caspofungin; to avoid increased risk of side effects, do not use these medicines together.
- Do not take red yeast rice extract while taking cyclosporine because of an increased risk of damage to your muscles.
- Cyclosporine increases blood potassium and should not be used with potassium-sparing diuretics (spironolactone) or

potassium supplements. Very high blood-potassium levels may also be reached if cyclosporine is taken with angiotensin-converting enzyme (ACE) inhibitors such as captopril; use with caution.

- Cyclosporine should be used carefully with other kidney-toxic drugs, including antibiotics (ciprofloxacin, gentamicin, tobramycin, vancomycin), antifungals (amphotericin B, ketoconazole), cimetidine, diclofenac, fenofibrate, melphalan, naproxen, nonsteroidal anti-inflammatory drugs (NSAIDs; e.g., ibuprofen), ranitidine, and sulfanamides (sulfadiazine, sulfasalazine, trimethoprim-sulfamethoxazole), sulindac, and tacrolimus.
- Mixing sirolimus and cyclosporine can increase kidney damage. This effect can often be reversed by reducing cyclosporine dosage or separating the doses by at least 4 hours.
- The risk of skin cancer is increased in psoriasis patients when cyclosporine is combined with coal tar, psoralen plus ultraviolet A light, methotrexate, and other immunosuppressive agents.
- Blood levels of both cyclosporine and corticosteroids such as methylprednisolone are increased when these drugs are used together. The chance of kidney damage or convulsions may be increased. Your doctor should closely monitor your health status while you take these medicines.
- Drugs and herbal products that may increase blood levels of cyclosporine include allopurinol, amiodarone, androgens (danazol, methyltestosterone), antibiotics (azithromycin, clarithromycin, erythromycin, telithromycin), antifungal agents (fluconazole, itraconazole, ketoconazole, posaconazole, voriconazole), beta blockers (carvedilol), bortezomib, bromocriptine, calcium channel blockers (diltiazem, nicardipine, verapamil), chamomile, chloramphenicol, chloroquine, clonidine, contraceptive drugs, ezetimibe, foscarnet, imatinib, imipenem-cilastatin, methoxsalen, metoclopramide, metronidazole, mibefradil, micafungin, nefazodone, propafenone, quercetin, quinupristin-dalfopristin, selective serontonin reuptake inhibitors (SSRIs; fluoxetine, fluvoxamine, sertraline), sulfonylureas (glipizide, glyburide), tigecycline, and vitamin E. Ketoconazole may be used by your doctor in order to reduce the dosage of cyclosporine that you take.
- Protease inhibitors, including indinavir, nelfinavir, ritonavir, and saquinavir, may also increase cyclosporine blood levels

because they slow liver enzymes responsible for cyclosporine breakdown.

- Drugs that decrease cyclosporine blood levels and may lead to organ rejection include aluminum salts, antibiotics (nafcillin, rifabutin, rifampin), anticonvulsants (carbamazepine, oxcarbazepine, phenobarbital, phenytoin), clindamycin, efavirenz, gemfibrozil, griseofulvin, nafacilin, octreotide, orlistat, probucol, St. John's wort, terbinafine, and ticlopidine.
- Cyclosporine interferes with the body's ability to clear digoxin, doxorubicin, etoposide, everolimus, and statin drugs (lovastatin, simvastatin), and vinca alkaloids (vinblastine, vincristine). People taking any of these medications who start on cyclosporine should be aware of possible drug side effects and have their drug dosage reduced.
- Cyclosporine can prolong the effects of muscle relaxants such as vecuronium; your doctor may need to reduce the dose of the muscle relaxant.
- Cyclosporine may increase the amount of nateglinide or repaglinide in the blood, increasing the risk of low blood sugar. A dosage reduction may be needed if you take this combination.
- Combining cyclosporine and nifedipine may lead to gum overgrowth.
- Omeprazole may alter the absorption of cyclosporine, increasing or decreasing blood levels. Your doctor should closely monitor your health status while you take both drugs.
- Cyclosporine substantially increases the amount of methotrexate in the blood. The importance of this interaction is not yet known, but they should be used together with caution.
- Cyclosporine prevents the body's normal response to live vaccines (See "Cautions and Warnings").

Food Interactions

Cyclosporine may be taken with food if it upsets your stomach. For optimal effectiveness, avoid eating a fatty meal within 30 minutes of taking Neoral or Gengraf.

You may mix Neoral or Gengraf in a glass—not a paper or plastic cup—with room-temperature orange or apple juice or chocolate milk to make it taste better. Drink immediately after mixing, then put more juice or chocolate milk in the glass and drink it to be sure that the entire dose has been taken. These medications may be unpalatable if taken with unflavored milk.

Do not drink or eat grapefruit, pomelo, or starfruit products because they increase the amount of cyclosporine in the blood.

Avoid red wine while taking cyclosporine, as it may decrease the effects of your medicine.

Do not use salt substitutes or eat foods high in potassium but low in sodium while taking cyclosporine, as this may lead to dangerously high levels of potassium in your body.

Usual Dose

In general, the usual dosage of Neoral or Gengraf is lower than Sandimmune, but dosage must be individualized for you by your doctor. Do not substitute one brand for the other. The first dose of cyclosporine is given 4–12 hours before the transplant operation or immediately after surgery. With 1–2 weeks after surgery, the dosage is slowly reduced to maintain a target amount of cyclosporine in the body.

Cyclosporine Eye Emulsion

Adult and Child (age 16 and over): One drop in the affected eye(s) every 12 hours. Before using, rotate and turn the vial over a few times until you have a uniform, white, opaque fluid inside. If you use artificial tears, allow 15 minutes between products. Discard the open vial immediately after use.

Gengraf and Neoral

Organ Transplant

Adult and Child: Initial dose for organ transplant—3–4 mg per lb. of body weight a day divided into 2 doses. The maintenance dose is lower and varies according to the organ transplanted.

Rheumatoid Arthritis or Psoriasis: 1.1–1.8 mg per lb. of body weight.

Sandimmune

Adult and Child: Maintenance dose—2.3–4.5 mg per lb. of body weight a day, although larger and more frequent doses may be needed for children.

Overdosage

Overdose victims may be expected to develop side effects, including decreased liver and kidney function and symptoms of extreme immunosuppression. Induce vomiting with ipecac syrup—available at any pharmacy—which is recommended up to 2 hours after the overdose was taken. Contact your doctor, hospital emergency room, or local poison control center before inducing vomiting; they may recommend a stomach pump procedure instead. If you seek treatment, ALWAYS bring the prescription bottle or container.

Special Information

Contact your doctor at the first sign of fever; sore throat; tiredness; weakness; nervousness; unusual bleeding or bruising; tender or swollen gums; convulsions; irregular heartbeat; confusion; numbness or tingling of your hands, feet, or lips; breathing difficulties; severe stomach pain with nausea; or blood in the urine. Other side effects such as shaking or trembling of the hands, increased hair growth, acne, headache, leg cramps, nausea, or vomiting are less serious but should be brought to your doctor's attention, particularly if they are bothersome or persistent.

Maintain good dental hygiene while taking cyclosporine and use extra care when brushing and flossing because the drug increases your risk of oral infection. See your dentist regularly.

Continue taking your medication as long as your doctor prescribes it. Do not stop taking it without your doctor's knowledge. If you cannot take one of the oral forms, cyclosporine can be given by injection.

Do not keep either brand of the oral liquid in the refrigerator. After the bottle is opened, use the medication within 2 months. At temperatures below 68°F, Neoral can form a gel and a light sediment can form in Sandimmune. These do not affect the potency of either product. They can still be used and are effective.

Cyclosporine may increase the risk of skin cancer. Wear protective clothing and use sunscreen while taking this drug.

If you forget a dose, take it as soon as you remember if it is within 12 hours of your regular dose. If not, skip the dose you forgot and continue with your regular schedule. Do not take a double dose.

For cyclosporine eye emulsion, each small plastic container is meant to be used once and then thrown away along with any remaining medication. Do not allow the tip of the disposable vial to touch the eye or any surface, as this may contaminate the emulsion.

Patients with decreased tear production typically should not wear contact lenses. But those who do must remove them before using cyclosporine eye emulsion. Lenses may be reinserted 15 minutes after using the medicine.

Special Populations

Pregnancy/Breast-feeding: In animal studies cyclosporine damages the fetus. Though a small number of pregnant women have taken cyclosporine without major problems, it is recommended that pregnant women avoid cyclosporine. Cyclosporine should be taken during pregnancy only if your doctor determines that the potential benefit outweighs the risks.

Cyclosporine passes into breast milk. Nursing mothers who must take cyclosporine should use infant formula.

Seniors: Due to decreased kidney, liver, and heart function, seniors are more susceptible to the side effects of this drug. Use with caution.

Cymbalta *see **Venlafaxine,** page 1204*

Generic Name

Dalfampridine (dal-FAM-prih-deen)

Brand Names

Ampyra

Type of Drug

Potassium channel blocker.

Prescribed For

Multiple sclerosis (MS).

General Information

Dalfampridine is the first potassium channel blocker approved in the United States. Its approval was based on improvement in the walking ability of people with MS. Multiple sclerosis is a disabling condition affecting the central nervous system, in which myelin, the protective sheath covering nerves, is damaged. Blocking potassium channels increases the ability of these nerves to carry impulses.

Cautions and Warnings

Do not take dalfampridine if you are **allergic** or **sensitive** to any of its ingredients.

This drug can cause **seizures**. People who have a history of seizures should not take dalfampridine.

People with moderate to severe **kidney disease** should not take dalfampridine.

Urinary infections are twice as common in people taking dalfampridine.

Possible Side Effects

- ▼ Most common: urinary infection.
- ▼ Common: sleeplessness, dizziness, headache, muscle weakness, back pain, and difficulty maintaining your balance.
- ▼ Less common: MS relapse; tingling, burning, or itching; common cold symptoms, including inflamed nose and throat; throat pain; constipation; and upset stomach.
- ▼ Rare: Seizures are rare at normal doses. Contact your doctor if you experience anything unusual while taking any medication.

Drug Interactions

There are no interactions between dalfampridine and interferon, glatiramer, or natalizumab, drugs often taken by people with MS.

- Dalfampridine can also be called 4AP, 4-aminopyridine, or fampridine. Do not mix dalfampridine with any other 4AP product.
- Alcoholic beverages and isoniazid can increase the breakdown of dalfampridine in the blood.
- Disulfiram slows the breakdown of dalfampridine, raising the risk of a drug side effect.

Food Interactions

Dalfampridine may be taken with food or meals.

Usual Dose

Adult: 10 mg every 12 hours.

Child: not recommended.

Overdosage

Symptoms include mental changes, seizures, confusion, tremors, sweating, and memory loss. One overdose equal to 30 dalfampridine pills caused a condition resembling brain damage. Take the overdose victim to a hospital emergency room for treatment. If you seek treatment, ALWAYS bring the prescription bottle or container.

Special Information

If you have a seizure, call your doctor or go to a hospital emergency room.

Tell your doctor if you have ever had kidney problems or a seizure or have ever taken a medicine for epilepsy or another seizure disorder.

You must take this drug every 12 hours. If you forget a dose, take it as soon as you remember, but do not take more than 2 pills in any 24-hour period. Taking just 1 extra tablet a day increases seizure risk by 4 times.

Do not crush, cut, or mix these pills with water before you take them. They are specifically designed to last 12 hours and must be swallowed whole. Crushing, cutting, or dissolving them releases too much medicine at once.

Special Populations

Pregnancy/Breast-feeding: Animal studies show this drug can damage a developing fetus. Dalfampridine should be taken during pregnancy only if your doctor determines that the potential benefit outweighs the risks.

Dalfampridine may pass into breast milk. Nursing mothers who must take it should use infant formula.

Seniors: Seniors taking dalfampridine are more likely to have seizures or other drug side effects because of normal declines in kidney function.

Generic Name

Deferasirox (deh-fur-ASS-sih-rox)

Brand Names

Exjade

Type of Drug

Iron chelating agent.

Prescribed For

Chronic iron overload.

General Information

Deferasirox binds with iron stored in the liver. It can also bind small amounts of zinc and copper, but the importance of these effects are not known. Almost ¾ of every dose is absorbed into the bloodstream. Most of the drug is broken down in the liver and passes out of the body in the feces. Women clear this drug from their bodies 17.5% slower than men, but this has not affected how it is used or the doses given.

Cautions and Warnings

Do not take deferasirox if you are **allergic** or **sensitive** to any of its ingredients. Most reactions occur within the first month of treatment.

Liver function should be checked regularly while taking deferasirox.

Kidney failure has developed in people taking deferasirox with fatal results in some cases. People with or those who are at risk of kidney failure should have routine kidney monitoring while taking this medication. People who are at risk for kidney failure include seniors, those with kidney disease, and people taking medicines that affect kidney function. Dose adjustment may be needed.

Deferasirox has been associated with potentially severe reduced white-blood-cell and platelet counts, usually in people with pre-existing **blood disorders**.

Rarely, deferasirox has caused hearing loss and eye problems. You should have a full hearing and eye exam before starting on this drug and once a year thereafter.

Gastrointestinal (GI) bleeding and ulcers have occurred in people taking this medicine, including some children and teens. Mixing this with blood thinners or other drugs that are irritating to the GI tract, such as corticosteroids and bisphosphonates, increases the risk.

Skin rash can occur with this medicine. If it is severe, the drug may have to be temporarily stopped. It may be restarted at a lower dosage.

Possible Side Effects

- ▼ Most common: fever, headache, abdominal pain, cough, sore throat, nasal irritation, diarrhea, flu-like symptoms, nausea, and vomiting.
- ▼ Common: respiratory infections, bronchitis, runny nose, rash, upper abdominal pain, joint pain, back pain, tonsillitis, and ear infection.
- ▼ Less common: itching.

Possible Side Effects *(continued)*

▼ Rare: stomach pain, swelling in the arms or legs, sleep disorder, skin color changes, dizziness, anxiety, gallstones, fatigue, early-onset cataracts or hearing loss, some visual haziness, and other eye disorders. Contact your doctor if you experience anything unusual while taking any medication.

Drug Interactions

- Do not mix antacids containing aluminum with deferasirox. They can prevent it from being absorbed.
- Ritonavir, rifampicin, phenytoin, and phenobarbital increase the release of deferasirox from the body. Your drug must be increased to account for this interaction.
- Deferasirox may interfere with the breakdown of amodiaquine, cerivastatin, paclitaxel, sorafenib, and torsemide, increasing drug concentrations in the blood and the risk for excess drug effects or side effects.
- Deferasirox interferes with the breakdown of repaglinide. Repaglinide dosages may need to be reduced.
- Use deferasirox with caution with drugs that may cause GI ulcers such as nonsteroidal anti-inflammatory drugs (NSAIDs), corticosteroids, oral bisphosphonates, or anticoagulants.

Food Interactions

This drug should be taken at the same time every day on an empty stomach, 30 minutes before eating.

Usual Dose

Adult and Child (age 2 and over): 9–13.6 mg per lb. of body weight once a day. Dose adjustments will be made according to your response. See "Special Information" for specific instructions on how to take these tablets.

Overdosage

Large doses of 2–3 times the prescribed amount taken for several weeks with no adverse effects have occurred. Overdose symptoms include hepatitis (mild fever, muscle or joint aches, nausea, vomiting, appetite loss, slight abdominal pain, diarrhea, and fatigue) and some drug side effects. Take the victim to a hospital emergency room for treatment because the heart may be affected. If you seek treatment, ALWAYS bring the prescription bottle or container.

Special Information

Contact your doctor at once if you develop a severe skin rash.

You must have regular vision and hearing tests while taking deferasirox.

Deferasirox tablets should not be chewed or swallowed whole. They must first be mixed completely in ½–1 glass of water, orange juice, or apple juice. The tablet will not dissolve but tablet particles will become suspended in the liquid. Drink the resulting suspension immediately. If there is anything left in the glass after drinking the suspension, add a small amount of liquid, mix it with the remaining tablet particles, and drink it.

This drug can cause dizziness. Be cautious while driving, operating machinery, or doing anything that requires intense concentration.

If you forget a dose, take it as soon as you remember. If it is almost time for the next dose, skip the one you forgot and continue with your regular schedule. Do not take a double dose.

Special Populations

Pregnancy/Breast-feeding: There are no studies of deferasirox in pregnant women or of its effect on the developing fetus. Deferasirox should be used during pregnancy only if your doctor determines that the potential benefit outweighs the risks.

This drug may pass into breast milk. Nursing mothers should use infant formula.

Seniors: Seniors with MDS (a blood disorder) may experience severe or deadly side effects due to greater chances of reduced kidney, liver, and heart function, other diseases, or drug side effects.

Generic Name

Denosumab (den-OH-suh-mab)

Brand Names

Prolia Injection
Xgeva Injection

Type of Drug

RANKL inhibitor.

Prescribed For

Osteoporosis; prevention of bone fractures in men being treated for prostate cancer, women being treated for breast cancer, and people with bone cancer.

General Information

Denosumab is a synthetic biological antibody that binds to a specific receptor (receptor activator of nuclear factor kappa-B ligand [RANKL]) on cells called osteoclasts. Osteoclasts are instrumental in the bone-thinning process, and denosumab prevents osteoclasts from forming and surviving. It is prescribed for postmenopausal women who are at a particularly high risk of developing osteoporosis and cannot take another osteoporosis medicine or have used other osteoporosis medicines but developed osteoporosis anyway. Studies have shown denosumab increases bone mineral density and reduces fractures of the hip, spine, and other bones.

Cautions and Warnings

Do not use denosumab if you are **allergic** or **sensitive** to any of its ingredients.

Do not use this medicine if you have **low blood calcium**. Blood-calcium levels must be corrected before you begin to take this medicine. Severe **kidney disease**, **thyroid problems**, and **poor nutrient absorption** through your intestines can lower blood-calcium levels.

Infections, including skin infection, may occur while you are on this medicine and may be serious enough to require hospital treatment.

Skin rash, dermatitis, and eczema can develop while taking denosumab. Your doctor may consider stopping the medicine if your skin reactions are severe.

Death of jaw bone tissue has occurred while taking this medicine. Known as osteonecrosis of the jaw (ONJ), it may not have a specific cause but generally occurs after tooth removal or local infections that do not heal properly. Your doctor and dentist should examine your mouth before starting denosumab.

Longer-term potential risks of denosumab include unusual bone fractures and delayed fracture healing. Bone tissue is constantly being recycled. Denosumab interferes with this process and can alter the makeup and structure of newly formed bone, but the long-term importance of this fact is not yet known.

Denosumab is a biological product that can, rarely, stimulate the formation of antibodies that can either counter its effectiveness or cause you to experience a drug reaction.

Possible Side Effects

- ▼ Most common: back pain and pain in the arms and legs.
- ▼ Common: rash, high blood cholesterol, muscle pain, bladder infection, and dizziness.
- ▼ Less common: upper-respiratory infections, arm or leg swelling, sciatica (leg pain, burning or tingling down the leg, constant pain on one side of your buttocks, leg weakness, or a sharp pain that makes it hard to stand up or walk), pneumonia, bone pain, abdominal pain, anemia, sleeplessness, sore throat, weakness, itching, stomach gas, spinal osteoarthritis, gastroesophageal reflux disease, abnormal heart rhythms, chest pain, shingles (herpes zoster), and reduced blood calcium.
- ▼ Rare: Other side effects, including pancreas inflammation, may occur. Contact your doctor if you experience anything unusual while taking any medication.

Drug Interactions

None known.

Food Interactions

This drug can be taken without regard to food or meals. Take a daily calcium and vitamin D supplement (see "Special Information").

Usual Dose

Prolia

Adult: 60 mg injected every 6 months.
Child: not recommended.

Xgeva

Adult: 120 mg injected every 4 weeks.
Child: not recommended.

Overdosage

There is no information on denosumab overdose.

Special Information

This medication is usually given by a health care professional. If you miss your regular denosumab injection, it should be taken as soon as possible. Schedule your next injection 6 months from the actual date when you received your last dose.

You must take calcium (1000 mg) and vitamin D (400 IU) every day while on denosumab; tell your doctor if you are unable to do this for any reason.

Tell your doctor if you experience pain, swelling, or infection of the gums or jaw; poor healing in your gums; dramatic loss of gum tissue; loose teeth; numbness or heaviness of the jaw; the appearance of exposed bone in your mouth; or oozing. These can be signs of ONJ that demand immediate dental attention. Pay careful attention to your oral health while taking denosumab. See your dentist regularly.

Special Populations

Pregnancy/Breast-feeding: Animal studies show denosumab may harm the developing fetus. Denosumab should be taken during pregnancy only if your doctor determines that the potential benefit outweighs the risks. You can enroll in a program sponsored by the drug maker to monitor women who become pregnant while taking this medicine.

It is not known if this drug passes into breast milk. Denosumab can interfere with normal development of the glands that produce breast milk. Nursing mothers who must take this drug should use infant formula.

Seniors: Most women studied with denosumab were 65 years or older. Seniors responded in the same way as younger adults, but some older adults may be more sensitive to denosumab.

Generic Name

Desmopressin (dez-moe-PRES-in) G

Brand Names

DDAVP
Minirin
Stimate

Type of Drug

Pituitary hormone replacement.

Prescribed For

Nighttime bed-wetting (children), nocturia (frequent nighttime urination in adults), and diabetes insipidus (central or cranial diabetes); also used to control bleeding in certain forms of hemophilia A and von Willebrand's disease.

General Information

Desmopressin is a synthetic version of antidiuretic hormone (ADH). When ADH is lacking, the body has difficulty retaining fluid. People lacking ADH experience excessive thirst, increased urination, and dehydration; desmopressin controls these symptoms. When used for nighttime bed-wetting, desmopressin should be used in conjunction with behavioral or other nondrug therapies.

Cautions and Warnings

Do not take desmopressin if you are **allergic** or **sensitive** to any of its ingredients.

People with moderate or severe **kidney disease** should not use this drug.

Do not use desmopressin if you have **hyponatremia** (low blood sodium) or a history of hyponatremia.

Desmopressin can cause water intoxication and hyponatremia if you drink too much water; this can result in seizures, coma, or death. Therefore, people taking this drug, especially **children** and **seniors** and people with **cystic fibrosis**, **heart failure**, and **electrolyte imbalances**, should drink only enough fluid to satisfy their thirst. People who drink excessive amounts of fluid out of habit or for psychiatric reasons must use this drug with caution. Excess fluid intake can also occur during hot weather and following strenuous exercise or when you are sick with severe vomiting and diarrhea, fever, the flu, or a severe cold.

People with **coronary artery disease**, **heart disease**, or **high blood pressure** should use this drug with caution. Heart attacks and strokes after treatment with desmopressin have been reported in people at risk for them, but there is no definite link to desmopressin use.

Possible Side Effects

- ▼ Most common: headache, runny nose.
- ▼ Less common: nasal congestion, flushing, abdominal pain, weakness, chills, dizziness, nosebleeds, nostril pain, nausea, red and swollen eyes, tearing, chest pain, upset stomach, sleeplessness and sleepiness, heart rhythm changes, warm feeling, and diarrhea.

Possible Side Effects *(continued)*

▼ Rare: slight increases in blood pressure, loss of sodium, and water intoxication. Contact your doctor if you experience anything unusual while taking any medication.

Drug Interactions

- Desmopressin may increase the effects of other drugs that raise blood pressure. This only happens with large dosages.
- Carbamazepine, chlorpromazine, lamotrigine, nonsteroidal anti-inflammatory drugs (NSAIDs; e.g., naproxen), opiate drugs (e.g., methadone), selective serotonin reuptake inhibitors (SSRIs; e.g., fluoxetine), and tricyclic antidepressants (e.g., amitriptyline) may increase the effects of desmopressin and raise the risk of hyponatremia (low blood sodium).
- Mixing desmopressin with any drug that can make your mouth dry or make you thirsty, such as an antidepressant, painkiller, or a seizure medicine, can increase the risk of hyponatremia (low blood sodium).

Food Interactions

None known.

Usual Dose

Nasal Solution—Diabetes Insipidus

Adult and Child (age 13 years and over): 10–40 mcg a day in 1–3 doses.

Child (age 3 months–12 years): 5–30 mcg a day in 1–2 doses.

Tablets—Diabetes Insipidus

Adult and Child (age 4 and over): 0.05–1.2 mg a day in 2–3 divided doses.

Child (under age 4): Begin with 0.05 mg and adjust according to individual need.

Tablets—Nighttime Bed-Wetting

Adult and Child (age 6 and over): 0.2–0.6 mg at bedtime.

Child (under age 6): not recommended.

Overdosage

Symptoms include confusion, drowsiness, problems passing urine, rapid weight gain, and headache. Contact your doctor or a hospital emergency room if you suspect an overdose. Because there is no known antidote to desmopressin, your dosage may be temporarily reduced until overdose symptoms subside. If you seek treatment, ALWAYS bring the prescription bottle or container.

Special Information

Contact your doctor if you or your child develop headache; nausea; vomiting; muscle weakness, spasms, or cramps; weight gain; restlessness; fatigue; lethargy; disorientation; depressed reflexes; appetite loss; irritability; and mental changes, including hallucinations, loss of consciousness, and confusion. Severe symptoms of hyponatremia may include seizures, coma, not breathing, and death.

Contact your doctor if you or your child is thirstier than usual while taking desmopressin.

Minimize the amount of water or other fluids you drink from 1 hour before to 8 hours after you take desmopressin tablets.

While you are taking desmopressin your doctor will periodically check your urine. Your doctor should also check for nasal swelling, congestion, and scarring.

Desmopressin nasal solution spray pumps must be primed before first use. To prime the pump, press down 4 times. DDAVP delivers 50 doses per bottle, and Stimate delivers 25 doses. Throw away the bottle after these doses have been used, because anything remaining afterward is unlikely to deliver the necessary amount of drug.

If your child uses a desmopressin spray, be sure to supervise him/her to be sure the correct dose is taken.

If you forget a dose of desmopressin, take it as soon as you remember. If it is almost time for your next dose, skip the forgotten dose and continue with your regular schedule. Do not take a double dose.

Special Populations

Pregnancy/Breast-feeding: The safety of using desmopressin during pregnancy is not known, although it has been used to treat diabetes insipidus in pregnant women without apparent harm to the fetus. Desmopressin should be taken during pregnancy only if your doctor determines that the potential benefit outweighs the risks.

Desmopressin may pass into breast milk. Nursing mothers who must use this drug should use infant formula.

Seniors: Seniors should start desmopressin at lower doses than younger people because of the greater chances of heart, kidney, liver, and other diseases that might affect blood-sodium levels.

Detrol *see **Overactive Bladder Drugs,** page 884*

Dexilant *see **Proton-Pump Inhibitors,** page 956*

Generic Name

Dicyclomine (dih-SYE-kloe-meen) G

Brand Names

Bemote
Bentyl
Byclomine
Dibent
Dilomine
Di-Spaz
OR-Tyl

Type of Drug

Antispasmodic and anticholinergic.

Prescribed For

Irritable bowel, spastic colon, and similar digestive problems; also prescribed for colic in children over age 6 months.

General Information

Dicyclomine has been used for many years to calm "nervous stomach." It and other anticholinergics work by blocking the effects of the neurohormone acetylcholine in the gastrointestinal (GI) tract. This reduces the mobility of the GI tract and slows the production of enzymes and other secretions.

Cautions and Warnings

Do not take dicyclomine if you are **allergic** or **sensitive** to any of its ingredients.

Dicyclomine should not be used by those with **obstructive disease of the GI or urinary tract** (often indicated by diarrhea), severe **ulcerative colitis, reflux esophagitis, acute bleeding with unstable heart function, myasthenia gravis**, or **glaucoma**.

Dicyclomine should not be used in **infants less than age 6 months** or by **breast-feeding mothers**.

This drug should be used with caution if you have **heart disease, Down's syndrome, spastic paralysis, reduced mobility of**

the stomach and lower esophagus, **fever**, **urinary difficulties**, **enlarged prostate**, **hiatal hernia**, **intestinal paralysis**, **kidney or liver disease**, **rapid heartbeat**, **hyperthyroidism** (overactive thyroid gland), **high blood pressure**, or **ulcerative colitis**.

Dicyclomine reduces your ability to sweat and may lead to heat exhaustion and heatstroke, which can be life-threatening. Avoid extended heavy exercise and limit your exposure to high temperatures.

Anticholinergenic psychosis has been reported by those taking anticholinergenics, but it usually resolves within 24 hours after discontinuation of the drug.

Possible Side Effects

- ▼ Common: dry mouth, dizziness, blurred vision, nausea, and lightheadedness.
- ▼ Less common: drowsiness, weakness, nervousness, constipation, and decreased sweating.
- ▼ Rare: drug allergy (symptoms include rash, itching, hives, and breathing difficulties), confusion, eye pain, dizziness when rising quickly from a sitting or lying position, a bloated feeling, difficult or painful urination, headache, memory loss, and vomiting. Contact your doctor if you experience anything unusual while taking any medication.

Drug Interactions

- Antacids containing calcium or magnesium, citrates, sodium bicarbonate, and carbonic anhydrase inhibitor drugs may increase dicyclomine's therapeutic effect and side effects.
- Combining dicyclomine with other anticholinergic drugs, including atropine, belladonna, clidinium, glycopyrrolate, hyoscyamine, isopropamide, propantheline, and scopolamine may intensify side effects.
- Dicyclomine may reduce stomach acidity and blood levels of oral ketoconazole (an antifungal).
- Dicyclomine may decrease the therapeutic effects of antiglaucoma medications. Taking dicyclomine with corticosteroids used to treat glaucoma may be hazardous.
- Dicyclomine may counteract the effect of metoclopramide in reducing nausea and vomiting.
- Taking dicyclomine with a narcotic pain reliever may cause severe constipation.

- Taking this or any drug that slows the movement of stomach and intestinal muscles with a potassium chloride supplement—especially one in wax-matrix tablet form—may lead to excessive irritation of the stomach.
- Combining dicyclomine with amantadine, certain drugs to control heart rhythm, antihistamines, nitrates, or nitrites, may increase dicyclomine side effects.
- Dicyclomine may increase the effects of atenolol and digoxin.
- Phenothiazine drugs, monoamine oxidase inhibitor (MAOI) antidepressants, benzodiazepines, and tricyclic antidepressants may increase side effects of dicyclomine. The effectiveness of phenothiazines to control psychotic symptoms may be decreased.

Food Interactions

Take dicyclomine on an empty stomach, ½ hour before or 2 hours after a meal.

Usual Dose

Adult: 80–160 mg a day in 4 divided doses. Seniors should receive the lowest possible dosage and increase only as needed.

Child (age 3 and over): 5–10 mg 3–4 times a day.

Child (age 6 months–2 years): 5–10 mg of syrup 3–4 times a day.

Child (under 6 months): not recommended.

Overdosage

Symptoms include blurred vision; clumsiness; confusion; breathing difficulties; dizziness; drowsiness; dry mouth, nose, or throat; rapid heartbeat; fever; hallucinations; weakness; slurred speech; excitement, restlessness, or irritability; warmth; and dry or flushed skin. Take the victim to a hospital emergency room at once. If you seek treatment, ALWAYS bring the prescription bottle or container.

Special Information

Children taking dicyclomine may be more likely to develop high body temperature in hot weather and other side effects and should be carefully watched for side effects. Dicyclomine should not be given to infants or children unless the doctor decides that its use is absolutely necessary.

Contact your doctor if you develop diarrhea, rash, flushing, eye pain, dry mouth, urinary difficulties, constipation, increased sensitivity to light, or any bothersome or persistent side effect.

Brush and floss your teeth regularly while taking this drug. Because dicyclomine may cause dry mouth, you may be more likely to develop cavities or other dental problems. Ice or hard candy may relieve dry mouth.

Constipation may be treated by using a laxative.

Dicyclomine may make you drowsy or tired and cause blurred vision. Be careful when driving or doing any task that requires concentration.

If you forget a dose, take it as soon as you remember. If it is almost time for your next dose, skip the dose you forgot and continue with your regular schedule. Do not take a double dose.

Special Populations

Pregnancy/Breast-feeding: A few cases of human malformation were linked to dicyclomine, but studies have shown that the drug has no effect on the fetus. Dicyclomine should be used during pregnancy only if your doctor determines that the potential benefit outweighs the risks.

Dicyclomine can reduce the amount of milk produced. Infants given dicyclomine may faint, go limp, and develop breathing problems and seizures. Nursing mothers who must take this drug should use infant formula.

Seniors: Seniors may be more susceptible to side effects, especially memory loss, changes in mental state, and glaucoma. Seniors may obtain maximum benefit with smaller dosages.

Generic Name

Digoxin (dih-JOX-in) G

Brand Names

Lanoxin

Type of Drug

Cardiac glycoside.

Prescribed For

Congestive heart failure (CHF) and other heart conditions involving a very rapid heartbeat.

General Information

Digoxin works directly on heart muscle. It improves the heart's pumping ability or helps to control its beating rhythm. People with heart failure often develop swelling of the lower legs, feet, and ankles; digoxin improves these symptoms by improving blood circulation. Digoxin is generally used as part of the lifelong treatment of CHF.

Cautions and Warnings

Do not take digoxin if you are **allergic** or **sensitive** to any of its ingredients. Digoxin allergies are rare.

Digoxin should not be used in people with **ventricular fibrillation**.

Digoxin should be used with caution in people with **sinus node disease** or **incomplete atrioventricular (AV) block**, as it may cause a worsening of these conditions.

Digoxin has been used to treat **obesity**. The risk of fatal heart rhythms associated with such treatment makes it extremely dangerous as weight-loss medication.

Kidney disease may increase blood levels of digoxin. Your dosage may need adjustment.

Low levels of blood potassium or magnesium can increase digoxin's effects on the heart. For this reason, be sure to eat a balanced diet and include foods rich in potassium and magnesium—bananas, citrus fruits, melons, tomatoes, and green vegetables such as broccoli and spinach. Digoxin should be used with caution in those with pre-existing low blood potassium or magnesium.

Digoxin requirements vary with **thyroid status**. If you are taking digoxin and your thyroid status changes, your doctor will need to alter your digoxin dosage.

Possible Side Effects

Adult and Senior

▼ Common: dizziness, headache, nausea, and diarrhea.

▼ Less common: appetite loss, vomiting, weakness, apathy, drowsiness, blurred or yellow-tinted vision, seeing halos around bright lights, depression, psychoses, confusion or disorientation, restlessness, hallucinations, delirium, seizure, nerve pain, abnormal heart rhythms, and slow pulse.

▼ Rare: Enlargement of the breasts has been reported after long-term use of digoxin. Contact your doctor if you experience anything unusual while taking any medication.

Child

▼ Children are more likely to develop abnormal heart rhythms before they see yellow or green halos or spots and before they develop nausea, vomiting, diarrhea, or stomach pain.

Possible Side Effects *(continued)*

Any abnormal heart rhythms that develop while a child is taking digoxin should be assumed to be a side effect.

Drug Interactions

- Drugs that may increase the effect of digoxin are beta blockers, calcium, calcium channel blockers (such as verapamil), succinylcholine, sympathomimetics, and thiazide and loop diuretics. These combinations increase the risks of cardiac arrhythmias.
- Other drugs that increase blood levels of digoxin include alprazolam, amiodarone, amphotericin B, anticholinergics such as diphenoxylate and propantheline, azole antifungals such as itraconazole and ketoconazole, cyclosporine, dronedarone, epoprostenol, ginseng, macrolide antibiotics (such as clarithromycin, erythromycin, and telithromycin), nefazodone, nonsteroidal anti-inflammatory drugs (NSAIDs) such as ibuprofen and indomethacin, omeprazole, propafenone, protease inhibitors such as ritonavir and saquinavir, quinidine, quinine, rabeprazole, ranolazine, selective serotonin reuptake inhibitor (SSRI) antidepressants (such as fluoxetine, paroxetine, and sertraline), spironolactone, tetracycline, tramadol, and vasopressin receptor antagonists such as conivaptan.
- Drugs that may decrease blood levels of digoxin include acarbose, albuterol, aluminum salts, amiloride, certain anticancer drugs, cholestyramine, colestipol, esomeprazole, lansoprazole, metoclopramide, penecillamine, rifampin, St. John's wort, sucralfate, sulfasalazine, and thyroid hormones such as levothyroxine. Monitoring and dosage adjustments, separation of dosages, or stopping of one or both of the drugs may be necessary.
- Variable effects may be seen when digoxin is combined with hydantoins such as phenytoin or aminoglycosides such as neomycin. Digoxin levels may be increased or decreased and should be monitored for adjustments.
- Digoxin may increase the effects of dofetilide, adding to the risk of dangerous heart rhythm disorders.

Food Interactions

Digoxin can generally be taken without regard to food or meals. Taking your medication after a high-fiber meal reduces the amount of drug absorbed into your blood.

Usual Dose

Adult and Child (age 10 and over): starting dose—known as the digitalizing or loading dose—is about 4–7 mcg per lb. of body weight. Digitalization may also be accomplished with a lower dose over 7 days. Maintenance dose—0.125–0.5 mg once a day; it must be corrected for kidney function. For seniors, a lower dose is required.

Child (under age 10): starting dose—9–27 mcg per lb. of body weight. Maintenance dose—20–35% of the starting dose. Careful measurement of your child's digoxin dose is crucial to safe and effective treatment.

Overdosage

Adult: Symptoms include appetite loss, nausea, vomiting, diarrhea, headache, weakness, apathy, blurred vision, yellow or green spots or halos before the eyes, yellowing of the skin or whites of the eyes, and changes in heartbeat.

Senior: Vomiting, diarrhea, and eye trouble are frequently seen.

Child: An early sign is a change in heart rhythms.

Contact your doctor immediately if any of these symptoms appear. Take the victim to a hospital emergency room. If you seek treatment, ALWAYS bring the prescription bottle or container.

Special Information

Take each day's dose at the same time of day.

Do not stop taking digoxin without your doctor's knowledge.

Avoid over-the-counter diet and cold medications containing stimulants.

Contact your doctor at once if you develop side effects.

There may be some variation between digoxin tablets from different manufacturers. Do not change drug brands without telling your doctor.

Check your pulse every day—your doctor will teach you how—and contact your doctor if it drops below 60 beats per minute.

If you forget a dose and remember at least 12 hours before your next dose, take it right away. If you do not remember until it is less than 12 hours before your next dose, skip the one you forgot and continue with your regular schedule. Do not take a double dose. Contact your doctor if you miss a dose for 2 or more days.

Special Populations

Pregnancy/Breast-feeding: Digoxin crosses into the fetal circulation. Although digoxin is sometimes used during pregnancy to treat fetal heart disease, women who are or might be pregnant should not take digoxin without their doctor's approval. Digoxin should be taken during pregnancy only if your doctor determines that the potential benefit outweighs the risks.

Small amounts of digoxin pass into breast milk. Nursing mothers who must take digoxin should use infant formula.

Seniors: Seniors are more sensitive to digoxin's effects, especially appetite loss. Seniors with impaired renal function may need lower dosages.

Generic Name

Dimenhydrinate (dye-men-HYE-drih-nate) G

Brand Names

Dramamine
Driminate
Trav-Tabs
Triptone

The information in this profile also applies to the following drugs:

Generic Ingredients: Meclizine G
Antivert
Bonine
Meni-D
Ru-Vert-M
TH Motion Relief
UniVert
Vertin-32

Type of Drug

Antihistamine and antiemetic (an agent that prevents or relieves nausea and vomiting).

Prescribed For

Nausea, vomiting, vertigo, and dizziness associated with motion sickness.

General Information

Dimenhydrinate, which depresses middle-ear function, is a mixture of diphenhydramine—an antihistamine believed to be the active ingredient—and another ingredient. Meclizine is an antihistamine. It takes a little longer to start working than dimenhydrinate, but its effects last much longer. Meclizine does a better job of preventing motion sickness than treating its symptoms. It takes 30 minutes to 1 hour to work and lasts for 12–24 hours.

Cautions and Warnings

Do not take these medications if you are **allergic** or **sensitive** to any of their ingredients. Newborn babies should not be given this drug.

People who have difficulty urinating due to an **enlarged prostate gland**, those with **asthma or other breathing difficulties**, and people with **glaucoma** should take these medications with caution.

Because it controls nausea and vomiting, dimenhydrinate may hide the symptoms of appendicitis or overdoses of other drugs.

Possible Side Effects

- ▼ Most common: drowsiness.
- ▼ Less common: confusion; nervousness; excitation; restlessness; headache; sleeplessness, especially in children; tingling; heavy or weak hands; fainting; dizziness; tiredness; rapid heartbeat; low blood pressure; heart palpitations; blurred or double vision; difficult or painful urination; increased sensitivity to the sun; appetite loss; nausea; vomiting; diarrhea; upset stomach; constipation; nightmares; rash; drug reaction (symptoms include rash, itching, hives, and breathing difficulties); ringing or buzzing in the ears; dry mouth, nose, or throat; stuffy nose; wheezing; and increased chest phlegm or chest tightness.

Drug Interactions

- Taking these medications with an alcoholic beverage, other antihistamine, sedative, or other central-nervous-system depressant may cause excessive dizziness, drowsiness, or other signs of depression.
- Combining dimenhydrinate and certain antibiotics that cause dizziness or other ear-related side effects may mask early signs of these side effects, especially in infants and children.

Food Interactions

Take dimenhydrinate with food or milk if it upsets your stomach.

Usual Dose

Dimenhydrinate

Adult and Child (age 12 and over): 50–100 mg 30 minutes prior to travel; then every 4–6 hours; do not take more than 400 mg a day.

Child (age 6–11): 25–50 mg every 6–8 hours; do not take more than 150 mg a day.

Child (age 2–5): 12.5–25 mg every 6–8 hours; do not take more than 75 mg a day.

Child (under age 2): Consult your doctor.

Meclizine

Adult and Child (age 13 and over): 25–50 mg 1 hour before travel; repeat every 24 hours for duration of journey. Up to 100 mg a day in divided doses may be needed to control dizziness from other causes.

Child (under age 13): not recommended.

Overdosage

Symptoms of overdose include drowsiness; clumsiness; unsteadiness; feeling faint; facial flushing; and dry mouth, nose, or throat. Convulsions, coma, and breathing difficulties may also develop. Overdose victims should be taken to a hospital emergency room for treatment. If you seek treatment, ALWAYS bring the prescription bottle or container.

Special Information

For maximum effectiveness against motion sickness, take these medications 1–2 hours before traveling; they may still be effective if taken 30 minutes before traveling.

These drugs may cause drowsiness. Be extremely cautious when driving, operating hazardous machinery, or doing anything that requires concentration.

Dimenhydrinate and meclizine may cause dry mouth, nose, or throat. Sugarless candy, gum, or ice chips can usually relieve these symptoms. Constant dry mouth may increase the likelihood of developing tooth decay or gum disease. Pay special attention to oral hygiene while you are taking these medications, and contact your doctor if dry mouth lasts more than 2 weeks.

If you forget to take a dose of dimenhydrinate or meclizine, take it as soon as you remember. If it is almost time for your next dose, skip the one you forgot and continue with your regular schedule. Do not take a double dose.

Special Populations

Pregnancy/Breast-feeding: Animal studies suggest that meclizine may cause birth defects. Do not take any antihistamine without your doctor's knowledge if you are or might be pregnant—especially during the last 3 months of pregnancy, because newborns may have severe reactions to antihistamines.

Small amounts of dimenhydrinate may pass into breast milk. Dimenhydrinate may also slow milk production. Nursing mothers who must take dimenhydrinate should use infant formula.

Seniors: Seniors are more sensitive to antihistamine side effects and should take the lowest effective dose.

Diovan *see **Angiotensin II Blockers,** page 97*

Generic Name

Diphenhydramine Hydrochloride

(dye-fen-HYE-druh-mene hye-droe-KLOR-ide) G

Brand Names

There are many brand-name diphenhydramine products, most of which are available over the counter. Check with your pharmacist about which specific brands are available alcohol- or sugar-free.

Type of Drug

Antihistamine.

Prescribed For

Stuffy and runny nose, itchy eyes, and scratchy throat caused by seasonal allergy and for other symptoms of allergy such as itching, rash, and hives; insomnia; and Parkinson's disease; also prescribed for motion sickness.

General Information

Antihistamines generally work by blocking the release of histamine (a chemical released by body tissue during an allergic reaction), drying the nose, throat, and eye secretions. Diphenhydramine is the most common active ingredient found in nonprescription sleep aids.

Cautions and Warnings

Do not take this drug if you are **allergic** or **sensitive** to any of its ingredients. It should be avoided or used with extreme care if you have **narrow-angle glaucoma**, **stomach ulcer**, **intestinal**

obstruction, **other stomach problems**, **difficulty urinating**, or **enlarged prostate**. It should not be used by people who have **sleep apnea** or **deep-breathing problems** such as **asthma**. Use with care if you have a history of **thyroid disease**, **heart disease**, **emphysema**, **chronic bronchitis**, or **high blood pressure**.

Possible Side Effects

▼ Common: drowsiness and weakness.

▼ Less common: itching; rash; sensitivity to bright light; perspiration; fever; chills; lowering of blood pressure; headache; rapid heartbeat; sleeplessness; dizziness; disturbed coordination; confusion; restlessness; nervousness; irritability; euphoria (feeling "high"); tingling and weakness of the hands or feet; blurred or double vision; ringing in the ears; upset stomach; appetite loss; nausea; vomiting; constipation; diarrhea; urinary difficulties; thickening of lung secretions; tightness of the chest; wheezing; nasal stuffiness; and dry mouth, nose, or throat.

Drug Interactions

- This drug should not be taken with a monoamine oxidase inhibitor (MAOI) antidepressant.
- The effects of sedatives, sleeping medications, and other central-nervous-system depressants will be intensified when combined with diphenhydramine hydrochloride; it is extremely important that doses of these drugs are properly adjusted.
- This drug increases the intoxicating and sedating effects of alcohol.

Food Interactions

Take this drug with food if it upsets your stomach.

Usual Dose

Allergy

Adult: 25–50 mg 3–4 times a day.

Child (over 20 lbs.): 12.5–25 mg 3–4 times a day.

Cough Syrup

Adult and Child (age 12 and over): 25 mg every 4 hours; do not take more than 150 mg in 24 hours.

Child (age 6–11): 12.5 mg every 4 hours; do not take more than 75 mg in 24 hours.

Child (age 2–5): 6.25 mg every 4 hours; do not take more than 25 mg in 24 hours.

Nighttime Sedation

Adult and Child (age 12 and over): 25–50 mg at bedtime.

Thin Strips

TheraFlu

Adult and Child (age 12 and over): 1 strip every 4 hours; do not take more than 6 strips in 24 hours.

Triaminic

Child (age 6–11): 1 strip every 4 hours; do not take more than 6 strips in 24 hours.

Overdosage

Symptoms of overdose include depression or stimulation, especially in children; dry mouth; fixed or dilated pupils; flushing; and upset stomach. Overdose victims should be made to vomit with ipecac syrup, which is available at any pharmacy. Take the overdose victim to a hospital emergency room immediately if you cannot induce vomiting. If you seek treatment, ALWAYS bring the prescription bottle or container.

Special Information

This drug may cause drowsiness. Be extremely cautious when driving or operating hazardous equipment.

If you are taking this medication for motion sickness, take the first dose at least 30 minutes prior to exposure.

If you forget to take a dose of diphenhydramine, take it as soon as you remember. If it is almost time for your next dose, skip the one you forgot and continue with your regular schedule. Do not take a double dose.

Special Populations

Pregnancy/Breast-feeding: Animal studies have shown that some antihistamines may cause birth defects. Do not take any antihistamine without your doctor's knowledge if you are or might be pregnant—especially during the last 3 months of pregnancy—because newborns may have severe reactions to antihistamines.

Small amounts of antihistamine pass into breast milk. Nursing mothers who must take this drug should use infant formula.

Seniors: Seniors are more sensitive to antihistamine side effects and may require lower dosages.

Type of Drug

Direct-Acting Anticoagulants

Brand Names

Generic Ingredients: Apixaban
Eliquis

Generic Ingredients: Dabigatran
Pradaxa

Generic Ingredients: Rivaroxaban
Xarelto

Prescribed For

Stroke or blood clot and pulmonary embolism prevention.

General Information

These drugs are the first of an important new class of medications used to thin the blood as an alternative to warfarin, previously the gold standard of anticoagulants. They are seen by many as a replacement for warfarin because they are safer and do not require regular blood testing. Blood clotting is a complicated process and these drugs work at different points in this process. Dabigatran directly inhibits the clotting factor thrombin. Apixaban and rivaroxaban inhibit factor Xa. Dabigatran is approved to reduce stroke risk and blood clots in people with the abnormal heart rhythm atrial fibrillation. Rivaroxaban is approved for people undergoing knee or hip replacement surgery to prevent the formation of a blood clot in a deep vein that can lead to a dangerous blood clot in the lung. As time passes, more studies will be completed and additional approved uses will be added.

Cautions and Warnings

Do not use these drugs if you are **allergic** or **sensitive** to any of their ingredients.

These drugs carry a risk of bleeding that can be serious and, rarely, fatal.

Most of each dose of these drugs passes out of the body through the kidneys. Dosage must be reduced in those with moderate **kidney disease** and should not be used by people with severe kidney disease. Dose reduction is not necessary in mild kidney disease. Apixaban and rivaroxaban should be avoided in those with moderate to severe **liver disease**. It may be used in people with mild liver disease unless the condition is associated with abnormal blood clotting.

Do not take these medicines if you have an active major **bleeding problem**, as it will make it harder to manage the bleeding. They can also cause serious and possibly fatal bleeding. Clinical studies with these drugs have revealed a small risk of severe and possible deadly bleeding episodes in people taking them.

These medicines may need to be stopped to prevent a stroke due to excessive blood thinning.

Your doctor may not use one of these drugs if you have a history of **spinal or epidural punctures** due to the risk of pools of blood forming in the central nervous system.

Healthy Japanese people taking rivaroxaban have about 50% more medication in their blood than adults of other ethnic groups. Women taking apixaban tend to have higher levels of the drug in their blood than men.

Possible Side Effects

Apixaban

- ▼ Most common: anemia, bleeding, confusion, and nausea.
- ▼ Rare: major or life-threatening bleeding. Contact your doctor if you experience anything unusual while taking any medication.

Dabigatran

- ▼ Most common: upset stomach, gastroesophageal reflux disease, throat irritation, stomach bleeding, gastrointestinal ulcer, and generalized bleeding.
- ▼ Common: difficulty breathing, dizziness, swelling in the arms or legs, fatigue, cough, joint pains, back pain, common cold symptoms, diarrhea, and abnormal heart rhythms.
- ▼ Less common: urinary infections and upper-respiratory infections.
- ▼ Rare: major or life-threatening bleeding. Drug-sensitivity reactions are very rare. Contact your doctor if you experience anything unusual while taking any medication.

Rivaroxaban

- ▼ Common: bleeding in hip replacement patients.
- ▼ Less common: urinary infections and upper-respiratory infections.

Possible Side Effects *(continued)*

▼ Rare: major or life-threatening bleeding. Drug-sensitivity reactions are very rare. Contact your doctor if you experience anything unusual while taking any medication.

Drug Interactions

- Avoid mixing these drugs with another blood-thinning anticoagulant or antiplatelet drug such as clopidogrel; prasugrel; ticagrelor; nonsteroidal anti-inflammatory drugs (NSAIDs), including the regular use of aspirin; and high doses of fish oil, as they will increase the risk of bleeding.
- Do not mix rifampin or St. John's wort with these drugs because they speed their breakdown, making them less effective. Phenytoin and rifampin also speed the breakdown of rivaroxaban. If absolutely needed, your dose of rivaroxaban may be raised to 20 mg a day.
- Amiodarone, calcium channel blockers, clarithromycin, cyclosporine, erythromycin, indinavir, itraconazole, ketoconazole, quinidine, saquinavir, sirolimus, and tacrolimus slow the breakdown of apixaban and dabigatran. Caution is recommended.
- Amiodarone, cyclosporine, indinavir, itraconazole, ketoconazole, quinidine, saquinavir, sirolimus, and tacrolimus should not be mixed with rivaroxaban because they significantly increase the risk of serious bleeding. No precaution is needed if you mix clarithromycin with rivaroxaban.
- People with reduced kidney function taking rivaroxaban should not take azithromycin, calcium channel blockers, dronedarone, erythromycin, quinidine, or ranolazine because of the increased risk of bleeding. This caution does not apply if your kidney function is normal.

Food Interactions

These drugs can be taken without regard to food or meals in their normal doses. If your dose of rivaroxaban is increased above 10 mg per day, take it with food.

Usual Dose

Apixaban

Adult: 2.5–5 mg twice a day.
Child: not recommended.

Dabigatran

Adult: 150 mg twice a day. Moderate kidney disease and people taking dronedarone or ketoconazole: 75 mg twice a day.

Child: not recommended.

Rivaroxaban

Clot Prevention with Atrial Fibrillation

Adult: 20 mg once a day with your evening meal. Moderate kidney disease: 15 mg once a day. Severe kidney disease: Do not use.

Child: not recommended.

Deep Vein Thrombosis

Adult: 10 mg once a day with or without food for 12 days after knee replacement and 35 days after hip replacement. The first dose is taken 6–10 hours after surgery. Dosage is reduced in moderate kidney disease; do not use if you have severe kidney disease. Dose modification is not required for people under 100 or over 240 lbs.

Child: not recommended.

Overdosage

Overdose with these drugs can lead to bleeding. There is no antidote for them, as there is for warfarin. Overdose victims must be taken to an emergency room as soon as possible. If you seek treatment, ALWAYS bring the prescription bottle or container.

Special Information

Take these medicines exactly as directed by your doctor, especially if you are switching from warfarin or another anticoagulant to dabigatran.

If you forget a dose of your medicine, take it if you remember within 6 hours of the scheduled time. Otherwise, skip the forgotten dose and continue with your regular schedule. Do not take a double dose. If you forget a dose of rivaroxaban, take it as soon as you remember and then continue with your regular schedule. Do not take a double dose of rivaroxaban.

Contact your doctor if you develop unusual bruises, pink or dark stools, abdominal pain, indigestion, appetite loss, nausea, coughing, or vomiting, especially of blood or coffee-ground-like material.

Other important reasons to contact your doctor include pain or swelling in a joint, headache, dizziness or weakness, gum bleeding, extended time to heal from a minor cut or bruise, and heavier than normal periodic bleeding.

Do not chew or open dabigatran capsules.

Dabigatran capsules lose their strength very quickly when exposed to moisture. For this reason, your pharmacist will provide them in the original bottle, not in a pharmacy vial. They must stay in the manufacturer's original bottle until you take them. Moving the capsules to another container increases the chances of taking a sub-potent product. They must be used within 60 days of opening the bottle.

Regular blood monitoring is *not* required as it is with warfarin. The anticoagulant effect is best checked with the ECT (ecarin clotting time) test. The activated partial thromboplastin time (APTT), the standard for warfarin, is a less accurate measure of dabigatran's anticoagulant effect.

Special Populations

Pregnancy/Breast-feeding: These drugs are not recommended for pregnant women. They should be taken during pregnancy only if your doctor determines that the potential benefit outweighs the risks. Other anticoagulants are preferred because these drugs cannot be monitored with standard lab tests and their effects cannot be easily reversed by other medicines.

It is not known if these drugs pass into breast milk. Nursing mothers who must take one of these medicines should use infant formula because of possible bleeding in the nursing infant.

Seniors: Seniors taking apixaban tend to have 30% more drug in their blood due to normal declines in kidney function that accompany age.

Dabigatran was studied mainly in people over age 65. Stroke risk and bleeding is increased in older patients taking dabigatran. However, it still offers substantial benefits.

Rivaroxaban studies included a majority of people age 65 and over. Bleeding risk may be greater due to normal age-related losses of kidney function.

Generic Name

Disopyramide (die-soe-PIE-rah-mide) G

Brand Names

Norpace Norpace CR

Type of Drug

Antiarrhythmic.

Prescribed For

Abnormal heart rhythms.

General Information

Disopyramide slows the rate at which nerve impulses are carried through heart muscle, reducing the response of heart muscle to those impulses. It acts on the heart similarly to the more widely used antiarrhythmic medication quinidine sulfate. Disopyramide is often prescribed for people who do not respond to other antiarrhythmic drugs, but should only be used in cases that are life-threatening.

Cautions and Warnings

Do not take disopyramide if you are **allergic** or **sensitive** to any of its ingredients or if you have **heart block**, unless you have a cardiac pacemaker.

This drug can worsen **heart failure** or trigger severely low blood pressure. It should be used in combination with another antiarrhythmic agent or beta blocker with caution.

In rare instances, disopyramide has caused a reduction in blood-sugar levels. Therefore, the drug should be used with caution by **diabetics**, **older adults**—who are more susceptible to this effect—and people with **poor kidney or liver function**. Ask your doctor if you should have your blood-sugar levels checked while taking this drug.

Because of its anticholinergic effects, men with a severe **prostate condition** and people who have **glaucoma**, **myasthenia gravis** (a neuromuscular disease), or severe **difficulty urinating** should use disopyramide with caution.

People with **liver or kidney disease** must take a reduced dose of disopyramide.

Potassium levels affect the action of disopyramide. People with **abnormal blood-potassium levels** must correct this imbalance before starting disopyramide.

Possible Side Effects

- ▼ Most common: dry mouth, urinary difficulty, and constipation.
- ▼ Common: blurred vision; dry eyes, nose, and throat; frequent urination; nausea; stomach pain or bloating; gas; dizziness; fatigue; headache; and nervousness.
- ▼ Less common: itching, rashes, muscle weakness, generalized aches and pains, not feeling well, low blood-potassium

Possible Side Effects *(continued)*

levels, increases in blood-cholesterol and triglyceride levels, heart failure, and low blood pressure.

▼ Rare: Rare side effects can occur in almost any part of the body. Contact your doctor if you experience anything unusual while taking any medication.

Drug Interactions

- Phenytoin and rifampin may increase the rate at which the body removes disopyramide from the blood. Your disopyramide dose may need alteration if this combination is used. Other drugs known to increase drug breakdown by the liver, such as barbiturates and primidone, may also have this effect.
- Other antiarrhythmic drugs, such as quinidine, may increase the effect of disopyramide, making dosage reduction necessary. At the same time, disopyramide may reduce the effectiveness of quinidine.
- When disopyramide is combined with a beta-blocker drug, increased disopyramide effects, additive effects, or depression of heart function may result.
- Azole antifungals, clarithromycin, diclofenac, doxycycline, erythromycin, imatinib, isoniazid, nefazodone, nicardipine, propofol, protease inhibitors, telithromycin, and verapamil may increase the amount of disopyramide in your blood, causing abnormal heart rhythms or other cardiac effects.
- Disopyramide may reduce the effectiveness of oral anticoagulant (blood thinning) drugs. Your doctor should check your anticoagulant dosage to be sure you are getting the right amount.
- Hydantoins may cause a decrease in the effectiveness of disopyramide.
- Disopyramide may increase the amount of digoxin in your blood, though the amount of the increase is not likely to affect your heart.
- St. John's wort may decrease disopyramide levels.

Food Interactions

Disopyramide should be taken on an empty stomach at least 1 hour before or 2 hours after meals.

Usual Dose

Adult: 400–800 mg a day (divided into 2 or 4 doses for the immediate-release form). In severe cases, 400 mg every 6 hours may be required. This level of dosage should be monitored in the hospital. The sustained-release preparation is taken every 12 hours. People with reduced kidney function should receive a lower dosage, depending on the degree of kidney function present. People with liver failure should take 400 mg a day.

Child (age 13–17): 2.5–7 mg a day per lb. of body weight.

Child (age 5–12): 4.5–7 mg a day per lb. of body weight.

Child (age 1–4): 4.5–9 mg a day per lb. of body weight.

Child (under age 1): 4.5–13.5 mg a day per lb. of body weight.

Overdosage

Overdose symptoms are breathing difficulties, abnormal heart rhythms, and unconsciousness. In severe cases, overdosage can lead to death. Overdose victims should be made to vomit with ipecac syrup—available at any pharmacy—to remove any remaining drug from the stomach. Contact your doctor or poison control center before doing this. If you seek treatment, ALWAYS bring the prescription bottle or container. Prompt and vigorous treatment can mean the difference between life and death in severe overdosage.

Special Information

Disopyramide may cause symptoms of low blood sugar: anxiety, chills, cold sweats, drowsiness, excessive hunger, nausea, nervousness, rapid pulse, shakiness, unusual weakness, tiredness, or cool, pale skin. If this happens to you, eat some chocolate, candy, or other high-sugar food and contact your doctor at once.

Disopyramide can cause dry mouth, urinary difficulty, constipation, or blurred vision. Contact your doctor if these symptoms become severe or intolerable, but do not stop taking the medication without your doctor's approval.

If disopyramide is required for a child and capsules are not appropriate, your pharmacist can make a liquid product. Do not do this at home: This medication requires special preparation. The liquid should be refrigerated and protected from light and should be thrown away after 30 days.

Do not crush, chew, or open sustained-release capsules.

If you forget to take a dose of disopyramide, take it as soon as possible. However, if it is within 4 hours of your next dose, skip the dose you forgot and go back to your regular schedule. Do not take a double dose.

Special Populations

Pregnancy/Breast-feeding: Do not take this drug if you are pregnant or planning to become pregnant while using it, because it will pass into the fetus and may affect its development. Disopyramide should be taken during pregnancy only if your doctor determines that the potential benefit outweighs the risks.

Disopyramide passes into breast milk. Nursing mothers who must take this drug should use infant formula.

Seniors: Seniors, especially those with liver or kidney disease, are more sensitive to the effects of this drug.

Generic Name

Dofetilide (DOH-fet-a-lyed)

Brand Names

Tikosyn

Type of Drug

Antiarrhythmic.

Prescribed For

Specific abnormal heart rhythms.

General Information

Dofetilide is used to establish and maintain normal sinus rhythm in the heart. Dofetilide is available only to hospitals and doctors who receive specific training and education on how to use this drug because of the risks associated with using it.

Cautions and Warnings

Do not take dofetilide if you are **allergic** or **sensitive** to any of its ingredients.

Dofetilide is reserved for people whose abnormal heart rhythms have not responded to other drugs. People taking dofetilide must be in a hospital or other facility for at least 3 days where appropriate blood tests can be performed to monitor kidney and heart function.

This drug is cleared through the kidneys. **Poor kidney function** increases the amount of dofetilide in the body. Liver disease has no effect on dofetilide blood levels.

Dofetilide, like other antiarrhythmic drugs, can cause severe and sometimes fatal abnormal rhythms of its own.

If you have **low blood levels of potassium or magnesium**, do not take dofetilide without first alerting your doctor of this condition.

Women may be at a greater risk for some arrhythmias caused by dofetilide.

Possible Side Effects

Serious heart arrhythmias can develop in up to 3.5% of patients taking up to 1000 mcg a day of dofetilide. People taking daily doses above 1000 mcg a day are at up to 5 times greater risk for arrhythmias.

- ▼ Most common: headache, chest pain, and respiratory infection.
- ▼ Common: difficulty breathing, nausea, and dizziness.
- ▼ Less common: flu; sleeplessness; accidental injury; back pain; diarrhea; abdominal pain; angina; anxiety; joint pain; weakness; atrial and ventricular arrhythmia; high blood pressure; pain; heart palpitations; swollen legs, ankles, or arms; sweating; and urinary infections.
- ▼ Rare: some arrhythmias, heart attack, hives, slow heartbeat, stroke, facial or other paralysis, tingling in the hands or feet, cough, liver damage, migraine, fainting, and sudden death. Contact your doctor if you experience anything unusual while taking any medication.

Drug Interactions

Dofetilide should not be given with drugs that are known to interact with it. Dofetilide must be stopped at least 2 days before any potentially interacting drug is taken.

- Do not mix dofetilide with any product containing verapamil (a calcium channel blocker) or trimethoprim (used for urinary infections). These combinations can substantially raise the amount of dofetilide in the blood.
- Some drugs may increase the amount of dofetilide in the blood by inhibiting enzymes that break it down in the liver. These include amiodarone, cannabis, cimetidine, ciprofloxacin, clarithromycin, delavirdine, diltiazem, erythromycin, fluconazole, fluvoxamine, indinavir, itraconazole, ketoconazole, mifepristone, nefazodone, norfloxacin, mibefradil, ritonavir, saquinavir, selective serotonin reuptake inhibitors (SSRIs), and zafirlukast.

- Some drugs may reduce the amount of dofetilide in the blood by stimulating enzymes that break it down in the liver, including carbamazepine, corticosteroids, efavirenz, modafanil, nevirapine, phenobarbital and other barbiturates, phenytoin, pioglitazone, and rifampin. Amiloride, megestrol, metformin, and triamterene can interfere with the elimination of dofetilide via the kidney, raising blood levels of the drug.
- Other drugs that can increase the effects of dofetilide are other antiarrhythmic drugs, bepridil, phenothiazines, and tricyclic antidepressants.
- Mixing dofetilide with digoxin may lead to a ventricular arrhythmia called torsade de pointes. Thiazides, furosemide, and other potassium-depleting diuretics can also increase the risk of this arrhythmia.

Food Interactions

Grapefruit juice may increase dofetilide blood levels.

Usual Dose

Adult: 125–500 mcg twice a day.
Child: not recommended.

Overdosage

Dofetilide overdose is likely to cause significant heart rhythm problems. Overdose victims must be treated symptomatically by their cardiologist.

Special Information

Read all information supplied to you before you begin taking this medication and read it again if anything in your treatment program changes.

Tell your doctor about any changes in your prescription or nonprescription drug use or in your use of vitamins, minerals, and other dietary supplement products.

Be sure that any other doctor or hospital that treats you and might prescribe another drug knows you are taking dofetilide.

Contact your doctor at once if you develop any signs of altered electrolyte balance, including excessive or prolonged diarrhea, sweating, vomiting, appetite changes, or excessive thirst.

If you forget to take a dose, take it as soon as you remember. If it is almost time for your next dose, skip the dose you forgot and continue with your regular schedule. Do not take a double dose.

Special Populations

Pregnancy/Breast-feeding: Dofetilide causes birth defects in animal studies. Dofetilide should be taken during pregnancy only if your doctor determines that the potential benefit outweighs the risks.

It is unknown whether dofetilide passes into breast milk. Nursing mothers who take it should use infant formula.

Seniors: Older adults may take this drug without special precaution.

Brand Names

Donnatal

Generic Ingredients

Atropine Sulfate + Hyoscyamine Sulfate + Phenobarbital + Scopolamine Hydrobromide G

Other Brand Names

Antispas
Antispasmodic
Barbidonna
Bellatal
Donnapine
Donnatal Extentabs
Hyosophen
Spasmolin

The information in this profile also applies to the following drugs:

Generic Ingredients: Hyoscyamine Sulfate G

Anaspaz
Colidrops
Cytospaz
Ed-Spaz
HyoMax DT
HyoMax FT
HyoMax SL
HyoMax SR
Hyosyne
IB-Stat
Levbid
Levsin
Levsinex Timecaps
NuLev
Oscimin
Spasdel
Symax

Generic Ingredients: Propantheline G

Type of Drug

Anticholinergic combination.

Prescribed For

Stomach spasm and gastrointestinal cramps.

General Information

Donnatal is a mild antispasmodic sedative. Its principal action is to counteract the effect of acetylcholine, an important neurohormone. Donnatal is used only to relieve symptoms, not to treat the underlying condition, and there is considerable doubt among medical experts that this drug lives up to its claims. In addition to the brand names listed above, there are about 50 other anticholinergic combinations with similar properties. All are used to relieve cramps and all are about equally effective. Some have additional ingredients to reduce or absorb excess gas in the stomach, to coat the stomach, or to control diarrhea. Donnatal and products like it should not be used for more than the temporary relief of symptoms.

Cautions and Warnings

Do not take Donnatal if you are **allergic** or **sensitive** to any of its ingredients.

Donnatal should not be used by people with **glaucoma**, **urinary difficulties**, **acute bleeding** with unstable heart function, **severe ulcerative colitis**, **obstruction or inflammation of the gastrointestinal tract**, **myasthenia gravis**, **acute intermittent porphyria** (a rare blood disorder), or **hiatal hernia**. Donnatal should be used with caution or not at all by people with **diarrhea** who have had a portion of their **lower gastrointestinal tract removed**. The diarrhea may be a sign of partial intestinal obstruction.

Phenobarbital may be habit-forming and should not be administered to people with a history of **drug dependence**.

Donnatal should be used with caution in **children** and in people with **brain damage**, **heart disease**, **high blood pressure**, **hyperthyroidism** (overactive thyroid gland), **kidney or liver disease**, **autonomic neuropathy**, or **gastric ulcer**.

Donnatal can reduce your ability to sweat and may lead to heat exhaustion. Avoid extended heavy exercise and limit your exposure to high temperatures.

Possible Side Effects

- ▼ Most common: blurred vision, dry mouth, urinary difficulties, flushing, and dry skin.
- ▼ Less common: rapid or unusual heartbeat, increased sensitivity to bright light, loss of the sense of taste, headache, nervousness, tiredness, weakness, dizziness, sleeplessness,

Possible Side Effects *(continued)*

nausea, vomiting, fever, stuffy nose, heartburn, loss of sex drive, decreased sweating, constipation, feeling bloated, and allergic reactions such as fever and rash.

Drug Interactions

- Although Donnatal contains only a small amount of phenobarbital, it is wise to avoid alcohol or other sedative drugs.
- Some phenothiazine drugs, sedatives, tricyclic antidepressants, antihistamines, and narcotics may increase the side effects of the atropine sulfate ingredient in these drugs, causing dry mouth, urinary difficulties, and constipation. The effectiveness of phenothiazines to control psychotic symptoms may be decreased. These interactions are possible with hyoscyamine and propantheline also.
- Donnatal may counteract the effects of anticoagulant (blood thinning) medications.
- Mixing Donnatal with haloperidol may lead to a worsening of symptoms of schizophrenia.
- Antacids may decrease hyoscyamine effectiveness; do not take antacids within 1 hour of taking hyoscyamine.

Food Interactions

Take Donnatal 30–60 minutes before meals.

Usual Dose

Donnatal

Adult: 1–2 tablets or capsules or 5–10 mL of elixir 3–4 times a day, or 1 extended-release tablet every 12 hours.

Child: 0.5–5 mL of elixir (as determined by body weight) every 4–6 hours.

Hyoscyamine

Adult and Child (age 12 and over): tablets: 1–2 tablets every 4 hours or as needed, not to exceed 12 a day. Extended-release tablets or capsules: 1–2 tablets or capsules every 12 hours, not to exceed 4 a day. Elixir: 1–2 tsp. of elixir every 4 hours or as needed, not to exceed 12 tsp. a day. Oral solution or spray: 1–2 mL or sprays every 4 hours or as needed, not to exceed 12 mL or sprays a day.

Child (age 2–11): tablets: ½–1 tablet every 4 hours or as needed, not to exceed 6 tablets a day. Oral solution: 0.25–1 mL every 4 hours or as needed, not to exceed 6 mL a day.

Child (under age 2): 4–8 drops of oral solution determined by body weight every 4 hours or as needed.

Propantheline

Adult: 15 mg 3 times a day before meals, and 30 mg at bedtime.

Senior: 7.5 mg 3 times a day.

Overdosage

Symptoms of overdose include dry mouth; difficulty swallowing; thirst; blurred vision; sensitivity to bright light; flushed, hot, or dry skin; rash; fever; abnormal heart rate; high blood pressure; urinary difficulties; restlessness; confusion; delirium; and breathing difficulties. The victim should be taken to a hospital emergency room immediately. If you seek treatment, ALWAYS bring the prescription bottle or container.

Special Information

Contact your doctor if you experience persistent diarrhea, bloating, fever, heart palpitations, rash, flushing, or eye pain.

Do not crush or chew Donnatal tablets.

Dry mouth usually can be relieved by chewing gum or sucking hard candy or ice chips. Constipation can be treated with a stool-softening laxative.

Donnatal may reduce the amount of saliva in your mouth, making it easier for bacteria to grow there. Pay special attention to dental hygiene while taking this medication to prevent cavities and gum disease.

Donnatal may cause drowsiness and blurred vision. Be careful when driving or operating hazardous equipment.

If you forget to take a dose of Donnatal, take it as soon as you remember. If it is almost time for your next dose, skip the one you forgot and continue with your regular schedule. Do not take a double dose.

Special Populations

Pregnancy/Breast-feeding: Donnatal may cause drug dependency or breathing problems in newborns and may interfere with labor and delivery. Donnatal should be taken during pregnancy only if your doctor determines that the potential benefit outweighs the risks.

Donnatal may pass into breast milk and may reduce the amount of milk produced. It may cause tiredness, shortness of breath, and a slower-than-normal heartbeat in infants. Nursing mothers who must take this medication should use infant formula.

Seniors: Seniors are often more sensitive to the side effects of Donnatal, such as excitement, confusion, drowsiness, agitation, constipation, dry mouth, and urinary difficulties. Memory may be impaired and glaucoma worsened.

Generic Name

Doxercalciferol (dox-er-kal-SIH-fer-ahl) G

Brand Names

Hectorol Capsules

The information in this profile also applies to the following drugs:

Generic Ingredients: Ergocalciferol
Drisdol Liquid

Generic Ingredients: Paricalcitol
Zemplar

Type of Drug

Vitamin D analog.

Prescribed For

Elevated parathyroid hormone levels in patients undergoing kidney dialysis.

General Information

Doxercalciferol is a synthetic form of vitamin D that is processed in the body to form calcitriol, the active form of vitamin D. Paricalcitol is synthetic calcitriol that supplements the production of calcitriol in kidney failure. Vitamin D and parathyroid hormone are key elements of the calcium-regulating system in the body. Normally, your body releases parathyroid hormone if blood-calcium levels are too low. Parathyroid hormones move calcium from the place where it is found in greatest quantity—your bones—into the bloodstream. This can have disastrous effects for a wide variety of body functions in which calcium is crucial, including muscle contraction, nervous system function, bone density, and blood clotting. Doxercalciferol helps to stabilize the system and normalize parathyroid hormone levels that can be artificially elevated in dialysis patients.

Cautions and Warnings

Do not take these medications if you are **allergic** or **sensitive** to any of their ingredients.

Do not take any other vitamin D supplement while taking this drug.

People with a tendency toward **high blood levels of calcium or vitamin D** should not take doxercalciferol. Symptoms of high calcium can include tiredness, confusion, appetite loss, nausea, vomiting, constipation, thirst, increased urination, and weight loss. High blood calcium also increases the risk of abnormal heart rhythms.

Before taking this medication, tell your doctor if you have **liver disease**. You may not be able to take doxercalciferol, or you may require a dosage adjustment or special monitoring during treatment. Paricalcitol dosage does not need to be adjusted for mild or moderate liver disease. Dose modification may be needed if you have severe liver disease.

Dialysis patients experience increases in blood calcium and phosphate while taking this drug.

Possible Side Effects

Doxercalciferol

▼ Common: swelling, headache, general discomfort, nausea, vomiting, dizziness, difficulty breathing, and itching.

▼ Less common: loss of appetite, indigestion, weight gain, joint pain, constipation, sleepiness, and slowed heart rate.

Paricalcitol

The risk of drug side effects increases as you take more paricalcitol, particularly diarrhea.

▼ Common: diarrhea, nausea, arm or leg swelling, drug-sensitivity reactions, high blood pressure, virus, infections, and common cold symptoms.

▼ Less common: dizziness, fainting, headache, depression, vomiting, abdominal discomfort, constipation, chest pain, pain, fungal infections, sinusitis, stomach irritation, urinary infection, dehydration, arthritis, back pain, muscle spasm, cough, mouth or throat pain, low blood pressure, itching, skin sores, low blood sugar, and sleeplessness.

Possible Side Effects *(continued)*

▼ Rare: Other side effects such as dry mouth, taste changes, and hives can occur. Contact your doctor if you experience anything unusual while taking any medication.

Drug Interactions

- Do not take antacids that contain magnesium while you are taking doxercalciferol.
- Cholestyramine and other bile acid sequestrants may reduce the absorption of these medications.
- Prolonged use of mineral oil may reduce the absorption of these drugs.
- Do not combine any other over-the-counter or prescription medicines or vitamin supplements with doxercalciferol without first talking with your doctor.
- The following medicines can slow the transformation of doxercalciferol to its active form in the body, reducing its effectiveness: amiodarone, aprepitant, chloramphenicol, cimetidine, ciprofloxacin, clarithromycin, delavirdine, diltiazem, erythromycin, fluconazole, fluvoxamine, gestodene, indinavir, itraconazole, ketoconazole, mibefradil, mifepristone, nefazodone, nelfinavir, norfloxacin, ritonavir, and verapamil.
- The following drugs can increase the breakdown of doxercalciferol in the liver, possibly reducing its effectiveness: barbiturates, carbamazepine, efavirenz, glucocorticoids, modafinil, nevirapine, oxcarbazepine, phenobarbital, phenytoin, pioglitazone, rifabutin, rifampin, and St. John's wort. Dosage adjustment may be needed.
- Ketoconazole increases the amount of time that paricalcitol stays in the body, possibly increasing its effects. Other drugs that may have the same effect include: atazanavir, clarithromycin, indinavir, itraconazole, nefazodone, nelfinavir, ritonavir, saquinavir, telithromycin, and voriconazole.
- Paricalcitol should be combined cautiously with digoxin.

Food Interactions

Avoid grapefruit products as they can slow the transformation of doxercalciferol to its active form in the body, reducing its effectiveness. Paricalcitol can be taken without regard to food or meals.

It is important to get the right amount of calcium and vitamin D from your food. Follow the dietary plan given by your doctor.

Usual Dose

Doxercalciferol

Adult: starting dose—10 mcg 3 times a week during kidney dialysis treatment. Dosage may be adjusted to 2.5 mcg at 8-week intervals if necessary.

Paricalcitol

Adult: 1–4 mcg taken once a day or 3 times a week depending on your blood-calcium levels.

Overdosage

Symptoms include weakness, headache, drowsiness, nausea, vomiting, dry mouth, metallic taste in the mouth, constipation, muscle pain, bone pain, and irregular heartbeat. The overdose victim should be taken to a hospital emergency room. If you seek treatment, ALWAYS bring the prescription bottle or container.

Special Information

Compliance with dosage instruction, diet, and calcium supplementation is important while taking these medications.

Lab tests are required to monitor therapy while taking doxercalciferol and paricalcitol.

These medications may cause dizziness. Use caution while driving or performing other tasks requiring alertness, coordination, or physical dexterity.

If you take one of these medicines every other day and forget your dose, take it as soon as you remember if it is on the same day. If you do not remember until the next day, take the forgotten dose but you must then skip a day before your next dose.

If you take paricalcitol every day and forget a dose, take it as soon as you remember. If you do not remember until your next scheduled dose, skip the one you forgot and continue with your regular schedule.

Special Populations

Pregnancy/Breast-feeding: The safety of using doxercalciferol or paricalcitol during pregnancy is not known. These medications should be taken during pregnancy only if your doctor determines that the potential benefit outweighs the risks.

It is not known if doxercalciferol passes into breast milk. Paricalcitol passes into breast milk. Nursing mothers who must use these drugs should use infant formula.

Seniors: Seniors may be more sensitive to drug side effects.

Type of Drug

DPP-4 Inhibitors

Brand Names

Generic Ingredients: Linagliptin
Tradjenta

Generic Ingredients: Saxagliptin
Onglyza

Generic Ingredients: Sitagliptin
Januvia

Combination Products
Generic Ingredients: Saxagliptin + Metformin Hydrochloride Extended Release
Kombiglyze XR

Generic Ingredients: Sitagliptin + Metformin Hydrochloride
Janumet Janumet XR

Generic Ingredients: Sitagliptin + Simvastatin
Juvisync

Prescribed For

Type 2 diabetes.

General Information

DPP-4 inhibitors prevent the breakdown of the incretin hormone glucagon-like peptide 1 (GLP-1) by interfering with the enzyme dipeptidyl peptidase 4 (DPP-4). GLP-1, which plays a role in the body's blood-sugar management system, is released in the intestine after a meal and helps increase the secretion of insulin and also helps prevent the release of the hormone glucagon from the pancreas. Glucagon helps the liver maintain enough sugar in the blood to meet the body's needs between meals. By stopping the breakdown of GLP-1, DPP-4 inhibitors have clinical effects that are similar to, but less potent than, the injectable incretin mimetic drugs, which directly stimulate GLP-1 receptors in the pancreas to increase insulin and decrease glucagon production.

These drugs have been studied alone and in combination with metformin, glitazones, sulfonylureas, and insulin, and may be used with these antidiabetic medicines to achieve better control of blood sugar. Saxagliptin and sitagliptin are eliminated primarily through the kidneys, although about ¼ of saxagliptin is broken down in the liver, and linagliptin leaves the body in feces through the biliary system. These drugs do not affect blood sugar in non-diabetic people. Sitagliptin increases the number of beta cells (that produce insulin) in animals and may have the same effect in humans. This could help reduce the need for other medicines and improve diabetes control.

Individual antidiabetes drugs and therapies have not been proven to reduce your chance of developing heart disease or stroke. However, in some studies, good blood-glucose control has been associated with a better chance of avoiding those complications.

Cautions and Warnings

Do not take these medicines if you are **allergic** or **sensitive** to them. Severe drug reactions have been reported, including swelling of the tongue, lips, face, or throat. Contact your doctor if you experience any of these symptoms.

Saxagliptin and sitagliptin should be used with caution in people with **kidney disease**, and a lower dosage may be prescribed.

These medicines do not work in people with **type 1 diabetes**.

Do not use these drugs if you are in a state of **diabetic ketoacidosis** (see "Special Information"). This condition should be treated with insulin.

Inflammation of the pancreas (acute pancreatitis) has developed in a small number of people taking these drugs. This can be a serious and disabling condition characterized by sudden very sharp pain in the abdomen.

Do not use Janumet if you have **heart failure** or **liver or kidney disease**. These conditions increase the risk for lactic acidosis, a rare, potentially fatal condition that can occur with metformin treatment.

Possible Side Effects

The overall risk of side effects with DPP-4 inhibitors is very low.

Linagliptin

Most linagliptin side effects were reported in studies where it was combined with another diabetes medicine.

- ▼ Common: joint pain, back pain, and headache.
- ▼ Less common: common cold symptoms, increased cholesterol or triglycerides, and weight gain.

Possible Side Effects *(continued)*

▼ Rare: drug reactions (itching, skin reactions, swollen lips and eyelids, difficulty breathing), low blood sugar, muscle aches, and irritation of the pancreas. Contact your doctor if you experience anything unusual while taking any medication.

Saxagliptin

▼ Most common: urinary infections, respiratory infections, and headache.

▼ Less common: sinus irritation, abdominal pain, stomach irritation, vomiting, leg and ankle swelling (see "Drug Interactions"), hives and itching, and swollen face.

▼ Rare: reduced white-blood-cell count, rash, reduced kidney function, broken bones, and low platelet count. Contact your doctor if you experience anything unusual while taking any medication.

For more information about Kombiglyze XR, see Metformin, page 731.

Sitagliptin

▼ Most common: upper-respiratory infection, common cold symptoms, and headache.

▼ Less common: abdominal pain, nausea, and diarrhea.

▼ Rare: elevated liver enzymes. Contact your doctor if you experience anything unusual while taking any medication.

For more information about Janumet, see Metformin, page 731, and for Juvisync, see Statin Cholesterol-Lowering Agents, page 1065.

Drug Interactions

- If taken with sulfonylurea drugs or insulin injections, these medicines may cause very low blood sugar (below 50 mg/dL as measured on your blood-glucose meter). You may need to take less sulfonylurea after starting one of these medicines.
- These medicines can cause a slight increase in the amount of digoxin absorbed into the system, but no dose adjustment is needed.
- Mixing these medicines with atazanavir, clarithromycin, cyclosporine, erythromycin, indinavir, itraconazole, ketoconazole, nefazodone, nelfinavir, nicardipine, propaphenone, quinidine, ritonavir, saquinavir, tacrolimus, tamoxifen, or telithromycin causes a large increase in blood levels of DPP-4 inhibitors.

Your dose should be reduced if you are taking one of these combinations. Your normal dose may be restored after the second drug is stopped.

- Amiodarone, aprepitant, chloramphenicol, cimetidine, ciprofloxacin, delavirdine, diltiazem, fluconazole, fluvoxamine, gestodene, imatinib, mibefradil, mifepristone, norfloxacin, norfluoxetine, verapamil, and voriconazole can also raise blood levels of DPP-4 inhibitors, but dose adjustments are usually not needed.
- Barbiturates, carbamazepine, corticosteroid drugs, efavirenz, glitazone antidiabetes drugs, modafinil, nevirapine, oxcarbazepine, phenobarbital, phenytoin, rifabutin, rifampin, and St. John's wort can speed the breakdown of DPP-4 inhibitors in the liver, but dose adjustments are not required.
- Mixing saxagliptin with a glitazone antidiabetes drug triples the risk of leg and ankle swelling.

For more information about Janumet or Kombiglyze XR, see Metformin, page 731, and for Juvisync, see Statin Cholesterol-Lowering Agents, page 1065.

Food Interactions

These drugs can be taken without regard to food or meals. Do not eat or drink large quantities of grapefruit or starfruit products with saxagliptin.

Usual Dose

Adult

Linagliptin: 5 mg once a day.

Saxagliptin: 2.5–5 mg once a day; 2.5 mg is prescribed in moderate to severe kidney disease.

Saxagliptin + Metformin: 2.5/1000–5/2000 mg once a day.

Sitagliptin: 25–100 mg once a day; 25 mg is prescribed for severe kidney disease and 50 mg for moderate kidney disease.

Sitagliptin + Metformin: 50/500–50/1000 mg twice a day.

Sitagliptin + Metformin Extended Release: 100/1000–100/2000 mg once a day.

Sitagliptin + Simvastatin: 100/10, 100/20, 100/40, 50/10, 50/20, 50/40, once a day in the evening.

Child: None of the DPP-4 inhibitors are recommended for children.

Overdosage

Clinical studies used daily doses of linagliptin up to 600 mg, sitagliptin up to 800 mg, and saxagliptin up to 400 mg. At these doses, there were no clinically important effects. Overdose victims should be taken to a hospital emergency room. If you seek treatment, ALWAYS bring the prescription bottle or container.

Special Information

If you forget a dose, take it as soon as you remember. If it is almost time for the next dose, skip the one you forgot and continue with your regular schedule. Do not take a double dose.

Contact your doctor at once if you suddenly begin to feel ill, have muscle aches, have difficulty breathing, become increasingly tired, or have pain or discomfort in your abdomen while taking Janumet or Kombiglyze XR. These could be signs of a condition called diabetic ketoacidosis.

Contact your doctor at once if your legs and ankles start swelling with fluid.

As a person with diabetes, you cannot depend on medicine alone to control your condition. Regular exercise, dietary management, and monitoring of your blood sugar are also necessary to achieve your goals.

Special Populations

Pregnancy/Breast-feeding: Animal studies using high doses of DPP-4 inhibitors have shown they cross into the blood circulation of the developing fetus and can cause some fetal malformations. A DPP-4 inhibitor should be taken during pregnancy only if your doctor determines that the potential benefit outweighs the risks. Pregnant women with diabetes are usually treated with insulin.

Saxagliptin passes into breast milk; it is not known if linagliptin or sitagliptin pass into breast milk. Nursing mothers who must take a DPP-4 inhibitor should use infant formula.

Seniors: Seniors can take these drugs without special restriction. Less sitagliptin may be required due to normal age-related changes in kidney function.

Generic Name

Dronabinol (droe-NAB-ih-nol) G

Brand Names

Marinol

Type of Drug

Antinauseant.

Prescribed For

Nausea and vomiting associated with cancer chemotherapy, and appetite stimulation and weight-loss prevention in people with acquired immunodeficiency syndrome (AIDS).

General Information

Dronabinol is a legal form of marijuana. The psychoactive chemical in marijuana is delta-9-THC. Dronabinol has all of the psychological effects of marijuana and is therefore considered to have a high potential for abuse. It can cause personality changes, feelings of detachment, hallucinations, and euphoria (feeling "high"). Younger adults have reported a greater success rate with dronabinol, probably because they are better able to tolerate these effects.

Most people start taking dronabinol while in the hospital so their response to the drug and its possible adverse effects can be monitored. Dronabinol has also been studied as a glaucoma treatment.

Cautions and Warnings

Do not take dronabinol if you are **allergic** or **sensitive** to any of its ingredients, to marijuana, or to sesame oil.

Dronabinol should not be used to treat nausea and vomiting caused by anything other than cancer chemotherapy.

Dronabinol should be used with caution in those with a history of **seizure disorders** or **substance abuse**.

Dronabinol has a profound effect on mental states; it will impair your ability to operate complex equipment or engage in any activity that requires intense concentration, sound judgment, or coordination—such as driving a car.

Dronabinol produces withdrawal symptoms when the drug is stopped. These may develop within 12 hours of the drug's discontinuation and include restlessness, sleeplessness, and irritability. Within a day after the drug has been stopped, stuffy nose, hot flashes, sweating, loose stools, hiccups, or appetite loss may occur. The symptoms usually subside within a few days.

Dronabinol should be used with caution by people with **heart disease** or **high blood pressure**. Dronabinol should be used with caution by people with a **manic-depressive or schizophrenic history** because it may aggravate the underlying disease.

Possible Side Effects

- ▼ Most common: drowsiness, euphoria, dizziness, anxiety, muddled thinking, perceptual difficulties, poor coordination, irritability, a separation in time and space, depression, weakness, sluggishness, nausea and vomiting, headache, hallucinations, memory lapses, loss of muscle coordination, unsteadiness, paranoia, depersonalization, disorientation, confusion, rapid heartbeat, and dizziness when rising from a sitting or lying position.
- ▼ Less common: difficulty talking or slurred speech, facial flushing, excessive perspiration, nightmares, ringing or buzzing in the ears, fainting, diarrhea, loss of bowel control, and muscle pain.

Drug Interactions

- Dronabinol increases the effects of alcohol, sleeping pills, sedatives, and other depressants. It also enhances the effects of psychoactive drugs, including tricyclic antidepressants, amphetamines, cocaine, and other stimulants.
- Dronabinol may increase the effects of fluoxetine and disulfiram.
- The effects of theophylline drugs are reduced by dronabinol.
- Combining dronabinol and antihistamines or anticholinergic drugs may cause either rapid heartbeat or excessive drowsiness.

Food Interactions

This drug can be taken without regard to food or meals; as an appetite stimulant, it is often taken before meals.

Usual Dose

Antiemetic: 5 mg 1–3 hours before starting chemotherapy treatment and repeated every 2–4 hours after treatment, for a total of 4–6 doses a day. Dosage may be increased up to 15 mg per dose if needed; psychiatric side effects increase greatly at higher dosages.

Appetite Stimulant: 2.5 mg before lunch or dinner, or 2.5 mg at bedtime. Dosage may be increased to 20 mg a day.

Overdosage

Overdose symptoms may occur at usual dosages or at higher dosages if the drug is being abused. The primary symptoms of overdose are the psychological symptoms listed above (see "Possible Side Effects"). In some cases, overdose may lead to panic reactions or seizure. Contact a hospital or local poison control center for more information. If you seek treatment, ALWAYS bring the prescription bottle or container.

Special Information

Be careful when driving or performing any task that requires concentration. Avoid alcohol and other central-nervous-system depressants.

Dronabinol may cause acute psychiatric or psychological side effects. Contact your doctor if any develop.

The capsules must be stored in the refrigerator.

If you forget a dose, take it as soon as you remember. If it is almost time for your next dose, skip the one you forgot and continue with your regular schedule. Do not take a double dose.

Special Populations

Pregnancy/Breast-feeding: Animal studies have shown adverse effects on the fetus. Dronabinol should be taken during pregnancy only if your doctor determines that the potential benefit outweighs the risks.

Dronabinol passes into breast milk. Nursing mothers who must take this drug should use infant formula.

Seniors: Seniors may be more sensitive to this drug, especially its psychological effects.

Generic Name

Dronedarone (droh-NED-ah-rown)

Brand Names

Multaq

Type of Drug

Antiarrhythmic.

Prescribed For

Atrial arrhythmias.

General Information

Dronedarone is a unique treatment for people with or who have had abnormal heart rhythms, atrial fibrillation, or atrial flutter. By preventing a recurrence of the arrhythmia, dronedarone helps reduce the chances that you will have to be re-hospitalized. It is safe for people who also have other risk factors, such as advanced age (over 70 years old), high blood pressure, diabetes, a previous stroke, or some kinds of heart disease.

Cautions and Warnings

Do not take dronedarone if you are **allergic** or **sensitive** to any of its ingredients.

Dronedarone doubles the rate of stroke, heart failure, and death due to cardiovascular events when taken by people who cannot be converted from atrial fibrillation to normal rhythm. You must have your heart rhythm checked by your doctor at least every 3 months to make sure your heart is beating normally.

This drug may not be used by people with Class II, III, or IV **heart failure** who have recently been hospitalized because of their heart condition. These people have twice the risk of dying if they take dronedarone. Others who should not take dronedarone are those with a **very slow heart rate** (below 50 beats per minute), **heart block** and other defects in the ability of electrical signals to travel efficiently through heart muscle, or severe **liver disease**. People taking dronedarone have suffered severe liver injury due to the medicine.

Do not take dronedarone if you are taking any drug or herbal product that can affect the breakdown of dronedarone or that can affect the heart (see "Drug Interactions").

People taking dronedarone should also take a blood-thinning medicine to prevent blood clots from forming.

Pregnant women and **nursing mothers** should not take dronedarone.

Blood levels of potassium and magnesium can fall while taking dronedarone and must be monitored.

Possible Side Effects

- ▼ Most common: slight changes in kidney function.
- ▼ Common: diarrhea, nausea, abdominal pain, vomiting, upset stomach, and weakness.
- ▼ Less common: heart rate below 50 beats per minute, abnormal heart rhythms, rash, itching, eczema, and dry skin.
- ▼ Rare: unusual sensitivity to bright light. Other side effects of dronedarone can affect almost any part of the body. Contact your doctor if you experience anything unusual while taking any medication.

Drug Interactions

- Do not take dronedarone with antiarrhythmic medicines, including amiodarone, disopyramide, dofetilide, flecainide, propafenone, quinidine, or sotalol.
- Mixing beta-blocker drugs with dronedarone can result in excessive slowing of the heartbeat. Your doctor will use a low dose of beta blocker to start and increase gradually if needed.
- Calcium channel blockers should be started at a low dose and increased slowly to gauge their effect on heart rate.
- Mixing dronedarone with clarithromycin, ketoconazole, itraconazole, nefazodone, indinavir, ritonavir, saquinavir, or telithromycin increases the amount of both dronedarone and the interacting drug in the blood. Do not mix dronedarone with these drugs because they can increase dronedarone blood levels by up to 1700%!
- Amiodarone, aprepitant, chloramphenicol, cimetidine, ciprofloxacin, delavirdine, diltiazem, erythromycin, fluconazole, fluvoxamine, gestodene, imatinib, mibefradil, mifepristone, norfloxacin, norfluoxetine, verapamil, and voriconazole can also raise dronedarone blood levels, but less than the drugs listed above. These drugs should be avoided if you are taking dronedarone.
- Barbiturates, carbamazepine, corticosteroid drugs, efavirenz, glitazone antidiabetes drugs, modafinil, nevirapine, oxcarbazepine, phenobarbital, phenytoin, rifabutin, rifampin, and St. John's wort can speed the breakdown of dronedarone in the liver, reducing its effectiveness. Dose adjustments may be required.
- Diuretics and other medicines that reduce blood potassium should only be taken if prescribed by your doctor. Abnormal potassium levels can affect your heart.
- Digoxin can increase the effects of dronedarone on your heart. Dronedarone also slows the breakdown of digoxin, increasing the chance of digoxin-related gastrointestinal side effects. If you stay on digoxin, your dose is likely to be cut in ½.
- Phenothiazine drugs, tricyclic antidepressants, and erythromycin increase the risk of a particular abnormal heart rhythm called torsade de pointes.
- Dronedarone increases blood levels of warfarin. Your warfarin dose may have to be modified.
- Dronedarone increases blood levels of the statin cholesterol-lowering drugs tacrolimus and sirolimus (but not pravastatin

and rosuvastatin) by slowing their breakdown in the liver. Other drugs whose blood levels, clinical effects, and side effects can also be increased by dronedarone in this way are: alfentanil, alprazolam, amlodipine, astemizole, buspirone, cafergot, caffeine, cilostazol, cisapride, cocaine, cyclosporine, dapsone, dexamethasone, diazepam, docetaxel, domperidone, eplerenone, estradiol, felodipine, fentanyl, finasteride, hydrocortisone, irinotecan, lercanidipine, methadone, midazolam, nateglinide, nifedipine, nisoldipine, nitrendipine, paclitaxel, pimozide, progesterone, quetiapine, quinidine, quinine, salmeterol, sildenafil, sorafenib, sunitinib, terfenadine, testosterone, torisel, trazodone, triazolam, vincristine, zaleplon, ziprasidone, and zolpidem. Your drug dose may be adjusted.

- Dronedarone may increase blood levels of the following drugs by interfering with their breakdown in the liver; your dose may need to be modified: alprenolol, amitriptyline, amphetamine, aripiprazole, atomoxetine, carvedilol, chlorpheniramine, chlorpromazine, clomipramine, codeine, debrisoquine, desipramine, dextromethorphan, donepezil, duloxetine, encainide, flecainide, fluoxetine, haloperidol, imipramine, lidocaine, metoclopramide, metoprolol, mexiletine, nebivolol, nortriptyline, ondansetron, oxycodone, paroxetine, perhexiline, perphenazine, phenacetin, phenformin, promethazine, propafenone, propranolol, risperidone, sparteine, tamoxifen, thioridazine, timolol, tramadol, and venlafaxine.

Food Interactions

Take each dose with a meal. Dronedarone must be taken with food because it is very poorly absorbed into the blood when taken on an empty stomach. It takes 3–6 hours for each dose to reach maximum concentration in the blood. Do not eat or drink grapefruit and starfruit products while you are taking dronedarone, as they can substantially increase the amount of drug in your blood.

Usual Dose

Adult: 400 mg with breakfast and dinner.
Child: not recommended.

Overdosage

Overdose symptoms can be expected to affect your heart. Overdose victims must be taken to a hospital emergency room. If you seek treatment, ALWAYS bring the prescription bottle or container.

Special Information

Women of childbearing age must use an effective contraceptive method while taking dronedarone. Contact your doctor at once if you think you are pregnant.

Contact your doctor if any of the following symptoms develop while you are taking dronedarone, as they can be signs of worsening heart failure: difficulty breathing or wheezing; chest tightness or coughing up frothy sputum; trouble sleeping or waking up at night because of breathing problems; using more pillows to prop yourself up at night so you can breathe more easily; gaining more than 5 lbs. very quickly; or increased swelling in your feet, ankles, or legs.

Make sure your doctor knows all the medicine you are taking and that you report this new medicine to all other doctors who might prescribe additional medicines.

Contact your doctor right away if you develop any of the following: appetite loss, nausea, vomiting, fever, feeling sick, fatigue, pain in the upper right side of your abdomen, yellowing of the skin or whites of the eyes, dark urine, or severe itching. These symptoms can be signs of severe liver injury.

If you forget to take a dose of dronedarone with your meal, skip it and take your next regular dose. Do not take a double dose.

Special Populations

Pregnancy/Breast-feeding: Dronedarone causes birth defects and can affect a nursing infant. This drug should not be taken by women who are or might be pregnant. Women of childbearing age taking dronedarone must use an effective contraception method.

Nursing mothers who must take dronedarone must use infant formula.

Seniors: Seniors can take dronedarone with no special precautions.

Brand Names

Dyazide

Generic Ingredients

Hydrochlorothiazide + Triamterene G

Other Brand Names

Maxzide Maxzide-25

The information in this profile also applies to the following drugs:

Generic Ingredients: Hydrochlorothiazide + Amiloride G
Moduretic

Generic Ingredients: Hydrochlorothiazide + Spironolactone G
Aldactazide

Type of Drug

Diuretic (an agent that increases urination).

Prescribed For

Hypertension (high blood pressure) or any condition where it is desirable to eliminate excess water from the body.

General Information

Dyazide combines a thiazide diuretic and a potassium-sparing diuretic. The latter, triamterene, helps the body retain potassium while producing a diuretic effect. This balances the other ingredient, hydrochlorothiazide, which normally causes a loss of potassium. Different products contain differing concentrations of these 2 drugs. Dyazide should be used only when you need its exact proportion of ingredients and should not be used for initial therapy of hypertension or edema. It may be used alone or with other antihypertensive drugs such as beta blockers. Dosage adjustment may be necessary.

Cautions and Warnings

Do not take Dyazide if you are **allergic** or **sensitive** to any of its ingredients or to any sulfa drug or if you have a history of allergy.

Taking a diuretic such as Dyazide can cause high blood-potassium levels. This potentially serious effect is more likely in those with **diabetes** or **kidney disease**, the **elderly**, and the **severely ill**. It is important to have blood-potassium levels regularly monitored while taking Dyazide.

Do not use Dyazide if you have **severe kidney disease** or **hyperkalemia** (high blood-potassium levels).

Do not combine any **potassium supplement** and Dyazide without your doctor's knowledge. Dyazide may reduce blood levels of sodium and potassium and raise blood-calcium levels.

Dyazide should be used with caution in people with **diabetes**, **liver disease**, a history of **kidney stones**, or an **electrolyte imbalance**.

Possible Side Effects

- ▼ Most common: appetite loss, drowsiness, lethargy, headache, gastrointestinal upset, cramping, and diarrhea.
- ▼ Less common: rash (possibly severe), mental confusion, fever, feeling unwell, impotence, bright red tongue, burning sensation in the tongue, tingling in the toes and fingers, restlessness, anemia or other effects on blood components, increased sensitivity to sunlight, and dizziness when rising quickly from a sitting position. Dyazide may also produce muscle spasms, gout, weakness, and blurred vision.

Drug Interactions

- Dyazide increases the effect of other blood-pressure-lowering drugs. This is why other blood-pressure drugs are often prescribed with Dyazide, but dosage adjustments may be required.
- Combining Dyazide and digitalis drugs, amphotericin B, or adrenal corticosteroids increases the risk of an electrolyte imbalance.
- If you are taking insulin or an oral antidiabetic drug and begin taking Dyazide, the insulin or antidiabetic dosage may need to be modified.
- Antigout drug dosage may need to be modified because Dyazide raises uric-acid levels.
- Lithium carbonate taken with Dyazide should be monitored carefully by a doctor due to an increased risk of lithium side effects.
- Cholestyramine and colestipol prevent Dyazide from being absorbed. Dyazide should be taken at least 2 hours before cholestyramine or colestipol.
- Methenamine and other urinary agents may reduce the effect of Dyazide.
- Some nonsteroidal anti-inflammatory drugs (NSAIDs), particularly indomethacin, may reduce the effect of Dyazide. Sulindac, another NSAID, may increase its effect.
- Potassium-sparing diuretics should be used with caution in combination with ACE inhibitors.
- Chronic or overuse of laxatives may interfere with the potassium-retaining effects of triamterene.

Food Interactions

Take Dyazide with food if it upsets your stomach.

Usual Dose

Adult

Hydrochlorothiazide + Amiloride: 1–2 tablets a day with meals.

Hydrochlorothiazide + Spironolactone: 25–200 mg of each component once a day or in divided doses.

Hydrochlorothiazide + Triamterene: 1–2 capsules or tablets a day.

Child: not recommended.

Overdosage

Symptoms may include tingling in the arms or legs, weakness, fatigue, changes in heartbeat, a sickly feeling, dry mouth, restlessness, muscle pain or cramps, urinary difficulties, nausea, and vomiting. In some cases, low blood pressure and decreased respiration may occur. Take the victim to a hospital emergency room immediately. If you seek treatment, ALWAYS bring the prescription bottle or container.

Special Information

Dyazide causes excess urination at first, but this subsides after several weeks of use. Diuretics are usually taken early in the day to prevent excessive nighttime urination that may interfere with sleep.

Dyazide may make you drowsy. Be careful when driving or performing any task that requires concentration.

Contact your doctor if you develop muscle pain, sudden joint pain, weakness, cramps, nausea, vomiting, restlessness, excessive thirst, tiredness, drowsiness, increased heart or pulse rate, diarrhea, dizziness, headache, or rash.

People with diabetes may experience an increased blood-sugar level and require dosage adjustments of their antidiabetic medications.

Avoid other drugs while taking Dyazide unless otherwise directed by your doctor. Avoid alcohol.

If you are taking Dyazide for the treatment of hypertension or congestive heart failure, avoid over-the-counter cough, cold, or allergy medications, which may contain stimulants.

Take Dyazide exactly as prescribed. Be aware that all hydrochlorothiazide-triamterene products are not equal to each other and should not be freely substituted. Check with your doctor and pharmacist before switching brands.

If you forget a dose, take it as soon as you remember. If it is almost time for your next dose, skip the dose you forgot and continue with your regular schedule. Do not take a double dose.

Special Populations

Pregnancy/Breast-feeding: Dyazide may enter the fetal circulation, though it is sometimes used to treat specific conditions in pregnant women. Dyazide should be taken during pregnancy only if your doctor determines that the potential benefit outweighs the risks.

The thiazide diuretic in Dyazide passes into breast milk. Nursing mothers who must take Dyazide should use infant formula.

Seniors: Seniors are more sensitive to the effects of Dyazide.

Effexor *see **Venlafaxine,** page 1204*

Generic Name

Eflornithine (eh-FLOOR-nih-thene)

Brand Names

Vaniqa

Type of Drug

Hair growth retardant.

Prescribed For

Removal of unwanted facial hair by women.

General Information

This drug has only been studied for its ability to prevent hair growth on the face and chin and should not be used on other body areas. It works by interfering with enzymes in the skin necessary for hair growth, slowing the rate at which hair will grow. Improvement may be seen as soon as 4–8 weeks after you start using eflornithine, but the condition will return within 8 weeks after you stop using it.

Cautions and Warnings

Do not use eflornithine if you are **allergic** or **sensitive** to any of its ingredients.

For external use only; do not ingest.

Possible Side Effects

Eflornithine side effects are similar to those of a placebo (sugar pill).

Possible Side Effects *(continued)*

- ▼ Most common: acne, bumps, or small pustules on the skin.
- ▼ Common: stinging.
- ▼ Less common: headache, dizziness, burning, itching, redness, tingling, irritation, rash, hair loss, upset stomach, and appetite loss.
- ▼ Rare: fainting, ingrown hairs, inflamed hair follicles, facial swelling, nausea, bleeding, contact dermatitis, inflammation of one or both lips, herpes breakout, numbness, and dilated blood vessels and pores on the nose and cheeks.

Contact your doctor if you experience anything unusual while taking any medication.

Drug Interactions

None known.

Usual Dose

Adult and Child (age 12 and over): Apply a thin layer of cream to affected areas and rub in thoroughly twice a day at least 8 hours apart. Do not wash your face until at least 4 hours after you have applied eflornithine cream. Wait at least 5 minutes after hair removal to apply eflornithine.

Child (under age 12): not recommended.

Overdosage

Little is known about the effects of eflornithine overdose or accidental ingestion. Contact your local poison control center for more information. If you seek treatment, ALWAYS bring the prescription container.

Special Information

If you forget to apply a dose of eflornithine, apply it as soon as you remember. Bear in mind that at least 8 hours must elapse between doses and you cannot wash the area for another 4 hours after application. If it is almost time for your next dose, skip the dose you forgot and continue with your regular schedule.

This product slows hair growth. It is not a depilatory. You will have to continue shaving, tweezing, or using another hair removal technique.

Wait several minutes after application of eflornithine before applying cosmetics or sunscreen.

Use only on your face and neck.

Contact your doctor if your skin becomes irritated or if you develop other side effects. If skin irritation continues, you may have to stop using eflornithine.

Special Populations

Pregnancy/Breast-feeding: Eflornithine cream may cause birth defects. Eflornithine cream should be used during pregnancy only if your doctor determines that the potential benefit outweighs the risks.

It is not known if this drug passes into breast milk. Nursing mothers should use infant formula.

Seniors: Seniors may use eflornithine without special precaution.

Generic Name

Eltrombopag (el-TROM-bo-pahg)

Brand Names

Promacta

Type of Drug

Thrombopoietin receptor agonist.

Prescribed For

Idiopathic thrombocytopenia purpura (ITP) that has not responded to other treatments.

General Information

ITP is a condition in which platelet count is abnormally low. In ⅔ of people, ITP develops when antibodies against their own platelets are created. Ordinarily, blood-platelet count is about 150,000–400,000 for most people. The actual platelet count necessary for an ITP diagnosis is not fixed, but is often around 50,000. Half of all new cases of ITP in the United States (150–300 a year) are children, almost ¾ of which get better in 6 months, with or without treatment. Adult ITP affects about 60,000 American adults and is usually diagnosed between age 50 and 60. Usual ITP symptoms include bruising, black-and-blue marks, and nose and gum bleeding. A very low platelet count can lead to blood blisters in the mouth or mucous membranes. Bleeding in the brain, gastrointestinal tract, or other internal sites, though rare, can be fatal. Platelet counts below 20,000 can be treated with a number of possible therapies, but eltrombopag is one of the few oral treatments available. Your doctor will try another treatment if your platelet count does not improve after 4 weeks of treatment.

Cautions and Warnings

Do not take eltrombopag if you are **allergic** or **sensitive** to any of its ingredients.

This drug can cause liver damage and should be stopped at the first sign of liver inflammation or hepatitis. People with **mild to moderate liver disease** may take this drug at a reduced dosage. It should not be taken by anyone with **severe liver disease**. Because of the risk of liver disease, this drug is not available from neighborhood pharmacies, only through a special distribution program managed by the drug's manufacturer.

People with **kidney disease** should use this medicine with caution. Report anything unusual to your doctor.

People of **East Asian ancestry** (such as Chinese, Japanese, Taiwanese, or Korean) treated with eltrombopag typically have blood levels of the drug about 70% higher than other ethnic groups and generally require a lower dose of eltrombopag.

Drugs of this type can increase the risk for bone marrow fibers to form.

Stopping eltrombopag may result in a rapid and even more severe drop in blood platelets and risk of bleeding than was present before treatment. Do not suddenly stop treatment.

This drug can increase the chances of blood cancers.

Eltrombopag should be used with extreme caution in **children**.

Possible Side Effects

▼ Common: nausea.

▼ Less common: vomiting, vaginal bleeding, muscle aches, tingling in the hands or feet, upset stomach, cataracts, eye bleeding, black-and-blue marks, hemorrhage, elevated platelet counts, and liver irritation.

Drug Interactions

- Aluminum, calcium, iron, magnesium, selenium, and zinc interfere with the absorption of eltrombopag into the blood. Separate each dose of eltrombopag by 4 hours from any food, medicine (such as antacids), or supplement product that contains a mineral.
- Eltrombopag may increase the amount of cyclosporine, rifampicin, rosuvastatin, and, to a lesser extent, sildenafil in

the blood by interfering with their ability to enter liver cells where they are broken down. Dose adjustments may be needed.

- This drug is broken down by several enzyme systems in the liver, but the importance of possible interactions with other drugs broken down by the same systems is not yet known.

Food Interactions

This drug should be taken on an empty stomach, at least 1 hour before or 2 hours after eating. Allow 4 hours to pass after eating any food containing any mineral before you take your medicine. Minerals prevent this drug from being absorbed into the bloodstream.

Usual Dose

Adult: 25–50 mg a day. Dosage adjustments are based on platelet count response, with a maximum daily dose of 75 mg.

Child: not recommended.

Overdosage

One person took 5000 mg of eltrombopag and developed a rash, slow heart rate, liver irritation, and fatigue. Eltrombopag overdose can also lead to excessively high platelet counts and unwanted blood clot formation. In this case, high platelet counts took 3 weeks to go down. Overdose victims should be taken to a hospital emergency room. If you seek treatment, ALWAYS bring the prescription bottle or container.

Special Information

This drug can cause liver damage. Contact your doctor at once if you develop yellowing of the skin or whites of the eyes, unusually dark urine, pain in the right upper stomach area, or if you become unusually tired.

Eltrombopag should only be used for the management of ITP with bleeding symptoms. It should not be used to normalize low platelet counts not related to ITP.

Regular blood tests are necessary after your dose adjustment is completed to be sure your blood counts remain in a normal range.

Avoid any activities that may cause bruising or injury while taking eltrombopag. Report anything unusual to your doctor, especially if you are taking any other medicine.

Special Populations

Pregnancy/Breast-feeding: This drug can damage the developing fetus and should be avoided by pregnant women. The drug's manufacturer has established a registry to collect such information as the drug is taken during pregnancy.

Nursing mothers who must take it should use infant formula because it can affect the newborn.

Seniors: Seniors may be sensitive to the side effects of this drug.

Generic Name

Enfuvirtide (en-FUV-ir-tide)

Brand Names

Fuzeon

Type of Drug

Antiviral fusion inhibitor.

Prescribed For

Human immunodeficiency virus (HIV) infection.

General Information

Enfuvirtide is the first of a new class of anti-HIV drugs. Unlike all other anti-HIV medicines, it works by preventing the HIV virus from fusing to healthy CD_4 cells, a key part of the human immune system. This helps fight HIV by having fewer HIV-infected cells as well as a healthier immune system to fight off the HIV virus. Enfuvirtide is always prescribed in combination with other antiviral medicines. It is possible for the HIV virus to become resistant to enfuvirtide, but this drug can work against types of the virus that have become resistant to other anti-HIV therapies.

Cautions and Warnings

Do not take enfuvirtide if you are **allergic** or **sensitive** to any of its ingredients. Symptoms of drug allergy can include generalized itching, rash, severe chills, and low blood pressure. In rare cases, enfuvirtide triggers severe hypersensitivity. Patients experiencing symptoms (a combination of rash, fever, nausea, and/or respiratory distress) should stop using enfuvirtide and seek medical attention immediately.

People taking enfuvirtide may be more likely to develop bacterial pneumonia. See your doctor regularly and report any breathing difficulties or unusual respiratory reactions.

Enfuvirtide may raise blood-sugar levels, worsen diabetes, or trigger latent diabetes. People with **diabetes** who take this drug may need to have the dosage of their antidiabetes medication adjusted.

Possible Side Effects

- ▼ Most common: allergic skin reaction at the site of injection (symptoms include itching, rash, and swelling of tissue under the skin), diarrhea, nausea, fatigue, and sleeplessness.
- ▼ Common: tingling in the hands or feet, depression, anxiety, cough, sinusitis, herpes infection, weight loss, appetite loss, weakness, itching, and muscle ache.
- ▼ Less common: taste changes, small skin tumors, influenza, constipation, abdominal pain, pancreas inflammation, conjunctivitis (pinkeye), and lymph gland inflammation.
- ▼ Rare: Rare side effects can affect the blood, immune system, kidneys, urinary tract, and central nervous system. Contact your doctor if you experience anything unusual while taking any medication.

Drug Interactions

Enfuvirtide is not broken down in the liver and does not affect liver enzyme systems, so it is not likely to be involved in common drug interactions.

- Enfuvirtide raises blood levels of tipranavir. Dosage adjustments are not likely to be necessary.

Food Interactions

None known.

Usual Dose

Adult and Child (age 17 and over): 90 mg injected under the skin into the upper arm, thigh, or abdomen twice a day.

Child (age 6–16): 0.91 mg per lb. of body weight twice a day, up to 90 mg per injection. Be sure to increase enfuvirtide dosage as your child's weight increases.

Child (under age 6): not recommended.

Overdosage

Little is known about the effects of enfuvirtide overdose. Take the victim to a hospital emergency room. If you seek treatment, ALWAYS bring the prescription bottle or container.

Special Information

Enfuvirtide is not a cure for HIV. It will not prevent you from transmitting the HIV virus to another person; you must still practice safe sex. People taking this drug may still develop opportunistic infections and other complications associated with HIV infection.

This drug is given by injection under the skin. For information on how to properly administer this drug, see page 1242.

Do not use a vial of enfuvirtide if the final solution has particles floating in it. It should be completely clear, colorless, and have no bubbles in the vial.

You may keep solutions of enfuvirtide in the refrigerator and use them for up to 24 hours after they have been mixed. After that, they must be thrown away.

Tell your doctor if you are pregnant, have become pregnant, or plan to become pregnant.

Do not stop taking enfuvirtide, or any other anti-HIV medicine, without first consulting your doctor.

Special Populations

Pregnancy/Breast-feeding: Although animal studies of enfuvirtide reveal no damage to the fetus, this drug should be taken during pregnancy only if your doctor determines that the potential benefit outweighs the risks. A national registry has been established to gather information on pregnant women who take this drug.

It is not known if enfuvirtide passes into breast milk. Nursing mothers with HIV should always use infant formula, regardless of whether they take this drug, to avoid transmitting the virus to their child.

Seniors: The effects of enfuvirtide in seniors are unknown.

Generic Name

Entacapone (in-TACK-a-pohn)

Brand Names

Comtan

Type of Drug

Antiparkinsonian.

Prescribed For

Parkinson's disease patients for whom levodopa + carbidopa loses its effectiveness between doses.

General Information

Entacapone is always used in combination with levodopa + carbidopa. Some patients experience signs and symptoms of an end-of-dose "wearing-off" effect with these drugs. Entacapone enhances the effect of levodopa + carbidopa by reversing the action of an enzyme known as catechol-O-methyltransferase (COMT), which is primarily responsible for breaking down levodopa in the body.

Cautions and Warnings

Do not take entacapone if you are **allergic** or **sensitive** to any of its ingredients.

People with **liver disease** should use entacapone with caution as they may accumulate twice as much of this drug in their blood as people with normal liver function.

Entacapone has been rarely associated with the formation of fibrous tissues in unusual places such as the urinary tract and lungs. It has also caused fluid in the lungs.

Entacapone may cause kidney toxicity.

Entacapone may increase the risk of dizziness or fainting when rising from a sitting or lying position.

Hallucinations have been reported with other Parkinson's disease drugs.

Possible Side Effects

- ▼ Most common: difficulty performing voluntary muscle functions, excessive muscle activity, nausea, urine discoloration, and diarrhea.
- ▼ Common: reduced muscle activity, dizziness, fatigue, constipation, and abdominal pain.
- ▼ Less common: low blood pressure and fainting when rising from a sitting or lying position, hallucinations, anxiety, agitation, gastritis or other stomach disorders, dry mouth, vomiting, increased sweating, back pain, taste changes, shortness of breath, easy bruising, weakness, and bacterial infection.

Possible Side Effects *(continued)*

▼ Rare: muscle damage or death, high fever, and confusion.

Contact your doctor if you experience anything unusual while taking any medication.

Drug Interactions

- Do not mix entacapone with the monoamine oxidase inhibitor (MAOI) antidepressants phenelzine or tranylcypromine. Entacapone may be taken with the MAOI selegiline.
- Other drugs broken down by COMT will also be affected by entacapone. Apomorphine, dobutamine, dopamine, epinephrine, isoproterenol, methyldopa, and norepinephrine will interact with entacapone, even when taken by inhalation. The result may be increased heart rate, arrhythmias, and excessive changes in blood pressure.
- Ampicillin, chloramphenicol, cholestyramine, erythromycin, probenecid, and rifampin may interfere with the elimination of entacapone from the body.
- Entacapone may enhance the effects of sedatives and other nervous system depressants.

Food Interactions

This drug can be taken without regard to food.

Usual Dose

Adult: 200 mg with each levodopa + carbidopa dose, up to 1600 mg a day.

Child: not recommended.

Overdosage

Theoretically, a massive entacapone overdose could prove lethal by completely inhibiting COMT throughout the body. There have been no reports of significant entacapone overdose. Doses up to 800 mg have been taken and side effects were mainly abdominal pain and loose stools. Other effects that might be expected include difficulty breathing, loss of muscle coordination, reduced level of activity, and convulsions. Overdose victims should be taken to a hospital emergency room as soon as possible. If you seek treatment, ALWAYS bring the prescription bottle or container.

Special Information

Always take your entacapone dose together with your levodopa + carbidopa dose. If you forget a dose, take it as soon as you remember. If it is within 2 hours of your next dose, skip the dose you forgot and continue with your regular schedule.

This drug can cause dizziness, nausea, sweating, or fainting when rising quickly from a sitting or lying position, especially at the beginning of treatment.

Increased body movements and twitching, twisting, or uncontrolled tongue, lip, face, arm, or leg movement may occur. If this happens, your doctor may need to adjust your dose of levodopa + carbidopa.

Exercise caution when performing tasks that require coordination and concentration, such as driving, until your body has become accustomed to the effects of entacapone.

Gradually reducing the dose of entacapone decreases some drug side effects.

Rapid withdrawal can cause high fever, sweating, unstable blood pressure, stupor, and muscular rigidity. Patients who stop using entacapone should be monitored.

Entacapone can cause your urine to turn a brownish-orange color. This change is harmless.

Special Populations

Pregnancy/Breast-feeding: Entacapone causes birth defects, miscarriage, and abortion in pregnant animals. Entacapone should be taken during pregnancy only if your doctor determines that the potential benefit outweighs the risks.

Entacapone passes into the breast milk of animals but no information on humans is available. Nursing mothers who must take this drug should use infant formula.

Seniors: Seniors may take this drug without special precaution.

Brand Names

Entex PSE

Generic Ingredients

Guaifenesin + Pseudoephedrine Hydrochloride G

Other Brand Names

Altarussin-PE
Ambifed G
Anatuss LA
Coldmist
Congestac
Despec Tab

Dynex
ExeFen IR
Guaifed PD
Guaifenex PSE
Guaimax-D
Iosal II
Maxifed
Medent LDI
Mucinex D
Nasatab LA
Nomuc PE
PolyVent
Q-Tussin PE
Respa-1st
Respaire
Rydex G
Sinutab
Stamoist E
SudaTex
Touro LA

The information in this profile also applies to the following drugs:

Generic Ingredients: Guaifenesin + Ephedrine Hydrochloride G

Broncholate
Bronkaid
Primatene

Generic Ingredients: Guaifenesin + Phenylephrine Hydrochloride G

Crantex
Deconex
Deconsal II
Despec
Donatussin
D-Phen 1000
D-Tab
Duratuss
Dynex LA
ED Bron GP
Entex LQ
ExeFen PD
ExeTuss
Extendryl G
Gentex LA
Gilphex TR
Guaifen PE
Guiatex PE
J-Max
Liquibid
Lusair
Medent PE
Mucinex
MyDex
Nariz
Norel EX
PE-GuaiDrops
PhenaVent D
Reluri
Rescon-GG
Robitussin PE
Siltex
Sinuvent PE
Sitrex PD
Sudafed PE Non-Drying Sinus
Supress PE
Triaminic
TussBid
Zinx GP
Zotex GPX
Zyrphen

Type of Drug

Decongestant and expectorant combination.

Prescribed For

Cold or allergy and for nasal congestion, runny nose, and cough associated with other upper-respiratory conditions.

General Information

The decongestant ingredient in Entex PSE, pseudoephedrine, dramatically reduces congestion and stuffiness. The decongestant ingredients ephedrine and phenylephrine act similarly. The expectorant, guaifenesin, is used to help loosen thick mucus that may contribute to chest congestion; the effectiveness of guaifenesin and other expectorants has not been established. There are other drugs on the market using this same general formula—an expectorant plus a decongestant—but they use different decongestant ingredients or a combination of decongestants plus guaifenesin. Nothing cures a cold or allergy, but Entex PSE may provide relief from symptoms.

Cautions and Warnings

Do not take Entex PSE if you are **allergic** or **sensitive** to any of its ingredients.

Entex PSE may cause anxiety or nervousness or interfere with sleep.

Do not use Entex PSE if you have **ventricular tachycardia** (quickened heart rate) or **hypertension** (high blood pressure).

Entex PSE should be used with extreme caution in those with **heart disease**, other **heart rhythm disorders**, **thyroid disease**, **diabetes**, **glaucoma**, **stomach ulcer**, **urinary blockage**, or a **prostate condition**.

Entex PSE should not be used over extended periods of time to treat **persistent or chronic cough**, especially one that may be caused by cigarette smoking, asthma, or emphysema.

Possible Side Effects

- ▼ Most common: anxiety, restlessness, sleeplessness, tension, excitation, dizziness, drowsiness, and headache.
- ▼ Less common: nausea, vomiting, upset stomach, low blood pressure, heart palpitations, chest pain, rapid or slow heartbeat, abnormal heart rhythms, irritability, euphoria (feeling

Possible Side Effects *(continued)*

"high"), eye irritation and tearing, hysterical reaction, appetite loss, kidney stones, urinary difficulties in men with a prostate condition, weakness, loss of facial color, and breathing difficulties.

Drug Interactions

- Entex PSE should be avoided if you are taking a monoamine oxidase inhibitor (MAOI) antidepressant for depression or hypertension because the MAOI may cause a very rapid rise in blood pressure or increase side effects such as dry mouth or nose, blurred vision, and abnormal heart rhythms. You should not take Entex PSE for 14 days after stopping an MAOI antidepressant.
- Taking Entex PSE with furazolidone may increase the risk of Entex PSE side effects. You should separate doses of furazolidone and Entex PSE by 14 days.
- Beta-blocker medications may increase the side effects of Entex PSE.
- Tricyclic antidepressants such as amitriptyline may decrease the effects of Entex PSE.
- The risk of irregular heartbeat or heart attack may be increased by mixing digoxin or droxidopa with Entex PSE.
- Guanadrel, guanethidine, mecamylamine, or reserpine may have their effectiveness decreased by Entex PSE. The effectiveness of Entex PSE may also be decreased when taken with guanethidine or reserpine.
- If Entex PSE is taken with methyldopa, methyldopa effects are decreased and Entex PSE effects are increased.
- The decongestant in Entex PSE may interfere with blood-pressure-lowering medication.

Food Interactions

Take Entex PSE with food if it upsets your stomach.

Usual Dose

Adult and Child (age 12 and over): 1 tablet or capsule twice a day or 2 tsp. of liquid 4 times a day.

Child (age 6–11): ½–1 tablet or 1 capsule twice a day or 1 tsp. of liquid 4 times a day.

Child (under age 6): not recommended.

Overdosage

Most cases of overdose are not severe. Symptoms include sedation, sleepiness, increased sweating, and increased blood pressure. Hallucinations, convulsions, nervous system depression, and breathing difficulties are more prominent in older adults. Induce vomiting with ipecac syrup, which is available at any pharmacy. Contact your local poison control center or a hospital emergency room before doing this. If you seek treatment, ALWAYS bring the prescription bottle or container.

Special Information

Contact your doctor if your side effects are severe or gradually become intolerable.

If you forget a dose, take it as soon as you remember. If it is almost time for your next dose, skip the one you forgot and continue with your regular schedule. Do not take a double dose.

Special Populations

Pregnancy/Breast-feeding: Women who are or might be pregnant should avoid this medication. Entex PSE should be taken during pregnancy only if your doctor determines that the potential benefit outweighs the risks.

The decongestant in Entex PSE may pass into breast milk. Nursing mothers who must take Entex PSE should use infant formula.

Seniors: Seniors are more sensitive to the effects of Entex PSE.

Generic Name

Epoetin (EE-poh-eh-tin)

Brand Names

Epogen Procrit

The information in this profile also applies to the following drugs:

Generic Ingredients: Darbepoetin Alfa
Aranesp

Type of Drug

Red-blood-cell growth stimulator.

Prescribed For

Treating anemia and reducing the need for red-blood-cell transfusions due to bone marrow suppression caused by drug treatment. Some cancer patients may receive 1 of these drugs, but only when cure of the cancer is not anticipated. If prescribed for a cancer patient, chemotherapy must continue for at least 2 more months and should not be continued or restarted after chemotherapy is completed. These drugs should never be used in some cancers (see "Cautions and Warnings") and may be prescribed for some people with kidney failure and in people taking the HIV medication zidovudine (also known as AZT).

General Information

Epoetin is a natural hormone that stimulates the bone marrow to produce red blood cells. It is used for anemia that does not respond to iron supplements. In most cases of anemia, there are plenty of red blood cells circulating, but they lack iron. People who need epoetin do not have enough red blood cells. Epoetin stimulates the production of new red blood cells to carry needed oxygen. Studies of these drugs have generally not shown them to improve quality of life or well-being in people receiving them.

Cautions and Warnings

Do not use epoetin if you are **allergic** or **sensitive** to any of its ingredients, or to albumin or products manufactured from animal cells.

These drugs should not be used by people with **cervical**, **breast**, **non-small-cell lung**, **lymph**, **or head and neck cancers** because they can increase the risk of tumor growth and shorten survival.

These drugs should not be prescribed for **cancer patients being treated with hormones**, **biologic products**, **or radiation** unless they are also taking a medicine that suppresses the bone marrow.

If your hemoglobin levels become too high, the risk of heart attack, stroke, heart failure, blood clots, and death is increased. It is important to have your blood tested to manage your epoetin or darbepoetin dosage throughout treatment.

People with **uncontrolled high blood pressure** should not use epoetin.

Some people with **chronic kidney failure** and severe **anemia** should not take epoetin. Epoetin is not a replacement for emergency blood transfusion.

Epoetin should never be used for **anemia caused by folate or iron deficiency, hemolysis, or gastrointestinal bleeding**.

People using epoetin may require anticoagulant medicine to prevent **blood clotting** during treatment. Tell your doctor if you have any blood-clotting disorders.

In rare cases, people taking epoetin may have seizures. Avoid driving or any other activities where a sudden seizure could be dangerous. Do not take epoetin if you have a history of **seizures** or **strokes**.

Possible Side Effects

Side effects reported in studies of epoetin were similar to those reported with an inactive placebo (sugar pill).

- ▼ Most common: high blood pressure, headache, constipation, diarrhea, nausea, joint pain, fever, fatigue, itching, rash, and difficulty breathing.
- ▼ Common: swelling, vomiting, chest pain, skin reactions at the site of injection, weakness, dizziness, urinary infections, diarrhea, upset stomach, blood clots, anxiety, tingling in the hands or feet, and trunk pain.
- ▼ Rare: stroke and heart attack. Contact your doctor if you experience anything unusual while taking any medication.

Drug Interactions

None known.

Usual Dose

Dosage varies with condition, underlying disease, and response to treatment. The target blood-hemoglobin level should not be above 11 g/dL.

Adult: starting dose—23–69 units per lb. of body weight 3 times a week by intravenous or subcutaneous injection. Adult cancer patients may receive 40,000 units per week during chemotherapy. Final dose is based on response and need, with a maximum dose of 136 mg per lb. Surgery patients take 138 units per lb. for 10 days before surgery or 276 units per lb. once a week for 3 weeks before surgery and another dose on the day of surgery. Dialysis patients take epoetin once a week.

Child on Dialysis (age 1 month–16 years): 23–180 units per lb. of body weight 3 times a week by intravenous or subcutaneous injection. Final dose is based on response and need.

Child with HIV (age 8 months–17 years): 23–180 units per lb. of body weight 3 times a week by intravenous or subcutaneous injection. Final dose is based on response and need.

Child on Chemotherapy (age 5–17 years): 272–409 units per lb. of body weight once a week by intravenous or subcutaneous injection. Maximum dose 60,000 units per week.

Premature Infant: 90 units per lb. a day for 2 weeks, or 180 units per lb. 3 times a week for 2 weeks.

Overdosage

Little is known about the effects of epoetin overdose. Contact your local poison control center or a hospital emergency room for information. If you seek treatment, ALWAYS bring the prescription container.

Special Information

People taking epoetin should have regular blood tests to ensure the drug is working well. Your doctor may want to take blood samples twice a week for several weeks and then test your blood regularly. Doctors and hospitals prescribing this medicine for any cancer patient must first enroll in a company-sponsored program in order to provide information on the progress of these patients.

Epoetin has been used by athletes to enhance physical performance. This is called blood doping and has resulted in several deaths due to hazardous percentages of red blood cells.

Epoetin must be stored in a refrigerator.

Multiple-dose vials should not be used to prepare an infant's dose of this medicine because of dangerous reactions associated with the benzyl alcohol preservative used in them.

Most patients will need to take iron supplements with this drug.

This drug can be given by injection under the skin. For more information on how to properly administer this drug, see page 1242.

Special Populations

Pregnancy/Breast-feeding: Animal studies suggest that epoetin may enter fetal circulation. Epoetin should be taken during pregnancy only if your doctor determines that the potential benefit outweighs the risks.

It is not known if epoetin passes into breast milk. Nursing mothers who must take this drug should use infant formula.

Seniors: Seniors may use this product without special precaution.

Type of Drug

Erectile Dysfunction Drugs

Brand Names

Generic Ingredients: Sildenafil Citrate
Revatio
Viagra

Generic Ingredients: Tadalafil
Adcirca
Cialis

Generic Ingredients: Vardenafil
Levitra
Staxyn

Prescribed For

Erectile dysfunction (ED). Sildenafil and tadalafil are also prescribed for pulmonary arterial hypertension. Tadalafil is also prescribed for benign prostatic hyperplasia (BPH; enlarged prostate).

General Information

The chemical nitric oxide is released in the penis during sexual stimulation. Nitric oxide causes the release of an enzyme called cyclic guanosine monophosphate (cGMP), which increases blood flow into the penis, producing an erection. cGMP is broken down by the enzyme phosphodiesterase type 5 (PDE5). In men with low levels of cGMP, these medicines help achieve and maintain an erection by inhibiting PDE5, thus causing higher levels of cGMP. ED can be the result of nerve, blood vessel, or psychological problems. These drugs, which are effective in about 70% of men, only help when poor blood flow is the cause of the dysfunction. These medicines start working in 30–60 minutes and their effects usually last from 2–4 hours, although some have noted an effect for 24 hours or more. Some drug interactions and kidney or liver diseases extend this time. Tadalafil begins working in 30–60 minutes and can remain in the body for more than 2 days, much longer than the other medicines in this group. Low-dose tadalafil may be taken every day for chronic ED.

Pulmonary arterial hypertension, a rare disease in which the blood flow between the heart and lungs is reduced because the vessels have become stiff and narrow, is also treated with sildenafil and tadalafil.

Cautions and Warnings

Do not take these drugs if you are **allergic** or **sensitive** to any of their ingredients.

These medicines lower **blood pressure** and should be avoided if you have high (greater than 170/100) or low (less than 90/50) blood pressure. Several people have died from a sudden blood-pressure drop after combining ED medications with other medications that can reduce blood pressure.

These medicines should never be taken by those taking heart medications called **nitrates**, as fatal reactions have occurred.

Sexual activity may be a cardiac risk in men with pre-existing **heart disease**. People with heart disease for whom sexual activity is not recommended should not take these medications.

Avoid these medicines if you have had a **heart attack**, **stroke**, or life-threatening **abnormal heart rhythms** in the past 6 months, or if you have **heart failure**, unstable **angina pectoris**, **damage to the penis**, or a progressive eye disease called **retinitis pigmentosa**. Vision and hearing loss have rarely been reported with use of these medications. Contact your doctor immediately if you experience any kind of vision or hearing disturbance while taking one of these medications.

People taking sildenafil or vardenafil have experienced difficulties seeing blue or green colors and may see things with a blue tinge surrounding them. This happens because they affect an enzyme in the eye. The effect clears up after the drug passes out of the body.

People with **kidney or liver damage** retain these medicines in their bodies longer than people whose kidneys and liver function normally. People with kidney or liver problems should always begin with the lowest possible dosage. Those with severe disease should avoid these medicines.

Rarely, people have experienced **priapism** (a persistent, painful erection) after using ED drugs. Patients with a condition that predisposes them to priapism—such as **leukemia, multiple myeloma**, or **sickle cell anemia**—should be cautious about taking these medicines.

Vardenafil and sildenafil should be avoided by people with **stomach or bleeding ulcers** because its effect on these conditions is not known.

Possible Side Effects

Sildenafil

▼ Most common: headache and flushing.

▼ Less common: upset stomach, stuffy nose, urinary tract infection, diarrhea, rash, dizziness, seizure, anxiety, double

Possible Side Effects *(continued)*

vision, visual changes, bloodshot eyes, burning eyes, swelling in the eye, and blood vessel diseases in the retina.

- ▼ Rare: priapism (a persistent, painful erection). Other rare side effects can occur in almost any part of the body. Contact your doctor if you experience anything unusual while taking any medication.

Tadalafil

- ▼ Most common: headache.
- ▼ Common: upset stomach. Back pain and muscle aches can develop 12–24 hours after taking tadalafil and go away on their own after 2 days.
- ▼ Less common: flushing, nasal congestion, and arm or leg pain.
- ▼ Rare: priapism (a persistent, painful erection). Other rare side effects can occur in almost any part of the body. Contact your doctor if you experience anything unusual while taking any medication.

Vardenafil

- ▼ Most common: headache and flushing.
- ▼ Less common: upset stomach, sinus infection, flu-like symptoms, dizziness, and nausea.
- ▼ Rare: priapism (a persistent, painful erection). Other rare side effects can occur in almost any part of the body. Contact your doctor if you experience anything unusual while taking any medication.

Drug Interactions

- Do not combine any of these drugs with nitrates (such as nitroglycerin) and other drugs that lower blood pressure. The combination can cause a sudden, rapid drop in blood pressure.
- Do not combine sildenafil, tadalafil, and vardenafil. The effects of combining these drugs are not known.
- Do not take vardenafil if you are taking any medicine to treat an abnormal heartbeat, including amiodarone, quinidine, and sotalol.
- Caution should be used when combining one of these medications with an alpha blocker (such as alfuzosin, doxazosin, prazosin, tamsulosin, or terazosin).

- Macrolide antibiotics such as erythromycin, azole antifungals such as itraconazole or ketoconazole, and protease inhibitors such as ritonavir or saquinavir (used to combat HIV) can cause blood levels of these medications to increase substantially. Your ED medication dosage may need reducing if you are taking one of these drugs.
- Rifampin can be expected to reduce the effect of these medicines by reducing the amount of drug in the blood. Other drugs that may reduce the effects of these drugs are bosentan, carbamazepine, phenobarbital, and phenytoin. Sildenafil may increase levels of bosentan.
- Combining sildenafil with cimetidine, ciprofloxacin, or delavirdine may lead to a substantial increase in the amount of sildenafil in the blood. Ciprofloxacin and other quinolones may increase levels of vardenafil.
- Selective serotonin reuptake inhibitor (SSRI) antidepressants and tacrolimus may increase sildenafil concentrations in the blood. Dosage reductions of sildenafil may be necessary if you are taking these medications.
- Substantial alcohol consumption (more than 5 drinks) adds to the blood-pressure-lowering effects of these medicines.

Food Interactions

Grapefruit juice may increase the amount of these drugs in the blood. Taking sildenafil with a high-fat meal reduces the amount of drug absorbed. Tadalafil and vardenafil can be taken without regard to food or meals.

Usual Dose

Sildenafil

Erectile Dysfunction

Adult: 50 mg taken about 1 hour before sexual activity. Individual doses can range from 25–100 mg. The maximum dosing frequency is once a day.

Senior: Begin with 25 mg and gradually increase dosage as needed.

Pulmonary Arterial Hypertension

Adult: 20 mg taken 3 times a day, every 4–6 hours.

Tadalafil

BPH

Adult: 5 mg taken once a day.

Erectile Dysfunction

Adult: for occasional use, 10 mg taken about 1 hour before sexual activity. Individual doses can range from 5–20 mg. Do not take more than 1 dose of tadalafil a day. For chronic ED, 2.5 mg a day.

Senior: Begin with 5 mg and gradually increase dosage as needed.

Pulmonary Arterial Hypertension

Adult: 40 mg taken once a day.

Vardenafil

Adult: 10 mg taken about 1 hour before sexual activity. Individual doses can range from 5–20 mg.

Senior: Begin with 5 mg and gradually increase dosage as needed.

Overdosage

Sildenafil and tadalafil overdose are likely to produce exaggerated drug side effects. Vardenafil overdose may cause neck pain, muscle aches, or vision changes. Contact your local poison control center or hospital emergency room for more information. If you seek treatment, ALWAYS bring the prescription bottle or container.

Special Information

Contact your doctor and do not engage in sexual activity if the erection produced by ED drugs is painful or lasts 4 or more hours, or if you experience dizziness, nausea, or chest pain after taking an ED drug. In rare cases, men taking ED drugs have reported a sudden decrease or loss of vision and/or hearing. Contact your doctor right away if you experience this adverse side effect.

People who use organic nitrates for gardening or other purposes can experience a severe and dangerous blood pressure drop if they take sildenafil or vardenafil. It is not known how long you have to wait to resume nitrate use.

These drugs do not protect against sexually transmitted diseases.

Special Populations

Pregnancy/Breast-feeding: There is no evidence that these drugs harm the fetus; however, they are not intended for pregnant women or nursing mothers.

Seniors: Men age 65 and over eliminate these drugs more slowly than younger men and should begin with the lowest possible dosage.

Generic Name

Ergoloid Mesylates

(ER-goe-loid MES-il-ates) G

Brand Names

Hydergine

Type of Drug

Psychotherapeutic agent.

Prescribed For

Age-related decline in mental capacity.

General Information

Ergoloid mesylates are used to treat decreased mental capacity of unknown cause in people over age 60. These drugs should not be used for any condition that is treatable with another drug or that may be reversible. People who respond to ergoloid mesylates are likely to have Alzheimer's disease or some other cause of dementia. Nobody knows exactly how ergoloid mesylates produce their effect, but they improve the supply of blood to the brain in test animals, reduce their heart rate, and improve muscle tone in blood vessels. Some studies show the drugs to be very effective in relieving mild symptoms of mental impairment, while others find it to be only moderately effective. They are most beneficial in people whose symptoms are due to the effects of high blood pressure in the brain.

Cautions and Warnings

Do not take ergoloid mesylates if you are **allergic** or **sensitive** to any of their ingredients or you have **psychotic symptoms** or **psychosis**.

Ergoloid mesylates should be used with caution in people with **liver disease**, **low blood pressure**, or **slow heartbeat**.

Possible Side Effects

Ergoloid mesylates do not produce serious side effects.

▼ Common: When taken under the tongue, these drugs may cause irritation, nausea, or upset stomach. Other side effects are drowsiness, slow heartbeat, and rash.

Drug Interactions

None known.

Food Interactions

Do not eat, drink, or smoke while you have an ergoloid mesylate pill under your tongue.

Usual Dose

Starting dose is 1–2 mg 3 times a day. Increase as needed. Do not exceed 12 mg a day.

Overdosage

Symptoms include blurred vision, dizziness, fainting, flushing, headache, appetite loss, nausea, vomiting, stomach cramps, and stuffy nose. Take the victim to a hospital emergency room. If you seek treatment, ALWAYS bring the prescription bottle or container.

Special Information

The effects of ergoloid mesylates are gradual and frequently not seen for up to 6 months. A 6-month period of treatment with ergoloid mesylates is recommended before your doctor can fully evaluate your response to the drug. Your doctor should periodically reevaluate your condition to determine if ergoloid mesylate treatment is still needed and that it is working for you.

Dissolve sublingual tablets under the tongue. Do not chew or crush them; they are not effective if swallowed whole.

If you forget a dose, skip it and go back to your regular schedule. Do not take a double dose. Contact your doctor if you miss 2 or more consecutive doses.

Special Populations

Pregnancy/Breast-feeding: Ergoloid mesylates may interfere with fetal development. Ergoloid mesylates should be taken during pregnancy only if your doctor determines that the potential benefit outweighs the risks.

Ergoloid mesylates pass into breast milk. Nursing mothers who must take these drugs should use infant formula.

Seniors: Seniors are more likely to develop side effects, especially hypothermia (low body temperature).

Generic Name

Erythromycin (eh-rith-roe-MYE-sin) G

Brand Names

Akne-Mycin
E-Glades
Eryc
Erygel
Ery-Tab
Erythra-Derm
Erythro-Statin
PCE

The information in this profile also applies to the following drugs:

Generic Ingredients: Clarithromycin G
Biaxin
Biaxin XL

Generic Ingredients: Erythromycin Ethylsuccinate G
E.E.S.
EryPed
Pediamycin

Generic Ingredients: Erythromycin Stearate G
Erythrocin Stearate

Combination Products
Generic Ingredients: Clarithromycin + Amoxicillin + Lansoprazole
Prevpac

Generic Ingredients: Clarithromycin + Amoxicillin + Omeprazole G

Generic Ingredients: Erythromycin Ethylsuccinate + Sulfisoxazole G

Type of Drug

Macrolide antibiotic.

Prescribed For

Infections of virtually any part of the body, including upper- and lower-respiratory tract; urinary tract; intestinal tract; skin; mouth, gums, or teeth; and nose, ears, or sinuses; as well as sexually transmitted diseases, acne, diphtheria, dysentery, ulcers, and stomach inflammation. Also prescribed for Legionnaires' disease, rheumatic fever, whooping cough, bacterial endocarditis, and pelvic inflammatory disease. The eye ointment is used to prevent newborn gonococcal or chlamydial eye infections.

General Information

Erythromycin and other macrolide antibiotics are either bactericidal (bacteria-killing) or bacteriostatic (inhibiting bacterial growth), depending on the organism in question and amount of antibiotic present. Clarithromycin is used to fight *Helicobacter pylori* infection, which is present in almost all ulcers and most cases of stomach inflammation. Erythromycin is deactivated by stomach acid, so the tablet form is made to bypass the stomach and dissolve in the intestine.

Erythromycin is used instead of penicillin for mild to moderate infections in people who are allergic to penicillin. Erythromycin is not the antibiotic of choice for severe infections.

Cautions and Warnings

Do not take these drugs if you are **allergic** or **sensitive** to any of their ingredients or to any macrolide antibiotic. Serious allergic reactions are possible.

These drugs are excreted primarily through the liver. People with **jaundice** or **liver disease or damage** resulting from previous treatment with clarithromycin should not take it again, and anyone with liver disease should consult their doctor before taking erythromycin. Those on long-term therapy with erythromycin should have periodic blood tests. If you restart erythromycin after having experienced liver damage, it is likely that symptoms will recur within 48 hours. Liver failure is rare.

A serious condition known as infantile hypertrophic pyloric stenosis (IHPS) has occurred in babies treated with erythromycin. This condition may require intestinal surgery.

Colitis (bowel inflammation) has been associated with all antibiotics and can range from mild to life-threatening (see "Possible Side Effects"). Clarithromycin may be gentler on the digestive tract than erythromycin.

Patients with impaired kidney function require reduced dosages of clarithromycin.

After using topical erythromycin for acne treatment, skin irritation may occur, especially if abrasive agents to remove dead skin cells are used concurrently.

Erythromycin can worsen symptoms of **myasthenia gravis** and bring on new ones.

Possible Side Effects

- ▼ Most common: loss of appetite; abnormal taste; diarrhea; nausea; vomiting; stomach cramps, pain, or upset; and headache. Colitis (symptoms include severe abdominal cramps and severe, persistent, and possibly bloody diarrhea) may develop. Side effects of the topical erythromycin include peeling, dryness, itching, and oiliness.
- ▼ Less common: hairy tongue, itching, irritation of the anal or vaginal region, eye irritation, and skin tenderness. If any of these symptoms appear, contact your physician immediately.
- ▼ Rare: abnormal heart rhythms; allergic reactions; convulsions; inflammation of the pancreas; liver damage; mental status changes, including anxiety, confusion, and hallucinations; changes in levels of red and white blood cells and platelets; and hearing loss, which reverses itself after the drug is stopped and occurs most often in people with liver and kidney problems. Contact your doctor if you experience anything unusual while taking any medication.

For more information on combination products, see Proton-Pump Inhibitors, page 956, and Sulfa Drugs, page 1075.

Drug Interactions

- Do not combine these drugs with astemizole, cisapride, diltiazem, eletriptan, pimozide, ranolazine, or terfenadine. Serious side effects, including death, have occurred with some of these combinations. Doses of macrolide antibiotics and eletriptan should be separated by at least 72 hours.
- Colchicine should not be mixed with erythromycin at all and should not be used with clarithromycin if you have liver or kidney disease.
- Combining these drugs with carbamazepine may lead to serious side effects. Do not combine them unless there is no alternative.
- When these medications are combined with medications to treat heart rhythm disorders (antiarrhythmics, including amiodarone, bretylium, disopyramide, dofetilide, quinidine, and sotalol), the risk of dangerous, abnormal heart rhythms may be increased.

- Combining these drugs with alfentanil (an injectable pain reliever), benzodiazepines (such as alprazolam, diazepam, midazolam, and triazolam), bromocriptine, buspirone, cabergoline, cilostazol, cyclosporine, digoxin, erectile dysfunction medications (sildenafil, tadalafil, vardenafil), methylprednisolone (a corticosteroid), quetiapine, repaglinide, tacrolimus, verapamil, or warfarin may increase the effects of these drugs. Your doctor should monitor your condition closely.
- Mixing these medicines with a statin cholesterol-lowering drug increases the risk of developing a potentially fatal condition involving severe muscle pain and destruction.
- These medications may reduce the beneficial effects of clopidogrel.
- Mixing these drugs with rifabutin or rifampin can interfere with the antibiotic's effect and increase the risk of intestinal side effects.
- Do not combine clarithromycin with conivaptan, dihydroergotamine, eplerenone, or ergotamine.
- People who have had porphyria in the past (symptoms include abdominal pain, light sensitivity, rash, and convulsions) should not take clarithromycin with ranitidine.
- Do not mix erythromycin with the fluoroquinolone levofloxacin to avoid severe, possibly fatal, abnormal heart rhythms. Moxifloxicin should be used with caution.
- The effects of the following drugs may be increased when combined with erythromycin: clozapine, ergotamine and dihydroergotamine, felodipine, or vinblastine. Your doctor should monitor your condition closely.
- Mixing erythromycin with aminophylline and theophylline may decrease the antibacterial effects of erythromycin as well as interfere with the elimination of theophylline from the body, possibly leading to theophylline overdose.
- Erythromycin may neutralize the effects of chloramphenicol and the antibiotics clindomycin and lincomycin.
- Combining clarithromycin and omeprazole raises the amount of both drugs in the blood. Blood levels of other proton-pump inhibitors such as esomeprazole and lansoprazole may be increased when given with clarithromycin as well.
- Combining zidovudine (an HIV drug also known as AZT) and clarithromycin may affect the amount of zidovudine in the bloodstream.

- Cimetidine may reduce the beneficial effects of clarithromycin.
- Taking clarithromycin with fluconazole and ritonavir increases blood levels of clarithromycin. Your clarithromycin dosage should be reduced if you have moderate or severe kidney disease and require ritonavir.

For more information on combination products, see Proton-Pump Inhibitors, page 956, and Sulfa Drugs, page 1075.

Food Interactions

Grapefruit juice slows the breakdown of erythromycin, increasing the amount of drug in the blood. For optimum effectiveness, take erythromycin base and erythromycin stearate on an empty stomach with a 6–8 oz. glass of water at least 30 minutes (and preferably 2 hours) before meals. Other forms of erythromycin can be taken without regard to food or meals.

Clarithromycin can be generally taken without regard to food or meals; however, Biaxin XL should be taken with food.

Usual Dose

Infection

Clarithromycin

Adult: 250–500 mg every 12 hours (1000 mg once a day for Biaxin XL) for 7–14 days. Dosage must be reduced in people with severe kidney disease.

Child (age 6 months and over): 3.4 mg per lb. of body weight every 12 hours, up to 500 mg a dose, depending on the infecting organism, for 10 days.

Erythromycin

Eye Ointment: ½ in. 2–6 times a day.

Tablet and Suspension

Adult: 250–500 mg every 6–12 hours for 10–14 days for most conditions. Maximum dose is 4 g a day.

Child: 14–23 mg per lb. of body weight a day in divided doses depending on age, weight, and severity of infection.

Topical Solution: Apply morning and night.

Ulcer

Clarithromycin + Amoxicillin + Lansoprazole

Adult: 500/1000/30 mg every 12 hours for 10–14 days.

Child: not recommended.

Clarithromycin + Amoxicillin + Omeprazole

Adult: 500/1000/20 mg every 12 hours for 10 days. Omeprezole 20 mg may need to be continued for an additional 18 days to aid ulcer healing.

Child: not recommended.

Overdosage

Overdose may cause severe side effects, especially nausea, vomiting, stomach cramps, and diarrhea. Mild hearing loss, ringing or buzzing in the ears, or fainting may also occur. Contact your local poison control center or a hospital emergency room for more information. If you seek treatment, ALWAYS bring the prescription bottle or container.

Special Information

Since the action of this antibiotic depends on its concentration in the invading bacteria, it is crucial that you follow your doctor's directions regarding the spacing of doses as well as the number of days you must take the medication—otherwise, this antibiotic may be much less effective. Erythromycin products should be stored at room temperature, except for oral liquids, which should be kept in the refrigerator. Clarithromycin suspension must be shaken well before each dose. Do NOT store it in the refrigerator.

Contact your doctor if you develop nausea; vomiting; diarrhea; stomach cramps; severe abdominal pain; rash, itching, or redness; dark or amber-colored urine; yellowing of the skin or whites of the eyes; or any severe or persistent side effect.

If you forget a dose of oral erythromycin, take it as soon as you remember. If it is almost time for your next dose, space the next 2 doses over 4–6 hours, then continue with your regular schedule. Do not take a double dose.

Remember to complete the full course of therapy prescribed even if you feel well before you finish the medication.

Special Populations

Pregnancy/Breast-feeding: Erythromycin passes into the fetal circulation but has been used safely. In general, these drugs should be taken during pregnancy only if your doctor determines that the potential benefit outweighs the risks. Clarithromycin should not be used during pregnancy unless absolutely necessary. The extended-release version has been shown to harm a developing fetus.

Erythromycin passes into breast milk; it is not known whether clarithromycin does as well. Nursing mothers who must take these drugs should use infant formula.

Seniors: Seniors with liver disease should use caution when taking erythromycin. Seniors taking high doses of erythromycin may be at an increased risk of hearing loss. Seniors with severe kidney disease need a lower dose of clarithromycin than those with normally functioning kidneys.

Type of Drug

Estrogens (ES-troe-jens)

Brand Names

Generic Ingredients: Conjugated Estrogens G

Premarin
Premarin Cream

Generic Ingredients: Conjugated Estrogens (Synthetic) G

Cenestin
Enjuvia

Generic Ingredients: Conjugated Estrogens + Medroxyprogesterone

Premphase
Prempro

Generic Ingredients: Esterified Estrogens

Menest

Generic Ingredients: Estradiol G

Alora
Climara
Divigel
Elestrin
Estrace
Estraderm
Estrasorb
Estring
Estrogel
Evamist Transdermal Spray
Femring
Femtrace
Menostar
Vagifem
Vivelle
Vivelle-Dot

Generic Ingredients: Estradiol + Drospirenone

Angeliq

Generic Ingredients: Estradiol + Levonorgestrel

Climara Pro

Generic Ingredients: Estradiol + Norethindrone G

Activella
Combipatch

Generic Ingredients: Estradiol + Norgestimate G
Prefest

Generic Ingredients: Estropipate G
Ortho-Est

Generic Ingredients: Ethinyl Estradiol + Etonogestrel
NuvaRing

Generic Ingredients: Ethinyl Estradiol + Norethindrone G
FemHRT 1/5

Prescribed For

Moderate to severe menopausal symptoms such as hot flashes, night sweats and sleep problems, and vaginal dryness and irritation (creams and gels); also prescribed for ovarian failure, osteoporosis prevention, male breast cancer, advanced prostate cancer, abnormal bleeding of the uterus, female castration, Turner's syndrome, and birth control.

General Information

Six estrogens have been identified in women but only 3 are present in large amounts: estradiol, estrone, and estriol. Estradiol is the most potent and most important. Other estrogens are produced by chemical conversions in the body. Estradiol, for example, is transformed into estrone, which in turn becomes estriol. Estrogens all have the same actions and side effects; only potency varies. More potent types require smaller dosages to produce the same effect.

Millions of women have taken hormone replacement therapy (HRT) to manage menopausal symptoms, but studies show that HRT does not improve quality of life for most. Women who experience severe menopause symptoms must weigh the benefits of prolonged HRT against its risks.

Estrogens are largely responsible for the growth and maintenance of the female reproductive system and sex characteristics. They affect the release of hormones from the pituitary gland (controller of hormone production and regulator of basic bodily functions). These hormones control the functioning of capillaries (smallest blood vessels), may cause fluid retention, affect protein breakdown in the body, prevent ovulation and breast engorgement after childbirth, and influence the shaping and maintenance of the skeleton through an effect on calcium.

Estrogen products differ in their hormone content and dosage. Some may affect one part of the body more than another. Generally, though, estrogens are interchangeable as long as dosage differences are taken into account.

The results of a very large study called the Women's Health Initiative (WHI), first published in 2002 and since updated with new reports, have drastically changed the face of estrogen replacement therapy by shedding new light on the risks and benefits of this treatment. In terms of heart disease and stroke, the results are mixed. Among women age 50–59 taking estrogen who had had menopause for less than 10 years, the study showed a small but unimportant reduction in heart disease risk, but the study also revealed a small but insignificant increase in the risk of nonfatal heart attacks among all postmenopausal women. In contrast, in the women age 50–79 taking an estrogen without a progestin (e.g., medroxyprogesterone), the risk of a stroke was increased by 36% in the WHI study. Moreover, the risk of spontaneous blood clot formation increased by 53% in women taking an estrogen-only product and doubled in women taking an estrogen-progestin product.

The risk of cancer in women's reproductive organs is generally increased with estrogen treatment, especially if the estrogens have been taken for long periods of time. In the WHI, the risk of invasive breast cancer was increased 24% among women taking estrogen—which meant over 1 year, there were 8 more cases of invasive breast cancer among women taking estrogens for every 10,000 women in the study. However, the risk of invasive breast cancer probably does not increase until estrogen replacement has been taken for at least 7 years. Another study of women with breast cancer found those who took estrogens were 86% more likely to have breast cancer, an increase of 21 cases per 10,000 women studied for 1 year. In the WHI, breast cancer tumors were also harder to detect in women taking estrogen. Several studies have shown that using estrogen without a progestin increases the risk of endometrial cancer by 4.5–24 times in postmenopausal women taking them for 10 years or more; the actual increase in risk depends on the dosage and how long you take the drug. What's more, the risk remains 8–15 years after the estrogen treatment is stopped. The risk does not appear to be increased if an estrogen-only product is used for a year or less.

The WHI study did show some benefits of long-term hormone replacement in colon cancer and osteoporosis, but these benefits may not outweigh the risks of HRT.

Cautions and Warnings

Do not take estrogens if you are **allergic** or **sensitive** to any of their ingredients.

Do not use an estrogen product if you currently have or have had in the past one of the following conditions: **estrogen-dependent cancer**, **breast cancer** (unless you are being treated for **breast cancer that has spread**), **stroke**, **heart attack**, **blood-clotting problems**, **liver damage or disease**, **thrombophlebitis**, or **abnormal vaginal bleeding** with an unknown cause.

Stop taking estrogen at the first sign of a stroke, heart attack, or blood-clotting problem. Estrogen-containing products should be stopped 4–6 weeks before **surgery** or if you will be unable to **get out of bed or move** for an extended period of time.

Products containing an estrogen and a progestin should not be used for the prevention or treatment of **bladder-control problems**, **heart disease**, or **mental decline (dementia)**. In fact, estrogen use increases the risk of dementia.

Women who choose HRT for menopausal symptoms should take the lowest effective dose for the shortest possible time to minimize the risks associated with these medicines, which include breast, endometrial, and ovarian cancer; stroke and blood clots; and nonfatal heart attacks (but not heart disease). Using estrogen without a progestin increases the risk of endometrial cancer.

Women who have had a **hysterectomy** and are taking an estrogen-progestin product have a greater risk of breast cancer than those taking estrogen alone.

Estrogens may lead to abnormal mammograms.

Women who smoke cigarettes, especially those over age 35, and take estrogen have a greater risk of cardiovascular side effects, including stroke, hardening of the arteries, and blood clots. The risk increases with age and tobacco use.

Women with a strong **family history of breast cancer** or those who have **breast nodules or cysts** or an **abnormal mammogram** should be cautious about using estrogens. Women taking an estrogen for **breast cancer that has spread to their bones** can develop large increases in blood calcium. On the other hand, women with an **underactive parathyroid gland**, which produces a hormone essential to calcium balance in the body, risk developing low blood calcium if they take an estrogen.

Postmenopausal women taking estrogen are 2–4 times more likely to develop gallbladder disease.

Estrogens can cause significant increases in blood triglycerides and cause pancreas inflammation in women with **inherited blood-fat disorders**. Estrogens can also increase blood-glucose levels and should be used with caution in people with **diabetes**.

Estrogens can sometimes raise blood pressure. Pressure usually returns to normal when the drug is stopped.

Other conditions that may be worsened by estrogens include **asthma**, **epilepsy**, **migraine**, or **porphyria**.

Estrogens should not be used to treat painful **breast enlargement** that sometimes develops after giving birth.

Vaginal estrogen cream may stimulate bleeding of the uterus. It may also cause breast tenderness, vaginal discharge, and withdrawal bleeding if the product is suddenly stopped. Women with **endometriosis** may experience heavy vaginal bleeding, unless the estrogen is used for a year or less.

Estrogens can cause visual problems, including blindness, double vision, or bulging of the eye. They may also cause migraines.

Drospirenone, a progestin and an ingredient in Angeliq, can raise blood-potassium levels in some people because it opposes the hormone aldosterone. It should not be used in people with conditions that can lead to high blood potassium such as **kidney disease** or a **poorly functioning adrenal gland**. Your doctor may want to check your blood-potassium level if you might be at risk of high blood potassium.

Possible Side Effects

- ▼ Most common: breast enlargement or tenderness, ankle and leg swelling, appetite loss, weight changes, water retention and bloating, nausea, vomiting, and abdominal cramps. The estrogen patch may cause rash, irritation, and redness where it is applied.
- ▼ Less common: bleeding gums, breakthrough vaginal bleeding, vaginal spotting or discharge, changes in menstrual flow, painful menstruation, premenstrual syndrome, absence of menstrual periods during and after estrogen use, uterine fibroid enlargement, vaginal *Candida* infection,

Possible Side Effects *(continued)*

cystitis, mild diarrhea, yellowing of the skin or whites of the eyes, eye lesions, contact lens intolerance, rash, hair loss, development of new hairy patches, migraine, mild dizziness, depression, increased sex drive (women), and decreased sex drive (men).

▼ Rare: stroke, blood-clot formation, dribbling or sudden passage of urine, loss of coordination, chest pain, leg pain, breathing difficulties, slurred speech, and changes in vision. Women using a vaginal ring product rarely develop toxic shock syndrome or bowel obstruction, and the ring may stick to the vaginal wall. Men who take large estrogen dosages for prostate cancer have a greater risk of heart attack, phlebitis, and blood clots in the lungs.

Drug Interactions

- Tranexamic acid increases the risk of a blood-clotting event in women taking estrogen-progestin combinations. Avoid mixing these drugs unless there is a strong medical need.
- Drosperinone should be used with caution by women who are also taking other medicines that raise blood potassium, such as nonsteroidal anti-inflammatory drugs (NSAIDs), potassium-sparing diuretics, potassium supplements, angiotensin-converting enzyme (ACE) inhibitors, AII-receptor antagonists, and heparin.
- Estrogen may interfere with hydantoin anticonvulsants (e.g., phenytoin) and make them less effective, and estrogen-progestin combinations may reduce the effectiveness of lamotrigine and valproic acid; dosage adjustments may be necessary to control seizures.
- Hydantoins and topiramate may interfere with estrogen's effects.
- Estrogens may reduce the effect of oral anticoagulant (blood thinning) drugs such as warfarin. Your anticoagulant dosage may need an adjustment.
- Estrogens may increase the side effects of antidepressants.
- Estrogens may increase corticosteroid blood levels. Dosage adjustments may be needed.
- Estrogens may reduce the effectiveness of thyroid replacement therapy.

- Blood levels and side effects of estrogen may be increased by the following drugs: itraconazole, ketoconazole, macrolide antibiotics, and ritonavir.
- Rifampin, barbiturates, carbamazepine, St. John's wort, and other drugs that stimulate the liver to break down drugs may reduce estrogen blood levels.
- Aprepitant, felbimate, griseofulvin, nevirapine, penicillins, and tetracycline may reduce the effectiveness of estrogen-progestin combinations.
- Estrogen-progestin combination products may increase the effects of beta blockers, cyclosporine, selegiline, tacrolimus, theophyllines, and tizanidine. Dosage adjustments may be necessary.
- Estrogens interfere with many diagnostic tests. Make sure your doctor knows you are taking estrogen before conducting any blood tests or other diagnostic procedures.

Food Interactions

Estrogens may be taken with food to reduce nausea and upset stomach. Avoid drinking grapefruit juice if you are taking this drug.

Usual Dose

Dosage varies. All of these products, including the transdermal skin patch, may be taken continuously or on a cyclic schedule of 3 weeks on, 1 week off.

Estradiol Gel: Spread 1 pumpful (1.25 g) of the gel as thinly as possible over the entire area on the inside and outside of your arm from wrist to shoulder, once a day at the same time every day.

Estradiol Ring

Insert once every 3 months.

Estradiol Transdermal Patch (0.014, 0.025, 0.0375, 0.05, 0.06, 0.075, or 0.1 mg)

Alora, Estraderm, Vivelle, and Vivelle-Dot: 1 patch twice a week; or use 1 patch twice a week for 3 weeks, stop for 1 week, then start again.

Climara and Menostar: 1 patch every week; or use 1 patch once a week for 3 weeks, stop for 1 week, then start again.

Estradiol Transdermal Spray: 1–3 sprays (1.53 mg estradiol in each spray) applied next to each other every morning on the inner surface of the forearm, starting near the elbow. Do not allow the sprays to overlap each other. Allow the spray to dry for about 2 minutes and do not wash the arm for 30 minutes. Do not apply the spray to any other part of the body. Take care to avoid accidentally exposing your children or pets to this product. It is absorbed through the skin and will exert an effect on their bodies.

Tablets

Conjugated Estrogens: 0.3–30 mg a day.
Conjugated Estrogens, Synthetic: 0.3–1.25 mg a day.
Esterified Estrogens: 0.3–30 mg a day.
Estradiol: 0.5–30 mg a day.
Estropipate: 0.75–9 mg a day.

Vaginal Cream

Conjugated Estrogens: 0.5–2 g a day for 3 weeks, stop for 1 week, then start again.

Estradiol: 2–4 g a day for 1–2 weeks, 1–2 g a day for another 1–2 weeks, then 1 g 1–3 times a week.

Overdosage

Symptoms may include nausea and vaginal bleeding in adult women. Contact your local poison control center or a hospital emergency room for information. If you seek treatment, ALWAYS bring the prescription bottle or container.

Special Information

Contact your doctor if you develop breast pain or tenderness, swelling of the feet and lower legs, rapid weight gain, chest pain, breathing difficulties, pain in the groin or calves, unusual or persistent vaginal bleeding, missed menstrual period, lumps in the breast, sudden severe headache, migraine, dizziness or fainting, disturbances in speech or vision, weakness or numbness in the arms or legs, abdominal pain, sudden severe vomiting, depression, yellowing of the skin or whites of the eyes, or jerky or involuntary muscle movement.

Women taking estrogens or combined estrogen and progestin therapy should have yearly breast exams, perform monthly breast self-examinations, and have regular mammograms.

Talk to your health care provider about ways to reduce risk factors for heart disease (blood-pressure control, improving your diet, stopping tobacco use) and osteoporosis (an appropriate diet, vitamin D and calcium supplements, weight-bearing exercise).

Your doctor should reevaluate your need for estrogen vaginal cream every 36 months. Do not stop using the drug suddenly because this may increase your risk of developing unpredicted or breakthrough vaginal bleeding.

Estrogen skin patches should be applied to a clean, dry, non-oily, hairless area of intact skin, preferably on the abdomen. Do not apply it to your breasts or waist, or to any area where tight-fitting clothes may loosen the patch from your skin. The application site should be rotated to prevent irritation, and each site should have a patch-free period for 7 days.

Good dental hygiene is important while taking estrogen because estrogen may increase your risk of oral infection. Dental work should be completed prior to starting estrogen, if possible.

Vaginal estrogen cream should be inserted high into the vagina, about ⅔ of the length of the applicator.

Press the vaginal ring into an oval and insert as deeply as possible in the upper ⅓ of the vagina.

Some of these products contain tartrazine (a commonly used orange dye and food coloring). If you are allergic to tartrazine or have asthma, check with your pharmacist to find out if your estrogen product contains this coloring agent.

If you forget a dose, take it as soon as you remember. If it is almost time for your next dose, skip the one you forgot and continue with your regular schedule. Do not take a double dose.

Authorities note that the risk of serious complications for an individual woman taking HRT is very small. Thus, you may decide to take hormones but your decision should be based on a complete discussion of the facts and your individual situation with your doctor. Continue to talk with your doctor regularly about weighing the risks against the benefits of taking estrogen.

Special Populations

Pregnancy/Breast-feeding: Estrogens harm the fetus and should never be used during pregnancy for any reason.

Estrogens pass into breast milk and reduce its flow. Nursing mothers who must take them should use infant formula.

Seniors: The risk of side effects increases with age, especially if you smoke. Women age 65 or older taking estrogens may be more likely to develop a stroke, blood clot, or dementia.

Generic Name

Etanercept (eh-TAN-er-sept)

Brand Names

Enbrel

Type of Drug

Immune system modulator.

Prescribed For

Rheumatoid arthritis, juvenile rheumatoid arthritis, psoriatic arthritis, ankylosing spondylitis, and psoriasis.

General Information

Etanercept binds to a specific protein in the body known as tumor necrosis factor (TNF) and blocks it from interacting with cell surfaces. TNF is involved in normal inflammatory and immune responses and the inflammatory processes of rheumatoid arthritis, juvenile rheumatoid arthritis, and other conditions. Etanercept can also interfere with biological actions that are either caused or regulated by TNF.

Cautions and Warnings

Do not use etanercept if you are **allergic** or **sensitive** to any of its ingredients.

Serious infections (including tuberculosis), blood and other cancers, and psoriasis are more likely to occur in people using etanercept because of its ability to suppress the immune response. Infections may be more common in people with other conditions, such as advanced or uncontrolled **diabetes**, or those who are taking other medications that predispose them to infections. People who have previously been infected with **tuberculosis** or **hepatitis B** are at higher risk for reinfection or activation of dormant illness.

Do not take etanercept if you have a bacterial infection of the blood or tissues called **sepsis**.

Levels of blood platelets and some white blood cells may be reduced in rare cases, leading to persistent fever, bruising, bleeding, and pale skin. Contact your doctor if any of these symptoms develop. Etanercept should be used with caution by those with existing **blood disorders**.

Etanercept may increase the risk of some nervous system disorders, including multiple sclerosis.

Etanercept may cause or worsen **congestive heart failure**.

Etanercept should be used with caution by those with moderate to severe **liver disease**.

In rare cases, people taking etanercept have developed a lupus-like syndrome that may disappear when the drug is discontinued.

People taking etanercept should not receive any live vaccines, because the body may not be able to respond as expected to the vaccine. Patients being treated for **juvenile idiopathic arthritis** should be brought up to date with their childhood vaccinations before beginning therapy with etanercept.

People taking a medication for **diabetes** may experience a drop in blood glucose while taking etanercept. Monitor blood-glucose levels and adjust your antidiabetes medication as needed.

Possible Side Effects

Reactions may develop at the site where etanercept is injected. Injection sites should be rotated among the thigh, abdomen, and upper arm to avoid excessive bruising or other skin damage.

- ▼ Most common: infection, injection-site reactions, upper-respiratory infection, headache, and runny nose.
- ▼ Common: nausea, dizziness, sore throat, cough, weakness, abdominal pain, rash, and respiratory problems.
- ▼ Less common: upset stomach, sinus irritation, vomiting, swelling in the legs or feet, mouth sores, and hair loss.
- ▼ Rare: malignancy, stroke, seizure, tingling in the hands or feet, nervous system irritation similar to multiple sclerosis, eye inflammation, joint pain, generalized pain, appetite loss, blood vessel inflammation in the skin, dry eyes, lumps under the skin, fever, flu-like symptoms, weight gain, chest pain, flushing, diarrhea, taste changes, difficulty breathing, worsening of existing lung conditions, itching, and skin reactions. Contact your doctor if you experience anything unusual while taking any medication.

Drug Interactions

- Do not mix etanercept in the same syringe as another drug.
- Etanercept should not be taken with anakinra, abatacept, cyclophosphamide, or tocilizumab. Serious infections are possible with these combinations.
- The use of etanercept in people with Wegener granulomatosis (a rare blood vessel disorder) who are receiving immunosuppressive agents such as corticosteroids or methotrexate is not recommended.

Food Interactions

None known.

Usual Dose

Adult: rheumatoid arthritis, psoriatic arthritis, ankylosing spondylitis—50 mg a week; plaque psoriasis—50 mg twice a week, reducing to 50 mg a week after 3 months.

Child (age 2–17): 0.36 mg per lb. of body weight, up to 50 mg a week.

Child (under age 2): not recommended.

Overdosage

In one study, a patient accidentally self-administered 62 mg of etanercept twice a week for 3 weeks with no ill effects. Contact your local poison control center or a hospital emergency room for more information. If you seek treatment, ALWAYS bring the prescription container.

Special Information

Etanercept is taken by injection under the skin. You must be trained in proper injection technique by your doctor. Self-injection should be permitted only after your doctor has made sure you know how to do it properly. For more information on how to properly administer this drug, see page 1242.

To mix and inject etanercept: Withdraw all the water supplied with the medicine into a syringe and slowly inject it into the vial containing etanercept. Swirl the mixture gently to avoid excess foaming in the vial. *Do not shake the vial.*

Do not combine etanercept with any other injectable drug.

Etanercept may be stored in a refrigerator for up to 14 days after it is mixed.

Single-use pre-filled syringes must be refrigerated. Do not use past the provided expiration date.

If you forget to administer a dose, do so as soon as you remember. Remember that etanercept doses must be administered at least 3 days apart. Contact your doctor or pharmacist if you have any questions about how to time your etanercept doses.

Special Populations

Pregnancy/Breast-feeding: The safety of using etanercept during pregnancy is not known. Etanercept should be taken during pregnancy only if your doctor determines that the potential benefit outweighs the risks.

It is not known if this drug passes into breast milk. Nursing mothers who must take etanercept should use infant formula.

Seniors: Seniors are more likely to develop infections while using etanercept.

Evista *see **Raloxifene,** page 975*

Generic Name

Exemestane **(ex-eh-MES-tane)** G

Brand Names

Aromasin

Type of Drug

Aromatase inhibitor.

Prescribed For

Breast cancer. Also prescribed for prostate cancer prevention.

General Information

Some breast cancers depend on the presence of the hormone estrogen to stimulate their growth. Depriving these cancers of estrogen is an effective way of treating the condition. Exemestane significantly reduces the amount of estrogen in the blood by binding permanently to an enzyme called aromatase, an essential element in the conversion of androgen (male hormones) to estrogen in premenopausal and postmenopausal women. Exemestane does not affect other hormones in the body. Exemestane is broken down in the liver.

Cautions and Warnings

Do not take exemestane if you are **allergic** or **sensitive** to any of its ingredients.

Exemestane may be prescribed for men and postmenopausal women only.

Possible Side Effects

- ▼ Most common: hot flashes and muscle pain.
- ▼ Common: sweating, hair loss, high blood pressure, sleeplessness, nausea, fatigue, abdominal pain, depression, diarrhea, dizziness, skin rash, headache, anxiety, flu-like

Possible Side Effects *(continued)*

symptoms, high blood pressure, vomiting, leg swelling or other fluid retention, appetite loss, constipation, and coughing.

▼ Less common: increased appetite, fever, weakness, tingling in the hands or feet, broken bones, bronchitis, sinusitis, itching, urinary infection, and swollen lymph glands.

▼ Rare: chest pain; confusion; reduced sensitivity to stimulation; upset stomach; joint, back, or other bone pain; respiratory infection; sore throat; and runny nose. Contact your doctor if you experience anything unusual while taking any medication.

Drug Interactions

- Estrogen-containing drugs reduce the effectiveness of exemestane. Do not combine these drugs.
- Rifampin, phenytoin, carbamazepine, phenobarbital, and St. John's wort may potentially reduce the effectiveness of exemestane.

Food Interactions

Take this drug with a meal. The amount of exemestane absorbed into the blood is increased by 40% when taken with a high-fat meal.

Usual Dose

Adult: 25 mg once a day with or just after a meal. Dose adjustment is not needed in people with kidney or liver disease.

Child: not recommended.

Overdosage

Doses as large as 600 mg have been well tolerated by women with advanced breast cancer. Overdose victims should be taken to a hospital emergency room for evaluation and treatment. If you seek treatment, ALWAYS bring the prescription bottle or container.

Special Information

If you forget a dose, skip the forgotten dose and continue with your regular schedule. Contact your doctor if you skip more than 1 dose.

Special Populations

Pregnancy/Breast-feeding: Exemestane is intended only for postmenopausal women. It can cause birth defects and miscarriage and should not be used by pregnant women or women who may become pregnant.

Exemestane may pass into breast milk. Nursing mothers who must take it should use infant formula.

Seniors: Seniors may take this drug without special precaution.

Exforge *see **Calcium Channel Blockers,** page 224*

Generic Name

Ezetimibe (eh-ZEH-tim-ibe)

Brand Names

Zetia

Combination Product

Generic Ingredients: Ezetimibe + Simvastatin

Vytorin

Type of Drug

Cholesterol-lowering agent.

Prescribed For

High blood cholesterol; also prescribed for two rare genetic disorders called homozygous familial hypercholesterolemia and homozygous sitosterolemia.

General Information

Unlike statin drugs, ezetimibe interferes with the absorption of cholesterol through the intestine and into the bloodstream. Cholesterol-lowering medicines should always be used together with appropriate diet and exercise.

Ezetimibe may be taken alone but is often taken in combination with a statin drug (generally simvastatin), especially in people whose low-density lipoprotein (LDL) cholesterol (i.e., the "bad" cholesterol) remains high despite statin treatment. Vytorin is a brand-name combination of these 2 medications. See Statin Cholesterol-Lowering Agents, page 1065. Your doctor might also prescribe ezetimibe with a fibrate.

Cautions and Warnings

Do not take this drug if you are **allergic** or **sensitive** to any of its ingredients.

Ezetimibe may increase liver enzymes if given with a statin. Your doctor should monitor your liver enzyme levels while you take this medication. People with moderate or severe **liver disease** should not take ezetimibe.

There may be a risk of myopathy (skeletal muscle disorder) with ezetimibe; contact your doctor if you experience any unexplained muscle pain, tenderness, or weakness. Ezetimibe + simvastatin has the same risk of myopathy as simvastatin alone, and this risk increases with increasing simvastatin dosage; see Statin Cholesterol-Lowering Agents, page 1065.

Some people may develop an allergic drug reaction. Symptoms include rash; swelling of the face, lips, and throat; breathing difficulties; fever; a general ill feeling; itching; joint aches; bloodshot or dry eyes; eye burning, itching, or pain; vision changes; or sores that can appear in the mouth or on the skin almost anywhere on the body. Stop taking ezetimibe and contact your doctor immediately if you experience any of these symptoms.

Possible Side Effects

Ezetimibe side effects are similar to those reported by people taking a placebo (sugar pill).

- ▼ Most common: respiratory infection, headache, and muscle ache.
- ▼ Less common: sinus irritation, joint pain, back pain, diarrhea, chest pain, abdominal pain, sore throat, and fatigue.
- ▼ Rare: allergic reactions (see "Cautions and Warnings"). Contact your doctor if you experience anything unusual while taking any medication.

For more information about ezetimibe + simvastatin, see Statin Cholesterol-Lowering Agents, page 1065.

Drug Interactions

- Cholestyramine reduces the amount of ezetimibe absorbed in the blood. Separate these drugs by 2 hours or more.
- Mixing cyclosporine and ezetimibe increases blood levels of both drugs. This combination must be monitored closely by your doctor.

- Fibrates (gemfibrozil, fenofibrate) increase the amount of ezetimibe in the blood, and the use of ezetimibe with fibrates also increases the risk of gallstones. Fibrates other than fenofibrate should not be used with ezetimibe because the risks are not well defined.

For more information about ezetimibe + simvastatin, see Statin Cholesterol-Lowering Agents, page 1065.

Food Interactions

This drug can be taken without regard to food or meals.

Usual Dose

Ezetimibe

Adult and Child (age 10 and over): 10 mg once a day.
Child (age 9 and under): not recommended.

Ezetimibe + Simvastatin

Adult: 10/10–10/40 mg once a day in the evening.

Overdosage

Ezetimibe overdose leads to increased side effects. Contact your local poison control center or a hospital emergency room for information. If you seek treatment, ALWAYS bring the prescription bottle or container.

Special Information

If you are taking more than 1 drug to lower cholesterol or another blood fat, consider the side effects of all of those drugs combined.

If you forget a dose of ezetimibe, take it as soon as you remember. If it is almost time for your next dose, skip the dose you forgot. Do not take more than 1 dose of ezetimibe a day.

Special Populations

Pregnancy/Breast-feeding: Little is known about the effects of ezetimibe during pregnancy. Ezetimibe should be taken during pregnancy only if your doctor determines that the potential benefit outweighs the risks.

It is not known if ezetimibe passes into breast milk. Nursing mothers who must take it should use infant formula.

Seniors: Seniors may use this drug without special precaution.

Generic Name

Ezogabine (ee-ZOE-gah-bean)

Brand Names

Potiga

Type of Drug

Anticonvulsant.

Prescribed For

Adult partial seizures.

General Information

Ezogabine opens calcium channels, stabilizing nerve endings and reducing brain excitability. It may also share the ability to support the activity of gamma-aminobutyric acid (GABA), the major inhibitor of nerve transmission in the brain and spinal cord with several other anticonvulsant medicines. It is broken down by liver enzymes and eliminated from the body through the kidneys.

Cautions and Warnings

Do not take ezogabine if you are **allergic** or **sensitive** to any of its ingredients.

This medicine can cause urinary difficulty and hesitation, sometimes requiring the insertion of a urinary catheter to allow urine to flow.

Ezogabine is broken down by liver enzymes and removed from the body via your kidneys. People with moderate to severe **liver or kidney disease** should receive a reduced dosage of this medication.

Confusion, hallucinations, and psychosis can occur in people taking this medicine. Most people who experience this effect had no previous history of psychological issues.

Ezogabine can make you dizzy or tired. This effect becomes less of a problem as you stay on the medication.

Ezogabine can change your heart rhythm. People with **heart failure** or other **heart condition** or **low blood potassium or magnesium** may be more likely to experience heart rhythm changes.

All seizure-control medicines can increase the risk of depression or suicide. People with a history of **depression** or **suicidal thoughts or actions** should be carefully monitored.

Suddenly stopping ezogabine can lead to withdrawal seizures.

Ezogabine can cause euphoria (feeling "high"), hallucinations, and disorientation. It may be possible to become psychologically dependent on this medication.

Possible Side Effects

Chances of experiencing side effects increase with increased dosages.

- ▼ Most common: tiredness, fatigue, dizziness, and blurred vision (at dosages of 1200 mg a day).
- ▼ Common: double or blurred vision, nausea, weakness, tremors, fainting, confusion, behavior or mood changes, poor coordination, and difficulty focusing or paying attention.
- ▼ Less common: constipation, upset stomach, infections, weight gain, unusual walk, memory loss, partial or complete loss of the ability to speak or read, joint pain, loss of balance, anxiety, disorientation, urinary pain or hesitation, blood in the urine, and change in urine color.
- ▼ Rare: Rare side effects may include psychosis, increased appetite, hallucinations, muscle spasms, arm or leg swelling, dry mouth, difficulty swallowing, excessive sweating, loss of mobility, not feeling well, and liver irritation. Contact your doctor if you experience anything unusual while taking any medication.

Drug Interactions

- Combining ezogabine with carbamazepine or phenytoin lowers ezogabine blood levels.
- Ezogabine may raise digoxin levels.
- Avoid alcohol while taking ezogabine.

Food Interactions

Ezogabine can be taken without regard to food or meals.

Usual Dose

Adult: starting dose—100 mg 3 times a day. Dosage may be increased gradually to 300 mg 3 times a day or a maximum of 400 mg 3 times a day. Reduced dosages are necessary in people with kidney or liver disease.

Child: not recommended.

Overdosage

Symptoms can include abnormal heart rhythms, hallucinations, disorientation, and euphoria. Overdose victims should be taken to a hospital emergency room for evaluation and treatment. If you seek treatment, ALWAYS bring the prescription bottle or container.

Special Information

Patients and caregivers should be alert to signs of suicidal thoughts or behavior. These can be a result of treatment with this or any other medicine to control seizures. Contact your doctor if you act on dangerous impulses or attempt suicide or if you experience suicidal thoughts; new or worsened anxiety or depression; agitation or restlessness; panic attacks; difficulty sleeping; irritability; aggressive, angry, or violent behavior; or other mood changes.

Do not stop taking this medication suddenly; the dose should be gradually reduced over 3 or more weeks to prevent withdrawal seizures.

Report any urinary hesitation, pain, or other changes in your urinary habits to your doctor. Make sure your doctor knows if you have any risk factors for urinary retention, including enlarged prostate or if you are taking medications that can affect urine flow.

If you forget to take a dose of ezogabine, take it as soon as you remember. If it is almost time for your next dose, skip the one you forgot and continue with your regular schedule. Do not take a double dose. Call your doctor if you forget 2 or more doses.

Special Populations

Pregnancy/Breast-feeding: Animal studies suggest that ezogabine causes fetal injury. Seizure disorder itself also increases the risk of birth defects. Ezogabine should be taken during pregnancy only if your doctor determines that the potential benefit outweighs the risk. The manufacturer has established a registry for women who do decide to take this medicine while pregnant to gather more information on this subject. Only patients may enroll in this registry.

Ezogabine may pass into breast milk. Nursing mothers who must take it should consider using infant formula.

Seniors: Seniors with reduced kidney or liver function need reduced dosages.

Generic Name

Felbamate (FEL-bam-ate) G

Brand Names

Felbatol

Type of Drug

Anticonvulsant.

Prescribed For

Partial seizures and Lennox-Gastaut syndrome in children.

General Information

Felbamate is related to the older sedative meprobamate. Exactly how felbamate works is not known, but it raises the seizure threshold and prevents the seizure impulse from spreading in the brain, as do other anticonvulsants. Because of the risks associated with it, felbamate should only be used when other seizure drugs have failed. About ½ of each dose passes out of the body through the kidneys; the other ½ is broken down and eliminated by the liver.

Cautions and Warnings

Do not take felbamate if you are **allergic** or **sensitive** to any of its ingredients or to any related drugs such as meprobamate.

People taking this drug are more likely to have suicidal thoughts or actually attempt suicide.

Felbamate is associated with an increase in the risk of aplastic anemia, a potentially fatal condition. People with a history of any **blood disorder** should not take felbamate.

Possibly fatal liver failure occurs in people taking felbamate much more often than normal. Regular liver function tests are recommended. People with **liver disease** should not take felbamate.

Felbamate is not recommended as first-line **epilepsy** treatment. Felbamate should be used only by those with severe epilepsy for whom the benefits outweigh the risks. Doctors prescribing felbamate should be thoroughly familiar with the drug and must obtain written, informed consent from patients before prescribing.

Felbamate should never be suddenly stopped, otherwise seizures may become more frequent. Dosage should be gradually reduced or replaced by another anticonvulsant.

Felbamate may cause increased sensitivity to the sun. Wear protective clothing and use sunscreen while taking this drug.

People with **kidney disease** may require lower doses.

Possible Side Effects

Adult

▼ Most common: sleeplessness, sleepiness, headache, dizziness, vomiting, nausea, and appetite loss.

▼ Common: fatigue, nervousness, upset stomach, constipation, anxiety, tremors, unusual walk, depression, tingling in the hands or feet, diarrhea, liver inflammation, abdominal pain, respiratory infections, abnormal vision, and taste changes.

▼ Less common: weakness, dry mouth, stupor, abnormal thinking, rash, sinus irritation, sore throat, muscle aches, fever, and chest pain.

▼ Rare: Rare side effects can occur in almost any part of the body. Contact your doctor if you experience anything unusual while taking any medication.

Child

▼ Most common: appetite loss, sleeplessness, vomiting, headache, respiratory infections, and sleepiness.

▼ Common: abdominal pain, fever, nervousness, constipation, black-and-blue marks, hiccups, sore throat, coughing, middle ear infections, fatigue, weight loss, temporary loss of urine control, pain, unusual walk, weakness, abnormal thinking, emotional instability, pinpoint pupils, rash, upset stomach, and low white-blood-cell count.

▼ Rare: Rare side effects can occur in almost any part of the body. Contact your doctor if your child experiences anything unusual while taking any medication.

Drug Interactions

- Combining felbamate and carbamazepine reduces blood levels of both drugs by roughly ½. Dosage adjustments are necessary.
- Combining phenobarbital and felbamate increases the amount of phenobarbital in the blood and decreases felbamate levels. Dosage adjustments are necessary.

- If you combine felbamate and phenytoin, your phenytoin dosage may have to be reduced by as much as 40%. This combination also decreases felbamate blood levels by almost 50%.
- Felbamate increases blood levels of valproic acid.

Food Interactions

Felbamate is best taken on an empty stomach but may be taken with food if it causes upset stomach.

Usual Dose

Adult and Child (age 14 and over): 1200–3600 mg a day, divided into 3–4 doses.

Child (age 2–13): 6.8–20.5 mg per lb. of body weight a day, divided into 3–4 doses.

Overdosage

Overdose symptoms may include upset stomach, increased heart rate, and felbamate side effects. Contact your local poison control center or a hospital emergency room for more information. If you seek treatment, ALWAYS bring the prescription bottle or container.

Special Information

Do not take more felbamate than your doctor has prescribed.

Felbamate can cause drowsiness; be careful when driving or performing tasks that require concentration.

Avoid prolonged exposure to the sun while taking felbamate.

Contact your doctor if you develop any bothersome or persistent side effect.

Maintain good dental hygiene while taking felbamate and use extra care when brushing or flossing because this drug can cause swollen gums. See your dentist regularly.

If you forget a dose, take it as soon as you remember. If it is almost time for your next dose, take 1 dose right away and another in 3 or 4 hours, then go back to your regular schedule. Do not take a double dose.

Special Populations

Pregnancy/Breast-feeding: This drug may cross into fetal circulation. Felbamate should be taken during pregnancy only if your doctor determines that the potential benefit outweighs the risks.

Felbamate passes into breast milk. Nursing mothers who must take this drug should consider using infant formula.

Seniors: Seniors, especially those with liver, kidney, or heart disease, may be more sensitive to the effects of this drug and should receive lower doses.

Generic Name

Fenofibrate (fen-oe-FIH-brate) G

Brand Names

Antara	Lofibra
Fenoglide	TriCor
Lipofen	Triglide

The information in this profile also applies to the following drugs:

Generic Ingredients: Fenofibric Acid

Fibricor	Trilipix

Type of Drug

Anti-hyperlipidemic (blood-fat reducer).

Prescribed For

High blood cholesterol, high triglycerides, and low high-density lipoprotein (HDL) cholesterol; also prescribed for gout.

General Information

These drugs work by interfering with the body's ability to make triglycerides and by increasing their breakdown by enzymes in the body. They also reduce levels of uric acid, total cholesterol, low-density lipoprotein (LDL) cholesterol—the "bad" cholesterol—and other blood lipids. HDL cholesterol—the "good" cholesterol—levels are increased. Their impact on heart disease is still in question. A study of almost 10,000 diabetics, who are at significant risk for heart disease, showed an insignificant reduction in coronary artery disease and heart attack over 5 years, but there was a significant 11% reduction in all heart and blood-vessel-related disease experienced during the study. In people with type 2 diabetes, adding fenofibrate to a statin reduces the number of heart attacks, strokes, and blocked blood vessels requiring surgery but does not reduce the risk of dying from heart disease. Studies of fenofibric acid in people with type 2 diabetes have shown that it does not reduce the risk of a heart attack or stroke.

Fenofibrate is broken down in the liver to fenofibric acid, the active form of this medicine. A single fenofibrate 200-mg capsule or 145-mg tablet or three 48-mg tablets all provide the same blood level of fenofibric acid as a single 135-mg dose of Trilipix. These drugs are prescribed only for people with very high triglyceride levels who have not responded to diet, weight loss, and other medicines, including statin drugs. High triglyceride levels can cause inflammation of the pancreas. These drugs are often part of a treatment program designed to reverse this inflammation by lowering triglycerides and cholesterol.

Cautions and Warnings

Do not take these medicines if you are **allergic** or **sensitive** to any of their ingredients.

People taking fenofibrate, fenofibric acid, and gemfibrozil may develop pancreatitis (inflammation of the pancreas).

People with **liver, gallbladder, or severe kidney disease** should avoid these drugs. People with less severe kidney disease should take a lower dosage of these medicines. Your doctor should monitor your liver and kidney function with regular blood tests.

People taking these medicines are more likely to develop **gallbladder disease** or **gallstones.**

These drugs can destroy muscle cells, leading to kidney failure, especially when combined with a statin cholesterol-lowering drug (see "Drug Interactions").

Possible Side Effects

▼ Common: abnormal liver function and respiratory problems.

▼ Less common: abdominal pain, back pain, headache, nausea, diarrhea, runny nose, weakness, flu-like symptoms, abnormal muscle and kidney tests, and constipation.

▼ Rare: Other side effects can occur in any part of the body. Contact your doctor if you experience anything unusual while taking any medication.

Drug Interactions

- Combining these drugs and cyclosporine increases the risk of kidney damage. This combination should only be used if it is absolutely necessary and the lowest effective dosage is taken.
- Combining these medicines and a statin cholesterol-lowering drug (atorvastatin, fluvastatin, lovastatin, pravastatin,

rosuvastatin, or simvastatin) can lead to myopathy, the symptoms of which are severe muscle pain, muscle cell destruction, and kidney failure. If you have extremely high blood-fat levels, the potential benefits of this combination may outweigh the risks. However, if your doctor prescribes both drugs, your statin dose will likely be reduced, and muscle and kidney health must be monitored regularly via blood tests.

- These drugs increase the effects of anticoagulant (blood thinning) drugs. Your anticoagulant dosage will need adjustment.
- If you are taking a bile acid sequestrant (cholestyramine, colestipol, or colesevelam) in addition to fenofibrate or fenofibric acid, take the fenofibrate at least 1 hour before or 4–6 hours after the bile acid sequestrant.

Food Interactions

Some forms of fenofibrate should be taken with food to get the best effect. Fenofibric acid, Antara, TriCor, or Triglide may be taken without regard to food or meals.

Usual Dose

These products may not be substituted for each other because of important dosage differences. None of these products are recommended for children; dosages given are for adults only. Seniors and people with kidney disease should start with the lowest dose.

Antara: 43–130 mg a day.

Fenoglide: 40–120 mg a day with food.

Fibricor: 35–105 mg a day.

Lipofen: 50–150 mg a day with food.

Lofibra Capsules: 67–200 mg a day with food.

Lofibra Tablets: 54–160 mg a day with food.

TriCor: 48–145 mg a day.

Triglide: 50–160 mg a day. This product must be protected from light and moisture. Do not remove it from the special protective container it comes in and do not transfer any Triglide pills to another holder.

Trilipix: 45–135 mg a day.

Overdosage

Little is known about the effects of an overdose of these drugs. Victims should be taken to a hospital emergency room. If you seek treatment, ALWAYS bring the prescription bottle or container.

Special Information

People should take these medicines only after a triglyceride-lowering, low-fat, low-cholesterol diet and other medications have failed. Continue your low-fat, low-cholesterol diet while you are taking this medicine.

Contact your doctor if you cannot swallow your fenofibric acid capsule, as you may have to be switched to a different medicine. Do not crush, chew, or break the fenofibric acid capsule.

If you forget a dose, take it as soon as you remember. If it is almost time for your next dose, skip the forgotten dose and continue with your regular schedule.

Special Populations

Pregnancy/Breast-feeding: Fenofibrate causes fetal injury and death in animal studies. Fenofibric acid did not cause damage in animal studies where doses similar to those taken by people were used, but damage occurs when larger doses are used. Fenofibrate should be taken during pregnancy only if your doctor determines that the potential benefit outweighs the risks.

Nursing mothers who must take this drug should use infant formula.

Seniors: Seniors are more likely to experience side effects because of normal age-related loss of kidney function and should start with the lowest effective dosage.

Generic Name

Fidaxomicin (fih-DAX-oh-MYE-sin)

Brand Names

Dificid

Type of Drug

Antibacterial.

Prescribed For

Clostridium difficile–associated diarrhea (CDAD).

General Information

Fidaxomicin is a member of the macrolide antibiotics, the same drug class as erythromycin, clarithromycin, and others. It was developed specifically to fight the bacterium *Clostridium difficile*

(*C. difficile* or C diff). C diff has been a problem since the 1970s, when it was found to be the cause of severe diarrhea in people being treated with antibiotics that wiped out other intestinal bacteria. Over the years, various medicines have been used against it, and C diff has continually evolved to develop resistance against these products. For this reason, fidaxomicin should only be used for diarrhea proven or strongly suspected to be caused by C diff. Fidaxomicin works by interfering with the process of creating new C diff bacteria. After you take fidaxomicin, most of the medicine stays in the gastrointestinal (GI) tract, though some is absorbed into the bloodstream. It mainly passes out of the body in the feces.

Cautions and Warnings

Do not use fidaxomicin if you are **allergic** or **sensitive** to any of its ingredients.

Fidaxomicin should be used only for diarrhea and GI infection with C diff. It cannot be used to treat blood infections or infections in other parts of the body. Improper or inappropriate use of fidaxomicin is likely to lead to the development of C diff resistance.

Possible Side Effects

- ▼ Most common: nausea.
- ▼ Common: vomiting and abdominal pain.
- ▼ Less common: GI bleeding, anemia, and reduced white blood cell count.
- ▼ Rare: Other side effects include rash, itching, high blood sugar, and those that primarily affect the GI tract, including bloating, gas, and difficulty swallowing. Contact your doctor if you experience anything unusual while taking any medication.

Drug Interactions

- Cyclosporine may slightly raise blood levels of fidaxomicin, but the effect is not significant and does not require a change in dose.

Food Interactions

This drug can be taken without regard to food or meals.

Usual Dose

Adult: 200 mg twice a day for 10 days.

Child: not recommended.

Overdosage

There have been no reported cases of fidaxomicin overdose. Overdose symptoms could be expected to be similar to drug side effects, primarily affecting the GI tract. In case of an accidental overdose, call your hospital emergency room or poison control center for more information. If you seek treatment, ALWAYS bring the prescription bottle or container.

Special Information

If you forget a dose, take it as soon as you remember. If it is almost time for your next dose, skip the forgotten dose and continue with your regular schedule, but be sure to take all the fidaxomicin your doctor prescribed. Do not take a double dose.

Fidaxomicin is only for C diff infections. It should not be used for diarrhea caused by any other bacteria or virus.

Special Populations

Pregnancy/Breast-feeding: Fidaxomicin has been studied in animals and has not caused any damage to the developing fetus. Nevertheless, fidaxomicin should be taken during pregnancy only if your doctor determines that the potential benefit outweighs the risks.

It is not known if fidaxomicin passes into breast milk. Nursing mothers who must take it should use infant formula.

Seniors: Seniors may take fidaxomicin without special precaution.

Generic Name

Finasteride (fin-ASS-ter-ide) G

Brand Names

Propecia Proscar

The information in this profile also applies to the following drugs:

Generic Ingredients: Dutasteride
Avodart

Generic Ingredients: Dutasteride + Tamsulosin
Jalyn

Type of Drug

Alpha-reductase inhibitor and androgen hormone inhibitor.

Prescribed For

Benign prostatic hyperplasia (BPH; Proscar, dutasteride, and dutasteride + tamsulosin) and male-pattern baldness (Propecia). May also play a role in preventing prostrate cancer.

General Information

Finasteride works by interfering with the action of the enzyme alpha-reductase, which converts testosterone into 5-dihydrotestosterone (DHT). By suppressing DHT levels, finasteride reduces the size of the prostate in most men who take the drug for BPH. You may need to take finasteride for 6–12 months before its effects can be assessed.

Urine flow improves in about 60% of men taking finasteride for BPH, and symptoms improve in about 30%. In one study, men experienced a significant regression in prostate size after 3 months, and the reduction was maintained through the 12-month study period; these men experienced a significant improvement in urine flow that could be maintained for up to 36 months.

Studies of finasteride for hair loss on the top and back-middle of the scalp show new hair growth in 65–80% of men taking the drug continuously for 2 years. The drug must be taken for 3 months or more before it begins to have an effect and must be taken continuously to maintain hair growth. Once you stop taking this drug, any new hair you have grown is likely to fall out in the next 12 months. Between 14 and 17% of men taking the drug continued to lose hair throughout the study period.

Finasteride has been studied as therapy following radical prostatectomy surgery and in the prevention of first-stage prostate cancer, acne in women, and unusual hairiness.

Cautions and Warnings

Do not take these medications if you are **allergic** or **sensitive** to any of their ingredients. Severe drug reactions can include swelling of the tongue, face, and lips, and choking.

These drugs should not be used in **women** or **children**. Pregnant women must not handle the tablets and capsules because of the risk to the fetus. Men should not donate blood while taking dutasteride or dutasteride + tamsulosin or for 6 months following their cessation to avoid contaminating a pregnant female.

People who do not respond to these medications may have a condition that causes BPH-like symptoms, such as prostate cancer, bladder or nerve disorders, or physical obstruction of the urinary tubes. Finasteride and dutasteride cannot be used to treat these conditions.

Because it is broken down in the liver, finasteride must be used with caution by people with **liver disease**.

Men taking these drugs for BPH may have a reduced risk of prostate cancer, but those that do develop prostate cancer while taking them are slightly more likely to have the more aggressive form known as high-grade prostate cancer.

Possible Side Effects

Side effects are generally mild and often subside with continued use of the drug.

▼ Common: impotence, loss of sex drive, decreased amount of semen, breast tenderness and enlargement, testicular pain, and drug-sensitivity reactions such as lip swelling and rash.

Drug Interactions

- Finasteride affects the prostate-specific antigen (PSA) blood test used for prostate cancer screening. Be sure your doctor knows you are taking this drug if you have a PSA test done or are being tested for prostate cancer.
- Dutasteride blood levels may increase when mixed with ritonavir, ketoconazole, cimetidine, and ciprofloxacin, all of which are inhibitors of a liver enzyme called CYP3A4. Blood levels of dutasteride also increase with verapamil and diltiazem.

Food Interactions

You may take finasteride or dutasteride with food if it upsets your stomach. Dutasteride + tamsulosin should be taken 30 minutes after the same meal every day.

Usual Dose

Dutasteride

Adult: 0.5 mg (1 capsule) once a day.
Child: not recommended.

Dutasteride + Tamsulosin

Adult: 1 capsule 30 minutes after the same meal once a day.
Child: not recommended.

Finasteride

Adult: BPH—5 mg once a day. Male-pattern baldness—1 mg once a day.

Child: not recommended.

Women should not take finasteride.

Overdosage

Side effects are unlikely. Doses of dutasteride as high as 400 mg a day have been taken with no adverse side effects. Contact your local poison control center or a hospital emergency room for more information. If you seek treatment, ALWAYS bring the prescription bottle or container.

Special Information

Women who are or might be pregnant should not handle crushed tablets because small amounts of the drug may be absorbed into the blood, possibly affecting the fetus.

Obtain medical help if you have trouble breathing or your throat, tongue, and/or face swells noticeably. These may be signs of a severe drug reaction.

If your sexual partner is or might be pregnant and you start taking one of these medications, you must wear a condom during sex to avoid directly exposing her to the drug in the semen.

Semen volume may decrease while taking one of these medications. Impotence or reduced sex drive is also a risk.

If you forget a dose, take it as soon as you remember. If it is almost time for your next dose, skip the one you forgot and continue with your regular schedule. Do not take a double dose. Contact your doctor if you miss a dose for 2 or more days.

Special Populations

Pregnancy/Breast-feeding: These drugs are not intended for women. They will harm the fetus even if absorbed in small amounts through the skin by a woman handling them.

Seniors: Seniors with liver disease should use this drug with caution.

Generic Name

Fingolimod (fin-GOH-lih-mod)

Brand Names

Gilenya

Type of Drug

S1P receptor antagonist.

Prescribed For

Multiple sclerosis (MS).

General Information

Fingolimod reduces the number of MS attacks and delays the worsening of physical disabilities associated with MS. It antagonizes the enzyme sphingosine 1-phosphate (S1P). S1P is important throughout the body but is a major regulator of the vascular and immune systems and may have a role in the multiplication of skin cells. In MS, it prevents lymph cells from moving into the central nervous system, probably protecting it against some further damage.

Cautions and Warnings

Do not use fingolimod if you are **allergic** or **sensitive** to any of its ingredients.

Fingolimod may slow your heart or slow the movement of electrical signals around the heart. People taking a **beta blocker, calcium channel blocker, or other drug for abnormal heart rhythms** are at greater risk of developing heart block or bradycardia. Your doctor should monitor you for 6 hours after your first dose in case your heart slows unexpectedly. If fingolimod treatment is stopped for more than 2 weeks, the same heart effects may develop if it is restarted.

This medicine may increase the risk of infection. Your doctor should check your blood for infection during fingolimod treatment and for 2 months after you have stopped.

People taking fingolimod have developed the eye condition macular edema. Macular edema can lead to blindness and may develop without symptoms. Your doctor and your ophthalmologist should regularly check your eyes. People with **diabetes** and a history of the eye condition **uveitis** have a greater chance of developing macular edema with this medicine.

Fingolimod can lead to an increase in liver enzymes. Treatment with this medicine must be stopped if significant liver injury occurs.

Fingolimod is broken down by liver enzymes and stays in the body for more than 2 months. People with severe **liver damage** can have twice as much drug in their blood and the risk of side effects goes up.

Blood levels of some of the breakdown products of fingolimod increase up to 13 times in severe kidney damage. The importance of this effect is not yet known.

Fingolimod may reduce lung function, making it harder to breathe. This can develop as soon as 1 month after starting fingolimod but reverses a month or 2 after the drug is stopped.

People taking fingolimod may develop relatively small increases in blood pressure, which may be significant over time.

One person passed away within 24 hours of taking their first dose of fingolimod; however, there is no definite link between the medicine and sudden death.

Possible Side Effects

- ▼ Most common: headache, influenza, back pain, cough, diarrhea, and increased liver enzyme levels.
- ▼ Common: difficulty breathing, depression, herpes infection, bronchitis, sinusitis, stomach virus, dizziness, and high blood pressure.
- ▼ Less common: slow heart rate, gastroenteritis (stomach flu), fungal infection, tingling in the hands or feet, migraines, weakness, hair loss, eczema, itching, blurred vision, eye pain, reduced white-blood-cell and lymph cell counts.
- ▼ Rare: Stroke, lymphoma, and other side effects may occur. Contact your doctor if you experience anything unusual while taking any medication.

Drug Interactions

- Live virus vaccines should be avoided while you are taking fingolimod due to the increased infection risk.
- Mixing this medicine with anticancer drugs or drugs that affect the immune system can be expected to raise the risks of immune system suppression. People switching from mitoxantrone and natalizumab, which have long-acting immune system effects, are of special concern.
- Mixing a beta blocker or calcium channel blocker with fingolimod can lead to unusual slowing of heart rate. People starting a beta blocker while on this medicine must be monitored for this effect. The risk is reduced when dosage of the beta blocker is established.
- Mixing this drug with amiodarone, quinidine, sotalol, and similar drugs for abnormal heart rhythms can lead to unusual slowing of the heart.

- The chance of fingolimod side effects increases if you take it with aprepitant, clarithromycin, delavirdine, diltiazem, erythromycin, fluconazole, indinavir, itraconazole, ketoconazole, nefazodone, nelfinivir, ritonavir, saquinavir, telithromycin, and verapamil. The combination slows the clearance of fingolimod and your doctor may reduce your fingolimod dose.

Food Interactions

This drug can be taken without regard to food or meals.

Usual Dose

Adult: One 0.5-mg tablet once a day.
Child: not recommended.

Overdosage

Fingolimod overdose has not led to any important side effects. Some people taking 40 mg of this drug felt chest tightness and discomfort. If you seek treatment, ALWAYS bring the prescription bottle or container.

Special Information

Take this medicine exactly as directed. If you forget a dose, take it as soon as you remember and contact your doctor. Do not take a double dose. Do not stop taking this medicine without first contacting your doctor.

Contact your doctor if you develop a fever, chills, or other sign of possible blood infection. The risk of infection lasts for 2 months after you have stopped taking this medicine.

Contact your doctor if you develop mild to moderate dizziness, fatigue, heart palpitations, or chest pain. These symptoms can be a sign of bradycardia, an unusual slowing of heart rate.

Contact your doctor if you develop nausea, vomiting, abdominal pain, fatigue, appetite loss, yellowing of the skin or whites of the eyes, or dark urine. These are signs of liver damage.

Contact your doctor if you develop blurriness or shadows in the center of your vision, a blind spot at the center of your vision, or light sensitivity. These can be signs of macular edema and must be addressed quickly.

This is a specially formulated product. Do not split, crush, chew, or dissolve the fingolimod tablet.

It is not known if racial background affects individual response to fingolimod.

Special Populations

Pregnancy/Breast-feeding: The S1P enzyme is involved in blood vessel formation in the growing fetus. Not surprisingly, fingolimod caused birth defects in animal studies. Women of childbearing age who take this medicine must use effective contraception while they are taking it and for 2 months after it is stopped. Fingolimod should be taken during pregnancy only if your doctor determines that the potential benefit outweighs the risks. You or your doctor can enroll in a registry that has been created to gather information on pregnant women who decide to take fingolimod.

Fingolimod may pass into breast milk. Nursing mothers who must take it should use infant formula.

Seniors: Seniors may be at a greater risk of drug side effects because of normal reductions in liver and kidney function and the likelihood that seniors will be taking other medicines.

Brand Names

Fioricet

Generic Ingredients

Acetaminophen + Butalbital + Caffeine G

Other Brand Names

Alagesic LQ
Capacet
Dolgic Plus
Esgic
Esgic-Plus
Margesic
Medigesic
Orbivan
Repan
Zebutal

Type of Drug

Barbiturate and analgesic (pain reliever) combination.

Prescribed For

Symptom relief of tension headache.

General Information

Fioricet is one of many combination products containing a barbiturate—butalbital—and an analgesic—acetaminophen. Products of this kind also often contain a sedative or a narcotic. Other analgesic combinations, such as Fiorinal, substitute aspirin for acetaminophen.

Cautions and Warnings

Do not take Fioricet if you are **allergic** or **sensitive** to any of its ingredients.

Use this drug with caution if you have **kidney or liver disease** or a history of **porphyria** (a rare blood disorder). The use of high-dose acetaminophen (over 4000 mg a day) has been associated with liver failure.

Chronic (long-term) use of Fioricet may lead to drug dependence or addiction. It is not recommended for multiple or recurrent headaches.

Butalbital is a respiratory depressant and affects the central nervous system (CNS), producing drowsiness, tiredness, and an inability to concentrate. Alcohol increases the CNS depression caused by this drug.

The safety and effectiveness of these medications have not been established in children under age 12.

For more information see Acetaminophen, page 16.

Possible Side Effects

- ▼ Most common: lightheadedness, dizziness, sedation, shortness of breath, nausea, vomiting, upset stomach, and a feeling of intoxication.
- ▼ Less common: weakness, headache, agitation, tremor, uncoordinated muscle movement, disorientation, dry mouth, constipation, facial flushing, changes in heart rate, palpitations, feeling faint, urinary difficulties, rash, and itching.

For more information see Acetaminophen, page 16.

Drug Interactions

- Combining Fioricet with alcohol, sedatives, barbiturates, sleeping pills, antihistamines, monoamine oxidase inhibitor (MAOI) antidepressants, or other CNS depressants may cause tiredness, drowsiness, and trouble concentrating.
- These medications may reduce the effectiveness of corticosteroids, contraceptives containing estrogen, beta blockers such as propranolol, doxycycline, felodipine, griseofulvin, nifedipine, phenylbutazone, quinine, theophylline, warfarin, and tricyclic antidepressants.
- Combining Fioricet with carbamazepine or sulfinpyrazone increases your risk for liver damage.

For more information see Acetaminophen, page 16.

Food Interactions

Fioricet is best taken on an empty stomach but may be taken with food if it upsets your stomach.

Usual Dose

Adult (age 12 and over): 1–2 tablets or capsules every 4 hours or as needed. Do not exceed 6 doses a day.

Child (under age 12): not recommended.

Overdosage

Symptoms include breathing difficulties, nervousness progressing to stupor or coma, pinpoint pupils, cold and clammy skin and lowered heart rate or blood pressure, nausea, vomiting, dizziness, ringing in the ears, facial flushing, sweating, and thirst. Take the victim to a hospital emergency room immediately. If you seek treatment, ALWAYS bring the prescription bottle or container.

Special Information

Fioricet may cause drowsiness. Be careful when driving or performing any task that requires concentration.

You should avoid alcohol while taking this medication.

Do not take Fioricet for longer or in amounts greater than prescribed.

If you have been taking this medication for more than a few weeks, do not stop taking it without your doctor's instruction. Suddenly stopping Fioricet may lead to withdrawal symptoms.

Contact your doctor if your headache or pain persists or gets worse, or if you develop side effects that are bothersome or persistent.

If you forget a dose, take it as soon as you remember. If it is almost time for your next dose, skip the one you forgot and continue with your regular schedule. Do not take a double dose.

For more information see Acetaminophen, page 16.

Special Populations

Pregnancy/Breast-feeding: Fioricet should not be taken during pregnancy. It is associated with birth defects, prolonged labor and delayed delivery, and breathing problems in newborns. Regular use of Fioricet during the last 3 months of pregnancy may also cause drug dependency in the newborn.

Fioricet passes into breast milk. Breast-feeding while using Fioricet may cause babies to become tired, short of breath, or have a slow heartbeat. Nursing mothers who must take this drug should use infant formula.

Seniors: Fioricet may have a greater depressant effect on seniors. Seniors are also more likely to experience stimulation and disorientation.

Brand Names

Fiorinal

Generic Ingredients

Aspirin + Butalbital + Caffeine G

Other Brand Names

Lanorinal

Type of Drug

Barbiturate and analgesic (pain reliever) combination.

Prescribed For

Symptom relief of tension headache.

General Information

Pain relief products often combine an analgesic with a sedative. The analgesic ingredient in Fiorinal is aspirin; other brand-name products, such as Esgic and Fioricet, contain acetaminophen. The sedative ingredient in pain relief combinations may be a barbiturate, narcotic, or other sedative. Fiorinal contains the barbiturate butalbital. Fiorinal also contains caffeine, which is often used in analgesic combinations that treat headache because it enhances the pain-relieving effect of aspirin.

Cautions and Warnings

Do not take Fiorinal if you are **allergic** or **sensitive** to any of its ingredients or to any nonsteroidal anti-inflammatory drugs (NSAIDs). Serious allergic reactions are possible in people who have had nasal polyps, swelling, or an asthma-like reaction to aspirin or NSAIDs.

Do not give Fiorinal to **children** or **teenagers with chickenpox or flu-like symptoms** due to the aspirin content and danger of Reye's syndrome. The safety and efficacy of Fiorinal use in children under age 12 has not been established.

Use Fiorinal with extreme caution or not at all if you have

peptic ulcer, problems with **blood clotting** or other **bleeding disorders**, a history of **porphyria** (a rare blood disorder), or are about to have **surgery**.

This drug should be used with caution if you have **kidney or liver disease** or **diabetes**.

Long-term use of this drug may cause drug dependence and addiction. It is not recommended for the treatment of multiple recurrent headaches.

Butalbital is a respiratory depressant and affects the central nervous system (CNS), producing drowsiness, tiredness, and an inability to concentrate. Alcohol increases the CNS depression caused by butalbital.

For more information see Aspirin, page 125.

Possible Side Effects

▼ Most common: lightheadedness, dizziness, and sedation.

▼ Less common: nausea, vomiting, flatulence, and rash.

For more information see Aspirin, page 125.

Drug Interactions

- Combining Fiorinal with alcohol, sedatives, barbiturates, sleeping pills, antihistamines, monoamine oxidase inhibitor (MAOI) antidepressants, or other CNS depressants may cause tiredness, drowsiness, and trouble concentrating.
- Use of corticosteroids and Fiorinal may decrease the effects of both medications. Stopping corticosteroids suddenly may lead to aspirin toxicity.
- The effects of beta blockers (such as propranolol), doxycycline, estrogens (including contraceptive drugs), felodipine, griseofulvin, nifedipine, phenylbutazone, quinidine, and theophylline may be increased when combined with these medications.
- Fiorinal may decrease the effects of tricyclic antidepressants.
- Fiorinal may enhance the effects of oral anticoagulants (blood thinners), oral antidiabetes drugs, insulin, and NSAIDs.
- Fiorinal may decrease the effectiveness of medications taken for gout, including probenecid and sulfinpyrazone.

For more information see Aspirin, page 125.

Food Interactions

Fiorinal is best taken on an empty stomach but may be taken with food if it upsets your stomach.

Usual Dose

Adult (age 12 and over): 1–2 tablets or capsules every 4 hours or as needed. Do not exceed 6 doses a day.

Child (under age 12): not recommended.

Overdosage

Symptoms include breathing difficulties, nervousness progressing to stupor or coma, pinpoint pupils, cold and clammy skin, lowered heart rate or blood pressure, nausea, vomiting, stomach pain, dizziness, ringing in the ears, flushing, sweating, and thirst. Symptoms of mild overdose are rapid and deep breathing, nausea, vomiting, dizziness, ringing or buzzing in the ears, flushing, sweating, thirst, headache, drowsiness, diarrhea, and rapid heartbeat. Severe overdose may cause fever, excitement, confusion, convulsions, liver or kidney failure, coma, and bleeding. Take the victim to a hospital emergency room immediately. If you seek treatment, ALWAYS bring the prescription bottle or container.

Special Information

Fiorinal may cause drowsiness. Be careful when driving or performing any task that requires concentration.

Avoid alcohol while taking Fiorinal.

If you have been taking this medication for more than a few weeks, do not stop taking it without your doctor's instruction. Suddenly stopping this drug may lead to withdrawal symptoms.

Do not take Fiorinal for longer or in amounts greater than prescribed.

Contact your doctor if your headache pain persists or gets worse, or if you develop any bothersome or persistent side effect.

If you forget a dose, take it as soon as you remember. If it is almost time for your next dose, skip the dose you forgot and continue with your regular schedule. Do not take a double dose.

For additional information see Aspirin, page 125.

Special Populations

Pregnancy/Breast-feeding: Fiorinal should not be taken during pregnancy. Pregnant women taking it may experience prolonged labor, delayed delivery, and bleeding problems. Fiorinal increases the risk of birth defects and may cause breathing or bleeding problems in newborns. Regular use of Fiorinal during the last 3 months of pregnancy may also cause drug dependency in the newborn.

Fiorinal passes into breast milk. Breast-feeding while using Fiorinal may cause tiredness, shortness of breath, or slowed heartbeat in the baby. Nursing mothers who must take Fiorinal should use infant formula.

Seniors: Fiorinal may have a greater depressant effect on seniors. Seniors are also more likely to experience stimulation and disorientation.

Generic Name

Flecainide (FLEH-kan-ide) G

Brand Names

Tambocor

Type of Drug

Antiarrhythmic.

Prescribed For

Abnormal heart rhythm.

General Information

Flecainide is prescribed in situations where the abnormal heart rhythm is so severe as to be life-threatening and the patient does not respond to other drug treatments. Like other antiarrhythmic drugs, flecainide works by affecting the movement of nervous impulses within the heart. Flecainide's effects may not become apparent for 3–4 days after you start taking it.

Cautions and Warnings

Do not take flecainide if you are **allergic** or **sensitive** to any of its ingredients or if you have **heart block**, unless you have a cardiac pacemaker. As with other antiarrhythmic drugs, there is no proof that flecainide helps people live longer or avoid sudden death.

Flecainide causes or worsens **arrhythmias** in 7% of people who take it; this risk increases with certain kinds of underlying heart disease and higher doses of the drug. Flecainide causes or worsens **heart failure** in about 5% of people taking it because it tends to reduce the force and rate of each heartbeat.

Flecainide is extensively broken down in the liver. People with **poor liver function** should not take flecainide unless the benefits clearly outweigh the risks.

Changes in the pH of urine may affect the effectiveness of flecainide.

Possible Side Effects

▼ Most common: dizziness, fainting, lightheadedness, unsteadiness, visual disturbances such as blurred vision and seeing spots before the eyes, breathing difficulties, headache, nausea, fatigue, heart palpitations, chest pain, tremors, weakness, constipation, bloating, a bad taste in the mouth, and abdominal pain.

▼ Less common: new or worsened heart arrhythmias or heart failure; heart block; slowed heart rate; vomiting; diarrhea; upset stomach; loss of appetite; stomach gas; dry mouth; tingling in the hands or feet; partial or temporary paralysis; loss of muscle control; flushing; sweating; ringing or buzzing in the ears; anxiety; sleeplessness; depression; not feeling well; twitching; weakness; convulsions; speech disorders; stupor; memory loss; personality loss; nightmares; apathy; eye pain; unusual sensitivity to bright light; sagging eyelids; reduced white-blood-cell or blood-platelet counts; impotence; reduced sex drive; frequent urination; urinary difficulty; itching; rash; fever; muscle ache; closing of the throat; and swollen lips, tongue, or mouth.

Drug Interactions

- The combination of propranolol and flecainide may cause an exaggerated lowering of heart rate. Other drugs that slow the heart may also interact with flecainide to produce an excessive slowing of heart rate.
- Avoid megadoses of vitamin C while taking this drug.
- The amount of flecainide in your blood and its effect on your heart may be increased if it is taken together with cimetidine, disopyramide, or verapamil.
- Your dose of flecainide should be halved when given with amiodarone.
- Smokers may need a larger dose of flecainide than nonsmokers.
- Flecainide may increase the amount of digoxin in the bloodstream, increasing the chance of side effects.

Food Interactions

A strict vegetarian diet and anything that makes urine less acid interferes with flecainide's elimination from the body, increasing drug toxicity.

Usual Dose

Adult: starting dose—50–100 mg every 12 hours, increased in increments of 50 mg per dose. Maximum dosage is 400 mg a day. Do not increase dosage more frequently than once every 4 days. Dosage may be reduced once arrhythmia is under control.

Child: not recommended.

Overdosage

Flecainide overdose affects heart function, causing slower heart rate, low blood pressure, and possible death from respiratory failure. Victims of flecainide overdose should be taken to a hospital emergency room. If you seek treatment, ALWAYS bring the prescription bottle or container.

Special Information

Flecainide can make you dizzy, lightheaded, or disoriented. Take care while driving or performing complex tasks.

Contact your doctor if you develop chest pains, an abnormal heartbeat, breathing difficulties, bloating in your feet or legs, tremors, fever, chills, sore throat, unusual bleeding or bruising, yellowing of the whites of your eyes, or any other intolerable side effect.

Take exactly as prescribed, and try not to skip doses. If you forget to take a dose of flecainide and remember within 6 hours, take it as soon as possible. If you do not remember until later, skip the dose you forgot and continue with your regular schedule. Do not take a double dose, and do not increase or decrease your dose without your doctor's supervision.

Special Populations

Pregnancy/Breast-feeding: At high doses, flecainide damages an animal fetus. Flecainide should be taken during pregnancy only if your doctor determines that the potential benefit outweighs the risks.

Flecainide passes into breast milk. Nursing mothers who must take this drug should use infant formula.

Seniors: Seniors with reduced kidney or liver function are more likely to develop side effects and require a lower dosage.

Flomax *see **Alpha Blockers,** page 70*

Flovent HFA *see* ***Corticosteroids, Inhalers,*** *page 334*

Generic Name

Flucytosine (floo-SYE-toe-seen) G

Brand Names

Ancobon

Type of Drug

Antifungal.

Prescribed For

Serious blood-borne fungal infections.

General Information

Flucytosine is meant for fungal infections—*Candida, chromomycoses,* and *cryptococcus*—carried in the blood that affect the urinary tract, respiratory tract, central nervous system, heart, and other organs. It is not meant for fungal infections of the skin, such as common athlete's foot.

Cautions and Warnings

Do not take this drug if you are **allergic** or **sensitive** to any of its ingredients.

People with **kidney disease** must be closely monitored by their doctors and should take this medication with extreme caution; daily dosage must be reduced. Liver and kidney function and blood composition should be monitored while you are taking this drug. Flucytosine can cause the death of liver tissue.

Flucytosine can worsen **bone-marrow depression** in people whose immune systems are already compromised. Several people have died from this effect.

The safety and efficacy of flucytosine have not been established in **children**.

Possible Side Effects

▼ Most common: unusual tiredness or weakness, liver inflammation, yellowing of the eyes or skin, abdominal pain, diarrhea, loss of appetite, nausea, vomiting, rash, redness, itching, sore throat, fever, and unusual bleeding or bruising.

Possible Side Effects *(continued)*

▼ Less common: chest pain, breathing difficulties, sensitivity to the sun or bright light, dry mouth, duodenal ulcers, severe bowel irritation, stomach bleeding, colitis, destruction of liver tissue, interference with kidney function, kidney failure, reduced red- and white-blood-cell counts or other changes in blood composition, headache, hearing loss, confusion, dizziness, weakness, shaking, sedation, psychosis, hallucinations, heart attack, and low levels of blood sugar and potassium.

Drug Interactions

- Amphotericin B increases flucytosine's effectiveness; this combination is generally used to produce better results.
- Flucytosine may interfere with some routine blood tests.
- Cytosine may inactivate the antifungal activity of flucytosine.

Food Interactions

Take flucytosine with food if it upsets your stomach.

Usual Dose

22–68 mg per lb. of body weight a day, in divided doses.

Overdosage

Little is known about the effects of flucytosine overdose, but it may cause exaggerated drug side effects. If you seek treatment, ALWAYS bring the prescription bottle or container.

Special Information

Take the capsules a few at a time over 15 minutes to avoid nausea and vomiting.

Contact your doctor if you develop unusual tiredness or weakness; yellowing of the skin or whites of the eyes; rash, redness, or itching; sore throat or fever; unusual bleeding or bruising; or any persistent or intolerable side effect.

Maintain good dental hygiene while taking flucytosine. Use extra care when using your toothbrush or dental floss because of the risk that flucytosine will make you more susceptible to infection. Dental work should be completed prior to starting on this drug.

Exposure to sunlight may cause rash, itching, redness, discoloration of the skin, or severe sunburn. Stay out of direct sunlight when taking flucytosine.

If you forget a dose, take it as soon as you remember. If it is almost time for your next dose, take 1 dose right away and another in 3 or 4 hours, then go back to your regular schedule. Do not take a double dose.

Special Populations

Pregnancy/Breast-feeding: Flucytosine causes birth defects in animals and crosses the placenta. Flucytosine should be taken during pregnancy only if your doctor determines that the potential benefit outweighs the risks.

It is not known if flucytosine passes into breast milk. Nursing mothers who must take this drug should use infant formula.

Seniors: Dosage adjustment may be required due to age-related loss of kidney function.

Type of Drug

Fluoroquinolone Anti-infectives

(flor-oe-QUIN-oe-lone)

Brand Names

Generic Ingredients: Besifloxacin
Besivance Eye Drops

Generic Ingredients: Ciprofloxacin G
Cetraxal Ear Drops
Ciloxan Eye Drops
Ciloxan Eye Ointment
Cipro
Cipro HC Ear Drops
Cipro XR
Ciprodex Ear Drops

Generic Ingredients: Gatifloxacin G
Zymar Eye Drops

Generic Ingredients: Gemifloxacin
Factive

Generic Ingredients: Levofloxacin G
Iquix Eye Drops
Levaquin
Quixin Eye Drops

Generic Ingredients: Moxifloxacin
Avelox
Vigamox Eye Drops

Generic Ingredients: Norfloxacin
Noroxin

Generic Ingredients: Ofloxacin G
Floxin Otic Ear Drops
Ocuflox Eye Drops

Prescribed For

Infections of the lower-respiratory tract, sinuses, urinary tract, pelvis, skin, bone and joints, stomach and intestine, and prostate; also prescribed for sexually transmitted diseases, infectious diarrhea, bronchitis, pneumonia, typhoid fever, anthrax, tularemia (rabbit fever), and traveler's diarrhea. The eye drops are used to treat ocular infections; the ear drops are for ear infections.

General Information

Fluoroquinolone anti-infectives work against many organisms that traditional antibiotics have trouble killing. They do not work against the common cold, flu, or other viral infections. The fluoroquinolones were first used as treatment for urinary infections and then other uses developed over the years. The new uses depend on how well the specific drug penetrates different body tissues as well as on how they have been tested in the laboratory. Individual fluoroquinolones are not all equally effective in treating all infections.

Cautions and Warnings

Do not take a fluoroquinolone if you are **allergic** or **sensitive** to any of its ingredients, or to any drug in this group, or have had a reaction to related medications such as nalidixic acid. Severe, possibly fatal, allergic reactions can occur even after the very first dose. These reactions include kidney damage, cardiovascular collapse, loss of consciousness, jaundice (yellowing of the skin or whites of the eyes), joint or muscle aches, tingling, swelling of the face or throat, breathing difficulties, anemia, bleeding, bruising, itching, and rash. Stop taking the drug if you experience allergic symptoms and seek medical help at once.

Avoid fluoroquinolones if you currently have **tendinitis** or a **ruptured tendon** in your body. These drugs carry an increased risk of damaged tendons, which may require surgery or lead to extended disability. Contact your doctor if you experience joint pain, swelling, or inflammation, or if you cannot use a joint or it becomes difficult to use. Rest, avoid exercise, and stop taking the medicine.

Do not take a fluoroquinolone if you have or have ever had **myasthenia gravis**, as your condition may worsen.

Levofloxacin, moxifloxacin, and gatifloxacin should be avoided by people with **heart rhythm problems** or those taking drugs that can affect heart rhythm.

Fluoroquinolones may cause increased pressure on parts of the brain, leading to convulsions and psychotic reactions. Other possible effects include tremors, restlessness, lightheadedness, confusion, and hallucinations. Fluoroquinolones should be used with caution in people with **head trauma**, **seizure disorders**, or other **nervous system conditions**.

Moxifloxacin should be used with caution by people with **liver disease**.

People with **kidney disease** require reduced dosage of these drugs, except in the case of moxifloxacin.

People taking fluoroquinolones may be unusually sensitive to the **sun**. Avoid the sun while taking this drug and for several days following therapy, even if you are using sunscreen. Contact your doctor if you become sensitive to the sun.

People taking a fluoroquinolone may develop colitis that could range from mild to very serious. Contact your doctor if you develop diarrhea or cramps.

Fluoroquinolones may change blood-sugar levels. People with **diabetes** who must take fluoroquinolones should carefully monitor their blood sugar while taking the antibiotic.

Some people taking fluoroquinolones have developed tingling or loss of sensation in the hands and feet.

Prolonged fluoroquinolone use can lead to fungal overgrowth.

Possible Side Effects

Side effects are rarely serious.

- ▼ Common: nausea, vomiting, and diarrhea (may be least likely with norfloxacin).
- ▼ Less common: dizziness, abdominal pain, headache, unusual sun sensitivity (skin rash or sunburn), itching, vaginal irritation, and liver inflammation.
- ▼ Rare: Rare side effects, including some severe drug reactions, can occur in almost any part of the body. Contact

Possible Side Effects *(continued)*

your doctor if you experience anything unusual while taking any medication.

Drug Interactions

- People taking drugs to correct abnormal heart rhythms should avoid fluoroquinolones.
- Levofloxacin, gatifloxacin, and moxifloxacin can increase the risk of abnormal heart rhythms. Combining these drugs with bepridil, cisipride, erythromycin, tricyclic antidepressants, and antipsychotics also increases the risk of abnormal heart rhythms. Do not mix moxifloxacin and ziprasidone, and use phenothiazines with caution.
- Nitrofurantoin may interfere with norfloxacin's antibacterial effects. Do not take these drugs together.
- Nonsteroidal anti-inflammatory drugs (NSAIDs) and other anti-inflammatory drugs should not be combined with fluoroquinolones because of the increased risk of nervous system stimulation and seizures.
- The risk of seizures is also increased when tramadol and moxifloxacin are taken together.
- Ciprofloxacin, norfloxacin, and ofloxacin may increase theophylline blood levels and the risk of seizures and other side effects.
- Avoid mixing tretinoin and moxifloxacin; this combination increases the risk of sun sensitivity.
- Blood levels of both fluoroquinolones and corticosteroids are increased when these drugs are taken together, which may increase the risk of tendon damage.
- Rifamycin and rifampin may decrease the effectiveness of moxifloxacin.
- Cimetidine may increase fluoroquinolone blood levels and raise the risk of side effects.
- Fluoroquinolones may increase the effect of oral anticoagulant drugs such as warfarin. Your anticoagulant dosage may need to be reduced.
- Fluoroquinolones may increase the toxic effects of cyclosporine (used for organ transplants) on your kidneys.
- Azlocillin may increase the risk of ciprofloxacin side effects.
- Separate your fluoroquinolone dose from that of antacids, didanosine, iron supplements, or zinc by 2–6 hours, and

take your fluoroquinolone at least 4 hours before or 8 hours after sucralfate. These drugs decrease the amount of fluoroquinolone absorbed. Moxifloxacin must be taken 4 hours before or 8 hours after antacids, iron, or zinc.

- Ciprofloxacin and norfloxacin may increase caffeine's effects.

Food Interactions

Gemifloxacin, levofloxacin, moxifloxacin, and ofloxacin may be taken with or without food. Take norfloxacin at least 1 hour before or 2 hours after meals or dairy products. Ciprofloxacin is best taken 1 hour before or 2 hours after meals, but may be taken with food. Dairy products and calcium-fortified orange juice interfere with the absorption of ciprofloxacin and should be avoided.

Usual Dose

Check with your doctor if you suffer from kidney disease, as your fluoroquinolone dosage may need to be reduced.

Ear Drops

Ciprofloxacin: Place contents of single-use container in affected ear twice a day for 7 days.

Ofloxacin: 5–10 drops in the affected ear twice a day for 7–14 days.

Eye Drops

Besifloxacin: 1 drop in the affected eye 3 times a day, at least 4 hours apart for 7 days.

Ciprofloxacin: bacterial conjunctivitis—days 1–2, place 1–2 drops in the affected eye every 2 hours while awake; days 3–7, place 1–2 drops in the affected eye every 4 hours while awake. Bacterial corneal ulcer—first 6 hours, 2 drops in affected eye every 15 minutes; next 18 hours, 2 drops in affected eye every 30 minutes; day 2, place 2 drops in the affected eye hourly; days 3–14, place 2 drops in affected eye every 4 hours. Your doctor may decide it is necessary to continue treatment after day 14.

Gatifloxacin: days 1–2, place 2 drops in affected eye every 2 hours while awake, up to 8 times a day; days 3–7, place 2 drops in affected eye 4 times a day.

Levofloxacin: bacterial conjunctivitis—days 1–2, place 1–2 drops in affected eye every 2 hours while awake, up to 8 times a day; days 3–7, place 1–2 drops in affected eye every 4 hours while awake, up to 4 times a day. Bacterial corneal ulcer—days

1–3, place 1–2 drops in the affected eye every 30 minutes to 2 hours while awake; awaken 4–6 hours after going to sleep for one more dose; day 4 until end of treatment course, 1–2 drops every 1–4 hours while awake.

Moxifloxacin: 1 drop in the affected eye 3 times a day for 1 week.

Ofloxacin: bacterial conjunctivitis—days 1–2, place 1–2 drops in the affected eye every 2–4 hours while awake; days 3–7, place 1–2 drops in the affected eye 4 times a day. Bacterial corneal ulcer—days 1–2, place 1–2 drops in the affected eye every 30 minutes while awake; awaken 4–6 hours after you go to sleep for one more dose; days 3–7, place 1–2 drops in the affected eye every hour while awake; days 7–9, or through the end of treatment, place 1–2 drops in the affected eye 4 times a day.

Eye Ointment

Ciprofloxacin: ½ in. ribbon in the affected eye 3 times a day for 2 days, then twice a day for next 5 days.

Tablets

Adult

Ciprofloxacin: 250–750 mg every 12 hours for 3–60 days, depending on condition.

Ciprofloxacin (Extended Release): 500–1000 mg once a day for 3–14 days.

Gemifloxacin: 320 mg once a day for 5–7 days.

Levofloxacin: 250–750 mg once a day for 3–60 days.

Moxifloxacin: 400 mg once a day for 5–14 days.

Norfloxacin: 400 mg every 12 hours for 3–28 days; a single dose of 800 mg may be taken for gonorrhea.

Ofloxacin: 200–400 mg every 12 hours for 3 days–6 weeks; a single dose of 400 mg may be taken for gonorrhea.

Child

Ciprofloxacin: 4.5 mg per lb. of body weight up to 750 mg twice a day.

Levofloxacin: Under 110 lbs.—3.6 mg per lb. of body weight, up to 250 mg, once a day. Over 110 lbs.—500 mg once a day.

Overdosage

Overdose symptoms generally mimic drug side effects. Overdose may cause kidney failure and, in the case of moxifloxacin, abnormal heart rhythms. Contact your local poison control center or a hospital emergency room for more information. You may be told to induce vomiting with ipecac syrup—available at any pharmacy—before taking the victim to an emergency room. If you seek treatment, ALWAYS bring the prescription bottle or container.

Special Information

Take each dose with a full glass of water. Be sure to drink at least 8 glasses of water a day while taking any of these drugs to help avoid kidney side effects.

Follow your doctor's directions exactly. Complete the full course of drug therapy, even if you feel well.

Fluoroquinolones can cause temporary changes in vision, dizziness, drowsiness, and lightheadedness. Be careful when driving or performing any task that requires concentration.

If you forget to administer a dose, do so as soon as you remember. If it is almost time for your next dose, skip the missed dose and continue with your regular schedule. Do not take a double dose.

Eye Drops

To avoid infection, do not let the eyedropper tip touch your finger, eyelid, or any surface. Wait 5 minutes before using another eye drop or eye ointment.

Do not use contact lenses while you have conjunctivitis or while you are using an anti-infective eye drop to treat the conjunctivitis.

Allergic reactions to eye drops are uncommon but they can occur.

Contact your doctor at once if your vision declines or if eye stinging, itching or burning, redness, irritation, swelling, or pain worsens.

Special Populations

Pregnancy/Breast-feeding: Animal studies have shown that fluoroquinolones may damage the fetus or reduce the likelihood of a successful pregnancy. A fluoroquinolone should be taken during pregnancy only if your doctor determines that the potential benefit outweighs the risks.

Fluoroquinolones pass into breast milk. Nursing mothers who must take them should use infant formula.

Seniors: With the exception of moxifloxacin, seniors may require reduced dosage due to age-related decreases in kidney function. The risk of a ruptured tendon may increase in seniors, especially those also taking a corticosteroid. In the case of eye drops, seniors may also need less medication.

Generic Name

Fluoxymesterone

(flue-OX-ee-MES-ter-one) G

Brand Names

Androxy

Type of Drug

Androgen (male hormone).

Prescribed For

Men: hormone replacement or augmentation and male menopause; also prescribed as male contraception for up to 12 months, and for delayed puberty.

Women: some breast cancer types; may also be used for breast pain or fullness.

General Information

Fluoxymesterone is an androgen. Androgens are responsible for the normal growth and development of male sex organs and for maintaining secondary sex characteristics such as hair distribution, vocal cord thickening, muscle development, and fat distribution.

Cautions and Warnings

Do not use fluoxymesterone if you are **allergic** or **sensitive** to any of its ingredients.

Androgens do not improve athletic performance and may cause serious side effects.

Women taking any androgen may develop deepening of the voice, oily skin, acne, hairiness, increased sex drive, and menstrual irregularities. Women who are **pregnant** should not take fluoxymesterone.

Androgens should be used with caution in **boys** with **delayed puberty**. Androgens can accelerate bone growth without accelerating height to compensate. Bone measurements of the wrist and hand should be conducted every 6 months during therapy with this medication.

Fluoxymesterone may cause gynecomastia (swollen male breast tissue).

Men with known or suspected **prostate cancer** or **prostate destruction**, or **breast cancer** should not use fluoxymesterone, nor should anyone with severe **liver, heart, or kidney disease**.

High blood-calcium levels may develop in those taking fluoxymesterone who are **immobile** or have **breast cancer**.

Patients with **benign prostatic hypertrophy (BPH)** may develop serious urinary obstruction while taking this medication. Other risks include priapism (a persistent, painful erection) or excessive sexual stimulation.

Long-term, high-dose androgen therapy may cause severe liver disease, including hepatitis and cancer, reduced sperm count, and water retention.

Blood cholesterol may be raised by androgens. This can be a problem for people who have **heart disease**.

Androgens may cause or worsen **sleep apnea** (intermittent cessation of breathing during sleep).

For patients with **diabetes**, this drug may affect blood-sugar levels.

Possible Side Effects

Men

▼ Most common: inhibition of testicle function, impotence, chronic erection, and painful enlargement of breast tissue.

Women

▼ Most common: unusual hairiness, male-pattern baldness, deepening of the voice, and enlargement of the clitoris. These changes may be irreversible if they are not noticed in mild stages and treatment discontinued. Increased blood calcium and menstrual irregularities may also develop.

Men and Women

▼ Most common: changes in sex drive, headache, anxiety, depression, a tingling feeling, sleep apnea, flushing, rash, acne, habituation (the drug may be habit-forming), excitation, chills, sleeplessness, water retention, nausea, vomiting, diarrhea, hepatitis (symptoms include yellowing of the skin or whites of the eyes), liver inflammation, and liver cancer. Symptoms resembling those of a stomach ulcer may also develop.

Drug Interactions

- Fluoxymesterone may increase the effect of an oral anticoagulant (blood thinner); dosage of the anticoagulant may need to be reduced.
- Fluoxymesterone may raise blood levels of oxyphenbutazone.
- Androgens may decrease insulin requirements.

Food Interactions

Take fluoxymesterone with meals if it upsets your stomach.

Usual Dose

Adult: Hormone replacement for men: 5–20 mg a day. Breast cancer treatment for women: 10–40 mg a day.

Child: 2.5–20 mg a day for a duration of no more than 6 months.

Overdosage

Symptoms include nausea, vomiting, and diarrhea. Contact your local poison control center or a hospital emergency room for more information. If you seek treatment, ALWAYS bring the prescription bottle or container.

Special Information

Androgens must be taken only under the close supervision of your doctor. The dosage and clinical effects of fluoxymesterone vary widely and require constant monitoring.

Contact your doctor if you develop nausea or vomiting, swelling of the legs or feet, yellowing of the skin or whites of the eyes, or a painful or persistent erection. Women should contact their doctor immediately if they develop a deep or hoarse voice, acne, hairiness, male-pattern baldness, or menstrual irregularities.

If you forget a dose, take it as soon as you remember. If it is almost time for your next dose, skip the one you forgot and continue with your regular schedule. Do not take a double dose.

Special Populations

Pregnancy/Breast-feeding: Fluoxymesterone should never be taken by pregnant or nursing women because it can affect the developing fetus and nursing infant.

Seniors: Seniors are more likely to develop prostate enlargement or prostate cancer. A marked increase in sex drive may also occur.

Focalin XR *see **Methylphenidate,** page 742*

Generic Name

Fosfomycin (fos-foe-MYE-sin)

Brand Names

Monurol

Type of Drug

Urinary anti-infective.

Prescribed For

Uncomplicated urinary infections.

General Information

Fosfomycin kills a variety of bacteria. It works by preventing bacteria from sticking to the wall of the urinary tract and by interfering with bacterial cell division. In the body, it is converted to its active form—free fosfomycin. Generally, bacteria that are resistant to other antibiotics are not resistant to fosfomycin, so this drug may work when others have failed.

Cautions and Warnings

Do not take fosfomycin if you are **allergic** or **sensitive** to any of its ingredients.

Fosfomycin is meant to be taken once, in a single dose. Taking more than 1 packet of fosfomycin only increases side effects; it does not improve the drug's effectiveness.

Possible Side Effects

- ▼ Less common: diarrhea, vaginal irritation, runny nose, nausea, and headache.
- ▼ Rare: Rare side effects can occur in almost any part of the body. Contact your doctor if you experience anything unusual while taking any medication.

Drug Interactions

- Metoclopramide reduces fosfomycin blood levels.

Food Interactions

You can take fosfomycin without regard to food or meals.

Usual Dose

Adult (age 12 and over): 1 packet mixed with water.
Child (under age 12): not recommended.

Overdosage

Little is known about the effects of fosfomycin overdose. Contact your local poison control center or a hospital emergency room for more information. If you seek treatment, ALWAYS bring the prescription container.

Special Information

Do not take fosfomycin powder in its dry form. Mix the contents of the packet with 3–4 oz. of cool or cold water until it dissolves. Then drink the solution immediately.

Contact your doctor if your infection does not improve within 2 or 3 days.

Special Populations

Pregnancy/Breast-feeding: The safety of using fosfomycin during pregnancy is not known. Fosfomycin should be taken during pregnancy only if your doctor determines that the potential benefit outweighs the risks.

It is not known if fosfomycin passes into breast milk. Nursing mothers who must take this drug should use infant formula.

Seniors: Seniors may take fosfomycin without special restriction.

Generic Name

Gemfibrozil (jem-FI-broe-zil) G

Brand Names

Lopid

Type of Drug

Anti-hyperlipidemic (blood-fat reducer).

Prescribed For

High blood triglycerides and prevention of heart disease.

General Information

Gemfibrozil consistently reduces blood triglycerides and reduces the risk of heart disease in people with high levels of triglycerides, low levels of high-density lipoprotein (HDL) cholesterol—the "good" cholesterol—and high levels of low-density lipoprotein (LDL) cholesterol—the "bad" cholesterol. It works by affecting the breakdown of body fats and by reducing the amount of triglyceride manufactured by the liver. It is usually prescribed only for people with very high blood-fat levels who have not responded to dietary changes or other therapies. Gemfibrozil usually has little effect on blood-cholesterol levels, although it may reduce blood cholesterol in some people.

Cautions and Warnings

Do not take gemfibrozil if you are **allergic** or **sensitive** to any of its ingredients.

People with **gallbladder disease** or severe **liver or kidney disease** should not take gemfibrozil. Some people taking gemfibrozil have experienced worsening liver or kidney function, and gemfibrozil users may have an increased risk of developing gallbladder disease and gallstones.

People taking gemfibrozil and fenofibrate may develop pancreatitis (inflammation of the pancreas).

People taking gemfibrozil may develop muscle aches and inflammation. Tell your doctor if you experience muscle tenderness or weakness.

Gemfibrozil may cause a moderate rise in blood sugar and mild decreases in white-blood-cell counts.

Possible Side Effects

▼ Most common: abdominal and stomach pain, fatigue, heartburn, and diarrhea.

▼ Less common: nausea, vomiting, rash, itching, dizziness, blurred vision, anemia, reduced levels of white blood cells, increased blood sugar, and muscle pain—especially in the arms or legs.

▼ Rare: dry mouth, constipation, appetite loss, upset stomach, sleeplessness, tingling in the hands or feet, ringing or buzzing in the ears, back pain, swollen or painful joints, feeling unwell, reduction in blood potassium, and abnormal liver function. Contact your doctor if you experience anything unusual while taking any medication.

Drug Interactions

- Do not use gemfibrozil if you take repaglinide because of the risk of dangerously low blood sugar. If you take a sulfonylurea antidiabetic drug and gemfibrozil together, the sulfonylurea dosage may need to be reduced.

- Combining gemfibrozil with a statin cholesterol-lowering drug (atorvastatin, fluvastatin, lovastatin, pravastatin, rosuvastatin, or simvastatin) has led to the destruction of skeletal muscles. Avoid this combination unless your doctor determines it is absolutely necessary, in which case your doctor should frequently monitor your condition.
- Gemfibrozil increases the effects of oral anticoagulant (blood thinning) drugs. These drugs should not be used together unless there is no alternative. The anticoagulant dosage should be reduced.
- Gemfibrozil increases the risk of side effects with bexarotene, glitazone antidiabetes drugs, loperamide, montelukast, and tiagabine. Lower dosages of these drugs may be necessary.
- Combining gemfibrozil and cyclosporine may decrease the effectiveness of cyclosporine. Your doctor may need to increase the dose of cyclosporine and should carefully monitor your condition.
- Colestipol may decrease the effectiveness of gemfibrozil. Separate doses by at least 2 hours.

Food Interactions

Gemfibrozil is best taken on an empty stomach 30 minutes before meals but may be taken with food if it upsets your stomach. It is important that you follow your doctor's dietary instructions.

Usual Dose

Adult: 1200 mg a day, divided into 2 doses taken 30 minutes before breakfast and dinner.

Child: not recommended.

Overdosage

Symptoms reported with gemfibrozil overdose were abdominal cramps, abnormal liver function tests, diarrhea, joint and muscle pain, nausea, and vomiting. Induce vomiting with ipecac syrup—available at any pharmacy—but contact your doctor or local poison control center before doing this. If you seek treatment, ALWAYS bring the prescription bottle or container.

Special Information

Your doctor should perform periodic blood counts during the first year of gemfibrozil treatment to check for anemia or other changes in blood components. Liver-function tests are also necessary.

Gemfibrozil may cause dizziness or blurred vision. Be careful when driving or doing any task that requires concentration.

Gemfibrozil is less effective if you are greatly overweight.

Contact your doctor if side effects become severe or intolerable, especially diarrhea, nausea, vomiting, or stomach pain or gas. These may disappear if your doctor reduces the dosage.

If you forget a dose, take it as soon as you remember. If it is almost time for your next dose, skip the one you forgot and continue with your regular schedule. Do not take a double dose.

Special Populations

Pregnancy/Breast-feeding: The safety of using gemfibrozil during pregnancy is not known. Gemfibrozil should be taken during pregnancy only if your doctor determines that the potential benefit outweighs the risks.

It is not known if gemfibrozil passes into breast milk. Nursing mothers who must take this drug should use infant formula.

Seniors: Seniors are more likely to develop drug side effects due to normal declines in kidney function.

Geodon *see **Ziprasidone,** page 1013*

Generic Name

Glatiramer (glah-TYE-ram-er)

Brand Names

Copaxone

Type of Drug

Relapsing-remitting multiple sclerosis (MS) therapy.

Prescribed For

Multiple sclerosis.

General Information

Glatiramer is a mixture of several amino acids. It is thought to work by modifying the immune processes responsible for MS. In studies, people who took the drug for over a year were twice as likely to be relapse-free as those who took a placebo (sugar pill).

Cautions and Warnings

Do not use this drug if you are **allergic** or **sensitive** to any of its ingredients or to mannitol.

About 10% of people who self-administer glatiramer experience a post-injection reaction with symptoms that include flushing, chest pain, heart palpitations, anxiety, breathing difficulties, closing of the throat, and an itchy rash. These symptoms usually go away without treatment. This reaction generally occurs after several months of drug therapy, though it may occur earlier.

About 21% of the people who took glatiramer in drug studies had transient chest pain (usually lasting several minutes), but the exact relationship of this pain to use of glatiramer could not be determined. Report any chest pain to your doctor at once, particularly if it lasts longer than a few minutes.

Glatiramer may make you more sensitive to sunlight.

Because it interferes with immune response, glatiramer may increase your risk of developing infections and tumors.

Glatiramer may interfere with kidney function.

Possible Side Effects

- ▼ Most common: infections, weakness, pain, chest pain, flu-like symptoms, back pain, flushing, heart palpitations, anxiety, muscle stiffness or spasticity, an urgent need to urinate, swollen lymph glands, injection-site reactions (including pain, inflammation, itching, an unknown mass at the injection site, welts, skin marks, and bleeding), breathing difficulties, runny nose, and joint pain.
- ▼ Common: fever, neck pain, facial swelling, bacterial infection, migraine, rapid heartbeat, tremors, fainting, appetite loss, vomiting, general stomach disorders, vaginal infection, painful menstruation, black-and-blue marks, swelling in the arms or legs, bronchial irritation, spasm of the larynx, and ear pain.
- ▼ Less common: chills, cysts, agitation, foot drop, nervousness, rolling eyeballs, rapid eye movement, confusion, speech problems, cold sores, redness, itchy rash, skin nodules, stomach pain and irritation, and weight gain.

Possible Side Effects *(continued)*

▼ Rare: Other side effects can occur in almost any part of the body, including the heart and blood vessels, digestive system, blood and lymph systems, muscles and bones, respiratory system, kidney, reproductive system, and eyes. Contact your doctor if you experience anything unusual while taking any medication.

Drug Interactions

None known.

Usual Dose

Adult: 20 mg a day by injection under the skin.

Child: not recommended.

Overdosage

Little is known about the effects of glatiramer overdose. Contact your local poison control center or a hospital emergency room for information. If you seek treatment, ALWAYS bring the prescription bottle or container.

Special Information

This medication is given by injection. For information on how to properly administer this drug, see page 1242.

Store unused glatiramer in the refrigerator before it is mixed with the diluent supplied by the manufacturer. Do not use any other diluent. The mixed injection must be used right away.

Suggested injection sites are the arms, abdomen, hips, and thighs. Be sure to rotate injection sites.

Glatiramer works best if given at the same time each day.

If you forget to administer a dose, do so as soon as you remember. If it is almost time for your next dose, skip the dose you forgot and continue with your regular schedule. Do not take a double dose. Contact your doctor if you miss more than 2 doses in a row.

Special Populations

Pregnancy/Breast-feeding: The safety of using glatiramer during pregnancy is not known. Glatiramer should be taken during pregnancy only if your doctor determines that the potential benefit outweighs the risks.

It is not known if glatiramer passes into breast milk. Nursing mothers who must take it should use infant formula.

Seniors: Seniors may use glatiramer without special restriction.

Type of Drug

Glitazone Antidiabetes Drugs

(GLIT-uh-zone)

Brand Names

Generic Ingredients: Pioglitazone Hydrochloride
Actos

Generic Ingredients: Rosiglitazone Maleate
Avandia

Combination Products
Generic Ingredients: Pioglitazone Hydrochloride + Metformin Hydrochloride G
ACTOplus Met ACTOplus Met XR

Generic Ingredients: Pioglitazone Hydrochloride + Glimepiride
Duetact

Generic Ingredients: Rosiglitazone Maleate + Metformin Hydrochloride
Avandamet

Generic Ingredients: Rosiglitazone Maleate + Glimepiride
Avandaryl

Prescribed For

Type 2 diabetes; not to be used by people with type 1 diabetes. These drugs may also be prescribed for the treatment of polycystic ovary syndrome (PCOS).

General Information

The glitazones reduce the amount of sugar produced by the liver and increase insulin sensitivity of muscle, liver, and fat cells. Pioglitazone (but not rosiglitazone) may also help to control blood-fat levels, which are often elevated in diabetes. Glitazones work by affecting genes responsible for controlling the use of sugar and fat in the body, making cells more sensitive to insulin. They are effective for people with type 2 diabetes, whose cells do not respond well to insulin. Glitazones only work when insulin is present. They do not increase the amount of insulin made in the pancreas. Glitazones can be used alone or combined with other diabetes drugs. Studies have indicated that taking these medicines can delay or prevent type 2 diabetes in people with prediabetes.

Studies specifically testing the effects of pioglitazone on the heart and blood vessels have shown no increased risk of cardiac side effects but also only modest benefits to the heart, whereas rosiglitazone may be harmful. People with diabetes are at increased risk of heart disease. Contact your doctor if you have chest pain or feel chest pressure.

Cautions and Warnings

Do not take these drugs if you are **sensitive** or **allergic** to any of their ingredients or to related drugs.

Do not take these drugs if you are being treated for **heart failure**. Glitazones may cause or worsen fluid retention and can lead to heart failure. This effect is more common when these drugs are combined with insulin.

Rosiglitazone may increase the risk of heart attack and other cardiovascular events. Rosiglitazone use is now restricted to patients who are already taking this drug and have not experienced any harmful side effects.

Glitazones are broken down in the liver; people with **liver disease** should not take them. Liver enzyme monitoring is recommended for all people taking a glitazone. People taking pioglitazone and rosiglitazone have experienced liver failure, though no direct causal effect of the drug has been established.

Pioglitazone has been associated with an increased risk of **bladder cancer** and should be used with caution if you have or have had bladder cancer.

Broken bones are more common in **women** taking a glitazone.

Glitazones may cause macular edema, or swelling within the eye. The symptoms of this condition include blurred and less acute vision.

These drugs can trigger ovulation. Premenopausal women with **PCOS** or another medical **condition that prevents ovulation** may be at risk of becoming pregnant. Contraception should be used to prevent unwanted pregnancy.

Glitazones can cause weight gain, which increases with dosage.

Rosiglitazone may raise blood levels of cholesterol and other blood fats.

Women may achieve maximum benefit with smaller dosages.

Possible Side Effects

Pioglitazone

▼ Most common: upper-respiratory infections, headaches, and sinus irritation.

▼ Common: muscle aches, tooth problems, and sore throat.

▼ Less common: anemia and swollen legs or arms.

▼ Rare: swelling below the surface of the skin, especially around the eyes and lips; yellowing of the skin or whites of the eyes; hepatitis; and liver failure. Contact your doctor if you experience anything unusual while taking any medication.

For more information on ACTOplus Met, see Metformin, page 731. For more information on Duetact, see Sulfonylurea Antidiabetes Drugs, page 1081.

Rosiglitazone

The risk of leg and ankle swelling, weight gain, and anemia increases with larger doses.

▼ Common: upper-respiratory infections, accidental injuries, and headache.

▼ Less common: fatigue, sinus irritation, swollen legs or arms, and back pain.

▼ Rare: hives, anemia, blurry or distorted vision, heart attack, and low blood sugar. Swelling below the surface of the skin, especially around the eyes and lips, may also affect the hands, feet, and throat. Contact your doctor if you experience anything unusual while taking any medication.

For more information on Avandamet, see Metformin, page 731. For more information on Avandaryl, see Sulfonylurea Antidiabetes Drugs, page 1081.

Drug Interactions

- Do not mix a glitazone with any nitrate drug, typically used to treat angina. This combination increases the risk of heart attack and angina.
- Taking a glitazone and insulin may increase the risk of fluid retention and heart failure.

- Do not use a glitazone with gatifloxacin, as there is a risk of dangerously low blood sugar with this combination.
- Mixing gemfibrozil with a glitazone increases the amount of the glitazone absorbed into the body. A reduction in the dose of the glitazone may be needed if you start taking gemfibrozil.
- Rifampin can reduce the amount of a glitazone that is absorbed by the body, possibly leading to higher blood-sugar levels.
- Ketoconazole and trimethoprim may significantly increase the amount of glitazone in the body.
- Mixing pioglitazone with atorvastatin may reduce the amount of either drug in the body.
- Pioglitazone may reduce the effectiveness of contraceptive drugs containing norethindrone and ethinyl estradiol. Higher-dose contraceptives or another contraceptive method may be needed.
- Glitazones may reduce blood levels of midazolam, nevirapine, and nifedipine.

For additional drug interactions for Avandamet and ACTOplus Met, see Metformin, page 731. For additional drug interactions for Avandaryl and Duetact, see Sulfonylurea Antidiabetes Drugs, page 1081.

Food Interactions

These drugs can be taken without regard to food or meals, except for Avandaryl, which should be taken with the first meal of the day.

Usual Dose

Adult

ACTOplus Met: 15/500–45/2550 mg once a day or in divided doses.

ACTOplus Met XR: 15/1000–45/2000 mg once a day.

Avandamet: 2/500–4/1000 mg twice a day.

Avandaryl: 4/1–8/4 mg with the first meal of the day.

Duetact: 30/2–30/4 mg once a day.

Pioglitazone: 15–45 mg once a day.

Rosiglitazone: 4–8 mg once a day or in divided doses.

Child: not recommended.

Overdosage

Little is known about the effects of glitazone overdose. Take the victim to a hospital emergency room. If you seek treatment, ALWAYS bring the prescription bottle or container.

Special Information

Diet, calorie control, exercise, and weight loss are essential to controlling type 2 diabetes. Do not depend solely on this drug to manage your condition.

Contact your doctor if you develop symptoms of liver disease, including nausea, vomiting, abdominal pain, fatigue, appetite loss, or dark-colored urine; or if you have symptoms suggestive of heart failure, including swelling, especially in the legs or ankles; shortness of breath or difficulty breathing, especially when you lie down; unusually rapid weight gain; or feeling unusually tired. Your diabetes medicine will be changed if this happens.

See your doctor for regular monitoring of blood sugar, glycosylated hemoglobin (a more sensitive indicator of long-term diabetes control), and liver function.

If you forget a dose of any of these medicines, take it as soon as you remember. If it is almost time for your next dose, skip the dose you forgot and continue with your regular schedule.

Special Populations

Pregnancy/Breast-feeding: The safety of using glitazones during pregnancy is not known. A glitazone should be taken during pregnancy only if your doctor determines that the potential benefit outweighs the risks. Diabetes during pregnancy is usually treated with insulin.

It is not known if glitazones pass into breast milk. Nursing mothers who must take a glitazone should use infant formula.

Seniors: Seniors may take this drug without special restriction.

Generic Name

Guanabenz (GWAN-uh-benz) G

Brand Names

Only available in generic form.

Type of Drug

Antihypertensive.

Prescribed For

High blood pressure.

General Information

Guanabenz works by depressing the central nervous system (CNS) by stimulating certain receptors. Initially, guanabenz reduces blood pressure without a major effect on blood vessels; however, long-term use of guanabenz may result in the dilation (widening) of blood vessels and a slight slowing of pulse rate. Guanabenz may be taken alone or with a thiazide diuretic.

Cautions and Warnings

Do not take guanabenz if you are **allergic** or **sensitive** to any of its ingredients.

People with severe **kidney or liver disease** should take this drug with caution. Guanabenz should also be used with caution by people who have had a recent **heart attack** or **stroke**.

Possible Side Effects

Risk and severity of side effects increase with dosage.

- ▼ Most common: drowsiness, sedation, dry mouth, dizziness, weakness, and headache.
- ▼ Less common: chest pain; swelling in the hands, legs, or feet; heart palpitations or abnormal heart rhythms; stomach or abdominal pain or discomfort; nausea; diarrhea; vomiting; constipation; anxiety; poor muscle control; depression; difficulty sleeping; stuffy nose; blurred vision; muscle aches and pains; breathing difficulties; frequent urination; decreased sex drive; impotence; unusual taste in the mouth; and swollen and painful breasts in men.

Drug Interactions

- Other blood-pressure-lowering agents such as beta blockers increase the effect of guanabenz.
- The sedating effects of guanabenz are increased by combining it with sedatives, sleeping pills, or other CNS depressants, including alcohol.
- People taking this drug for high blood pressure should avoid over-the-counter drugs that might aggravate their condition, including decongestants, cold and allergy remedies, and diet pills—all of which may contain stimulants.

Food Interactions

This drug is best taken on an empty stomach, but it may be taken with food if it upsets your stomach.

Usual Dose

4 mg twice a day to start, increased gradually to a maximum dose of 32 mg twice a day—though doses this large are rarely needed.

Overdosage

Overdose causes sleepiness, lethargy, low blood pressure, irritability, pinpoint pupils, and reduced heart rate. Overdose victims should be made to vomit with ipecac syrup—available at any pharmacy—but contact your doctor or poison control center first. If you seek treatment, ALWAYS bring the prescription bottle or container.

Special Information

Take guanabenz exactly as prescribed for maximum benefit. If any side effect becomes severe or intolerable, contact your doctor.

Guanabenz often causes tiredness or dizziness; avoid alcohol because it increases these effects. Take care when driving or doing anything that requires concentration.

Do not stop taking guanabenz without your doctor's approval. Suddenly stopping this drug may cause a rapid increase in blood pressure. Dosage must be gradually reduced by your doctor.

If you forget a dose, take it as soon as you remember. If it is almost time for your next dose, skip the one you forgot and continue with your regular schedule. Do not take a double dose. Contact your doctor if you miss 2 or more consecutive doses.

Special Populations

Pregnancy/Breast-feeding: Guanabenz may affect the fetus. It should be avoided by women who are or might be pregnant. Guanabenz should be taken during pregnancy only if your doctor determines that the potential benefit outweighs the risks.

It is not known if guanabenz passes into breast milk. Nursing mothers who must take this drug should use infant formula.

Seniors: Seniors are more sensitive to the sedating and blood-pressure-lowering effects of guanabenz.

Generic Name

Haloperidol (hal-oe-PER-ih-dol) G

Brand Names

Only available in generic form.

Type of Drug

Butyrophenone antipsychotic.

Prescribed For

Psychotic disorders; Tourette syndrome; severe behavioral problems in children; and short-term treatment of hyperactive children. May also be prescribed for prevention of nausea and vomiting associated with cancer treatment, obsessive-compulsive disorder, hiccups, and phencyclidine psychosis.

General Information

Haloperidol is one of many nonphenothiazine agents used to treat psychosis. These drugs are equally effective when given in therapeutically equivalent doses. The major differences are in the type and severity of side effects. Some people may respond well to one and not at all to another. Haloperidol acts on a portion of the brain called the hypothalamus. It affects parts of the hypothalamus that control metabolism, body temperature, alertness, muscle tone, hormone balance, and vomiting. Haloperidol is available in liquid form for those who have trouble swallowing tablets.

Cautions and Warnings

Haloperidol should not be used by people who are **allergic** or **sensitive** to any of its ingredients.

People with **severe central-nervous-system depression** or who are in a **coma** and those with **Parkinson's disease** should not take haloperidol.

Haloperidol has been associated with increased mortality in seniors with **dementia**-related psychosis events or infection, mostly pneumonia.

Caution is advised when haloperidol is given to those with **heart or heart rhythm abnormalities**, **high blood-calcium or -magnesium levels**, or **hypothyroidism** (underactive thyroid gland). Sudden death due to heart rhythm problems has occurred in those taking haloperidol even without these predisposing conditions.

A serious set of side effects known as neuroleptic malignant syndrome (NMS) may occur while taking haloperidol. Symptoms include high fever, convulsions, difficult or fast breathing, rapid heartbeat, rapid or irregular pulse or blood pressure, increased sweating, muscle rigidity, and mental changes. NMS can be fatal and requires immediate medical attention. This condition has been associated with most antipsychotic medicines.

Tardive dyskinesia (a group of severe side effects associated with antipsychotic and other drugs) may occur while taking haloperidol and is often considered a reason to stop taking this drug. Symptoms include lip smacking or puckering, puffing of the cheeks, rapid or wormlike movements of the tongue, uncontrolled chewing motions, and uncontrolled arm or leg movements. Symptoms can increase with the length and dosage of antipsychotic drug therapy and may become permanent. Report any of these side effects to your doctor.

People with severe **heart disorders**, very **low blood pressure**, or a history of **seizures** should take this medication with caution.

If haloperidol is used to control mania in **bipolar disorder**, a rapid depressive mood swing may occur.

Possible Side Effects

- ▼ Most common: drowsiness, blurred vision, constipation, diarrhea, dizziness, dry mouth, headache, loss of appetite, nausea, stomach pain, or sleeplessness.
- ▼ Less common: jaundice (yellowing of the skin or whites of the eyes), which may occur in the first 2–4 weeks. The jaundice usually goes away when the drug is discontinued, but there have been cases in which it did not. If you notice this effect, develop fever, or generally feel unwell, contact your doctor immediately. Other less common side effects are changes in components of the blood, including anemias; raised or lowered blood pressure; abnormal heartbeat; restlessness; anxiety; euphoria (feeling "high"); depression; confusion; acne-like skin reactions; excessive salivation; breast engorgement; development of breast tissue in males; vomiting; excessive sweating; menstrual irregularities; impotence; and breathing difficulties.
- ▼ Rare: neurological effects such as spasms of the neck muscles, severe stiffness of the back muscles, rolling back of the eyes, convulsions, difficulty swallowing, and symptoms associated with Parkinson's disease. These effects usually disappear after the drug has been withdrawn; however, symptoms of the face, tongue, or jaw may persist for years, especially in seniors with a long history of brain disease. If you experience any of these effects, contact your doctor immediately. Other rare side effects can occur in almost any part of the body. Contact your doctor if you experience anything unusual while taking any medication.

Drug Interactions

- Be cautious about taking haloperidol with barbiturates, sleeping pills, narcotics or other sedatives, tricyclic antidepressants, alcohol, or any other medication that may produce a depressive effect.
- When haloperidol is combined with amiodarone, arsenic trioxide, bretylium, chloroquine, chlorpromazine, cisapride, disopyramide, dofetilide, dolasetron, droperidol, erythromycin and related antibiotics, flecainide, halofantrine, lapatinib, maprotiline, mefloquine, mesoridazine, methadone, moxifloxacin, nilotinib, paliperidone, pentamidine, perflutren, pimozide, propafenone, quinidine, sotalol, tacrolimus, tetrabenazine, thioridazine, or ziprasidone, serious heart rhythm disorders are possible.
- Haloperidol should not be used with medications to treat Parkinson's disease.
- Anticholinergic drugs may reduce the effectiveness of haloperidol and increase the risk of side effects.
- Risk of seizures is increased if haloperidol is combined with antiseizure medication or tramadol. Haloperidol should not be taken with tramadol.
- The use of azole antifungal agents (fluconazole, itraconazole, ketoconazole, posaconazole, and voriconazole) may cause an increase in haloperidol side effects, possibly requiring adjustments in haloperidol doses.
- Severe low blood pressure or heartbeat irregularities may occur if haloperidol is combined with a beta blocker such as propranolol.
- The efficacy of cabergoline is decreased if taken with haloperidol. This combination should be avoided.
- Combining haloperidol with carbamazepine may decrease the effectiveness of haloperidol, requiring a dosage adjustment.
- Haloperidol may inhibit the blood-pressure-lowering effects of guanethidine. This combination should be avoided.
- Taking lithium together with haloperidol may lead to disorientation, loss of consciousness, or uncontrolled muscle movements.
- Careful dosage monitoring is required if haloperidol is taken with rifampin.
- Selective serotonin reuptake inhibitors (SSRIs) such as fluoxetine may increase haloperidol's effects. Careful monitoring is necessary with this combination.

Food Interactions

Haloperidol is best taken on an empty stomach, but you may take it with food if it upsets your stomach.

Usual Dose

Psychotic Disorders

Adult: starting dose—0.5–2 mg 2 or 3 times a day. Some patients may need 3–5 mg 2 or 3 times a day. Rarely, some patients may require up to 100 mg a day.

Child (age 3–12 or 33–88 lbs.): starting dose—0.5 mg a day. Dosage may be increased in 0.5-mg steps every 5–7 days. The maintenance dose is 0.02–0.07 mg per lb. of body weight a day in divided doses, reduced once the desired effect is reached.

Child (under age 3): not recommended.

Tourette Syndrome

Adult: starting dose—0.5–1.5 mg 3 times a day; up to 10 mg a day may be needed.

Child (age 3–12 or 33–88 lbs.): starting dose—0.5 mg a day. Dosage may be increased in 0.5-mg steps every 5–7 days. The maintenance dose is 0.02–0.03 mg per lb. of body weight a day in divided doses, reduced once the desired effect is reached. The same dosages apply to children with behavioral disorders or hyperactivity.

Overdosage

Symptoms of overdose are depression, extreme weakness, tiredness, desire to sleep, coma, lowered blood pressure, uncontrolled muscle spasms, agitation, restlessness, convulsions, fever, dry mouth, and abnormal heart rhythm. The patient should be taken to a hospital emergency room immediately. If you seek treatment, ALWAYS bring the prescription bottle or container.

Special Information

This medication may cause drowsiness. Use caution when driving or operating hazardous equipment; also, avoid alcoholic beverages while taking it.

Haloperidol may cause unusual sensitivity to the sun. It may also turn your urine reddish-brown or pink.

If dizziness occurs, avoid sudden changes in posture and avoid climbing stairs.

Avoid extreme heat while taking haloperidol. This medication may make you more prone to heat stroke.

If you forget to take a dose of haloperidol, take it as soon as you remember. Take the rest of the day's doses evenly spaced throughout the day. Do not take a double dose.

Special Populations

Pregnancy/Breast-feeding: Newborns whose mothers are taking any antipsychotic medicine are more likely to experience agitation, abnormally increased or decreased muscle tone, tremor, sleepiness, severe difficulty breathing, and difficulty in feeding. In some newborns, the symptoms subside within hours or days and do not require specific treatment; other newborns may require longer hospital stays. If you are or might be pregnant, do not stop taking this medication without talking to your doctor, because suddenly stopping antipsychotic medications can cause significant treatment complications.

Haloperidol passes into breast milk. Nursing mothers who must use this medication should use infant formula.

Seniors: Seniors are more sensitive to the effects of this medication and usually require ¼–½ the usual adult dose. Seniors are also more likely to develop side effects.

Brand Names

Helidac

Generic Ingredients

Bismuth Subsalicylate + Metronidazole + Tetracycline

The information in this profile also applies to the following drugs:

Generic Ingredients: Bismuth Subcitrate Potassium + Metronidazole + Tetracycline
Pylera

Type of Drug

Antibacterial combination.

Prescribed For

Duodenal ulcers.

General Information

Research has shown that the bacterium *Helicobacter pylori* is usually present in ulcer disease and some forms of gastritis. Drugs used to treat the *H. pylori* infection are prescribed along with a drug that alleviates ulcer symptoms by blocking stomach acid. There are a variety of approaches to treating ulcers by using combinations of various antibiotic and acid-blocking drugs. Helidac combines 3 drugs with antibacterial or antibiotic action. This combination generally works by disrupting the cell walls of the bacterium and interfering with its ability to make proteins or duplicate itself. It is often prescribed together with ranitidine, cimetidine, or another acid blocker. Other treatments use other drug combinations.

Cautions and Warnings

Do not take Helidac if you are **allergic** or **sensitive** to any of its ingredients. If you are allergic to aspirin, do not take Helidac.

Children or **teenagers** who have or are recovering from **chickenpox** should not use Helidac because it contains a small amount of salicylate, which is related to aspirin. Children or teenagers who take aspirin or a salicylate during chickenpox may develop Reye's syndrome, which involves brain and liver damage; symptoms include nausea and vomiting.

Children under age 8 should not take Helidac because its tetracycline component may negatively affect tooth development.

Do not take Helidac if you have severe **liver or kidney disease**. People with less severe liver disease may require a reduced dosage.

Metronidazole, one of the ingredients in Helidac, has been shown to cause cancer in animal studies. This medication should be used cautiously and only for approved conditions.

Rarely, bismuth causes severe nervous system toxicity. Symptoms go away after the drug is stopped.

Metronidazole can cause convulsive seizures and nervous system effects, including numbness or tingling in the arms, legs, hands, or feet. The risk of developing these effects increases with dosage and duration of use. Contact your doctor at once if you experience any of these effects.

Metronidazole should be taken with caution by people who have had **blood diseases** or **nervous system disorders**, such as seizure disorders.

Other infections, called superinfections, can develop while you are taking tetracycline or metronidazole. Superinfections may be caused by fungi, including *Candida*, or other bacteria. If this happens, your doctor will discontinue Helidac and prescribe a different drug to treat your *H. pylori* infection, as well as another drug to treat the superinfection.

People taking tetracycline can develop pseudotumor cerebri (increased pressure in the brain), the symptoms of which are usually headache and blurred vision. Symptoms usually go away when the drug is stopped, but permanent damage can result.

Tetracycline may increase your sensitivity to the sun; use sunscreen and wear protective clothing.

Possible Side Effects

- ▼ Most common: nausea, abdominal pain, stool discoloration, and diarrhea.
- ▼ Less common: blood in the stool, changes in taste, headache, anal discomfort, vaginal irritation, appetite loss, dizziness, tingling in the hands or feet, vomiting, muscle weakness, constipation, sleeplessness, pain, and respiratory infections.

For more information see Metronidazole, page 750, and Tetracycline Antibiotics, page 1122.

Drug Interactions

- Metronidazole should not be used if you are currently taking disulfiram (a drug used to maintain alcohol abstinence) or have taken it within 2 weeks of starting Helidac because the combination can cause confusion and psychotic reactions. Likewise, do not drink alcohol while using Helidac and for at least 1 day after finishing treatment, as you may experience heart rhythm changes, flushing, abdominal cramps, nausea, or vomiting.
- Tetracycline should not be used with methoxyflurane due to the risk of a fatal toxic interaction.
- Tetracycline antibiotics, which are bacteriostatic, may interfere with the action of bactericidal (bacteria-killing) agents such as penicillin. You should not take both kinds of antibiotics for the same infection.
- If bismuth subsalicylate is taken with aspirin, a ringing in the ears may occur. Treatment should be discontinued if this happens.
- Antacids, mineral supplements, and multivitamins containing bismuth, calcium, zinc, magnesium, and iron can reduce the effectiveness of tetracycline. Separate doses of your antacid,

mineral supplement, vitamin with minerals, or sodium bicarbonate and Helidac by at least 2 hours.

- Bismuth subsalicylate, tetracycline, and metronidazole may each increase the effect of anticoagulant (blood thinning) drugs such as warfarin. An adjustment in the anticoagulant dosage may be required.
- Cimetidine may increase metronidazole blood levels.
- Urinary alkalinizers such as potassium citrate, sodium bicarbonate, and tromethamine may reduce the effectiveness of tetracycline. Separate doses by 3–4 hours.
- Bismuth subsalicylate may increase the effects of medications to treat diabetes. If you are using this combination, be sure to carefully monitor your blood-sugar level.
- Metronidazole raises lithium blood levels, effects, and toxicity.
- Phenobarbital and other barbiturates and phenytoin can decrease metronidazole's effectiveness.
- Tetracycline may interfere with the actions of contraceptive drugs.

Food Interactions

Do not take this drug with milk or dairy products. Helidac should be taken at least 1 hour after meals.

Usual Dose

Helidac

Adult: Each dose consists of 4 pills. Take all 4 pills, 4 times a day for 14 days with a full glass of water after meals and at bedtime. Take your acid blocker according to your doctor's directions.

Child: not recommended.

Pylera

Adult: 3 pills 4 times a day for 10 days with a full glass of water. Take your acid blocker according to your doctor's directions.

Child: not recommended.

Overdosage

All 3 ingredients in Helidac can be dangerous if taken in overdose, but salicylate poisoning is the most threatening. Symptoms of salicylate toxicity are rapid or heavy breathing, nausea, vomiting, ringing or buzzing in the ears, high fever, lethargy, rapid heartbeat, and confusion. Other more serious symptoms may develop. Take the victim to a hospital emergency room at once. If you seek treatment, ALWAYS bring the prescription bottle or container.

Special Information

Women should use non-hormonal contraception while taking Helidac to avoid unwanted pregnancy. Breakthrough bleeding is also possible.

Bismuth can cause a temporary darkening of your tongue or stool. This is a harmless effect. Stool darkening should not be confused with blood in the stool, which turns it black.

Avoid alcohol while taking Helidac and for 1 day after you stop taking it.

Contact your doctor if you develop ringing in the ears. This can be a sign of salicylate toxicity from the bismuth.

If you forget a dose, take it as soon as you remember. If it is almost time for your next dose, skip the dose you forgot and continue with your regular schedule. Never take a double dose.

Special Populations

Pregnancy/Breast-feeding: Helidac should not be taken by pregnant women. Tetracycline affects bone and tooth development in the fetus.

Tetracycline and metronidazole pass into breast milk. Tetracycline interferes with the development of the child's skull, bones, and teeth, and metronidazole also may cause side effects in the baby. Nursing mothers who must take Helidac should use infant formula.

Seniors: Seniors may take this drug without special restriction.

Type of Drug

Hepatitis C Protease Inhibitors

Brand Names

Generic Ingredients: Boceprevir
Victrelis

Generic Ingredients: Telaprevir
Incivek

Prescribed For

Chronic hepatitis C virus (HCV).

General Information

Boceprevir and telaprevir, approved within 3 days of each other, are the first of a new type of drugs for HCV. They work by inhibiting an enzyme needed for the formation of proteins required for the production of the mature hepatitis C virus particle. They are intended for adults with chronic HCV and compensated liver disease, in which the liver is still able to carry out all of its functions in spite of the disease, including cirrhosis due to the infection. These drugs should never be taken by themselves because of the very high chances the virus will quickly become resistant. They must be taken with interferon alpha and ribavirin, 2 other antiviral medicines. These medicines may be prescribed for people who have either not responded to other treatments or who have never been treated for HCV.

Cautions and Warnings

Do not use boceprevir or telaprevir if you are **allergic** or **sensitive** to any of their ingredients or have had a previous reaction to them.

These drugs have not been studied in people who have already taken them, or another member of this drug class, without success. Poor interferon responders are less likely to respond fully when one of these medicines is added.

The combination of boceprevir or telaprevir with peginterferon and ribavirin can cause anemia. Tell your doctor about any unusual weakness or tiredness. Substantial reduction in white-blood-cell count may cause dosage reduction or even discontinuation of drug treatment.

People taking telaprevir may experience serious and potentially fatal skin reactions, including DRESS syndrome (rash, fever, inflammation of internal organs, swollen lymph glands, and blood changes) and Stevens-Johnson syndrome, in which the upper layer of skin peels away from your body.

Thromboembolism (blood clots) occurred in clinical trials of boceprevir, but they were most likely due to interferon alpha.

This combination of drug therapy also suppresses one type of white blood cell and can make you more likely to develop a serious infection. Use special caution if you have had or are being treated for a **chronic infection**. Your doctor will check your blood for infection during boceprevir treatment. Tell your doctor if you develop a fever or any other sign of infection.

The safety of these drugs has not been studied in people with **decompensated cirrhosis**, severe **liver disease**, or who have received an **organ transplant**. Their safety has also not been established in people who are coinfected with **hepatitis B virus** or **HIV**.

These drugs interact with many other drugs. See "Drug Interactions" for more information.

Possible Side Effects

Boceprevir

▼ Most common: fatigue, chills, weakness, anemia, reduced white-blood-cell count, nausea, headache, diarrhea, vomiting, taste changes, appetite loss, dry mouth, joint pains, sleeplessness, irritability, hair loss, dry skin, and rash.
▼ Common: difficulty breathing.
▼ Rare: Other rare side effects can occur. Contact your doctor if you experience anything unusual while taking any medication.

Telaprevir

▼ Most common: rash, itching, anemia, nausea, hemorrhoids, diarrhea, rectal discomfort, taste changes, fatigue, and vomiting.
▼ Common: rectal itch.
▼ Rare: Other rare side effects can occur. Contact your doctor if you experience anything unusual while taking any medication.

Drug Interactions

- Do not mix boceprevir or telaprevir with carbamazepine, dexamethasone, efavirenz, modafinil, nevirapine, phenobarbital and other barbiturates, phenytoin, pioglitazone, rifabutin, rifampin, rifapentine, ritonavir, and St. John's wort, as they can substantially lower blood levels of boceprevir by stimulating the production of enzymes that break them down in the blood. This can negate the effect of boceprevir.
- These drugs interfere with the breakdown of and should not be mixed with alfentanil, amiodarone, astemizole, benzodiazepines, bepridil, calcium channel blockers, cisapride, cyclosporine, digoxin, drosperinone, erectile dysfunction drugs, ergot-based migraine medicines, fentanyl, flecainide, lidocaine, pimozide, propaphenone, quinidine, rifabutin, salmeterol, sirolimus, tacrolimus, and terfenadine. These combinations can lead to substantially increased blood levels of the interacting drugs and possible toxicities and drug side effects.

- Mixing telaprevir with HIV antiviral drugs and protease inhibitors reduce telaprevir levels, interfering with its effectiveness. This combination can also affect blood levels of the HIV medicines. These drugs should not be mixed.
- Do not mix telaprevir with any corticosteroid medicine. Corticosteroid blood levels are significantly increased. Also, dexamethasone reduces telaprevir blood levels. Boceprevir should be mixed with the inhaled corticosteroids budesonide and fluticasone with caution.
- These medicines can either raise or lower blood levels of warfarin and the narcotic pain relievers. Close monitoring is needed.
- These medicines can increase blood levels of trazadone, desipramine, and erectile dysfunction drugs, leading to drug side effects. Reduced drug dose may help avoid this problem.
- Telaprevir reduces blood levels of escitalopram. More escitalopram may be needed to maintain its effect.
- Mixing boceprevir and telaprevir with the antifungal drugs itraconazole, ketoconazole, posaconazole, and voriconazole can raise blood levels of all of these drugs. Itraconazole and ketoconazole should be limited to 200 mg a day. Clinical monitoring is recommended for all other combinations.
- Mix these drugs and bosentan with caution, due to the possibility of higher bosentan drug levels.
- These drugs cause significant increases in colchicine blood levels. People with gout and liver or kidney disease should not be given both medicines. Individual gout flares may be treated with individual colchicine doses.
- Statin drug levels are raised by boceprevir. Low daily doses of atorvastatin may be used with careful monitoring for side effects. Lovastatin and simvastatin should not be mixed with boceprevir.
- Boceprevir and telaprevir affect blood levels of the hormone ingredients of contraceptive drugs. For this reason, women taking boceprevir should not rely on hormonal contraceptive drugs in any form. See "Pregnancy/Breast-feeding" for more information.

Food Interactions

These drugs should be taken with food or meals (not low-fat) for maximum absorption into the blood.

Usual Dose

Boceprevir

Adult: 800 mg (four 200-mg capsules) 3 times a day, every 7–9 hours. Depending on how well you respond and whether you have been previously treated with other medicines, you may take boceprevir for 12–48 weeks.

Child: not recommended.

Telaprevir

Adult: 750 mg (two 375-mg tablets) 3 times a day, every 7–9 hours. Depending on how well you respond and whether you have been previously treated with other medicines, you may take telaprevir for 12–48 weeks.

Child: not recommended.

Overdosage

Doses up to 3600 mg a day of boceprevir have been safely taken by healthy volunteers for 5 days. In a study of healthy volunteers taking 5600 mg a day of telaprevir for 4 days, side effects were nausea, headache, diarrhea, vomiting, appetite loss, and taste changes. In the event of an overdose, take the victim to a hospital emergency room. If you seek treatment, ALWAYS bring the prescription bottle or container.

Special Information

Contact your doctor if you develop any rash, with or without itching, blisters or skin lesions, mouth sores or ulcers, red or inflamed eyes (such as "pink eye"), fever, or facial swelling while taking telaprevir. These can be early signs of a serious skin reaction and are a cause for stopping drug treatment. Dizziness, difficulty breathing, shortness of breath, tiredness, and weakness may be signs of anemia.

Your doctor will occasionally take blood samples to measure your response to these medicines.

If you forget a dose of boceprevir, take it as soon as you remember with food. If it is 2 hours or less until your next dose is due, skip the forgotten dose and continue with your regular schedule.

If you forget a dose of telaprevir, take it as soon as you remember with food. If it is 4 hours or less before your next dose, skip the forgotten dose and take your next dose at the regular time.

Talk to your pharmacist or doctor if you have trouble remembering your medicine. They may be able to help set up medication reminders.

The effect of treating HCV infection on your ability to transmit the virus is not known. Caution is recommended.

Before starting treatment, make sure your doctor knows if you are pregnant or nursing, or if you have any other medical condition, including anemia, any other form of liver disease, HIV infection, gout or high blood levels of uric acid, if you have had an organ transplant, or if you plan to have surgery sometime soon.

These drugs must not be taken by themselves. They must be taken with other HCV treatment. Do not stop taking any of these medicines without your doctor's approval. If your doctor does tell you to stop, do not restart again on your own.

Boceprevir may be kept at room temperature for up to 3 months. For longer storage, boceprevir capsules must be refrigerated. Throw the refrigerated capsules away once their expiration date has passed. Telaprevir can be stored at room temperature. Once a bottle of telaprevir capsules is open, they should be discarded after 4 weeks.

For more information about the drugs that must always be taken along with boceprevir and telaprevir see Interferon Alpha, page 634, and Ribavirin, page 997.

Special Populations

Pregnancy/Breast-feeding: Ribavirin causes birth defects or death of the fetus. Neither boceprevir nor telaprevir has been shown to affect a developing fetus. However, women who must take this combination of medicines must obtain a negative pregnancy test before starting treatment and use at least 2 types of birth control—such as an intrauterine device (IUD) and a barrier method—while taking these drugs and for 6 months after completing treatment. You should NOT rely on birth control pills or other hormonal contraceptives. Since boceprevir enters male semen, female partners of men taking it must also take the same precautions. A registry has been created by the drug maker for women exposed to boceprevir while pregnant. You or your doctor may enroll.

These drugs may pass into breast milk but it is not known if it can be absorbed if swallowed by a nursing infant. Nursing mothers who must take it should use infant formula during treatment.

Seniors: Seniors should use this medicine with caution because of the chances of some loss of liver function, other diseases, and concurrent drug therapies.

Type of Drug

Histamine H_2 Antagonists

Brand Names

Generic Ingredients: Cimetidine

Tagamet
Tagamet HB

Generic Ingredients: Famotidine

Pepcid
Pepcid Complete
Pepcid AC

Generic Ingredients: Nizatidine

Axid
Axid AR

Generic Ingredients: Ranitidine

Zantac

Prescribed For

Acute treatment and maintenance of ulcers of the stomach and duodenum (upper intestine), gastroesophageal reflux disease (GERD), heartburn, prevention of upper gastrointestinal (GI) bleeding in critically ill patients, and certain conditions related to oversecretion of bodily fluids (Zollinger-Ellison syndrome, systemic mastocytosis, multiple endocrine adenomas). These medicines may also be used to prevent bleeding in the stomach and upper intestines, stress ulcers, stomach damage caused by nonsteroidal anti-inflammatory drugs (NSAIDs), and to stop the production of stomach acid during surgery.

General Information

Histamine H_2 antagonists work by turning off the system that produces stomach acid and other secretions. Cimetidine is effective in treating the symptoms of ulcer and preventing complications of the disease, although an ulcer that does not respond to another histamine H_2 antagonist will probably not respond to cimetidine. Histamine H_2 antagonists differ only in their potency. Cimetidine is the least potent; 1000 mg are roughly equal to 300 mg of either nizatidine or ranitidine, or 40 mg of famotidine. These drugs are roughly equal in their ability to treat ulcer disease and their risk of side effects.

Cautions and Warnings

Do not take these drugs if you are **allergic** or **sensitive** to any of their ingredients or any histamine H_2 antagonist. If you are allergic to one of these, there is a good chance you will also react to other members of this group.

Cimetidine has a mild antiandrogen effect, which probably causes the painful, swollen breasts that some people experience after taking this drug for a month or more.

People with **kidney or liver disease** should take these medicines with caution because ⅓ of each dose is broken down in the liver and passes out of the body through the kidneys.

Reducing stomach acid levels in a person with **compromised immune function** may increase the risk of intestinal worm infection.

Ranitidine should not be used in people with **acute porphyria** (a rare blood disorder).

Do not self-treat with over-the-counter forms of these medicines for anything besides heartburn without first consulting your doctor. The fact that symptoms are alleviated does not preclude the possibility of more serious problems, including stomach cancer, which can have symptoms similar to other GI disorders. Make sure your doctor tests you for other conditions.

Some people—mostly the very ill—experience confusion, agitation, psychosis, hallucinations, depression, anxiety, or disorientation, usually within 2–3 days of starting cimetidine. Normally these symptoms stop 3–4 days after discontinuing the drug. Contact your doctor if this happens to you.

Possible Side Effects

Cimetidine

Serious side effects are uncommon.

- ▼ Most common: mild diarrhea, dizziness, rash, painful breast swelling, nausea and vomiting, headache, confusion, drowsiness, hallucinations, and impotence.
- ▼ Less common: liver inflammation, peeling or red and swollen rash, breathing difficulties, tingling in the hands or feet, feeling delirious, and oozing from the nipples.
- ▼ Rare: Cimetidine may affect white blood cells or blood platelets. Some symptoms of these effects are unusual bleeding or bruising, unusual tiredness, and weakness. Other rare side effects are inflammation of the pancreas, hair loss (reversible), abnormal heart rhythms, heart attack, muscle or joint pain, and drug reactions. Contact your doctor if you experience anything unusual while taking any medication.

Possible Side Effects *(continued)*

Famotidine

- ▼ Most common: headache.
- ▼ Less common: dizziness, mild diarrhea, and constipation.
- ▼ Rare: Rare side effects can occur in almost any part of the body. Contact your doctor if you experience anything unusual while taking any medication.

Nizatidine

Side effects noted in clinical studies were similar to placebo (sugar pill).

- ▼ Most common: low red-blood-cell count and hives.
- ▼ Common: headache, abdominal pain, diarrhea, upset stomach, nausea, runny nose, flatulence, weakness, dizziness, and sore throat.
- ▼ Less common: anxiety, sleeplessness, nervousness, sleepiness, itch, rash, weight loss, constipation, and dry mouth.
- ▼ Rare: Rare side effects can affect the heart, liver, kidneys, stomach and intestines, blood, joints and muscles, mental status, and sexual function. Contact your doctor if you experience anything unusual while taking any medication.

Ranitidine

Side effects with ranitidine are rare.

- ▼ Most common: nausea, vomiting, constipation, diarrhea, abdominal discomfort, and headache.
- ▼ Rare: joint pain, hair loss, blurred vision, sleeplessness, dizziness, confusion, agitation or anxiety, depression, hallucinations, inflammation of the pancreas, painful breast swelling, impotence, loss of sex drive, rash, rapid or irregular heartbeat, reversible reduction in white-blood-cell or blood-platelet count, and hepatitis. Contact your doctor if you experience anything unusual while taking any medication.

Drug Interactions

- Separate cimetidine and ranitidine from antacids by about 3 hours to avoid reducing cimetidine's effectiveness.
- H_2 antagonists may increase the side effects of a variety of drugs, possibly leading to drug toxicity. These drugs include chlordiazepoxide, diazepam, glipizide, lidocaine, metronidazole, midazolam, nifedipine, phenytoin, propranolol, theophylline, triazolam, certain tricyclic antidepressants, and

warfarin-type anticoagulants. Close monitoring is necessary when an H_2 antagonist and warfarin are given together.

- Atazanavir, delavirdine, gefitinib, and ketoconazole absorption may be decreased by these drugs. If these drugs are both prescribed, ketoconazole should be given 2 hours before cimetidine.
- Enteric-coated tablets should not be taken with famotidine. The change in stomach acidity that famotidine produces causes the tablets to disintegrate prematurely in the stomach.
- Antacids, anticholinergics, and metoclopramide may slightly reduce the amount of nizatidine absorbed into the blood, but no precaution is needed.
- Nizatidine may increase blood levels of aspirin in people taking very large doses of aspirin.

Food Interactions

Take these drugs up to 1 hour before eating to prevent heartburn, acid indigestion, or sour stomach. Otherwise you can take them without regard to food or meals.

Usual Dose

Over-the-counter forms of these medicines should only be used for the temporary relief of heartburn and are not recommended for children under 12 years of age. Do not take more than 2 capsules or chewable tablets in 24 hours.

Cimetidine

Adult: 400–800 mg at bedtime; 300 mg 4 times a day with meals and at bedtime; or 400 mg twice a day. To treat GERD—400 mg 4 times a day. Do not exceed 2400 mg a day. Users of Tagamet HB should not take more than 400 mg a day. Smaller doses may be as effective for seniors or those with impaired kidney function.

Famotidine

Adult and Child (age 17 and over): 20–40 mg at bedtime, or 20 mg twice a day for 4–12 weeks. Dosage should be reduced in people with severe kidney disease.

Child (age 1–16): 0.23–0.90 mg per lb. of body weight, at bedtime or in 2 divided doses, up to 80 mg a day.

Child (age 3–11 months): 0.23 mg per lb. of body weight of oral suspension twice a day for up to 8 weeks.

Child (under age 3 months): 0.23 mg per lb. of body weight of oral suspension once a day for up to 8 weeks.

Nizatidine

Adult: 300 mg at bedtime or 150 mg twice a day. Maintenance dose is 150 mg at bedtime. Dosage is reduced in people with kidney disease.

Child: not recommended.

Ranitidine

Adult and Child (age 17 and over): 150–300 mg a day. People with severe conditions may require up to 600 mg a day. People with severe kidney disease need less medication.

Child (age 1 month–16 years): 0.9–1.8 mg per lb. of body weight every 12 hours up to the 150–300 mg a day maintenance dose.

Overdosage

Little is known about the effects of H_2 antagonist overdose, but victims may experience exaggerated side effects. Two deaths have occurred. Your local poison control center may advise giving ipecac syrup—available at any pharmacy—to induce vomiting and remove any drug remaining in the stomach. Victims who have definite symptoms should be taken to a hospital emergency room. If you seek treatment, ALWAYS bring the prescription bottle or container.

Special Information

Take these medications exactly as directed and follow your doctor's instructions regarding diet and other treatment in order to get the maximum benefit from the drug. It may take several days to relieve stomach pain. Antacids may be taken with these drugs, if needed.

Do not take the maximum dose continuously for more than 2 weeks without the consent and supervision of your doctor.

Cigarette smoking is associated with stomach ulcers and reduces the effectiveness of these drugs.

If you empty the nizatidine capsule and mix it with juice before taking it, you may keep it in the refrigerator. Do not store it for more than 2 days because the drug may lose potency.

Contact your doctor at once if you develop any unusual side effects such as bleeding or bruising, tiredness, diarrhea, dizziness, rash, or hallucinations. Black, tarry stools or vomiting material that resembles coffee grounds may indicate your ulcer is bleeding.

If you miss a dose of medicine, take it as soon as possible. If it is almost time for your next dose, skip the dose you forgot and continue with your regular schedule. Do not take a double dose.

Special Populations

Pregnancy/Breast-feeding: Animal studies reveal no damage to the fetus, although these medicines can pass into the fetal blood. Cimetidine should be taken during pregnancy only if your doctor determines that the potential benefit outweighs the risks.

Large amounts of cimetidine and ranitidine pass into breast milk. Small amounts of famotidine and nizatidine may also enter breast milk. Nursing mothers who must take one of these drugs should use infant formula.

Seniors: Seniors may need lower medication doses due to loss of kidney function and be more susceptible to side effects, especially confusion and other nervous system effects (see "Cautions and Warnings").

Type of Drug

HIV Antivirals

Brand Names

Generic Ingredients: Abacavir
Ziagen

Generic Ingredients: Delavirdine
Rescriptor

Generic Ingredients: Didanosine G
Videx EC

Generic Ingredients: Efavirenz
Sustiva

Generic Ingredients: Emtricitabine
Emtriva

Generic Ingredients: Etravirine
Intelence

Generic Ingredients: Lamivudine
Epivir

Generic Ingredients: Nevirapine
Viramune Viramune XR

Generic Ingredients: Rilpivirine
Edurant

Generic Ingredients: Stavudine G
Zerit

Generic Ingredients: Tenofovir
Viread

Generic Ingredients: Zidovudine G
Retrovir

Combination Products
Generic Ingredients: Abacavir + Lamivudine
Epzicom

Generic Ingredients: Abacavir + Lamivudine + Zidovudine
Trizivir

Generic Ingredients: Efavirenz + Emtricitabine + Tenofovir
Atripla

Generic Ingredients: Emtricitabine + Rilpivirine + Tenofovir
Complera

Generic Ingredients: Emtricitabine + Tenofovir
Truvada

Generic Ingredients: Lamivudine + Zidovudine
Combivir

Prescribed For

Human immunodeficiency virus (HIV) infection.

General Information

Zidovudine (also known as azidothymidine, or AZT) was the first drug approved for treating HIV infection. Over the years, AZT use has been expanded from adults to children to the prevention of HIV transmission between a pregnant woman and her developing fetus.

These drugs, nucleoside and non-nucleoside antiviral agents, slow the reproduction of the HIV virus by interfering with and altering an enzyme called HIV reverse transcriptase, essential to the virus' ability to reproduce. When infected cells try to build more HIV virus with the altered reverse transcriptase, the result is an inactive molecule. This reduces the total viral load and helps the body's immune system deal with the remaining HIV virus.

People with HIV infection always take these drugs in combination with at least one protease inhibitor and another antiviral.

Combination pills of HIV antivirals have been developed because they reduce the number of required pills each day, making it easier to follow an anti-HIV regimen. Some drugs, such as tenofovir, are eliminated through the urine while others, such as abacavir, etravirine, and nevirapine, are broken down in the liver. This difference is important because it affects how each drug interacts both with other antivirals and other medicines, and how it is affected by liver and kidney disease.

Cautions and Warnings

Do not take any of these drugs if you are **allergic** or **sensitive** to any of their ingredients. Stop taking abacavir or the combination product Trizivir at the first sign of drug allergy, as people have died from sensitivity reactions. Another treatment should be started immediately. Contact your doctor at once if you develop signs of a reaction (fever, skin rash, fatigue, nausea, vomiting, diarrhea, pain, sore throat, difficulty breathing, or cough). Up to 8 of every 100 people who take abacavir may develop a severe reaction to it, and if you have a reaction to abacavir, you must never take it again. Restarting abacavir can result in very severe, possibly fatal reactions. Your doctor may screen your blood for a specific genetic variation that has been associated with this reaction.

People with **kidney disease** require lower dosages of emtricitabine, lamivudine, stavudine, and tenofovir than people with normal kidney function. Rilpivirine may be used by people with mild or moderate kidney disease, but should be used with caution by people with severe or end-stage kidney disease because of substantial increases in drug blood levels.

People with **liver disease** may require lower doses of abacavir, didanosine, efavirenz, and nevirapine. Rilpivirine may be taken by people with mild or moderate liver disease but has not been studied in people with severe liver disease. People taking tenofovir may develop severe, sometimes fatal liver disease. Didanosine has been associated with a rare liver complication.

People with **kidney or liver disease** should not use any fixed-dose combination antiviral product because the dosage of individual ingredients cannot be changed. Individual medicines must be used in this case. AZT should be used with caution by these patients.

Up to 50% of patients who take didanosine experience symptoms of nervous system inflammation, and about 33% need to reduce their dosage to control these symptoms. Some symptoms are numbness, tingling, and pain in the hands and feet. People who already have signs of **nerve damage** should not take didanosine.

People with HIV taking abacavir or delavirdine have a higher risk of heart attack than those who have not taken these medicines. Rilpivirine should be used with caution if you have **torsade de pointes**, an unusual heart rhythm.

The HIV virus can become resistant to HIV antiviral drug combinations. Resistance patterns are constantly changing and are an important reason for the creation of new antiviral medicines. People with both **HIV and hepatitis B** should not use emtricitabine due to a large increase in the risk of liver damage. These people should also use caution if discontinuing use of lamivudine or tenofovir; worsening of hepatitis B virus infection has been reported when either lamivudine or tenofovir was stopped. Special monitoring and follow-up of anti–hepatitis B therapy may be necessary.

Efavirenz can raise blood cholesterol by 10–20%.

Etravirine can lead to severe, life-threatening skin reactions. In clinical studies, most rashes were mild to moderate and occurred within 2–4 weeks of starting treatment. Other HIV antivirals can also be associated with a rash, but it is much less severe and not a reason to stop the medicine.

HIV antivirals can rarely cause liver enlargement and lactic acidosis (a potentially fatal metabolic imbalance). People with a history of **alcohol abuse** or **hepatitis** should use these drugs with caution. This mainly occurs in **women**, but **obesity** and long-term treatment may also be risk factors; however, people with no known risk factors have also developed these problems. Symptoms of liver problems include yellow skin, dark urine, pale stool, lower abdominal pain, and loss of appetite. Symptoms of lactic acidosis include heart problems, bluish discoloration of the skin, cold hands or feet, rapid heartbeat, low blood pressure, dehydration, rapid or difficulty breathing, lethargy, stupor or coma, vomiting, and/or abdominal pain. Contact your doctor immediately if you develop these or any other unusual symptoms.

Lamivudine and didanosine have rarely caused fatal inflammation of the pancreas. Symptoms include major changes in blood-sugar levels, increased triglyceride levels, a drop in blood calcium, nausea, vomiting, and abdominal pain. People who develop pancreatic inflammation must stop taking these drugs.

Severe depression can develop in people taking rilpivirine or efavirenz. People with a history of **depression** or **suicidal ideation** should contact their doctor if they experience any change in or worsening of depression symptoms who will determine whether the risk of continuing therapy outweighs the benefit.

Trizivir is associated with liver toxicity. People with HIV who also have chronic **liver disease** due to **hepatitis B** infection are especially likely to be affected.

Trizivir and AZT may cause muscle irritation and abnormalities similar to those caused by HIV infection.

HIV antivirals can cause a significant reduction in bone mineral density, increasing the risk of bone fractures.

AZT has been associated with low white-blood-cell count and anemia.

People taking HIV antivirals may experience unusual fat accumulation or redistribution, leading to buffalo hump, breast enlargement, abnormal thinness, or a round, moon-shaped face. The exact reasons for this are not known.

People taking combination HIV antiviral therapy may develop immune reconstitution syndrome, in which your body starts reacting to opportunistic infections that have found their way into your system. As the immune system rebounds, it starts fighting off these organisms by developing an inflammation around them that may then require further treatment.

Possible Side Effects

Abacavir

Abacavir is always taken with other drugs, so the side effects listed here are those of the drugs in combination.

Adult

- ▼ Most common: nausea, headache, fatigue, vomiting, diarrhea, and appetite loss.
- ▼ Common: sleep disturbances.

Child

- ▼ Most common: nausea, vomiting, fever, headache, diarrhea, and rash.
- ▼ Common: appetite loss.

Delavirdine and Efavirenz

More than ½ of people who take these drugs experience some nervous system and psychiatric side effects and rash. About 2% have to stop treatment because of them. Children are more likely than adults to develop rash.

Possible Side Effects *(continued)*

- Most common: nausea, dizziness, sleeplessness, headache, and temporary rash.
- Common: abnormal dreaming, poor concentration, tiredness, and diarrhea.
- Less common: itching, sweating, stomach pain or gas, upset stomach, reduced sensitivity to stimulation, depression, appetite loss, hallucinations, and nervousness.
- Rare: blisters, wet ulcers, peeling skin, blood in the urine, delusions, inappropriate behavior, and severe depression. Blood cholesterol can rise 10–20%. Other rare side effects can occur in almost any part of the body. Contact your doctor if you experience anything unusual while taking any medication.

Didanosine

Adult

- Most common: diarrhea, nervous system inflammation, fever, chills, itching, rash, abdominal pain, weakness, headache, nausea, vomiting, infection, pneumonia, and pancreatic inflammation.
- Less common: tumors, muscle pain, appetite loss, dry mouth, convulsions, abnormal thought patterns, breathing difficulties, drug allergy, anxiety, nervousness, twitching, confusion, depression, and blood component abnormalities.
- Rare: Rare side effects can occur in almost any part of the body. Contact your doctor if you experience anything unusual while taking any medication.

Child

Almost all children who take didanosine experience side effects. They are likely to experience many of the same reactions as adults, most commonly chills, fever, weakness, appetite loss, nausea and vomiting, diarrhea, liver dysfunction, headache, nervousness, sleeplessness, cough, runny nose, asthma or breathing difficulties, rash, and skin problems. Four children taking didanosine developed severe eye disease, resulting in some loss of sight. The progress of the eye disease slowed or stopped when dosage was reduced. Children taking this drug should have an eye examination every 6 months or if vision starts to worsen.

Possible Side Effects *(continued)*

Emtricitabine

Because this drug is always taken with other antiviral drugs, the listed side effects are those of the drugs in combination. The risk of developing specific side effects can be different depending on the exact drug combination you are taking. The long-term effects of emtricitabine are not known.

- ▼ Most common: rash, itching, allergic reactions, cough, runny nose, nausea, weakness, diarrhea, abdominal pain, depression, and headache.
- ▼ Common: discoloration of the soles of the feet or palms of the hands, upset stomach, vomiting, joint or muscle pain, unusual dreams, dizziness, sleeplessness, and tingling or pain in the hands or feet.
- ▼ Rare: Rare side effects can occur in almost any part of the body. Contact your doctor if you experience anything unusual while taking any medication.

Etravirine and Stavudine

Most common side effects apply to both etravirine and stavudine. Common and less common side effects apply to stavudine only.

- ▼ Most common: peripheral neuropathy, which can produce tingling, burning, numbness, or pain in the hands, arms, feet, or legs; diarrhea; nausea; vomiting; headache; fever; chills; weakness; abdominal pain; back pain; muscle or joint ache; generalized pain; not feeling well; sleeplessness; anxiety; depression; nervousness; breathing difficulties; appetite and weight loss; rash; itching; and sweating.
- ▼ Common: allergic reactions; flu-like symptoms; swollen lymph glands, usually felt under the arms or in the neck; chest pain; constipation; upset stomach; and dizziness.
- ▼ Less common: pelvic pain, tumors, hypertension (high blood pressure), swelling, flushing, stomach ulcers, confusion, migraine headache, sleepiness, tremors, nerve pain, asthma, pneumonia, skin tumors, conjunctivitis (pinkeye), visual disturbances, painful urination, genital pain, painful menstruation, and vaginitis.
- ▼ Rare: frequent urination, blood in the urine, impotence, fainting, paralysis, inflammation of the pancreas, worsening of

Possible Side Effects *(continued)*

diabetes or high blood sugar, nerve pain, and peeling skin. Contact your doctor if you experience anything unusual while taking any medication.

Lamivudine

Because this drug is always taken with AZT, the listed side effects are those of the drugs in combination. The long-term effects of lamivudine are not known.

- ▼ Most common: headache, not feeling well, fever, chills, rash, nausea, vomiting, diarrhea, appetite loss, abdominal pain or cramps, nervous system problems such as tingling and poor coordination, sleeplessness, dizziness, depression, stuffy or runny nose, cough, and muscle pain.
- ▼ Common: upset stomach, joint pain, and tingling in the hands or feet in children. Lamivudine may affect the results of a variety of blood tests.
- ▼ Rare: pancreas irritation, more often seen in children than adults. Contact your doctor if you experience anything unusual while taking any medication.

Nevirapine

- ▼ Most common: rash, fever, nausea, headache, hypersensitivity, and changes in liver function tests.
- ▼ Less common: abdominal pain, mouth or throat sores, tingling in the hands or feet, muscle aches, and liver inflammation.
- ▼ Rare: diarrhea, pain, and changes of sensation in the arms or legs. Contact your doctor if you experience anything unusual while taking any medication.

Rilpivirine

In clinical studies, rilpivirine was compared to efavirenz and was found to have fewer side effects.

- ▼ Most common: fever, nausea, headache, hypersensitivity reactions (symptoms include itching, rash, swelling, bronchospasms, and breathing difficulties), and changes in liver function tests.
- ▼ Less common: abdominal pain, mouth or throat sores, tingling in the hands or feet, muscle aches, and liver inflammation.

Possible Side Effects *(continued)*

- Rare: diarrhea, pain, and changes of sensation in the arms or legs. Contact your doctor if you experience anything unusual while taking any medication.

Tenofovir

- Most common: nausea, diarrhea, weakness, and headache.
- Common: vomiting, stomach gas, abdominal pain, and loss of appetite.

Trizivir

- Most common: anemia, reduced white-blood-cell counts, chills, rash, nausea, vomiting, diarrhea, appetite loss, abdominal pain or cramps, nervous system problems such as tingling and poor coordination, sleeplessness, dizziness, depression, stuffy or runny nose, cough, muscle pain, fever, headache, feeling or being sick, and weakness.
- Common: sensitivity reaction, upset stomach, joint pain, tingling in the hands or feet, and sleep disturbances. Trizivir may affect the results of a variety of blood tests.
- Less common: blood infection, nervousness, and irritability.
- Rare: pancreas irritation, weight loss, seizures, heart failure and other cardiac abnormalities, blood in the urine, and bladder infections. Contact your doctor if you experience anything unusual while taking any medication.

Zidovudine (AZT)

Adult

- Most common: anemia, reduced white-blood-cell counts, headache, fatigue, loss of appetite, vomiting, nausea, sleeplessness, skin yellowing, and muscle aches.
- Less common: Less common side effects can occur in almost any part of the body. Contact your doctor if you experience anything unusual while taking any medication.

Child

- Most common: anemia, reduced white-blood-cell counts, vomiting, abdominal pain, fever, cough, liver enlargement, brownish and itchy skin rash, diarrhea, nausea, and sleeplessness.
- Less common: headache, blood infection, nervousness, and irritability.

Possible Side Effects *(continued)*

▼ Rare: weight loss; fainting; seizures; heart failure, rapid heartbeat, and other cardiac abnormalities; blood in the urine; and bladder infections. Contact your doctor if you experience anything unusual while taking any medication.

Drug Interactions

Abacavir

- Alcohol interferes with the elimination of abacavir through the liver and can lead to a 40% increase in the amount of drug in the blood.
- Abacavir can increase blood levels of acetaminophen, amitriptyline, bumetanide, chloral hydrate, chlorpheniramine, chlorpromazine, chlorzoxazone, doxepin, fluconazole, imipramine, ketoconazole, labetalol, lamotrigine, miconazole, morphine, naloxone, nonsteroidal anti-inflammatory drugs (NSAIDs), oxazepam, promethazine, propofol, propranolol, and valproic acid.
- Cigarette smoking may reduce the amount of abacavir in the blood.
- Combining abacavir with isoniazid may decrease abacavir levels and increase isoniazid levels in the blood.
- Abacavir levels in the blood may be decreased if you are also taking phenobarbital, phenytoin, or T3 thyroid hormone replacement.
- Abacavir may increase the speed with which methadone is cleared from the body. Changes in methadone dose are usually not required.

Delavirdine and Efavirenz

- Combining delavirdine or efavirenz with astemizole; midazolam, triazolam, or other benzodiazepine sedatives; or ergot-containing products can lead to life-threatening abnormal heart rhythms, excessive sedation, or severe breathing difficulties. Do not combine these drugs.
- Delavirdine or efavirenz increases the nervous system effects of alcohol, sedatives, antidepressants, and other psychoactive drugs.
- Combining delavirdine or efavirenz with ritonavir increases blood levels of both drugs. This interaction increases the

effectiveness of anti-HIV therapy as well as the risk of side effects.

- Delavirdine or efavirenz reduces indinavir blood levels. Your indinavir dosage may need to be increased.
- Delavirdine or efavirenz significantly reduces saquinavir blood levels.
- The antifungal drugs itraconazole, ketoconazole, and voriconazole increase the amount of delavirdine or efavirenz in the blood by about 50% while the concentration of the antifungals is significantly reduced. These drugs should not be mixed.
- Combining delavirdine or efavirenz with clarithromycin, ethinyl estradiol, nelfinavir, or rifampin can alter blood levels of either drug. The importance of these interactions is unclear; dosage adjustments are unnecessary.
- Anticonvulsants and rifabutin decrease blood levels of delavirdine or efavirenz. Dosage adjustments may be necessary.
- Nevirapine decreases blood levels of delavirdine or efavirenz.
- Antacids and didanosine may reduce the amount of delavirdine or efavirenz in the blood by interfering with its absorption; take these drugs and delavirdine or efavirenz at least 1 hour apart.
- Delavirdine or efavirenz decreases blood levels of methadone. The methadone dose may need to be altered.
- Combining delavirdine or efavirenz and warfarin may increase the risk of excessive bleeding.
- The effect of delavirdine or efavirenz on contraceptive drugs is not known. People combining these drugs should use an additional contraceptive method for at least 12 weeks after discontinuing treatment.
- Delavirdine or efavirenz should not be combined with St. John's wort.

Didanosine

- Other drugs that may cause inflammation of the nervous system such as chloramphenicol, cisplatin, disulfiram, ethionamide, glutethimide, gold, hydralazine, isoniazid, metronidazole, nitrofurantoin, ribavirin, and vincristine should be avoided while you are taking didanosine.
- Use extreme caution when combining didanosine with stavudine in pregnant women, as fatal lactic acidosis has been reported with this combination.

- Drugs that may cause inflammation of the pancreas, including intravenous pentamidine, should not be taken with didanosine.
- Do not mix allopurinol or ribavirin with didanosine, as they raise didanosine blood levels. People mixing didanosine and ribavirin have developed fatal liver failure, nerve disease, pancreas inflammation, and metabolic conditions.
- Methadone increases blood levels of didanosine. If this combination is necessary, didanosine dose may have to be altered.
- Quinolone anti-infectives, tetracycline antibiotics, and other drugs whose absorption into the bloodstream may be affected by antacids should not be taken within 2 hours of taking didanosine because of its high magnesium and aluminum content.

Emtricitabine

- Do not mix emtricitabine or an emtricitabine combination with lamivudine or adefovir (for hepatitis B) or any combination drug containing lamivudine.

Etravirine

- Etravirine blood levels are increased when taken with atazanavir, lopinavir + ritonavir, and atazanavir + ritonavir. These drugs should not be mixed with etravirine.
- Atazanavir + ritonavir, darunavir + ritonavir, tipranavir + ritonavir, ritonavir, and saquinavir + ritonavir reduce etravirine blood levels. Dose adjustment may be required, especially with a tipranavir + ritonavir.
- Fluconazole, itraconazole, ketoconazole, and posaconazole increase etravirine blood levels. When etravirine and voriconazole are mixed, blood levels of both drugs are increased. In both cases, dose adjustments are required.
- Etravirine reduces blood levels of the antifungal drugs itraconazole and ketoconazole.
- When etravirine + protease inhibitors are mixed with rifabutin, rifabutin levels will be drastically reduced; another antibiotic should be used with this combination. If no protease inhibitors are used, then 300 mg a day of rifabutin is appropriate.
- Statin drugs have no effect on etravirine but etravirine affects some statins. The dose of atorvastatin, lovastatin, and simvastatin may need to be raised and fluvastatin may need to be reduced. Rosuvastatin and pravastatin are unaffected.

- Etravirine reduces blood levels of sildenafil and other drugs for erectile dysfunction. Larger doses may be needed to achieve the same effect. Etravirine levels are not affected when they are mixed.
- Carbamazepine, dexamethasone, phenobarbital, phenytoin, rifampin, rifapentine, and St. John's wort drastically reduce etravirine blood levels. They should not be mixed with etravirine.
- Etravirine reduces clarithromycin blood levels. Another antibiotic should be substituted while you are on etravirine.
- Etravirine reduces blood levels of the immune suppressants cyclosporin, sirolimus, and tacrolimus. It also reduces levels of some drugs for abnormal heart rhythms (amiodarone, bepridil, disopyramide, flecainide, systemic lidocaine, mexiletine, propafenone, and quinidine). All these drugs should be combined with etravirine with caution. Your doctor will check blood levels of the heart drug to make sure they are high enough.
- Etravirine increases blood levels of diazepam and warfarin, the most widely used oral blood-thinning drug. Dose adjustments may be required.
- When etravirine is taken by people in a methadone maintenance program, the methadone dose may need to be adjusted.

Lamivudine

- Lamivudine increases maximum blood levels of AZT by 39%, which is helpful in fighting the HIV virus.
- Trimethoprim-sulfamethoxazole, taken for opportunistic AIDS-related infections, increases the amount of lamivudine in the blood.

Nelfinavir

- Anticonvulsant medication such as carbamazepine, phenytoin, or phenobarbital may reduce the amount of nelfinavir in the blood.
- Nelfinavir interferes with the liver's ability to break down triazolam, midazolam, statin drugs (except pravastatin and simvastatin), ergot derivatives, amiodarone, and quinidine. Do not combine nelfinavir with any of these drugs, as severe side effects may result.
- Combining nelfinavir with indinavir or saquinavir, other protease inhibitors, results in large increases in the amounts of

both drugs in the blood. Other drugs that increase the amount of nelfinavir in the blood are ketoconazole and ritonavir.

- Combining rifabutin with nelfinavir lowers the amount of nelfinavir in the blood and raises the amount of rifabutin. Rifabutin dosage should be cut in ½ when this combination is used.
- Do not combine rifampin or pimozide and nelfinavir. Combine nelfinavir and sildenafil or vardenafil with extreme caution.
- Nelfinavir reduces the amount of contraceptive hormones in your bloodstream (see "Special Information").
- If you combine nelfinavir, lamivudine, and AZT, your AZT dosage may have to be increased.
- St. John's wort may decrease the effectiveness of nelfinavir. Avoid this combination.

Nevirapine

- Rifampin and rifabutin may stimulate liver enzymes that break down nevirapine, reducing the amount of nevirapine in the blood. Neither of these drugs should be combined with nevirapine.
- Nevirapine may reduce the effectiveness of ketoconazole. Ketoconazole should not be combined with nevirapine.
- The enzyme systems that break down protease inhibitors are stimulated by nevirapine. Combining nevirapine and a protease inhibitor may reduce the amount of protease inhibitor in the blood, reducing its effectiveness and increasing the risk of protease inhibitor resistance.
- Combining nevirapine with a contraceptive drug may reduce the effectiveness of the contraceptive by lowering the amount of hormone in the blood.
- Nevirapine may interact with many medications, both prescription and over-the-counter, including herbal products such as St. John's wort.

Rilpivirine

- Do not mix rilpivirine with carbamazepine, dexamethasone (more than 1 dose), esomeprazole, lansoprazole, omeprazole, oxcarbazepine, phenobarbital, phenytoin, rabeprazole, rifabutin, rifampin, rifapentine, or St. John's wort supplements. They can reduce blood levels of rilpivirine, making it less effective against the HIV virus.
- Do not mix rilpivirine with non-nucleotide reverse transcriptase inhibitors (NNRTI) HIV antivirals (efavirenz, etravirine,

or nevirapine) because they can reduce rilpivirine blood levels, reducing its effectiveness. The NNRTI delavirdine raises rilpivirine blood levels and is also not recommended.

- Mixing rilpivirine with protease inhibitors raises rilpivirine blood levels but the increases are not enough to require dose reduction.
- Antacids can interfere with the absorption of rilpivirine into the blood. Take your antacids at least 2 hours before or 4 hours after you take your daily rilpivirine dose.
- Cimetidine, famotidine, nizatidine, and ranitidine can substantially reduce the amount of rilpivirine absorbed into the blood. These drugs should be taken at least 12 hours before or 4 hours after rilpivirine.
- Fluconazole, ketoconazole, itraconazole, posaconazole, and voriconazole raise rilpivirine blood levels, but no dose adjustment is needed.
- Do not mix rilpivirine with clarithromycin, or erythromycin because of significant increases in rilpivirine blood levels. Azithromycin may be taken instead.
- Mixing rilpivirine with any drug that can also cause torsade de pointes arrhythmia should be done with extreme caution. These drugs include: amiodarone, arsenic trioxide, astemizole, chloroquin, chlorpromazine, cisapride, clarithromycin, disopyramide, dofetilide, domperidone, droperidol, erythromycin, halofantrine, haloperidol, ibutilide, levomethadyl, mesoridazine, methadone, moxifloxacin, pebridil, pentamidine, pimozide, probucol, quinidine, sotalol, sparfloxacin, terfenadine, and thioridazine.

Stavudine

- Combining stavudine with didanosine or hydroxyurea increases the risk of lactic acidosis, peripheral neuropathy, inflamed pancreas, or liver toxicity.
- Methadone and AZT may reduce blood levels of stavudine by more than 25%.
- Doxorubicin and ribavirin may affect stavudine; use with caution.

Tenofovir

- Tenofovir may reduce the breakdown of acetaminophen, amitriptyline, caffeine, clomipramine, clozapine, cyclobenzaprine, estradiol, fluvoxamine, haloperidol, imipramine, mexiletine, naproxen, propranolol, riluzole, ropivacaine, theophylline, verapamil, warfarin, zileuton, and zolmitriptan, modestly increasing the amount of these drugs in the blood.

- Do not mix tenofovir with adefovir (for hepatitis B).
- Tenofovir increases blood levels of didanosine, which increases the risk of side effects. People taking both of these drugs must take tenofovir either 2 hours before or 1 hour after taking didanosine.
- Tenofovir decreases the amount of ritonavir and lopinavir (with higher tenofovir doses) absorbed into the bloodstream.
- At higher tenofovir doses, the blood concentration of lamivudine may be reduced.
- The effect of tenofovir on contraceptive drugs is not known, but it can increase the amount of estradiol (a contraceptive hormone) in the blood. People combining these drugs should use an additional contraceptive method.
- Tenofovir may decrease blood levels of atazanavir.

Trizivir

- Trizivir slows the elimination of alcohol from the body and can lead to a large increase of alcohol in the blood.
- Aspirin, indomethacin, interferon beta-1b, methadone, probenecid, trimethoprim + sulfamethoxazole (an anti-infective combination), trimethoprim, and valproic acid increase the amount of Trizivir in the blood and the risk of Trizivir side effects.
- Cigarette smoking, phenobarbital, liothyronine, isoniazid, acetaminophen, and rifampin may reduce the amount of Trizivir in the blood.
- Trizivir should not be used with stavudine, doxorubicin, or ribavirin because the 2 drugs may antagonize each other.
- Mixing Trizivir with anticancer drugs or drugs that suppress the immune system increases the risk of blood toxicity.
- Mixing clarithromycin or fluconazole with Trizivir can increase the amount of Trizivir in the blood, but the importance of this interaction is not known.
- Atovaquone increases the amount of Trizivir in the blood by interfering with its breakdown in the liver. Trizivir dosage reduction may be necessary.
- Combining Trizivir with other drugs that can damage your kidneys, including adriamycin, amphotericin B, flucytosine, interferon alpha and beta, pentamidine, vinblastine, and vincristine, increases the risk of loss of some kidney function.

- Trizivir can increase blood levels of acetaminophen, amitriptyline, bumetanide, chloral hydrate, chlorpheniramine, chlorpromazine, chlorzoxazone, doxepin, fluconazole, imipramine, ketoconazole, labetalol, lamotrigine, miconazole, morphine, naloxone, NSAIDs, oxazepam, promethazine, propofol, and propranolol.
- Combining Trizivir and isoniazid may increase isoniazid levels in the blood.
- Acyclovir is used in combination with Trizivir to combat opportunistic infections in AIDS patients; however, this combination may cause severe drowsiness or lethargy.
- Other drugs that can cause anemia, including interferon alpha and ganciclovir, should be used carefully in combination with Trizivir because of the risk of worsening drug-related anemia.
- Taking phenytoin and Trizivir together may affect the amounts of both drugs in the blood, usually increasing the amount of Trizivir. The effect on phenytoin blood levels varies. This combination can result in either too much phenytoin (leading to increased phenytoin side effects) or too little phenytoin (leading to a possible increase in the number of seizures). Your doctor should check your phenytoin levels if you are also taking Trizivir.

Zidovudine (AZT)

- Combining AZT with other drugs that can damage your kidneys, such as pentamidine, amphotericin B, flucytosine, vincristine, vinblastine, adriamycin, and interferon alpha and beta, increases the risk of some kidney function loss.
- Avoid using AZT with stavudine, ribavirin, and doxorubicin.
- Probenecid may reduce the rate at which your body eliminates AZT, increasing the amount of the drug in your blood and the risk for side effects. Other drugs that can reduce the liver's ability to break down AZT are acetaminophen, aspirin, indomethacin, and trimethoprim; combining any of these drugs with AZT may lead to increased side effects.
- Acyclovir is often used in combination with AZT to combat opportunistic infections in AIDS patients; however, this combination may cause lethargy or seizures.
- Other drugs that can cause anemia, including ganciclovir, should be used carefully in combination with AZT because of the risk of worsening drug-related anemia.

- Taking AZT together with rifampin may reduce the amount of AZT absorbed into the blood.
- Taking phenytoin and AZT together may affect the amounts of both drugs in the blood, usually increasing the amount of AZT. The effect on phenytoin blood levels varies. This combination can result in either too much phenytoin (leading to phenytoin side effects) or too little phenytoin (leading to a possible increase in the number of seizures). Your doctor should check your phenytoin levels if you are also taking AZT.
- Atovaquone, fluconazole, methadone, probenecid, trimethoprim, and valproic acid may increase blood levels of AZT.

Food Interactions

Most of these drugs can be taken without regard to food or meals.

Food may prevent the absorption of a dose of didanosine by up to 50%. Take didanosine either 30 minutes before or 2 hours after eating. Efavirenz may be taken with or without food, but do not take efavirenz with a high-fat meal because it will increase the amount of efavirenz absorbed by about 50%, raising the risk of adverse effects. Symptoms may be more severe if taken with alcohol. Lamivudine is absorbed more slowly when taken with food, but not enough to affect the total amount of drug that reaches the blood. Rilpivirine must be taken with food.

Usual Dose

Abacavir

Adult (age 17 and over): 300 mg twice a day. For mild hepatic impairment—200 mg twice a day. Oral solution—15 mL twice a day.

Child (age 3 months–16 years): 3.6 mg per lb. of body weight twice a day, up to a maximum of 300 mg in each dose.

Child (under 3 months): not recommended.

Atripla

Adult: 1 tablet a day on an empty stomach. Taking the combination at bedtime may make it easier to tolerate.

Child: not recommended.

Combivir

Adult and Child (age 12 and over): 1 tablet—lamivudine 150 mg + zidovudine 300 mg—twice a day. Poor kidney or liver function requires reducing the dosage of both drugs. In this situation, it is preferable to take the individual drugs separately so that you retain maximum dosage flexibility.

Child (under age 12): not recommended.

Complera

Adult: 1 tablet—200 mg emtricitabine + 25 mg rilpivirine + 300 mg tenofovir—once a day with a meal.

Child: not recommended.

Delavirdine

Adult: 400 mg 3 times a day.

Didanosine

Adult: 250–400 mg a day (tablets); 167–250 mg every 12 hours (powder).

Child (age 2 weeks and over): Dose is based on weight and height, up to the maximum adult dose.

Efavirenz

Adult: 600 mg once a day, preferably at bedtime at first.
Child (88 lbs. and over): 600 mg a day.
Child (71.5–87 lbs.): 400 mg a day.
Child (55–71.5 lbs.): 350 mg a day.
Child (44–54 lbs.): 300 mg a day.
Child (33–43 lbs.): 250 mg a day.
Child (22–32 lbs.): 200 mg a day.
Child (under age 3 or less than 22 lbs.): not recommended.

Emtricitabine

Capsules

Adult: 200 mg once a day. People with reduced kidney function may take as little as 200 mg once every 4 days. Dialysis patients take 1 dose after dialysis is complete.

Child (over 68 lbs.): 200 mg once a day.

Oral Solution

Adult: 240 mg (24 mL) once a day.
Child: 2.7 mg per lb. of body weight up to 240 mg a day.

Epzicom

Adult: 1 tablet—abacavir 600 mg + lamivudine 300 mg—once a day.

Child: not recommended.

Etravirine

Adult: 200 mg twice a day with food.
Child: not recommended.

Lamivudine

Adult and Child (age 16 and over): 150 mg twice a day combined with other antiretroviral agents. Adults who weigh less than 110 lbs. should receive about 1 mg per lb. of body weight twice a day. Dosage is reduced as kidney function decreases. For hepatitis B, take 100 mg once a day.

Child (age 3 months to 16 years): about 1.4–2 mg per lb. of body weight twice a day, no more than 150 mg per dose.

Child (under 3 months): not recommended.

Nevirapine

Adult and Child (age 9 and over): starting dose—200 mg a day for 2 weeks; maintenance dose—200 mg twice a day in combination with a nucleoside-type antiviral such as didanosine or AZT.

Child (age 2 months–8 years): starting dose—about 2 mg per lb. of body weight a day for 2 weeks; maintenance dose—3 mg per lb. of body weight twice a day. The total daily dose should not exceed 400 mg.

Child (under 2 months): not recommended.

Nevirapine Extended-Release (XR)

Adult: 400 mg once a day in combination with a nucleoside antiviral such as didanosine or AZT.

Child: not recommended.

Rilpivirine

Adult: 25 mg once a day with food.

Child: not recommended.

Stavudine

Immediate-Release

Adult and Child (66 lbs. and over): 30–40 mg every 12 hours. Dosage reduction may be needed in seniors.

Child (under 66 lbs.): 0.5 mg per lb. of body weight every 12 hours.

Extended-Release

Adult: 75–100 mg once a day.

Child: not recommended.

Tenofovir

Adult: 300 mg once a day. If you are taking tenofovir and didanosine, take your tenofovir 2 hours before or 1 hour after taking didanosine.

Child (age 2–17): 3.6 mg per lb. of body weight, up to 300 mg, once a day.

Child (under age 2): not recommended.

Trizivir

Adult (88 lbs. and over): 1 tablet twice a day.

Adult (less than 88 lbs.): not recommended.

Child (age 13 and over, and 88 lbs. and over): 1 tablet twice a day.

Child (age 13 and over, but under 88 lbs.): not recommended.

Child (under age 13): not recommended.

Truvada

Adult: 1 tablet a day. People with mild kidney disease should take 1 tablet every other day.

Child: not recommended.

Zidovudine (AZT)

Adult and Child (age 13 and over): symptomatic AIDS—100 mg every 4 hours around the clock, even if sleep must be interrupted. Dosage may be reduced if side effects develop. Asymptomatic AIDS—100 mg every 4 hours during waking hours.

Child (age 3 months–12 years): up to 100 mg every 6 hours.

Child (under age 3 months): about 1 mg per lb. of body weight every 6 hours by mouth, starting within 12 hours of birth and continuing through 6 weeks of age. The drug may be given intravenously if necessary.

Pregnancy: AZT is used to prevent transmission of HIV infection to the fetus. After 14 weeks of pregnancy—100 mg 5 times a day until labor starts. During labor and delivery—intravenously, until the umbilical cord is clamped.

Overdosage

Little is known about the effects of abacavir, emtricitabine, etravirine, lamivudine, nevirapine, rilpivirine, and tenofovir overdose. Didanosine overdose will cause many of the drug's usual side effects, especially inflammation of the nervous system or pancreas, diarrhea, and liver failure. Efavirenz overdose may include dizziness, nausea, loss of concentration, and other nervous system effects. Chronic stavudine overdose can produce peripheral neuropathy (see "Special Information") and liver toxicity. The most serious effect of AZT overdose is suppression of the bone marrow and its ability to make red and white blood cells.

Contact your local poison control center or a hospital emergency room for more information. Overdose victims should be taken to a hospital emergency room. If you seek treatment, ALWAYS bring the prescription bottle or container.

Special Information

These drugs are not a cure for HIV. They will not prevent you from transmitting the HIV virus to another person; you must still practice safe sex. People taking these drugs may still develop opportunistic infections and other complications associated with HIV infection. It is very important to take these drugs exactly as prescribed. Remember, every dose of HIV medication you forget or skip can make it more difficult for the drugs to do their job and can also lead to the development of HIV resistance.

People with HIV infection must take especially good care of their teeth and gums to minimize the risk of developing oral infections.

Abacavir

Stop taking this drug and contact your doctor at the first sign of allergy or sensitivity. Symptoms include fever, rash, fatigue, nausea, vomiting, diarrhea, abdominal pain, sore throat, difficulty breathing, and coughing. Some patients who experienced a hypersensitivity reaction were thought to have a respiratory infection at first. If you continue to take abacavir and are allergic to it, more severe reactions such as a life-threatening drop in blood pressure could develop within hours. Report anything unusual to your doctor.

If you forget to take a dose and remember within 2–3 hours, take the medication. If you forget until it is almost time for your next dose, skip the forgotten dose and continue with your regular schedule.

Delavirdine

Delavirdine solution is somewhat better absorbed than the tablets. The amount of drug absorbed from delavirdine tablets can be increased by allowing the 100-mg tablet to disintegrate in water and then swallowing the mixture. 200-mg tablets do not dissolve in water.

Didanosine

If you are taking didanosine chewable tablets, be sure to thoroughly chew each tablet. You may also completely dissolve them in about ¼ cup of water and drink the entire mixture immediately. Do not mix didanosine tablets with juice or any other acidic drink. If you are using the powdered form of didanosine, make a solution by pouring the entire contents of a packet into ½ cup of water. Stir until dissolved and drink immediately. Do not mix didanosine powder with juice or any other acidic drink. For children, your pharmacist will prepare a mixture of 10 mg per mL of didanosine and an equal amount of Mylanta Double Strength Antacid or Maalox TC Antacid. This mixture must be stored in a refrigerator and can be kept for 30 days. Shake well before using.

Spilled didanosine should be cleaned immediately to prevent accidental poisoning.

If you forget to take a dose of didanosine, take it as soon as you remember. If it is almost time for your next dose, allow 4–8 hours to pass between the dose you took late and your next dose, and then continue with your regular schedule. Contact your doctor for more specific advice if you forget to take several doses.

Efavirenz

People with achlorhydria (absence of stomach acid) should take efavirenz with an acidic drink, such as orange or cranberry juice. About ½ of people taking efavirenz develop dizziness, loss of concentration, depression, delusions, or drowsiness. Contact your doctor if this occurs or if strange behavior develops. Do not combine efavirenz with alcohol, sedatives, or other psychoactive drugs. Be careful when driving or performing any task that requires concentration. Take your medication at bedtime to better tolerate the depressant effects of efavirenz. If you forget a dose, take it as soon as you remember. Contact your doctor if you forget your medication for 1 day.

Emtricitabine

Contact your doctor immediately if your child develops signs of pancreas inflammation while taking emtricitabine. Symptoms include severe abdominal pain, tense abdominal muscles, sweating, feeling very ill, shallow and rapid breathing, fever, and possible fainting.

If you forget a dose, take it as soon as you remember. If it is almost time for your next dose, skip the dose you forgot and continue with your regular schedule. Contact your doctor if you forget 2 or more doses in a row.

Etravirine

Contact your doctor immediately if you develop a rash or another skin reaction. You will have to stop etravirine if your reaction is severe.

If you cannot swallow whole etravirine tablets, mix them in a glass of water until you have a milky mixture. Stir the mixture and drink it right away. Then rinse the glass with water several times and drink each rinse to be sure you have taken the entire dose of etravirine.

If you forget to take a dose of etravirine and remember within 6 hours of your regular schedule, take it right away with a meal, then go back to your regular schedule. If more than 6 hours has passed, skip the forgotten dose and continue with your next regular dose. Do not take a double dose of this medicine.

Lamivudine

Contact your doctor at once if your child develops signs of pancreas inflammation while taking lamivudine. Symptoms include very severe abdominal pain, tense abdominal muscles, sweating, feeling very ill, shallow and rapid breathing, fever, and possible fainting.

If you forget a dose, take it as soon as you remember. If it is almost time for your next dose, skip the dose you forgot and continue with your regular schedule. Contact your doctor if you forget 2 or more doses in a row.

Nevirapine

Contact your doctor at once if you develop any rash or other skin side effect.

If you forget a dose of nevirapine, take it as soon as you remember. If it is almost time for your next dose, skip the dose you forgot and continue with your regular schedule. If you forget to take nevirapine for a week, you will have to start the treatment program all over again, beginning with 200 mg a day for 2 weeks.

You must take nevirapine 200 mg once a day before you can take the long-acting product. If you are already taking nevirapine 200 mg twice a day, you can be switched to the long-acting product. If you are taking nevirapine XR and forget your medicine for 7 days in a row, you must start again with the 2-week lead-in dosing.

Rilpivirine

Tell your doctor if you have had any mental health issues in the past and if you experience significant mood changes, negative thoughts, feelings of hopelessness, or thoughts of suicide. These can be signs of serious depression and should be tended to immediately.

Contact your doctor about any other side effects that are particularly bothersome or persistent.

If you forget a dose of rilpivirine, take it as soon as you remember. If you do not remember until 12 hours before your next regular dose, skip the forgotten dose and continue with your regular schedule. Do not take a double dose.

Rilpivirine is intended for adults who have not been previously treated for HIV with other medicines.

Rilpivirine interacts with many other medicines (see "Drug Interactions"). Check with your doctor and pharmacist about any possible interactions with rilpivirine and inform them of any other medicines you are taking, including herbal supplements such as St. John's wort.

Rilpivirine can be stored at room temperature but should be kept in the original bottle to protect against being exposed to light.

Stavudine

Peripheral neuropathy (symptoms include tingling, pain, or numbness in the hands, arms, legs, or feet) occurs in 15–20% of people who take stavudine. If the drug is stopped, symptoms may disappear, although they can actually worsen for a time after you stop taking stavudine. If the symptoms do go away, your doctor may restart stavudine treatment at a lower daily dosage.

Your stavudine dosage will be reduced if you develop symptoms of neuropathy or if you have reduced kidney function.

Tell your doctor immediately if you have symptoms of extreme weakness, nausea, difficulty breathing, or weight loss.

If you forget a dose of stavudine, take it as soon as you remember. If it is almost time for your next dose, take the dose you forgot, take the next 2 doses 8 hours apart, and then go back to your regular schedule. Do not take a double dose. Contact your doctor if you skip more than 2 consecutive doses.

Tenofovir

If you forget a dose of tenofovir, take it as soon as you remember. If it almost time for your next dose, skip the dose you forgot and continue with your regular schedule. Do not take a double dose. Skipping doses of this drug increases the risk that your HIV will become resistant to its effects.

Trizivir

Stop taking Trizivir and contact your doctor at the first sign of allergy or drug sensitivity (fever, rash, fatigue, nausea, vomiting, diarrhea, or abdominal pain). See your doctor if any significant change in your health occurs. Periodic blood counts are very important while taking Trizivir to detect possibly serious side effects.

If you miss a dose of Trizivir, take it as soon as possible. If it is almost time for your next dose, skip the dose you forgot and continue with your regular schedule. Contact your doctor if you forget 2 or more doses in a row. Do not take more Trizivir than your doctor prescribed.

Zidovudine (AZT)
If you miss a dose of AZT, take it as soon as possible. If it is almost time for your next dose, allow 2–4 hours to pass between the dose you took late and your next dose, and then continue with your regular schedule. Do not take a double dose.

Protect AZT capsules and liquid from light.

Special Populations

Pregnancy/Breast-feeding: These drugs should be taken during pregnancy only if your doctor determines that the potential benefit outweighs the risks.

Most of these drugs pass into breast milk. HIV-positive nursing mothers should use infant formula instead of breast milk to avoid transmitting the virus to their child.

Abacavir
Abacavir passes into the fetal circulation. In animal studies, it caused low birth weight and increased the risk of stillbirth. The effect of abacavir in pregnant women is not known.

Didanosine
Didanosine was slightly toxic to pregnant animals receiving doses 12 times human levels. There are no studies of pregnant women taking this drug; however, women who are or might become pregnant should only take didanosine if absolutely necessary and should use effective contraception to avoid passing on the virus.

Efavirenz
This drug may cause birth defects if taken during the first 3 months of pregnancy. Women taking this medicine and its combinations should avoid becoming pregnant and should be tested to ensure they are not pregnant before starting treatment. Birth defects are much less likely if it is taken in the final 6 months of pregnancy. Your doctor may consider efavirenz if you are pregnant and have no other treatment options, but you should discuss the risks and benefits of treatment with him or her.

Emtricitabine
Emtricitabine enters the fetal circulation. A national registry has been established to gather information on pregnant women who must use this drug.

Etravirine
Etravirine should be taken during pregnancy only if your doctor determines that the potential benefit outweighs the risks.

Lamivudine
Lamivudine passes into the blood circulation of the fetus. Some animal studies of lamivudine indicate that it may be dangerous to the fetus, but others showed no effect. There is no information about the effect of lamivudine in pregnant women.

Nevirapine
Studies of nevirapine in pregnant women have shown a significant decrease in fetal body weight.

Rilpivirine
Animal studies revealed no effects of rilpivirine on the developing fetus but there are no human studies. A registry has been established by the manufacturer to collect information about pregnant women taking rilpivirine. You or your doctor may enroll.

Stavudine
Animal studies show that stavudine passes to the fetus and causes birth defects, but there is no direct information on what happens in humans.

Tenofovir
Animal studies of tenofovir using up to 19 times the human dose have revealed no birth defects. There are no studies in pregnant women.

Trizivir
Animal studies of all 3 ingredients of Trizivir harmed developing fetuses. Notify your doctor at once if you do become pregnant.

Zidovudine (AZT)
If you are HIV-positive and pregnant, talk to your doctor about taking or continuing this drug. AZT treatment in HIV-positive women who are pregnant has been shown to sharply reduce the risk of transmitting the HIV virus to babies. Treatment should begin by the 14th week of pregnancy and continue through delivery. The baby should also be given AZT for the first 6 weeks of life. Studies have shown that the risk of birth defects is not increased by taking AZT during pregnancy.

Seniors: Seniors may require lower doses of these drugs because of reduced liver, kidney, or cardiac function.

Type of Drug

HIV Protease Inhibitors

Brand Names

Generic Ingredients: Atazanavir
Reyataz

Generic Ingredients: Darunavir
Prezista

Generic Ingredients: Fosamprenavir
Lexiva

Generic Ingredients: Indinavir
Crixivan

Generic Ingredients: Nelfinavir
Viracept

Generic Ingredients: Ritonavir
Norvir

Generic Ingredients: Saquinavir
Invirase

Generic Ingredients: Tipranavir
Aptivus

Combination Products
Generic Ingredients: Ritonavir + Lopinavir
Kaletra

Prescribed For

Human immunodeficiency virus (HIV) infection. Darunavir may be reserved for HIV that has not responded to other protease inhibitors.

General Information

Protease inhibitors are a class of drugs used to prevent HIV and Hepatitis C virus infections. Protease inhibitors have revolutionized HIV treatment because, when taken in combination, they reduce the amount of HIV virus in the bloodstream to levels that are often undetectable by current methods—CD_4 (immune system cell) counts and viral load (amount of virus in the blood) measurements. Multiple-drug therapy has transformed HIV from a fatal disease to a manageable chronic illness.

Protease inhibitors must be accompanied by at least 2 other HIV antivirals. These drugs work at the end of the virus' reproduction process, when proteins are "cut" into strands of exactly the correct size to duplicate HIV. An enzyme known as protease cuts the protein. Protease inhibitors prevent the mature virus from being formed by inhibiting this cutting process. Viral proteins that are cut to the wrong length or that remain uncut are inactive. As with other antivirals, it is possible for the HIV virus to develop resistance to a particular protease inhibitor.

Some protease inhibitors are combined with ritonavir to extend their action against the HIV virus. When atazanavir is prescribed for an adult or child who has been previously treated with other HIV therapy, it should always be combined with up to 100 mg of ritonavir to extend its action against the HIV virus. Darunavir must be taken with a low dose of ritonavir to extend the action of darunavir in the body. Without ritonavir, darunavir would be eliminated too rapidly to be effective.

Cautions and Warnings

Do not take these medicines if you are **allergic** or **sensitive** to any of their ingredients or to sulfa drugs. Darunavir can cause a severe or life-threatening rash. If a serious toxic reaction occurs while taking darunavir, you should stop the drug until your doctor can determine the cause or until the reaction resolves itself. Then treatment can be resumed.

Protease inhibitors are metabolized by the liver, so regular liver function tests are needed to monitor possible liver impairment. These drugs should not be used if you have severe **liver disease**. They should be taken with caution with mild to moderate liver disease; however, no dose adjustments are necessary. Protease inhibitors can worsen **hepatitis**.

These drugs may raise your blood sugar, worsen your **diabetes**, or bring out latent diabetes. People with diabetes who take protease inhibitors may need the dosage of their antidiabetes medication adjusted.

People with **hemophilia** may be more likely to bleed while taking a protease inhibitor.

The HIV virus may become resistant to protease inhibitors. For this reason it is essential that you take these drugs exactly according to your doctor's directions.

Protease inhibitors can cause body fat redistribution, including increased fat deposits in the upper back and neck, breast and around the back, chest, and stomach. Fat may be lost from the legs, arms, and face.

These drugs can affect nerve impulse flow in the heart, leading to abnormal heart rhythms.

Some people with HIV and a history of an opportunistic infection may develop signs and symptoms of the infection soon after anti-HIV treatment is started. This is called immune reconstitution syndrome.

Each protease inhibitor has many drug interactions. Check with your doctor before adding anything new to your treatment program.

Possible Side Effects

Atazanavir

Most side effects are mild. Other side effects become more prominent when atazanavir is taken together with antiretroviral drugs; these include weakness, muscle pain, and mouth ulcers.

▼ Most common: nausea and headache.
▼ Common: vomiting, diarrhea, abdominal pain, rash, infection, drowsiness, insomnia, and jaundice (yellowing of the skin or whites of the eyes).
▼ Less common: fever, fat accumulation, joint pain, depression, dizziness, and tingling or other unusual sensation in the arms, hands, legs, or feet.
▼ Rare: Rare side effects can occur in almost any part of the body. Contact your doctor if you experience anything unusual while taking any medication.

Darunavir

▼ Most common: diarrhea, nausea, headache, and common cold symptoms.
▼ Less common: vomiting, abdominal pain, and constipation.
▼ Rare: Rare side effects can occur in almost any part of the body. Contact your doctor if you experience anything unusual while taking any medication.

Fosamprenavir

Fosamprenavir is always taken with other drugs, so the side effects listed here are associated with multiple-drug therapy rather than fosamprenavir taken alone. Fosamprenavir has been studied in children age 4–12 and side effects are the same as in adults.

Possible Side Effects *(continued)*

- Most common: nausea, vomiting, diarrhea, mild rash, itching, high blood sugar, and high blood-triglyceride levels.
- Common: changes in sense of taste and tingling in or around the mouth or in the hands or feet.
- Less common: depression and high blood-cholesterol levels.
- Rare: life-threatening rash, diabetes, and buffalo hump. Contact your doctor immediately if you notice signs of a worsening rash, especially if it is accompanied by fever, flu-like symptoms, swelling, blisters, red eyes, or if you experience anything unusual while taking any medication.

Indinavir

- Most common: nausea, abdominal pain, and headache.
- Common: kidney stones, itching, weakness or fatigue, pain in the side, diarrhea, vomiting, changes in sense of taste, acid regurgitation, and sleeplessness.
- Less common: dizziness, drowsiness, and back pain.
- Rare: Rare side effects can occur in almost any part of the body. Contact your doctor if you experience anything unusual while taking any medication.

Nelfinavir

- Most common: diarrhea.
- Common: liver inflammation and nausea.
- Less common: abdominal pain, gas, weakness, nightmares, agitation, gallstones, and rash.
- Rare: Rare side effects can occur in almost any part of the body, including the blood, muscles and joints, gastrointestinal tract, kidneys, and eyes, and can affect mental state and sexual function. Contact your doctor if you experience anything unusual while taking any medication.

Ritonavir

- Most common: weakness, tiredness, nausea, abnormal stools, diarrhea (more common with once-daily dosage), vomiting, appetite loss, abdominal pains, taste changes, and tingling around the mouth and in the hands or feet.
- Less common: increased levels of cholesterol and other blood fats, rash, diabetes, and high blood sugar, and

Possible Side Effects *(continued)*

increased fat deposits in some areas of the body, including the back of the neck.

- ▼ Rare: Rare side effects can occur in almost any part of the body, including muscles and joints, blood components, the mouth, stomach and intestines, nervous system, skin, kidneys, liver, and urinary and respiratory tracts. Changes in mental state and sexual function may also occur. Contact your doctor if you experience anything unusual while taking any medication.

Saquinavir

Most side effects are mild. Other side effects become more prominent when saquinavir is taken together with antiretroviral drugs; these include weakness, muscle pain, and mouth ulcers.

- ▼ Most common: diarrhea, dyspepsia, nausea, and abdominal discomfort.
- ▼ Less common: upset stomach, abdominal pain, headache, tingling or numbness in the hands or feet, dizziness, nerve damage, changes in appetite, and rash.
- ▼ Rare: Rare side effects can occur in almost any part of the body. Contact your doctor if you experience anything unusual while taking any medication.

Tipranavir

Side effects may become more prominent when tipranavir is combined with antiretroviral drugs.

- ▼ Most common: diarrhea.
- ▼ Common: nausea.
- ▼ Less common: vomiting, abdominal pain, fever, fatigue, weakness, headache, depression, sleeplessness, and rash.
- ▼ Rare: Rare side effects can occur in almost any part of the body. Contact your doctor if you experience anything unusual while taking any medication.

Drug Interactions

Atazanavir

- Rifampin and St. John's wort substantially reduce atazanavir blood levels. Do not mix these drugs.
- If you are also taking didanosine, take your atazanavir dose 2 hours before or 1 hour after didanosine.

- Nevirapine may reduce the effects of atazanavir; they should not be taken together.
- H_2 antagonists (cimetidine, famotidine, and ranitidine) reduce atazanavir blood levels. Take atazanavir at least 2 hours before or 10 hours after these drugs.
- Both atazanavir and indinavir cause elevated levels of bilirubin in the blood. Do not combine these medicines.
- Atazanavir increases levels of cisapride, diltiazem, ergot drugs, irinotecan (an injectable anticancer drug), midazolam, pimozide, and triazolam, leading to potentially serious or fatal drug toxicities. These drugs should not be mixed with atazanavir.
- Combining atazanavir with the antibiotic clarithromycin may lead to an increased chance of clarithromycin-related cardiac toxicity. Clarithromycin dose should be halved.
- Taking atazanavir and cisapride together can lead to serious or fatal abnormal heart rhythms.
- Atazanavir increases the blood levels and side effects of the statin-type blood-cholesterol drugs, increasing the risk of muscle pain and breakdown. Use the lowest possible dosage of atorvastatin, lovastatin, rosuvastatin, or simvastatin. Pravastatin and fluvastatin are less affected because of the way in which they are broken down in the body. Do not mix pitavastatin with a protease inhibitor.
- If you also take other buffered medications or use antacids, take atazanavir with food, 1 hour before or 2 hours after you take the other medications.
- If you must take efavirenz and atazanavir, your doctor should also be prescribing ritonavir to increase the effectiveness of atazanavir.
- Atazanavir can increase blood levels of the hormones in contraceptive drugs. Your doctor should prescribe the lowest effective dose to avoid undesirable hormone side effects.
- Atazanavir may raise blood levels of amiodarone, calcium channel blockers, cyclosporine, lidocaine, quinidine, rifabutin, sirolimus, tacrolimus, tricyclic-type antidepressants, and warfarin. It may be necessary for your doctor to reduce drug dosage by as much as ½ to avoid drug side effects if you start taking atazanavir.
- Protease inhibitors, including atazanavir, may drastically increase blood levels of the erectile dysfunction (ED) drugs sildenafil, tadalafil, and vardenafil, increasing the risk of side

effects, including low blood pressure, visual changes, and persistent, painful erection. Reduce ED drug dose by ½ and use with caution.

- Atazanavir should be used with caution in people taking atenolol. Serious cardiac adverse events may occur.
- Prolonged or increased sedation or breathing difficulties may occur if atazanavir is mixed with benzodiazepine drugs.

Darunavir

- Do not take any of the following medicines with darunavir + ritonavir: astemizole, cisapride, ergot-based drugs for migraine headache, midazolam, pimozide, terfenidine, or triazolam. Mixing these drugs with darunavir + ritonavir can result in very high blood levels and serious side effects.
- Carbamazepine, phenobarbital, phenytoin, rifampin, and St. John's wort can substantially reduce protease inhibitor blood levels. Do not mix these medicines.
- Ritonavir + lopinavir and saquinavir can significantly reduce blood levels of darunavir. Darunavir significantly increases blood levels of ritonavir + lopinavir. Do not mix these drugs.
- Mixing darunavir with indinavir can increase blood levels of both drugs.
- Darunavir + ritonavir does not appear to affect blood levels of atazanavir, nor does atazanavir appear to affect blood levels of darunavir + ritonavir. It may be possible to combine these two protease inhibitors.
- Taking darunavir with tenofovir can increase blood levels of both drugs. These drugs can be combined with no dose adjustments, though it is necessary to watch carefully for kidney damage related to tenofovir.
- Darunavir can increase blood levels of efavirenz, and efavirenz reduces darunavir levels. These medicines should be mixed with caution.
- Darunavir increases nevirapine blood levels but the combination can be taken with no dose adjustment.
- If didanosine is a part of a darunavir + ritonavir treatment program, it must be taken on an empty stomach, 1 hour before or 2 hours after darunavir + ritonavir, which should be taken with food.
- Darunavir increases blood levels of clarithromycin, itraconazole, and ketoconazole. Daily dosage of itraconazole and

ketoconazole should not exceed 200 mg. No clarithromycin adjustment is necessary in people with normal kidney function.

- Darunavir + ritonavir may reduce voriconazole levels in the blood. Do not mix these medicines.
- Darunavir + ritonavir can increase rifabutin levels in the bloodstream. Rifabutin can also reduce darunavir levels in the bloodstream. If rifabutin is mixed with darunavir + ritonavir, the rifabutin dose should be 150 mg every other day.
- Caution should be exercised when combining darunavir + ritonavir with calcium channel blockers such as felodipine, nifedipine, and nicardipine.
- Darunavir increases blood levels of the heart antiarrhythmic drugs bepridil, lidocaine, and quinidine. These drugs should be used together with caution and only in situations where blood levels of the heart drugs can be monitored regularly.
- Darunavir + ritonavir can reduce blood levels of warfarin. It is necessary to monitor warfarin levels while taking this combination.
- Darunavir + ritonavir can raise blood levels of the tricyclic antidepressant desipramine and the tetracyclic antidepressant trazodone. Dosage reduction is recommended.
- Darunavir + ritonavir may reduce blood levels of the selective serotonin reuptake inhibitor (SSRI) antidepressants sertraline and paroxetine. SSRI doses may need to be increased to account for this effect.
- Darunavir + ritonavir can drastically increase the blood levels of some statin-type cholesterol-lowering drugs, substantially increasing the risk of statin side effects. Simvastatin, pravastatin, and lovastatin should not be mixed with darunavir + ritonavir. It is also possible to take darunavir + ritonavir with atorvastatin, although it can increase the level of atorvastatin in the bloodstream. If atorvastatin is prescribed, it is best to begin with 10 mg a day and slowly increase the dose as necessary. Little is known about how darunavir + ritonavir affects rosuvastatin. The safest statin to take with darunavir + ritonavir is fluvastatin.
- Darunavir + ritonavir can increase blood levels of the inhaled corticosteroids dexamethasone and fluticasone, and the anti-rejection drugs cyclosporine, tacrolimus, and sirolimus. The corticosteroids reduce darunavir blood levels, interfering with its effectiveness.

- Darunavir + ritonavir can reduce methadone levels in the bloodstream. Methadone dose adjustment may be needed.
- Darunavir + ritonavir reduces the effectiveness of some contraceptive drugs by decreasing the amount of the hormones ethinyl estradiol and norethindrone in the bloodstream. Women mixing these medicines should use additional contraceptive measures (e.g., condoms).
- Protease inhibitors, including darunavir, may drastically increase blood levels of the ED drugs sildenafil, tadalafil, and vardenafil, increasing the risk of side effects, including low blood pressure, visual changes, and persistent, painful erection. Reduce ED drug dose by ½ and use with caution.
- Dexamethasone may reduce blood levels of darunavir.

Fosamprenavir

- Astemizole, bepridil, dihydroergotamine, ergot derivatives, ergotamine, lidocaine injection, midazolam, quinidine, triazolam, and tricyclic antidepressants should never be combined with fosamprenavir because of the risk of severe, life-threatening reactions.
- St. John's wort should not be used with fosamprenavir because it can cause fosamprenavir resistance.
- You may require dosage adjustments of amiodarone and warfarin when you start taking fosamprenavir.
- Do not combine rifampin with fosamprenavir because it reduces drug levels by 90%. Rifabutin reduces the amount of fosamprenavir in the blood by 15%.
- Protease inhibitors, including fosamprenavir, may drastically increase blood levels of the ED drugs sildenafil, tadalafil, and vardenafil, increasing the risk of side effects, including low blood pressure, visual changes, and persistent, painful erection. Reduce ED drug dose by ½ and use with caution.
- Fosamprenavir can reduce the effectiveness of contraceptive drugs. Use another means of contraception while taking fosamprenavir.
- Fosamprenavir must be taken at least 1 hour before or after antacids.
- Combining fosamprenavir with statin cholesterol-lowering drugs increases the risk of drug toxicity.

- Carbamazepine, phenytoin, and phenobarbital reduce the effectiveness of fosamprenavir.
- Other drugs that could interact with fosamprenavir and should be used with caution are alprazolam, calcium channel blockers, clorazepate, clozapine, corticosteroids, delavirdine, diazepam, efavirenz, erythromycin, estrogens, flurazepam, loratadine, nevirapine, pimozide, and progestogens.
- Ritonavir must be added to the combination of fosamprenavir and nevirapine, a non-nucleoside reverse transcriptase inhibitor–type antiviral; they are prescribed together to obtain maximum benefit.
- Fosamprenavir should be used with caution with antacids, antiarrhythmic drugs, anticonvulsant drugs, bepridil, dexamethasone, diltiazem, felodipine, immune suppressants, itraconazole, ketoconazole, methadone, nicardipine, nifedipine, nimodipine, rifabutin, trazodone, and verapamil because of the increased risk of drug side effects.
- Fosamprenavir oral solution form should not be combined with disulfiram or metronidazole because of the risk of serious side effects.
- Fosamprenavir reduces blood levels of lopinavir. Dose adjustments may be needed.
- Fosamprenavir capsules and oral solution contain large amounts of vitamin E. Do not take a vitamin E supplement while taking this drug.

Indinavir

- Rifampin reduces the amount of indinavir in the blood. Do not combine these drugs.
- Indinavir should not be used with amiodarone, as amiodarone toxicity may result.
- Indinavir interferes with the liver's ability to break down terfenadine and sedatives such as triazolam and midazolam. Do not combine indinavir with any of these drugs, as severe side effects may result.
- Combining indinavir with clarithromycin or with zidovudine (AZT) increases the amount of each drug in the blood.
- Combining indinavir with isoniazid increases the amount of isoniazid in the blood.
- Combining indinavir with rifabutin can reduce the amount of indinavir absorbed into the blood by ⅓ and double the amount of rifabutin absorbed.

- Didanosine interferes with the absorption of indinavir into the body. If you need both of these medications, take them at least 1 hour apart.
- Combining fluconazole with indinavir reduces the amount of indinavir in the blood by about 20%.
- Combining indinavir with ketoconazole increases the amount of indinavir in the blood by about 65%.
- Combining indinavir with quinidine raises indinavir levels by about 10%.
- Taking indinavir with AZT and lamivudine results in ⅓ more AZT in the blood and small decreases in lamivudine blood levels.
- Indinavir raises the amount of stavudine absorbed into the blood by 25% and the amount of trimethoprim by about 20%.
- Delavirdine increases the effects of indinavir.
- St. John's wort and efavirenz decrease the effects of indinavir. Do not mix these drugs.
- Indinavir substantially increases the blood levels and potential side effects of ritonavir and fentanyl.
- Protease inhibitors, including indinavir, may drastically increase blood levels of the ED drugs sildenafil, tadalafil, and vardenafil, increasing the risk of side effects, including low blood pressure, visual changes, and persistent, painful erection. Reduce ED drug dose by ½ and use with caution.
- Do not mix indinavir with lovastatin, simvastatin, or rosuvastatin. Atorvastatin may be used with caution. This combination can increase the risk of painful muscle damage.
- Combining indinavir with contraceptive drugs can result in higher blood-hormone levels. This may lead to an excess of hormone-related side effects. If this happens to you, your doctor may be able to lower the dose of your contraceptive drug.

Nelfinavir

- Anticonvulsant medication such as carbamazepine, phenobarbital, or phenytoin may reduce the amount of nelfinavir in the blood.
- Nelfinavir interferes with the liver's ability to break down amiodarone, azithromycin, ergot derivatives, fluticasone (inhaled), immunosuppressants, midazolam, quinidine, sildenafil, statin

drugs (except pravastatin), trazodone, and triazolam. These drugs should be mixed with caution.

- Combining nelfinavir with indinavir or saquinavir, other protease inhibitors, results in large increases in the amounts of both drugs in the blood. Other drugs that increase the amount of nelfinavir in the blood are ketoconazole and ritonavir.
- Combining rifabutin with nelfinavir lowers the amount of nelfinavir in the blood and raises the amount of rifabutin. Rifabutin dosage should be cut in ½ when this combination is used.
- Do not combine rifampin or pimozide and nelfinavir.
- Protease inhibitors, including nelfinavir, may drastically increase blood levels of the ED drugs sildenafil, tadalafil, and vardenafil, increasing the risk of side effects, including low blood pressure, visual changes, and persistent, painful erection. Reduce ED drug dose by ½ and use with caution.
- Nelfinavir reduces the amount of hormonal contraceptive in your bloodstream (see "Special Information").
- If you combine nelfinavir, lamivudine, and AZT, your AZT dosage may need to be increased.
- St. John's wort may decrease the effectiveness of nelfinavir. Avoid this combination.

Ritonavir + Lopinavir

- Combining ritonavir + lopinavir with statin-type cholesterol-lowering drugs can result in serious reactions. Pravastatin and fluvastatin are not subject to this interaction and may be used instead.
- Ritonavir can be expected to substantially raise the blood levels of amiodarone, astemizole, bepridil, bupropion, clozapine, encainide, flecainide, meperidine, piroxicam, propafenone, quinidine, rifabutin, and sildenafil, possibly leading to serious drug side effects. In some cases, these drugs can be mixed with ritonavir, but drug blood levels and drug side effects must be monitored.
- Combining ritonavir with any of the following drugs may cause excessive sedation and breathing difficulties: alprazolam, clorazepate, diazepam, estazolam, flurazepam, midazolam, triazolam, and zolpidem. These drug combinations should be avoided.

- The effectiveness of some other sedative-hypnotics is likely to be reduced by ritonavir. Ritonavir may interact with narcotic pain relievers, but the exact interaction is not predictable.
- Rifampin substantially decreases the amount of ritonavir + lopinavir absorbed into the blood and should be avoided.
- Ritonavir should not be used with the antimigraine drugs dihydroergotamine and ergotamine.
- Ritonavir + lopinavir should not be combined with pimozide.
- Combining ritonavir with clarithromycin, itraconazole, or ketoconazole raises the amount of these drugs in the blood. High doses of itraconazole and ketoconazole are not recommended. People with reduced kidney function should take less clarithromycin.
- Ritonavir + lopinavir should not be taken with voriconazole, because voriconazole blood levels are substantially reduced, decreasing its chances of working.
- Mixing ritonavir with isoniazid increases the amount of isoniazid in the blood.
- Combining ritonavir with didanosine may reduce the amount of didanosine in the blood by about 15%. Take didanosine 1 hour before or 2 hours after taking ritonavir.
- Combining fluconazole or fluoxetine with ritonavir increases the amount of ritonavir in the blood.
- Combining ritonavir with trazodone substantially increases the amount of these drugs in the blood. Dosage adjustment may be required.
- Combining ritonavir with methadone and with contraceptive drugs containing ethinyl estradiol can lower blood levels, possibly reducing their effectiveness.
- Combining ritonavir with saquinavir, another protease inhibitor, slows the breakdown of saquinavir and increases its blood levels.
- Ritonavir lowers the amount of sulfamethoxazole absorbed into the blood by about 20% and raises trimethoprim by about 20%.
- Combining ritonavir with theophylline reduces the amount of theophylline absorbed by about 40%.
- Ritonavir is likely to increase the absorption of these drugs into the blood: alpha blockers, antiarrhythmics, anticancer drugs, antidepressants, antiemetics, antifungals, antimalarials, beta blockers, blood-fat reducers, calcium entry blockers,

cimetidine, desipramine, ergot alkaloids, erythromycin, immunosuppressants, indinavir, methylphenidate, pentoxifylline, phenothiazines, and warfarin. Dose adjustments may be needed to take this effect into account.

- Ritonavir + lopinavir increases the amount of calcium-channel-blocker drugs in the blood. People mixing these medicines must be monitored for potentially serious side effects. Dose reduction may be needed.
- Ritonavir is likely to reduce the amount of these drugs absorbed into the blood: atovaquone, daunorubicin, diphenoxylate, theophylline, and metoclopramide. Dose adjustments may be needed.
- St. John's wort significantly reduces blood levels of ritonavir. Do not mix these drugs.
- Efavirenz and nevirapine reduce the amount of lopinavir in the blood. An increase in the ritonavir + lopinavir dose is needed if you are taking either of those drugs. The ritonavir + lopinavir combination must be taken more than once a day if you are using either efavirenz or nevirapine.
- Tipranavir reduces the amount of lopinavir absorbed into the blood. Do not mix these drugs.
- Delavirdine increases the amount of lopinavir in the blood. Proper dosing of this drug combination has not been established.
- Blood levels of tenofovir are increased by the ritonavir + lopinavir combination. The chance of tenofovir side effects is increased.
- Ritonavir + lopinavir increases blood levels of the anticancer drugs vinblastine and vincristine, increasing the risk of drug side effects.
- Ritonavir + lopinavir increases blood levels of maraviroc. People using this combination should take no more than 150 mg twice a day.
- Ritonavir + lopinavir can reduce blood levels of abacavir and AZT. The importance of this interaction is not yet known.
- Ritonavir + lopinavir reduces blood levels of the antianxiety drug bupropion, possibly reducing its effectiveness.
- Indinavir, nelfinavir, or saquinavir blood levels are increased and lopinavir blood levels reduced when indinavir, nelfinavir, or saquinavir is taken with ritonavir + lopinavir. Dosage adjustments are necessary. You will have to take ritonavir + lopinavir more than once a day.

- The anticonvulsant drugs carbamazepine, phenobarbital, and phenytoin reduce blood levels of ritonavir + lopinavir and should be mixed with caution. If you take one of these drugs, your ritonavir + lopinavir dosage may have to be increased, and you will have to take it more than once a day.
- Ritonavir + lopinavir increases blood levels of felodipine, nifedipine, and nicardipine. Caution should be exercised when mixing these drugs because of the risk of an excessive blood-pressure drop.
- Dexamethasone reduces the amount of lopinavir in the blood, reducing its effectiveness.
- Protease inhibitors, including ritonavir + lopinavir, may drastically increase blood levels of the ED drugs sildenafil, tadalafil, and vardenafil, increasing the risk of side effects, including low blood pressure, visual changes, and persistent, painful erection. Reduce ED drug dose by ½ and use with caution.
- Ritonavir + lopinavir increases blood levels of immune suppressants (cyclosporine, tacrolimus, and sirolimus—also called rapamycin).
- Blood levels of the inhaled corticosteroid fluticasone are increased when used with ritonavir or lopinavir. The combination is not recommended unless the potential benefit outweighs the risks.
- Because ritonavir formulas contain alcohol, mixing some cephalosporin antibiotics, chloral hydrate, chloramphenicol, disulfiram, griseofulvin, metronidazole, some edible mushrooms nitrofurantoin, or sulfa drugs may cause a severe reaction.

Saquinavir

- Do not combine rifampin or rifabutin with saquinavir, as they reduce saquinavir blood levels by 80% and 40%, respectively. Rifabutin levels are increased. Another protease inhibitor may be added to compensate for the interaction's effect. Dexamethasone, carbamazepine, garlic capsules, nevirapine, phenobarbital, and phenytoin may also reduce blood levels of saquinavir.
- Blood levels of saquinavir may be elevated by terfenadine, astemizole, ketoconazole, and itraconazole. Other drugs that may lead to serious side effects when combined with saquinavir are amiodarone, bepridil, cisapride, calcium channel

blockers, clarithromycin, clindamycin, delavirdine, ergot derivatives, flecainide, midazolam, propafenone, quinidine, rifampin, and triazolam. Do not combine these medications.

- Saquinavir increases blood levels of the benzodiazepines, cyclosporine, pimozide, rapamycin, tacrolimus, and tricyclic antidepressants (amitriptyline, imipramine). Dose reductions of these medicines may be needed.
- Saquinavir reduces blood levels of the narcotic analgesics and the estrogen part of contraceptive drugs. Talk to your doctor about additional or different contraceptive protection.
- Ritonavir increases blood levels of saquinavir and increases the risk of side effects. This combination is often used to boost the effects of saquinavir.
- Combining rifampin with ritonavir + saquinavir can lead to hepatitis and serious increases in liver enzymes.
- Do not mix lovastatin or simvastatin with saquinavir or ritonavir + saquinavir. The combination leads to muscle pain and damage and to kidney damage. Atorvastatin and other statin drugs may also produce this reaction and should be used with caution.
- St. John's wort decreases the effectiveness of saquinavir. Do not combine these medications.
- Protease inhibitors, including saquinavir, may drastically increase the blood levels of the ED drugs sildenafil, tadalafil, and vardenafil, increasing the risk of side effects such as low blood pressure, visual changes, sudden hearing loss, and persistent, painful erection. Reduce ED drug dose by ½ and use with caution.
- People taking warfarin with saquinavir should have their blood tested periodically to be sure that their anticoagulant dose is correct.

Tipranavir

- Do not take amiodarone, astemizole, cisapride, flecainide, pimozide, propafenone, quinidine, or terfenadine with tipranavir because of the possibility of serious and potentially life-threatening effects such as abnormal heart rhythms.
- Rifampin can increase resistance to all protease inhibitors, including tipranavir, reducing their effectiveness.
- Do not take migraine medicines such as dihydroergotamine, ergonovine, ergotamine, or methylergonovine with

tipranavir, because of the possibility of serious and possible life-threatening reactions due to ergot toxicity.

- Do not take the statin-type drugs simvastatin or lovastatin with tipranavir because of the risk of severe reactions such as muscle damage and breakdown. Atorvastatin may be taken, but the lowest effective dose should be used.
- Blood levels of tipranavir may be raised by enfuvirtide, terfenadine, ketoconazole, and itraconazole. Dose adjustments may not be needed.
- If you take tipranavir and also take oral antidiabetes drugs, you must carefully monitor blood-sugar levels, as dose adjustments may be required.
- Tipranavir cuts levels of ethinyl estradiol, an ingredient in many contraceptive drugs, by ½ and can lead to contraceptive failure. Women taking any contraceptive with an estrogen ingredient should use an alternative means of birth control. Women taking estrogen replacement therapy and tipranavir may find they need to increase their hormone dose to maintain the same benefit.
- Other drugs that may interact with tipranavir and should be carefully monitored by your doctor are calcium channel blockers, clarithromycin, clindamycin, delavirdine, desipramine, and rifabutin.
- If you must take an antacid, take it at least 1 hour before or after you take tipranavir.
- St. John's wort decreases the effectiveness of all protease inhibitors, including tipranavir. Do not combine them.
- Protease inhibitors, including tipranavir, may drastically increase blood levels of the ED drugs sildenafil, tadalafil, and vardenafil, increasing the risk of side effects, including low blood pressure, visual changes, and persistent, painful erection. Reduce ED drug dose by ½ and use with caution.
- Carbamazepine, dexamethasone, nevirapine phenobarbital, and phenytoin may reduce blood levels of protease inhibitors such as tipranavir.
- Tipranavir can drastically increase the effects of benzodiazepine sedatives such as midazolam and triazolam, leading to prolonged sedation or severe breathing difficulties. Do not take these drugs with tipranavir.
- Blood levels of SSRI antidepressants may be increased with tipranavir. SSRI dosage reductions may be needed.

- Immune system suppressants (cyclosporine, sirolimus, and tacrolimus) may be affected by tipranavir. Dosage adjustments may be necessary until blood levels of the immune suppressant have been stabilized.
- Tipranavir reduces the amount of methadone in the blood by ½. Methadone dosage increases may be needed.
- Tipranavir affects meperidine and long-term use of meperidine with tipranavir is not recommended because of the possibility of seizure activity.
- Frequent blood monitoring is suggested if you are taking warfarin, aspirin, or any blood-thinning drug and begin taking tipranavir.
- Tipranavir solution contains a lot of vitamin E. If you use the oral solution, do not take more vitamin E than is recommended for daily intake (30 IU a day for adults or 10 IU a day for children).

Food Interactions

Generally, protease inhibitors should be taken with food or right after a meal to maximize the amount of medicine absorbed into the blood.

Indinavir is best taken with water—or liquids such as skim milk or juice—at least 1 hour before or 2 hours after a meal. You should not eat meals that are high in calories, fat, and protein from 1 hour before to 2 hours after taking indinavir. You may take indinavir with a light meal.

Nelfinavir oral powder form may be mixed with a small amount of water, milk, soy milk, or dairy foods such as pudding or ice cream. If the entire dose is not consumed, it may be refrigerated for up to 6 hours. Do not heat the mixed dose after refrigeration.

Ritonavir oral solution should be taken on an empty stomach, 1 hour before or 2 hours after meals. The taste of the oral liquid may be improved by mixing it with chocolate milk or Ensure. Do not mix earlier than 1 hour before you take your dose.

Usual Dose

Atazanavir

Adult: 300 mg once a day with 100 mg ritonavir, taken with food. Do not open atazanavir capsules before taking them. People unable to tolerate ritonavir should receive 400 mg atazanavir once a day, taken with food.

If you are also taking efavirenz: 400 mg atazanavir and 100 mg ritonavir once a day. Take efavirenz on an empty stomach at bedtime.

If you are also taking tenofovir and an H_2 antagonist: 400 mg atazanavir and 100 mg ritonavir once a day with food and/or at least 10 hours after the H_2 antagonist.

Patients with moderate liver disease should take no more than 300 mg a day.

Additional dose adjustments may be needed with other drug combinations, or if you have a kidney or liver condition.

Child (age 6–17): Dosage is based on body weight, up to 150–300 mg once a day with food. Previously untreated children who cannot tolerate ritonavir should take 400 mg atazanavir once a day with food. Consult your doctor for more information.

Darunavir

Adult: 600–800 mg (two 300- or 400-mg tablets) with 100 mg ritonavir once or twice a day. Do not chew these tablets.

Child: not recommended.

Fosamprenavir

Adult: first-time treatment—1400 mg twice a day (without ritonavir); or 1400 mg once a day with 100–200 mg ritonavir once a day; or 700 mg twice a day with 100 mg ritonavir twice a day. Previous treatment with another protease inhibitor—700 mg twice a day plus 100 mg ritonavir twice a day.

Child: not recommended.

Indinavir

Adult: 800 mg every 8 hours, around the clock. People with cirrhosis should take 600 mg every 8 hours.

Child: not recommended.

Nelfinavir

Adult and Child (age 14 and over): 1250 mg twice a day or 750 mg 3 times a day.

Child (age 2–13): 9–13 mg per lb. of body weight 3 times a day.

Child (under age 2): not recommended.

Ritonavir

Adult: 600 mg twice a day. You may start with a lower dosage and increase gradually to avoid upset stomach.

Child (age 1 month and over): 250–400 mg per m^2 of body surface area (BSA) twice a day. BSA is calculated by your doctor using height and weight.

Ritonavir + Lopinavir

Adult and Child (88 lbs. or more or age 12 and over): 2–4 capsules twice a day.

Child (age 6 months–11 years): Consult your doctor.

Saquinavir

Adult and Child (age 16 and over): 200 mg 5 times a day (administered with 100 mg ritonavir twice a day), within 2 hours after a full meal.

Child (under age 16): Consult your doctor.

Tipranavir

Adult and Child (age 16 and over): 500 mg taken with 200 mg ritonavir twice a day.

Child (under age 16): Consult your doctor

Overdosage

Protease inhibitor overdose is likely to result in exaggerated drug side effects, though the risk varies between members of this group. Overdose victims should be taken to a hospital emergency room for evaluation and treatment. If you seek treatment, ALWAYS bring the prescription bottle or container. Contact your local poison center or hospital emergency room for more information.

Special Information

These medicines do not cure HIV and will not prevent you from giving the HIV virus to another person; you must still practice safe sex. You may still develop opportunistic infections or other complications associated with advanced HIV disease.

Protease inhibitors may cause the redistribution or accumulation of body fat, leading to buffalo hump, breast enlargement, abnormal thinness, or a round, moon-shaped face.

Oral solutions of these products may be absorbed differently from the capsules. They cannot be interchanged for each other on a milligram for milligram basis. Avoid alcohol while taking fosamprenavir oral solution.

Loperamide, an over-the-counter remedy, may control diarrhea associated with some of these drugs.

It is imperative for you to take this medication exactly according to your doctor's instructions. Do not skip any doses. Skipping doses of a protease inhibitor increases the risk that your virus will become resistant to the drug. Contact your doctor if you skip several doses.

Saquinavir should be used only when combined with ritonavir (though it is sometimes combined with lopinavir + ritonavir). It is imperative for you to take this medication exactly according to your doctor's instructions. Missing doses of saquinavir increases the risk that you will become resistant to the drug. If you forget a dose of atazanavir, nelfinavir, saquinavir, or tipranavir, take it as soon as you remember and then continue with your regular schedule. Do not take a double dose.

If you forget a dose of darunavir or ritonavir and remember within 6 hours, take it as soon as you remember and then continue with your regular schedule. If 6 hours have passed since the time when you should have taken your medicine, skip the forgotten dose and take your next dose at the regular time. Do not take a double dose.

If you forget a dose of fosamprenavir, take it as soon as you remember. If you miss a dose by more than 4 hours, skip the forgotten dose and continue with your regular schedule. Never take a double dose.

If you forget a dose of indinavir and remember within 2 hours, take it. Otherwise skip the forgotten dose and wait until your next regular dose.

Special Populations

Pregnancy/Breast-feeding: Protease inhibitor-based therapy is generally safe for mother and child and has been proven to be effective in reducing transmission of the HIV virus from mother to child. Follow your doctor's instructions when considering a protease inhibitor during pregnancy.

These drugs pass into breast milk in varying amounts. However, nursing mothers with HIV should always use infant formula to avoid transmitting the virus, regardless of whether they are taking a protease inhibitor. Breast-feeding by an HIV-positive mother is discouraged.

Seniors: Seniors may take protease inhibitors without special precaution.

Humalog *see **Insulin,** page 628*

Generic Name

Hydralazine (hye-DRAL-uh-zene) G

Brand Names

Only available in generic form.

Type of Drug

Antihypertensive.

Prescribed for

High blood pressure. Also prescribed for aortic insufficiency after heart valve replacement and congestive heart failure.

General Information

Although its mechanism of action is not completely understood, hydralazine hydrochloride is believed to lower blood pressure by relaxing vascular smooth muscles throughout the body. This also helps to improve heart function and blood flow to the kidneys and brain.

Cautions and Warnings

Do not use hydralazine if you are **allergic** or **sensitive** to any of its ingredients.

You should not use hydralazine if you have **coronary artery disease** or **rheumatic heart disease**.

Long-term administration of more than 200 mg a day of hydralazine may produce the symptoms of lupus erythematosus (a chronic autoimmune disease), including muscle and joint pain, skin reactions, fever, kidney inflammation, and anemia, although they usually disappear when the drug is discontinued. Report any fever, chest pain, feelings of ill health, or other unexplained symptoms to your doctor. The risk of developing lupus increases with higher dosages; approximately 5% of people taking 100 mg a day and 10% of people taking 200 mg a day of hydralazine develop lupus.

Hydralazine may actually improve kidney blood flow and kidney function in people who have below-normal function. It should be used with caution in people with advanced **kidney damage**.

Hydralazine may worsen heart problems and should be used with care in people with a history of **heart disease**. It can cause angina and may cause heart attacks. This medication should also be used with caution in people with **pulmonary hypertension**.

Tingling in the hands or feet caused by hydralazine may be relieved by taking pyridoxine (vitamin B_6).

People taking hydralazine may develop reduced hemoglobin and red-blood-cell counts. Reduced white-blood-cell and platelet counts may also occur. Periodic blood counts are recommended while taking hydralazine.

Possible Side Effects

- ▼ Most common: headache, appetite loss, nausea, vomiting, diarrhea, rapid heartbeat, and chest pain.
- ▼ Less common: stuffy nose; flushing; tearing, itching, or redness of the eyes; numbness or tingling in the hands or feet; dizziness; tremors; muscle cramps; depression; disorientation; anxiety; itching; rash; fever; chills; occasional hepatitis (symptoms include yellowing of the skin or whites of the eyes); constipation; urinary difficulties; and adverse effects on normal blood composition.

Drug Interactions

- Taking hydralazine with the beta blockers metoprolol or propranolol may result in increased blood levels of both hydralazine and the beta blocker.
- Monoamine oxidase inhibitor (MAOI) antidepressants should be used with caution by those taking hydralazine.
- Nonsteroidal anti-inflammatory drugs (NSAIDs) may reduce the effects of hydralazine.
- Do not use over-the-counter cough, cold, or allergy medications, or appetite suppressants. These products often contain stimulant ingredients that can increase blood pressure.

Food Interactions

Take hydralazine with food.

Usual Dose

Adult: 10 mg 4 times a day for the first 2–4 days, increased to 25 mg 4 times a day for the rest of the first week. Dosage is then increased until desired effect is seen to a maximum of 300 mg a day.

Child: 0.34 mg per lb. of body weight a day, in 4 divided doses, increased up to 200 mg a day.

Overdosage

Symptoms include extreme lowering of blood pressure, rapid heartbeat, headache, flushing, chest pain, and abnormal heart rhythms. If you experience any of these symptoms, contact your doctor immediately. If you seek treatment, ALWAYS bring the prescription bottle or container.

Special Information

Take hydralazine exactly as prescribed.

Contact your doctor if you experience prolonged and unexplained tiredness, fever, muscle or joint aches, or chest pain while taking this drug.

If you forget a dose, take it as soon as you remember. If it is almost time for your next dose, skip the one you forgot and continue with your regular schedule. Do not take a double dose.

Special Populations

Pregnancy/Breast-feeding: High doses of hydralazine caused birth defects in animal studies, and temporary blood-related problems have been seen in newborns whose mothers took hydralazine during pregnancy. Hydralazine should be taken during pregnancy only if your doctor determines that the potential benefit outweighs the risks.

Hydralazine passes into breast milk. Nursing mothers who must take this drug should consider using infant formula.

Seniors: Seniors are more sensitive to the blood-pressure-lowering effects of hydralazine and its side effects, especially low body temperature.

Generic Name

Hydroxyzine (hye-DROK-suh-zene) G

Brand Names

Vistaril

Type of Drug

Antihistamine and antianxiety agent.

Prescribed For

Itching caused by allergy, sedation preceeding or following general anethesia, and anxiety.

General Information

Hydroxyzine is an antihistamine with antianxiety, muscle-relaxing, antiemetic (antivomiting), bronchial-dilating, pain-relieving, and antispasmodic properties. Hydroxyzine has been used to treat a variety of problems, including stress related to dental or other minor surgical procedures, acute emotional problems, anxiety associated with heart disease, skin problems, and behavioral difficulties in children.

Cautions and Warnings

Hydroxyzine should not be used if you are **allergic** or **sensitive** to any of its ingredients, or to cetirizene.

Possible Side Effects

Wheezing, chest tightness, and breathing difficulties are signs of a drug-sensitivity reaction.

▼ Most common: dry mouth and drowsiness. These usually disappear after a few days of continuous use or when the dose is reduced.

▼ Rare: occasional tremors or convulsions at higher doses. Contact your doctor if you experience anything unusual while taking any medication.

Drug Interactions

- Hydroxyzine depresses the nervous system, producing drowsiness and sleepiness. Do not take this drug with alcohol, sedatives, or other antihistamines or central-nervous-system depressants. When hydroxyzine is taken with one of these drugs, the dose of the latter should be cut in ½.

Food Interactions

Take hydroxyzine with food if it upsets your stomach.

Usual Dose

Adult: 25–100 mg 3–4 times a day for anxiety and allergic reactions; 50–100 mg for sedation.

Child (age 6 and over): 50–100 mg a day in divided doses for anxiety and allergic reactions; 0.27 mg per lb. of body weight for sedation.

Child (under age 6): 50 mg a day in divided doses for anxiety and allergic reactions; 0.27 mg per lb. of body weight for sedation.

Overdosage

The most common sign of overdose is sleepiness. Overdose victims should be taken to a hospital emergency room for treatment.

If you seek treatment, ALWAYS bring the prescription bottle or container.

Special Information

Hydroxyzine may cause drowsiness: Be careful when driving, operating hazardous machinery, or doing anything that requires concentration.

The dry mouth associated with taking hydroxyzine may increase your risk of dental cavities and decay. Pay attention to dental hygiene while taking this drug.

Contact your doctor if you develop a drug-sensitivity reaction to hydroxyzine (symptoms include wheezing, chest tightness, and breathing difficulties).

If you forget a dose of hydroxyzine, take it as soon as you remember. If it is almost time for your next dose, skip the one you forgot and continue with your regular schedule. Do not take a double dose.

Special Populations

Pregnancy/Breast-feeding: Animal studies have shown that regular treatment with hydroxyzine during the first few months of pregnancy may cause birth defects. Do not take this drug without your doctor's knowledge if you are or might be pregnant.

Hydroxyzine may reduce the amount of breast milk you produce and may pass into breast milk. Nursing mothers who must take hydroxyzine should use infant formula.

Seniors: Seniors are more sensitive to side effects and may require lower dosages.

Hyzaar *see **Angiotensin II Blockers,** page 97*

Generic Name

Icatibant (ih-CAT-ih-bahnt)

Brand Names

Firazyr

Type of Drug

Bradykinin B2 inhibitor.

Prescribed For

Hereditary angioedema (HAE).

General Information

HAE is a very rare and potentially life-threatening genetic disease accounting for 0.4% of all cases of angioedema. HAE symptoms include edema (swelling) in various body parts, including the hands, feet, genitals, face, and airway or throat. Swelling in the intestinal wall can cause severe abdominal pain, nausea, and vomiting. There are 3 types of HAE. Type I HAE is defined by low blood levels of a protein in the body called C1 inhibitor. Type II HAE is characterized by the normal or high blood levels of a dysfunctional form of C1 inhibitor. Type III HAE is an estrogen-dependent inherited form of angioedema occurring mainly in women; C1 inhibitor proteins function normally and are present in normal amounts in type III HAE.

Icatibant is injected subcutaneously (under the skin) and is used to treat all 3 forms of HAE attacks; it is not effective for prevention of attacks. It works by widening blood vessels in the areas affected by the attack, which helps to relieve swelling, pain, and inflammation.

Cautions and Warnings

Do not use this product if you are **allergic** or **sensitive** to any of its ingredients.

Laryngeal edema (throat closing) is the most dangerous of all HAE symptoms. If you must treat yourself for a laryngeal attack, contact your doctor immediately afterward.

If you have recently had a **stroke** or **heart attack** or currently have unstable **angina** (brief attacks of chest pain), you should use icatibant only if your doctor determines that the potential benefit outweighs the risk, as this drug may further damage your heart and blood vessels.

Possible Side Effects

- ▼ Most common: injection reactions, including bruising, burning, swelling, irritation, pain, and numbness.
- ▼ Less common: fever, increased liver enzymes, and dizziness.
- ▼ Rare: rash, nausea, headache, and drowsiness. Contact your doctor if you experience anything unusual while taking any medication.

Drug Interactions

- This drug may interfere with the blood-pressure-lowering effects of angiotensin-converting enzyme (ACE) inhibitor drugs. Your doctor should monitor your blood pressure and condition if you must take these medicines together.

Usual Dose

Adult: 30 mg (1 syringe) injected under the skin of the abdomen. Additional doses may be given every 6 hours if needed, up to 3 doses in 24 hours.

Children: not recommended.

Overdosage

Overdose symptoms include itching, redness, and low blood pressure, which usually do not require medical treatment. In case of an overdose, contact your local poison control center or a hospital emergency room for information. If you seek treatment, ALWAYS bring the prescription bottle or container.

Special Information

Contact your doctor if you experience hives, itching, chest tightness, wheezing, low blood pressure, dizziness or fainting after injecting icatibant. These can be signs of a drug hypersensitivity reaction.

Talk to your doctor when planning a trip. Make sure to take a sufficient supply of your medicine with you and prepare for proper medication storage (refrigeration) at your destination. This medication may be stored in the refrigerator or at room temperature up to 77°F. Do not freeze it.

Patients and caregivers who give this medicine must be trained to recognize HAE symptoms and when and how to use it.

Icatibant is clear and colorless. Do not use if it is cloudy or has any color or particles floating in it. Your doctor will instruct you in the proper administration of this medicine, but for more information on injections see page 1242.

Use caution when operating machinery or driving a car after you take icatibant, as it may cause drowsiness or dizziness.

Special Populations

Pregnancy/Breast-feeding: The effect of this drug on a growing fetus is not known. Icatibant has affected fetal growth and development in animal studies. Make sure your doctor knows if you are pregnant or intend to become pregnant while using this medication.

This drug should be taken during pregnancy only if your doctor determines that the potential benefit outweighs the risks.

It is not known if this drug passes into breast milk. Nursing mothers who must take this medicine should use infant formula.

Seniors: Seniors eliminate icatibant more slowly from their bodies than younger adults.

Generic Name

Iloperidone (eye-low-PER-ih-doan)

Brand Names

Fanapt

Type of Drug

Atypical antipsychotic.

Prescribed For

Schizophrenia.

General Information

Iloperidone is a potent antipsychotic that blocks several different chemical receptors in the brain. Exactly how iloperidone works is unknown. But, like other atypical or second-generation antipsychotics, iloperidone probably works by affecting a combination of dopamine and serotonin receptors in the brain. Iloperidone is eliminated mainly through the liver.

Cautions and Warnings

Do not use this product if you are **allergic** or **sensitive** to any of its ingredients.

Antipsychotic drugs have been associated with increased mortality in seniors with **dementia** or **Alzheimer's disease**. The specific causes of death related to iloperidone and other atypical antipsychotic drugs were mostly due to either a heart-related event or infection, mostly pneumonia.

People taking iloperidone are more likely to have a stroke or transient ischemic attack (TIA)—mini-stroke—than those taking other atypical antipsychotics, such as aripiprazole, olanzapine, or risperidone.

Iloperidone affects how electrical signals pass through the heart, exposing you to possibly fatal arrhythmias. People with a history of **abnormal heart rhythms**, **recent heart attack**, or other **heart disease**, including some inborn heart conditions, should not take this medicine. The chances of an arrhythmia are greater if you are also taking a medicine that can increase the amount of iloperidone in the blood or cause abnormal heart rhythms on their own. (See "Drug Interactions.")

Iloperidone can cause rapid heartbeat, dizziness, or fainting when rising from a sitting or lying position, especially when you first start taking it. For this reason, people are generally started at a low dose that is gradually increased until the dizziness is intolerable or a maximum effect is achieved.

A serious set of side effects known as neuroleptic malignant syndrome (NMS), which includes symptoms of a high fever, convulsions, difficult or fast breathing, rapid heartbeat, and rapid pulse has been associated with antipsychotic medicines. Other symptoms of NMS include muscle rigidity, mental changes, irregular pulse or blood pressure, and increased sweating. NMS can be fatal and requires immediate medical attention.

Tardive dyskinesia (symptoms include lip smacking or puckering, puffing of the cheeks, rapid or wormlike movements of the tongue, uncontrolled chewing motions, and uncontrolled arm or leg movements) can occur and is often considered a reason to stop taking this drug. Report any of these side effects to your doctor.

Iloperidone, like other antipsychotic medicines, has been associated with obesity, high cholesterol, high blood sugar, and diabetes and can cause significant weight gain over time. People with **diabetes** should have regular monitoring of blood-glucose control while taking iloperidone.

Seizures occur in a small number of people taking iloperidone. Iloperidone should be taken with care if you have had **seizures** or are at increased risk due to other medications.

Antipsychotic medicines have been linked to reduced white-blood-cell counts. Your doctor will periodically check your blood and may exchange iloperidone for a different medication if your white counts go down.

Iloperidone raises levels of prolactin—a hormone involved with reproduction, estrogen and testosterone levels, and the immune system. Increased prolactin can interfere with reproductive function in both men and women and cause an absence of monthly periods, spontaneous breast milk flow, painful breast enlargement, and impotence (men). Eventually, increased prolactic levels can lead to bone density loss in men and women.

Avoid being exposed to extreme heat. Antipsychotics can upset your body's temperature-regulating mechanism.

Antipsychotics may cause swallowing difficulty, leading to pneumonia caused by inhaled food, especially in those with advanced Alzheimer's disease.

Suicide is a danger with all psychotics and antidepressants. To reduce risk of possible overdose, people taking iloperidone should have no more than a 30-day supply of medication in their possession at any time.

Priapism (a persistent, painful erection), possibly requiring surgery, can occur while taking this medication.

Women eliminate iloperidone about 30% more slowly than men, but this effect is not considered a problem. Women may respond to lower doses than men.

People with **liver disease** should not use iloperidone.

Possible Side Effects

Side effects increase with larger doses.

- ▼ Most common: weight gain, rapid heartbeat, dizziness, being tired or sleepy, nausea, dry mouth, and diarrhea.
- ▼ Common: stuffy nose; uncontrolled shaking; spastic movements; restlessness; slowing of the ability to start or continue normal motions; difficulty performing ordinary movements or becoming contorted or twisted when attempting them; repetitive movements; sustained muscle contractions causing twisting; abnormal or unusual postures; and difficulty talking.
- ▼ Less common: joint pain, stiffness, blurred vision, abdominal discomfort, nose and/or throat irritation, upper-respiratory infection, tremors, lethargy, difficulty reaching ejaculation (men), breathing difficulties, skin rash, dizziness when arising from a chair or bed, and low blood pressure.
- ▼ Rare: Rare side effects can occur in almost any part of the body. Contact your doctor if you experience anything unusual while taking any medication.

Drug Interactions

- Iloperidone increases the effects of blood-pressure-lowering drugs and nervous system depressants. Dosage adjustments may be needed if you add iloperidone to one of these medicines.

- Combinations of iloperidone with another drug that can affect the heart in the same way (antiarrhythmic agents such as amiodarone, bretylium, disopyramide, dofetilide, quinidine, or sotalol; arsenic trioxide; chlorpromazine; cisapride; dolasetron; droperidol; mefloquine; mesoridazine; moxifloxacin; pentamidine; pimozide; tacrolimus; thioridazine; and ziprasidone) should be avoided.
- Mixing iloperidone with bupropion, fluoxetine, atazanavir, indinavir, nelfinavir, ritonavir, saquinavir, clarithromycin, telithromycin, paroxetine, ketoconazole, itraconazole, or nefazodone causes a large increase in blood levels of iloperidone. Your iloperidone dose should be cut in ½ if you are taking one of these combinations.
- Aprepitant, celecoxib, chlorpheniramine, chlorpromazine, cimetidine, cinacalcet, ciprofloxacin, citalopram, clemastine, clomipramine, cocaine, delavirdine, diphenhydramine, doxepin, doxorubicin, duloxetine, erythromycin, escitalopram, fluconazole, fluvoxamine, gestodene, halofantrine, haloperidol, hydroxyzine, imatinib, levomepromazine, methadone, metoclopramide, mibefradil, midodrine, mifepristone, moclobemide, norfloxacin, norfluoxetine, perphenazine, ranitidine, sertraline, terbinafine, ticlopidine, tripelennamine, verapamil, and voriconazole can also raise iloperidone blood levels but dose adjustments may not be needed.
- Iloperidone may increase the effects of medications to treat high blood pressure and dextromethorphan.

Food Interactions

Grapefruit juice and starfruit slow the breakdown of this drug by the liver. Avoid large amounts of these fruit products while you are taking this drug.

Usual Dose

Adult and Child (age 17 and over): 1 mg twice a day to start, increasing gradually to 6–12 mg twice a day.

Child (under age 17): not recommended.

Overdosage

Individual doses up to 576 mg at once and 292 mg over 3 days have been reported without any deaths. Overdose symptoms can be expected to be drowsiness, sedation, rapid heartbeat, dizziness, fainting, and others found under "Possible Side Effects." Overdose victims should be taken to a hospital emergency room for treatment. If you seek treatment, ALWAYS bring the prescription bottle or container.

Special Information

Contact your doctor at once if you become dizzy, faint, or have heart palpitations. These symptoms can be indicators of an abnormal heart rhythm. Also, report any changes in condition, especially if you start or stop another medicine.

Sleepiness occurs in about 12% of people who take 10 mg a day or more of iloperidone. Take extreme care when engaging in activities, such as driving, that require concentration or coordination.

Avoid alcohol and other nervous system depressants while taking iloperidone.

Be sure your doctor knows all the medication you are taking, including over-the-counter products.

If you forget to take a dose of iloperidone, take it as soon as you remember. If it is almost time for your next dose, skip the dose you forgot, and continue with your regular schedule. Do not take a double dose.

If you stop taking iloperidone for any reason and then restart it, your doctor may begin again with the lowest dose and gradually increase it.

Special Populations

Pregnancy/Breast-feeding: Animal studies have shown this drug may have the potential to affect a developing fetus, but there is no information on how pregnant women are affected. Iloperidone should be taken during pregnancy only if your doctor determines that the potential benefit outweighs the risks.

Iloperidone may pass into breast milk. Nursing mothers who must take this medication should use infant formula.

Seniors: Studies of iloperidone included too few seniors and none age 75 or older to determine if there is an important difference between seniors and others. Seniors with Alzheimer's disease are at a greater risk of stroke, TIA, and dying.

Generic Name

Iloprost (EYE-low-prahst)

Brand Names

Ventavis

Type of Drug

Synthetic prostacyclin.

Prescribed For

Pulmonary hypertension.

General Information

Pulmonary hypertension occurs when blood pressure rises in the arteries that supply blood to the lungs. This condition can develop by itself, but it also occurs among children with congenital heart problems, people with heart valve damage, and people with heart failure. People with pulmonary hypertension tend to become dizzy and tired, and easily lose their breath. Exercise becomes very difficult as the condition worsens. Iloprost improves the symptoms of pulmonary hypertension by dilating (opening) blood vessels in the lungs and throughout the body. It also affects the normal function of blood platelets in the clotting process. In clinical studies, many people taking iloprost were able to maintain their condition at an acceptable level while using the medicine.

Cautions and Warnings

Do not take iloprost if you are **allergic** or **sensitive** to any of its ingredients.

People with moderate to severe **liver disease** should be cautious about using this drug because it is eliminated from the body through the liver.

The effects of **dialysis** on iloprost are not known.

Dizziness or fainting may occur when you first start taking this medicine. Your doctor should monitor your blood pressure, heart rate, and breathing when you start using this medicine.

Do not swallow this medicine or allow it to get into your eyes.

This medicine has not been studied in people with **chronic obstructive pulmonary disease**, **severe asthma**, or **active lung infections**.

If signs of pulmonary edema occur (difficulty breathing, wheezing, cough, feeling of "drowning," or gurgling or grunting sounds with breathing), stop treatment immediately.

Possible Side Effects

- ▼ Most common: flushing, coughing, headache, nausea, and low blood pressure.
- ▼ Common: lockjaw, sleeplessness, vomiting, flu-like symptoms, back pain, heart palpitations, dizziness or fainting

Possible Side Effects *(continued)*

when rising from a lying or sitting position, muscle cramps, vomiting blood, and increased liver enzymes and other abnormal lab tests.

- ▼ Less common: tongue pain and pneumonia.
- ▼ Rare: Rare side effects can include congestive heart failure, chest pain discomfort or tightness, rapid heartbeat, difficulty breathing, swelling in the arms or legs, and kidney failure. Contact your doctor if you experience anything unusual while taking any medication.

Drug Interactions

- Iloprost may increase the blood-pressure-lowering effects of some blood-pressure-lowering drugs, especially those that work by dilating (widening) blood vessels.
- Iloprost may increase the risk of bleeding in people taking oral blood-thinning (anticoagulant) drugs.

Usual Dose

Adult: 2.5–5 mcg by inhalation 6–9 times a day while awake, with a maximum daily dose of 45 mcg. Do not inhale this drug more than once every 2 hours even though its effect may not last for 2 hours.

Child: not recommended.

Overdosage

There are no known cases of iloprost overdose, but symptoms should mimic the known effects of this drug, including headache, flushing, nausea, vomiting, and diarrhea. Take the overdose victim to a hospital emergency room at once. If you seek treatment, ALWAYS bring the prescription bottle or container.

Special Information

This drug has only been studied with the nebulizer provided by its manufacturer. Using it with any other type or brand of nebulizer may result in the incorrect dose of iloprost being inhaled.

Do not mix any other drug with iloprost when you inhale it.

Do not allow this product to come into contact with your skin or eyes. Do not swallow it.

You must use a fresh ampule of iloprost for each inhalation. Place all the liquid in the ampule into the medication chamber, choose your inhaler dose (2.5 or 5 mcg), inhale the medicine, and throw away any remaining medication from that iloprost ampule.

Contact your doctor at once if your symptoms get worse despite using this medicine. Other treatments may be needed.

Special Populations

Pregnancy/Breast-feeding: Animal studies indicate that iloprost given by intravenous injection may cause birth defects. Iloprost should be taken during pregnancy only if your doctor determines that the potential benefit outweighs the risks.

It is not known if this drug passes into breast milk. Nursing mothers who must take it should use infant formula.

Seniors: Seniors should use the lowest possible dose of this medicine because of normal declines in kidney and liver function.

Generic Name

Imiquimod (ih-MIH-kwih-mod) G

Brand Names

Aldara Zyclara

The information in this profile also applies to the following drugs:

Generic Ingredients: Ingenol Mebutate G
Picato

Type of Drug

Immune modifier.

Prescribed For

Genital warts, perianal warts, actinic keratosis, and superficial basal cell carcinoma (sBCC). Ingenol is used only for actinic keratosis.

General Information

Imiquimod has no direct antiviral activity. Animal studies suggest that it stimulates the skin to produce cytokines, potent natural chemicals that fight the warts, but its actual effect on genital warts and condyloma is not known. In studies, 50% of people who used it had complete clearance of their warts. Imiquimod does not cure genital warts—new ones may develop while others are being treated. Only minimal amounts of imiquimod enter the bloodstream. Ingenol kills affected skin cells and is used for only 2–3 days.

Cautions and Warnings

Do not use imiquimod if you are **allergic** or **sensitive** to any of its ingredients.

Imiquimod has not been studied in other viral diseases of the skin, such as papilloma virus, and should not be used to treat them, since its effect is unknown.

Do not apply imiquimod to any area until it has healed from any previous drug or surgery. Imiquimod can worsen skin that is already inflamed or sunburnt.

Imiquimod may increase your sun sensitivity. Avoid exposure to sunlight.

Imiquimod is not recommended for patients with **lowered immune response**.

Possible Side Effects

- ▼ Most common: redness, itching, erosion of the skin, burning, flaking, abrasions, swelling, and fungal infections in women. Ingenol may cause headaches.
- ▼ Common: pain, marks on the skin, ulcers, skin scabbing, and headache.
- ▼ Less common: skin soreness, flu-like symptoms, skin discoloration, muscle aches, fungal infections in men, and diarrhea.

Drug Interactions

- Do not apply these drugs with others that may also cause skin irritation.

Usual Dose

Actinic Keratosis

Imiquimod

Adult: Wash and let the treatment area dry thoroughly. Apply twice a week—for example, Monday and Thursday—to the face or neck, but not both, before bedtime for 16 weeks. After 8 hours, remove the cream with mild soap and water.

Child: not recommended.

Ingenol

Adult: Face and scalp—apply 0.015% gel once a day for 3 days and then stop. Body, arms, and legs—apply 0.05% gel once a day for 2 days and then stop.

Child: not recommended.

Genital Warts

Adult and Child (age 12 and over): At bedtime, apply a thin layer of the cream to external warts and rub it in until the cream disappears.

Do not bandage. Leave it on the skin for 6–10 hours, then remove the cream with mild soap and water. Do this 3 times a week—for example, Monday, Wednesday, and Friday. Continue treatment for up to 16 weeks or until the warts go away.

Child (under age 12): not recommended.

Superficial Basal Cell Carcinoma

Adult: Wash and let the treatment area dry thoroughly. Apply 5 times per week at bedtime for 6 weeks to the sBCC, including the 1 cm surrounding the tumor. After 8 hours, wash the areas with mild soap and water.

Child: not recommended.

Overdosage

Overdose is not likely because such a small amount of imiquimod is absorbed through the skin. Accidental ingestion of imiquimod may cause low blood pressure. Anyone who has swallowed imiquimod should be taken to a hospital emergency room. If you seek treatment, ALWAYS bring the prescription bottle or container.

Special Information

Wash your hands before each application.

Most skin reactions are mild. If you develop a severe skin reaction to these drugs, contact your doctor and remove the product with a mild soap and water. You can resume treatment after the reaction has completely subsided.

Imiquimod may weaken condoms and vaginal diaphragms. These birth control methods may prove undependable while you are using imiquimod cream. Avoid sexual contact while the cream is on your skin.

Uncircumcised men who use imiquimod to treat warts under the foreskin should retract the foreskin and cleanse the area every day.

These drugs are meant to be applied to the skin only. Do not let them get into your eyes, mouth, nose, or vagina. If you forget to apply a dose of imiquimod, do it as soon as you remember. If you don't remember until your next scheduled application, space the remaining doses equally throughout the rest of the week and continue with your regular schedule.

Throw away unused and partially used packets.

Special Populations

Pregnancy/Breast-feeding: The safety of using these drugs during pregnancy is not known. They should be taken during pregnancy only if your doctor determines that the potential benefit outweighs the risks.

It is not known if these drugs pass into breast milk. Nursing mothers who must use them should use infant formula.

Seniors: Seniors may use these drugs without special precaution.

Type of Drug

Incretin Mimetics

Brand Names

Generic Ingredients: Exenatide

Bydureon Byetta

Generic Ingredients: Liraglutide

Victoza

Prescribed For

Type 2 diabetes.

General Information

Incretin mimetics improve blood-sugar control in people with type 2 diabetes. They may be used alone or added to existing therapy, including insulin. These drugs have many of the same actions as glucagon-like peptide 1 (GLP-1), a natural incretin hormone. They differ chemically and work differently from other diabetes medications, including insulin.

Exenatide begins working about 30 minutes after injection and continues to work for at least 8 hours, necessitating 2 injections a day. A weekly formulation of exenatide suspension is also available. Liraglutide continues to work for a longer period and is suitable for 1 daily injection. They help the pancreas to release insulin into the blood in response to sugar levels, so insulin rises when blood sugar is high and declines as blood sugar goes down. They also reduce the production of a hormone called glucagon, which raises blood sugar. They keep food in the stomach longer, which in turn helps reduce the amount of sugar absorbed from dietary sources, and they increase chemical signals in the brain that tell you when you are full, effectively reducing the amount of food you eat. Incretin mimetics increase the number of pancreatic beta cells (which produce insulin) in animals, and may have the same effect in humans. This could help reduce the need for other medicines and improve diabetes control.

Cautions and Warnings

Do not take these medicines if you are **allergic** or **sensitive** to any of their ingredients.

People with severe **stomach or intestinal disease** should not use exenatide.

Liraglutide has caused some thyroid tumors in rat studies using 8 times the human dose. It is not known whether these tumors also develop in people taking liraglutide, although a few have developed nonmalignant thyroid growths. Liraglutide should not be used by people with a personal or family history of **multiple endocrine neoplasia syndrome type 2 (MEN2)** or **medullary thyroid carcinoma**.

People with severe **kidney disease** should not use exenatide, and anyone with kidney disease should use liraglutide with caution. Some people taking exenatide have experienced kidney failure or worsening of kidney disease. Contact your doctor if you develop signs of kidney disease, including changes in urine color, less frequent urination or smaller amounts of urine, unexplained swelling of your hands or feet, fatigue, changes in appetite or digestion, or a dull ache in the mid- to lower back. Kidney function may return to normal with supportive care and stopping the medicine.

Severe inflammation of the pancreas (pancreatitis) has developed in a small number of people taking these drugs, some of whom were hospitalized and several died. Pancreatitis symptoms include nausea, vomiting, tenderness when touching your abdomen, and pain in the upper abdomen. This pain can spread to your back, feel worse after eating, and feel better when you lean forward or curl into a ball. Contact your doctor if you experience any of these symptoms.

These drugs are not a substitute for insulin.

People with **liver disease** should use liraglutide with caution.

Low blood sugar may occur if you are taking an incretin mimetic with another drug for type 2 diabetes, including sulfonylurea antidiabetes drugs or glitazones. Call your doctor if you develop signs of low blood sugar, including shakiness, sweating, headache, drowsiness, weakness, dizziness, irritability, confusion, hunger, rapid heartbeat, or a jittery feeling.

Antibodies to these drugs may develop, but antibody levels generally go down with time. Most people who develop antibodies still have good sugar control and experience similar types of side effects to those who do not develop antibodies.

Possible Side Effects

Exenatide

▼ Most common: nausea, vomiting, diarrhea, and low blood sugar (when mixed with a sulfonylurea or metformin plus a sulfonylurea).

▼ Less common: low blood sugar (when mixed with a glitazone), feeling jittery, dizziness, headache, upset stomach, weakness, and excessive sweating.

▼ Rare: rash, abdominal swelling and pain, constipation, and kidney failure. Contact your doctor if you experience anything unusual while taking any medication.

Liraglutide

▼ Most common: nausea, vomiting, diarrhea, and appetite loss.

▼ Common: constipation, upset stomach, flu, common cold and other upper-respiratory infections, headache, urinary infections, dizziness, sinus infection, back pain, and fatigue.

▼ Less common: injection site reactions.

▼ Rare: low blood sugar (especially when mixed with a sulfonylurea or metformin plus a sulfonylurea) and kidney/urinary problems. Contact your doctor if you experience anything unusual while taking any medication.

Drug Interactions

- Combining incretin mimetics with a sulfonylurea or meglitinide antidiabetes drug may lead to hypoglycemia (low blood sugar). Carefully monitor your blood-sugar levels and contact your doctor if you experience low blood sugar. A dosage change may be needed.
- These drugs extend the time it takes for the stomach to empty and may reduce the amount of medication absorbed by mouth. Take ALL oral medicines (including over-the-counter drugs such as acetaminophen) at least 1 hour before or 4 hours after you inject to ensure maximum absorption. If you are using exenatide and must take oral drugs with food or meals, take them with a snack or meal at a time when exenatide is not being injected.
- Exenatide may reduce the effectiveness of digoxin and lovastatin. Your doctor may decide a dose increase of these medications is necessary.

- Exenatide may reduce the effectiveness of hormone ingredients in some contraceptive drugs. Take them at least 1 hour before you take an exenatide injection.
- Exenatide may increase the amount of warfarin in the body and increase the risk of bleeding.

Food Interactions

Do not eat too fast while taking an incretin mimetic, and stop eating when you feel full. If you overeat while taking exenatide, you may feel nauseous or throw up. Liraglutide may be injected at any time of the day, without regard to food or meals.

Usual Dose

Exenatide

Adult: 5 or 10 mcg twice a day by subcutaneous injection up to 1 hour before breakfast and dinner. Exenatide comes in a pre-filled pen injection device. Exenatide suspension—2 mg by subcutaneous injection once a week.

Child: not recommended.

Liraglutide

Adult: 0.6–1.8 mg once a day by subcutaneous injection. Liraglutide comes in a pre-filled pen.

Child: not recommended.

Overdosage

Symptoms of an incretin mimetic overdose are severe nausea, severe vomiting, and severe rapid drops in blood-sugar levels. An oral sugar source may help, but overdose victims should be taken to a hospital emergency room for evaluation and treatment. If you seek treatment, ALWAYS bring the medication pen with you.

Special Information

Each dose of incretin mimetic must be given as a subcutaneous injection under the skin of the thigh, abdomen, or upper arm. Do not inject into a muscle or vein.

If you forget a dose, skip the dose you forgot and continue with your regular schedule. Do not take a double dose.

These injections are clear and colorless. Do not use if they are cloudy or have any color or particles floating in them. For more information on how to properly administer these drugs, see page 1242.

Keep these drugs in the refrigerator, and do not use them after the expiration date has passed. DO NOT freeze the medication, but do protect it from heat and sunlight.

Keep the cap on your pen when not using it. Do not store your pen with the needle attached to it.

This drug may lead to a loss of appetite and loss of body weight. Do not change your regular dosage if this happens to you.

Special Populations

Pregnancy/Breast-feeding: In animal studies of these medicines, the growth of the fetus was affected. They should be taken during pregnancy only if your doctor determines that the potential benefit outweighs the risks. Diabetes during pregnancy is usually treated with insulin.

Small amounts of exenatide may pass into breast milk and may affect a nursing infant. It is not known if liraglutide passes into breast milk. Nursing mothers who must take these drugs should use infant formula.

Seniors: Seniors may take these drugs without special restriction, though seniors may be more sensitive to their effects.

Generic Name

Indomethacin (IN-doe-METH-uh-sin) G

Brand Names

Indocin

Type of Drug

Nonsteroidal anti-inflammatory drug (NSAID).

Prescribed For

Rheumatoid arthritis; osteoarthritis; ankylosing spondylitis; menstrual pain; tendinitis; bursitis; painful shoulder; gout—except extended-release form; sunburn; and migraine and cluster headache—except extended-release form. Indomethacin has been used to prevent premature labor, to treat a rare condition in premature infants called patent ductus arteriosus, and (in eye-drop form) to treat a severe and unusual inflammation in the retina.

General Information

Indomethacin and other NSAIDs are used to relieve pain and inflammation. We do not know exactly how NSAIDs work, but they may achieve their effects by blocking the body's production of a hormone called prostaglandin and the action of other body chemicals. Pain relief comes about 30 minutes after taking the first dose of indomethacin and lasts for 4–6 hours, but its anti-inflammatory effect takes a week to become apparent and may take 2 weeks to reach maximum effect. Indomethacin is broken down in the liver and eliminated through the kidneys. Indomethacin is available in capsule, oral suspension, and rectal suppository forms. Because of its adverse effects, indomethacin should only be used at the lowest possible dosage and when other NSAID therapy has not been effective.

Cautions and Warnings

Do not take indomethacin if you are **allergic** or **sensitive** to any of its ingredients or to any other NSAID. Those with a history of **asthma** attacks brought on by an NSAID, iodides, or aspirin should not take indomethacin.

Indomethacin may cause gastrointestinal (GI) bleeding, ulcers, and stomach perforation, which can occur at any time, with or without warning, in people who take indomethacin regularly. People with a history of **active GI bleeding** should be cautious about taking any NSAID. People who develop bleeding or ulcers and continue NSAID treatment may develop more serious side effects. Indomethacin should not be used by people who have had **ulcers or other stomach lesions**.

Indomethacin may affect platelets and blood clotting at high doses and should be avoided by people with **clotting problems** and **those taking warfarin**.

NSAIDs may cause an increased risk of serious cardiovascular reactions such as heart attack or stroke that are sometimes fatal. People with **cardiovascular disease** have an increased risk of adverse heart effects. People with **heart failure** who use indomethacin may experience swelling in their arms, legs, or feet.

Indomethacin may worsen **depression or other psychiatric disorders**, **epilepsy**, and **parkinsonism**.

Indomethacin should never be used as "first therapy" for any disorder, with the possible exception of ankylosing spondylitis, because of the severe side effects associated with this drug.

Indomethacin may cause severe toxic effects to the kidney. Report any unusual side effects to your doctor, who might need to periodically test your kidney function. People with advanced **kidney disease** should avoid taking indomethacin.

Indomethacin may make you unusually sensitive to the effects of the sun.

Possible Side Effects

- ▼ Most common: headache, dizziness, diarrhea, nausea, vomiting, constipation, stomach gas, stomach upset or irritation, and appetite loss, especially during the first few days of treatment.
- ▼ Less common: stomach ulcers, GI bleeding, hepatitis, gallbladder attacks, painful urination, poor kidney function, kidney inflammation, blood and protein in the urine, dizziness, fainting, nervousness, depression, hallucinations, confusion, disorientation, tingling in the hands or feet, lightheadedness, itching, increased sweating, dry nose and mouth, heart palpitations, chest pain, breathing difficulties, and muscle cramps.
- ▼ Rare: severe allergic reactions—including closing of the throat, fever, and chills—changes in liver function, jaundice (yellowing of the skin or whites of the eyes), and kidney failure. People who experience such effects must be promptly treated in a hospital emergency room or doctor's office. NSAIDs have caused severe skin reactions; if this happens to you, see your doctor immediately. Contact your doctor if you experience anything unusual while taking any medication.

Drug Interactions

- Indomethacin may increase the effects of oral anticoagulant (blood thinning) drugs such as warfarin. Your anticoagulant dose may need to be reduced.
- Combining diflunisal and indomethacin has resulted in fatal GI hemorrhage.
- Indomethacin may reduce the blood-pressure-lowering effect of angiotensin-converting enzyme (ACE) inhibitor drugs, beta blockers, and loop, potassium-sparing, or thiazide diuretics.
- Taking indomethacin with cyclosporine may increase the kidney-related side effects of both drugs. Methotrexate side effects may be increased in people also taking indomethacin.
- Indomethacin may increase digoxin levels in the blood.
- Indomethacin may increase the body's absorption of penicillamine.
- Combining indomethacin with phenylpropanolamine—found in many over-the-counter drug products—may cause an increase in blood pressure.

- Combining indomethacin and dipyridamole may increase water retention.
- Indomethacin may increase phenytoin's side effects.
- Lithium blood levels may be increased by indomethacin.
- Combining indomethacin with selective serotonin reuptake inhibitors (SSRIs) may increase the risk of GI bleeding.
- Indomethacin blood levels may be affected by cimetidine.
- Cholestyramine may decrease the effectiveness of indomethacin.
- Probenecid may increase the risk of indomethacin side effects.
- Aspirin and other salicylates should never be combined with indomethacin to treat arthritis.
- Do not take indomethacin and triamterene concurrently, as this combination may cause acute kidney failure.

Food Interactions

Take indomethacin with a glass of water, food, or a magnesium/aluminum antacid to avoid an upset stomach.

Usual Dose

Adult and Child (age 15 and over): 50–200 mg a day, individualized to your needs.

Child (under age 15): not recommended.

Overdosage

People have died from NSAID overdoses. Common signs of overdose are drowsiness, nausea, vomiting, diarrhea, abdominal pain, rapid breathing, rapid heartbeat, increased sweating, ringing or buzzing in the ears, confusion, disorientation, stupor, and coma. Take the victim to a hospital emergency room at once. If you seek treatment, ALWAYS bring the prescription bottle or container.

Special Information

Take each dose with a full glass of water and do not lie down for 15–30 minutes afterward.

Indomethacin can make you drowsy or tired: Be careful when driving or operating hazardous equipment. Do not take any over-the-counter products containing acetaminophen or aspirin while taking indomethacin. Avoid alcohol.

Contact your doctor if you develop rash or itching, visual disturbances, weight gain, breathing difficulties, fluid retention, hallucinations, black or tarry stools, persistent headache, or any unusual or intolerable side effect.

If you forget a dose of indomethacin, take it as soon as you remember. If you take indomethacin once a day and it is within 8 hours of your next dose, or if you take several doses a day and it is within 4 hours of your next dose, skip the dose you forgot and continue with your regular schedule. Never take a double dose.

Special Populations

Pregnancy/Breast-feeding: Indomethacin may affect the developing fetal heart if used during the second ½ of pregnancy. Pregnant women should not take indomethacin without their doctor's approval. Indomethacin should be taken during pregnancy only if your doctor determines that the potential benefit outweighs the risks.

Indomethacin may pass into breast milk. There is a possibility that the heart of a nursing baby could be affected by indomethacin. Nursing mothers who must take indomethacin should use infant formula.

Seniors: Seniors may be more susceptible to side effects, especially ulcer disease.

Generic Name

Insulin (IN-suh-lin)

Most Common Brand Names

Generic Ingredients: Regular Insulin
Humulin R
Oral-lyn Oral Spray

Generic Ingredients: Insulin Aspart
Novolog
Novolog Mix 70/30

Generic Ingredients: Insulin Detemir
Levemir

Generic Ingredients: Insulin Glargine
Lantus

Generic Ingredients: Insulin Glulisine
Apidra

Generic Ingredients: Insulin Lispro
Humalog
Humalog Mix 50/50
Humalog Mix 75/25

Generic Ingredients: NPH Insulin
Humulin N

Generic Ingredients: NPH Insulin + Insulin
Humulin 70/30

Type of Drug

Antidiabetic.

Prescribed For

Type 1 and type 2 diabetes mellitus; also prescribed for gestational diabetes and hyperkalemia (high blood-potassium levels) and for severe complications of diabetes such as ketoacidosis or diabetic coma. Insulin may be prescribed in combination with oral antidiabetes drugs for people with type 2 diabetes who do not respond to pills alone.

General Information

Insulin, a hormone made in the pancreas, helps the body turn sugar into energy. Insulin works by helping sugar enter body cells. Also, insulin helps us store energy that we can use later. Between meals, insulin helps us use the fat, sugar, and protein we have stored. In type 1 diabetes, the body does not make any insulin naturally. People with type 2 diabetes often eventually need insulin as the insulin-producing cells in the pancreas die off as their disease gets worse. Without insulin, glucose cannot get into body cells and the cells will not work properly. Insulin dosage must be balanced against the amount and type of food eaten and the amount of exercise you do. Blood glucose can drop too low or rise too high if your insulin dose is not changed with diet and exercise patterns.

The most widely used variety is human insulin. It is identical to natural human insulin, but it is manufactured by semisynthetic or recombinant DNA methods. Older products were made with animal insulin but had some impurities. No animal-based products are currently available in the United States. Insulin is not available in pill form because it is destroyed by stomach acid.

Rapid-acting insulins: Regular insulin starts to work in 30–60 minutes and lasts only 8–12 hours. Insulin aspart, glulisine, and lispro are all very short-acting insulins designed to control mealtime blood sugar spikes in both type 1 and type 2 diabetes. They begin working in 15 minutes and last for 2–5 hours. Oral insulin spray is absorbed into the blood directly from the mouth and starts working within minutes. The spray is currently available only for people with type 1 or 2 diabetes who are unable to receive insulin in any other way and who cannot qualify for the company's Phase III study.

Intermediate-acting insulins: NPH insulin starts working in 60–90 minutes and lasts for 12–16 hours.

Long-acting insulins: Insulin glargine starts working in about an hour and lasts for at least 24 hours. Insulin detemir lasts between 6 and 24 hours, depending on the dose. Larger doses last for longer periods of time. Other factors that influence insulin response include diet, exercise, and the use of other drugs.

Cautions and Warnings

Low blood sugar (see "Overdosage" for symptoms) can result from taking too much insulin, doing excess physical work or exercise without eating, not absorbing food normally because meals are postponed or skipped, or because of illness with vomiting, fever, or diarrhea. You may be able to correct the imbalance by eating sugar, food with sugar, or a commercial 40% glucose product. For severe low blood sugar, you may require a glucagon injection.

Hypersensitivity reactions to injected insulin can develop at the site of injection, such as redness, swelling, and itching, and may indicate a need to change the type of insulin you use. Reactions such as difficulty catching your breath, feeling your throat closing, fast pulse, sweating, low blood pressure with or without fainting, and skin eruptions may be life-threatening.

Thyroid disease can affect the clearance of insulin from the body.

You may need less insulin if you have **liver or kidney disease**.

All insulin products cause potassium to move from the blood into body cells, possibly leading to low blood-potassium levels. Left untreated, this can lead to an inability to breathe, abnormal heart rhythms, and death. Your doctor will monitor your blood-potassium levels. This is especially important if you use a potassium-lowering medication or take a medication such as digoxin that is sensitive to serum potassium concentrations.

Several insulin overdose deaths have been caused by **incorrect glucose meter readings**, which showed a normal result when blood sugar was actually very low. The **nonglucose sugars maltose, galactose, and xylose** can falsely increase blood sugar readings with glucose meters that use technology known as *GDH-PQQ* (glucose dehydrogenase pyrroloquinoline quinone). This technology is employed in ACCU-CHEK, TRUEtest, TRUEresult, and TRUE2go test strips and meters. Your meter or strips should be labeled with either the brand or the letters *GDH-PQQ*. If not, consult your pharmacist or meter provider. These sugars can be found in some drug products and are also used in no-sugar or no-sugar-added food products. If your meter reading is normal but you feel like you have low blood sugar, pay attention to your body and contact your doctor for instructions before taking insulin. If you experience this reaction, change to another meter that does not use *GDH-PQQ* technology.

Possible Side Effects

- ▼ Most common: low blood sugar (see "Overdosage" for symptoms), weight gain, and low blood potassium.
- ▼ Less common: redness, swelling, itching, or rash at the site of injection; changes in the distribution of body fat; allergic reactions; salt and water retention; and swelling in the hands and feet.
- ▼ Rare: worsening of eyesight due to breakdown of the retina of the eye.

Drug Interactions

- Drugs that reduce the effect of insulin include acetazolamide, albuterol, HIV antivirals, asparaginase, atypical antipsychotics, calcitonin, contraceptive drugs, corticosteroids, cyclophosphamide, danazol, dextrothyroxine, diazoxide, diltiazem, diuretics, dobutamine, epinephrine, estrogens, ethacrynic acid, glucagon, isoniazid, morphine, niacin, nicotine, phenothiazines, phenytoin, protease inhibitors, somatropin, terbutaline, and thyroid hormones. Dosage increases may be required.
- Substances that increase the effects of insulin include other antidiabetes drugs, ACE inhibitors, anabolic steroids, calcium, chloroquine, disopyramide, fenugreek, fibrates, fluoxetine, guanethidine, mebendazole, monoamine oxidase inhibitor (MAOI) antidepressants, pentamidine, pentoxifylline, phenylbutazone, pyridoxine, salicylates (including aspirin), somatostatin analogues, sulfa drugs, sulfinpyrazone, and tetracycline. Dosage reductions may be required.
- The following drugs may either increase or decrease the effects of insulin: alcohol, beta-blocker drugs, clonidine, and

lithium. Use caution when taking these medications with insulin, and avoid alcohol altogether.

- Nonselective beta blockers, clonidine, guanathidine, and reserpine may mask the symptoms of low blood sugar and thus increase the risk of this side effect. Cardioselective beta blockers are preferred. Check your blood sugar regularly while you take these medications with insulin.
- Quitting smoking—regardless of whether you are using a nicotine patch or gum, or another smoking deterrent—can also lower blood sugar. A lower insulin dosage may be necessary once you stop smoking.
- Insulin reduces blood-potassium levels, which can affect digitalis drugs.

Food Interactions

Follow your doctor's instructions on diet.

Usual Dose

Dosage must be individualized. Regular insulin is generally injected 30 minutes before meals. Puffs of insulin spray are applied to the inside lining of the mouth 10 minutes before each meal. Aspart, glulisine, and lispro are injected 15 minutes before meals or within 20 minutes after you start eating. NPH insulin may be taken 30 minutes before breakfast and/or at night, according to your doctor's instructions. Glargine is usually taken once a day at bedtime; detemir may be given once or twice a day. Premixed insulins are given twice a day, before the morning and evening meals.

Overdosage

Accidentally swallowing insulin has little or no effect. Injecting too much insulin causes an insulin reaction or low blood sugar. Symptoms occur suddenly and include weakness, fatigue, nervousness, confusion, headache, double vision, convulsions, dizziness, psychosis, unconsciousness, rapid and shallow breathing, numbness or tingling around the mouth, hunger, nausea, loss of skin color, dry skin, and pulse changes. Overdose victims should immediately eat high-sugar, low-fat foods such as fruit juice or a glucose product for diabetics to raise blood-sugar levels. (Such foods should be carried with you at all times.) If victims are unable to eat or drink (due to a seizure, unconsciousness, or other debilitating condition), they should be given an injection of glucagon immediately, and taken to a hospital emergency room. If the signs of low blood sugar do not clear up within 30 minutes, contact your doctor. You may need further treatment.

Special Information

Use the same brand and strength of insulin and insulin syringes or administration devices to avoid dosage errors. Rotate injection sites every 1–2 weeks. For information on how to properly administer injectable insulin, see page 1242.

Diabetic ketoacidosis occurs when your body has no insulin to help utilize sugar for energy and the body switches to breaking down fat for fuel instead. Blood sugar increases, and you urinate frequently and become dehydrated. This can happen over hours or days and leads to excessive potassium loss and dangerous abnormal heart rhythms. Report any of the following symptoms of diabetic ketoacidosis to your doctor: very high blood sugar; being very thirsty; urinating frequently; a sense of generalized weakness; fever; vomiting; appetite loss; confusion; abdominal pain; being short of breath; looking sickly; dry skin; dry mouth; rapid heartbeat; rapid breathing; an odd, fruity odor that smells like nail-polish remover on your breath; and low blood pressure. If your doctor is not available, go to a hospital emergency room for treatment.

Mix insulins only according to your doctor's directions; do not change the method or order of mixing. Insulin glargine and insulin detemir should not be mixed with anything else, including another insulin product. Your pharmacist may also mix your insulins to ensure accuracy.

Take the exact dose of insulin prescribed. Too much insulin will excessively lower blood sugar, and too little will not control diabetes. Follow the diet prescribed by your doctor and avoid alcohol.

Your insulin requirements may change if you get sick, especially if you vomit or have a fever.

If your insulin is in suspension form, you must gently rotate the vial and turn it over several times to evenly distribute the particles throughout the liquid before withdrawing the dose. Do not shake the vial.

People with diabetes must maintain good dental hygiene because of their increased risk of developing oral infections. Be sure your dentist knows you have diabetes. Visit your doctor every 3–6 months and have your eyes checked annually.

Read and follow all patient information provided with insulin products. Monitor your blood and urine regularly for sugar and ketones.

Insulin products are generally stable at room temperature for about 2 years. They must be kept away from direct sunlight and extreme temperatures. Most manufacturers recommend that insulin be stored in a refrigerator or another cool place, although it should not be put in a freezer. Partly used vials of insulin should be thrown away after several weeks if not used. Do not use any insulin that looks different from the way it did when you purchased it.

If you forget a dose, take it as soon as you remember. If it is almost time for your next dose, or if you completely forget 1 or more doses, contact your doctor for exact instructions.

Special Populations

Pregnancy/Breast-feeding: Pregnant women must follow their doctor's directions for insulin use exactly, because insulin requirements normally decrease during the first ½ of pregnancy and then increase during the second ½.

Insulin does not pass into breast milk. Breast-feeding can reduce your insulin needs, so your doctor should closely monitor your insulin dosage during this period.

Seniors: Seniors may use insulin without special restriction. However, seniors may be less likely than younger people to recognize the symptoms of low blood sugar. Use your meter regularly to monitor your blood sugar.

Generic Name

Interferon Alpha (in-ter-FEER-on AL-fuh)

Brand Names

Alferon N
Infergen
Intron A
Pegasys
PegIntron

Type of Drug

Antiviral.

Prescribed For

Chronic hepatitis B and C, hairy cell leukemia, malignant melanoma, and AIDS-related Kaposi's sarcoma; also used to treat laryngeal papillomatosis (growths in the respiratory tract) in children, genital warts, bladder cancer, carcinoid tumors, chronic myelocytic leukemia, kidney cancer, non-Hodgkin's lymphoma, multiple myeloma, mycosis fungoides, ovarian cancer, polycythemia vera (a cancer of the blood), skin cancer, and thrombocytosis (high blood-platelet count).

General Information

Interferon alpha attaches to the surface of an infected cell and stimulates a complicated set of reactions. These reactions lead to the production of enzymes inside the cell that prevent the hepatitis C virus (HCV), for example, from reproducing. Other causes of hepatitis do not respond to interferon treatment. Hepatitis C infection can be especially serious in people with HIV. Interferon alpha or a long-acting (pegylated) interferon called Pegasys, taken either alone or in combination with the antiviral ribavirin, can be given to people coinfected with chronic HCV and HIV who are at greatest risk for progression to serious disease. Treatment does not always work, but HIV-infected patients may benefit from treatment with this combination.

Cautions and Warnings

Do not take interferon alpha if you are **allergic** or **sensitive** to any of its ingredients. Serious and life-threatening allergic or drug-sensitivity reactions can develop, including an itchy rash, swelling, and breathing difficulties.

Alpha interferons may cause life-threatening bacterial, viral, or fungal infections, and may require anti-infective treatment. They have also been associated with the development or exacerbation of autoimmune diseases.

People taking this drug must be closely monitored by their doctors and receive periodic blood tests and liver and thyroid function tests.

People with **kidney or heart disease** should use this drug with caution. If heart disease worsens during treatment, the drug should be discontinued.

Bleeding and stroke have occurred in people using this drug.

Interferon alpha may worsen **liver disease**.

Interferon alpha can affect the nervous system in many ways, including causing seizures, coma, dizziness, memory loss, agitation, psychosis, and complete loss of sensation. These effects generally go away when the drug is stopped.

Interferon alpha may cause menstrual problems or interfere with ovulation.

Depression and suicidal behavior has been reported in association with interferon alpha treatment. People who develop severe side effects or become depressed while taking this drug should have their dosage temporarily lowered. The drug should be stopped if depression is severe. Patients with an existing **psychiatric condition**, or a history of depression or other psychiatric disorders, should not be treated with interferon alpha.

It is not known if this drug is safe for **children**.

Possible Side Effects

- ▼ Most common: anxiety, sleep disturbances, depression, hair loss, nausea, diarrhea, abdominal pain, muscle or joint pain, weakness, headache, fever, chills, injection-site reactions, back pain, and generalized pain.
- ▼ Common: dizziness, confusion, abnormal thought patterns, memory loss, tingling in the hands or feet, rash, dry skin, sweating, vomiting, appetite loss, weight loss, cough, bronchitis, breathing difficulties, pneumonia, pleurisy, lung problems, runny nose, and sore throat.
- ▼ Less common: poor vision, abnormal heart rhythms, high blood pressure, chest pain, high blood sugar, thyroid problems, urinary infection, low sex drive, accidental injury, liver problems, migraine, increased sensitivity to the sun, psoriasis, attempted suicide, seizures, and a ruptured spleen.
- ▼ Rare: blood in the urine, eye problems, rheumatoid arthritis, lupus and other autoimmune conditions, painful spasms of blood vessels in the legs, and worsening of diabetes and thyroid problems. Contact your doctor if you experience anything unusual while taking any medication.

Drug Interactions

- Interferon alpha may interfere with the breakdown of vinblastine, zidovudine (also known as AZT), and theophylline.

Usual Dose

All dosages are for adults (age 18 and over). Administration in children is not recommended.

Alferon N: 0.05 mL (250,000 IU) per wart twice weekly for up to 8 weeks. The maximum recommended dose per treatment session is 0.5 mL (2.5 million IU).

Infergen: 9 mcg in a single subcutaneous injection 3 times a week for 24 weeks. Allow at least 2 days between doses.

Intron A: 2–5 million units by subcutaneous or intramuscular injection 3 times a week for 6–18 months. Larger doses (10–20 million units) are given by intravenous infusion.

Pegasys: 180 mcg once a week for 48 weeks. Dosage reduction to 135 mcg may be necessary, depending on reaction.

PegIntron: 1–1.5 mcg for every 2.2 lbs. of body weight by subcutaneous injection once a week for 1 year.

Overdosage

Symptoms may include increased side effects and changes in lab test results. Seizures have occurred at high dosages. Repeated overdose may cause lethargy or coma. Contact your local poison control center or a hospital emergency room for more information. If you seek treatment, ALWAYS bring the prescription bottle or container.

Special Information

This drug does not prevent you from giving hepatitis C to others through unprotected sex or contact with blood or other body fluids.

People who have a seizure disorder or other nervous system problem, low white-blood-cell or blood-platelet count, or asthma or other breathing problems, or who take drugs that depress bone marrow function may be especially sensitive to the effects of interferon alpha.

This medication is given by injection under the skin. For information on how to properly administer this drug, see page 1242.

Ibuprofen, aspirin, and other anti-inflammatory drugs may alleviate some of the discomfort associated with starting interferon alpha.

Your doctor may instruct you to drink extra fluids while taking interferon alpha. This will help prevent low blood pressure due to excess loss of water.

This drug must be stored in the refrigerator and protected from light. Do not shake or freeze it.

Special Populations

Pregnancy/Breast-feeding: Animal studies suggest that interferon alpha may harm the fetus and cause spontaneous abortion. Interferon alpha should be taken during pregnancy only if your doctor determines that the potential benefit outweighs the risks.

It is not known if this drug passes into breast milk. Nursing mothers who must take it should use infant formula.

Seniors: Seniors with liver, kidney, or heart conditions should use this drug with caution.

Generic Name

Interferon Beta (in-ter-FEER-on BAY-tuh)

Brand Names

Avonex (interferon beta-1a)
Betaseron (interferon beta-1b)
Extavia (interferon beta-1b)
Rebif (interferon beta-1a)

Type of Drug

Multiple sclerosis (MS) therapy; biological response modifier.

Prescribed For

MS; also used for HIV infection, AIDS-related Kaposi's sarcoma, metastatic renal-cell carcinoma, herpes of the lips or genitals, malignant melanoma, cutaneous T-cell lymphoma, and acute non-A/non-B hepatitis.

General Information

The interferons are a family of natural proteins produced in response to viral infection and other biological inducers. Three major classes of interferons have been identified: alpha, beta, and gamma; they each have overlapping, yet distinct, biological activities. Interferon beta has antiviral effects, slows cell growth, and helps regulate the immune system. The way it works in MS is not clearly understood. However, it is known that interferon beta interacts with specific receptors on the surface of human cells. Binding causes the production of a number of gene products believed to mediate the biological actions of interferon beta. People receiving this drug may be vaccinated, but the effectiveness of the vaccination is unpredictable.

Cautions and Warnings

Do not take interferon beta if you are **allergic** or **sensitive** to any of its ingredients or to human albumin. Rare severe allergic reactions have been reported.

The safety and benefit of interferon beta in **chronic progressive MS** is unproven.

Some people taking interferon beta in studies had severe depression and suicidal tendencies. People with **depression**, **suicidal ideation**, or severe **psychiatric symptoms** should use any interferon product with caution and report any changes in their emotions or behavior to a doctor.

People with **seizure disorders** may be more likely to develop a seizure while taking interferon beta.

Up to 75% of people who take interferon beta are likely to develop flu-like symptoms, including fever, chills, muscle aches, sweating, and feeling unwell. These symptoms may prove stressful to people with **heart disease**.

In rare cases, severe liver disease has occurred while taking interferon beta. People with **liver or thyroid disease** should not use this drug.

Interferon beta can cause reductions in white-blood-cell and platelet counts.

People with a history of **latex allergy** should use caution, as some of this drug's packaging may contain latex.

Interferon beta may cause increased sensitivity to the sun. Wear protective clothing and use sunscreen.

Possible Side Effects

In general, interferon beta-1a has fewer side effects than interferon beta-1b.

Interferon Beta-1a

- ▼ Most common: respiratory infection, sinusitis, headache, fever, weakness, chills, dizziness, muscle aches, abdominal pain, flu-like symptoms, depression, painful menstruation, diarrhea, nausea, upset stomach, and sleeping difficulties. Pain, burning, or stinging at the injection site may also occur.
- ▼ Less common: swelling, pelvic pain, cyst, thyroid goiter, heart palpitations, bleeding, laryngitis, breathing difficulties,

Possible Side Effects *(continued)*

joint pain, stiffness, tiredness, speech problems, convulsions, uncontrolled movements, hair loss, urinary urgency, and cystitis (bladder infection).

- ▼ Rare: Rare side effects can occur in almost any part of the body. Contact your doctor if you experience anything unusual while taking any medication.

Interferon Beta-1b

- ▼ Most common: pain, burning, or stinging at the injection site; sinusitis; headache; migraine; fever; weakness; chills; muscle ache; abdominal pain; flu-like symptoms; depression; menstrual disorders; painful menstruation; constipation; diarrhea; vomiting; liver inflammation; sweating; and reduced white-blood-cell count.
- ▼ Less common: itching, swelling, pelvic pain, cyst, thyroid goiter, heart palpitations, high blood pressure, rapid heartbeat, bleeding, laryngitis, breathing difficulties, muscle weakness, stiffness, tiredness, speech problems, convulsions, uncontrolled movements, visual disturbances or conjunctivitis (pinkeye), urinary urgency, cystitis (bladder infection), breast pain, cystic breast disease, breast cancer, and weight changes.
- ▼ Rare: Rare side effects can occur in almost any part of the body. Contact your doctor if you experience anything unusual while taking any medication.

Drug Interactions

None known.

Usual Dose

Adult

Avonex: 30 mcg into a large muscle once a week.

Betaseron: usual dose—0.25 mg injected under the skin every other day. Patients are started at ¼ of the usual dose and increased gradually over 7 weeks to the regular dose. Betaseron comes with a special solution with which to mix the product before injection.

Extavia: starting dose—0.0625 mg (¼ mL) injected under the skin every other day. The dose is increased gradually over 6 weeks to 0.25 mg (1 mL) injected under the skin every other day.

Rebif: usual dose—44 mcg injected 3 times a week, 2 days apart, usually late in the day. Patients are started on injections of 8.8 mcg 3 times a week. Dosage is increased over 4 weeks to the usual dose.

Child: not recommended.

Overdosage

Little is known about the effects of interferon beta overdose. Symptoms may include exaggerated side effects. Contact your local poison control center or a hospital emergency room for more information. If you seek treatment, ALWAYS bring the prescription bottle or container.

Special Information

Interferon beta-1a and interferon beta-1b may be associated with severe depression. Mood swings or changes, lack of interest in daily activities, excessive sleep, and other possible signs of depression should be reported to your doctor at once.

This medication is given by injection. For information on how to administer this drug, see page 1242.

If you forget to administer a dose, do so as soon as you remember. If it is almost time for your next dose, skip the one you forgot and continue with your regular schedule. Do not take a double dose.

Special Populations

Pregnancy/Breast-feeding: Animal studies show that interferon beta may cause abortion. Women who are or might be pregnant should not use this drug.

It is not known if interferon beta passes into breast milk. Nursing mothers who must take it should use infant formula.

Seniors: Seniors may use this drug without special restriction.

Generic Name

Ipilimumab (ih-pill-IM-u-mab)

Brand Names

Yervoy

Type of Drug

Monoclonal antibody.

Prescribed For

Malignant melanoma.

General Information

Ipilimumab is prescribed for severe skin cancer that has spread to other parts of the body or which cannot be surgically removed. It is a human monoclonal antibody that helps build immune system cells so they can fight the melanoma.

Cautions and Warnings

Do not use ipilimumab if you are **allergic** or **sensitive** to any of its ingredients.

Treatment with this biological product can result in severe, possibly fatal, immune reactions. Mild to moderate reactions may be treated with a corticosteroid medicine and you may restart the medicine once the reaction subsides, but you should stop ipilimumab treatments after suffering a severe reaction. Severe reactions usually occur any time from 3–17 weeks after your dose and can take 4 months to resolve. During clinical studies, a few people died after experiencing a severe ipilimumab reaction.

Ipilimumab reactions can cause damage to the liver, skin, nervous system, and thyroid and other glands. The most common signs of a severe ipilimumab reaction are fever; abdominal swelling; nausea and vomiting; rectal or intestinal bleeding; more frequent bowel movements or inability to control them; sluggishness; mouth sores; skin rashes; blisters and other reactions, including peeling of large sections of skin; pain; numbness; tingling; blurry vision, double vision, or other vision problems; eye pain or redness; and unexplained weakness. Yellowing of the skin or whites of the eyes, tea-colored urine, bleeding or bruising easily and pain on the right side of your stomach are signs of liver inflammation (hepatitis). Signs of glandular inflammation include persistent or unusual headaches, sluggishness, weight gain, feeling cold all the time, dizziness, and fainting. Severe reactions can also affect any other part of the body. Contact your doctor if you experience anything unusual.

A small number of people receiving ipilimumab will develop antibodies against the drug that make it less effective.

Possible Side Effects

- ▼ Common: diarrhea, itching, fatigue, and rash.
- ▼ Less common: colitis, reduced thyroid activity, and reduced pituitary gland activity.

Possible Side Effects *(continued)*

▼ Rare: hives, ulcer, irritated esophagus, sudden and severe breathing difficulties, kidney inflammation and failure, infusion site reactions, liver toxicity, skin reactions, blood toxicity, and irritation of tissues surrounding the heart. Contact your doctor if you experience anything unusual while taking any medication.

Drug Interactions

None known.

Usual Dose

Adult: 1.3 mg per lb. of body weight by intravenous infusion over 90 minutes every 3 weeks for 4 doses.

Child: not recommended.

Overdosage

There is no information on ipilimumab overdose, although it would be unlikely since it is given only by a health care provider. Call your doctor if you experience anything unusual.

Special Information

If you experience a moderate or severe drug reaction, your doctor may hold the next dose until reaction symptoms subside. If you do not fully recover from the reaction or are unable to receive a full course of treatment by 16 weeks after your first dose, your doctor will stop ipilimumab treatments. Treatment will also be stopped if your liver enzyme levels are very high.

Make sure your doctor knows if you have had an organ transplant; any autoimmune condition, including ulcerative colitis, Crohn's disease, lupus, or sarcoidosis; or liver disease or damage.

Special Populations

Pregnancy/Breast-feeding: Animal studies have shown ipilimumab can damage the developing fetus. Ipilimumab should be taken during pregnancy only if your doctor determines that the potential benefit outweighs the risks.

Ipilimumab may pass into breast milk. Nursing mothers who must take this drug should use infant formula.

Seniors: More than 25% of people studied with ipilimumab were 65 years or older and responded in the same way as younger adults.

Generic Name

Ipratropium (ipe-ruh-TROE-pee-um) G

Brand Names

Atrovent
Atrovent HFA

Combination Products
Generic Ingredients: Ipratropium Bromide + Albuterol Sulfate G
Combivent
DuoNeb
Combivent Respimat

The information in this profile also applies to the following drugs:

Generic Ingredients: Tiotropium Bromide
Spiriva

Type of Drug

Anticholinergic.

Prescribed For

Bronchospasm associated with bronchitis, emphysema, and other chronic lung diseases; also prescribed for runny nose.

General Information

Ipratropium is related to atropine, another anticholinergic drug. Ipratropium works against natural acetylcholine in the bronchial muscles, causing them to dilate. It has little effect on other parts of the body. Much of each inhaled dose is swallowed and passes out of the body in the stool. Like all anticholinergic drugs, ipratropium has a drying effect; the nasal spray provides relief from runny nose.

Cautions and Warnings

Do not use ipratropium if you are **allergic** or **sensitive** to any of its ingredients or to atropine, soy lecithin, or any related product.

Ipratropium should be used with caution if you have **glaucoma**, **prostate disease**, or **bladder obstruction**.

Ipratropium is not meant for the treatment of acute bronchospasm. This drug should be used only to prevent bronchospasm associated with chronic lung diseases.

Patients may experience a temporary blurring of vision or worsening of **narrow-angle glaucoma** if the solution comes into direct contact with the eyes.

Possible Side Effects

Generally, ipratropium side effects are infrequent and mild.

Inhalation

- ▼ Most common: bronchitis, upper-respiratory infection, nervousness, dizziness, headache, nausea, upset stomach, blurred vision, sensitivity to bright light, dry mouth, throat irritation, cough, worsening of symptoms, rash, and mouth irritation.
- ▼ Less common: rapid heartbeat, heart palpitations, urinary difficulties, tingling in the hands or feet, poor coordination, itching, hives, flushing, loss of hair, constipation, tremors, fatigue or sleeplessness, and hoarseness.
- ▼ Rare: worsening of glaucoma, eye pain, low blood pressure, and severe skin reactions. Contact your doctor if you experience anything unusual while taking any medication.

Nasal Spray

- ▼ Most common: headache, upper-respiratory infection, nosebleeds, and nasal dryness.
- ▼ Less common: dry mouth or throat and stuffy nose.
- ▼ Rare: changes in sense of taste, nasal burning, red and itchy eyes, coughing, dizziness, hoarseness, heart palpitations, rapid heartbeat, thirst, ringing or buzzing in the ears, blurred vision, and difficulty urinating. Contact your doctor if you experience anything unusual while taking any medication.

Drug Interactions

- Ipratropium should be administered with caution when taking other anticholinergic-containing medications.

Food Interactions

Do not inhale a dose of ipratropium if you have any food in your mouth.

Usual Dose

Ipratroprium

Inhalation

Adult: 2 inhalations 4 times a day to a maximum of 12; or one 500-mcg vial 3–4 times a day, 6–8 hours apart.

Child (age 12 and over): 1 vial 3–4 times a day, 6–8 hours apart.
Child (under age 12): not recommended.

Nasal Spray

Adult: 2 sprays of 0.03% solution per nostril up to 2–3 times a day, or 2 sprays of 0.06% solution 3–4 times a day.

Child (age 6 and over): 2 sprays of 0.03% solution per nostril up to 2–3 times a day.

Child (under age 6): not recommended.

Ipratropium + Albuterol

Adult: Combivent—2 inhalations 4 times a day to a maximum of 12 a day. Combivent Respimat—1 inhalation 4 times a day to a maximum of 6 a day. DuoNeb—one 3-mL vial 4 times a day to a maximum of 6 vials a day.

Tiotropium

Adult: 2 inhalations of the contents of 1 capsule once a day.

Overdosage

The risk of overdose is small because very little ipratropium is absorbed into the bloodstream. Ipratropium accidentally sprayed into the eye will cause blurred vision. If you seek treatment, ALWAYS bring the prescription bottle or container with you.

Special Information

Use this product according to your doctor's instructions. Do not stop taking ipratropium without your doctor's approval even if you feel well.

Contact your doctor if you develop rash or hives, sores on the mouth or lips, blurred vision, or other side effects that are bothersome or persistent.

Contact your doctor if you stop responding to your usual dose of ipratropium: This may be a sign that your condition has worsened.

Prolonged use of ipratropium may decrease or stop the flow of saliva produced in your mouth. This can expose you to an increased chance of cavities, gum disease, oral infections, and other problems. Dry mouth can be relieved with hard candies or regular fluids. Increased attention to dental hygiene is important.

If, in addition to ipratropium, you use a corticosteroid inhaler or cromolyn sodium for lung disease, use ipratropium about 5 minutes before using the other inhaler.

If you take ipratropium and albuterol, metaproterenol, or another beta-stimulating aerosol product for bronchial disease, use the beta stimulator about 5 minutes before ipratropium unless otherwise instructed by your doctor. Ipratropium solution for inhalation can be mixed with albuterol or metaproterenol for inhalation as long as the mixture is used within 1 hour. The combination product Combivent (a mixture of ipratropium and albuterol) is also available.

The first use of each ipratropium nasal pump requires 2 pumps to prime the spray. Regular use of the spray should prevent the need to prime the pump again. If you do not use the spray for 3 days, you will have to prime the spray again with 2 pumps.

If you forget to administer a dose of ipratropium, do so as soon as you remember. If it is almost time for your next dose, skip the one you forgot and continue with your regular schedule. Do not take a double dose.

Store this product at room temperature—59°–86°F—and avoid freezing. Unused vials of the solution for inhalation should be stored in their foil wrapper.

Special Populations

Pregnancy/Breast-feeding: Massive oral doses of ipratropium have caused birth defects in animals. Ipratropium should be taken during pregnancy only if your doctor determines that the potential benefit outweighs the risks.

It is not known if ipratropium passes into breast milk. Nursing mothers who must take this drug should use infant formula.

Seniors: Seniors may use ipratropium without special precaution.

Type of Drug

Iron Supplements

Brand Names

Generic Ingredients: Carbonyl Iron, 100% Iron

Feosol
Icar
Ircon
Iron Chews
Wee Care

Generic Ingredients: Ferrous Fumarate G*, 33% Iron*

Femiron
Feostat
Ferretts
Ferro-Sequels
Hemocyte
Nephro-Fer S
Vitron-C S

Generic Ingredients: Ferrous Gluconate G, *12% Iron*
Ferate
Fergon

Generic Ingredients: Ferrous Sulfate G, *20–30% Iron*
Feosol
Fer-In-Sol
Slow-FE

Generic Ingredients: Polysaccharide Iron Complex
EZFE
Ferrex
iFerex
Myferon
Nu-Iron
Poly-Iron

Prescribed For

Iron-deficiency anemia.

General Information

Iron supplements are used to treat anemias that result from iron deficiency. Iron is incorporated into red blood cells, which carry oxygen throughout the body. Iron is absorbed only in a small section of the gastrointestinal tract called the duodenum, the upper part of the small intestine. Sustained-release iron products should be used only to help minimize the stomach discomfort that iron supplements can cause, as some of the drug in these forms may bypass the duodenum and not be absorbed. Other products combining iron with vitamins or special extracts may also be used to treat iron-deficiency anemia. Iron supplements are available in many different forms and they all have different amounts of iron. When choosing an iron supplement, you must be sure to take one that gives you the amount of elemental iron you need.

Cautions and Warnings

Do not take an iron supplement if you are **allergic** or **sensitive** to any of its ingredients or if you have **hemochromatosis**, **hemosiderosis**, or a **hemolytic anemia**.

Accidental overdose of iron-containing products is a leading cause of fatal poisoning in children under the age of 6. Keep all iron supplements out of reach of children. See "Overdose" for more information.

Do not take iron supplements if you have a history of **stomach problems**, **peptic ulcer**, or **ulcerative colitis**. People with normal iron levels should not take any iron product on a regular basis.

Possible Side Effects

- ▼ Common: stomach upset or irritation, nausea, diarrhea, constipation, appetite loss, darkened stools, and leg cramps.
- ▼ Less common: heartburn, darkened urine, and staining of the teeth.

Drug Interactions

- Iron and tetracycline interfere with each other. Iron may also interfere with the absorption of cephalosporin-type antibiotics. Separate doses of these by at least 2 hours.
- Doses of iron and trientine or captopril should be separated by 2 hours.
- Iron interferes with the absorption of levodopa + carbidopa, methyldopa, mycophenolate mofetil, penicillamine, and quinolone antibacterials.
- Antacids, calcium salts, digestive enzymes, histamine$_2$ antagonists, proton-pump inhibitors, and acetohydroxamic acid interfere with iron absorption.
- Ascorbic acid (vitamin C) and chloramphenicol increase the amount of iron absorbed.
- Iron reduces the effectiveness of levothyroxine, a thyroid replacement hormone. Combining these 2 drugs may lead to symptoms of hypothyroidism (underactive thyroid gland).

Food Interactions

Iron supplements are best taken on an empty stomach, but they may be taken with food if they upset your stomach. Eggs and milk interfere with iron absorption. Coffee or tea consumed with a meal or within an hour of eating reduces the amount of iron absorbed into the blood. Do not take iron products together with calcium supplements and food. If you need both iron and calcium, take calcium carbonate (Tums) and use it between meals.

Usual Dose

Iron dosage is the same regardless of type. Read the product label to determine iron content.

Adult

Iron Replacement Therapy: 150–300 mg a day divided in 3 doses.

Prevention of Iron Deficiency: 60 mg a day can be given in 1 or 2 divided doses.

Pregnancy: 30 mg a day. Do not take with food or meals.

Child

Iron Replacement Therapy: 1.4–2.7 mg per lb. of body weight a day, given in 1–3 divided doses.

Prevention of Iron Deficiency: 0.45–0.9 mg per lb. of body weight a day, given in 1–3 divided doses.

For both indications, the maximum dosage is 15 mg a day.

Premature Infant

Iron Replacement Therapy: 0.9–1.8 mg per lb. of body weight a day, given in 1–2 divided doses.

Prevention of Iron Deficiency: 0.9 mg per lb. of body weight a day, given in 1–3 divided doses.

For both indications, the maximum dosage is 15 mg a day.

Overdosage

Iron overdosage can be fatal. Accidental overdose of iron-containing products is a leading cause of fatal poisoning in children under age 6. Always keep iron supplements out of the reach of children. Overdose symptoms usually appear after 30 minutes to several hours; they include tiredness, vomiting, diarrhea, upset stomach, weak and rapid pulse, and lowered blood pressure or, after massive doses, shock, black and tarry stools due to massive bleeding in the stomach or intestine, and pneumonia. In case of overdose, contact your local poison control center or a hospital emergency room. You may be told to induce vomiting with ipecac syrup—available at any pharmacy—and to give the victim eggs and milk before seeking treatment. Time is a critical factor in emergency care: Stomach pumping should not be performed after the first hour of iron ingestion due to the risk of stomach perforation. If you seek treatment, ALWAYS bring the prescription bottle or container.

Special Information

Iron often causes black discoloration of stools and is slightly constipating. However, stools that are black or tarry may also indicate bleeding in the stomach or intestine. If you experience this symptom, discuss it with your doctor at once.

Do not chew or crush sustained-release iron products. Liquid iron products may stain your teeth. Mix water or juice with them and sip the iron through a straw to prevent tooth contact.

Nausea may be minimized by slowly increasing to the recommended dosage.

If you forget a dose, take it as soon as you remember. If it is almost time for your next dose, skip the one you forgot and continue with your regular schedule. Do not take a double dose.

Special Populations

Pregnancy/Breast-feeding: This drug is safe for use during pregnancy and breast-feeding and is frequently prescribed for pregnant and nursing women. If you are pregnant, however, you should check with your doctor before taking any medication.

Seniors: Seniors may require larger dosages.

Generic Name

Isosorbide Dinitrate

(eye-soe-SORE-bide dih-NYE-trate) G

Brand Names

Dilatrate-SR	Isordil
Isochron	Isordil Tembids
IsoDitrate ER	Isordil Titradose

The information in this profile also applies to the following drugs:

Generic Ingredients: Isosorbide Mononitrate G

Imdur	Isotrate ER
ISMO	Monoket

Type of Drug

Antianginal agent.

Prescribed For

Heart or chest pain associated with angina pectoris; also prescribed in congestive heart failure and similar conditions to prevent the recurrence of chest or heart pain and to reduce stress on the heart.

General Information

Isosorbide dinitrate and other nitrates are used to treat pain associated with heart problems. Although the exact nature of their action is not fully understood, they are believed to relax vascular smooth muscles. Isosorbide dinitrate sublingual tablets begin working in 2–5 minutes and last for 1–3 hours. The regular tablets begin working in 20–40 minutes and continue for 4–6 hours. The sustained-release form may take up to 4 hours to begin working and lasts for 6–8 hours. Isosorbide mononitrate begins working in 30–60 minutes and lasts for an undetermined period of time.

Cautions and Warnings

Do not take isosorbide dinitrate if you are **allergic** or **sensitive** to any of its ingredients or to another nitrate product, such as nitroglycerin.

If you have or recently have had a **head injury**, use this drug with caution.

This drug may be inappropriate for you if you have had a recent **heart attack** or have severe **anemia**, severe **kidney or liver disease**, **overactive thyroid**, **cardiomyopathy** (loss of blood-pumping ability due to damaged heart muscle), **glaucoma**, or **low blood pressure**, especially postural low blood pressure (symptoms include dizziness or fainting when rising from a sitting or lying position).

If you have been taking isosorbide for several weeks or longer, do not suddenly stop using it.

Possible Side Effects

- ▼ Common: headache and flushing, which should disappear after your body adjusts to the drug. You may experience lightheadedness, dizziness, and weakness during this process. There is a risk of blurred vision and dry mouth; if either occurs, stop taking the drug and contact your doctor.
- ▼ Less common: rapid heartbeat; low blood pressure; fainting; nausea; vomiting; weakness; trouble urinating; bronchitis; sweating; and rash with itching, redness, and peeling. If these symptoms appear, discontinue the medication and consult your doctor.

Drug Interactions

- If you take isosorbide dinitrate, do not self-medicate with over-the-counter appetite suppressants and cough, cold, and allergy remedies, because many contain ingredients that may aggravate heart disease.
- Taking this drug with large amounts of alcohol may rapidly lower blood pressure, resulting in weakness, dizziness, and fainting.
- Nitrates raise dihydroergotamine blood levels, which may elevate blood pressure or block isosorbide's effects.

- Calcium channel blockers and large doses of aspirin can increase isosorbide blood levels and the risk of side effects.
- Do not take sildenafil, tadalafil, or vardenafil if taking isosorbide or another nitrate drug. The combination can result in a rapid and potentially fatal drop in blood pressure.

Food Interactions

Take isosorbide on an empty stomach with a glass of water. If you get a persistent headache, the drug can be taken with meals.

Usual Dose

Adult

Isosorbide Dinitrate: starting dose—5–20 mg 2–3 times a day; maintenance dose—10–40 mg every 6 hours. Sustained-release starting dose—40 mg; maintenance dose—40–80 mg every 8–12 hours. Sublingual tablets starting dose—2.5–5 mg; increased gradually until angina is relieved. All dosing should include a daily dose-free interval of at least 14 hours to prevent the development of drug tolerance.

Isosorbide Mononitrate: 20 mg twice a day, with the 2 doses taken 7 hours apart. Usually, the first dose is taken upon waking and the second dose is taken 7 hours later. Extended-release tablets should begin with 30–60 mg once a day; after several days this may be increased to 120 mg once a day. Although it is rare, 240 mg may be required.

Child: not recommended.

Overdosage

Overdose can result in low blood pressure; very rapid heartbeat; flushing; perspiration followed by cold, bluish, and clammy skin; headache; heart palpitations; blurred vision and other visual disturbances; dizziness; nausea; vomiting; difficult, slow breathing; slow pulse; confusion; moderate fever; and paralysis. Take the victim to a hospital emergency room at once. If you seek treatment, ALWAYS bring the prescription bottle or container.

Special Information

If you take this drug sublingually (under the tongue), be sure the tablet is fully dissolved before you swallow the drug. Do not crush or chew sustained-release capsules or tablets. Avoid alcohol.

Do not switch brands of isosorbide without consulting your doctor or pharmacist—they may not be equivalent.

Contact your doctor if you develop a persistent headache, dizziness, facial flushing, blurred vision, or dry mouth.

You may develop a tolerance to the effects of isosorbide, in which case you may have to schedule your doses so that there is no isosorbide in your body for a period of time every 24 hours. Follow your doctor's instructions.

If you take isosorbide on a regular schedule and forget a dose, take it as soon as you remember. If you take isosorbide more than once a day and it is within 2 hours of your next dose, skip the dose you forgot and continue with your regular schedule. If you take the sustained-release form once a day and it is within 6 hours of your next dose, skip the dose you forgot and continue with your regular schedule. Never take a double dose.

Special Populations

Pregnancy/Breast-feeding: Isosorbide crosses into the fetal circulation. It should be taken during pregnancy only if your doctor determines that the potential benefit outweighs the risks.

This drug passes into breast milk. Nursing mothers who must take it should use infant formula.

Seniors: Seniors may be more sensitive to the effects and side effects of isosorbide because of the greater chance of reduced liver, kidney, or cardiac function, and the increased likelihood of concurrent diseases and drug therapies.

Generic Name

Isotretinoin (eye-soe-TRET-ih-noin)

Brand Names

Amnesteem	Claravis	Sotret

Type of Drug

Antiacne.

Prescribed For

Severe cystic acne that has not responded to other treatment.

General Information

It is not known exactly how isotretinoin, which is related to vitamin A, works in cases of severe cystic acne. It reduces the amount of sebum (the skin's natural oily lubricant), shrinks the skin glands that produce sebum, and inhibits keratinization (hardening of the skin cells)—key to the problem of severe acne because it leads to the buildup of sebum within skin follicles and causes the formation of closed comedones (whiteheads). Sebum production may be permanently reduced after isotretinoin treatment.

Isotretinoin is also being studied as a treatment for keratinization and mycosis fungoides.

Cautions and Warnings

Do not take isotretinoin if you are **allergic** or **sensitive** to any of its ingredients, to vitamin A (or any vitamin A product), or to paraben preservatives.

Isotretinoin greatly increases the risk of severe birth defects (including very low IQs as well as multiple physical defects), abortion, and premature birth. Not every fetus exposed to isotretinoin will be affected, but women who are **pregnant or nursing** must not take isotretinoin.

Isotretinoin has been associated with depression, psychosis, and suicidal thoughts or attempts. Use with caution if you have a history of **psychiatric disorders**.

Isotretinoin has been associated with pseudotumor cerebri (increased pressure in the brain). The symptoms of this condition include severe headaches, nausea, vomiting, and visual disturbances.

Isotretinoin may cause an increased risk for pancreatitis, sometimes fatal, and low white-blood-cell counts.

Diabetics taking isotretinoin may have to have their diabetes drugs reevaluated by their doctors. Some new cases of diabetes were found in people taking isotretinoin, but no direct relationship to drug therapy has been found.

Isotretinoin may cause temporary opaque spots on the cornea of your eye, causing visual disturbances. These are usually gone within 2 months after the drug is stopped.

Difficulty seeing at night or in the dark can develop suddenly while taking isotretinoin.

Several cases of severe bowel inflammation (symptoms include abdominal discomfort and pain, severe diarrhea, or bleeding from the rectum) have developed in people taking isotretinoin.

About 25% of people who take isotretinoin develop high blood-triglyceride levels. Fifteen percent have lower high-density lipoprotein (HDL)—“good” cholesterol—and 7% have higher total cholesterol.

Several cases of hepatitis have been linked to this drug. Fifteen percent of people who take it develop signs of liver inflammation.

Isotretinoin may worsen **osteoporosis**, cause low bone density, and slow bone healing. Long-term treatment or multiple courses of therapy may worsen these problems.

Children age 13–17 may experience increased back pain while using isotretinoin. This drug has not been studied in children under age 12.

Isotretinoin causes extreme elevations of blood-triglyceride levels and milder elevations of other blood-fat levels, including cholesterol. It also can raise blood-sugar or uric-acid levels and can increase liver-function test values.

Possible Side Effects

Side effects increase with dosage.

▼ Most common: dry, chapped, or inflamed lips; dry mouth; dry nose; nosebleeds; eye irritation; conjunctivitis (pinkeye); dry or flaky skin; rash; itching; peeling skin on the face, palms, or soles; unusual sensitivity to the sun; temporary skin discoloration; brittle nails; inflammation of the nail bed or bone under toe- or fingernails; temporary hair thinning; nausea; vomiting; abdominal pain; tiredness; lethargy; sleeplessness; headache; tingling in the hands or feet; dizziness; protein, blood, or white blood cells in the urine; urinary difficulties; blurred vision; bone and joint aches or pains; and muscle pain or stiffness.

▼ Less common: wound crusting caused by an exaggerated healing response stimulated by the drug, hair problems other than thinning, appetite loss, upset stomach or intestinal discomfort, severe bowel inflammation, stomach or intestinal bleeding, weight loss, visual disturbances, contact lens intolerance, pseudotumor cerebri, mild bleeding or easy bruising, fluid retention, and lung or respiratory-system infection. Several people taking isotretinoin have developed widespread herpes simplex infections.

Drug Interactions

- Vitamin A supplements increase isotretinoin's side effects and must be avoided while taking this drug. Avoid alcohol because this combination can severely raise blood-triglyceride levels.
- Combining tetracycline antibiotics and isotretinoin may increase the risk of pseudotumor cerebri.

- Isotretinoin may reduce the amount of carbamazepine (an anticonvulsant) in the blood.
- Isotretinoin may decrease the effectiveness of microdosed progesterone contraceptive drugs ("mini-pills"). Use 2 forms of contraception instead of using this combination (see "Special Information").
- Do not use the herbal supplement St. John's wort while taking isotretinoin. There may be a possible interaction with hormonal contraceptives and St. John's wort, making them less effective and increasing the chance of accidental pregnancy.

Food Interactions

Isotretinoin should be taken with food or meals. Avoid eating beef or chicken liver while taking isotretinoin, because liver contains very large amounts of vitamin A. Limit your intake of foods containing moderate to large amounts of vitamin A.

Usual Dose

Adult and Child (age 13 and over): 0.22–0.9 mg per lb. of body weight a day in 2 divided doses for 15–20 weeks. Lower doses may be effective, but relapses are more common. Isotretinoin, like vitamin A, dissolves in body fat. Individuals who weigh more than 155 lbs. may need doses at the high end of the usual range.

If the total acne lesion count drops by 70% in 15–20 weeks, the drug may be discontinued. Stop taking isotretinoin for 2 months after 15–20 weeks of treatment. A second course of treatment may be needed if the acne does not clear.

Overdosage

Isotretinoin overdose is likely to cause nausea, vomiting, facial flushing, abdominal pain, lethargy, and other common drug side effects. Overdose victims must be made to vomit with ipecac syrup—available at any pharmacy—to remove any remaining drug from the stomach. Contact your doctor or local poison control center before doing this. If you seek treatment, ALWAYS bring the prescription bottle or container.

Special Information

Women of childbearing age should not take isotretinoin unless their severe, disfiguring acne has not responded to any other treatment, they are using 2 effective forms of contraception, they understand that it causes serious birth defects, and they have had 2 negative pregnancy tests during the 2 cycles before taking isotretinoin and after the last incidence of unprotected sex. You may have to take a pregnancy test each month of your treatment before another prescription is written. You should start taking isotretinoin on day 2 or 3 of your next period. Be sure your doctor knows if you are breast-feeding, diabetic, taking a vitamin A supplement—as a multivitamin or vitamin A alone—or if you or any family member has a history of high blood-triglyceride levels. Continue using contraceptives for at least 1 month after stopping isotretinoin.

If isotretinoin causes the side effect of depression, do not treat depression with the herbal supplement St. John's wort, as it may reduce the efficacy of hormonal contraceptives. Pregnancies have been reported by people using contraceptive drugs with some form of St. John's wort.

Your skin may become unusually sensitive to the sun while you are taking this drug. Use sunscreen and wear protective clothing until your doctor can determine if you are likely to develop this effect.

Contact your doctor if you develop any severe or unusual side effects, such as abdominal pain; bleeding from the rectum; severe diarrhea; headache; nausea or vomiting; visual difficulties; severe muscle, bone, or joint aches or pains; or unusual sensitivity to sunlight or to ultraviolet light.

Your acne may worsen when isotretinoin treatment begins, but then it should improve. Do not be alarmed if this happens, but tell your doctor.

Avoid using depilatories or waxing while using isotretinoin, and for 6 months after treatment.

Do not donate blood during isotretinoin treatment—or for at least 30 days after you have stopped—because of the risk to the fetus of a pregnant woman who may receive the blood.

If you forget a dose of isotretinoin, take it as soon as you remember. If it is almost time for your next dose, skip the one you forgot and continue with your regular schedule. Do not take a double dose.

Special Populations

Pregnancy/Breast-feeding: Pregnant women should never take isotretinoin because it will injure the fetus. Your doctor will confirm that you are not pregnant before starting isotretinoin (see "Special Information"). Accidental pregnancy during isotretinoin therapy

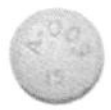

Abilify
15 mg
p. 121

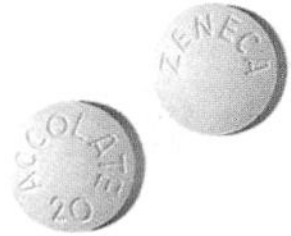

Accolate
20 mg
p. 679

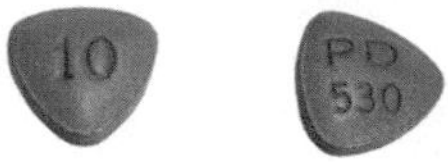

Accupril
10 mg
p. 7

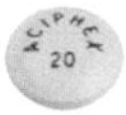

Aciphex
20 mg
p. 956

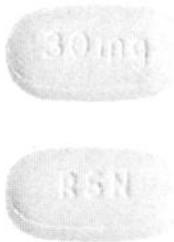

Actonel
30 mg
p. 188

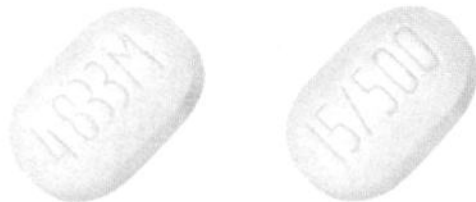

ACTOplus Met
15/500 mg
p. 529

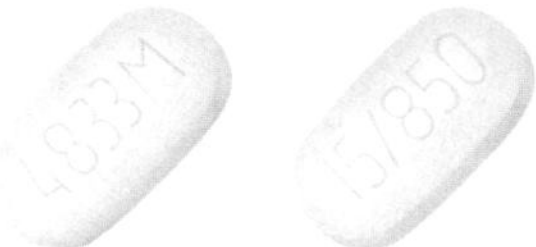

ACTOplus Met XR
15/850 mg
p. 529

Actos
30 mg
p. 529

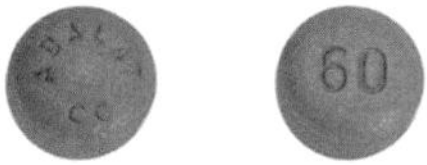

Adalat CC
60 mg
p. 224

Adderall
10 mg
p. 38

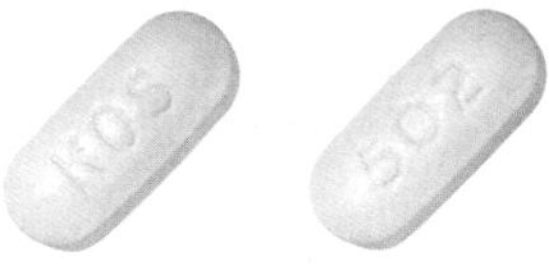

Advicor
500/20 mg
p. 1065

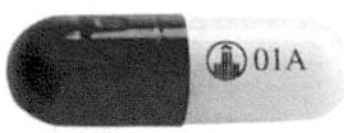

Aggrenox
25/200 mg
p. 48

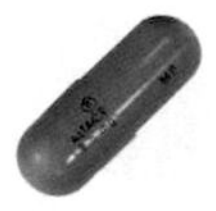

Altace
2.5 mg
p. 7

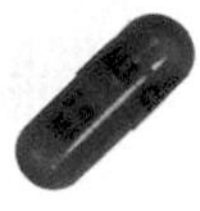

Altace
5 mg
p. 7

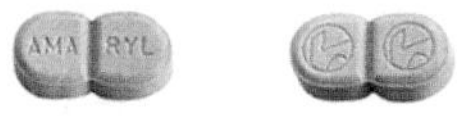

Amaryl
2 mg
p. 1081

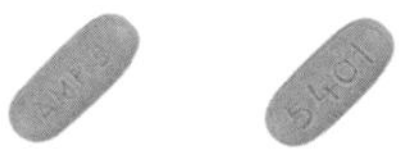

Ambien
5 mg
p. 1033

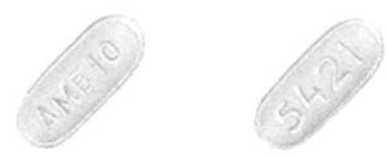

Ambien
10 mg
p. 1033

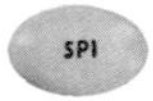

Amitiza
8 mcg
p. 709

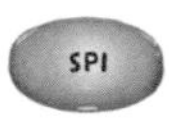

Amitiza
24 mcg
p. 709

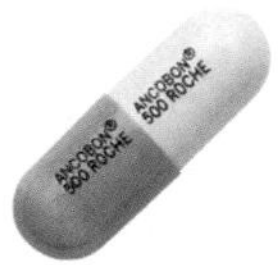

Ancobon
500 mg
p. 510

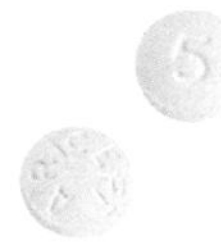

Aricept
5 mg
p. 286

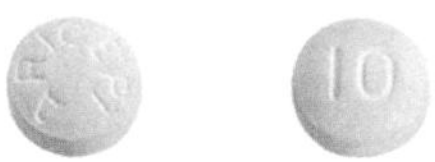

Aricept
10 mg
p. 286

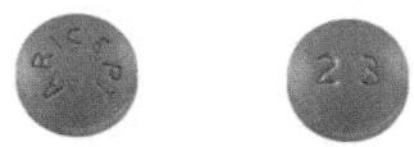

Aricept
23 mg
p. 286

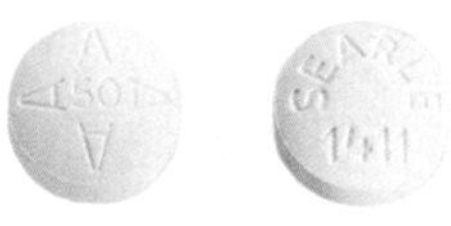

Arthrotec
50 mg
p. 863

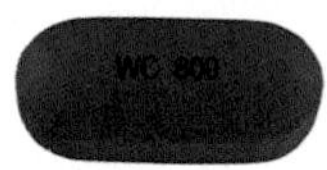

Asacol HD
800 mg
p. 199

B

	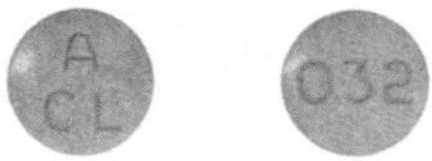
Atacand 16 mg p. 97	**Atacand** 32 mg p. 97
	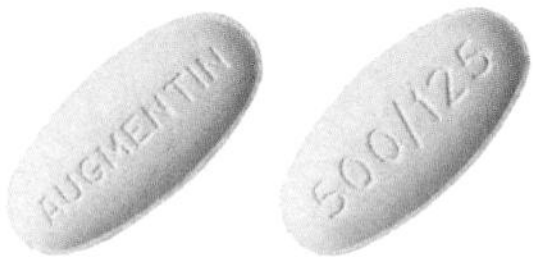
Ativan 0.5 mg p. 157	**Augmentin** 500 mg p. 899
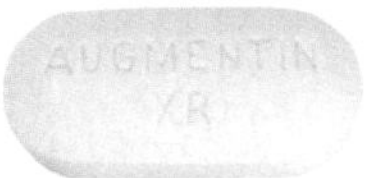	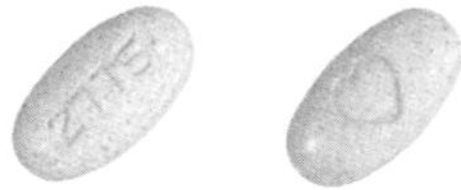
Augmentin XR 1000 mg p. 899	**Avalide** 150/12.5 mg p. 97
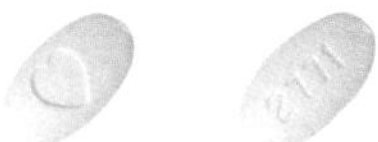	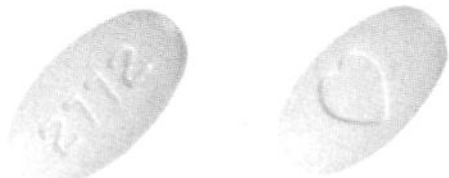
Avapro 75 mg p. 97	**Avapro** 150 mg p. 97
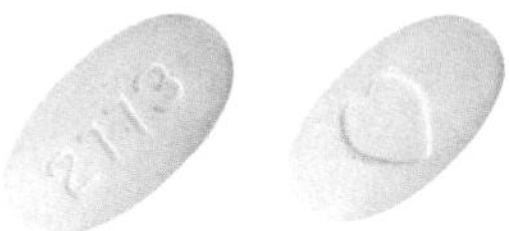	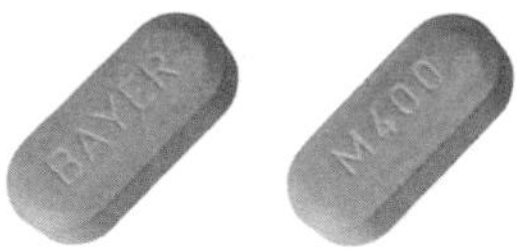
Avapro 300 mg p. 97	**Avelox** 400 mg p. 512

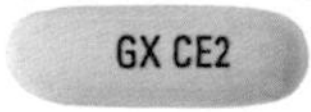

Avodart
0.5 mg
p. 494

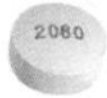

Axert
6.25 mg
p. 1187

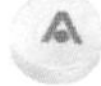

Axert
12.5 mg
p. 1187

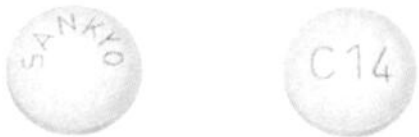

Benicar
20 mg
p. 97

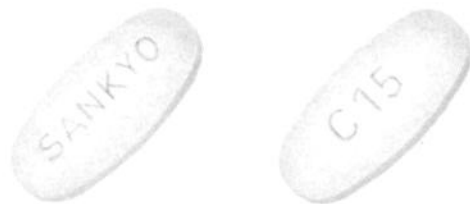

Benicar
40 mg
p. 97

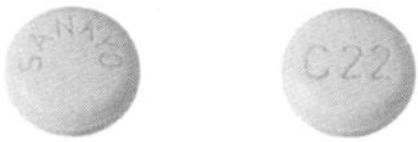

Benicar HCT
20/12.5 mg
p. 97

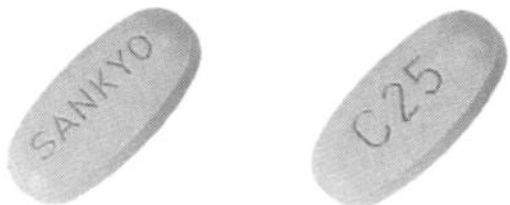

Benicar HCT
40/25 mg
p. 97

Biaxin XL
500 mg
p. 460

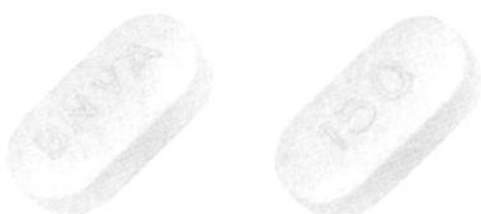

Boniva
150 mg
p. 188

BuSpar
5 mg
p. 211

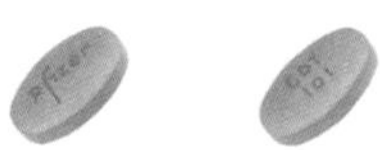

Caduet
10/10 mg
pp. 224, 1065

<table>
<tr><td>
</td><td>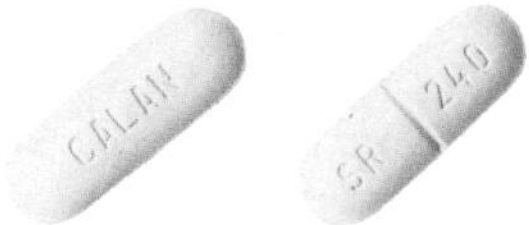
</td></tr>
<tr><td>Calan
40 mg
p. 224</td><td>Calan SR
240 mg
p. 224</td></tr>
<tr><td></td><td></td></tr>
<tr><td>Cardizem
30 mg
p. 224</td><td>Cardizem
60 mg
p. 224</td></tr>
<tr><td>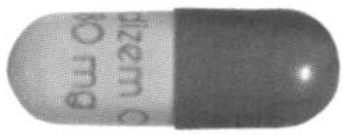</td><td>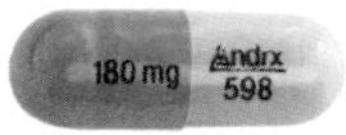
</td></tr>
<tr><td>Cardizem CD
180 mg
p. 224</td><td>Cartia XT
180 mg
p. 224</td></tr>
<tr><td>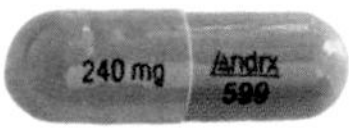
</td><td>
</td></tr>
<tr><td>Cartia XT
240 mg
p. 224</td><td>Casodex
50 mg
p. 181</td></tr>
<tr><td>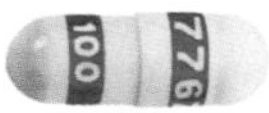
</td><td>
</td></tr>
<tr><td>Celebrex
100 mg
p. 255</td><td>Celebrex
200 mg
p. 255</td></tr>
</table>

E

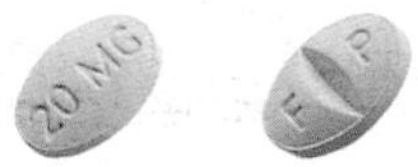

Celexa
20 mg
p. 1045

CellCept
250 mg
p. 813

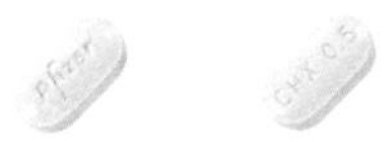

Chantix
0.5 mg
p. 1201

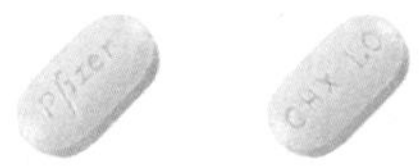

Chantix
1 mg
p. 1201

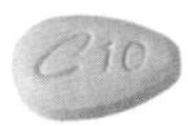

Cialis
10 mg
p. 453

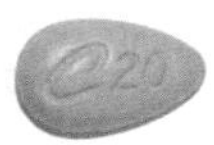

Cialis
20 mg
p. 453

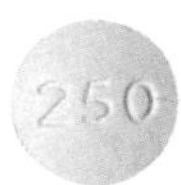

Cipro
250 mg
p. 512

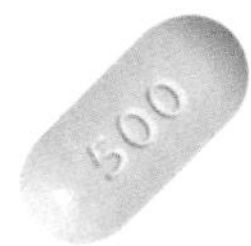

Cipro
500 mg
p. 512

Cipro
750 mg
p. 512

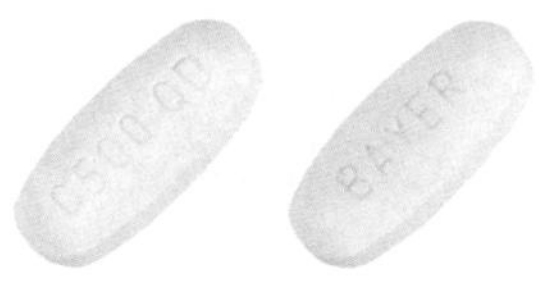

Cipro XR
500 mg
p. 512

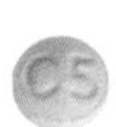

Clarinex
5 mg
p. 706

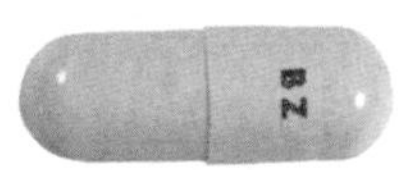

Colazal
750 mg
p. 199

Colcrys
0.6 mg
p. 311

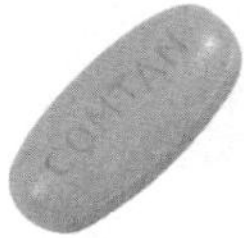

Comtan
200 mg
p. 442

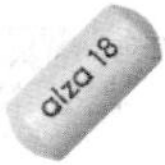

Concerta
18 mg
p. 742

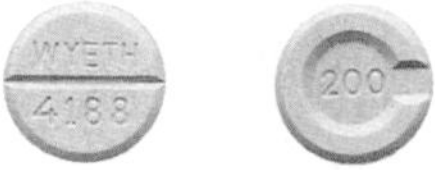

Cordarone
200 mg
p. 81

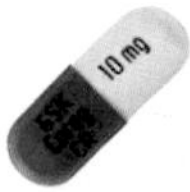

Coreg CR
10 mg
p. 250

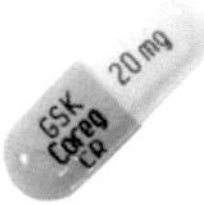

Coreg CR
20 mg
p. 250

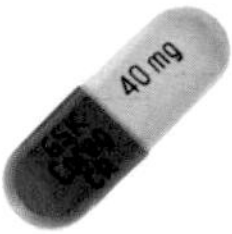

Coreg CR
40 mg
p. 250

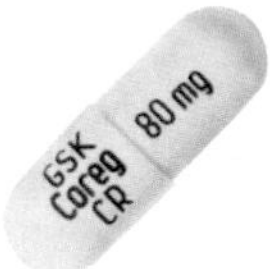

Coreg CR
80 mg
p. 250

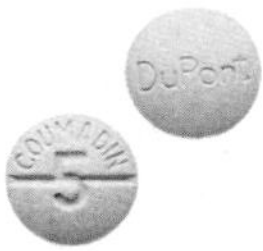

Coumadin
5 mg
p. 1224

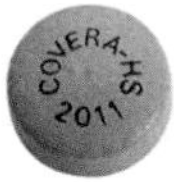

Covera-HS
180 mg
p. 224

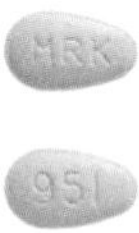

Cozaar
25 mg
p. 97

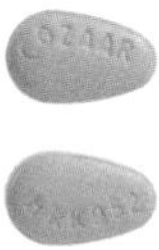

Cozaar
50 mg
p. 97

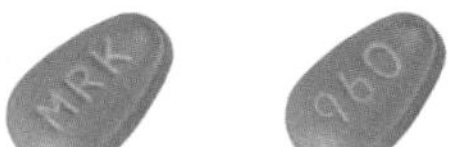

Cozaar
100 mg
p. 97

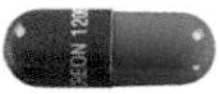

Creon
6,000 units
p. 891

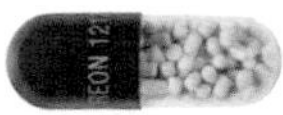

Creon
12,000 units
p. 891

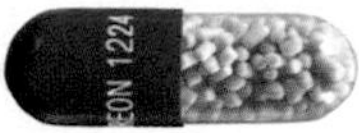

Creon
24,000 units
p. 891

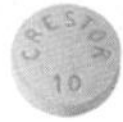

Crestor
10 mg
p. 1065

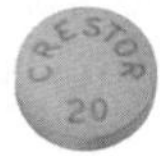

Crestor
20 mg
p. 1065

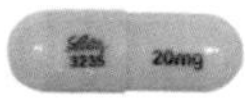

Cymbalta
20 mg
p. 1204

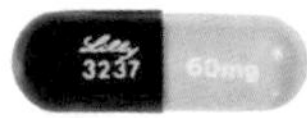

Cymbalta
60 mg
p. 1204

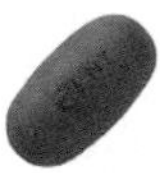

Depakote
125 mg
p. 1197

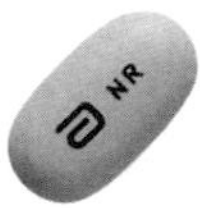

Depakote
250 mg
p. 1197

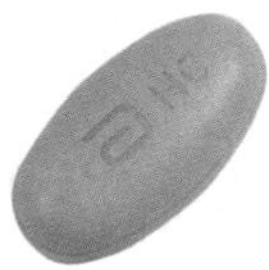

Depakote ER
500 mg
p. 1197

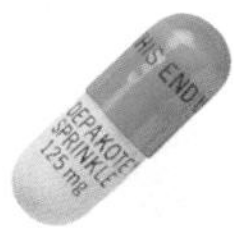

Depakote Sprinkle
125 mg
p. 1197

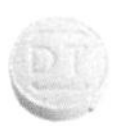

Detrol
2 mg
p. 884

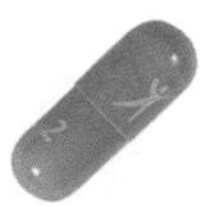

Detrol LA
2 mg
p. 884

DiaBeta
5 mg
p. 1081

Diflucan
100 mg
p. 142

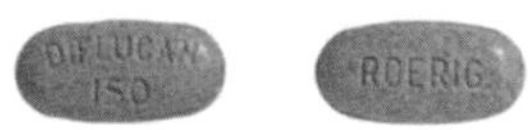

Diflucan
150 mg
p. 142

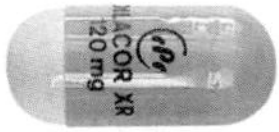

Dilacor XR
120 mg
p. 224

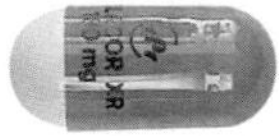

Dilacor XR
180 mg
p. 224

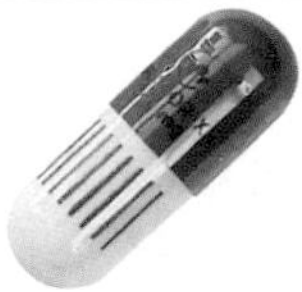

Dilacor XR
240 mg
p. 224

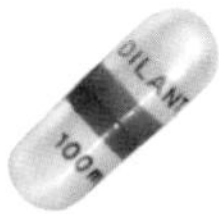

Dilantin
100 mg
p. 912

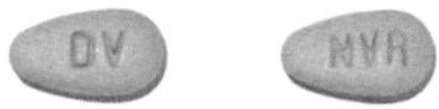

Diovan
80 mg
p. 97

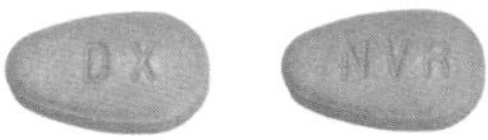

Diovan
160 mg
p. 97

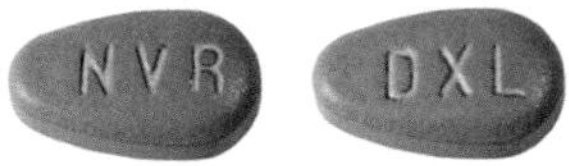

Diovan
320 mg
p. 97

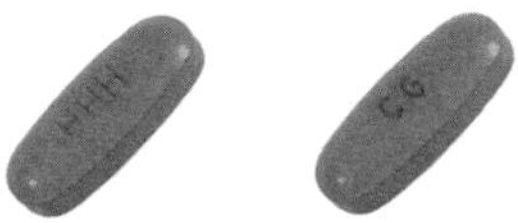

Diovan HCT
160/12.5 mg
p. 97

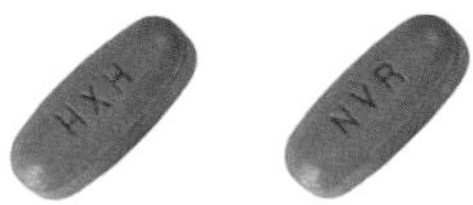

Diovan HCT
160/25 mg
p. 97

Ditropan
5 mg
p. 884

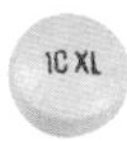

Ditropan XL
10 mg
p. 884

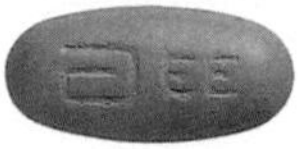

E.E.S.
400 mg
p. 460

Effexor
25 mg
p. 1204

Effexor
37.5 mg
p. 1204

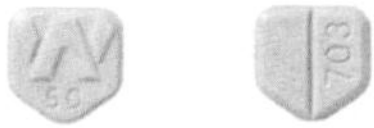

Effexor
50 mg
p. 1204

Effexor
75 mg
p. 1204

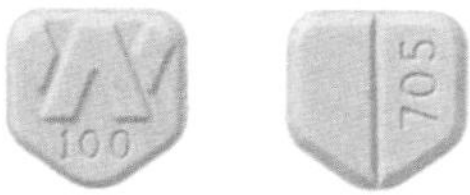

Effexor
100 mg
p. 1204

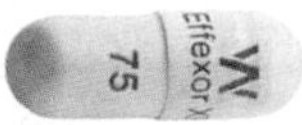

Effexor XR
75 mg
p. 1204

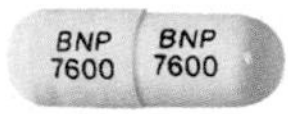

Elmiron
100 mg
p. 904

Enablex
7.5 mg
p. 884

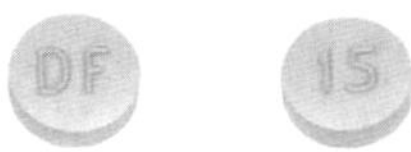

Enablex
15 mg
p. 884

Epzicom
600/300 mg
p. 555

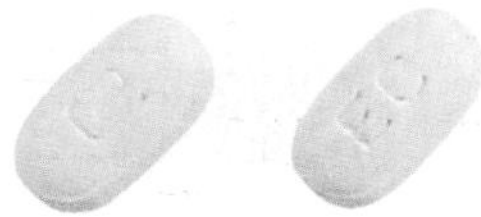

Ery-Tab
250 mg
p. 460

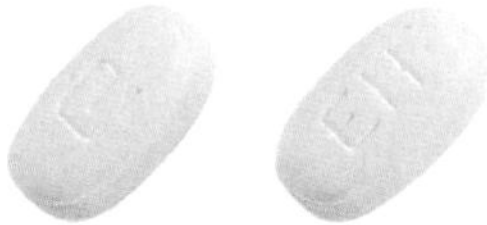

Ery-Tab
333 mg
p. 460

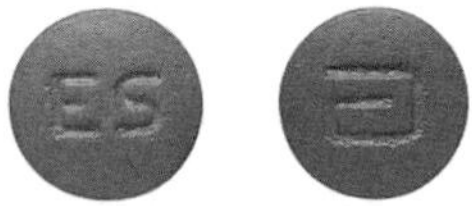

Erythrocin Stearate
250 mg
p. 460

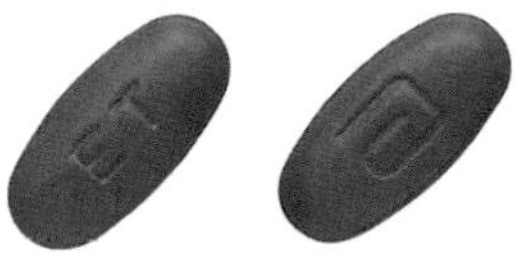

Erythrocin Stearate
500 mg
p. 460

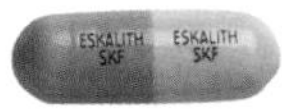

Eskalith
300 mg
p. 694

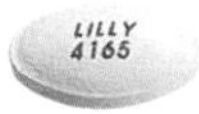

Evista
60 mg
p. 975

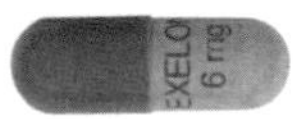

Exelon
6 mg
p. 286

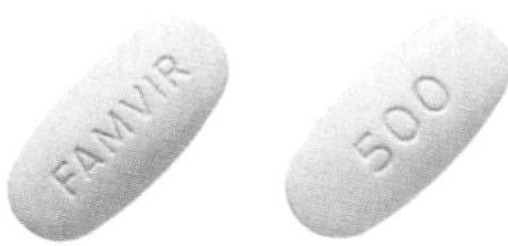

Famvir
500 mg
p. 26

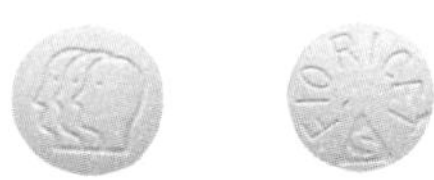

Fioricet
50/325/40 mg
p. 823

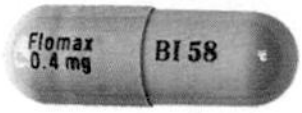

Flomax
0.4 mg
p. 70

Fosamax
10 mg
p. 188

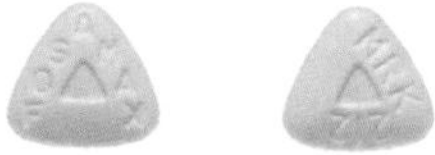

Fosamax
40 mg
p. 188

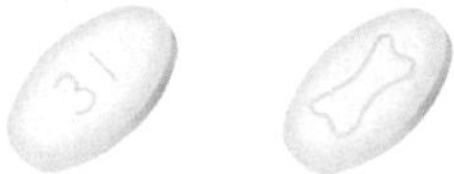

Fosamax
70 mg
p. 188

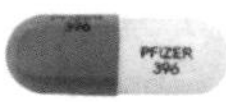

Geodon
20 mg
p. 1012

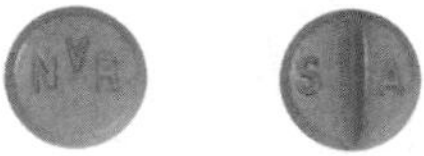

Gleevec
100 mg
p. 791

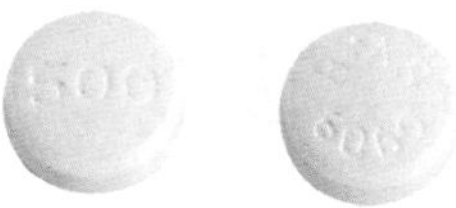

Glucophage
500 mg
p. 731

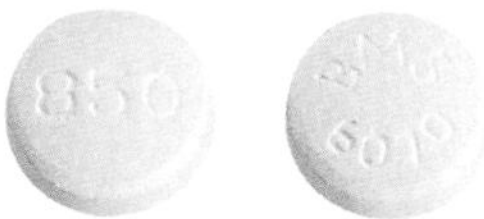

Glucophage
850 mg
p. 731

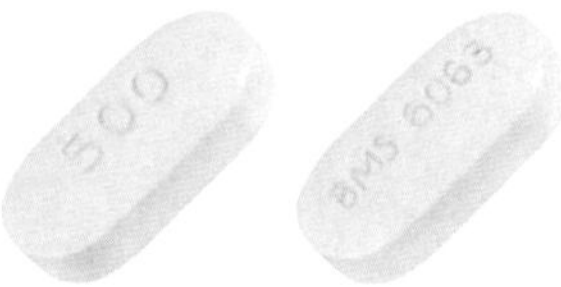

Glucophage XR
500 mg
p. 731

Glucotrol
5 mg
p. 1081

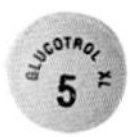

Glucotrol XL
5 mg
p. 1081

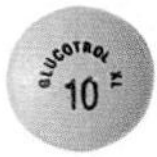

Glucotrol XL
10 mg
p. 1081

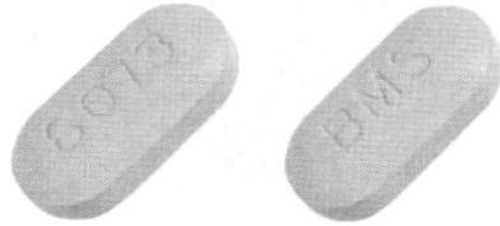

Glucovance
2.5/500 mg
p. 1081

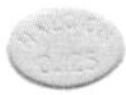

Halcion
0.125 mg
p. 1033

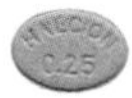

Halcion
0.25 mg
p. 1033

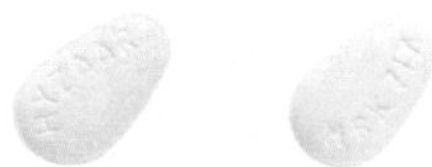

Hyzaar
50/12.5 mg
p. 97

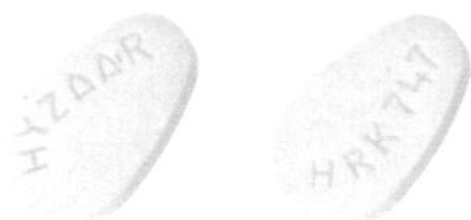

Hyzaar
100/25 mg
p. 97

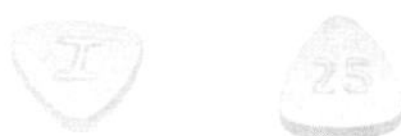

Imitrex
25 mg
p. 1187

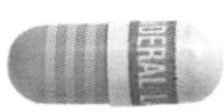

Inderal LA
60 mg
p. 166

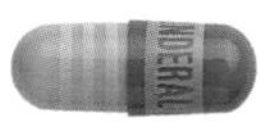

Inderal LA
120 mg
p. 166

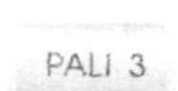

Invega
3 mg
p. 1012

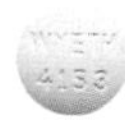

Isordil Titradose
10 mg
p. 651

<table>
<tr><td>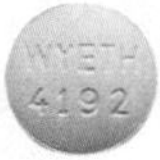
</td><td colspan="2">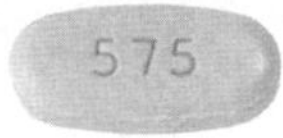
</td></tr>
<tr><td>Isordil Titradose
40 mg
p. 651</td><td colspan="2">Janumet
50/500 mg
p. 420</td></tr>
<tr><td>
</td><td>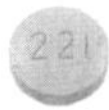
</td><td>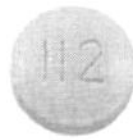
</td></tr>
<tr><td>Janumet
50/1000 mg
p. 420</td><td>Januvia
25 mg
p. 420</td><td>Januvia
50 mg
p. 420</td></tr>
<tr><td>
</td><td colspan="2">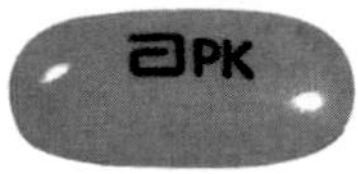
</td></tr>
<tr><td>Januvia
100 mg
p. 420</td><td colspan="2">Kaletra
133.3/33.3 mg
p. 582</td></tr>
<tr><td></td><td colspan="2">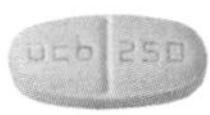
</td></tr>
<tr><td>K-Dur 20
20 mEq
p. 931</td><td colspan="2">Keppra
250 mg
p. 684</td></tr>
<tr><td>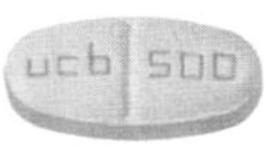
</td><td colspan="2">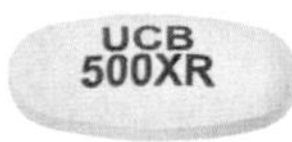
</td></tr>
<tr><td>Keppra
500 mg
p. 684</td><td colspan="2">Keppra XR
500 mg
p. 684</td></tr>
</table>

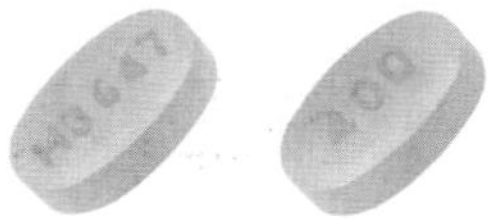

Ketek
400 mg
p. 1099

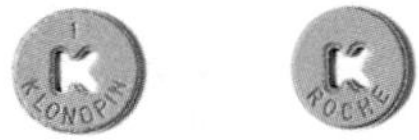

Klonopin
1 mg
p. 157

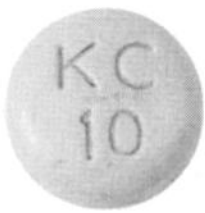

Klor-Con
10 mEq
p. 931

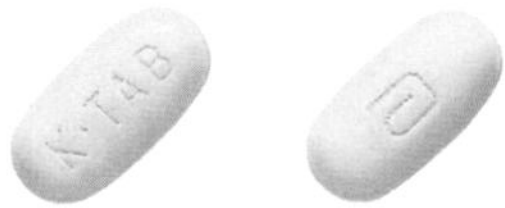

K-Tab
10 mEq
p. 931

Lanoxin
0.125 mg
p. 391

Lanoxin
0.25 mg
p. 391

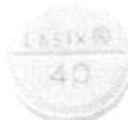

Lasix
40 mg
p. 698

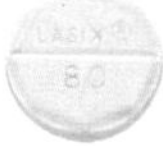

Lasix
80 mg
p. 698

Lescol
20 mg
p. 1065

Lescol
40 mg
p. 1065

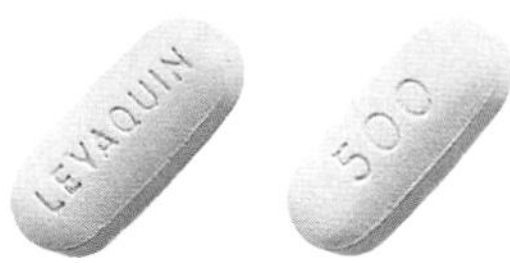

Levaquin
500 mg
p. 512

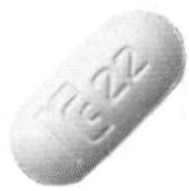	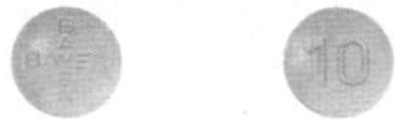
Levatol 20 mg p. 166	**Levitra** 10 mg p. 453
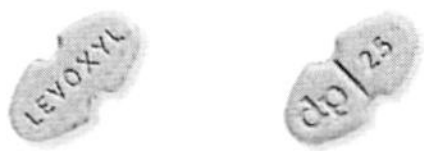	
Levoxyl 25 mcg p. 1136	**Levoxyl** 50 mcg p. 1136
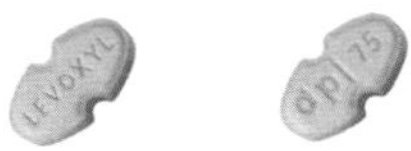	
Levoxyl 75 mcg p. 1136	**Levoxyl** 100 mcg p. 1136

Levoxyl 125 mcg p. 1136	**Levoxyl** 175 mcg p. 1136
	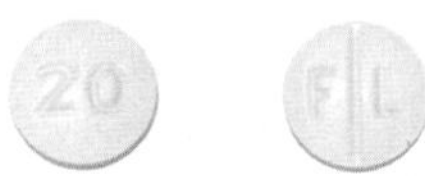
Lexapro 10 mg p. 1045	**Lexapro** 20 mg p. 1045

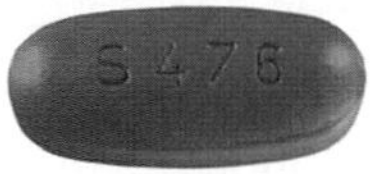

Lialda
1.2 g
p. 199

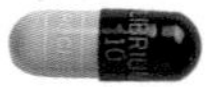

Librium
10 mg
p. 157

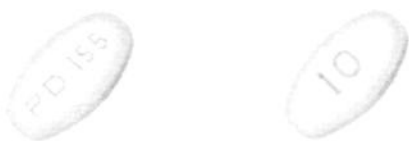

Lipitor
10 mg
p. 1065

Lipitor
20 mg
p. 1065

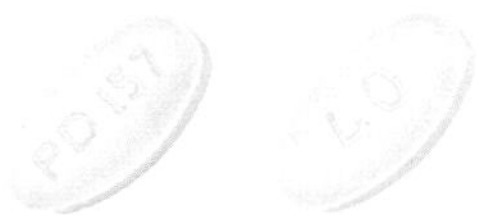

Lipitor
40 mg
p. 1065

Lipitor
80 mg
p. 1065

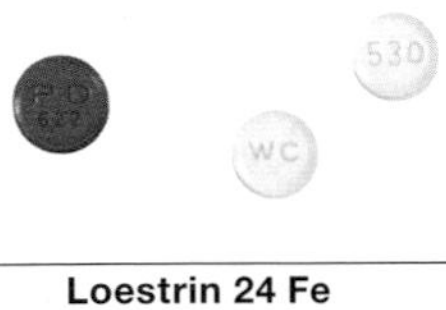

Loestrin 24 Fe
1 mg/20 mcg
p. 316

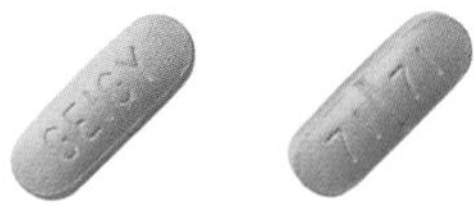

Lopressor
100 mg
p. 166

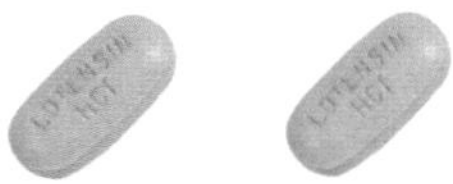

Lotensin HCT
20/12.5 mg
p. 7

Lotrel
5/10 mg
p. 224

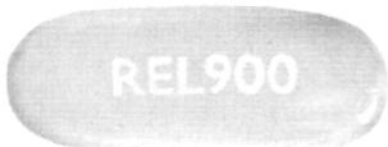

Lovaza
1 g
p. 876

Lunesta
3 mg
p. 1033

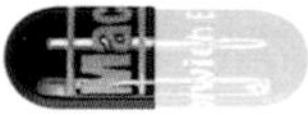

Macrobid
100 mg
p. 852

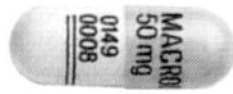

Macrodantin
50 mg
p. 852

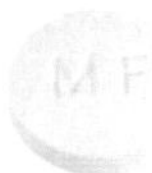

Mifeprex
1.25 mg
p. 760

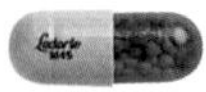

Minocin
50 mg
p. 1122

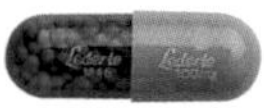

Minocin
100 mg
p. 1122

Mirapex
0.125 mg
p. 934

Mirapex
0.25 mg
p. 934

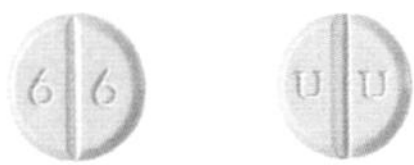

Mirapex
1 mg
p. 934

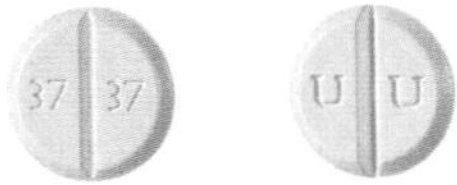

Mirapex
1.5 mg
p. 934

Mobic
15 mg
p. 863

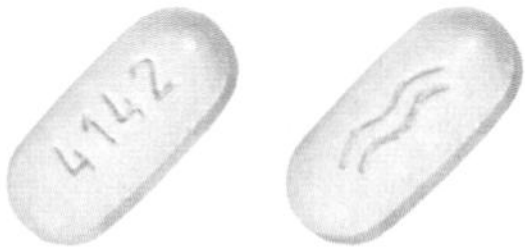

Multaq
400 mg
p. 427

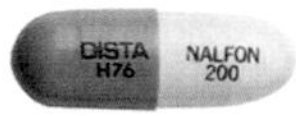

Nalfon
200 mg
p. 863

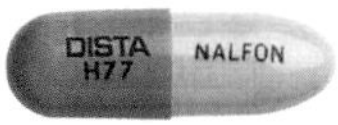

Nalfon
300 mg
p. 863

Namenda
5 mg
p. 725

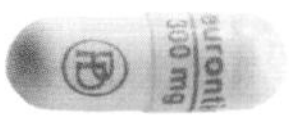

Neurontin
300 mg
p. 1141

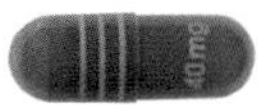

Nexium
40 mg
p. 956

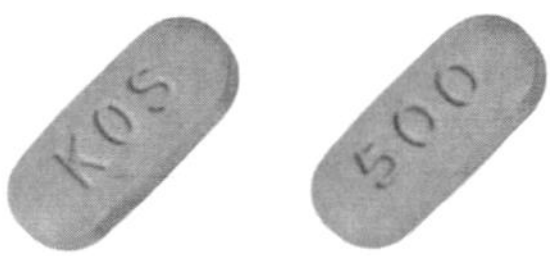

Niaspan
500 mg
p. 841

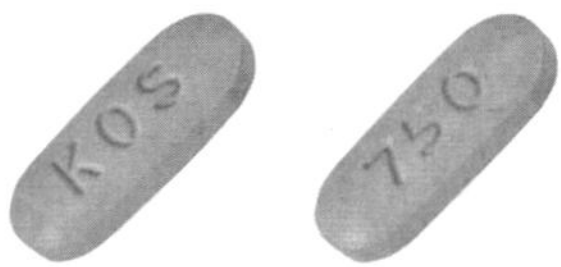

Niaspan
750 mg
p. 841

S

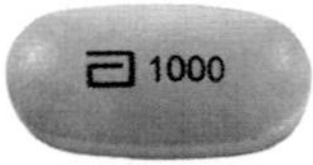

Niaspan
1000 mg
p. 841

Noroxin
400 mg
p. 512

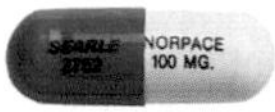

Norpace
100 mg
p. 405

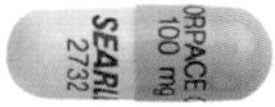

Norpace CR
100 mg
p. 405

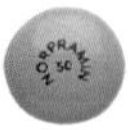

Norpramin
50 mg
p. 1180

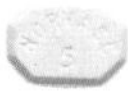

Norvasc
5 mg
p. 224

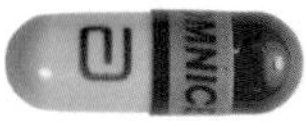

Omnicef
300 mg
p. 260

Onglyza
2.5 mg
p. 420

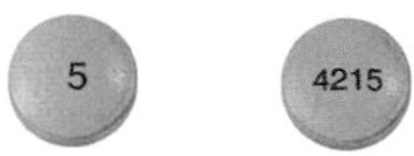

Onglyza
5 mg
p. 420

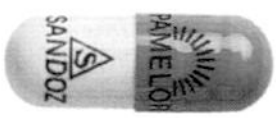

Pamelor
25 mg
p. 1180

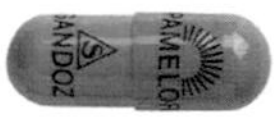

Pamelor
75 mg
p. 1180

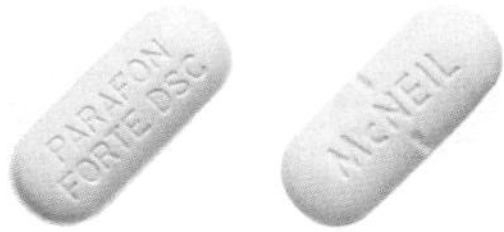

Parafon Forte DSC
500 mg
p. 281

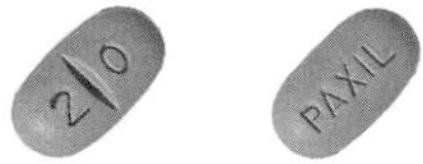

Paxil
20 mg
p. 1045

Paxil CR
12.5 mg
p. 1045

Paxil CR
25 mg
p. 1045

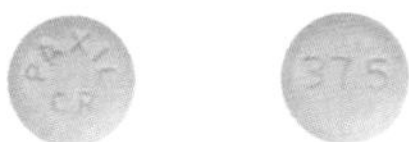

Paxil CR
37.5 mg
p. 1045

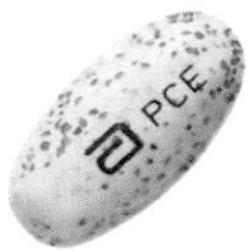

PCE
333 mg
p. 460

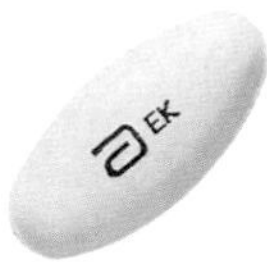

PCE
500 mg
p. 460

Pepcid
20 mg
p. 550

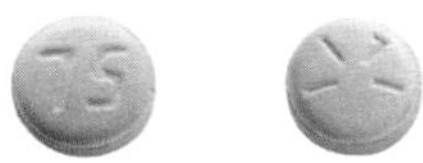

Plavix
75 mg
p. 920

Pletal
50 mg
p. 292

Pletal
100 mg
p. 292

Prandin
1 mg
p. 990

Pravachol
10 mg
p. 1065

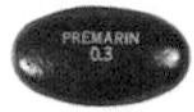

Premarin
0.3 mg
p. 466

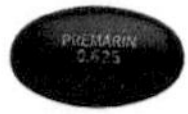

Premarin
0.625 mg
p. 466

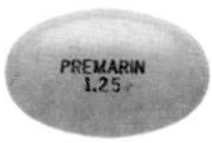

Premarin
1.25 mg
p. 466

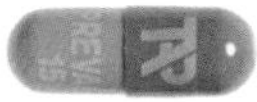

Prevacid
15 mg
p. 956

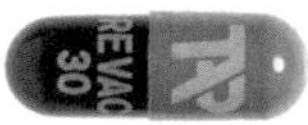

Prevacid
30 mg
p. 956

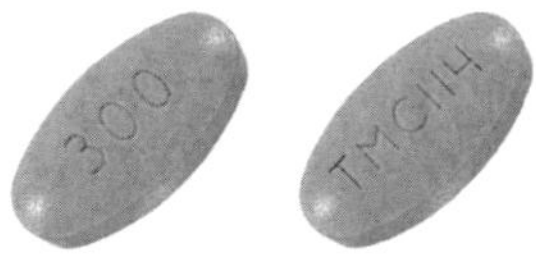

Prezista
300 mg
p. 582

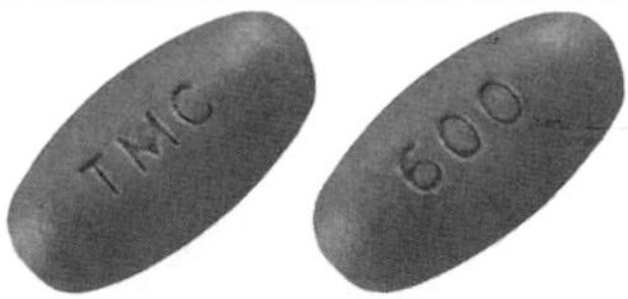

Prezista
600 mg
p. 582

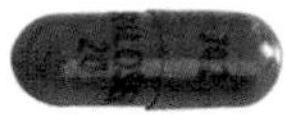

Prilosec
20 mg
p. 956

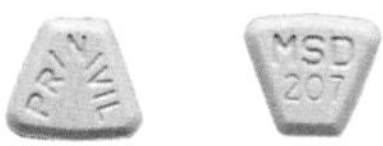

Prinivil
20 mg
p. 7

Pristiq
50 mg
p. 1204

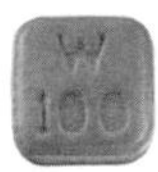

Pristiq
100 mg
p. 1204

ProAmatine
2.5 mg
p. 757

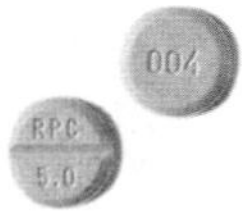

ProAmatine
5 mg
p. 757

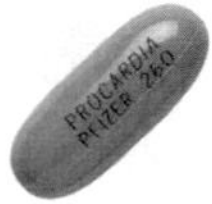

Procardia
10 mg
p. 224

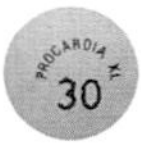

Procardia XL
30 mg
p. 224

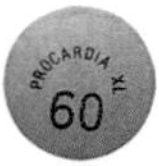

Procardia XL
60 mg
p. 224

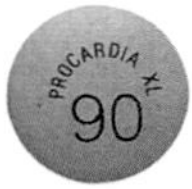

Procardia XL
90 mg
p. 224

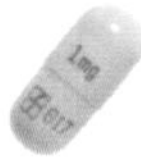

Prograf
1 mg
p. 1087

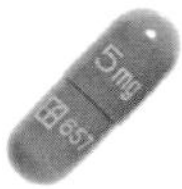

Prograf
5 mg
p. 1087

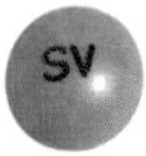

Prometrium
100 mg
p. 720

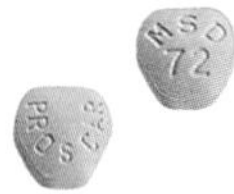

Proscar
5 mg
p. 494

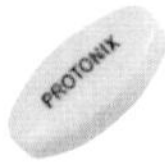

Protonix
40 mg
p. 956

Provera
2.5 mg
p. 720

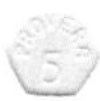

Provera
5 mg
p. 720

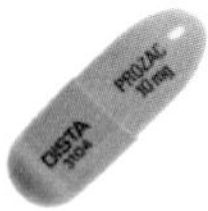

Prozac
10 mg
p. 1045

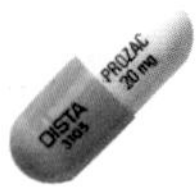

Prozac
20 mg
p. 1045

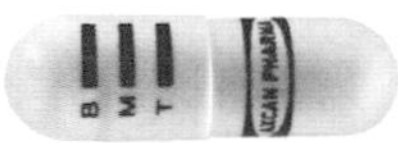

Pylera
140/125/125 mg
p. 540

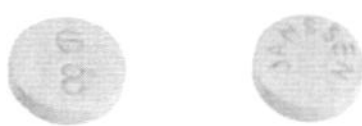

Razadyne
8 mg
p. 286

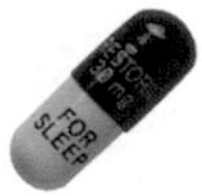

Restoril
30 mg
p. 1033

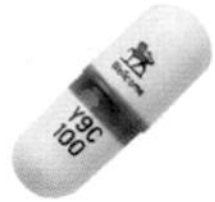

Retrovir
100 mg
p. 555

Risperdal
2 mg
p. 1012

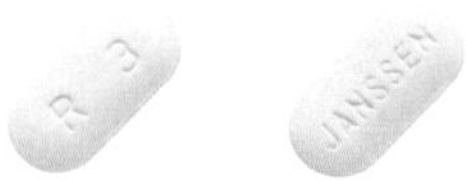

Risperdal
3 mg
p. 1012

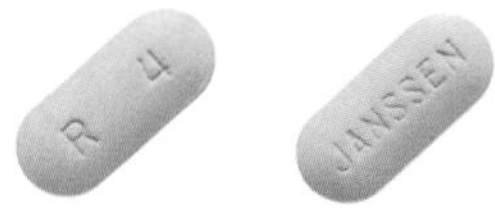

Risperdal
4 mg
p. 1012

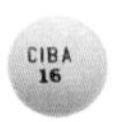

Ritalin-SR
20 mg
p. 742

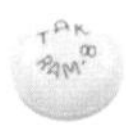

Rozerem
8 mg
p. 981

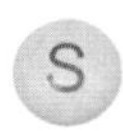

Sanctura
20 mg
p. 884

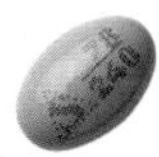

Sandimmune
25 mg
p. 369

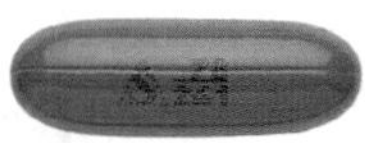

Sandimmune
100 mg
p. 369

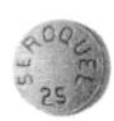

Seroquel
25 mg
p. 961

Seroquel
50 mg
p. 961

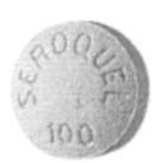

Seroquel
100 mg
p. 961

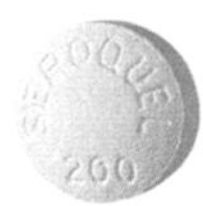

Seroquel
200 mg
p. 961

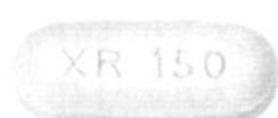

Seroquel XR
150 mg
p. 961

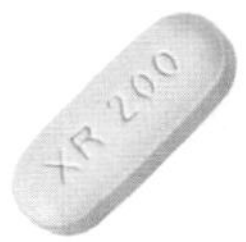

Seroquel XR
200 mg
p. 961

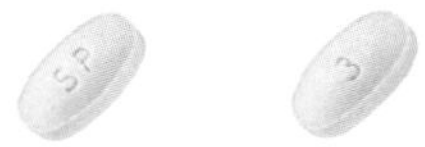

Silenor
3 mg
p. 1180

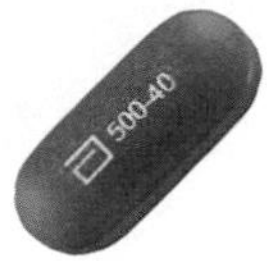

Simcor
40/500 mg
p. 1065

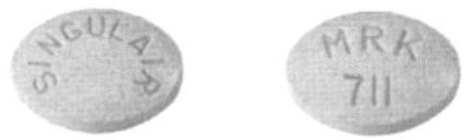

Singulair
4 mg
p. 679

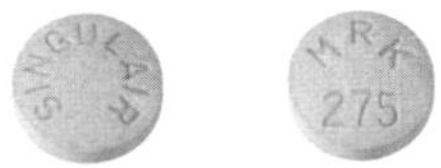

Singulair
5 mg
p. 679

Singulair
10 mg
p. 679

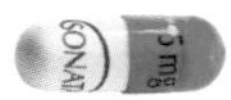

Sonata
5 mg
p. 1033

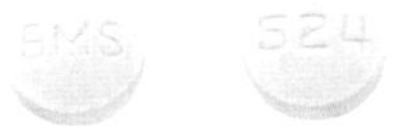

Sprycel
70 mg
p. 791

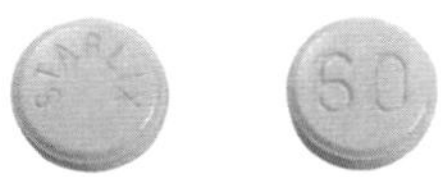

Starlix
60 mg
p. 990

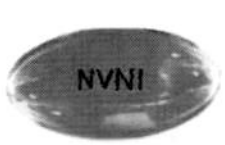

Stavzor
250 mg
p. 1197

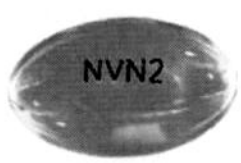

Stavzor
500 mg
p. 1197

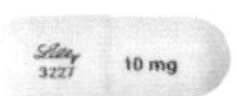

Strattera
10 mg
p. 130

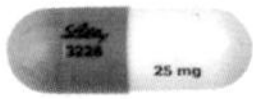	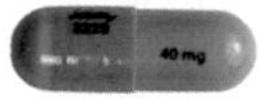
Strattera 25 mg p. 130	**Strattera** 40 mg p. 130

Synthroid 25 mcg p. 1136	**Synthroid** 50 mcg p. 1136

Synthroid 75 mcg p. 1136	**Synthroid** 100 mcg p. 1136

Synthroid 125 mcg p. 1136	**Synthroid** 150 mcg p. 1136
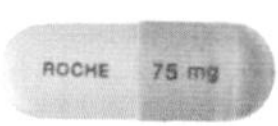	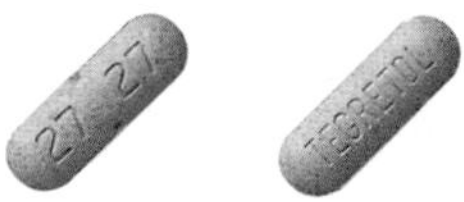
Tamiflu 75 mg p. 881	**Tegretol** 200 mg p. 241

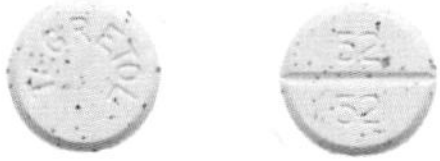

Tegretol (Chewable)
100 mg
p. 241

Tegretol-XR
100 mg
p. 241

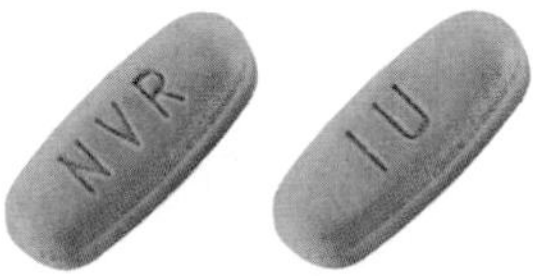

Tekturna
300 mg
p. 59

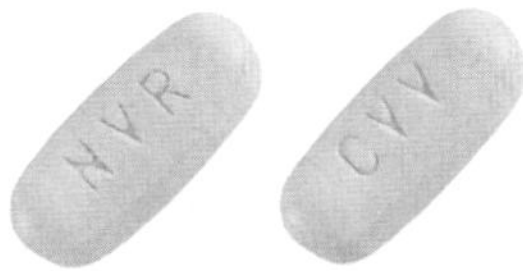

Tekturna HCT
300/25 mg
p. 59

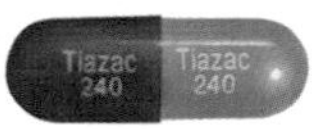

Tiazac
240 mg
p. 224

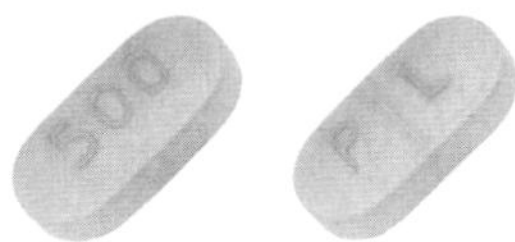

Tindamax
500 mg
p. 750

Topamax
25 mg
p. 1162

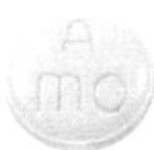

Toprol-XL
50 mg
p. 166

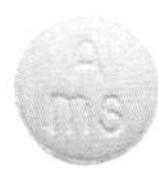

Toprol-XL
100 mg
p. 166

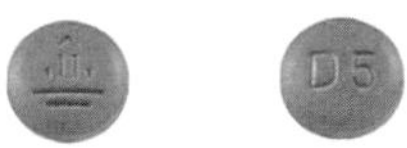

Tradjenta
5 mg
p. 420

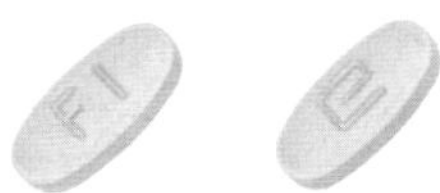

TriCor
48 mg
p. 489

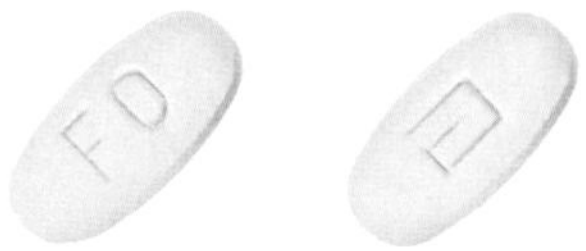	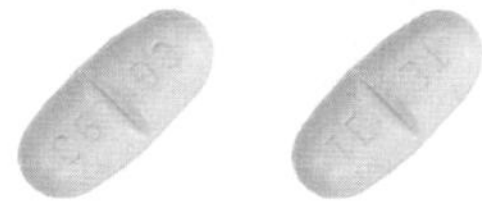
TriCor 145 mg p. 489	**Trileptal** 300 mg p. 241
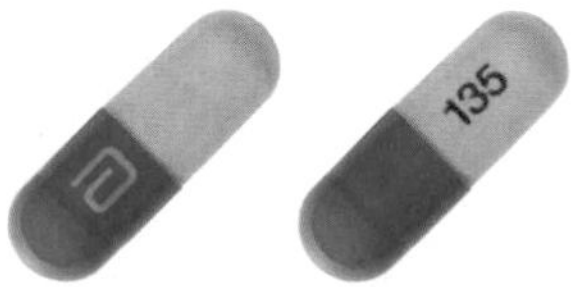	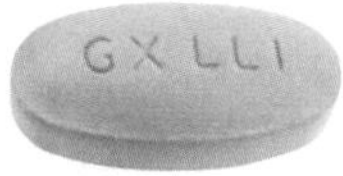
Trilipix 135 mg p. 489	**Trizivir** 300/150/300 mg p. 555
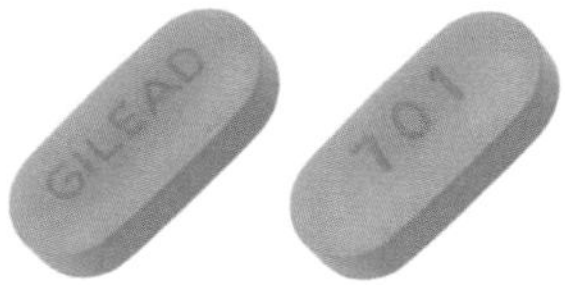	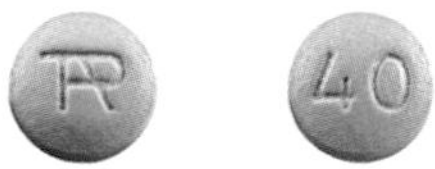
Truvada 200/300 mg p. 555	**Uloric** 40 mg p. 66
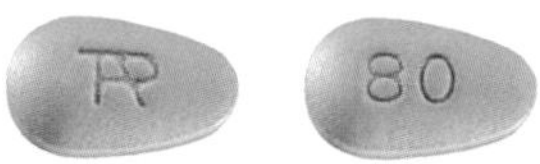	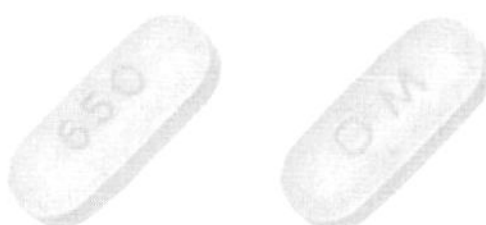
Uloric 80 mg p. 66	**Ultracet** 37.5/325 mg p. 823
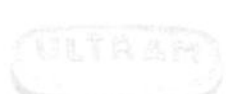	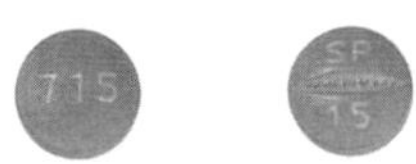
Ultram 50 mg p. 823	**Univasc** 15 mg p. 7

Valium
5 mg
p. 157

Valium
10 mg
p. 157

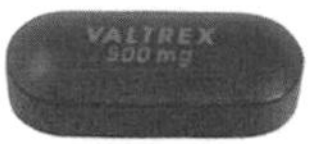

Valtrex
500 mg
p. 26

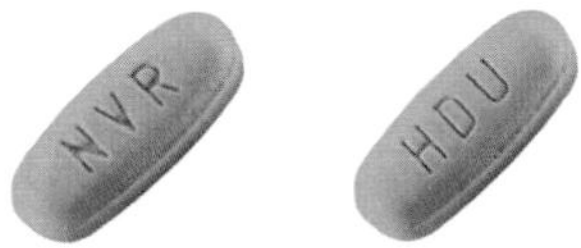

Valturna
150/160 mg
p. 59

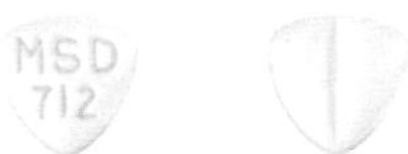

Vasotec
5 mg
p. 7

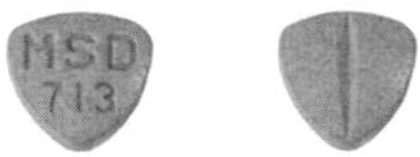

Vasotec
10 mg
p. 7

Verelan
240 mg
p. 224

VESIcare
5 mg
p. 884

VESIcare
10 mg
p. 884

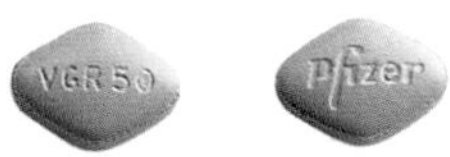

Viagra
50 mg
p. 453

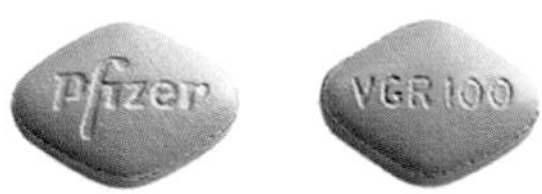

Viagra
100 mg
p. 453

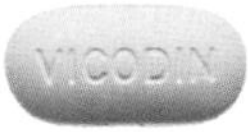

Vicodin
5/500 mg
p. 823

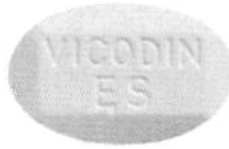

Vicodin-ES
7.5/750 mg
p. 823

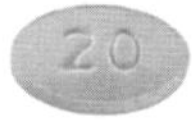

Viibryd
20 mg
p. 1217

Vytorin
10/20 mg
pp. 480, 1065

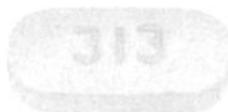

Vytorin
10/40 mg
pp. 480, 1065

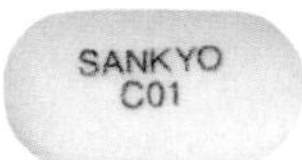

WelChol
625 mg
p. 283

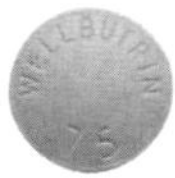

Wellbutrin
75 mg
p. 206

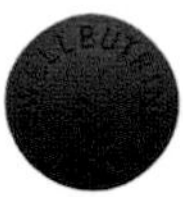

Wellbutrin
100 mg
p. 206

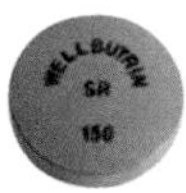

Wellbutrin SR
150 mg
p. 206

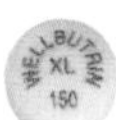

Wellbutrin XL
150 mg
p. 206

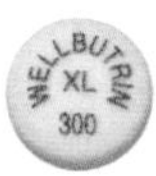

Wellbutrin XL
300 mg
p. 206

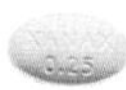

Xanax
0.25 mg
p. 157

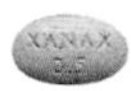

Xanax
0.5 mg
p. 157

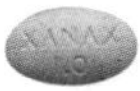

Xanax
1 mg
p. 157

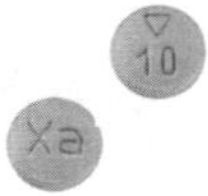

Xarelto
10 mg
p. 401

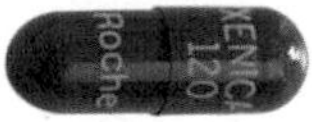

Xenical
120 mg
p. 878

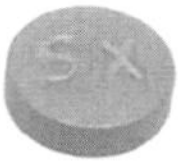

Xifaxan
200 mg
p. 1005

Yasmin
3/0.03 mg
p. 316

Yaz
3/0.02 mg
p. 316

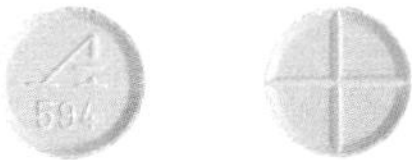

Zanaflex
4 mg
p. 1146

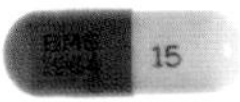

Zerit
15 mg
p. 555

Zerit
20 mg
p. 555

Zerit
30 mg
p. 555

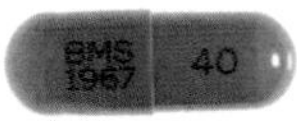

Zerit
40 mg
p. 555

	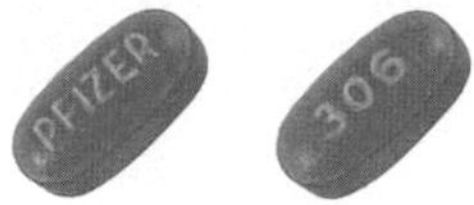
Zetia 10 mg p. 480	**Zithromax** 250 mg p. 138
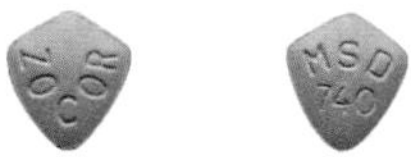	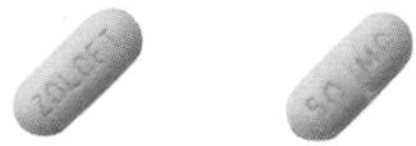
Zocor 20 mg p. 1065	**Zoloft** 50 mg p. 1045
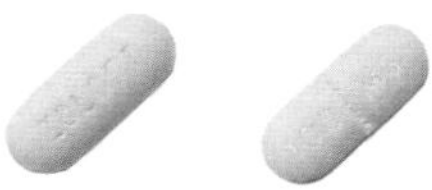	
Zoloft 100 mg p. 1045	**Zomig** 5 mg p. 1187
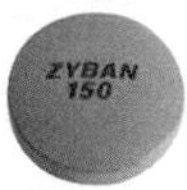	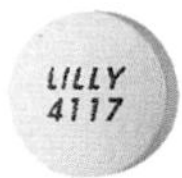
Zyban 150 mg p. 206	**Zyprexa** 10 mg p. 961
	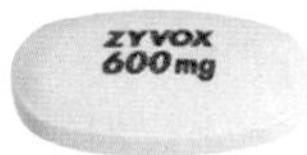
Zyrtec 5 mg p. 265	**Zyvox** 600 mg p. 691

may be grounds for an abortion due to the severe birth defects this drug will cause. Contact your doctor immediately.

It is not known if isotretinoin passes into breast milk. Nursing mothers who must take it should use infant formula.

Seniors: Seniors may take this medication without special restriction.

Janumet *see **Sitagliptin,** page 420*

Januvia *see **Sitagliptin,** page 420*

Kariva *see **Contraceptives,** page 316*

Generic Name

Ketotifen (kee-toe-TIH-fen) G

Brand Names

Alaway Eye Drops
Claritin Eye
Refresh Eye Itch Relief
Zaditor Eye Drops
ZyrTEC Itchy Eye

The information in this profile also applies to the following drug:

Generic Ingredients: Lodoxamide
Alomide Eye Drops

Type of Drug

Antihistamine.

Prescribed For

Conjunctivitis (pinkeye) caused by allergies, and itching of the eyes caused by allergic reaction.

General Information

Ketotifen relieves and prevents eye itchiness and irritation associated with seasonal allergies. Lodoxamide only treats itchiness and allergies. They achieve their effects by stabilizing mast cells in the eye, which prevents the release of chemicals such as histamine that cause redness and irritation during an allergic reaction. Ketotifen starts working within minutes after administering the drops. This drug has not been studied in children under age 3. Lodoxamide may be used in children age 2 and over.

Cautions and Warnings

Do not use this drug if you are **allergic** or **sensitive** to any of its ingredients.

Possible Side Effects

- ▼ Most common: eye redness, headache, and runny nose.
- ▼ Less common: a burning or stinging sensation in the eye, eye discharge, tearing, increased sensitivity to bright light, dilation of the pupil, allergic reactions, rash, flu-like symptoms, and sore throat.

Drug Interactions

If you use more than 1 eye-drop medication, separate doses of these drugs by at least 1 hour.

Usual Dose

Ketotifen

Adult and Child (age 3 and over): 1 drop in the affected eye every 8–12 hours.

Lodoxamide

Adult and Child (age 2 and over): 1–2 drops in the affected eye 4 times a day.

Overdosage

Accidental ingestion of an entire bottle of ketotifen is unlikely to cause side effects because it contains less than 2 mg of medicine. Contact your local poison control center or a hospital emergency room for more information. If you seek treatment, ALWAYS bring the prescription bottle or container.

Special Information

Do not wear contact lenses if your eyes are red, because they may worsen the irritation.

Ketotifen does not alleviate eye irritation caused by contact lenses.

Remove your soft contact lenses before using ketotifen eye drops; you may replace them 10 minutes after a dose.

To prevent contamination, do not allow the eyedropper to touch your fingers, eyelids, or any surface.

If you forget to administer a dose, do so as soon as you remember. If it is almost time for your next dose, skip the dose you forgot and continue with your regular schedule. Do not take a double dose.

Special Populations

Pregnancy/Breast-feeding: In animal studies, very large dosages of ketotifen caused bone malformations in the fetus. Ketotifen should be used during pregnancy only if your doctor determines that the potential benefit outweighs the risks.

Though unlikely, ketotifen may pass into breast milk. Nursing mothers who must use this drug should use infant formula.

Seniors: Seniors may use this drug without special precaution.

Generic Name

Labetalol (luh-BET-uh-lol) G

Brand Names

Trandate

Type of Drug

Adrenergic blocker and antihypertensive.

Prescribed For

Hypertension (high blood pressure).

General Information

Labetalol hydrochloride is unique because it selectively blocks both alpha- and beta-adrenergic impulses. This combination of actions contributes to its ability to reduce blood pressure. Other drugs can increase or decrease heart rate; labetalol has an advantage over other beta blockers because it rarely affects heart rate. Labetalol may be used alone or in combination with other antihypertensive drugs, especially loop and thiazide diuretics.

Cautions and Warnings

Do not take labetalol if you are **allergic** or **sensitive** to any of its ingredients. People with **asthma**, **chronic bronchitis**, **emphysema**, severe **heart failure**, **reduced heart rate**, and **heart**

block (disruption of the electrical impulses that control heart rate) should not take labetalol.

People with **angina** who take labetalol for hypertension risk aggravating their angina if they suddenly stop taking the drug. These people should have their dosage reduced gradually over 1–2 weeks.

Those with **diabetes** should take this medication with caution. Labetalol may mask symptoms of low blood sugar such as rapid heart rate and require dosage adjustments of antidiabetes medications.

Labetalol should be used with caution if you have **liver disease**.

Possible Side Effects

Side effects develop early and increase with dosage.

- ▼ Most common: dizziness, tingling of the scalp, nausea, upset stomach, distortion in the sense of taste, fatigue, sweating, impotence, urinary difficulties, bile-duct blockage, bronchial spasm, breathing difficulties, muscle weakness, cramps, dry eyes, blurred vision, rash, facial swelling, and hair loss.
- ▼ Less common: aggravation of lupus erythematosus (a chronic autoimmune disease), stuffy nose, headache, depression, confusion, disorientation, loss of short-term memory, emotional instability, colitis, drug allergy (symptoms include fever, sore throat, and breathing difficulties), and a reduction in levels of white blood cells and blood platelets.

Drug Interactions

- Labetalol may suppress normal signs of low blood sugar and interfere with the action of oral antidiabetes drugs.
- Combining labetalol and a tricyclic antidepressant may cause tremor.
- Labetalol may interfere with the effect of some antiasthma drugs; dosage increases may be necessary.
- In patients who are prone to severe allergic reactions, labetalol may interfere with the action of ephedrine, used to treat such reactions.
- Cimetidine increases the amount of labetalol absorbed into the bloodstream from oral tablets.

- Labetalol may increase the blood-pressure-lowering effect of nitroglycerin.
- Use caution when combining labetalol with calcium channel blockers, especially verapamil.
- Labetalol should not be combined with halothane anesthesia.
- Mixing labetalol with digoxin or another digitalis drug slows heart rate.

Food Interactions

This drug may be taken with food if it upsets your stomach. Food increases the amount of labetalol absorbed into the blood.

Usual Dose

Adult: starting dose—100 mg twice a day; may be increased by 100 mg twice a day every 2–3 days to as much as 1200 mg twice a day. Usual dose—200–400 mg twice a day.

Child: 0.45–1.3 mg per lb. divided in 2 doses a day. The maximum recommended dose is 1200 mg.

Seniors: 100–200 mg twice a day.

Overdosage

Overdose slows heart rate and causes an excessive drop in blood pressure. The possible consequences of these effects can be treated only in a hospital emergency room. If you seek treatment, ALWAYS bring the prescription bottle or container.

Special Information

You may experience scalp tingling, especially when you first start taking labetalol.

Labetalol should be taken on a continuing basis. Do not stop this drug unless instructed to do so by your doctor.

Weakness; swelling of your ankles, feet, or legs; breathing difficulties; or other side effects should be reported to your doctor as soon as possible. Most side effects are not serious, but about 7% of people have to switch to another drug because of them.

If you forget a dose, take it as soon as possible. If it is within 8 hours of your next dose, skip the dose you forgot and go back to your regular schedule. Do not take a double dose.

Special Populations

Pregnancy/Breast-feeding: Labetalol enters the fetal circulation. Women who are or might be pregnant should not take this drug without their doctor's approval. Labetalol should be taken during pregnancy only if your doctor determines that the potential benefit outweighs the risks.

This drug passes into breast milk. Nursing mothers who must take labetalol should use infant formula.

Seniors: Seniors may be more sensitive to the effects of labetalol. Your dosage must be individually adjusted by your doctor, especially if you have liver disease. Seniors may be more likely to suffer from cold hands and feet, reduced body temperature, chest pain, feeling unwell, sudden breathing difficulties, sweating, or changes in heartbeat.

Generic Name

Lacosamide (lah-KOS-ah-mide)

Brand Names

Vimpat

Type of Drug

Anticonvulsant.

Prescribed For

Partial onset seizures.

General Information

Partial onset seizures affect a specific area of the brain, unlike generalized seizures, which affect the entire brain. Partial seizure symptoms can include muscle spasms, twitching or jerking movements, and eyeball rolling. Sudden detachment, or staring into space, can also occur. Partial seizures can last for a few to 30 or more seconds. Partial seizures are generally treated with anticonvulsant drugs for prevention, but the primary goal is to prevent physical injury caused by the seizure itself. Lacosamide may be given either by mouth or as an intravenous injection, depending on the patient's circumstances. This drug can produce euphoria, but lacosamide dependence has not been reported.

Cautions and Warnings

Do not take lacosamide if you are **allergic** or **sensitive** to any of its ingredients. With some anticonvulsant medicines, sensitivity reactions can occur in more than 1 organ, such as the liver, kidney, heart, and/or lymph glands. This has not been reported with lacosamide, but your doctor may decide to stop the medication if multiple reactions develop.

Anticonvulsant medicines increase the risk of depression, suicidal thoughts, and attempted suicide. Anyone taking lacosamide or any other anticonvulsant medicine should be carefully watched for new or worsening mood changes or behaviors.

Lacosamide can affect heart function by causing atrioventricular block (a disturbance in the impulses between heart chambers). In studies of lacosamide, this was more common among people with nerve damage caused by **diabetes**. People with **heart disease** should use this drug with caution. Your doctor may take an electrocardiogram (ECG) immediately after you take the medicine to see how it affects your heart's electrical system.

People with mild to moderate **liver disease** should have their dosage increased very carefully. No more than 300 mg a day is recommended. People with severe liver disease should not use this medicine.

People with **kidney disease** do not need any dose adjustment, but their maximum recommended dose is 300 mg per day.

As with all anticonvulsant medicines, do not abruptly stop taking lacosamide. The drug dose should be gradually reduced over at least a week to reduce the chances of drug withdrawal seizures.

Possible Side Effects

Side effects increase in number with increasing drug dose.

- ▼ Most common: dizziness, headache, blurred or double vision, nausea, and vomiting.
- ▼ Common: poor coordination, diarrhea, fatigue, tiredness, tremors, rhythmic shaking or wobbling of the eyes, and difficulty maintaining balance.
- ▼ Less common: fainting when standing up, low blood pressure, unusual walk, weakness, memory loss, depression, and itching.
- ▼ Rare: heart palpitations; rapid pulse; difficulty breathing; hepatitis; euphoria; rash; and kidney, liver, and heart muscle inflammation. Other rare side effects can affect almost any part of the body. Contact your doctor if you experience anything unusual while taking any medication.

Drug Interactions

None known.

Food Interactions

Lacosamide can be taken without regard to food or meals.

Usual Dose

Adult and Child (age 17 and over): 50–200 mg twice a day.

Child: not recommended.

Overdosage

One person took 12,000 mg of lacosamide along with large doses of other anticonvulsant drugs. The patient went into a coma, was hospitalized, and released 2 days later. Smaller overdoses are expected to produce exaggerated drug side effects. Take the overdose victim to a hospital emergency room at once. If you seek treatment, ALWAYS bring the prescription bottle or container.

Special Information

Your doctor must balance the potential benefits of treatment with lacosamide against the risk of new or worsening depression or suicidal thoughts or actions. Report anything unusual to your doctor at once.

Lacosamide may cause dizziness and/or poor muscle coordination that can affect your fingers, hands, arms, legs, body, eye movements, and speech. Do not drive or do anything requiring intense concentration until you see how the medicine affects you.

Lacosamide can affect your heart. Contact your doctor at once if you experience heart palpitations, rapid pulse, or difficulty breathing.

Do not stop taking lacosamide unless your doctor tells you to do so. If you forget a dose, take it as soon as you remember. If you do not remember until it is almost time for your next dose, skip the forgotten dose and go back to your regular schedule. Contact your doctor if you forget 2 or more doses in a row. Do not take a double dose.

Special Populations

Pregnancy/Breast-feeding: In animal studies, lacosamide damaged the developing fetus, but there is no information on the effect of lacosamide on the developing fetus in humans. There is no information on the effect of lacosamide during pregnancy. Lacosamide should be taken during pregnancy only if your doctor determines that the potential benefit outweighs the risks.

This drug passes into breast milk. Nursing mothers who must take it should use infant formula.

Seniors: Seniors may be sensitive to the side effects of this drug, though too few were included in clinical studies to establish any meaningful differences. Care should be taken as the drug dose is increased.

Generic Name

Lamotrigine (lam-OE-trih-jene) G

Brand Names

Lamictal
Lamictal CD
Lamictal ODT
Lamictal XR

Type of Drug

Anticonvulsant.

Prescribed For

Adult epilepsy and partial seizures; tonic-clonic, temporal lobe, absence, and myoclonic seizures; bipolar disorder; and for infants and children with Lennox-Gastaut syndrome.

General Information

Much like phenytoin and carbamazepine, lamotrigine stabilizes voltage-dependent channels in the brain. This prevents the release of chemicals that would stimulate the nervous system and lead to seizure. It reaches maximum blood concentration in 1.5–5 hours. Lamotrigine is eliminated from the body by the liver.

Cautions and Warnings

Do not take lamotrigine if you are **allergic** or **sensitive** to any of its ingredients.

Lamotrigine may cause severe and possibly life-threatening rashes, nearly always within 2–8 weeks of use. Minor rashes also occur, but it is not possible to tell which ones may become life threatening. If you develop a rash or swollen glands while taking this drug, contact your doctor at once.

Five people taking lamotrigine died from acute liver failure or multi-organ failure before the drug was approved for general use. It is not known if the drug played a role in these deaths.

Antiepileptic medications have been associated with an increased risk of suicidal thoughts and behavior. Patients being treated with lamotrigine for bipolar disorder should be watched for signs of worsening **depression** or the emergence of suicidal thoughts or behavior.

Lamotrigine may increase the risk of developing meningitis, inflammation of the tissues lining the brain and spinal cord.

When you stop taking lamotrigine, the dose should be reduced gradually over a period of 2 weeks or more to prevent withdrawal seizures.

Status epilepticus, a severe seizure disorder, and worsening of existing **seizure disorders** may develop in a small number of people taking lamotrigine.

Twenty sudden and unexplained deaths occurred among 4700 people taking lamotrigine before it was approved for general use. As unexplained deaths are more common in people with epilepsy than in the general population, these deaths are thought to be unrelated to lamotrigine.

Lamotrigine binds to melanin, a body hormone found in the skin and eyes. The long-term effects of lamotrigine on the eyes are not known.

People with **kidney or liver disease** should use this drug with caution.

Lamotrigine may cause unusual sensitivity to the sun. Wear protective clothing and use sunscreen.

Possible Side Effects

▼ Most common: headache, dizziness, nausea, vomiting, weakness, tiredness, loss of coordination, double vision, and blurred vision.

▼ Common: accidental injury, flu-like symptoms, abdominal pain, infection, neck pain, feeling unwell, worsening of seizures, diarrhea, upset stomach, constipation, dental problems, sleeplessness, tremors, depression, anxiety, convulsions, irritability, itching, visual difficulties, painful menstruation, and vaginal irritation.

▼ Less common: chills, hot flashes, heart palpitations, appetite loss, dry mouth, joint ache, muscle weakness, speech disorders, sore throat, coughing, memory loss, confusion, loss of concentration, emotional upset, fainting, racing thoughts, rolling of the eyes, muscle spasm, breathing difficulties, hair loss, acne, ear pain, ringing or buzzing in the ears, and missed periods.

Possible Side Effects *(continued)*

▼ Rare: Rare side effects can occur in almost any part of the body. Contact your doctor if you experience anything unusual while taking any medication.

Drug Interactions

- Combining acetaminophen and lamotrigine can slightly increase the rate at which lamotrigine is broken down, but occasional use of the 2 drugs together is not likely to be a problem. Regular acetaminophen users may require more lamotrigine.
- Anti-folate drugs—often used in cancer treatment—can increase the effects of lamotrigine.
- Combining carbamazepine and lamotrigine increases carbamazepine blood levels, possibly leading to side effects, and reduces the amount of lamotrigine in the blood by 40%.
- Hormone replacement therapy and contraceptives decrease levels of lamotrigine by ½. The effectiveness of levonorgestrel may also be lowered when taken with lamotrigine.
- Phenobarbital, phenytoin, and primidone reduce concentrations of lamotrigine in the blood by 40%.
- Sertraline may elevate lamotrigine levels.
- Protease inhibitors (such as ritonavir and saquinavir), orlistat, oxcarbazepine, rifamycins (such as rifampin), and succinimides may reduce the effectiveness of lamotrigine.
- Clozapine and topiramate concentrations are increased when given with lamotrigine.
- Combining lamotrigine and sodium valproate doubles lamotrigine concentrations in the blood and reduces those of valproate by ¼. Dosage adjustments are necessary. Combining these drugs may also increase the risk of rash.

Food Interactions

None known.

Usual Dose

The safety and efficacy of treating children under age 18 for bipolar disorder with lamotrigine has not been established.

Adult and Child (age 12 and over): starting dose—25 mg every other day or 25–50 mg every day depending on other medications being taken concurrently for seizure control. Increase gradually to a maximum daily dose of 500 mg. Lamotrigine is usually taken twice a day; be sure to take your doses 12 hours apart. The chewable tablets can be swallowed whole, chewed, or dissolved in water or fruit juice.

Child (under age 12): Consult your doctor.

Overdosage

Symptoms include dizziness, headache, sleepiness, and coma. Take the victim to a hospital emergency room at once. If you seek treatment, ALWAYS bring the prescription bottle or container.

Special Information

Dosage increases may be required if your liver starts breaking down the drug faster over time. Periodic monitoring of lamotrigine blood levels is necessary to determine this.

People with impaired kidney or liver function may require smaller dosages.

Contact your doctor at once if you develop a rash or swollen glands, but do not change your lamotrigine dosage or stop taking it until your doctor tells you to do so. If you stop taking lamotrigine on your own, do not restart it without telling your doctor.

Call your doctor if you develop headache, fever, stiff neck, nausea, vomiting, rash, and sensitivity to light. These can be signs of meningitis, inflammation of the tissues that cover the spinal cord and brain.

Lamotrigine may cause drowsiness, dizziness, or blurred vision, effects that are increased by alcohol. Be careful while driving or engaging in any activity requiring concentration, alertness, and coordination.

If you take acetaminophen while you are taking lamotrigine, especially for a lamotrigine headache, do not take more acetaminophen than is recommended on the package.

If you take lamotrigine once a day and forget a dose, take it as soon as you remember. If it is within 8 hours of your next dose, skip the one you forgot and continue with your regular schedule. Do not take a double dose.

After the first 2 weeks of treatment, most people take lamotrigine twice a day. If you take it twice a day, be sure to take your medication every 12 hours. If you forget a dose, take it as soon as you remember. If it is within 4 hours of your next dose, take 1 dose as soon as you remember and another in 5 or 6 hours, then go back to your regular schedule.

Special Populations

Pregnancy/Breast-feeding: Animal studies suggest that lamotrigine causes fetal injury. It reduces the amount of folate in the fetus, an effect that is associated with birth defects. Seizure disorder itself also increases the risk of birth defects. Lamotrigine should be taken during pregnancy only if your doctor determines that the potential benefit outweighs the risks.

Lamotrigine passes into breast milk. Nursing mothers who must take it should use infant formula.

Seniors: Seniors may take lamotrigine without special restriction.

Generic Name

Lanthanum (LANTH-uh-num)

Brand Names

Fosrenol

Type of Drug

Phosphate binder.

Prescribed For

High blood-phosphate levels (hyperphosphatemia) in people with end-stage renal disease (ESRD).

General Information

People with ESRD, a form of kidney disease, tend to retain phosphorous. High phosphate levels, in turn, can affect calcium balance in the body and cause deposits of this mineral to build up in the wrong places. Lanthanum helps manage high blood-phosphate levels by binding to phosphate in food before it can be absorbed into the blood. This is the same mechanism used by other phosphate-lowering drugs (sevelamer and the antacids aluminum hydroxide and calcium carbonate). Lanthanum, like other phosphate binders, must be taken with meals so that it can bind phosphate ions in the stomach before they can be absorbed into the blood. Very little of this drug is absorbed into the blood and it is not broken down in the body.

Cautions and Warnings

Do not take lanthanum if you are **allergic** or **sensitive** to any of its ingredients.

People with an **active peptic ulcer**, **ulcerative colitis**, **Crohn's disease**, or **bowel obstruction** should use this medication with caution.

Researchers found no difference in bone fracture rates or overall survival for lanthanum than for other phosphate-binding treatments over 3 years. The study period was too short to assume that it would improve bone fractures or survival beyond 3 years.

Possible Side Effects

Side effects primarily affect the digestive tract and are similar to other phosphate-lowering treatments in type and frequency.

- ▼ Most common: nausea, vomiting, complications with the dialysis graft, diarrhea, constipation, abdominal pain, and low blood pressure.
- ▼ Common: bronchitis and runny nose.
- ▼ Less common: high blood-calcium levels.
- ▼ Rare: Other side effects may affect any organ or organ system. Contact your doctor if you experience anything unusual while taking any medication.

Drug Interactions

- Lanthanum strongly binds to phosphate in the stomach and might also bind to other medications in the stomach. However, no interaction was found in tests conducted with digoxin, enalapril, furosemide, metoprolol, phenytoin, or warfarin.
- Compounds known to interact with antacids should not be taken within 2 hours of taking lanthanum.

Food Interactions

Lanthanum must be taken with or immediately after meals.

Usual Dose

Adult: Initially, 750–1500 mg a day with or immediately after each meal, in divided doses. Effective daily dosage may be increased in increments of 750 mg every 2–3 weeks, up to 3000 mg, until normal blood-phosphate levels are reached. Completely chew each tablet before you swallow it. Do not swallow whole tablets.

Child: not recommended.

Overdosage

There have been no reports of lanthanum overdose, even with single doses up to 1000 mg per lb. of body weight. Symptoms of overdose are likely to occur in the digestive tract. Overdose victims may be taken to a hospital emergency room for evaluation. If you seek treatment, ALWAYS bring the prescription bottle or container.

Special Information

If you forget to take lanthanum with or immediately after a meal, skip the forgotten dose and continue with your regular schedule.

Be sure to follow the low-phosphate diet your doctor prescribes. It is a key element in helping to manage your blood-phosphate levels.

Special Populations

Pregnancy/Breast-feeding: Animal studies with doses several times the maximum human dose revealed some harm to the developing fetus. Pregnancy in a woman with ESRD, especially those on dialysis, is uncommon because of reduced fertility; ESRD carries serious risks for a pregnant woman and her baby, including anemia, uncontrolled high blood pressure, and infection. This drug is not recommended for pregnant women.

It is not known if lanthanum passes into breast milk. Nursing mothers who must take it should use infant formula.

Seniors: Seniors may use this medication without special restriction.

Lantus *see **Insulin,** page 628*

Generic Name

Leflunomide (leh-FLUE-noe-mide) G

Brand Names

Arava

Type of Drug

Anti-inflammatory and antiproliferative (slows cell growth).

Prescribed For

Rheumatoid arthritis.

General Information

Leflunomide can help relieve symptoms of rheumatoid arthritis and slow the structural damage and erosion of tissues in affected joints. In studies, it was found to be as effective as methotrexate and sulfasalazine. It takes about a month for leflunomide to begin working, and it reaches maximum effect in 3–6 months. The maximum effect is retained for as long as you take this medicine. Leflunomide is broken down in the liver.

Cautions and Warnings

Do not take leflunomide if you are **allergic** or **sensitive** to any of its ingredients.

This drug can reactivate dormant **tuberculosis**. Make sure your doctor knows if you have ever had tuberculosis before you start taking this medication.

Leflunomide may cause liver irritation and an increase in certain liver enzymes, as well as severe liver injury. Your dosage may need to be reduced or the drug discontinued if the effect is severe. People with **liver disease** or **hepatitis B or C** should not take this drug. People with **kidney problems** should use it with caution.

Leflunomide is not recommended for people with severely **depressed immune systems**, **abnormal bone marrow**, or severe and uncontrolled **infection**.

New or worsening cough and difficulty breathing with or without fever may be a sign of an important drug side effect. Contact your doctor at once if this happens.

Use of live virus vaccines is not recommended while taking leflunomide.

Rare, serious skin reactions can occur with this drug. Contact your doctor if you develop a skin rash or lesion in your mouth, nose, or rectum.

Possible Side Effects

- ▼ Most common: diarrhea, high blood pressure, nausea, hair loss, rash, and respiratory infection.
- ▼ Common: headache, upset stomach, stomach or abdominal pain, abnormal liver function, bronchitis, generalized pain, itching, back pain, urinary infection, and accidents or injuries.
- ▼ Less common: chest pain, dizziness, tingling in the hands or feet, eczema, mouth ulcer, tooth disorder, dry skin, appetite loss, vomiting, low blood potassium, weight loss, muscle pain, leg cramps, inflamed tendons, arthritis, cough, sore

Possible Side Effects *(continued)*

throat, pneumonia, runny nose, sinus irritation, allergic reaction, weakness, flu-like symptoms, and infections.

▼ Rare: Rare side effects can occur in almost any part of the body. Contact your doctor if you experience anything unusual while taking any medication.

Drug Interactions

- Cholestyramine and charcoal rapidly reduce leflunomide blood levels. Do not mix these medications.
- Leflunomide can increase the liver toxicity of other drugs that are toxic to the liver, such as methotrexate. Your doctor should carefully monitor your condition if you must take leflunomide with one of these medications.
- Rifampin increases the amount of leflunomide in the blood by 40%. These drugs should be mixed with caution.
- Leflunomide increases blood levels of nonsteroidal anti-inflammatory drugs (NSAIDs). The importance of this effect is unclear.
- Leflunomide increases the amount of tolbutamide (an anti-diabetes drug) in the blood by up to 50%. The importance of this effect is unclear.
- Leflunomide, in rare cases, can increase the effects of warfarin.

Food Interactions

Leflunomide can be taken without regard to food or meals.

Usual Dose

Adult: 100 mg once a day for 3 days, then 20 mg once a day. If the side effects are intolerable, the dose may be lowered to 10 mg a day.

Child: not recommended.

When you stop taking leflunomide, it is recommended that you follow a drug elimination procedure: Take 8 g of cholestyramine (ordinarily used to help lower blood cholesterol) 3 times a day for 11 days. Without this procedure, it may take up to 2 years to eliminate the drug and its breakdown products from your body.

Overdosage

Symptoms are likely to include drug side effects. Take the victim to a hospital emergency room at once. If you seek treatment, ALWAYS bring the prescription bottle or container.

Special Information

Your liver function must be monitored regularly while you take this drug. Likewise, your blood pressure should be checked before starting this medicine and regularly while you are on it.

Men who wish to father a child should not attempt to do so without following the drug elimination procedure (see "Usual Dose").

If you forget a dose, take it as soon as you remember. If it is almost time for your next dose, skip the one you forgot and continue with your regular schedule. Do not take a double dose.

Special Populations

Pregnancy/Breast-feeding: Leflunomide causes birth defects and should not be used during pregnancy. Women of childbearing age must be tested for pregnancy before taking leflunomide and use effective contraception during treatment and until the drug is completely eliminated from the body. Women who plan to become pregnant after discontinuing the drug must follow the drug elimination procedure (see "Usual Dose").

Leflunomide may pass into breast milk. Nursing mothers who must take it should use infant formula.

Seniors: Seniors may take this drug without special precaution.

Generic Name

Lenalidomide **(len-ah-LID-oh-mide)**

Brand Names

Revlimid

Type of Drug

Immune system modulator.

Prescribed For

Multiple myeloma and transfusion-dependent anemia.

General Information

Lenalidomide has a number of known actions, including antineoplastic and immune system modulating. It also stops cancerous tumors from growing the new blood vessels that feed them, therefore stopping the tumor's growth, and acts as an anti-inflammatory agent by decreasing inflammatory proteins and increasing anti-inflammatory proteins in the body. Its exact mechanism of action in multiple myeloma and anemia is not known. When prescribed for multiple myeloma, it is accompanied by dexamethasone, a corticosteroid drug. It is rapidly absorbed into the bloodstream and probably passes out of the body in the urine. Lenalidomide is available only through doctors and pharmacies that have registered with a special distribution program called RevAssist, designed to prevent pregnant women from taking it.

Cautions and Warnings

Do not take lenalidomide if you are **allergic** or **sensitive** to any of its ingredients.

Lenalidomide can cause birth defects and fetal death. Do not take it if you are **pregnant**. Women of childbearing age must have 2 negative pregnancy tests and use an effective form of birth control for 4 weeks prior to starting treatment with lenalidomide. Men taking this drug—even those who have had a vasectomy—must wear a condom to protect female partners from exposure to semen containing lenalidomide and continue this practice for 4 weeks after stopping the medicine. For more information, see "Pregnancy/Breast-feeding."

Lenalidomide is associated with significant reductions in white-blood-cell and platelet counts, so people taking it should have blood counts every week for the first 8 weeks of therapy.

Lenalidomide increases the risk of blood clots in the lungs and deep veins in the legs. Shortness of breath, chest pain, and arm or leg swelling can be signs a clot has formed.

Serious, possibly life-threatening skin reactions, including Stevens-Johnson syndrome, have occurred in children and adults taking this medicine. Tell your doctor at once if you develop any type of skin reaction to the drug.

People receiving this medicine may be more likely to develop new cancers.

People with **kidney disease** should receive reduced dosages of lenalidomide.

Possible Side Effects

▼ Most common: reduced white-blood-cell count without fever and reduced platelet count, itching, rash, dry skin, diarrhea, constipation, nausea, abdominal pain, vomiting, sore throat, nose and throat irritation, cough, difficulty breathing, nosebleeds, fatigue, fever, arm or leg swelling,

Possible Side Effects *(continued)*

generalized pain, joint pain, muscle cramps, leg pain, dizziness, and headache.

▼ Common: reduced white-blood-cell count with fever, dry mouth, bruising, night sweats, increase in overall sweating, nosebleeds, swelling, loose stools, shortness of breath after exercise, runny nose, bronchitis, shaking chills, muscle pain, reduced sense of touch, taste changes, tingling or pain in the hands or feet, low blood levels of potassium or magnesium, appetite loss, sleeplessness, depression, high blood pressure, pain on urination, heart palpitations, and low thyroid activity.

▼ Less common: fainting, respiratory and other infections, fluid in the lungs, multi-organ failure, weakness, and confusion.

▼ Rare: Rare side effects can affect almost any part of the body. Contact your doctor if you experience anything unusual while taking any medication.

Drug Interactions

- Lenalidomide can increase blood levels of digoxin by 14%. Periodic testing of digoxin blood levels with possible dose adjustment is recommended.

Food Interactions

Lenalidomide can be taken without regard to food or meals.

Usual Dose

Adult: starting dose—10–25 mg a day with water, reduced for those with kidney disease.

Child: not recommended.

Overdosage

There is no information on lenalidomide overdose. Take the overdose victim to a hospital emergency room at once for treatment. If you seek treatment, ALWAYS bring the prescription bottle or container.

Special Information

Do not break, chew, or open lenalidomide capsules.

Contact your doctor at once if you develop difficulty breathing, chest pain, or arm or leg swelling.

If you forget a dose of lenalidomide, take it as soon as you remember. If you do not remember until it is almost time for your next dose, skip the one you forgot and continue with your regular schedule. Do not take a double dose.

Special Populations

Pregnancy/Breast-feeding: Lenalidomide is related to thalidomide, a drug known to damage or kill a developing fetus. Pregnant women should not take lenalidomide. If you miss a period or have irregular bleeding, you may be pregnant. Women who suspect that they are pregnant must contact their doctor at once and stop taking lenalidomide immediately.

Women of childbearing age must have a negative pregnancy test within 10–14 days before treatment and again within a day before starting the drug, weekly for the first month and then once a month in women with regular cycles or every 2 weeks in women with irregular cycles. Women of childbearing age with no alternative to lenalidomide must use 2 contraceptive methods: a highly effective one such as a hormonal contraceptive, an intrauterine device (IUD), a surgical method such as a tubal ligation (tubes tied) or vasectomy for the male partner; and a less reliable one such as a condom, diaphragm, or cervical cap. These protective measures should begin 4 weeks before starting on lenalidomide and continue until at least 4 weeks after treatment has been completed.

It is not known whether this drug passes into breast milk. Nursing mothers who must take lenalidomide should use infant formula.

Seniors: Seniors are likely to have more drug side effects with the same drug effectiveness as younger adults, due to age-related reductions in kidney function.

Type of Drug

Leukotriene Antagonists/ Inhibitors (LUE-koe-treen)

Brand Names

Generic Ingredients: Montelukast Sodium

Singulair

Singulair Granules

Generic Ingredients: Zafirlukast G
Accolate

Generic Ingredients: Zileuton
Zyflo
Zyflo CR

Prescribed For

Asthma, seasonal allergic rhinitis (montelukast), and exercise-induced bronchial spasm (montelukast). May also be prescribed for itching (montelukast and zafirlukast).

General Information

Leukotrienes play an important role in the body's allergic response. They are associated with the swelling of tissues and tightening of muscles in the throat that cause the throat to close during an asthma attack. Leukotriene receptor antagonists (montelukast and zafirlukast) help to prevent attacks by blocking leukotrienes from binding to special tissue receptors. Zileuton interferes with the formation of leukotrienes and has no effect on the receptors. When taken on a regular basis, these drugs can reduce the number of asthma attacks you experience, but do not treat them once they occur; other drugs must be used to treat acute attacks.

Cautions and Warnings

Do not take leukotriene antagonists or inhibitors if you are **allergic** or **sensitive** to any of their ingredients. It may be possible to be sensitive to one drug and tolerate another. Avoid aspirin and other nonsteroidal anti-inflammatory drugs (NSAIDs) if they have triggered an asthma attack in the past.

Do not use these drugs to treat an **acute asthma attack**. Keep your regular inhalants and other asthma drugs handy at all times in case you have an asthma attack. Leukotrienes do not prevent all attacks.

Neuropsychiatric events have been reported in adults, adolescents, and children taking montelukast and zileuton. Symptoms include sleep disorders and behavior changes. Report any unusual thinking or behavior to your doctor right away.

People with **liver disease** should not take zafirlukast or zileuton. People taking these drugs should have their liver enzymes measured periodically by their doctor. Life-threatening liver failure and unexplained liver injury have developed in people taking zafirlukast.

Possible Side Effects

Montelukast

- ▼ Most common: headache.
- ▼ Less common: influenza, dizziness, upset stomach, gastroenteritis (inflammation of the mucous lining of the stomach and intestine), cough, stuffy nose, nosebleeds, abdominal pain, hypersensitivity reactions, tingling in the hands and feet, reduced sense of touch, dream abnormalities, drowsiness, irritability, and restlessness.
- ▼ Rare: dental pain, rash, fever, injuries, liver damage, weakness, and tiredness. Contact your doctor if you experience anything unusual while taking any medication.

Zafirlukast

- ▼ Most common: headache.
- ▼ Less common: nausea, diarrhea, infections, dizziness, abdominal pain, vomiting, generalized pain, weakness, accidental injury, muscle aches, fever, back pain, and upset stomach.
- ▼ Rare: liver inflammation or damage, low white-blood-cell count, rash, worsening asthma, heart problems, nerve damage, bleeding, bruising, swelling, joint or muscle pain, sleeplessness, itching, and not feeling well. Contact your doctor if you experience anything unusual while taking any medication.

Zileuton

- ▼ Most common: headache.
- ▼ Common: general pains, upset stomach, nausea, and liver inflammation.
- ▼ Less common: abdominal pain, weakness, accidental injury, and muscle aches.
- ▼ Rare: joint pain, chest pain, eye redness, constipation, dizziness, fever, gas, muscle stiffness, sleeplessness, swollen lymph glands, feeling unwell, neck pain or rigidity, nervousness, itching, tiredness, urinary infections, vaginal inflammation, vomiting, and jaundice. Contact your doctor if you experience anything unusual while taking any medication.

Drug Interactions

Montelukast

- Phenobarbital and rifampin can reduce blood levels of montelukast, but dosage adjustment is not needed.

- Gemfibrozil may increase levels of montelukast.
- The adverse effects of prednisone may be increased when combined with montelukast.

Zafirlukast

- Aspirin increases the amount of zafirlukast in the blood by 45%.
- Zafirlukast may increase the effects of other drugs broken down in the liver.
- Erythromycin and theophylline may reduce zafirlukast's effectiveness.
- Zafirlukast increases the effects of warfarin.

Zileuton

- Alcohol use and liver disease may increase the risk of serious side effects.
- Zileuton may increase the effects of pimozide, beta blockers such as propranolol, theophylline, and warfarin. Zileuton should not be given with pimozide. In other cases, dose adjustments and careful monitoring are necessary.

Food Interactions

Zileuton and montelukast may be taken with or without food. Zileuton extended-release tablets should be taken within an hour after breakfast and dinner. For optimal effectiveness, take each dose of zafirlukast at least 1 hour before or 2 hours after meals.

Usual Dose

Montelukast

Those with asthma doses should take this medicine every evening. Allergy patients may take this medicine at any time according to individual need.

Adult and Child (age 15 and over): 10 mg every evening.

Child (age 6–14): 5-mg chewable tablet every evening.

Child (age 2–5): 4-mg chewable tablet or one 4-mg packet of oral granules a day.

Child (age 6–23 months): 4-mg packet of oral granules a day.

Child (under age 6 months): not recommended.

Zafirlukast

Adult and Child (age 12 and over): 20 mg twice a day. Take this medication on an empty stomach, at least 1 hour before or 2 hours after meals.

Child (age 5–11): 10 mg twice a day.
Child (under age 5): not recommended.

Zileuton

Adult and Child (age 12 and over): 600 mg 4 times a day.
Child (under age 12): not recommended.

Zileuton Extended-Release

Adult and Child (age 12 and over): Two 600-mg tablets within an hour after breakfast and dinner.
Child (under age 12): not recommended.

Overdosage

The most common symptoms of montelukast overdose include thirst, tiredness, pupil dilation, excessive movement, and abdominal pain. Symptoms of zafirlukast overdose include rash and upset stomach. Contact your local poison control center or a hospital emergency room for more information. If you seek treatment, ALWAYS bring the prescription bottle or container.

Special Information

These drugs must be taken on a regular basis to prevent asthma attacks. You should continue taking them even if you are having an asthma attack, unless instructed by your doctor to stop.

Your dosage of inhaled corticosteroids, commonly used for asthma prevention, may be gradually reduced if you take these drugs. This reduction should be gradual and occur only under your doctor's supervision. Do not stop using your corticosteroid inhaler without your doctor's knowledge.

Contact your doctor if you develop pain in the upper right portion of your abdomen, nausea, fatigue, lethargy, severe itching, yellowing of the skin or whites of the eyes, flu-like symptoms, and loss of appetite. These may be signs of liver damage.

Contact your doctor if, after starting on a leukotriene antagonist/inhibitor, your need for your regular asthma drug increases.

If you are giving montelukast oral granules to your child, do not open the packet until you are ready to use it. After opening the packet, the full dose must be administered within 15 minutes. The granules can be swallowed directly, dissolved in a teaspoonful of cold or room temperature baby formula or breast milk, or mixed with a spoonful of certain foods at either cold or room temperature. Only applesauce, carrots, rice, or ice cream should be used. If mixed with baby formula, breast milk, or food, it must not be stored for future use. Throw away any unused portion.

If you forget a dose, take it as soon as you remember. If it is almost time for your next dose, skip the one you forgot and continue with your regular schedule. Do not take a double dose.

Special Populations

Pregnancy/Breast-feeding: Montelukast passes into fetal circulation. Zafirlukast and zileuton have harmed the fetus in animal studies using more than 400 times the human dose. A leukotriene antagonist/inhibitor should be taken during pregnancy only if your doctor determines that the potential benefit outweighs the risks.

These drugs pass into breast milk. Nursing mothers who must take any of these drugs should use infant formula.

Seniors: Seniors taking this drug may require reduced dosage.

Levaquin *see **Fluoroquinolone Anti-infectives,** page 512*

Levemir *see **Insulin,** page 628*

Generic Name

Levetiracetam (leh-veh-tir-AS-eh-tam) G

Brand Names

Keppra

Keppra XR

Type of Drug

Antiepileptic.

Prescribed For

Partial onset and other seizure disorders. Levetiracetam can also be prescribed for seizures due to traumatic brain injuries, anxiety, bipolar II disorder, migraine headaches, nerve pain, and substance abuse.

General Information

Levetiracetam works differently than other antiepileptic drugs. Though it does not affect any pathway known to either block or stimulate nerve transmissions, research shows that it can help prevent seizures in adults with epilepsy. Levetiracetam is always prescribed in combination with other antiepileptic medicines.

Cautions and Warnings

Do not take this drug if you are **allergic** or **sensitive** to any of its ingredients.

People with **kidney problems** require a reduced dosage and should use levetiracetam with caution.

Levetiracetam is a nervous system depressant and can cause fatigue, sleepiness, poor coordination, and behavioral changes (including aggression, agitation, anger, anxiety, apathy, depression, emotional instability, and psychosis) in adults, most commonly during the first 4 weeks of treatment. People taking this drug are more likely to have suicidal thoughts or actually attempt suicide.

Almost 40% of **children** taking this drug will become sleepy, fatigued, and develop unusual behaviors such as agitation, anxiety, apathy, depersonalization, depression, emotional instability, hostility, nervousness, neurosis, hyperactivity, and personality disorders.

Antiepileptic drugs, including levetiracetam, have been linked to an increase in suicidal behavior. All patients started on it should be closely monitored, especially in the first few months of treatment, for changes in behavior, worsening of symptoms, or suicidal tendencies.

Levetiracetam can cause reductions in white- and red-blood-cell counts in children and adults. Your doctor will evaluate your blood components periodically.

Possible Side Effects

Adult

- ▼ Most common: tiredness, headache, weakness, and infection.
- ▼ Common: dizziness, pain, and sore throat.
- ▼ Less common: appetite loss, memory loss, anxiety, poor muscle coordination, depression, emotional upset, hostility, nervousness, tingling in the hands or feet, fainting, cough, runny nose, sinus irritation, and double vision.
- ▼ Rare: muscle aches, diarrhea, constipation, stomach problems, chest pain, black-and-blue marks, fever, flu-like symptoms, convulsions, sleeplessness, rash, middle ear

Possible Side Effects *(continued)*

infection, tremors, swollen gums, weight gain, reduced platelet and white-blood-cell counts, inflammation of the pancreas, bone marrow suppression, and hair loss. Contact your doctor if you experience anything unusual while taking any medication.

Child

- ▼ Most common: hostility, sleepiness, nervousness, accidental injury, vomiting, appetite loss, runny nose, sore throat, and coughing.
- ▼ Common: weakness, pain, diarrhea, personality changes, dizziness, emotional instability, and agitation.
- ▼ Less common: itching, skin discoloration, flu-like symptoms and viral infections, facial swelling, neck pain, constipation, stomach pain, black-and-blue marks, depression, confusion, increased reflexes, conjunctivitis (pinkeye), reduced vision in one eye, ear pain, dehydration, and urine abnormalities.
- ▼ Rare: abdominal pain, allergic reaction, loss of muscle coordination, rash, sinus irritation, abnormal thinking, tremors, poor urinary control, convulsions, nosebleeds, fever, headache, hyperactivity, infection, insomnia, and nausea. Contact your doctor if your child experiences anything unusual while taking any medication.

Drug Interactions

Levetiracetam has been studied in adults with a number of other commonly used medicines, including valproate, phenytoin, contraceptive drugs, digoxin, warfarin, and probenecid. No important interactions have been found.

In children, levetiracetam had no effect on blood levels of carbamazepine, valproate, topiramate, or lamotrigine. Some other seizure-control medicines caused an apparent increase in the rate at which this drug is released from the body, but no dose adjustment is needed to account for this effect.

Food Interactions

None known.

Usual Dose

Total daily dose must be reduced for all people with reduced kidney function.

Adult and Child (age 16 and over): starting dose—500 mg twice a day (extended-release form is 1000 mg once a day). Dosage should be increased by 1000 mg a day every 2 weeks to a maximum of 3000 mg a day. Maintenance dose—1500 mg twice a day.

Child (age 6 months–15 years, 44 lbs. or more): 500–1500 mg twice a day, depending on body weight.

Child (age 6 months–15 years, less than 44 lbs.): 250–750 mg twice a day, depending on body weight.

Child (age 1–5 months): 3–9 mg per lb. of body weight twice a day.

Child (under 1 month): not recommended.

Overdosage

The largest known individual dose taken was 6000 mg of levetiracetam. Symptoms may include drowsiness, agitation, aggression, loss of consciousness, difficulty breathing, and coma. Take the overdose victim to a hospital emergency room. If you seek treatment, ALWAYS bring the prescription bottle or container.

Special Information

Levetiracetam must be discontinued gradually. Stopping the drug too suddenly can lead to withdrawal seizures.

Levetiracetam causes dizziness and tiredness. Be careful when driving or performing any task that requires concentration.

Contact your doctor if you become pregnant or are planning on becoming pregnant while taking this medication.

If you forget a dose, take it as soon as you remember. If it is almost time for your next dose, skip the one you forgot and continue with your regular schedule. Do not take a double dose.

Special Populations

Pregnancy/Breast-feeding: Animal studies show that levetiracetam can cause birth defects. Levetiracetam should be taken during pregnancy only if your doctor determines that the potential benefit outweighs the risks. The manufacturer of this drug sponsors a registry to keep track of women who take levetiracetam during pregnancy and their outcomes.

This drug passes into breast milk. Nursing mothers who must take it should use infant formula.

Seniors: Seniors may need less of this medicine than younger adults because of normal declines in kidney function.

Levitra *see **Erectile Dysfunction Drugs,** page 453*

Levoxyl *see **Thyroid Hormone Replacements,** page 1136*

Lexapro *see **Selective Serotonin Reuptake Inhibitors,** page 1045*

Generic Name

Lidocaine (lie-DOE-cane) G

Brand Names

Anecream
LidaMantle
Lidoderm

Combination Products

Generic Ingredients: Lidocaine + Prilocaine
EMLA

Type of Drug

Topical anesthetic.

Prescribed For

Skin pain.

General Information

The anesthetic ingredients in these products penetrate all layers of skin, dulling nerve endings and providing a local anesthetic effect comparable with that produced by injectable drugs. Lidocaine transdermal patch is approved for chronic nerve pain experienced after shingles, but is used for other types of skin pain as well. It alleviates pain specifically associated with postherpetic neuralgia (PHN), an extremely painful complication of the herpes virus. PHN can be severe and debilitating, and over 50% of shingles patients over age 60 and 75% of patients over age 70 experience long-term pain associated with PHN.

EMLA—which stands for eutectic mixture of local anesthetics—is a mixture of anesthetics that turns to liquid on contact with the skin. EMLA can prevent or treat virtually any kind of skin pain and may be used by people of almost any age. It has been used to relieve the pain of intravenous catheter placement, minor plastic and skin surgery, shingles, and injections. EMLA is also available in patch form.

Cautions and Warnings

Do not use these products if you are **allergic** or **sensitive** to any of their ingredients or to amide anesthetics.

People with **methemoglobinemia** (a rare blood condition) should not use these products (see "Drug Interactions").

People with a history of **drug sensitivities** should use these products with caution.

People with severe **liver disease** are more prone to developing toxic blood concentrations of anesthetics because of their impaired ability to metabolize these drugs.

Do not apply EMLA cream beyond the area prescribed by your doctor—otherwise, too much anesthetic may enter your blood and cause systemic side effects. Do not put EMLA cream in your eyes, ears, or mouth. EMLA may, however, be used on genital mucous membranes as an anesthetic for minor surgery. Do not apply either patches or cream to **open wounds**, **burns**, or **broken or inflamed skin**. Do not apply the patch for longer than the recommended wearing time, as it could lead to serious adverse reactions.

Keep out of the reach of children at all times, and dispose of used patches immediately.

Possible Side Effects

- ▼ Most common: blisters, bruising, irritation, redness, burning, and swelling of the area to which it is applied.
- ▼ Common: skin pallor, patches of white skin, itching, rash, and changes in how skin temperature is sensed.
- ▼ Rare: In rare cases when these topical anesthetic products are applied in excess, are used too often, or when too much anesthetic is absorbed, the following reactions may occur: nervous system excitation; nervousness; apprehension; lightheadedness; euphoria (feeling "high"); confusion; dizziness; drowsiness; ringing or buzzing in the ears; blurred or double vision; vomiting; feelings of warmth, coldness, or numbness; twitching; tremors; convulsions; unconsciousness; or a very slow breathing rate or cessation of breathing. Contact your doctor if you experience anything unusual while taking any medication.

Drug Interactions

- Combining lidocaine with antiarrhythmic drugs such as mexiletine, quinidine, and tocainide may increase the risk of serious side effects.
- Do not use more than 1 topical anesthetic at a time because of the risk of absorbing too much of these drugs.
- Drugs that can cause methemoglobinemia—including acetaminophen, benzocaine, chloroquine, nitrites (preservatives used in meats), oral antidiabetes drugs, phenacetin, phenobarbital, phenytoin, primaquine, quinine, sulfa drugs, and thiazide diuretics—should not be taken with lidocaine products. This interaction is generally limited to children under age 1.

Usual Dose

EMLA Cream

Adult and Child (age 1 month and over): Apply a thick layer—2.5 g or ½ tsp.—and cover with the dressing provided in the package or some other occlusive bandage. Leave in place for at least 1–2 hours. The cream should be wiped away immediately before any surgical procedure or injection.

EMLA Patch: Apply to designated area and leave in place for at least 1–2 hours before removing.

Lidocaine Cream

Adult and Child (age 2 and over): Apply a thin layer over affected area 2–3 times a day, or according to your doctor's instructions.

Lidoderm Patch: Use this product to cover the most painful area. Apply up to 3 patches once every 12 hours within a 24-hour period.

Overdosage

Accidental ingestion of these medicines may affect the heart by making it less efficient. Contact your local poison control center or a hospital emergency room for more information. If you seek treatment, ALWAYS bring the prescription container.

Special Information

Apply the patch immediately after removing it from its protective envelope. Patches may be cut into smaller pieces with scissors while the lining is still attached.

If irritation or burning occurs during application, remove the patch(es) and do not reapply until symptoms subside.

When you apply EMLA cream, place the entire dose in the center of the designated area. Then cover it with the occlusive dressing and allow the pressure of the dressing to spread the cream. Since the cream numbs the skin, be careful not to accidentally scratch or burn yourself after the product has been applied.

Wash your hands after handling the lidocaine patch or cream. Be sure to properly dispose of the patch immediately after use, as leftover amounts of lidocaine remain and can be accidentally ingested by children or pets.

Do not apply these products near the eyes or to open wounds.

Contact your doctor if you develop severe, persistent, or bothersome side effects.

Special Populations

Pregnancy/Breast-feeding: The safety of using the lidocaine patch or cream during pregnancy is not known, though animal studies have revealed no harm to the fetus. Lidocaine should be taken during pregnancy only if your doctor determines that the potential benefit outweighs the risks.

The anesthetics in these products pass into breast milk. Nursing mothers who must use these drugs should consider using infant formula.

Seniors: Seniors may be more sensitive to the side effects of lidocaine, and may require a smaller dose.

Lidoderm *see **Lidocaine,** page 688*

Generic Name

Linezolid (lie-NEZ-oh-lid)

Brand Names

Zyvox

Type of Drug

Antibiotic.

Prescribed For

Staphylococcus, streptococcus, and enterococcus infections.

General Information

Linezolid is the first of a new group of antibiotics for infections that cannot be treated by other antibiotics. It does not kill bacteria, but rather interferes with their reproduction. The oral form of this antibiotic can be directly substituted for the intravenous form. This is helpful for people who may have been started on linezolid in a hospital or emergency room with an intravenous dose, as they can then continue taking linezolid at home.

Cautions and Warnings

Do not use linezolid if you are **allergic** or **sensitive** to any of its ingredients.

Colitis has been associated with nearly all antibiotic drugs, including linezolid. Mild colitis usually abates when the drug is stopped, but it is possible for drug-associated colitis to be fatal.

Linezolid can cause tingling or pain in the hands or feet and visual problems. Blurred vision has occurred in some people who took this medicine for 28 days or less. Blindness has occurred in some people who took this medicine for more than 28 days. Contact your doctor immediately if you experience blurred or tunnel vision or any changes in the quality or color of your vision.

Linezolid may increase the risk of convulsions, particularly in people with a history of **seizures**.

Lactic acidosis, which causes repeated nausea and vomiting, has been reported with the use of linezolid. This condition can be very serious, even fatal. Report any symptoms to your doctor immediately.

Low levels of different blood cell types have developed in people taking linezolid, which can lead to anemia and a higher risk of bleeding. This effect usually reverses after the drug is stopped. Your doctor may do blood tests.

Possible Side Effects

- ▼ Common: diarrhea, headache, and nausea.
- ▼ Less common: vaginal fungal infection.
- ▼ Rare: dizziness, vomiting, upset stomach, abdominal or stomach pain, taste changes, tongue discoloration, high blood pressure, itching, abnormal liver function tests, and

Possible Side Effects *(continued)*

oral fungal infection. Contact your doctor if you experience anything unusual while taking any medication.

Drug Interactions

- Linezolid inhibits the enzyme monoamine oxidase (MAO). The following drugs should not be used with linezolid or for 2 weeks after finishing linezolid treatment: apraclonidine, atomoxetine, buproprion, cyclobenzaprine, ginseng, levodopa + carbidopa, other MAO inhibitors (phenelzine), methylphenidate, and tetrabenazine.
- People taking the following medications should not take linezolid at the same time, unless your doctor determines that treatment is absolutely necessary and closely monitors your condition: buspirone, dobutamine, dopamine, entacapone, meperidine, pseudoephedrine, selective serotonin reuptake inhibitors (SSRIs), tricyclic antidepressants, triptan-type antimigraine medicine, or vasopressive agents (epinephrine, norepinephrine). Serious and even fatal reactions may occur. Two weeks should elapse between stopping these drugs and starting linezolid.
- Linezolid should be used with caution by those taking beta blockers or tryptophan due to an increased risk of severe side effects in 1 or both medications.
- Rifampin may decrease the effects of linezolid.

Food Interactions

Avoid foods that have been fermented, pickled, aged, or smoked. These include pickles, tap beer, fava beans, cheddar cheese, red wine, soy sauce, sauerkraut, and smoked meats or fish. These foods contain tyramine and can cause very high blood pressure if mixed with linezolid.

Usual Dose

Adult and Child (age 12 and over): 400–600 mg every 12 hours for 10–28 days.

Child (under age 12): 4.5 mg per lb. of body weight every 8–12 hours for 10–28 days.

Overdosage

Overdose symptoms may include vomiting, tremors, poor muscle coordination, and reduced activity. Overdose victims should be taken to a hospital emergency room. If you seek treatment, ALWAYS bring the prescription bottle or container.

Special Information

Be sure to tell your doctor if you have or have had high blood pressure, and if you are taking or plan to take any cold remedies or decongestants.

Linezolid oral suspension contains phenylalanine. The intravenous and oral forms do not.

If you forget a dose of linezolid, take it as soon as you remember. If it is almost time for your next dose, skip the dose you forgot and continue with your regular schedule. Do not take a double dose.

Special Populations

Pregnancy/Breast-feeding: There is no information on the effect of linezolid during pregnancy. It should be taken during pregnancy only if your doctor determines that the potential benefit outweighs the risks.

Linezolid passes into the breast milk of laboratory animals but it is not known if the drug passes into human breast milk. Nursing mothers who must take this drug should use infant formula.

Seniors: Seniors may take this medication without special restriction.

Lipitor

*see **Statin Cholesterol-Lowering Agents,** page 1065*

Generic Name

Lithium Carbonate

(LITH-ee-um CAR-buh-nate) G

Brand Names

Cibalith-S
Eskalith
Lithobid

The information in this profile also applies to the following drugs:

Generic Ingredients: Lithium Citrate G

Type of Drug

Antipsychotic and antimanic.

Prescribed For

Bipolar (manic-depressive) disorder, especially suppression of manic attacks or reduction in their number and intensity; also prescribed to improve white-blood-cell count in those with cancer undergoing chemotherapy and in those with human immunodeficiency virus (HIV), and for premenstrual tension, bulimia, postpartum psychosis, overactive thyroid, and alcoholism, especially in people who are also depressed. Lithium lotion has been used for genital herpes and dandruff.

General Information

Lithium is the best and most widely used of all antimanic drugs. They reduce the levels of manic episodes and may produce normal activity within the first 3 weeks of treatment. Typical manic symptoms include rapid speech, elation, hyperactive movements, reduced need for sleep, grandiose ideas, poor judgment, aggressiveness, and hostility.

Cautions and Warnings

Do not take lithium if you are **allergic** or **sensitive** to any of its ingredients.

Lithium toxicity can occur at blood levels that are very close to those achieved by therapeutic doses. Blood-level monitoring should be arranged before initiating treatment.

Lithium should not be taken by people with **heart or kidney disease**, **dehydration**, **low blood sodium**, or those taking **diuretic drugs** or **angiotensin-converting enzyme (ACE) inhibitors**. If such people require lithium carbonate, they must be very carefully monitored by their doctors, and hospitalization may be needed until the lithium carbonate dose is stabilized.

A few people treated with both lithium carbonate and haloperidol or another antipsychotic have developed encephalopathic syndrome (symptoms include weakness, tiredness, fever, confusion, tremulousness, and uncontrollable muscle spasms). In addition, your doctor may find laboratory indicators of liver or kidney disease. Rarely, this combination of symptoms is followed by irreversible brain damage.

Up to 20% of people on long-term lithium carbonate treatment develop structural changes in their kidneys and reduced kidney function.

Long-term use of this drug may lead to reduced thyroid activity, enlargement of the thyroid gland, and increased blood levels of thyroid-stimulating hormone. All of these conditions may be treated with thyroid hormone replacement therapy. Overactive thyroid has occasionally occurred.

Frequent urination and thirst associated with lithium carbonate may be a sign of a condition known as diabetes insipidus, in which the kidney stops responding to a hormone called vasopressin. This causes the kidney to reabsorb water and make concentrated urine. Lithium carbonate may reverse the kidneys' ability to perform this function, but things usually go back to normal when lithium carbonate treatment is stopped, dosage is reduced, or small doses of a thiazide diuretic are taken.

Your lithium carbonate dosage may have to be temporarily reduced if you develop an infection or fever.

Some lithium carbonate products contain tartrazine dyes for coloring purposes. Tartrazine can stimulate allergic responses in some people, including asthma.

Possible Side Effects

Side effects of lithium carbonate are directly related to the amount of drug in the bloodstream.

▼ Most common: fine hand tremor, thirst, and excessive urination, especially when treatment is first started; mild nausea and discomfort during the first few days of treatment.

▼ Less common: diarrhea, vomiting, drowsiness, muscle weakness, poor coordination, giddiness, ringing or buzzing in the ears, and blurred vision.

▼ Rare: Rare side effects can affect muscles and nerves (blackouts, seizures, and dizziness), stomach and intestines, kidneys and urinary tract, skin, and thyroid function. Lithium carbonate can also affect tests used to monitor heart and brain function. Contact your doctor if you experience anything unusual while taking any medication.

Drug Interactions

- When lithium carbonate is combined with haloperidol, weakness, tiredness, fever, or confusion may result. In some people, these symptoms have been followed by permanent brain damage. Also, haloperidol may increase the effect of lithium carbonate.
- Lithium may interfere with the effectiveness of phenothiazine drugs. Combining these drugs can have serious side effects.

- Lithium carbonate is counteracted by acetazolamide, theophylline drugs, urea, and urinary alkalinizers such as sodium bicarbonate. Verapamil can raise or lower blood levels of lithium carbonate.
- Lithium's effect may be increased by ACE inhibitors, carbamazepine, fluoxetine and other selective serotonin reuptake inhibitors (SSRIs), methyldopa, metronidazole, nonsteroidal anti-inflammatory drugs (NSAIDs), and thiazide and loop diuretics. Lithium should not be taken with ACE inhibitors or diuretics, as serious lithium toxicity may occur.
- When lithium is combined with phenothiazides, the effects of both drugs are altered and the risk of toxicity is increased.
- Lithium carbonate may increase the effects of tricyclic antidepressant medications.
- Lithium may interfere with the effectiveness of stimulant drugs.
- Lithium may increase the effects of neuromuscular blocking agents, which can lead to severe respiratory side effects.
- Use of metronidazole with lithium can cause lithium toxicity. Careful monitoring is required with this combination.

Food Interactions

Lithium carbonate should be taken immediately after meals or with food or milk.

Usual Dose

Adult and Child (age 12 and over): Dosage must be individualized. Most people respond to 1800 mg a day at first in 2 or 3 divided doses. Once the person has responded, daily lithium dosage is reduced to the lowest effective level, usually 300 mg 3–4 times a day.

Child (under age 12): not recommended.

Overdosage

Toxic blood levels of lithium carbonate are only slightly above the levels required for treatment. Signs of drug toxicity may be diarrhea, vomiting, nausea, tremors, drowsiness, poor coordination, giddiness, weakness, blurred vision, ringing or buzzing in the ears, dizziness, fainting, confusion, muscle twitching, uncontrollable muscle movements, loss of bladder control, worsening of manic symptoms, overactive reflexes, and painful muscles or joints. If any of these symptoms occur, stop taking the medication and contact your doctor immediately. If you seek treatment, ALWAYS bring the prescription bottle or container.

Special Information

Lithium carbonate may cause drowsiness. Be cautious while driving or operating hazardous machinery.

Lithium carbonate causes your body to lose sodium (salt). You must maintain a well-balanced diet and drink 8–12 glasses of water a day while taking this drug. Excessive sweating or diarrhea may make you more sensitive to side effects.

Contact your doctor if you develop diarrhea, vomiting, unsteady walking, tremors, drowsiness, or muscle weakness.

To avoid side effects, your doctor may need to reduce your dosage once manic symptoms decline.

If you forget to take a dose of lithium carbonate, take it as soon as possible. However, if it is within 2 hours of your next dose, or 6 hours if you take the long-acting form, skip the missed dose and go back to your regular schedule. Do not take a double dose. Contact your doctor if you miss more than 1 dose.

Special Populations

Pregnancy/Breast-feeding: Lithium can cause heart and thyroid birth defects, especially if taken during the first 3 months of pregnancy. Lithium should be taken during pregnancy only if your doctor determines that the potential benefit outweighs the risks.

Lithium carbonate passes into breast milk. It may cause weak muscle tone, low body temperature, bluish discoloration of the skin, and abnormal heart rhythm in an infant. Nursing mothers who must take this drug should use infant formula.

Seniors: Seniors are more sensitive to the effects of lithium carbonate. Because seniors have a higher frequency of heart, liver, and kidney problems, they should be monitored carefully and started on the low end of the dosage range.

Loestrin 24 Fe *see **Contraceptives,** page 316*

Type of Drug

Loop Diuretics

Brand Names

Generic Ingredients: Bumetanide G

Generic Ingredients: Ethacrynic Acid
Edecrin

Generic Ingredients: Furosemide G
Lasix

Generic Ingredients: Torsemide G
Demadex

Prescribed For

Congestive heart failure (CHF), cirrhosis of the liver, fluid accumulation in the lungs, kidney dysfunction, high blood pressure, and other conditions in which it may be desirable to rid the body of excess fluid. Bumetanide can be used to treat people who urinate frequently at night.

General Information

Stronger than thiazide diuretics, loop diuretics work in a similar fashion. Not only do they affect the same part of the kidney as thiazide diuretics, they also act in another portion called the loop of Henle. This dual action is what makes loop diuretics so potent. All 4 loop diuretics can be used for the same purposes, but their dosages vary.

Cautions and Warnings

Do not take loop diuretics if you are **allergic** or **sensitive** to any of their ingredients. People allergic to sulfa drugs may also be allergic to bumetanide, furosemide, or torsemide.

Loop diuretics can cause depletion of water and electrolytes. They should not be taken without constant medical supervision. Frequent lab evaluations of electrolytes should be performed during therapy and periodically thereafter. You should not take these drugs if your urine production has been decreased abnormally by **kidney disease**. Low magnesium, calcium, and potassium levels in the blood may occur with these medications.

Excessive use of loop diuretics results in dehydration or reduction in blood volume, and may cause circulatory collapse or other related problems, particularly in **older adults**. Very low blood pressure with symptoms of dizziness or fainting may also occur.

Ringing or buzzing in the ears, hearing loss, deafness, fainting, and a sensation of fullness in the ears can occur with these drugs. Hearing usually returns within 24 hours, but some loss may be permanent.

These drugs may worsen systemic **lupus erythematosus** (a chronic autoimmune disease).

Diarrhea may occur with ethacrynic acid or furosemide solution.

Rarely, people taking bumetanide develop thrombocytopenia (low blood-platelet count).

People taking a loop diuretic may develop increased levels of total cholesterol, low-density lipoprotein (LDL) cholesterol, and triglycerides.

Increases in blood-glucose levels have been observed with these medications, in rare cases bringing on diabetes mellitus.

People with **liver disease** should take these medications with caution.

Possible Side Effects

- ▼ Common: Changes may occur in blood levels of potassium or other electrolytes. Hypokalemia (low blood potassium), may cause dry mouth, excessive thirst, weakness, lethargy, drowsiness, restlessness, muscle pain or cramps, muscular tiredness, low blood pressure, decreased frequency of urination and urine volume, abnormal heart rate, and upset stomach, including nausea and vomiting. Loop diuretics may alter sugar metabolism.
- ▼ Less common: abdominal discomfort, nausea, vomiting, diarrhea, rash, dizziness, lightheadedness, headache, blurred vision, fatigue, weakness, jaundice (symptoms include yellowing of the skin or whites of the eyes), acute gout attacks, dermatitis and other skin reactions, tingling in the extremities, dizziness when rising quickly from a sitting or lying position, and anemia.
- ▼ Rare: a sweet taste in the mouth, a burning sensation in the stomach or mouth, excessive thirst, increased perspiration, and frequent urination. Contact your doctor if you experience anything unusual while taking any medication.

Drug Interactions

- If you are taking lithium carbonate, you should not take a diuretic, which greatly increases the risk of lithium side effects.
- Loop diuretics increase the effects of other blood-pressure-lowering drugs. This is beneficial and is frequently used to help lower blood pressure in people with hypertension.
- Periodic hearing loss or ringing or buzzing in the ears may occur if a loop diuretic is taken with cisplatin (an anticancer drug) or an aminoglycoside antibiotic. Make sure your doctor

knows you are taking a loop diuretic before giving you an injection of either of these.

- Nonsteroidal anti-inflammatory drugs (NSAIDs) may decrease the effectiveness of loop diuretics. Bumetanide should not be taken with indomethacin.
- Thiazide diuretics increase the effect of loop diuretics.
- Combining ethacrynic acid and digoxin increases the risk of developing electrolyte imbalances. Digoxin use may increase levels of torsemide but dosage adjustments are not needed.
- Ethacrynic acid may increase the effect of warfarin; a dosage adjustment may be needed.
- If furosemide or torsemide are taken with aspirin or other salicylate drugs, the risk of salicylate toxicity is increased.
- Probenecid may decrease the effects of bumetanide or torsemide. Bumetanide and probenecid should not be mixed.
- The risk of serious heart rhythm disorders is increased if furosemide is taken with amiodarone, arsenic trioxide, bretylium, chlorpromazine, cisapride, disopyramide, dofetilide, dolasetron, droperidol, mefloquine, mesoridazine, moxifloxacin, pentamidine, pimozide, quinidine, sotalol, tacrolimus, thioridazine, or ziprasidone.
- Doses of furosemide and sucralfate should be separated by 2 hours.
- Furosemide may antagonize the skeletal muscle relaxing effect of tubocurarine and may increase this effect in succinylcholine.
- Doses of torsemide and cholestyramine should be separated.
- If you are taking a loop diuretic for high blood pressure or CHF, avoid over-the-counter (OTC) cough, cold, and allergy products, which often contain stimulant drugs that can raise your blood pressure. Check with your pharmacist before taking any OTC drug if you are taking a loop diuretic.

Food Interactions

Furosemide should be taken on an empty stomach at least 1 hour before or 2 hours after meals. The other loop diuretics may be taken with food if they upset your stomach.

Usual Dose

Bumetanide

Adult: 0.5–2 mg a day, up to 10 mg a day. It may also be taken every other day for 3–4 consecutive days, followed by 1–2 days off the drug.

Child (age 6 months and over): 0.007–0.045 mg per lb. a day or every other day, to a maximum of 10 mg a day.

Child (under age 6 months): 0.0045–0.022 mg per lb. a day or every other day.

Ethacrynic Acid

Adult: 50–200 mg taken every day or every other day.

Child (age 13 months and over): starting dose—25 mg; increase slowly.

Child (under age 13 months): not recommended.

Furosemide

Adult: 20–80 mg a day. Dosages of 600 mg or more a day have been prescribed.

Child: 0.9 mg per lb. of body weight in a single daily dose. If therapy is not successful, the dosage may be increased in small steps up to 2.7 mg per lb. of body weight a day.

Torsemide

Adult: 5–20 mg once a day. Dosages up to 200 mg have been prescribed.

Child: not recommended.

Maintenance dosages for all of the loop diuretics are adjusted to individual needs.

Overdosage

Symptoms include dehydration, reduced blood volume, high urine volume, weakness, dizziness, confusion, appetite loss, tiredness, vomiting, circulatory collapse, and cramps. Take the victim to a hospital emergency room. If you seek treatment, ALWAYS bring the prescription bottle or container.

Special Information

If the amount of urine you produce each day is dropping, or if you experience cramps, significant appetite loss, muscle weakness, tiredness, or nausea, contact your doctor immediately.

Loop diuretics are usually taken once a day after breakfast. If a second dose is needed, it should be taken no later than 2 p.m. to avoid nighttime urination.

To avoid the dizziness associated with these drugs, rise slowly and carefully from a sitting or lying position.

Loop diuretics rob your body of potassium. To counteract this effect, be sure to eat high-potassium foods such as bananas, citrus fruits, melons, and tomatoes.

Loop diuretics can increase your sensitivity to the sun. Use sunscreen and wear protective clothing.

If you forget a dose, take it as soon as you remember. If it is almost time for your next dose, skip the one you forgot and continue with your regular schedule. Do not take a double dose.

Special Populations

Pregnancy/Breast-feeding: Loop diuretics have been used to treat specific conditions in pregnancy, but they should be used only when absolutely necessary.

Furosemide passes into breast milk, and the other loop diuretics may pass into breast milk. Nursing mothers who must take any of these drugs should use infant formula.

Seniors: Seniors are more sensitive to the effects of these drugs.

Generic Name

Loperamide (loe-PER-uh-mide) G

Brand Names

Diamode
Diar-Aid
Imodium
Imodium A-D
Imotil
Imperim
K-Pek II
Neo-Diaral
Pepto Diarrhea Control

Type of Drug

Antidiarrheal.

Prescribed For

Acute and chronic diarrhea; also prescribed to reduce the amount of discharge in an ileostomy (surgical procedure in which a hole is made in the small intestine, usually through the abdominal wall).

General Information

Loperamide, which relieves diarrhea but does not address the underlying cause, should be used only for short periods. It works by slowing intestinal movement and affecting the movement of water and salts in the intestines. In some cases, antidiarrheals should not be used at all; these drugs may harm people with bowel, stomach, or other diseases. Loperamide is available in over-the-counter (OTC) form under a variety of brand names. OTC loperamide products are used to treat acute diarrhea and traveler's diarrhea.

Cautions and Warnings

Do not use loperamide if you are **allergic** or **sensitive** to any of its ingredients. Drug allergy to loperamide is rare.

Do not take loperamide if you suffer from diarrhea associated with **colitis** or you have an **intestinal infection** of *Escherichia coli, Salmonella,* or *Shigella,* or **abdominal pain** without diarrhea.

If you have **ulcerative colitis** and start taking loperamide, stop the drug at once and contact your doctor if you develop abdominal problems of any kind.

Do not use loperamide if you have bloody or black stools.

Do not use loperamide to treat infants younger than 2 years old.

Stop taking loperamide if you develop constipation, abdominal distention, or intestinal blockage.

Use this drug with caution if you have **liver disease**.

Possible Side Effects

Incidence of side effects is low. They are most likely to occur when loperamide is taken over longer periods to treat chronic diarrhea.

▼ Most common: stomach and abdominal pain; bloating or other discomfort; constipation; dry mouth; dizziness; tiredness; nausea and vomiting; and drug-sensitivity reactions, including rash.

Other side effects that have occurred with loperamide are itching; hives; swelling of the tongue, lips, or face; rare but serious skin reactions; gas; severe bowel reactions; and urinary difficulty.

Drug Interactions

- Loperamide increases the effects of alcohol, sedatives, and sleeping pills. Avoid these combinations.
- Loperamide should not be taken with clindamycin or lincomycin, agents that can cause severe and possibly fatal colitis.
- Quinidine and ritonavir can increase the effects of loperamide. These drugs should be mixed with caution.
- Loperamide reduces saquinavir levels by more than 50%, interfering with the effects of that drug. Saquinavir dose adjustment may be necessary.

Food Interactions

Loperamide should be taken on an empty stomach.

Usual Dose

Acute Diarrhea

Adult and Child (age 12 and over): 4 mg to start, followed by 2 mg after each loose stool, up to 16 mg a day maximum. Improvement should be seen in 2 days.

Child (age 9–11): 2 mg 3 times a day to start, followed by 1 mg per 22 lbs. of body weight after each loose stool, up to 6 mg a day maximum.

Child (age 6–8): 2 mg twice a day to start, followed by 1 mg per 22 lbs. of body weight after each loose stool, up to 4 mg a day maximum.

Child (age 2–5): 1 mg 3 times a day to start, followed by 1 mg per 22 lbs. of body weight after each loose stool, up to 3 mg a day maximum.

Child (under age 2): not recommended.

Chronic Diarrhea

Adult and Child (age 12 and over): 4 mg to start, followed by 2 mg after each loose stool, until symptoms are controlled. Then dosage should be tailored to individual needs—usually 4–8 mg a day. Loperamide is usually effective within 10 days or not at all.

Child (under age 12): not recommended.

Overdosage

Symptoms include constipation, difficulty urinating, irritation of the stomach, tiredness, and central-nervous-system (CNS) depression. Children may be more sensitive to loperamide overdose than adults. Large doses usually cause vomiting. Take the victim to a hospital emergency room immediately. If you seek treatment, ALWAYS bring the prescription bottle or container.

Special Information

Loperamide depresses the CNS, which may cause drowsiness. Be careful when driving or performing any task that requires concentration.

Loperamide may cause dry mouth. Drink plenty of water or other clear fluids to prevent dehydration due to diarrhea. It is important to maintain a proper diet and drink plenty of fluids to restore normal bowel function.

Contact your doctor if diarrhea persists after a few days of loperamide treatment or if you develop abdominal discomfort or pain, fever, or any bothersome or persistent side effect.

If you forget a dose, skip it and go back to your regular schedule. Do not take a double dose.

Special Populations

Pregnancy/Breast-feeding: Loperamide has not been found to cause birth defects; however, women who are or might be pregnant should not take this drug without their doctor's approval. Loperamide should be taken during pregnancy only if your doctor determines that the potential benefit outweighs the risks.

It is not known if loperamide passes into breast milk. Nursing mothers who must take this drug should use infant formula.

Seniors: Seniors may be more sensitive to the constipating effects of loperamide, but no dosage adjustment is necessary.

Generic Name

Loratadine (lor-AH-tuh-dene) G

Brand Names

Alavert
Alavert For Kids 6+
Children's Claritin
Claritin
Claritin Liqui-Gels
Claritin RediTabs 12-Hour
Claritin RediTabs 24-Hour
Claritin RediTabs for Kids 12-Hour
Claritin RediTabs for Kids 24-Hour
Triaminic Aller Chews

The information in this profile also applies to the following drugs:

Generic Ingredients: Desloratadine
Clarinex
Clarinex RediTabs

Type of Drug

Antihistamine.

Prescribed For

Stuffy and runny nose, itchy eyes, and scratchy throat caused by seasonal allergy, and for other symptoms of allergy such as rash, itching, and hives; also prescribed for asthma.

General Information

Antihistamines generally work by blocking the release of histamine (chemical released by body tissue during an allergic reaction) from cells at the H_1 histamine receptor site, drying up secretions of the nose, throat, and eyes. Loratadine causes less sedation than most antihistamines and appears to be just as effective.

Cautions and Warnings

Do not take loratadine if you are **allergic** or **sensitive** to any of its ingredients.

People with **liver or kidney disease** require reduced dosage.

Possible Side Effects

- ▼ Common: headache, sleepiness, dry mouth, and fatigue.
- ▼ Less common: sore throat, diarrhea, heart palpitations, drug-sensitivity reactions (rash, itching, hives, swelling, and difficulty breathing), nervousness, stomach pain, and earache.
- ▼ Rare: Rare side effects can occur in almost any part of the body. Contact your doctor if you experience anything unusual while taking any medication.

Drug Interactions

- Ketoconazole, erythromycin, and cimetidine cause increases in blood levels of loratadine, although these interactions do not appear to cause any unwanted effects.
- Combine loratadine with monoamine oxidase inhibitor (MAOI) antidepressants with caution, as it can increase side effects.
- Combining loratadine with alcohol or nervous system depressants can cause increased nervous system depression.

Food Interactions

Loratadine is best taken on an empty stomach 1 hour before or 2 hours after eating; it may be taken with food or milk if it upsets your stomach. Desloratadine can be taken without regard to food or meals.

Usual Dose

Desloratadine

Adult and Child (age 12 and over): 5 mg once a day. People with liver disease should take one 5-mg tablet every other day.

Child (age 6–11): 2.5 mg once a day.

Child (age 1–5 years): 1.25 mg once a day.

Child (age 6–11 months): 1 mg once a day.

Child (under age 6 months): not recommended.

Loratadine

Adult and Child (age 6 and over): 10 mg once a day. Children with kidney or liver disease should take 10 mg every other day.

Child (age 2–5): 5 mg a day of loratadine syrup or chewable tablets. Children with kidney or liver disease should take 5 mg every other day.

Child (under age 2): not recommended.

Overdosage

Overdose is likely to cause drowsiness, headache, rapid heartbeat, or severe side effects. Overdose victims should be given ipecac syrup—available at any pharmacy—to make them vomit and should be taken to a hospital emergency room for treatment. Contact your local poison control center or hospital emergency room for instructions. If you seek treatment, ALWAYS bring the prescription bottle or container.

Special Information

Dizziness or fainting may be the first sign of a serious side effect. Contact your doctor at once if this happens to you. Also report sore throat, difficulty swallowing or speaking, swelling of the tongue, wheezing, dizziness or fainting, swelling around the mouth, drooling, or any other unusual side effect.

If you forget to take a dose of loratadine, take it as soon as you remember. If it is almost time for your next dose, skip the one you forgot and continue with your regular schedule. Do not take a double dose.

Rapidly disintegrating loratadine tablets must be used as soon as they are removed from their foil package. Place on your tongue and allow to dissolve. You may drink water or another liquid with it, but it is not necessary.

Special Populations

Pregnancy/Breast-feeding: Do not take any antihistamine without your doctor's knowledge if you are or might be pregnant—especially during the last 3 months of pregnancy—because newborns may have severe reactions to antihistamines.

Loratadine passes into breast milk. Nursing mothers who must take loratadine should use infant formula.

Seniors: Seniors are unlikely to experience nervous system effects with loratadine as opposed to the older, more sedating antihistamines. However, seniors, especially those with liver disease, are more likely to experience side effects than are younger adults. Seniors should take the smallest effective dose.

Lotrel *see* ***Calcium Channel Blockers,*** *page 224*

Lovaza *see* ***Omega-3-Acid Ethyl Esters,*** *page 876*

Generic Name

Lubiprostone (lew-bee-PROSS-tone)

Brand Names

Amitiza

Type of Drug

Local chloride channel activator.

Prescribed For

Chronic constipation and irritable bowel syndrome (IBS) with constipation in adult women.

General Information

One way to treat chronic constipation is to add fluid to the insides of the gut. Lubiprostone accomplishes this by acting inside the gastrointestinal (GI) tract to increase intestinal fluid secretion. This increases intestinal movement and speeds stool passage through the GI tract, eliminating symptoms of chronic constipation. Lubiprostone improves intestinal fluid secretion without altering sodium and potassium concentrations in the serum. Other constipation treatments work in a similar way but can be associated with other potential problems.

Cautions and Warnings

Do not take lubiprostone if you are **allergic** or **sensitive** to any of its ingredients.

Do not take lubiprostone if you have or have had a **blockage in the stomach or intestinal area**.

People taking lubiprostone have experienced difficulty breathing or chest tightness starting 30–60 minutes after taking it. These symptoms usually go away within a few hours.

This drug has not been studied in people with **liver or kidney problems** and it has not been studied in **children**.

People with **diarrhea** should not take this medication.

Possible Side Effects

Side effects increase with higher doses.

- ▼ Most common: nausea, diarrhea, and headache.
- ▼ Common: stomach bloating and fullness, abdominal pain, headache, and gas.
- ▼ Less common: sinusitis, urinary tract infection, upper-respiratory infections, irritation of the nose and throat, influenza or other viral infections, vomiting, loose stools, stomach or abdominal discomfort, upset stomach, upper or lower abdominal pain, gastroesophageal reflux disease (GERD), dry mouth, constipation, dizziness, swelling in the arms and legs, fatigue, chest pain or discomfort, fever, joint pain, back pain, leg or arm pain, difficulty breathing, cough, pain in the lower part of the throat (larynx or pharynx), depression, anxiety, and sleeplessness.
- ▼ Rare: loss of the sense of touch, muscle cramps, weight gain, and high blood pressure. Contact your doctor if you experience anything unusual while taking any medication.

Drug Interactions

The chances of lubiprostone interacting with other medications after they have been absorbed is small because very little lubiprostone is absorbed into the blood. There is no information on the interaction of lubiprostone with other medications in the GI tract.

Food Interactions

This drug should be taken with food and water to minimize nausea.

Usual Dose

Adult: chronic constipation—24 mcg twice a day with food; irritable bowel syndrome with constipation—8 mcg twice a day with food.

Child: not recommended.

Overdosage

High doses of lubiprostone cause drug side effects or other reactions. Contact your local poison control center or a hospital emergency room for more information. If you seek treatment, ALWAYS bring the prescription bottle or container.

Special Information

Taking lubiprostone with food may lessen symptoms of nausea if they occur. If you experience severe diarrhea while taking lubiprostone, contact your doctor.

Men and women respond similarly to this drug.

Contact your doctor if you have trouble breathing or tightness in your chest.

If you forget a dose of lubiprostone, take it as soon as you remember. If it is almost time for the next dose, skip the one you forgot and continue with your regular schedule. Do not take a double dose.

Special Populations

Pregnancy/Breast-feeding: Animal studies have shown lubiprostone can damage a developing fetus. Women who might become pregnant and who are starting on this medicine must take a pregnancy test before starting treatment to be sure they are not pregnant. Women taking lubiprostone should use birth control while taking it.

It is not known if lubiprostone passes into breast milk; however, nursing mothers should use infant formula while using this drug because of the possibility of side effects appearing in the nursing infant.

Seniors: Seniors may use this drug with no special precaution.

Lumigan *see **Prostaglandin Agonists,** page 953*

Lunesta *see **Sedatives (Benzodiazepine Type),** page 1033*

Type of Drug

Luteinizing Hormone Inhibitors

Brand Names

Generic Ingredients: Cetrorelix
Cetrotide
Generic Ingredients: Ganirelix Acetate G

Prescribed For

Infertility.

General Information

Luteinizing hormone inhibitors are prescribed as part of a treatment program offered by fertility specialists to help stimulate the development of follicles into mature eggs in women who have had difficulty becoming pregnant. These drugs block the release of gonadotropin-releasing hormones, which stimulate the production and release of 2 other hormones: luteinizing hormone (LH) and follicle-stimulating hormone (FSH). LH and FSH levels return to normal within 48 hours after treatment is stopped.

A luteinizing hormone inhibitor may be taken once a day by subcutaneous (under the skin) injection during the several days after FSH is given, specifically on day 2 or 3 of the cycle. Treatment with an LH inhibitor continues until chorionic gonadotropin (hCG)—the final drug in the sequence—is given. Your doctor will determine when enough follicles have reached an adequate size by ultrasound. In some cases hCG is given to help the follicles develop into mature eggs.

Cautions and Warnings

Do not use luteinizing hormone inhibitors if you are **allergic** or **sensitive** to any of their ingredients, including mannitol. People with a **latex allergy** may react adversely to ganirelix. People who are allergic to **gonadotropin-releasing hormone** must be monitored carefully after the first injection. A severe reaction associated with cough, rash, and hypotension occurred in 1 patient after 7 months of treatment with cetrorelix, when taken at a dosage of 10 mg a day, in a study for a use unrelated to infertility.

People with severe **kidney impairment** should not use cetrorelix.

Possible Side Effects

▼ Less common: abdominal pain, headache, miscarriage, hyperstimulation of the ovary, vaginal bleeding, injection-site allergy (symptoms include redness, rash, bruising, itching, and swelling), and nausea.

Drug Interactions

Ganirelix can suppress the secretion of pituitary gonadotropins, and may require dose adjustments of exogenous gonadotropins.

Food Interactions

None known.

Usual Dose

Cetrorelix: single-dose regimen—one 3-mg subcutaneous dose, usually on stimulation day 7 (range: day 5–9). If hCG is not given within 4 days after injection of 3 mg cetrorelix, then cetrorelix 0.25 mg once a day is prescribed until the day of hCG administration.

Multiple-dose regimen—0.25 mg of cetrorelix, on either stimulation day 5 (morning or evening) or day 6 (morning). Continue every day until the day of hCG administration.

Ganirelix: 250 mcg once a day after starting FSH therapy on day 2 or 3 of the cycle. Treatment is continued until the day of hCG administration.

Overdosage

Very high doses of these medicines have been used in clinical trials without serious side effects. Contact your local poison center or a hospital emergency room for more information. If you seek treatment, ALWAYS bring the prescription bottle or container.

Special Information

This drug is given by injection under the skin. For more information on how to properly administer this drug, see page 1242.

If taking a multiple-dose regimen, change the injection site regularly to minimize irritation.

Cetrorelix powder for injection requires more manipulation than Cetrotide, which comes in pre-filled syringes. You must dissolve the powder with sterile water provided by the manufacturer before it is injected. Follow the directions for dilution in the package.

Special Populations

Pregnancy/Breast-feeding: Women who are pregnant should not take these drugs because they may harm a developing fetus.

It is not known if these drugs pass into breast milk. Nursing mothers who take luteinizing hormone inhibitors should use infant formula.

Seniors: These medicines are not intended for use by seniors.

Lyrica *see **Pregabalin,** page 941*

Generic Name

Malathion (MAL-uh-thye-on) G

Brand Names

Ovide

Type of Drug

Scabicide.

Prescribed For

Head lice.

General Information

Originally used as an agricultural insecticide; malathion is effective against common lice and the eggs they leave behind in the scalp. Malathion works by interfering with the breakdown of acetylcholine, a neurohormone that carries nervous system impulses. The excess acetylcholine produced by malathion kills lice and their eggs. Once applied to the hair, malathion binds with the hair shaft within 6–12 hours, providing some protection against future infestations.

Cautions and Warnings

Do not use malathion if you are **allergic** or **sensitive** to any of its ingredients.

Malathion is extremely toxic if swallowed (see "Overdosage").

Normally, less than 10% of the malathion applied to the skin is absorbed into the bloodstream; more may be absorbed if it is applied to **broken skin or open sores**—this may cause a toxic reaction.

Malathion lotion is flammable. Do not expose the lotion—or hair that is still wet with the lotion—to an open flame or an electric dryer because of the risk of fire. Do not smoke while applying malathion, and wash hands thoroughly after application. Allow hair to dry naturally after application.

Malathion can damage the eyes and cause conjunctivitis (pinkeye). If it gets into your eyes, flush them with water immediately.

People who have had a recent **heart attack** or who have any of the following conditions should be cautious when using malathion because it can precipitate an attack or worsen your condition: **asthma**, very **slow heartbeat**, **low blood pressure**, **stomach spasms or ulcer**, or **Parkinson's disease**.

Do not use malathion in **children under age 2**, as they may absorb too much of it through the scalp.

Malathion can worsen the following conditions: **severe anemia**, **dehydration**, **insecticide exposure effects**, **liver disease** or **cirrhosis**, **malnutrition**, **myasthenia** or other **neuromuscular diseases**, and **seizure disorders**.

People with recent **brain surgery** should be cautious about using this product because it can initiate toxic nervous system effects, including seizures.

Possible Side Effects

- ▼ Common: scalp irritation.
- ▼ Rare: Convulsions and other side effects can occur if too much of the drug is absorbed into the blood through the scalp (see "Overdosage"). Contact your doctor if you experience anything unusual while taking any medication.

Drug Interactions

- Large dosages of malathion may interact with aminoglycosides (injectable antibiotics) to cause breathing problems, with local anesthetics to cause systemic side effects, and with glaucoma eye drops—physostigmine, echothiophate, demecarium, and isoflurophate—to cause side effects.
- Combining malathion and anticholinesterase muscle stimulants used to treat myasthenia gravis may lead to increased side effects.

Usual Dose

Adult and Child (age 6 and over): Sprinkle the lotion onto dry hair and rub it in until the hair and scalp are wet. Pay special attention to the back of your head and neck. Avoid contact with the eyes. Immediately after applying the lotion, wash your hands. Allow the treated hair to dry naturally; do not cover it or use an electric dryer or other heat source. After 8–12 hours, wash your hair with a plain shampoo. Remove dead lice and eggs from the scalp with a fine-tooth comb. Repeat after 7–9 days if necessary.

Child (age 2–5): Consult your doctor.

Child (under age 2): not recommended.

Overdosage

Accidental ingestion or absorbing too much drug through the skin is serious and potentially fatal. Symptoms of malathion toxicity include abdominal cramps; anxiety; restlessness; clumsiness or unsteadiness; confusion; depression; diarrhea; dizziness; drowsiness; increased sweating; watery eyes or mouth; loss of bowel or bladder control; muscle twitching in the eyelids, face, or neck; pinpoint pupils; difficulty breathing; seizures; slow heartbeat; trembling; and weakness. People who swallow this drug may not experience toxic effects for up to 12 hours. In case of accidental ingestion, induce vomiting with ipecac syrup—available at any pharmacy. Take the victim to a hospital emergency room. If you seek treatment, ALWAYS bring the prescription bottle or container.

Special Information

Follow your prescription exactly, paying careful attention to dosage, duration of exposure, and frequency of application. Do not increase the chance of absorption through the skin, as it may lead to overtoxicity.

Malathion should only be used on scalp hair.

Pregnant women should not handle this medication or apply it to others.

Avoid exposure to other insecticides while being treated with malathion.

Head lice can be easily transferred to people in close contact. Be sure to examine and treat other family members if necessary.

Special Populations

Pregnancy/Breast-feeding: Animal studies of malathion have revealed no drug-related birth defects. Because animal studies may not predict human results and about 10% of malathion applied to the skin may be absorbed, pregnant women should not use it or apply it to others.

It is not known if this drug passes into breast milk. Nursing mothers who must use it should use infant formula.

Seniors: Seniors may use this drug without special restriction.

Generic Name

Maraviroc (muh-RAH-vih-roc)

Brand Names

Selzentry

Type of Drug

CCR5 co-receptor antagonist.

Prescribed For

Human immunodeficiency virus (HIV) infection in people whose virus is resistant to multiple-drug treatment, in combination with other HIV antiviral drugs.

General Information

Other HIV antivirals work inside white blood cells, but maraviroc prevents the virus from entering uninfected cells by blocking the virus' major route of entry, the CCR5 co-receptor found on the surface of the white blood cell. CCR5 blockers are prescribed together with other antiviral medications. Maraviroc has not been tested in adults or children who have not already been treated with another HIV antiviral.

Cautions and Warnings

Do not take maraviroc if you are **allergic** or **sensitive** to it. Drug allergy may appear before maraviroc affects the liver.

Maraviroc should be used with caution if you have **liver disease**, **heart disease**, or **hepatitis B**. People with **kidney disease** should use it with caution because about 25% of the drug passes out of the body through the kidneys.

A small number of people taking maraviroc have had chest pain, heart attacks, and other cardiac disease.

About 20% of people on combination antiretroviral therapies develop immune reconstitution syndrome within 1 or 2 months after starting treatment. If this happens, people start feeling worse even though their HIV is better because infections, hepatitis, or other conditions that may have been dormant now begin to express themselves. Maraviroc can increase the risk of infection.

People taking HIV antivirals may experience unusual fat accumulation or redistribution leading to buffalo hump, breast enlargement, abnormal thinness, or a round, moon-shaped face. The exact reasons for this are not known.

Possible Side Effects

- ▼ Most common: fever, cough, upper-respiratory infection, rash, dizziness, muscle and joint pain, and stomach and abdominal pain.
- ▼ Common: herpes infections, constipation, fainting when rising quickly from a sitting or lying position, sinusitis, bronchitis, appetite changes, sensory changes, changes in consciousness, and nerve pain.

Possible Side Effects *(continued)*

- ▼ Less common: high blood pressure, upset stomach, ulcers of the stomach or mouth, pain and discomfort, influenza, pneumonia, genital warts, infection of hair follicles, benign skin tumors, kidney problems, difficulty breathing, sinus disorders, respiratory disorders, bronchial spasm, itching, sweat gland disorders, eczema and dermatitis, and body fat redistribution.
- ▼ Rare: Other side effects can involve almost any body part, including the brain (stroke), heart (angina, heart failure, heart attack, and coronary artery occlusion), liver, and bile system. Contact your doctor if you experience anything unusual while taking any medication.

Drug Interactions

- The daily dosage of maraviroc is doubled to 600 mg in people taking other drugs that speed its breakdown in the liver, including carbamazepine, efavirenz, phenobarbital, phenytoin, and rifampin. Other drugs that can interact in the same way are barbiturates, glitazone antidiabetes drugs, modafinil, oxcarbazepine, and rifabutin.
- Do not take maraviroc with St. John's wort because it will unpredictably reduce maraviroc blood levels.
- The daily dose of maraviroc is reduced by ½ or to 150 mg a day in people also taking other drugs that slow its breakdown in the liver such as delavirdine, indinavir, or nelfinavir. Other drugs that inhibit the enzyme that breaks down maraviroc are amiodarone, aprepitant, chloramphenicol, cimetidine, clarithromycin, diltiazem, erythromycin, fluconazole, fluvoxamine, gestodene, imatinib, itraconazole, ketoconazole, mifepristone, nefazodone, norfloxacin, norfluoxetine, mibefradil, verapamil, and voriconazole.
- HIV antiviral drugs that do not dictate maraviroc dose adjustment include enfuvirtide; the protease inhibitors ritonavir and tipranavir; and the reverse transcriptase inhibitors abacavir, adefovir, azidothymidine, didanosine, emtricitabine, lamivudine, nevirapine, stavudine, tenofovir, and zidovudine (AZT).

Food Interactions

Maraviroc can be taken without regard to food or meals. Do not drink grapefruit juice or eat any grapefruit-containing product while taking this medicine. Grapefruit and starfruit slow the breakdown of maraviroc in the liver.

Usual Dose

Adult (age 16 and over): 150–600 mg twice a day, depending on specific drug combinations.

Child (under age 16): not recommended.

Overdosage

Overdose symptoms can be expected to include drug side effects, especially dizziness or fainting. Overdose victims should be taken to a hospital emergency room because of the possibility of an impact on the heart. If you seek treatment, ALWAYS bring the prescription bottle or container.

Special Information

Maraviroc is not a cure for HIV. It will not prevent you from transmitting the HIV virus to another person; you must still practice safe sex. People taking maraviroc may still develop opportunistic infections and other complications associated with HIV infection. It is very important that you take this drug exactly as prescribed.

Contact your doctor at once if you have an allergic reaction to maraviroc or signs of liver toxicity. Symptoms of hepatitis or allergy include abdominal pain, dark urine, rash, yellowing of the skin or whites of the eyes, and vomiting. Stop taking maraviroc at once if you develop these symptoms and immediately get medical care.

Your doctor should test your liver function regularly while you are taking maraviroc and should monitor you for signs of any infection.

Maraviroc can make you dizzy or lightheaded. Take extreme care while driving or operating any complex equipment or machinery.

If you forget a dose, take it as soon as you remember. If it is almost time for the next dose, skip the one you forgot and continue with your regular schedule. Do not take a double dose.

Special Populations

Pregnancy/Breast-feeding: Animal studies of maraviroc have not shown it to be toxic to a developing fetus. Maraviroc should be taken during pregnancy only if your doctor determines that the potential benefit outweighs the risks. Pregnant women who decide to take maraviroc can be included by their doctor in a company-sponsored registry to help track the drug's effect.

It is not known if maraviroc passes into breast milk; however, mothers with HIV should always use infant formula, regardless of whether they take this drug, to avoid transmitting the virus to their child.

Seniors: Seniors may experience more drug side effects than younger adults. Caution should be used when seniors take maraviroc.

Generic Name

Medroxyprogesterone

(med-rok-see-proe-JES-ter-one) G

Brand Names

Depo-Provera
depo-subQ provera 104
Provera

The information in this profile also applies to the following drugs:

Generic Ingredients: Levonorgestrel G
Mirena IUD
Next Choice
Plan B One-Step

Generic Ingredients: Megestrol G
Megace
Megace ES

Generic Ingredients: Norethindrone G
Aygestin

Generic Ingredients: Progesterone
Crinone
Endometrin Vaginal Insert
Prometrium

Type of Drug

Progestin.

Prescribed For

Absence of menstruation, abnormal uterine bleeding caused by fibroids or uterine cancer, and menopausal changes in the lining of the uterus—in conjunction with estrogen replacement therapy; also prescribed to stimulate breathing in people who suffer from sleep apnea and for other conditions in which breathing rate is abnormally slow or stops completely for short periods of time. Norethindrone may be used for endometriosis and birth control (also called the "mini-pill" when used alone and not in combination with estrogen). Progesterone has been used to treat premenstrual syndrome, prevent spontaneous abortion or premature labor, and support embryo implantation and help maintain pregnancy in some assisted reproductive technology (ART) procedures. The levonorgestrel intrauterine device (IUD) is placed as a long-term (up to 5 years) contraceptive. Levonorgestrel is also used as an emergency contraceptive, either as a 1- or 2-pill product. (See Contraceptives, page 316.)

General Information

Progesterone is the principal hormone involved in the process of pregnancy. It helps to prepare the womb to accept the fertilized egg and maintain the growth and development of the fetus. The decision to take medroxyprogesterone on a regular basis should be made carefully by you and your doctor because of this drug's risks.

Megestrol is used in advanced breast and endometrial cancer to reduce symptoms of the disease, and for weight loss and decreased appetite in people living with HIV.

The levonorgestrel IUD is recommended for women who have already had at least 1 child.

Cautions and Warnings

Do not take medroxyprogesterone if you are **allergic** or **sensitive** to any of its ingredients or to any progestin.

Combinations of a progestin with estrogens should NOT be used to prevent heart or blood vessel disease or dementia. Studies of women taking these combinations have shown them to increase the risk of these conditions. The risk of invasive breast cancer is also increased by this combination.

If you have a history of **stroke, blood clots or similar disorders, varicose veins, liver or gallbladder disease**, known or suspected **breast or genital cancer**, undiagnosed **vaginal bleeding**, or **miscarriage**, do not take medroxyprogesterone. Medroxyprogesterone and other progestins should not be used regularly to treat weight loss.

Smoking may increase the risk of a stroke or blood clot.

Although progestins have been used to prevent spontaneous abortion, such treatment can harm a fetus if given during the first 4 months of pregnancy.

Medroxyprogesterone use should be carefully considered if you have had **asthma**, **cardiac insufficiency**, **epilepsy**, **HIV infection**, **migraine**, **kidney problems**, **ectopic pregnancy**, **high blood cholesterol**, or **depression**. People with **diabetes** may experience a decrease in glucose tolerance, worsening their condition.

The levonorgestrel IUD should not be used if you are already **pregnant** or have unexplained vaginal **bleeding** or **infection**, uterine **fibroids** or other uterine abnormality, **pelvic inflammatory disease**, abnormal **Pap smear**, or **cervical or uterine cancer**. It must be removed if you become pregnant while it is in place.

Pregnancy is possible if the IUD penetrates or tears the wall of your uterus or your cervix. The device must be removed if this happens because it can move outside the uterus and be responsible for numerous complications. Penetration is more likely immediately after you give birth or are nursing. It should not be placed until at least 6 weeks after birth.

The levonorgestrel IUD should not be used if you have another IUD that has not yet been removed.

Possible Side Effects

There is a strong relationship between the use of progestin drugs and the development of blood clots in the veins, lungs, or brain.

Levonorgestrel IUD

▼ Most common: breakthrough bleeding, spotting, changes in or loss of menstrual flow, pelvic pain, and ovarian cysts.

Levonorgestrel Tablets

▼ Most common: nausea, abdominal pain, fatigue, headache, and changes in menstruation.

Medroxyprogesterone, Megestrol, and Norethindrone

▼ Most common: breakthrough bleeding, spotting, changes in or loss of menstrual flow, water retention, weight change, breast tenderness, jaundice, acne, rash with or without itching, and depression.

▼ Common: changes in sex drive, changes in appetite and mood, headache, nervousness, dizziness, tiredness, backache, loss of scalp hair, hair growth in unusual quantities or places, itching, symptoms similar to those of a urinary infection, and unusual rashes.

Possible Side Effects *(continued)*

▼ Rare: allergy, fatigue, fever, flu-like symptoms, bloating, asthma, back or leg pain, sinus inflammation, respiratory infection, upset stomach, stomach gas or noise, emotional instability, sleeplessness, acne, itching, painful urination, and urinary infections. Contact your doctor if you experience anything unusual while taking any medication.

Progesterone Gel

Side effects are less common if you use this drug once a day.

▼ Most common: pelvic or abdominal pain or cramps, sleepiness, tiredness, headache, nervousness, depression, reduced sex drive, constipation, nausea, breast enlargement, and nighttime urination.

▼ Common: bloating, dizziness, diarrhea, vomiting, painful intercourse, joint pain, itching, and vaginal infection or discharge.

Drug Interactions

- Rifampin and aminoglutethimide may reduce medroxyprogesterone acetate's effectiveness.

Food Interactions

You may take these drugs with food if they upset your stomach.

Usual Dose

Levonorgestrel Tablets: 1 or 2 tablets taken within 72 hours of unprotected intercourse. If taking the 2-pill product, the second tablet should be taken 12 hours after the first dose. Contact your doctor if you vomit within 1 hour after the first dose.

Medroxyprogesterone: 5–10 mg a day for 5–10 days.

Megestrol: breast cancer—40 mg 4 times a day; endometrial carcinoma—40–320 mg a day in divided doses; weight or appetite loss—400–800 mg a day.

Norethindrone: endometriosis—5 mg a day for 14 days, then increased gradually up to 15 mg a day; treatment may continue for 6–9 months. Abnormal menstrual bleeding or no period—2.5–10 mg a day for 5–10 days during the second ½ of the menstrual cycle.

Progesterone Capsules: 5–10 mg a day for 6–8 days.

Progesterone Gel: Apply a single-use disposable unit once or twice a day.

Progesterone Insert: 100 mg 2 or 3 times a day.

Overdosage

Symptoms may include severe side effects, though small overdoses generally do not cause unusual symptoms. Contact your local poison control center or a hospital emergency room for more information. If you seek treatment, ALWAYS bring the prescription bottle or container.

Special Information

Your need for medroxyprogesterone should be evaluated at least every 6 months.

This drug may make you drowsy. Be careful when driving or performing any tasks that require concentration.

Stop taking this drug immediately and contact your doctor if you experience sudden, partial, or complete loss of vision; double vision; sudden falling; calf pain, swelling, and redness; numbness in an arm or leg; leg cramp; water retention; unusual vaginal bleeding; migraine or a sudden and severe headache; depression; or if you think you have become pregnant.

An IUD can be lost, with or without your knowledge. Symptoms include increased menstrual flow, bleeding, or pain. Contact your doctor if this happens. The device can be replaced within a week after your period ends and if you have a negative pregnancy test result.

Medroxyprogesterone may increase your sensitivity to the sun. Use sunscreen and wear protective clothing.

Avoid excessive salt intake while taking medroxyprogesterone.

Medroxyprogesterone may mask symptoms of menopause.

If you forget a dose, take it as soon as you remember. If it is almost time for your next dose, skip the one you forgot and continue with your regular schedule. Do not take a double dose.

Special Populations

Pregnancy/Breast-feeding: These drugs may cause birth defects or interfere with fetal development; they are not considered safe for use during pregnancy, except under very specific circumstances. Progesterone gel is used to support embryo implantation and help maintain pregnancies in some ART procedures.

Medroxyprogesterone passes into breast milk. It may also increase the amount of milk produced and the duration of milk production when taken after childbirth. Nursing mothers who must take this drug should use infant formula.

Seniors: Seniors with severe liver disease are more sensitive to the effects of this drug.

Generic Name

Memantine (meh-MAN-teen)

Brand Names

Namenda Namenda XR

Type of Drug

N-methyl-D-aspartate (NMDA) receptor inhibitor.

Prescribed For

Moderate to severe Alzheimer's disease (AD). It is also used to treat vascular dementia.

General Information

Overstimulation of nerve cells in the brain by a chemical called glutamate, which causes nerve degeneration, is thought to be a cause of AD symptoms. Memantine hydrochloride blocks NMDA receptors in the brain, which decreases the effects of glutamate, but it does not stop the nerve degeneration that is a normal part of AD. Thus, the drug is not a cure for AD but can be expected to improve symptoms and delay a patient's mental decline. Other available AD treatments work differently and are only approved for mild to moderate AD, although they have been studied in people with severe AD.

Cautions and Warnings

Do not take this drug if you are **allergic** or **sensitive** to any of its ingredients.

People with **kidney disease** may retain more memantine in their bodies. People with severe kidney disease may need a dosage reduction.

Some memantine is broken down by the liver. People with severe **liver disease** may require lower doses of this medication and should use it with caution. Those with mild or moderate disease may use it without dose adjustment.

Memantine has not been studied in people with **seizure disorders**. A very small number of people taking memantine in drug studies had seizures, but the number was similar to that which occurred in people taking a placebo (sugar pill).

Possible Side Effects

In most cases, memantine side effects reported in clinical studies were similar to those reported by people who took a placebo.

- ▼ Common: dizziness, headache, confusion, and constipation.
- ▼ Less common: fatigue, hallucinations, vomiting, difficulty breathing, high blood pressure, and back pain.
- ▼ Rare: Other side effects, including chest pain, stroke, convulsions, liver failure, low blood sugar, high blood lipids, impotence, and severe allergic reactions, can affect almost any part of the body. Contact your doctor if you experience anything unusual while taking any medication.

Drug Interactions

- Carbonic anhydrase inhibitors (such as acetazolamide) and bicarbonate of soda (baking soda)—drugs that reduce the acidity of urine—can cause the body to eliminate about 80% less memantine through the kidneys.
- Dosages of thiazide diuretics may need adjusting when taken with memantine.
- Memantine does not interfere with the ability of donepezil and other cholinesterase inhibitors to function.
- Dextromethorphan, a common ingredient in over-the-counter cough medicines, should be avoided when you are taking memantine.

Food Interactions

Memantine can be taken without regard to food or meals.

Usual Dose

Adult: starting dose—5 mg a day. Dose is increased weekly in 5-mg increments up to 20 mg a day.

Child: not recommended.

Overdosage

Symptoms include restlessness, psychosis, hallucinations, sleepiness, stupor, and loss of consciousness. Take the victim to a hospital emergency room. If you seek treatment, ALWAYS bring the prescription bottle or container.

Special Information

Patient caregivers who are responsible for ensuring that medicines are taken correctly must understand how memantine is taken and its dosage regimen.

Special Populations

Pregnancy/Breast-feeding: Animal studies with memantine revealed no danger to a developing fetus, even at the highest dosage. Memantine should be taken during pregnancy only if your doctor determines that the potential benefit outweighs the risks.

It is not known if memantine passes into breast milk. Nursing mothers who must take it should use infant formula.

Seniors: Seniors may use this drug without special precaution. Those with kidney disease may require lower doses.

Generic Name

Meprobamate (meh-proe-BUH-mate) G

Brand Names

Only available in generic form.

Type of Drug

Antianxiety agent.

Prescribed For

Short-term anxiety and tension.

General Information

Meprobamate works by directly affecting several areas of the brain. It can relax you, relieve anxiety, and act as a muscle relaxant, anticonvulsant, or sleeping pill. This drug should be used for less than 4 months.

Cautions and Warnings

Do not take meprobamate if you are **allergic** or **sensitive** to any of its ingredients or to a related drug such as carbromal, carisoprodol, felbamate, or mebutamate.

Do not use meprobamate if you have **intermittent porphyria**.

People with **epilepsy** should use this drug with caution because it may cause seizures in these people.

Meprobamate should be used with caution by people with **kidney or liver disease**, who may need to take lower dosages.

Some people taking meprobamate have developed severe physical and psychological drug dependence. This drug can produce chronic intoxication after prolonged use or if used in greater than recommended doses. Symptoms include slurred speech, dizziness, general sleepiness, and depression. Suddenly stopping meprobamate after prolonged and excessive use may result in drug withdrawal symptoms, including severe anxiety, vomiting, appetite loss, sleeplessness, tremors, muscle twitching, confusion, hallucinations, and convulsions. Withdrawal symptoms usually begin 12–48 hours after meprobamate has been stopped and may last 1–4 days. When stopping treatment with meprobamate, the drug should be reduced gradually over 1 or 2 weeks.

Possible Side Effects

- ▼ Most common: drowsiness, sleepiness, dizziness, slurred speech, poor muscle coordination, headache, weakness, tingling in the arms and legs, and euphoria (feeling "high").
- ▼ Less common: nausea, vomiting, diarrhea, abnormal heart rhythm, excitement or overstimulation, low blood pressure, itching, rash, and changes in blood components.
- ▼ Rare: allergic reactions, including high fever, chills, bronchospasm (closing of the throat), and reduced urinary function. Contact your doctor if you experience anything unusual while taking any medication.

Drug Interactions

- Combining meprobamate with central-nervous-system (CNS) depressants, including alcohol, other sedatives, narcotics, sleeping pills, or antihistamines, can cause excess sedation, depression, sleepiness, or fatigue.

Food Interactions

Take meprobamate with food if it upsets your stomach.

Usual Dose

Adult and Child (age 13 and over): 1200–1600 mg a day in 3–4 doses; maximum daily dose—2400 mg.

Child (age 6–12): 100–200 mg 2–3 times a day.

Child (under age 6): not recommended.

Overdosage

Overdose symptoms include extreme drowsiness, lethargy, stupor, and coma, with possible shock and respiratory collapse.

If alcohol or another depressant has also been taken, small overdoses can be fatal. After a large overdose, the victim will go to sleep very quickly, and blood pressure, pulse, and breathing levels will drop rapidly. The overdose victim must immediately be taken to a hospital emergency room. If you seek treatment, ALWAYS bring the prescription bottle or container.

Special Information

Take this drug according to your doctor's direction. Do not change your dose without your doctor's approval. Do not crush or chew meprobamate tablets.

This drug causes drowsiness and poor concentration. Be careful when driving or performing complex activities. Avoid alcohol and other CNS depressants because they increase these effects.

Contact your doctor if you develop fever, sore throat, rash, mouth sores, nosebleeds, unexplained black-and-blue marks, or easy bruising or bleeding, or if you become pregnant.

If you forget a dose and remember within about 1 hour of your regular time, take it right away. If you do not remember until later, skip the dose you forgot and go back to your regular schedule. Do not take a double dose.

Special Populations

Pregnancy/Breast-feeding: Meprobamate increases the risk of birth defects, particularly during the first 3 months of pregnancy. Inform your doctor immediately if you are taking this drug and are pregnant. Meprobamate should be taken during pregnancy only if your doctor determines that the potential benefit outweighs the risks.

Large amounts of meprobamate pass into breast milk. Nursing mothers who must take this drug should use infant formula.

Seniors: Seniors are more sensitive to the sedative and other effects of this drug and should take the lowest effective dosage.

Generic Name

Metaxalone (meh-TAX-uh-lone) G

Brand Names

Skelaxin

Type of Drug

Skeletal muscle relaxant.

Prescribed For

Muscle spasms.

General Information

Metaxalone is prescribed as part of a coordinated program of rest, physical therapy, and other measures for the relief of acute, painful spasm conditions. Exactly how metaxalone works is unknown.

Cautions and Warnings

Do not take metaxalone if you are **allergic** or **sensitive** to any of its ingredients.

Do not take metaxalone if you have a tendency toward **anemia**, or have serious **kidney or liver disease**.

Possible Side Effects

- ▼ Most common: nausea, vomiting, upset stomach, stomach cramps, drowsiness, dizziness, headache, nervousness, and irritability.
- ▼ Less common: rash, itching, low white-blood-cell count, low red-blood-cell count (symptoms include chills, fatigue, pale skin color, shortness of breath, rapid or pounding heartbeat, and dark urine), liver inflammation, and yellowing of the skin or whites of the eyes.
- ▼ Rare: drug-sensitivity reactions (symptoms include hives, changes in facial color, and breathing difficulties). Contact your doctor if you experience anything unusual while taking any medication.

Drug Interactions

- Sedatives, alcohol, and other nervous system depressants may increase the depressant effects of metaxalone.

Food Interactions

Metaxalone may be taken with food or meals if it upsets your stomach. Avoid high-fat meals.

Usual Dose

Adult and Child (age 12 and over): 800 mg 3 or 4 times a day.
Child (under age 12): not recommended.

Overdosage

Symptoms are likely to be severe side effects but may include some less common reactions as well. Overdose victims should be taken to a hospital emergency room. If you seek treatment, ALWAYS bring the prescription bottle or container.

Special Information

Long-term metaxalone treatment may cause liver toxicity or damage. If you are using this medicine for an extended period, your doctor should check your liver function about every 1–2 months.

Metaxalone may cause tiredness, dizziness, and lightheadedness. Be careful when driving or performing tasks that require concentration and coordination.

Contact your doctor if you develop breathing difficulties, unusual tiredness or weakness, fever, chills, cough or hoarseness, lower back or side pain, painful urination, yellowing of the skin or whites of the eyes, rash, hives, itching, redness, or any other bothersome or persistent symptom.

If you miss a dose of metaxalone, take it as soon as you remember. If it is almost time for your next dose, take 1 dose as soon as you remember, another in 3 or 4 hours, and then go back to your regular schedule. Do not take a double dose.

Special Populations

Pregnancy/Breast-feeding: The safety of metaxalone in pregnant women is unknown. Metaxalone should be taken during pregnancy only if your doctor determines that the potential benefit outweighs the risks.

It is not known if metaxalone passes into breast milk. Nursing mothers who must take it should use infant formula.

Seniors: Seniors with reduced kidney or liver function may require less metaxalone.

Generic Name

Metformin (met-FOR-min) G

Brand Names

Fortamet
Glucophage
Glucophage XR
Glumetza
Riomet

Type of Drug

Biguanide antidiabetic.

Prescribed For

Type 2 diabetes; insulin-resistant and prediabetic conditions, including impaired glucose tolerance, obesity, polycystic ovary syndrome, and metabolic abnormalities associated with HIV disease.

General Information

Metformin lowers the amount of glucose (sugar) produced by the liver, reduces the amount of glucose you absorb from food, and helps cells use glucose. If metformin fails to control your blood sugar, combining it with another antidiabetic drug may control your diabetes. Metformin can also moderately lower blood fats.

Metformin is available in either tablet form or as an oral solution.

Cautions and Warnings

Do not take metformin if you are **allergic** or **sensitive** to any of its ingredients.

Do not take metformin if you have **heart failure**. If you experience a heart attack or other sudden heart damage that requires hospitalization, your doctor will stop your metformin until your condition improves and it is certain that your kidneys are functioning properly.

People with moderate to severe **kidney disease** should not take metformin. If you are having surgery or an X-ray that requires the injection of an iodine-based contrast material, you should temporarily stop taking metformin because the combination could result in acute kidney problems and increased risk of lactic acidosis.

Metformin is related to an older antidiabetes drug that was removed from the market because of the risk of a very rare but serious complication known as lactic acidosis. Lactic acidosis is fatal about 50% of the time. It may also occur in association with a number of conditions, including diabetes mellitus. The risk of lactic acidosis increases with age, the presence of heart failure, and worsening kidney function. Regular monitoring of kidney function minimizes the risk of developing lactic acidosis, as does using the minimum effective dosage of metformin. People with **acidosis**, including those with **diabetic ketoacidosis**, should not take metformin. Diabetic ketoacidosis should be treated with insulin.

People with **liver disease** should not take metformin because of the increased risk of lactic acidosis.

Metformin can interfere with the absorption of vitamin B_{12}, leading to a vitamin B_{12} deficiency. Symptoms can include tingling, pain, or loss of sensation in the hands or feet. Taking a B_{12} supplement can avoid this problem. Your doctor should periodically check your vitamin B_{12} levels while you take metformin.

Possible Side Effects

People who have been stabilized on metformin should not consider gastrointestinal symptoms to be related to the drug unless other causes or lactic acidosis have been excluded.

- ▼ Most common: diarrhea, nausea, vomiting, and gas. These symptoms tend to occur when you first start taking metformin but are generally transient and resolve on their own. Occasionally, temporary dosage reduction is useful.
- ▼ Less common: weakness, stomach pain and indigestion, and headache.
- ▼ Rare: an unpleasant or metallic taste in the mouth (this usually resolves on its own), abnormal stools, chills, lightheadedness, flushing, changes to finger- or toenails, rash, sweating, chest pain, breathing difficulties, flu-like symptoms, muscle pain, low blood sugar, and heart palpitations. Contact your doctor if you experience anything unusual while taking any medication.

Drug Interactions

- Metformin may reduce the effect of glyburide (a sulfonylurea) but this interaction is highly variable from 1 person to another.
- Alcohol increases the risk of developing lactic acidosis while taking metformin.
- The following drugs may decrease the effectiveness of metformin: calcium channel blockers, contraceptive drugs, corticosteroids, estrogens, isoniazid, nicotinic acid, phenothiazines, phenytoin, sympathomimetics (amphetamine), thiazide diuretics, and thyroid drugs.
- Metformin blood levels may be increased by amiloride, cephalexin, digoxin, morphine, quinidine, quinine, ranitidine, triamterene, trimethoprim, and vancomycin. Careful monitoring is necessary.
- Cimetidine, furosemide, nifedipine, and rofecoxib can cause a large increase in metformin blood levels and possible side effects. Furosemide levels are reduced by metformin.
- The following drugs can raise blood sugar: calcium channel blockers, contraceptives, corticosteroids, estrogens, isoniazid, nicotinic acid, phenothiazines, phenytoin,

sympathomimetics (amphetamine), thiazide diuretics, and thyroid drugs. This may make diabetes harder to control and may necessitate more or different diabetes medicine.

Food Interactions

Metformin may be taken with food to reduce upset stomach.

Usual Dose

Extended-Release Tablets

Adult: 500–2500 mg once a day.
Child: not recommended.

Immediate-Release Tablets

Adult: 500 mg twice a day or 850 mg once a day, increased gradually to a maximum daily dosage of 2550 mg in 2–3 divided doses. Older adults should start with the regular dosage but generally are not given the maximum.

Child (age 10 and over): 500–2000 mg in divided doses.

Overdosage

Lactic acidosis has occurred in some cases. Take the victim to a hospital emergency room at once. If you seek treatment, ALWAYS bring the prescription bottle or container.

Special Information

Diet and exercise are the mainstays of diabetes treatment. Be sure to follow your doctor's directions in these areas while taking your medication.

Lactic acidosis is a medical emergency. Metformin treatment must be stopped immediately if you develop it. This disease is often subtle and is accompanied only by nonspecific symptoms such as feeling unwell, muscle aches, breathing difficulties, tiredness, and nonspecific upset stomach. Low body temperature, low blood pressure, and slow heartbeat can develop with more severe acidosis. Contact your doctor at once if you develop these symptoms.

Stomach and intestinal side effects may be reduced by gradually increasing your dosage and by taking metformin with meals.

Metformin should be temporarily stopped if you have severe diarrhea or vomiting. However, do not stop taking your medication without first consulting your doctor.

If you forget a dose, take it as soon as you remember. If it is almost time for your next dose, skip the dose you forgot and continue with your regular schedule. Do not take a double dose.

Special Populations

Pregnancy/Breast-feeding: The safety of using metformin during pregnancy is not known. Pregnant women with diabetes should take insulin.

Metformin passes into breast milk. Nursing mothers who must take it should use infant formula.

Seniors: Seniors may require reduced dosage.

Generic Name

Methotrexate (meth-oe-TREK-sate) G

Brand Names

Rheumatrex Trexall

Type of Drug

Antimetabolite, antiarthritic, and anti-inflammatory agent.

Prescribed For

Cancer chemotherapy; psoriasis; and adult and juvenile rheumatoid arthritis. Also used for Reiter's disease and severe asthma.

General Information

Used effectively in cancer treatment since the late 1940s, methotrexate is also prescribed for other conditions that respond to immune system suppressants. Dosage varies widely depending on the disease being treated. Even relatively low dosages, such as those prescribed for rheumatoid arthritis, can be extremely toxic. Because of the risks associated with methotrexate, it should be used in noncancerous conditions only when the disease is severe and other treatments have failed. Only doctors who are familiar with methotrexate and its risks should prescribe it.

Cautions and Warnings

Do not take methotrexate if you are **allergic** or **sensitive** to any of its ingredients.

Methotrexate should not be used in **pregnant women** to treat psoriasis or rheumatoid arthritis. It should only be used in pregnant women for cancer treatment when the potential benefits outweigh the risks.

Methotrexate can trigger a unique and dangerous form of lung disease at any time during your course of therapy. It can occur at dosages as low as 7.5 mg per week—the antiarthritis dosage. Symptoms of this condition are cough, respiratory infection, difficulty breathing, abnormal chest X-ray, and low blood-oxygen levels. Report any changes in breathing or lung status to your doctor.

Methotrexate can cause severe liver damage; this usually occurs only after taking it over a long period. Changes in liver enzymes, as measured by a blood test, are common. People with chronic **liver disease** should not take methotrexate to treat noncancerous conditions.

People with **kidney disease** should use this drug with caution and receive a reduced dosage.

Methotrexate can severely lower red- and white-blood-cell and blood-platelet counts. Your doctor should periodically evaluate your kidney and liver function and blood components.

Methotrexate suppresses the immune system and can make you more likely to develop an opportunistic infection such as pneumocystis. Those with a **compromised immune system** should not take methotrexate.

Methotrexate can cause severe diarrhea, stomach irritation, and mouth or gum sores. Death can result from intestinal perforation caused by methotrexate.

Severe, occasionally fatal, skin reactions have occurred with doses of methotrexate. These reactions may be reversible after discontinuation of the medicine.

Methotrexate has been studied as an abortion drug in combination with misoprostol (see Misoprostol, page 775).

Possible Side Effects

- ▼ Most common: liver irritation, loss of kidney function, reduced blood-platelet count, nausea, vomiting, diarrhea, stomach upset and irritation, itching, rash, hair loss, dizziness, and risk of infection.
- ▼ Less common: reduced red-blood-cell count, unusual sensitivity to the sun, acne, headache, drowsiness, blurred vision, respiratory infection and breathing problems, appetite loss, muscle aches, chest pain, coughing, painful urination, eye discomfort, nosebleeds, fever, infection, blood in the urine, sweating, ringing or buzzing in the ears, defective sperm production, reduced sperm count, menstrual dysfunction, vaginal discharge, convulsions, and slight paralysis.

Drug Interactions

- Aspirin and other nonsteroidal anti-inflammatory drugs (NSAIDs), as well as low-dose corticosteroid treatment, may be continued in most cases while you are taking methotrexate for rheumatoid arthritis, although an increase in drug toxicity is possible. However, fatal reactions have developed in 4 people taking methotrexate and an NSAID—3 with ketoprofen, 1 with naproxen. Do not take methotrexate and an anti-inflammatory or antiarthritic drug—even over-the-counter drugs such as ibuprofen or naproxen sodium—without your doctor's knowledge.
- Anticancer drugs, aspirin and other salicylates, etretinate, penicillins, phenytoin, probenecid, sulfa drugs, and trimethoprim can increase the therapeutic and toxic effects of methotrexate.
- Combining phenylbutazone and methotrexate increases the risk of severe white-blood-cell count reductions, but may be medically necessary. In these cases, your doctor should monitor your health for signs of drug toxicity (see "Cautions and Warnings").
- Oral antibiotics such as chloramphenicol and tetracycline, oral aminoglycosides, charcoal, and folic acid may counteract the effects of methotrexate.
- Methotrexate may decrease blood levels of digoxin and phenytoin, requiring dosage adjustments.
- Methotrexate may raise theophylline and thiopurines (such as azathioprine) blood levels. Monitoring and dosage adjustments may be necessary with these combinations.

Food Interactions

For optimal effectiveness, take this drug on an empty stomach, at least 1 hour before or 2 hours after meals. It may be taken with food if it upsets your stomach.

Usual Dose

Cancer: Dosage varies. Some cancers are treated with 10–30 mg a day, while others require 100s or 1000s of mg given intravenously.

Psoriasis: 10–25 mg per week in a single dose or in 3 divided doses taken 12 hours apart, not to exceed 30 mg a week.

Rheumatoid Arthritis: starting dose—7.5 mg a week by mouth, either as a single dose or in 3 separate doses of 2.5 mg taken every 12 hours. Weekly dose may be increased gradually up to 20 mg. Dosages above 20 mg a week are more likely to cause severe side effects.

Overdosage

Methotrexate overdose can be serious and life-threatening. Victims should be taken to a hospital emergency room immediately. A specific antidote to the effects of methotrexate, calcium leucovorin, is available in every hospital. If you seek treatment, ALWAYS bring the prescription bottle or container.

Special Information

If you vomit after taking a dose of methotrexate, do not take a replacement dose unless instructed to do so by your doctor.

Women taking this drug must use effective birth control.

People at risk of liver or kidney damage must be regularly monitored by their doctor for possible damage caused by methotrexate.

To avoid birth defects, men should not conceive during treatment or for 3 months after treatment has been completed.

Contact your doctor immediately if you develop diarrhea, fever or chills, skin reddening, mouth or lip sores, stomach pain, unusual bleeding or bruising, blurred vision, seizures, cough, or breathing difficulties.

The following symptoms are less severe but should still be reported to your doctor: back pain, darkened urine, dizziness, drowsiness, headache, unusual tiredness or sickness, and yellowing of the skin or whites of the eyes.

If you forget a dose, skip it and continue with your regular schedule. Contact your doctor at once. Do not take a double dose.

Special Populations

Pregnancy/Breast-feeding: Methotrexate can cause spontaneous abortion, stillbirth, and severe birth defects. Pregnant women should take methotrexate only after discussing the potential benefits versus risks with their doctor. Methotrexate should not be given to pregnant women to treat psoriasis or rheumatoid arthritis. Do not attempt to achieve pregnancy during methotrexate treatment or for at least 1 menstrual cycle after the treatment is completed. Use effective birth control while taking this drug. To avoid birth defects, men should not conceive during treatment or for 3 months after treatment has been completed. Methotrexate reduces sperm counts and may compromise sperm health.

This drug passes into breast milk. Nursing mothers who must take methotrexate should use infant formula.

Seniors: Seniors may be more susceptible to side effects and may obtain maximum benefit with smaller dosages.

Generic Name

Methyldopa (meth-ul-DOPE-uh) G

Brand Names

Only available in generic form.

The information in this profile also applies to the following drugs:

Generic Ingredients: Methyldopa + Hydrochlorothiazide G

Type of Drug

Antihypertensive.

Prescribed For

High blood pressure.

General Information

How methyldopa works is not well understood. It may lower blood pressure by stimulating receptors in the central nervous system, and by inhibiting or reducing levels of important pressure-regulating hormones such as norepinephrine and serotonin. It takes about 2 days for methyldopa to reach its maximal antihypertensive (blood-pressure-lowering) effect. It is usually prescribed with one or more other antihypertensive drugs or a diuretic.

Cautions and Warnings

Do not take methyldopa if you are **allergic** or **sensitive** to any of its ingredients or any other ingredient in the formulation, including sulfites.

Do not take this drug if you have had a previous **liver-related reaction** to it, or if you have **liver disease** such as hepatitis or cirrhosis. People taking this drug may develop a fever with changes in liver function within the first 3 weeks of treatment. Some people develop jaundice (symptoms include yellowing of the skin or whites of the eyes) during the first 2 or 3 months of treatment. Your doctor should periodically evaluate your liver function during the first 3 months of methyldopa treatment, or if you develop an unexplained fever.

Methyldopa should be used with caution in people with severe **kidney disease**, who may need reduced dosage.

Methyldopa may increase the risk of hemolytic anemia.

Some people taking methyldopa experience swelling or weight gain. This can usually be controlled when methyldopa is combined with a diuretic. Do not continue taking methyldopa if swelling progresses or you experience signs of heart failure.

Possible Side Effects

Most people have little trouble with methyldopa, but it can cause temporary sedation in the first few weeks of treatment or when the dose is increased. Passing headache and weakness are other possible early side effects.

▼ Less common: headache; dizziness; lightheadedness; tingling in the extremities; muscle spasms or weakness; decreased mental acuity; psychological disturbances, including nightmares, mild psychosis, and depression; rash; changes in heart rate; increased angina; water retention, resulting in weight gain; nausea; vomiting; constipation; diarrhea; mild dry mouth; sore or black tongue; stuffy nose; male breast enlargement or pain; lactation in females; impotence or decreased sex drive in males; mild arthritis symptoms; and skin reactions.

▼ Rare: Methyldopa may affect white blood cells or blood platelets. It may also cause involuntary jerky movements, twitching, restlessness, and slow, continuous, wormlike movements of the fingers, toes, hands, or other body parts. Contact your doctor if you experience anything unusual while taking any medication.

Drug Interactions

- Do not combine methyldopa and a monoamine oxidase inhibitor (MAOI) antidepressant. This combination can cause excessive stimulation.
- Reduced doses of anesthetics may be required while taking methyldopa.
- Methyldopa increases the effect of other blood-pressure-lowering drugs. This is a desirable interaction for people with hypertension. However, the combination of methyldopa and propranolol or nadolol—2 beta blockers often prescribed for hypertension—has, rarely, caused an increase in blood pressure.
- Methyldopa in combination with haloperidol may lead to increased effects of haloperidol or produce irritability, aggressive behavior, or other psychiatric symptoms.
- Combining methyldopa with levodopa + carbidopa may increase all their effects.

- The combination of methyldopa and lithium may cause symptoms of lithium overdose—upset stomach, frequent urination, muscle weakness, tiredness, and tremors—even though blood levels of lithium have not changed.
- Combining methyldopa with stimulants or a phenothiazine-type drug may lead to a serious increase in blood pressure.
- If methyldopa is combined with tizanidine, excessively low blood pressure may result.
- Avoid over-the-counter cough medicines, cold and allergy remedies, and appetite suppressants. These products contain stimulant ingredients that can increase blood pressure.

Food Interactions

Methyldopa is best taken on an empty stomach, but you may take it with food if it upsets your stomach.

Usual Dose

Adult: starting dose—250-mg tablet 2–3 times a day for the first 2 days. Dosage may then be increased until lower blood pressure is achieved. Maintenance dose—500–2000 mg a day in 2–4 divided doses, depending on individual need.

Child: 4.5 mg per lb. of body weight a day in 2–4 divided doses, depending on individual need. Do not exceed 30 mg per lb. of body weight or 3 g a day, whichever is less.

Overdosage

Symptoms include sedation, very low blood pressure, weakness, dizziness, lightheadedness, fainting, slow heartbeat, constipation, abdominal gas or bulging, nausea, vomiting, and coma. Overdose victims should be made to vomit if they are still conscious by using ipecac syrup—available at any pharmacy—and then taken to a hospital emergency room. If some time has passed since the overdose was taken, take the victim directly to an emergency room. If you seek treatment, ALWAYS bring the prescription bottle or container.

Special Information

Take methyldopa exactly as prescribed to maintain maximum control of your hypertension. Do not stop taking this drug unless you are told to do so by your doctor.

A mild sedative effect is to be expected from methyldopa and will resolve within several days. Be careful when driving, operating hazardous machinery, or performing any task that requires concentration.

Your urine may darken if left exposed to air. This is normal and not a cause for alarm.

You may experience dizziness when rising suddenly from a sitting or lying position. However, contact your doctor if you develop fever, prolonged general tiredness, or general dizziness. If you develop involuntary muscle movements, fever, or jaundice, stop taking the drug and contact your doctor immediately. If these reactions are due to methyldopa, your temperature or liver abnormalities will begin to normalize as soon as you stop taking it.

If you forget a dose, take it as soon as you remember. If it is almost time for your next dose, skip the one you forgot and continue with your regular schedule. Do not take a double dose.

Special Populations

Pregnancy/Breast-feeding: Methyldopa crosses into the fetal circulation. Methyldopa should be taken during pregnancy only if your doctor determines that the potential benefit outweighs the risks.

Small amounts of methyldopa pass into breast milk. Nursing mothers who must take this drug should use infant formula.

Seniors: Seniors are more sensitive to the sedating and blood-pressure-lowering effects of methyldopa and may experience dizziness or fainting. Older adults should receive reduced dosage.

Generic Name

Methylphenidate (meth-ul-FEN-ih-date) G

Brand Names

Concerta
Daytrana Patch
Metadate
Metadate CD
Metadate ER
Methylin
Methylin ER
Ritalin
Ritalin LA
Ritalin-SR

The information in this profile also applies to the following drugs:

Generic Ingredients: Dexmethylphenidate G
Focalin
Focalin XR

Type of Drug

Mild central-nervous-system stimulant.

Prescribed For

Attention-deficit hyperactivity disorder (ADHD); also prescribed for psychological, educational, or social disorders; narcolepsy; and mild depression in the elderly. Methylphenidate is also used in cancer treatment and stroke recovery and for treating hiccups after anesthesia.

General Information

Methylphenidate is prescribed for the treatment of ADHD in children. It should be used only after conducting a complete evaluation of the child. Frequency and severity of symptoms and their appropriateness for the age of the child—not solely the presence of certain behavioral characteristics—determine whether drug therapy is required. Many experts believe that methylphenidate offers only a temporary solution because it does not permanently change behavioral patterns. Psychological measures must also be taken to ensure successful treatment in the long term.

Cautions and Warnings

Do not take methylphenidate if you are **allergic** or **sensitive** to any of its ingredients. Severe drug reactions can occur and include rash, blisters, swelling of the tongue, and choking. These reactions require immediate medical attention.

Do not take methylphenidate on the day of **surgery** because there is a risk of sudden blood increases.

Do not take methylphenidate if you have **glaucoma or other visual problems**, a **seizure disorder**, severe **depression**, **tics** or **Tourette syndrome**, or if you are extremely **tense or agitated**.

People with a history of **drug dependence** or **alcoholism** should use methylphenidate with caution. Chronic or abusive use of methylphenidate can lead to drug dependence or addiction. This drug can also cause severe psychotic episodes and worsen other psychiatric disorders. Do not use methylphenidate for the prevention or treatment of normal fatigue.

Methylphenidate should be used with caution if you have **high blood pressure**, and your doctor should monitor your blood pressure frequently while you take this drug.

Stimulants like methylphenidate are not effective in **children** whose symptoms are related to environmental factors or to primary psychiatric conditions, including psychosis. Children who take these medicines for ADHD may have a higher risk of sudden death. Further research is under way to better define this risk.

Methylphenidate should not be used to treat a **primary stress reaction**.

Possible Side Effects

Adult

▼ Most common: nervousness and inability to sleep, which doctors generally control by reducing or eliminating the afternoon or evening dose.

▼ Rare: rash, itching, fever, hallucinations, convulsions, symptoms resembling those of arthritis, appetite loss, nausea, dizziness, blurred vision or other visual disturbances, abnormal heart rhythm, headache, obsessive-compulsive disorder (OCD), drowsiness, changes in blood pressure or pulse, chest pain, stomach pain, psychotic reactions, changes in blood components, and loss of some scalp hair. Contact your doctor if you experience anything unusual while taking any medication.

Child

▼ Most common: headache; appetite loss; stomach pain; weight loss, especially during prolonged therapy; sleeping difficulties; and abnormal heart rhythm.

Drug Interactions

- Serious reactions can develop when methylphenidate is combined with clonidine.
- Methylphenidate reduces the effectiveness of guanethidine (an antihypertensive drug).
- Monoamine oxidase inhibitor (MAOI) antidepressants may significantly increase the effect of methylphenidate, which may lead to extreme high blood pressure. Do not take these drugs together, or take methylphenidate for 14 days after you stop taking an MAOI.
- Methylphenidate may slow the breakdown of tricyclic and selective serotonin reuptake inhibitor (SSRI) antidepressants, phenylbutazone, and warfarin (a blood thinner), raising the risk of side effects. Dose reduction may be needed.
- Methylphenidate may increase anticonvulsant blood levels.
- If you take methylphenidate regularly, avoid alcohol. This combination increases drowsiness.

Food Interactions

This medication is best taken 30–45 minutes before meals.

Usual Dose

Oral Tablets

Adult: Doses range from 10–30 mg a day but can be as high as 60–72 mg. The immediate-release drug is taken 2–3 times a day.

Child (age 6 and over): starting dose—5 mg before breakfast and lunch. Increase by 5–10 mg each week as required, not to exceed 60 mg a day.

Child (under age 6): not recommended.

Sustained-release (SR) and extended-release (ER) tablets are designed to last for 8 hours, and Concerta, Ritalin LA, and Metadate CD last 8–12 hours. These medications may be used in place of more frequent doses during the same period of time.

Skin Patch: The methylphenidate patch should be applied to the hip area about 2 hours before an effect is needed and should be removed 9 hours after application. Apply the patch as close to the same time every day as possible to obtain consistent daily dosing.

Overdosage

Symptoms include vomiting, agitation, uncontrollable twitching of the muscles, convulsions followed by coma, euphoria (feeling "high"), confusion, hallucinations, delirium, sweating, flushing, headache, high fever, abnormal heart rate, high blood pressure, and dryness of the mouth and nose. Take the victim to a hospital emergency room immediately. If you seek treatment, ALWAYS bring the prescription bottle or container.

Special Information

Methylphenidate can mask the signs of temporary drowsiness or fatigue. Be careful when driving or doing any task that requires concentration. Take your last daily dose no later than 6 p.m. to avoid sleeping difficulties.

Contact your doctor if you develop any persistent or bothersome side effect. Do not increase your dosage without your doctor's knowledge.

If improvement is not seen after 1 month of adequate dosage, discontinue use of this drug.

Suppression of growth in children has been reported with long-term use of this drug. Contact your doctor if your child does not grow or gain weight as expected.

ER and SR tablets must be swallowed whole, never crushed or chewed.

Use of the methylphenidate skin patch should be stopped if an intense local reaction (redness plus small, solid, rounded bumps and pustules) does not get much better within 48 hours or spreads beyond the patch site. Redness is common and, by itself, not a severe reaction. Contact your doctor if a skin reaction develops; you may need to take the oral form in this case.

If you miss a dose, take it as soon as possible. Space the remaining daily dosage evenly throughout the day. Go back to your regular schedule the next day.

Special Populations

Pregnancy/Breast-feeding: Methylphenidate crosses into the fetal circulation and should be taken during pregnancy only if your doctor determines that the potential benefit outweighs the risks.

It is not known whether this drug passes into breast milk. Nursing mothers who must take this drug should use infant formula.

Seniors: Seniors may take this drug without special precaution.

Generic Name

Metoclopramide (met-oe-KLOE-pruh-mide) G

Brand Names

Metazolv ODT
Reglan*

**Some products in this brand-name group are alcohol- or sugar-free. Consult your pharmacist.*

Type of Drug

Antiemetic and gastrointestinal (GI) stimulant.

Prescribed For

Diabetic gastroparesis (stomach paralysis associated with diabetes; symptoms include nausea, vomiting, heartburn, persistent feeling of fullness, and appetite loss), gastroesophageal reflux disease (GERD), stomach ulcer, anorexia nervosa, and bleeding from blood vessels in the esophagus—often associated with severe liver disease. It also facilitates diagnostic X-ray procedures and improves the absorption of antimigraine medication and narcotic pain relievers. Nursing mothers are occasionally given metoclopramide to increase milk production.

General Information

Metoclopramide stimulates movement of the upper GI tract without producing excess stomach acids or other secretions. Doctors believe that it prevents nausea and vomiting primarily by affecting dopamine receptors in the brain. Metoclopramide also affects the secretion of a variety of hormones and may improve the absorption of other drugs into the bloodstream.

Cautions and Warnings

Do not take metoclopramide if you are **allergic** or **sensitive** to any of its ingredients.

Metoclopramide has been associated with tardive dyskinesia, a condition characterized by involuntary, disjointed movements. The risk of developing this condition, which is potentially irreversible, increases with duration of treatment and cumulative dosage.

Do not take this drug if you have a **seizure disorder**.

Metoclopramide should not be taken by those with **pheochromocytoma** (adrenal gland tumor). Metoclopramide should not be used if you have a **bleeding ulcer** or any condition that makes stimulation of the GI tract dangerous.

People with **high blood pressure, asthma**, or **kidney disease** should use metoclopramide with caution.

Metoclopramide has been safely used in people with liver disease although those with **cirrhosis** of the liver or **congestive heart failure** may be at higher risk for excessive fluid retention.

Mild to severe **depression** has occurred with metoclopramide. People with a history of depression should use this drug with caution.

Uncontrollable motions similar to those associated with **Parkinson's disease** have developed as a side effect of this drug. These generally occur within 6 months after starting metoclopramide and subside within 2–3 months. Those with Parkinson's disease should use this medication with extreme caution or not at all.

This drug may cause extrapyramidal side effects similar to those associated with phenothiazine drugs. These effects, which occur in 0.2–1% of the people taking the drug, include restlessness and involuntary movements of the arms and legs, face, tongue, lips, and other parts of the body. Do not combine metoclopramide with a phenothiazine drug because this may increase the risk of extrapyramidal effects.

A serious set of side effects known as neuroleptic malignant syndrome (NMS) has rarely been reported in those taking metoclopramide. Symptoms include high fever, convulsions, difficult or fast breathing, rapid heartbeat, rapid or irregular pulse or blood pressure, increased sweating, muscle rigidity, and mental changes. NMS can be fatal and requires immediate medical attention.

Women taking this drug develop chronic elevations of the hormone prolactin. About 33% of breast tumors are prolactin-dependent, a factor that you should consider before taking metoclopramide.

Metoclopramide is only prescribed for short-term relief of symptoms. Treatment with metoclopramide lasting longer than 12 weeks has not been studied and is not recommended.

Possible Side Effects

Mild side effects occur in 20–30% of people. Side effects increase with dosage or prolonged use.

- ▼ Most common: restlessness, drowsiness, fatigue, sleeplessness, dizziness, anxiety, loss of muscle control, nausea, diarrhea, headache, muscle spasm, confusion, and severe depression.
- ▼ Less common: rash, diarrhea, blood-pressure changes, abnormal heart rhythms, slow heartbeat, oozing from the nipples, tender nipples, loss of regular menstrual periods, breast swelling and tenderness, impotence, reduced white-blood-cell counts, frequent urination, loss of urinary control, visual disturbances, worsening of bronchial spasm, convulsions, and hallucinations.
- ▼ Rare: People taking this drug may develop a group of possibly fatal symptoms collectively called neuroleptic malignant syndrome. These symptoms include very high fever, semi-consciousness, and rigid muscles. Flushing of the face and upper body as well as liver toxicity after high doses have also occurred. Contact your doctor if you experience anything unusual while taking any medication.

Drug Interactions

- Metoclopramide should not be combined with any other medication that causes extrapyramidal side effects.
- Some formulations of metoclopramide syrup contain alcohol. They should not be combined with disulfiram, a medication used to treat chronic alcoholism. Serious reactions are possible.

- Narcotics and anticholinergic drugs interfere with metoclopramide's effect on stomach acid.
- Metoclopramide decreases the effects of cabergoline and pergolide; they should not be combined.
- Metoclopramide may reduce the effects of cimetidine and digoxin.
- Metoclopramide may increase the sedative effects of nervous system depressants, including alcohol, sedatives, and sleeping pills.
- Metoclopramide may increase blood levels of cyclosporine and succinylcholine.
- Due to metoclopramide's effect on food absorption, injected insulin doses may need adjustment.
- Metoclopramide and levodopa + carbidopa interfere with each other. Metoclopramide should generally not be used by those with Parkinson's disease.
- Combining metoclopramide and a monoamine oxidase inhibitor (MAOI) antidepressant may cause very high blood pressure.
- If metoclopramide is combined with a selective serotonin reuptake inhibitor (SSRI) antidepressant (such as sertraline or venlafaxine), the actions of both drugs and the risk of toxicity are increased.

Food Interactions

Take metoclopramide 30 minutes before meals and at bedtime.

Usual Dose

Adult and Child (age 15 and over): 5–15 mg before meals and at bedtime. Single doses of 10–20 mg are used before X-ray diagnostic procedures.

Child (under age 15): 0.45–0.9 mg per lb. of body weight every 2–6 hours as an antiemetic. For GERD or gastrointestinal paralysis, children may be given 0.045–0.09 mg per lb. of body weight 4 times a day, with a maximum dose of 0.36 mg per lb. of body weight a day, over 30 days.

Senior: starting dose—5 mg.

Overdosage

Symptoms of overdose include drowsiness, disorientation, restlessness, or uncontrollable muscle movement. These usually disappear within 24 hours after the drug has been stopped. Anticholinergic drugs help control overdose symptoms. Contact your local poison control center or a hospital emergency room for more information. If you seek treatment, ALWAYS bring the prescription bottle or container.

Special Information

Contact your doctor if you develop chills; fever; sore throat; dizziness; severe or persistent headache; feeling unwell; rapid or irregular heartbeat; difficulty speaking or swallowing; loss of balance; stiffness of the arms or legs; a shuffling walk; a mask-like face; lip-smacking or puckering; puffing of the cheeks; rapid, wormlike tongue movement; uncontrollable chewing movement; uncontrolled arm and leg movement; or any persistent or intolerable side effect.

Metoclopramide may cause dizziness, confusion, and drowsiness. Be careful when driving or doing any task that requires concentration. Avoid alcohol and be cautious about taking sedatives or sleeping pills.

If you forget a dose, take it as soon as you remember. If it is almost time for your next dose, skip the dose you forgot and continue with your regular schedule. Do not take a double dose.

Special Populations

Pregnancy/Breast-feeding: Metoclopramide enters the fetal circulation. Metoclopramide should be taken during pregnancy only if your doctor determines that the potential benefit outweighs the risks.

This drug passes into breast milk. Nursing mothers occasionally receive metoclopramide to increase milk production. There appears to be no risk for the infant whose nursing mother takes 45 mg or less a day. Always consider possible effects on the nursing infant if breast-feeding while taking this drug.

Seniors: Seniors, especially women, are more sensitive to side effects (see "Cautions and Warnings"). Shuffling walk and shaking hands may be likely to occur in seniors after prolonged use of metoclopramide. Dose adjustments may be necessary.

Generic Name

Metronidazole (meh-troe-NYE-duh-zole) G

Brand Names

Flagyl	MetroCream
Flagyl ER	MetroGel

MetroLotion
Noritate
Vandazole

The information in this profile also applies to the following drugs:

Generic Ingredients: Tinidazole
Tindamax

Type of Drug

Amoebicide and antibiotic.

Prescribed For

Metronidazole is prescribed for acute amoebic dysentery, pneumonia, and infections of the vagina, bone, joint, brain, nervous system, heart, liver, intestines, abdomen, and skin; also prescribed for ulcers caused by *Helicobacter pylori,* colitis caused by other antibiotics, periodontal (gum) infection, Crohn's disease, sinus infections, persistent urinary tract infections, and complications of severe liver disease. The gel may be used to treat rosacea, acne, severe skin ulcers, and inflammation of the skin around the mouth.

Tinidazole is prescribed for bacterial vaginosis, vaginal infections with trichomonas, giardia infections in adults and children, and intestinal and liver infections caused by amoeba infection.

General Information

Metronidazole is an effective treatment for infections caused by a variety of fungi and some bacteria. Metronidazole kills these microorganisms by disrupting their DNA after they enter body cells. Tinidazole is a drug chemically related to metronidazole that has been proven to work on bacterial vaginosis, vaginal trichomonas, giardia, and amoeba infections of the bowel or liver. These drugs may be prescribed for symptomless diseases when the doctor feels that an underlying infection may be involved. For example, asymptomatic women may be treated with one of these drugs when vaginal examination shows evidence of trichomonas.

Cautions and Warnings

Do not take metronidazole if you are **allergic** or **sensitive** to any of its ingredients.

Do not take metronidazole if you have a history of **blood disease**.

Metronidazole has been found to cause cancer in lab animals. Unnecessary use of this drug should be avoided.

People taking metronidazole have experienced seizures and numbness or tingling in the hands or feet. This effect is rare with low dosages but may be more common in people taking larger dosages for long periods, as in **Crohn's disease**. If this occurs, stop taking the drug and contact your doctor at once.

Metronidazole should be taken with caution if you have active **nervous system disease**, including **epilepsy**, or severe **liver problems**.

Metronidazole may cause *Candida* vaginitis in women.

Possible Side Effects

Metronidazole

- ▼ Most common: nausea, headache, vaginal irritation, and metallic taste.
- ▼ Less common: genital itching, abdominal pain, dizziness, diarrhea, respiratory infections, nasal and sinus irritation, urine color changes, vaginal pain and fungal infections, dry mouth, and urinary tract infection.
- ▼ Rare: changes in levels of white blood cells or platelets, drug sensitivity (rash, itching, flushing, fever), clumsiness or poor coordination, seizure, increased urination and incontinence, and reduced sex drive. Contact your doctor if you experience anything unusual when taking any medication.

Skin creams containing metronidazole may cause redness, itching, irritation, or worsening of rosacea.

Tinidazole

The chance of side effects increases with the amount of medication taken.

- ▼ Most common: metallic or bitter taste and nausea.
- ▼ Less common: loss of appetite, upset stomach, cramps, vomiting, constipation, weakness, fatigue, not feeling well, dizziness, and headache.
- ▼ Rare: drug sensitivity (itching, rash, flushing, sweating, dry mouth, fever, burning sensation, thirst, salivation, and swelling around the eyes or lips), which may also affect the nervous system, kidneys, heart, blood, and other systems. Contact your doctor if you experience anything unusual when taking any medication.

Drug Interactions

- Do not use alcohol or take disulfiram with these drugs because of the risk of serious interactions. Neither should be taken within 2 weeks of taking disulfiram.

- Metronidazole may increase the side effects of fluorouracil. Do not combine these treatments. If you must take tinidazole and fluorouracil together, your doctor should carefully monitor your condition.
- Dosages of oral anticoagulants (blood thinners) such as warfarin must be reduced because these drugs increase their effect.
- These drugs may increase blood levels and side effects of cyclosporine, lithium, and tacrolimus. Your doctor should monitor your condition if you must take them together.
- Cimetidine and ketoconazole may increase blood levels of these drugs by interfering with their breakdown in the liver. Your dosage may need to be reduced.
- Fosphenytoin, phenytoin, phenobarbital and other barbiturates, and rifampin may reduce the effectiveness of these drugs by increasing the rate at which they are cleared from the body.
- The antibiotic oxytetracycline may antagonize the effects of these drugs.
- Cholestyramine reduces the amount of these drugs absorbed into the blood. Separate these medicines by at least 2 hours to avoid this interaction.

Food Interactions

Do not drink grapefruit juice while taking these medicines because it can interfere with the liver's ability to break them down. Metronidazole and tinidazole (when they must be taken for more than 1 day) should be taken with food to avoid upset stomach.

Usual Dose

Metronidazole

Adult: 250–750 mg 1–4 times a day for for 5–10 days, or 2 g in 1 day in a single or divided dose, depending on the condition treated.

Child (age 3 and over): 16–23 mg per lb. of body weight 3 times a day for 10 days or as prescribed by your child's doctor.

Skin creams should be applied 1–2 times a day. Vaginal creams should be used 1–2 times a day for 5 days.

Tinidazole

Adult: 1–2 g a day with food for 1–5 days, depending on the condition treated.

Child (age 3 and over): 22.7 mg per lb. of body weight up to 2 g, taken with food, for 1–5 days.

Overdosage

Symptoms may include nausea, vomiting, clumsiness, unsteadiness, seizures, and pain or tingling in the hands or feet. Contact your local poison control center or a hospital emergency room for more information. If you seek treatment, ALWAYS bring the prescription bottle or container.

Special Information

Contact your doctor if you become dizzy or lightheaded while taking metronidazole, or if you develop numbness, tingling, pain, or weakness in your hands or feet; seizures; clumsiness or unsteadiness; mood changes; unusual vaginal irritation, discharge, or dryness; frequent or painful urination; rash, hives, or itching; severe pain in the back or abdomen accompanied by vomiting, appetite loss, or nausea; or any bothersome or persistent side effect.

Avoid drinking alcohol while taking metronidazole.

These medicines may cause darkening of your urine; this is probably not an important side effect, but inform your doctor if it happens.

Follow your doctor's dosage instructions exactly. Complete the full course of drug therapy.

Metronidazole may cause dry mouth, which usually can be relieved with ice, hard candy, or gum. Contact your doctor or dentist if dry mouth persists for more than 2 weeks.

If you are taking these drugs for more than 1 day and forget a dose, take it as soon as you remember. If it is almost time for your next dose, skip the dose you forgot and continue with your regular schedule. Do not take a double dose.

Special Populations

Pregnancy/Breast-feeding: Metronidazole passes into the fetal circulation and should not be taken during the first 3 months of pregnancy. It should be taken during the last 6 months of pregnancy only if your doctor determines that the potential benefit outweighs the risks.

Metronidazole passes into breast milk. Nursing mothers who must take this drug should use infant formula.

Seniors: Seniors, particularly those with advanced liver disease, are more sensitive to the effects of metronidazole and may require lower dosages.

Micardis *see* ***Angiotensin II Blockers,*** *page 97*

Generic Name

Miconazole (mye-KON-uh-zole) G

Brand Names

Monistat
Monistat-Derm

The information in this profile also applies to the following drugs:

Generic Ingredients: Butoconazole Nitrate
Femstat-3
Mycelex-3
Gynazole-1

Generic Ingredients: Oxiconazole
Oxistat

Generic Ingredients: Terconazole G
Terazol-3
Zazole
Terazol-7

Generic Ingredients: Tioconazole
Monistat-1
Vagistat

Type of Drug

Antifungal.

Prescribed For

Fungal infections of the vagina, skin, and blood.

General Information

Miconazole is used to treat a variety of fungal infections. Monistat-Derm cream and related products are applied directly to the skin to treat common fungal infections of the skin, including ringworm, athlete's foot, and jock itch. Monistat and similar products are used to treat vaginal yeast infections. Terconazole is prescribed primarily for vaginal infections. Oxiconazole is prescribed only for fungal infections of the skin, including athlete's foot and jock itch. Little of the drug applied to the skin is absorbed into the bloodstream.

Cautions and Warnings

Do not use any of these drugs if you are **allergic** or **sensitive** to any of their ingredients. If a reaction (such as a sensitivity reaction or a chemical irritation) occurs while using miconazole, discontinue use and consult your doctor.

Proper diagnosis is essential for effective treatment. Do not use this product without first consulting your doctor.

Possible Side Effects

Topical Application

- ▼ Less common: headache (affects 1 in 4 people using terconazole) and skin irritation, burning, rash, and redness.
- ▼ Rare: painful menstruation; genital pain; body pain; abdominal pain; fever; chills; and vaginal burning, itching, or irritation. Application of terconazole cream to the skin can cause unusual sensitivity to the sun. Contact your doctor if you experience anything unusual while taking any medication.

Vaginal Administration

- ▼ Common: itching, burning, and irritation.
- ▼ Less common: pelvic cramps, hives, rash, and headache.

Drug Interactions

These interactions do not apply to drugs applied to the skin.

- Miconazole may increase the effect of warfarin (an anticoagulant drug), which may cause bleeding problems such as nosebleeds, bleeding gums, and bruising.
- The use of miconazole and related drugs with some anticonvulsants may cause serious side effects.
- Miconazole may interact with oral antidiabetes drugs to produce very low blood-sugar levels.

Usual Dose

Topical Cream, Lotions, and Powder: Apply to clean, dry, affected areas twice a day, morning and evening, for up to 1 month, or as directed by your doctor.

Vaginal Suppositories and Cream: 1 applicatorful or suppository into the vagina at bedtime for 1–7 days, depending on the product and how it is manufactured.

Overdosage

Accidental ingestion may cause upset stomach. Contact your local poison control center or hospital emergency room for more information. If you seek treatment, ALWAYS bring the prescription bottle or container.

Special Information

When using the vaginal cream, insert the whole applicator of cream high into the vagina and be sure to complete the full course of treatment. Contact your doctor if you develop burning or itching.

Refrain from sexual intercourse or use a condom to avoid reinfection while using this product. Using sanitary napkins even if you do not have your period may prevent the product from staining your clothing.

If you forget to administer a dose of one of these drugs, do so as soon as you remember. If it is almost time for your next dose, skip the dose you forgot and continue with your regular schedule. Do not apply a double dose.

Oxiconazole is meant only for application to the skin. Do not apply to your eyes or mouth.

Continue using these medicines for the prescribed time of treatment, even if symptoms improve.

Do not use a covered dressing unless instructed by your doctor.

Special Populations

Pregnancy/Breast-feeding: Pregnant women should not use the vaginal suppositories or tablets during the first trimester. Use during the following 6 months only if absolutely necessary and without an applicator (insert by hand). Creams applied to the skin are unlikely to be absorbed to the extent they would affect a pregnancy.

Miconazole has not been shown to cause problems in breast-fed infants. Nursing mothers using oxiconazole or terconazole should use infant formula.

Seniors: Seniors may use these medications without special restriction.

Generic Name

Midodrine (MYE-doe-dreen) G

Brand Names

Orvaten ProAmatine

Type of Drug

Alpha stimulant.

Prescribed For

Dizziness or fainting when rising from a sitting position. Midodrine is also used for poor urinary control and retrograde ejaculation.

General Information

Midodrine is recommended only if other treatments for dizziness or fainting have failed and symptoms are severely interfering with your daily routine. It stimulates nerve endings in small veins and arteries, "tightening" them slightly to raise blood pressure. This helps control dizziness and fainting caused by poor blood flow to the brain. Systolic blood pressure increases by 15–30 points 1 hour after taking 10 mg of midodrine. The effect lasts about 2–3 hours.

Cautions and Warnings

Do not take midodrine if you are **allergic** or **sensitive** to any of its ingredients.

High blood pressure—especially when lying down—can be the most serious side effect of midodrine. This problem may be prevented by not completely reclining, or by raising the head of your bed when you sleep. Midodrine should only be taken by those whose symptoms are considerably debilitating. It is essential to have your blood pressure regularly monitored both while sitting and lying down when taking this medication.

Do not take this drug if you have severe **heart disease**, severe **kidney disease**, **pheochromocytoma** (adrenal gland tumor), a severely **overactive thyroid gland**, or excessive and persistent **high blood pressure** when lying down. If you have **diabetes**, **difficulty urinating**, or **visual problems** for which you take fludrocortisone, use this drug with caution. People with kidney disease require reduced dosage.

People with **liver disease** should be cautious about using midodrine because it may be partially broken down in the liver. Your doctor should evaluate your kidney and liver function periodically.

Heart rate may decrease while taking midodrine.

Possible Side Effects

▼ Most common: tingling in the hands or feet, pain, itching, goose bumps, painful urination, urinary urge, urinary retention, urinary frequency, high blood pressure when lying down, and chills.

Possible Side Effects *(continued)*

▼ Less common: headache, sensation of pressure in the head, facial flushing, confusion, abnormal thinking, dry mouth, nervousness, anxiety, and rash.

▼ Rare: visual problems, dizziness, sensitive skin, sleeplessness, tiredness, canker sores, dry skin, weakness, backache, nausea, upset stomach, gas, heartburn, and leg cramps. Contact your doctor if you experience anything unusual while taking any medication.

Drug Interactions

- Alpha blockers such as prazosin, terazosin, and doxazosin can block midodrine's effects.
- Ephedrine, dihydroergotamine, phenylephrine, and pseudoephedrine may increase the effects of midodrine.
- Midodrine enhances the effects of cardiac glycosides, psychopharmacologics, and beta blockers.
- People taking fludrocortisone must have their dosage reduced or salt intake lowered before starting midodrine.

Food Interactions

None known.

Usual Dose

Dizziness or Fainting

Adult: 10 mg 3 times a day. People with kidney failure should start with 2.5 mg.

Child: not recommended.

Urinary Incontinence

Adult: 2.5–5 mg 2–3 times a day.

Child: not recommended.

Overdosage

Symptoms include high blood pressure, goose bumps, feeling cold, and difficulty urinating. Take the victim to a hospital emergency room. If you seek treatment, ALWAYS bring the prescription bottle or container.

Special Information

Your doctor may suggest that you take the medication about every 4 hours: when you get up, around noon, and in the late afternoon—but no later than 6 p.m. The drug may also be taken every 3 hours to control symptoms. Do not take midodrine after dinner or less than 4 hours before you go to bed.

If you experience symptoms of high blood pressure when lying down, such as headache, pounding in the ears, blurred vision, and an acute awareness of your heartbeat, contact your doctor immediately.

Continue taking midodrine only if it works for you. If you forget a dose, take it as soon as you remember. If it is almost time for your next dose, skip the dose you forgot and continue with your regular schedule. Contact your doctor if you miss 2 or more doses in a row.

Special Populations

Pregnancy/Breast-feeding: Midodrine may pass into fetal circulation. Midodrine should be taken during pregnancy only if your doctor determines that the potential benefit outweighs the risks.

It is not known if midodrine passes into breast milk. Nursing mothers who must take it should use infant formula.

Seniors: Seniors may take midodrine without special precaution.

Generic Name

Mifepristone (mif-ih-PRIS-tone)

Brand Names

Mifeprex

Type of Drug

Abortifacient.

Prescribed For

Termination of pregnancies of less than 7 weeks. Also used as a "morning after" contraceptive and for uterine fibroids, fetal deaths or fetuses that are not viable in the early stages of pregnancy, meningioma that cannot be treated surgically, endometriosis, and Cushing's syndrome.

General Information

Mifepristone is a prostaglandin that works by interrupting the supply of hormones that maintain the interior of the uterus where the fetus attaches to obtain nourishment and grow. Without these hormones, the uterus cannot support the pregnancy and the contents of the uterus are expelled. It is related to misoprostol, a drug used to prevent gastrointestinal tract ulcers caused by aspirin and other nonsteroidal anti-inflammatory drugs (NSAIDs). Misoprostol is usually given 2 full days after mifepristone to complete the medical abortion.

Cautions and Warnings

Do not take mifepristone if you are **allergic** or **sensitive** to any of its ingredients.

Surgery may be needed if mifepristone treatment does not produce a complete termination. The same pre-surgical precautions should be taken with mifepristone as are taken with a surgical termination.

Death due to blood infection has occurred following a mifepristone-induced termination. Nausea, vomiting, or diarrhea and weakness, with or without abdominal pain or fever, developing more than 24 hours after taking mifepristone can be signs of infection. Go to your doctor or a hospital emergency room immediately.

Vaginal bleeding or spotting should be expected for 9–16 days. Up to 8% of women who use mifepristone can bleed for 30 days or more, which may lead to anemia.

There is no information on the effect of this drug in liver or kidney disease. You should not take this drug if you have problems with your **adrenal glands** or if you have an **IUD**, **ectopic pregnancy**, or a **bleeding disorder**.

Possible Side Effects

This drug is designed to produce the vaginal bleeding and cramping necessary to produce pregnancy termination. Nearly all women who use mifepristone can be expected to have at least 1 side effect.

- ▼ Most common: headache, abdominal cramps, uterine cramps, vaginal bleeding, nausea, vomiting, diarrhea, fatigue, and back pain.
- ▼ Common: uterine hemorrhage.
- ▼ Less common: upset stomach, vaginitis, pelvic pain and infection, fever, viral infection, shaking chills, weakness, leg pain, anemia (reduced red-blood-cell count), sinus irritation, and fainting.
- ▼ Rare: liver irritation and increased white-blood-cell count. Contact your doctor if you experience anything unusual while taking any medication.

Drug Interactions

- Mifepristone may be less effective if given less than 2 days after taking misoprostol, which is often used to treat stomach ulcers.
- Do not take this drug if you are also taking an anticoagulant (blood thinning) drug (e.g., warfarin) or a corticosteroid.
- Erythromycin, itraconazole, and ketoconazole may increase blood levels of mifepristone.
- Carbamazepine, dexamethasone, phenobarbital, phenytoin, rifampin, and St. John's wort may reduce the amount of mifepristone in the blood.
- Mifepristone stays in the body for a week or more and stimulates a particular liver enzyme involved in drug metabolism. This may lead to increases in blood levels of some antibiotics and antiviral medications, benzodiazepine sedatives, caffeine, calcium channel blockers, cocaine, codeine and other narcotics, cortisone drugs, hormone supplements, statins, and other drugs broken down by this enzyme.

Food Interactions

Grapefruit juice may slow the breakdown of mifepristone in the liver, increasing drug levels in the blood.

Usual Dose

600 mcg of mifepristone on the first office visit; 400 mcg of misoprostol 2 days later.

Overdosage

No serious symptoms were reported in men and nonpregnant women who took up to 3 times the recommended dose of mifepristone. Massive overdose may lead to adrenal gland failure. If you seek treatment, ALWAYS bring the prescription bottle or container.

Special Information

Be sure to read all written information given to you by your doctor and that all your questions are answered before proceeding.

Tell your doctor if you have any clotting or bleeding problems, or if you are anemic.

You should have a follow-up visit with your doctor 2 weeks after treatment to make sure that a complete termination has occurred. Surgery may be needed if mifepristone results in an incomplete termination. When using this drug, be sure you know exactly what to do and where to go if something goes wrong.

Contact your doctor right away if you develop any symptoms of a serious infection (see "Cautions and Warnings").

You may become pregnant again after your pregnancy has been terminated and before your next period. Contraception may be started as soon as your doctor has confirmed the pregnancy termination.

Special Populations

Pregnancy/Breast-feeding: Pregnant women who are not interested in pregnancy termination may not take this drug for any reason. Failed mifepristone treatment may lead to birth defects.

Mifepristone may pass into breast milk. Nursing mothers who must take this drug should use infant formula for several days after taking mifepristone.

Generic Name

Miglitol (mig-LIH-tol)

Brand Names

Glyset

The information in this profile also applies to the following drugs:

Generic Ingredients: Acarbose G
Precose

Type of Drug

Antidiabetic.

Prescribed For

Type 2 diabetes.

General Information

Miglitol works differently from other oral antidiabetes drugs, which control blood-sugar levels by increasing the production of insulin or helping the body to use the hormone more efficiently. Miglitol delays the digestion of carbohydrates (sugars) by acting in the cells that line the small intestine, where sugar is absorbed. This results in less sugar being absorbed into the blood and, therefore, a lower blood-sugar level. Miglitol also has some effect against the enzyme lactase, but usually does not cause lactose intolerance. Hypoglycemia (very low blood sugar) is unlikely with miglitol because of the way the drug works in diabetes.

People taking miglitol should have their blood sugar checked periodically to see how well the drug is working. (Home glucose monitors are available.) Miglitol may be prescribed with another antidiabetic drug if single-drug therapy is not enough to adequately control blood-sugar levels.

Cautions and Warnings

Do not take miglitol or acarbose if you are **allergic** or **sensitive** to any of their ingredients.

Do not take miglitol or acarbose if you have **diabetic keto-acidosis**, **inflammatory bowel disease**, **ulcers in the colon**, **intestinal obstruction**, **absorption or digestion diseases**, or if **intestinal gas** will be a severe problem.

Acarbose may lead to liver inflammation. Do not take this drug if you have **cirrhosis**.

People with **kidney disease** retain higher levels of miglitol and acarbose in the blood, but this does not affect either drug's action because they act locally in cells lining the small intestine. Those with severe kidney disease should not take these drugs because of drug retention in the blood.

Possible Side Effects

Acarbose

Intestinal side effects of acarbose tend to improve or go away after a few weeks.

- ▼ Most common: stomach gas (in 75% of people who take it), abdominal pain, and diarrhea. These side effects may be worse if you do not restrict the amount of carbohydrate in your diet.
- ▼ Less common: skin rashes, itching, hepatitis or yellowing of the skin or whites of the eyes, abdominal distress, and abdominal obstruction.
- ▼ Rare: swelling and minor abnormalities in blood tests. Contact your doctor if you experience anything unusual while taking any medication.

Miglitol

Most side effects of miglitol go away with continued use of the drug.

- ▼ Most common: gas, diarrhea, and abdominal pain.
- ▼ Less common: rash and low blood iron.

Drug Interactions

- Calcium channel blockers, contraceptive drugs, corticosteroids, estrogens, isoniazid, nicotinic acid, phenothiazines, phenytoin, stimulants, thiazides and other diuretics, and thyroid drugs may increase blood-sugar levels. Your blood glucose should be carefully monitored if you add or withdraw any of these drugs while taking miglitol or acarbose.
- Miglitol and acarbose add to the blood-sugar-lowering effect of sulfonylureas, insulin, and other antidiabetes drugs and may increase the risk of hypoglycemia (low blood sugar) associated with these drugs.
- Miglitol may interfere with the absorption of several drugs into the blood, including digoxin, glyburide, metformin, propranolol, and ranitidine. Your doctor may need to adjust your dose of these drugs.
- Charcoal and digestive enzyme preparations—as well as other drugs intended to absorb stomach contents—reduce the effects of miglitol and acarbose. Separate dosing of these drugs by at least 2 hours.
- Combining acarbose and digoxin may decrease the effects of digoxin.

Food Interactions

Miglitol must be taken with the first bite of each main meal.

Usual Dose

Acarbose

Adult (132 lbs. or more): 25–100 mg with breakfast, lunch, and dinner.

Adult (less than 132 lbs.): 25–50 mg with breakfast, lunch, and dinner.

Child: not recommended.

Miglitol

Adult: 25–100 mg with breakfast, lunch, and dinner.

Child: not recommended.

Overdosage

Overdose symptoms are likely to include gas, diarrhea, and pain. Contact your local poison control center or hospital emergency room for more information. If you seek treatment, ALWAYS bring the prescription bottle or container.

Special Information

Follow your doctor's instructions for diet, exercise, and blood-sugar testing.

Miglitol prevents the breakdown of table sugar. If you take this drug in combination with insulin or a sulfonylurea drug, be sure to have a quick source of glucose (dextrose) with you to treat hypoglycemia (symptoms include tiredness, increased hunger, increased heart rate, sweating, and numbness in the arms and legs).

Read product labels carefully or check with your pharmacist before buying any nonprescription drug to be sure it is safe for diabetics to take with acarbose or miglitol.

Take your dose with the first bite of each meal. The drug has to be present in your intestine to prevent the absorption of sugar into your blood.

If you forget to take a dose of miglitol with your meal, skip the dose you forgot because it cannot work unless there is food in your stomach. Continue with your regular dose at the beginning of your next meal.

Special Populations

Pregnancy/Breast-feeding: The safety of using miglitol during pregnancy is not known. Miglitol should be taken during pregnancy only if your doctor determines that the potential benefit outweighs the risks. Diabetes during pregnancy is usually treated with insulin.

Small amounts of miglitol pass into breast milk. Nursing mothers who must take this drug should use infant formula.

Seniors: Blood levels of acarbose are higher in older adults, but this is not considered important. Seniors with severe kidney disease should avoid this medication.

Generic Name

Minoxidil (mih-NOX-ih-dil) G

Brand Names

Rogaine
Rogaine Extra Strength for Men

Type of Drug

Antihypertensive and hair-growth stimulant.

Prescribed For

Hypertension (high blood pressure), male-pattern baldness, and alopecia areata.

General Information

Oral minoxidil is prescribed for severe hypertension that has not responded to other drugs. It reduces blood pressure by dilating (widening) peripheral blood vessels, allowing more blood to flow through the arms and legs. This increased blood flow reduces resistance levels in central blood vessels—for example, in the heart, lungs, and kidneys—and therefore reduces blood pressure. Minoxidil's effect on blood pressure is seen 30 minutes after a dose is taken and lasts up to 3 days. Minoxidil, which is usually taken once or twice a day, reaches maximum effect in as little as 3 days if the dose is large enough—40 mg a day.

Topical minoxidil stimulates hair growth in men and women with hereditary hair loss. It is also used to treat alopecia areata, a condition in which patches of hair fall out all over the body. No one knows exactly how minoxidil produces this effect and it does not work for everyone. The ideal candidate is a man who has just started to lose hair. The drug is not effective unless hair in the balding area is at least ½ in. long, and it takes 4–6 months of applications before any effect can be expected. The application regimen must be followed carefully; stopping the drug will nullify its effects and new growth will be lost. In some men who used minoxidil for a year, hair loss was only slowed.

Cautions and Warnings

Do not take minoxidil if you are **allergic** or **sensitive** to any of its ingredients.

Oral minoxidil may cause severe adverse effects on the heart, including angina and fluid around the heart, which affects cardiac function. This drug is only indicated for extremely high blood pressure and should not be used for **mild hypertension** or **pulmonary arterial hypertension**. It is usually prescribed with a beta blocker to prevent rapid heartbeat and a diuretic to prevent fluid accumulation. Hospitalization may be recommended for some people when they start minoxidil to avoid an overly rapid drop in blood pressure.

People with **pheochromocytoma** (adrenal gland tumor) should not use this drug.

This drug has not been carefully studied in people who have suffered a **heart attack** within a month of beginning minoxidil;

cardiac side effects may be particularly serious in people with a history of **heart disease**. People who use minoxidil for hair growth must have a healthy scalp and no heart disease.

Minoxidil should be used with caution in those with **kidney failure**.

Possible Side Effects

Lotion

Not enough minoxidil is usually absorbed into the blood to affect blood pressure or cause serious side effects.

▼ Most common: People using 2% minoxidil lotion may experience irritation or itching.

▼ Less common: bronchitis or other respiratory infections; rash; eczema; fungal infection; itching; redness; dry skin or scalp; flaking; worsening of hair loss; diarrhea; nausea; headache; dizziness; fainting; back pain; broken bones; tendonitis; swelling of the arms or legs; chest pain; blood-pressure changes; heart palpitations; allergic reactions (symptoms include breathing difficulties, rash, and itching); hives; runny nose; facial swelling; conjunctivitis (pinkeye); ear infection; visual disturbances; urinary infection; inflammation of the prostate or urethra; vaginal discharge; pain during sex; anxiety; depression; menstrual changes; nonspecific breast symptoms; and pain, inflammation, or redness of the testes, vagina, or vulva.

Tablets

Water and sodium retention may develop (which can worsen heart failure) as well as fluid in the sacs surrounding the heart.

▼ Most common: 80% of people experience thickening, elongation, and darkening of body hair within 3–6 weeks, first noticed on the temples, between the eyebrows, on the forehead, or on the upper cheek. Later it may extend to the back, arms, legs, and scalp. This effect stops when the drug is stopped, and symptoms usually disappear in 1–6 months. Heart rhythm changes occur in 60% of people, but cause no symptoms. Some laboratory tests, such as blood, liver, and kidney tests, may be affected by minoxidil.

▼ Less common: severe rash, nausea, vomiting, chest pain, edema, breast tenderness, and changes in blood composition and heart function.

Drug Interactions

- Minoxidil may interact with guanethidine to produce severe dizziness when rising from a sitting or lying position. These drugs should not be taken together.
- Do not use the lotion in conjunction with other topical drugs.

Food Interactions

None known.

Usual Dose

Lotion: Apply to scalp twice a day.

Tablets

Adult and Child (age 12 and over): 5 mg a day to start; effective range is usually 10–40 mg a day. Do not exceed 100 mg a day.

Child (under age 12): 0.1 mg per lb. of body weight a day to start; may be increased to 0.5 mg per lb. of body weight a day. Do not exceed 50 mg a day. Children should be monitored closely, as pediatric experience of this drug's effects is limited.

Minoxidil is usually taken with a diuretic, such as 100 mg of hydrochlorothiazide, 50–100 mg of chlorthalidone, or 80 mg of furosemide daily; and a beta blocker, such as 80–160 mg daily of propranolol. People who cannot take beta blockers may take 250–750 mg of methyldopa or 0.1–0.2 mg of clonidine daily.

Overdosage

Symptoms include dizziness, fainting, and rapid heartbeat. Contact your local poison control center or a hospital emergency room for instructions. If you seek treatment, ALWAYS bring the prescription bottle or container.

Special Information

Oral minoxidil is usually prescribed with 2 other drugs—a beta blocker and a diuretic; do not discontinue any of these drugs unless told to do so by your doctor. Take all medications exactly as prescribed.

The effect of oral minoxidil on body hair (see "Possible Side Effects") is more of a nuisance than a risk and is not a reason to stop taking it.

Contact your doctor if you experience an increase in your pulse of 20 or more beats per minute; weight gain of more than 5 lbs.; swelling of your arms, legs, face, or stomach; chest pain; breathing difficulties; dizziness; or fainting spells.

Minoxidil lotion has an alcohol base that may cause burning and irritation of the eyes. In case of accidental contact with eyes or other sensitive areas, flush with large amounts of cool tap water. Accidental ingestion of the lotion may lead to whole-body adverse effects.

If you forget a dose of oral minoxidil or an application of the lotion, take it as soon as you remember. If it is almost time for your next dose, skip the dose you forgot and continue with your regular schedule. Do not take a double dose.

Special Populations

Pregnancy/Breast-feeding: Oral minoxidil crosses into the fetal circulation. Minoxidil should be taken during pregnancy only if your doctor determines that the potential benefit outweighs the risks.

Oral minoxidil passes into breast milk, as may the lotion. Nursing mothers who must take either form of minoxidil should use infant formula.

Seniors: Seniors may be more sensitive to the blood-pressure-lowering effect of the drug due to loss of kidney function.

Generic Name

Mirtazapine (mur-TAZ-uh-pene) G

Brand Names

Remeron Remeron SolTab

The information in this profile also applies to the following drugs:

Generic Ingredients: Maprotiline G

Type of Drug

Antidepressant.

Prescribed For

Depression and anxiety.

General Information

Mirtazapine blocks the passage of stimulant chemicals (serotonin and noradrenaline) in and out of nerve endings and has a sedative effect. It also moderately counteracts the effects of the neurohormone acetylcholine. Mirtazapine can elevate mood, increase physical activity and mental alertness, and improve appetite and sleep patterns 2–4 weeks after you start taking it. Mirtazapine is useful in treating mild forms of depression associated with anxiety. It can also significantly reduce tremors associated with Parkinson's disease and other causes, though the effect is lost soon after drug treatment is stopped. Mirtazapine is broken down in the liver. Women clear the drug more slowly than men.

Cautions and Warnings

Do not take these medications if you are **allergic** or **sensitive** to any of their ingredients.

Antidepressants have been associated with an increased risk of suicide, especially in **teenagers**. Suicide is always a risk in severely **depressed** people, who should only be allowed to have minimal quantities of medication in their possession.

Mirtazapine and maprotiline should be taken with care if you have **heart disease**. Mirtazapine should be taken cautiously if you are taking medications to treat **high blood pressure**.

Antidepressants may aggravate the condition of people who are **schizophrenic** or **paranoid** and may cause people with **bipolar (manic-depressive) disorder** to switch phase. These reactions are also possible when changing or stopping antidepressants.

People with **epilepsy** or a history of **seizures** should not use maprotiline, and care should be used when initiating mirtazapine in this patient group.

People taking mirtazapine may develop very low white-blood-cell counts, leading to infections, fever, and related problems. Contact your doctor at once if you develop a sore throat, fever, infection, or mouth sores while taking this drug.

Mirtazapine should be taken with care if you have **kidney or liver disease**.

Maprotiline should be taken with care if you have **glaucoma**, a history of **difficulty urinating**, **overactive thyroid gland**, or **kidney or liver disease**.

Mirtazapine may cause dizziness and sleepiness with potentially serious effects on performance of complex tasks.

Possible Side Effects

▼ Most common: tiredness, dizziness, dry mouth, constipation, abnormal dreams, increased appetite, weight gain, large increases in blood cholesterol or triglyceride levels, weakness, and flu-like symptoms.

Possible Side Effects *(continued)*

▼ Less common: back pain, nausea, vomiting, muscle ache, abnormal thinking, anxiety, agitation, confusion, tremors, itching, rash, breathing difficulties, and frequent urination.

▼ Rare: blood-pressure changes, weakness, hair loss, uncontrollable muscle spasms or movements, hallucinations, manic reactions, and liver function changes. Other rare side effects can occur in almost any part of the body. Contact your doctor if you experience anything unusual while taking any medication.

Drug Interactions

- Combining mirtazapine or maprotiline with a monoamine oxidase inhibitor (MAOI) antidepressant may cause high fevers, convulsions, or death. Do not take an MAOI until at least 2 weeks after mirtazapine or maprotiline has been stopped. Furazolidone works in a similar manner to MAOI antidepressants and should also be avoided, including separating doses by at least 2 weeks.
- Mirtazapine and maprotiline increase the effects of alcohol and other sedative drugs.
- Impairment of motor skills and risk of seizures are increased when these drugs are combined with benzodiazepines such as diazepam.
- Azole antifungals (such as itraconazole, ketoconazole, or voriconazole), cimetidine, fluvoxamine, macrolide antibiotics (such as erythromycin), nefazodone, and protease inhibitors (such as atazanavir, indinavir, saquinavir, and ritonavir) may increase the effects of mirtazapine and maprotiline.
- Carbamazepine, hydantoins such as phenytoin, and rifampin may decrease the effects of mirtazapine and maprotiline.

Maprotiline

- Cisapride should not be combined with maprotiline. The risk of life-threatening cardiac arrhythmias may be increased.
- Maprotiline should be used with caution with anticholinergic drugs.
- Maprotiline may block the effects of guanethidine (used to treat high blood pressure). Tell your doctor if you are taking any drug for high blood pressure.

- Combining maprotiline and a phenothiazine medication such as chlorpromazine or thioridazine may increase the risk of seizures.
- Sympathomimetics such as dopamine and maprotiline should be used together with caution. Dosage adjustments may be required.
- Combining a thyroid hormone such as levothyroxine and maprotiline enhances the effects of maprotiline and may cause unwanted effects on the heart.

Mirtazapine

- Lithium, L-tryptophan, rasagiline, selective serotonin reuptake inhibitors (SSRIs, such as fluoxetine and venlafaxine), St. John's wort, tramadol, tricyclic antidepressants such as amitriptyline, and triptans (such as almotriptan, eletriptan, and sumatriptan) increase the risk of serotonin syndrome (symptoms include changes in thinking or behavior, fever, high blood pressure, rapid heart rate, and tremor) when combined with mirtazapine.
- The blood-pressure-lowering effect of clonidine may be compromised when it is given with mirtazapine.
- The blood-thinning effect of warfarin may be increased when it is mixed with mirtazapine.

Food Interactions

You may take mirtazapine with food if it upsets your stomach.

Usual Dose

Maprotiline

Adult: 75–150 mg a day. Severely depressed patients may need up to 225 mg a day.

Senior: usually 50–75 mg a day.

Mirtazapine

Adult: 15 mg at bedtime to start. After the first 1–2 weeks of taking the drug, dosage may be increased up to 45 mg a day. Dosage must be tailored to your needs.

Overdosage

Symptoms of mirtazapine overdose include disorientation, drowsiness, memory loss, and rapid heartbeat. Symptoms of maprotiline overdose include confusion, inability to concentrate, hallucinations, drowsiness, lowered body temperature, abnormal heart rate, heart failure, enlarged pupils, seizures, convulsions, very low blood pressure, stupor, and coma; agitation, stiffening of muscles, vomiting, and high fever may also develop. The victim should be taken to a hospital emergency room immediately. If you seek treatment, ALWAYS bring the prescription bottle or container.

Special Information

Do not stop taking this drug without your doctor's knowledge. Abruptly stopping mirtazapine may cause nausea, headache, and feelings of ill health.

The following symptoms may occur early in treatment or when drug dosage is adjusted up or down: anxiety, agitation, panic attacks, sleeplessness, irritability, restlessness, hostility, aggressiveness, acting impulsively, a manic reaction, deepening of depression, other unusual changes in behavior, and suicidal thinking. Report any changes to your doctor at once.

These medications may cause drowsiness and dizziness. Be careful when driving or doing any task that requires concentration. Avoid alcohol and other depressant drugs. Avoid prolonged exposure to the sun.

Be careful when taking over-the-counter (OTC) medications because mirtazapine may interact with sedative ingredients in OTC products.

Contact your doctor at once if you develop chills, difficult or rapid breathing, fever, sweating, blood-pressure changes, muscle stiffness, loss of bladder control, or unusual tiredness or weakness.

If your symptoms are unchanged after 6–8 weeks of treatment with an antidepressant, contact your doctor.

If you forget a dose, skip it and go back to your regular schedule. Do not take a double dose.

Special Populations

Pregnancy/Breast-feeding: Mirtazapine crosses into the fetal circulation and may cause birth defects. Mirtazapine and maprotiline should be taken during pregnancy only if your doctor determines that the potential benefit outweighs the risks.

It is not known if mirtazapine passes into breast milk. Maprotiline is excreted in breast milk. Nursing mothers who must take these drugs should use infant formula.

Seniors: Seniors are more sensitive to side effects and may require reduced dosage. Older men may need less of the drug than women of the same age.

Generic Name

Misoprostol (mye-soe-PROS-tol) G

Brand Names

Cytotec

Type of Drug

Anti-ulcer.

Prescribed For

Prevention of stomach ulcer associated with nonsteroidal anti-inflammatory drug (NSAID) use. It may also be used to soften the cervix, inducing contractions to begin labor, and as part of a medical abortion drug regimen.

General Information

Like most anti-ulcer drugs, misoprostol suppresses stomach acid. It has a demonstrated ability to protect the stomach lining from damage, though the exact way misoprostol works is not known. It may increase production of stomach lining and the thickness of the protective gel layer lining the stomach. Misoprostol may also increase blood flow in and subsequent healing of the stomach lining in addition to increasing production of bicarbonate, a natural antacid found in the stomach.

Misoprostol is intended to prevent severe stomach irritation and ulcers in people taking an NSAID. It is helpful for seniors and others with a history of ulcer or stomach disease who require NSAID treatment for arthritis. It is often an effective ulcer treatment for people who do not respond to or cannot tolerate cimetidine, ranitidine, famotidine, or nizatidine.

Misoprostol is also used as a medical abortion drug along with mifepristone. It has additionally been used for labor induction, postpartum hemorrhaging, and chronic constipation.

Cautions and Warnings

Do not take misoprostol if you are **allergic** or **sensitive** to any of its ingredients or to any prostaglandin agent.

You should not take misoprostol for ulcer prevention if you are **pregnant**. It has been shown to cause abortion, premature birth, and birth defects. Vaginal misoprostol has been used to induce labor but is associated with a higher risk of uterine rupture. Tell your doctor if you have risk factors for uterine rupture such as prior **Cesarean delivery**, **uterine surgery**, or **5 or more previous pregnancies**.

People with **kidney disease** may require reduced dosages.

Possible Side Effects

- ▼ Most common: diarrhea and abdominal pain. Most cases of diarrhea are mild and last no more than 2–3 days.
- ▼ Less common: headache, nausea, vomiting, and stomach upset or gas.
- ▼ Rare: spotting, cramps, excessive menstrual bleeding, painful menstruation or other menstrual disorders, and vaginal bleeding. Rare side effects can occur in almost any part of the body. Contact your doctor if you experience anything unusual while taking any medication.

Drug Interactions

- Misoprostol stimulates contractions of the uterus and may not be used at the same time as other uterine stimulants such as dinoprostone inserts and mifepristone.
- Antacids interfere with the absorption of misoprostol, reducing its effectiveness. Magnesium-containing antacids may worsen misoprostol-induced diarrhea.

Food Interactions

Though food interferes with the absorption of misoprostol, it should be taken with or after meals (and at bedtime) to minimize gastrointestinal side effects.

Usual Dose

Adult: 100–200 mcg 4 times a day.

Child: not recommended.

Overdosage

Symptoms include sedation, tremors, convulsions, breathing difficulties, stomach pain, diarrhea, fever, changes in heart rate (either very fast or very slow), gastrointestinal lesions, testicular atrophy, liver damage, central-nervous-system depression, and low blood pressure. Take the victim to a hospital emergency room. If you seek treatment, ALWAYS bring the prescription bottle or container.

Special Information

Do not stop taking misoprostol, or take it for more than 4 weeks, without your doctor's knowledge.

Contact your doctor if side effects, especially diarrhea or abdominal or stomach pain, become severe or intolerable. Women who experience menstrual problems and postmenopausal women who experience vaginal bleeding should discuss these side effects with their doctor.

If you forget a dose, take it as soon as you remember. If it is almost time for your next dose, skip the dose you forgot and continue with your regular schedule. Do not take a double dose.

Special Populations

Pregnancy/Breast-feeding: Pregnant women should not take this drug. Women of childbearing age should take misoprostol only if they absolutely must take an NSAID and already have, or are at high risk of developing, stomach ulcers. Misoprostol causes spontaneous miscarriage. Within 2 weeks of starting treatment, you must receive a negative blood test result for pregnancy—an over-the-counter urine test is not sufficient. Start taking misoprostol on day 2 or 3 of your period and use effective contraception throughout drug therapy.

It is not known if misoprostol passes into breast milk, although it is unlikely. Nursing mothers who must take this drug should use infant formula.

Seniors: Seniors should receive lower dosages if intolerable side effects develop.

Generic Name

Modafinil (moe-DAF-ih-nil)

Brand Names

Provigil

The information in this profile also applies to the following drugs:

Generic Ingredients: Armodafinil
Nuvigil

Type of Drug

Stimulant.

Prescribed For

Narcolepsy (uncontrollable desire to sleep); obstructive sleep apnea; attention-deficit hyperactivity disorder in children and adolescents ages 6–17; shift-work sleep disorder.

General Information

Modafinil promotes wakefulness. Armodafinil is the active form of modafinil. Although some of these actions are similar to those of amphetamine and methylphenidate, it may have more to do with the fact that these medications increase the amount of free dopamine, a major neurotransmitter, in the brain by reducing the amount reabsorbed into nerve endings. People taking these medications who continue to experience excessive sleepiness may not be able to recover their normal sleep patterns. People being treated with these drugs may experience euphoria (feeling "high"), anxiety, and changes in mood, mental state, and behavior. They are classified as Schedule IV controlled substances.

Cautions and Warnings

Do not take modafinil if you are **allergic** or **sensitive** to any of its ingredients. Serious reactions such as rash and difficulty breathing and/or swallowing have been reported with armodafinil. Rarely, serious rash requiring hospitalization has occurred in both adults and children taking modafinil.

People with a history of **heart failure**, an **enlarged heart ventricle**, **angina**, **chest pain**, **abnormal heart rhythms**, or **mitral valve prolapse** should not take modafinil.

Modafinil has not been studied in people with **high blood pressure**. People with high blood pressure who take this drug must be closely monitored.

Prazosin, a drug normally prescribed for high blood pressure, can counteract the wakefulness produced by these drugs.

People taking these medications may develop mania, delusions, hallucinations, and suicidal thoughts.

People with **cirrhosis** or **liver failure** may require reduced dosages.

People who regularly take large doses (more than 400 mg a day) of modafinil may develop some resistance to its effects.

Possible Side Effects

▼ Most common: headache, nausea, and runny nose.

Possible Side Effects *(continued)*

▼ Common: back pain, nervousness, dizziness, diarrhea, dry mouth, appetite loss, and sore throat.

▼ Less common: depression, anxiety, cataplexy (extreme muscle weakness, often precipitated by laughter, a surprised feeling, or emotions of fear or anger), sleeplessness, anxiety, tingling in the hands or feet, unusual facial or mouth movements, muscle stiffness, blood-pressure changes, liver function problems, vomiting, lung problems, breathing difficulties, vision problems, chest pain, neck pain, chills, and high white-blood-cell counts.

▼ Rare: confusion, memory loss, emotional instability, euphoria (feeling "high"), changes in mood, manic behavior, delusions, hallucinations, suicidal thinking, flushing, fainting, dry skin, herpes infections, mouth sores, gum sores, thirst, difficulty urinating, abnormal urination, abnormal ejaculation, high blood sugar, nosebleeds, asthma, rigid neck, fever with chills, and joint problems. Contact your doctor if you experience anything unusual while taking any medication.

Drug Interactions

- Combining these drugs with a monoamine oxidase inhibitor (MAOI) antidepressant may increase the effects of both drugs. Use this combination with caution and only under your doctor's supervision.
- Methylphenidate can delay these drugs' effects.
- Carbamazepine, itraconazole, ketoconazole, phenobarbital, and rifampin may reduce these drugs' effects.
- These drugs may reduce the effects of contraceptive drugs, cyclosporine, and theophylline.
- These drugs may elevate blood levels of clomipramine, clozapine, diazepam, omeprazole, phenytoin, propranolol, tricyclic antidepressants, and warfarin, increasing the risk of side effects, some of which can be very serious.
- Stimulants in some over-the-counter decongestants, diet pills, and asthma drugs may cause excessive stimulation when combined with these medications.

Food Interactions

Food can slow the rate at which these drugs are absorbed into the blood but is unlikely to change the effect of modafinil. The action of armodafinil is more likely to be delayed and extended if it is taken with food.

Usual Dose

Armodafinil

Adult and Child (age 16 and over): 150–250 mg every morning.

Child (under age 16): not recommended.

Modafinil

Adult and Child (age 16 and over): 200 mg every morning, with a maximum dose of 400 mg; 100 mg a day for people with cirrhosis or liver failure.

Child (age 6–15): Dosage is individualized to each child, starting at 85 mg a day.

Child (under age 6): not recommended.

Overdosage

Symptoms include excitation, sleeplessness, sleep disturbances, anxiety, irritability, aggressiveness, confusion, nervousness, tremors, heart palpitations, nausea, diarrhea, and bleeding. Take the victim to a hospital emergency room. If you seek treatment, ALWAYS bring the prescription bottle or container.

Special Information

Contact your doctor at once if you develop a fever; rash; hives; swelling of the face, eyes, lips, tongue, or larynx; hoarseness; or other signs of a drug reaction or allergy.

Modafinil's beneficial effects on mood, thought, and perception may produce psychological dependence, though drug withdrawal symptoms have not been reported.

Be careful when driving or doing any task that requires concentration. Avoid alcohol.

Special Populations

Pregnancy/Breast-feeding: These drugs cause fetal malformation in animal studies. These drugs should be taken during pregnancy only if your doctor determines that the potential benefit outweighs the risks.

These drugs may pass into breast milk. Nursing mothers who must take them should use infant formula.

Seniors: Seniors with kidney or liver problems may require reduced dosage.

Type of Drug

Monoamine Oxidase Inhibitors (MAOIs)

Generic Ingredients: Phenelzine G
Nardil

Generic Ingredients: Rasagiline G
Azilect

Generic Ingredients: Selegiline G
Eldepryl
Emsam
Zelapar

Generic Ingredients: Tranylcypromine Sulfate G
Parnate

Prescribed For

MAOIs may be prescribed for atypical depression, depression that does not respond to other drugs, and Parkinson's disease; also prescribed for a variety of conditions, including bulimia, night terrors, bipolar depression, panic disorder, post-traumatic stress disorder, chronic migraine, and social anxiety disorder.

General Information

Monoamine oxidase (MAO) is a complex enzyme system found throughout the body. MAO is responsible for breaking down hormones that make the nervous system work. MAOIs interfere with MAO action, causing an increase in the amount of serotonin, dopamine, and norepinephrine stored throughout the nervous system. This increase is what gives these drugs their therapeutic effect, which is long lasting and may continue for up to 2 weeks after you stop the medicine.

MAOIs used for depression inhibit all forms of the enzyme and the larger doses used are much more likely to have drug and food interactions.

When combined with levodopa + carbidopa these drugs are used to control Parkinson's disease, particularly the symptoms that appear when there is a "wearing off" of the effects of levodopa + carbidopa. At the proper dosage they block the effects of the MAO-B form of MAO, found almost exclusively in the brain.

The resulting increase in brain levels of the neurohormone dopamine makes this an effective treatment for Parkinson's disease. Selegiline and rasagiline inhibit primarily MAO-B, and selegiline also stimulates dopamine receptors. The selegiline skin patch (Emsam) is prescribed only for severe depression. It releases its medicine through the skin over 24 hours.

Cautions and Warnings

Do not use an MAOI if you are **allergic** or **sensitive** to any of its ingredients.

The most severe reactions to these drugs, which can be deadly, involve very high blood pressure, which may result in bleeding in the brain. Serious, potentially fatal reactions may occur if phenelzine and another antidepressant, especially a **selective serotonin reuptake inhibitor** (SSRI), are taken together (see "Drug Interactions"). There is no benefit to taking doses of this drug higher than the maximum dose recommended by your doctor and the manufacturer; otherwise you risk a severe reaction, including possibly fatal high blood pressure.

Hallucinations may occur in a small number of people taking 1 of these drugs, particularly with selegiline; report any hallucinations to your doctor at once.

MAOIs should not be taken by anyone with **pheochromocytoma** (adrenal gland tumor). Be extremely cautious about taking an MAOI if you have **heart failure**, **liver disease** or **abnormal liver function**, severe **kidney function loss**, **heart disease**, or a history of **headaches**, **stroke**, **transient ischemic attack** ("mini-stroke"), or **high blood pressure**.

Antidepressants, including MAOIs, may increase suicidal thoughts or actions in **children**, **teens**, and **young adults**, especially within the first few weeks or months of treatment, or when the dose is increased or decreased. Warning signs may include agitation, irritability, and unusual behavior changes. These drugs are not recommended for use in children, though some are approved for use in age 16 and over.

While taking any MAOI you will need to watch your diet carefully. See "Food Interactions" for full details.

People with Parkinson's disease have 2–6 times the risk of developing skin cancer (melanoma). It is not known if the increased risk is due to the condition or the drugs used to manage it. People taking an MAOI should frequently check themselves for skin cancers and see a dermatologist regularly.

MAOIs may cause dizziness or fainting when rising from a sitting or lying position.

People who cannot take **phenylalanine** should know that Zelapar contains phenylalanine.

Possible Side Effects

Phenelzine

- ▼ Common: dizziness, especially when rising from a sitting or lying position; drowsiness; fatigue; sleep disturbances; twitching; constipation; weight gain; dry mouth; and sexual disturbances.
- ▼ Less common: jitteriness, euphoria (feeling "high"), rash, sweating, blurred vision, and electric-shock sensations.

Rasagiline

- ▼ Most common: headache.
- ▼ Common: joint pain, upset stomach, depression, falling, and flu-like symptoms.
- ▼ Less common: conjunctivitis (pinkeye), fever, inflammation of the stomach and/or intestines, runny nose, arthritis, black-and-blue marks, neck pain, not feeling well, tingling in the hands or feet, and dizziness.
- ▼ Rare: diarrhea, chest pain, protein in the urine, allergic reactions, hair loss, angina, appetite loss, asthma, hallucinations, erectile dysfunction, reduction in white-blood-cell count, reduced sex drive, abnormal liver function tests, skin cancer, fainting, rash, and vomiting. Contact your doctor if you experience anything unusual while taking any medication.

Selegiline

In Parkinson's disease, selegiline often increases the side effects of levodopa + carbidopa.

- ▼ Most common: nausea, vomiting, dizziness, lightheadedness or fainting, headache, and insomnia.
- ▼ Common: constipation, agitation, anxiety, and muscle problems.
- ▼ Less common: dry mouth, abnormal movements, and hallucinations.

Tranylcypromine

- ▼ Common: dizziness, restlessness, jitteriness, dry mouth, diarrhea, insomnia, headache, weight loss, and nausea.

Possible Side Effects *(continued)*

▼ Less common: fast heartbeat, drowsiness, constipation, blurred vision, electric-shock sensations, and jerkiness.

Drug Interactions

- MAOIs should not be used with meperidine, methadone, tramadol, or other narcotics because of the risk of severe, possibly fatal reactions, including coma, severe changes in blood pressure, severe reduction in breathing rate, convulsions, very high fever, excitation, collapsed blood vessels, and death. Allow at least 2 weeks to elapse between these medicines.
- Taking an SSRI antidepressant and an MAOI at the same time or too close together may result in a serious, sometimes fatal reaction characterized by very high fever, rigidity, muscle spasms, and changes in mental state, blood pressure, pulse, and breathing rate. Allow 2 weeks between stopping an MAOI and starting an SSRI. At least 2 weeks should usually elapse between stopping an SSRI and starting an MAOI; for fluoxetine, the wait is 5 weeks.
- A tricyclic antidepressant and an MAOI may be combined only under your doctor's direct supervision. If dosages are not strictly controlled, this combination can lead to seizures, sweating, coma, hyperexcitability, high fever, rapid heartbeat, rapid breathing, headache, dilated pupils, flushing, confusion, and low blood pressure. When severe, this reaction can be fatal. Generally, 2 weeks must pass between stopping phenelzine and taking a tricyclic antidepressant.
- Do not combine these drugs with any other MAOI, atomoxetine, bupropion, carbamazepine, mirtazapine, oxcarbazepine, or St. John's wort.
- Cimetidine, ciprofloxacin and other fluoroquinolones, fluvoxamine, and ticlopidine inhibit the enzyme that breaks down rasagiline. Mixing these drugs with rasagiline can cause a substantial increase in the amount of rasagiline in the blood.
- Tobacco smoking stimulates the enzyme system responsible for breaking down rasagiline and may increase the speed at which rasagiline is broken down by the liver.
- Do not combine selegiline with dextromethorphan, the most common cough suppressant included in over-the-counter

medicines, due to the risk of bizarre behavior or a psychotic reaction.

- MAOIs should not be taken with any stimulant drugs, including amphetamines or any over-the-counter or prescription medicine containing ephedrine, phenylephrine, phenylpropanolamine, or pseudoephedrine without first checking with your pharmacist or the doctor who prescribed the MAOI. Severe high blood pressure may result.
- Contraceptives may increase the effects of selegiline. Combine with caution.
- MAOIs interfere with the blood-pressure-lowering effect of guanethidine. Do not combine these drugs.
- MAOIs increase the effects of sulfonylurea-type antidiabetes drugs, barbiturates, beta blockers, levodopa + carbidopa, methyldopa, rauwolfia drugs, sulfa drugs, sumatriptan, stimulants, thiazide-type diuretics, and L-tryptophan. The combination of any of these drugs and phenelzine can result in severe reactions.
- Combining tranylcypromine and disulfiram may lead to delirium, agitation, disorientation, and hallucinations.
- Do not mix an MAOI with the herbal medicine ginseng.
- When taken with levodopa + carbidopa, rasagiline may worsen the difficulty or distortion experienced while performing voluntary muscle movements (associated with levodopa) and dizziness or fainting when rising from a sitting or lying position. Dizziness and fainting is most common during the first 2 months of treatment and then becomes less common.
- If you take levodopa + carbidopa and start taking selegiline, you may experience an increase in levodopa + carbidopa side effects. Your dosage of levodopa + carbidopa may need to be reduced.

Food Interactions

Do not eat or drink 5 minutes before or after taking Zelapar. Avoid the following foods while taking any MAOI:

Alcohol: imported beer and ale; red wine, especially chianti; sherry; vermouth; and distilled spirits.

Cheese and Dairy: processed American cheese, blue cheese, boursault, natural brick cheese, brie, camembert, cheddar, emmenthaler, gruyere, mozzarella, parmesan, romano, Roquefort, sour cream, stilton, Swiss cheese, and yogurt.

Fruits and Vegetables: avocados, especially when overripe; yeast extracts; canned figs; raisins; sauerkraut; soy sauce; miso soup; and bean curd.

Meat and Fish: beef or chicken liver, meats prepared with a tenderizer, summer sausage, bologna, pepperoni, salami, game, meat extracts, caviar, dried fish, anchovies, salted herring, pickled and spoiled herring, and shrimp paste.

Other: fava beans, ginseng, caffeine, and some chocolate.

Although reactions to these foods are unlikely, patients should be cautious, and those taking the higher MAOI doses used for depression should avoid them entirely.

Usual Dose

Phenelzine

Adult and Child (age 16 and over): 15 mg 3 times a day to start, increased gradually to 60–90 mg a day.

Child (under age 16): not recommended.

Senior: 15 mg in the morning. Dosage is increased very gradually.

Rasagiline

Adult: 1 mg a day. Adjunctive therapy—0.5–1 mg a day.

Child: not recommended.

People with Mild Liver Disease: no more than 0.5 mg a day.

Selegiline

Depression

Adult: 5 mg twice a day to start, increasing gradually as needed to 10–30 mg twice a day.

Child: not recommended.

Parkinson's Disease

Eldepryl

Adult: 5 mg at breakfast and lunch.

Child: not recommended.

Emsam

Adult: 6–12 mg a day. Apply the patch to dry, clean skin once every 24 hours.

Child: not recommended.

Zelapar (Oral Disintegrating Tablets)

Adult: 1.25–2.5 mg a day. Allow the tablet to dissolve on your tongue.

Child: not recommended.

Tranylcypromine

Adult and Child (age 16 and over): 10–60 mg a day. Usual dose is 30 mg a day.

Child (under age 16): not recommended.

Senior: starting dose—2.5–5 mg a day.

Overdosage

Symptoms may include excitement, irritability, anxiety, low blood pressure, sleeplessness, restlessness, dizziness, weakness, drowsiness, flushing, sweating, heart palpitations, and unusual movements, including grimacing and muscle twitching. Serious overdoses may lead to convulsions, incoherence or confusion, severe headache, high fever, heart attack, shock, and coma. Death is possible. Take the victim to a hospital emergency room. If you seek treatment, ALWAYS bring the prescription bottle or container.

Special Information

Report these or any bothersome or persistent side effect to your doctor: intense headache; heart palpitations; stiff or sore neck; nausea; vomiting; sweating, sometimes accompanied by fever or cold, clammy skin; dilated pupils; and sensitivity to bright light.

These drugs can cause a marked increase in blood pressure if mixed with a variety of other drugs (see "Drug Interactions") or foods rich in tyramine (see "Food Interactions"). This can be a medical emergency requiring immediate treatment or hospitalization. Some symptoms of this reaction are severe headache, blurred vision or visual disturbances, difficulty thinking, stupor or coma, seizures, chest pain, unexplained nausea or vomiting, or the signs or symptoms of a stroke.

People with diabetes should be cautious because MAOIs can lower blood-sugar readings.

Vivid nightmares, agitation, psychosis, and convulsions occasionally occur in 1–3 days if an MAOI is abruptly stopped. Gradually stopping the medicine should prevent these problems.

MAOIs may cause drowsiness and blurred vision. Be careful when driving or performing any task that requires concentration. Avoid alcohol.

After you have taken selegiline for 2–3 days, your doctor will probably adjust your levodopa + carbidopa dosage by 10–30%. If the disease is still under control, your dosage may be reduced further.

Do not stop taking selegiline or change your dosage without your doctor's knowledge.

These drugs can reduce saliva flow in the mouth, increasing the risk of cavities, gum disease, and oral infections. Use candy, ice, sugarless gum, or a saliva substitute to avoid dry mouth.

People taking these and other medicines for Parkinson's disease have experienced intense urges (e.g., sexual activity, gambling, or overeating), with difficulty controlling these and other urges. This may be due to the increase in brain dopamine produced by Parkinson's disease medicines. These urges can pass after the medicine is reduced or stopped. Report any changes to your doctor.

If you forget a dose, take it as soon as you remember. Do not take a double dose.

These drugs should be stopped at least 14 days before elective surgery. People taking an MAOI should not undergo elective surgery requiring general anesthesia. Be sure your doctor or dentist knows that you are taking an MAOI before administering any anesthetic drug. Also, they should not be given cocaine or local anesthesia containing epinephrine or another blood-vessel-constricting medicine.

For the selegiline skin patch, follow package insert directions for how to properly administer the patch. It should be applied at the same time every day to clean, dry skin.

Special Populations

Pregnancy/Breast-feeding: Some MAOIs can damage a developing fetus and they should be taken during pregnancy only if your doctor determines that the potential benefit outweighs the risks.

It is not known if these medicines pass into breast milk. Nursing mothers who must take one should use infant formula.

Seniors: Seniors should receive the lowest effective dosage to minimize side effects.

Brand Names

Motofen

Generic Ingredients

Difenoxin Hydrochloride + Atropine Sulfate

Type of Drug

Antidiarrheal.

Prescribed For

Acute and chronic diarrhea.

General Information

Difenoxin is an antidiarrheal agent related to meperidine, a narcotic analgesic (pain reliever) used in Demerol. Difenoxin, which can be addictive, works by slowing the contractions of intestinal-wall muscles. The atropine sulfate ingredient in Motofen guards against drug overdose or abuse by producing undesirable effects at small dosages, thus deterring users from taking larger amounts of Motofen, as this drug is a Schedule IV controlled substance. This drug, which relieves diarrhea but does not address the underlying cause, should only be used for short periods and in cases that do not respond to other treatment.

Cautions and Warnings

Do not take Motofen if you are **allergic** or **sensitive** to any of its ingredients or to Lomotil.

Some people should not use this drug even if diarrhea is present. Antidiarrheal drugs may harm people with **stomach or bowel conditions**.

Avoid Motofen if you have advanced **liver disease** or have **jaundice** (symptoms include yellowing of the skin or whites of the eyes), or if your diarrhea was caused by taking clindamycin or another antibiotic.

People with **ulcerative colitis** or a history of **drug addiction** should use Motofen with caution.

Possible Side Effects

▼ Most common: nausea, vomiting, dry mouth, dizziness, lightheadedness, drowsiness, and headache.

▼ Less common: constipation, upset stomach, bloating, confusion, nervousness, tiredness, and sleeplessness.

▼ Rare: a burning sensation in the eyes, blurred vision, dry skin, rapid heartbeat, elevated temperature, and urinary difficulties. Contact your doctor if you experience anything unusual while taking any medication.

Drug Interactions

- Motofen may increase the effects of alcohol, barbiturates, pain relievers, sedatives, and other nervous system depressants. Avoid these combinations.

- Monoamine oxidase inhibitor (MAOI) antidepressants may, in theory, produce a high-blood-pressure crisis in combination with Motofen. Do not use Motofen if you are taking an MAOI unless you are under a doctor's care.

Food Interactions

None known.

Usual Dose

Adult and Child (age 12 and over): Two 1-mg tablets to start, then 1 after each loose stool or every 3–4 hours, as needed, up to 8 tablets a day. Treatment for more than 2 consecutive days is usually not needed.

Child (under age 12): not recommended.

Overdosage

It is crucial to keep this medication out of the reach of children at all times because of the risk of accidental overdose. Symptoms include dry skin, mouth, and nose; flushing; fever; and rapid heartbeat. These symptoms may be followed by loss of reflexes, pinpoint pupils, droopy eyelids, difficulty breathing, and lethargy or coma, which in extreme cases can lead to brain damage or death. Take the victim to a hospital emergency room immediately. If you seek treatment, ALWAYS bring the prescription bottle or container.

Special Information

Motofen can make you tired, dizzy, or lightheaded. Be careful when driving or doing any task that requires concentration. Alcohol, sedatives, and other nervous system depressants increase the depressant effects of this drug.

Your doctor may prescribe fluid and salt mixtures to replace the body fluids you lose while taking Motofen.

Contact your doctor if you develop heart palpitations or your symptoms do not clear up in 2 days. You may need a different dosage or drug.

If you forget a dose, take it as soon as you remember. If it is almost time for your next dose, skip the one you forgot and continue with your regular schedule. Do not take a double dose.

Special Populations

Pregnancy/Breast-feeding: Animal studies with very large dosages of Motofen showed an increase in stillbirths. Motofen should be taken during pregnancy only if your doctor determines that the potential benefit outweighs the risks.

The ingredients in Motofen may pass into breast milk. Nursing mothers taking Motofen should use infant formula.

Seniors: Seniors with severe kidney or liver disease require reduced dosage.

Type of Drug

Multiple Kinase Inhibitors

Brand Names

Generic Ingredients: Crizotinib
Xalkori

Generic Ingredients: Dasatinib
Sprycel

Generic Ingredients: Erlotinib
Tarceva

Generic Ingredients: Everolimus
Afinitor

Generic Ingredients: Gefitinib
Iressa

Generic Ingredients: Imatinib
Gleevec

Generic Ingredients: Lapatinib
Tykerb

Generic Ingredients: Nilotinib
Tasigna

Generic Ingredients: Pazopanib
Votrient

Generic Ingredients: Ruxolitinib
Jakafi

Generic Ingredients: Sorafenib
Nexavar

Generic Ingredients: Sunitinib
Sutent

Generic Ingredients: Vandetanib
Caprelsa

Generic Ingredients: Vemurafenib
Zelboraf

Prescribed For

Crizotinib is prescribed for people with non-small-cell lung cancer (NSCLC). Dasatinib is for adults with leukemias that have not responded to other therapies and pancreatic cancer tumors that are inoperable or have spread to other parts of the body. Erlotinib is prescribed together with gemcitabine for pancreatic cancer and NSCLC that has not responded to other therapies. Everolimus is for kidney cancer that has not responded to other therapies. Gefitinib may be prescribed for NSCLC that has not responded to other therapies; it is also used for breast, colorectal, and prostate cancers. Imatinib is prescribed for chronic myeloid leukemia (CML), gastrointestinal (GI) tumors, and other cancers. Lapatinib is prescribed together with capecitabine for HER2-positive advanced or metastatic breast cancer and is being studied for lung cancer. Nilotinib is prescribed for chronic and accelerated Philadelphia chromosome–positive CML in adults resistant or intolerant to prior therapy that included imatinib. Pazopanib and sorafenib are prescribed for advanced kidney cancer. Ruxolitinib is prescribed for people with or at risk for myelofibrosis, a condition in which blood-cell-producing bone marrow tissue is replaced with fibrous tissue. Sunitinib is prescribed for advanced kidney cancer and for rare cancers of the stomach, bowel, or esophagus that do not respond to imatinib. Vandetanib is prescribed for medullary thyroid cancer, which accounts for 3–5% of all thyroid cancer cases. Vemurafenib is prescribed for BRAF-positive malignant melanoma (skin cancer) that is untreatable or has spread despite treatment. The cancer must have a specific tumor mutation that is established by a special diagnostic test before it can be used. These medicines are usually prescribed until the condition starts to progress or unacceptable drug side effects occur.

General Information

These drugs inhibit the kinase enzymes that are central switches to many processes within cancer cells. They can overcome drug resistance that involves a family of kinase proteins responsible for the uncontrolled growth of some cancer cells, several of which are known to drive tumor growth and progression. Crizotinib's effects are specific to those tumors that carry a specific gene, known as ALK, and is defined by a specific pretreatment lab test. Early results with crizotinib were spectacular, indicating that it substantially improves quality of life and might help you live longer, but there is no long-term proof for these outcomes. No studies of either dasatinib or sunitinib have proven that people taking them live longer, though the drugs can extend the time until the cancer gets worse. Erlotinib inhibits the activation of tyrosine kinase and is involved with an important cellular growth factor receptor but its exact mechanism is not well understood. Everolimus inhibits *mTOR kinase*, leading to a slowing of protein manufacturing in the cancer cell. It also reduces the amount of vascular endothelial growth factor (VEGF) produced by cancer cells. These actions slow cancer cell growth, the formation of new blood vessels to feed the tumor, and the use of glucose in cancer cell growth activities. Gefitinib inhibits the stimulation of the "epidermal growth receptor" found on the surface of many cancer cells. When stimulated, the receptor triggers processes inside the cell to make it grow and divide. Gefitinib interferes with this process. Pazopanib is an oral multiple kinase inhibitor that works directly on VEGF, which is needed to grow new blood vessels to feed a growing solid tumor. Sorafenib decreases the spread of tumor cells. In some studies, it was found to reduce the growth of new blood vessels that are necessary to feed the growth of a cancerous tumor. These drugs are rapidly absorbed into the bloodstream, are broken down by enzymes in the liver, and eliminated primarily in the stool.

Cautions and Warnings

Do not take these drugs if you are **allergic** or **sensitive** to any of their ingredients. Severe drug reactions can occur with vemurafenib that may require discontinuation of treatment.

Dasatinib should only be prescribed after you have been treated with **imatinib**.

People with **liver disease** should use these drugs with caution, and dosage reduction is usually recommended. If you are taking crizotinib and develop elevated liver enzymes, your doctor may suspend or stop treatment or reduce the dose until your enzymes return to normal. People with severe liver disease should not take erlotinib, everolimus, or sorafenib, but vemurafenib can be used with caution. Sunitinib should not be used if you have liver or **pancreatic failure**.

Erlotinib and sorafenib should not be used in those with severe **kidney disease**, but vemurafenib can be used with caution. Everolimus can reduce kidney function with potentially fatal consequences and raise blood-sugar and -fat levels. Reductions in red- and white-blood-cell and blood-platelet counts can also occur.

Everolimus suppresses the body's immune system and increases the risk of serious, possibly fatal infection. People taking everolimus can develop lung irritation as well as mouth, tongue, and cheek irritation and sores that can be very painful. Avoid live vaccines and close contact with people who have received a live vaccine. Some live virus vaccines include nasal influenza, measles, mumps, rubella, oral polio, BCG, yellow fever, varicella, and typhoid.

People taking dasatinib can develop pulmonary arterial hypertension (abnormally high blood pressure in the arteries of the lungs). Symptoms of this rare condition include shortness of breath, fatigue, and swollen ankles or legs.

Crizotinib, erlotinib, gefitinib, and vandetanib have been linked to severe and sometimes fatal lung disease. People with **pre-existing lung disease** are most likely to experience a decline in health while taking these drugs. Your doctor may stop treatment if you develop lung damage and inflammation related to the medicine.

Dasatinib may affect male and female fertility and the developing fetus. Sexually active men and women taking this drug should use effective birth control.

Imatinib and dasatinib can severely reduce the numbers of blood platelets and white and red cells. Internal bleeding can be associated with platelet reductions induced by these drugs. Bleeding has occurred in people taking vandetanib and was fatal in 3 of them. Bleeding can also occur while you are taking sorafenib or sunitinib, which may affect wound healing. Interrupt treatment if you are undergoing **major surgery**. Your doctor will check blood counts every week for the first 2 months and then once a month to monitor for changes. These effects are generally reversible by reducing drug dosage or temporarily stopping treatment.

Severe fluid retention can occur in people taking dasatinib and imatinib. This includes fluid in the lungs, around the heart, and in the abdomen.

These drugs can affect the heart by interfering with the conduction of electrical signals, which changes the heart's rhythm. Inform your doctor if you have **heart problems**, **low blood levels of potassium or magnesium**, or are taking drugs for **abnormal heart rhythms**. Be sure your cardiologist knows you are taking these medications. People taking nilotinib or vandetanib have died suddenly, possibly because of torsade de pointes, an effect on the heart's electrical system that changes the heart's rhythm. Imatinib, lapatinib, and sunitinib can worsen **heart failure**. There are more heart attacks and other cardiac problems in people taking sorafenib. Regular cardiograms are recommended. Vandetanib remains in the body for a long time and cardiograms should be started as soon as you start treatment and continued regularly. Your dose may be reduced if you show a change in heart status. People born with a heart condition called **long QT syndrome** should not take crizotinib or vandetanib. People with **high blood pressure** should use caution while taking sorafenib or vandetanib, because high blood pressure, sometimes severe, is a common side effect of these drugs. Blood pressure should be checked during the first 6 weeks of treatment.

Erlotinib can lead to GI bleeding and perforation. This complication can be fatal.

Erlotinib and vandetanib can cause possibly fatal severe blisters and skin peeling reactions. New **malignant melanoma** tumors have occurred while taking vemurafenib. These may need to be surgically removed and may necessitate dose changes. About ¼ of people taking vemurafenib for malignant melanoma will develop a different skin cancer called cutaneous squamous cell carcinoma. Risk factors for this cancer include chronic sun exposure and previous skin cancer. Your dermatologist will check for this type of cancer before and during the time you take vemurafenib.

Extreme sun sensitivity can occur in people taking vemurafenib. Avoid all sun exposure while taking it.

Some of these medicines can cause severe eye reactions. Erlotinib can cause ulcers and perforation of the cornea. Tell your doctor about any vision changes or eye pain. Vemurafenib can cause swelling of the middle layer of the eye and interfere with blood flow to the eye.

People with **pancreatic cancer** have experienced chest pain, heart attack, stroke, and anemia due to red-blood-cell destruction and very low blood-platelet count while taking erlotinib.

Strokes, sometimes fatal, have occurred in people taking vandetanib.

Tobacco use, especially cigarette smoking, reduces blood levels of erlotinib. You should not smoke while taking erlotinib because it can interfere with the drug's effectiveness.

People taking ruxolitinib may experience anemia, and low white-blood-cell and blood-platelet counts, increasing the bleeding risk. People taking ruxolitinib must be observed for signs of infection because their bodies may not respond appropriately.

These drugs have been associated with reduced thyroid activity. Your doctor should check your thyroid gland function before you start treatment with any of these drugs. People taking vandetanib are likely to already have reduced thyroid gland activity. Raising the dose of thyroid replacement medicine can offset this effect. Sunitinib has been associated with increased and reduced thyroid and adrenal gland function and high blood pressure.

These medicines have been linked to a group of symptoms known as PRES syndrome, which includes headache, confusion, seizures, and blindness.

Lapatinib and vandetanib can cause diarrhea. Contact your doctor if this happens to you because it should be treated aggressively to avoid losing large amounts of fluid and electrolyte. Your doctor may have you take medicine to prevent diarrhea from developing. If you develop severe diarrhea with vandetanib, the medicine should be stopped until the diarrhea can be resolved.

Possible Side Effects

Crizotinib

▼ Most common: visual difficulties (flashes of light, blurred vision, light sensitivity, and floaters); nausea; vomiting; esophageal disorders (upset stomach, swallowing difficulty, stomach pain or burning, gastroesophageal reflux disease [GERD]); diarrhea; constipation; arm or leg swelling; abdominal pain; painful sores and inflammation of the mouth, cheeks, gums, tongue, lips, and throat; fatigue; chest pain or discomfort; fever; upper-respiratory infections; elevated liver enzymes; appetite loss; joint and back pain; dizziness; headache; taste changes; nerve damage (burning sensation, abnormal sensations, changes in nerve response to stimulation, nerve pain, tingling in the hands or feet, cramps, weakness, and muscle twitching); sleeplessness; cough; difficulty breathing; and rash.

▼ Rare: severe or fatal lung damage and severe liver irritation. Contact your doctor if you experience anything unusual while taking any medication.

Dasatinib

▼ Most common: abdominal pain; pain; difficulty breathing; cough; fever; chills; pneumonia; infections, including herpes virus and blood infection; fluid retention; nausea; vomiting; diarrhea; constipation; appetite loss; weight loss;

Possible Side Effects *(continued)*

abdominal enlargement; headache; muscle and joint pain; fatigue; skin rashes; itching; weakness; inflammation and ulcers in the mouth, GI tract, or anus; chest pain; tingling in the hands or feet; nerve inflammation; and abnormal heart rhythms.

- ▼ Common: fluid in the lungs, fever with very low white-blood-cell count, GI bleeding, reduced blood-platelet count, upset stomach, dental disorders, colitis, stomach pain, anal fissure, not feeling well, sweating, hair loss, dry skin, acne, unusual sun sensitivity, nail disorders, skin color changes, asthma, taste changes, tiredness, fainting, tremors, convulsions, muscle inflammation, muscle stiffness, elevated blood level of uric acid, heart palpitations, angina, heart enlargement, heart attack, conjunctivitis (pinkeye), dry eye, flushing, blood-pressure changes, sleeplessness, depression, anxiety, confusion, changes in affect, male breast enlargement, bruising, dizziness, ringing or buzzing in the ears, frequent urination, and kidney failure.
- ▼ Less common: anemia, heart failure, bleeding in the brain, and reduced sex drive.
- ▼ Rare: Rare side effects can occur in almost any part of the body. Contact your doctor if you experience anything unusual while taking any medication.

Erlotinib

Side effects limited to pancreatic cancer patients are most likely due to gemcitabine. All other side effects are due to erlotinib and are likely to occur in all people taking it.

Pancreatic Cancer

- ▼ Most common: bone pain, muscle pain, constipation, dizziness, fever and chills, swelling due to water retention, depression, upset stomach, headache, sleeplessness, anxiety, hair loss, and tingling and pain.

Non-Small-Cell Lung Cancer

- ▼ Most common: rash; diarrhea; loss of appetite; fatigue; difficulty breathing; cough; nausea; infections; vomiting; inflammation of the inside of your cheeks, gums, tongue, or lips; itching; dry skin; conjunctivitis (pinkeye); dry eye; and abdominal pain.

Possible Side Effects *(continued)*

- ▼ Less common: blood-clotting problems, dizziness and fainting, abnormal heart rhythms, temporary slowing or stopping of bowel movement, GI ulcers or perforation, pancreas irritation, anemia and low blood-platelet counts, bleeding in the brain and stroke, nosebleeds, kidney damage, hairiness, cornea irritation and perforation, eye pain, visual changes, eyelash or eyebrow changes, brittle and loose nails, skin darkening, and severe blisters or skin peeling that may worsen with sun exposure.
- ▼ Rare: Rare side effects can occur in almost any part of the body. Contact your doctor if you experience anything unusual while taking any medication.

Everolimus

- ▼ Most common: oral ulcers; infections; weakness; fatigue; fever; swelling in the feet, legs, or ankles; cough; nausea; vomiting and diarrhea; nosebleed; lung irritation; rash; itching; dry skin; loss of appetite; headache; changes in taste; and arm or leg pain.
- ▼ Common: abdominal pain, dry mouth, hemorrhoids, sleeplessness, dizziness, weight loss, chest pain, fluid in the lungs, and tingling in the hands or feet.
- ▼ Less common: kidney failure, rapid heartbeat, heart failure, high blood pressure, trouble swallowing, chills, throat pain, runny nose, redness (looks like sunburn), tenderness, peeling or numbness of the palms and soles of the feet, skin lesions, acne, diabetes, swollen eyelids, conjunctivitis (pinkeye), and jaw pain and bleeding.
- ▼ Rare: Rare side effects can occur in almost any part of the body. Contact your doctor if you experience anything unusual while taking any medication.

Gefitinib

The risk of drug side effects increases when taking high doses of gefitinib.

- ▼ Most common: rash, acne, dry skin, nausea, and diarrhea.
- ▼ Common: vomiting, dry mouth, itching, appetite loss, and weakness.
- ▼ Less common: weight loss, swelling in the arms or legs, poor vision in one eye, conjunctivitis (pinkeye), mild rash, mouth ulcers, and difficulty breathing, with or without cough

Possible Side Effects *(continued)*

and fever, that may become severe in a very short period of time.

- ▼ Rare: eye pain, erosion of the cornea, eye ulcer, unusual eyelash growth, bleeding in the eye, severe skin reaction, and allergic reaction. Contact your doctor if you experience anything unusual while taking any medication.

Imatinib

Most side effects are mild to moderate, but are very common in patients experiencing a myeloid blast crisis. As many as 5% of people taking the drug in clinical studies stopped because of side effects. Women taking imatinib are likely to develop more swelling around the eyes, headache, and fatigue.

- ▼ Most common: nausea, diarrhea, vomiting, swelling around the eyes, leg swelling and muscle cramps, and upset stomach.
- ▼ Common: muscle pain, fever, cough, rash, and difficulty breathing.
- ▼ Less common: headache, fatigue, severe joint pain, weight gain, abdominal pain, appetite loss, constipation, irritation of the nose or nasal cavity, night sweats, and weakness.
- ▼ Rare: severe fluid retention, bleeding, easy bruising, and pneumonia. Contact your doctor if you experience anything unusual while taking any medication.

Lapatinib

- ▼ Most common: diarrhea, nausea, vomiting, stomach irritation and pain, upset stomach, dry skin, rash, peeling of the palms and soles of the feet, inflamed mucosal tissue, pain in the hands or feet, back pain, difficulty breathing, and sleeplessness.

Nilotinib

- ▼ Most common: rash, itching, nausea, constipation, diarrhea, vomiting, fatigue, headache, fever, swelling in the arms or legs, bone and joint pain, arm or leg pain, back pain, muscle spasms, cough, difficulty breathing, and nose and throat infections.
- ▼ Rare: Rare side effects can occur in almost any part of the body. Contact your doctor if you experience anything unusual while taking any medication.

Possible Side Effects *(continued)*

Pazopanib

- ▼ Most common: diarrhea, high blood pressure, hair graying, nausea, vomiting, appetite loss, fatigue, weakness, abdominal pain, and headache. Liver and blood chemistry changes, including blood-sugar reduction, are also very common.
- ▼ Common: protein in the urine, hair loss, chest pain, taste changes, upset stomach, rash, and weight loss.
- ▼ Less common: facial swelling, skin color changes, and hand-foot syndrome (sunburn-like redness, tenderness, and possible peeling of the palms and soles, with numbness or tingling), which can be uncomfortable and may interfere with daily activities.

Ruxolitinib

- ▼ Most common: bruising or bleeding, dizziness, low blood-platelet count, anemia, low white-blood-cell count, and liver irritation.
- ▼ Common: urinary infections, weight gain, and stomach gas.
- ▼ Less common: herpes zoster (shingles) infections.
- ▼ Rare: Rare side effects can occur in almost any part of the body. Contact your doctor if you experience anything unusual while taking any medication.

Sorafenib

- ▼ Most common: high blood pressure; fatigue; swelling; blisters; rash and other skin reactions, especially on the soles of the feet and palms; hair loss; itching; diarrhea; nausea; appetite loss; vomiting; constipation; bleeding; cough; and difficulty breathing.
- ▼ Common: weight loss, numbness, tingling in the hands or feet, sensitivity to bright light, joint pain, abdominal pain, headache, hoarseness, erectile dysfunction, depression, anemia, low levels of white blood cells, increased liver enzyme levels, flu-like symptoms, and fever.
- ▼ Less common: GI tract perforation.
- ▼ Rare: Rare side effects can occur in almost any part of the body. Contact your doctor if you experience anything unusual while taking any medication.

Possible Side Effects *(continued)*

Sunitinib

- ▼ Most common: fatigue; fever; weakness; diarrhea; nausea; vomiting; constipation; abdominal pain; upset stomach; inflammation and ulceration in the mouth and GI tract; dry mouth; cough; difficulty breathing; high blood pressure; rash; dry skin; pain, redness, tenderness, and peeling of the palms of the hands and soles of the feet; skin discoloration; taste changes; appetite loss; sleeplessness; and bleeding.
- ▼ Common: oral pain; hair color changes; hair loss; GERD with or without irritation and swelling of the esophagus; gas; tongue pain; swelling in the arms or legs; dizziness; and depression.
- ▼ Less common: blood clots possibly leading to stroke.

Vandetanib

- ▼ Most common: diarrhea, colitis, rash, acne, dry skin, abnormal heart rhythms, nausea, high blood pressure (possibly severe), headache, fatigue, reduced appetite, abdominal pain, vomiting, weakness, unusual sun sensitivity, sleeplessness, stuffy nose, upset stomach, itching, and bleeding.
- ▼ Common: weight loss, protein in the urine, depression, blurred vision, visual halos, and blood test changes.
- ▼ Rare: respiratory failure, pneumonia, heart failure with abnormal heart rhythm, blood infection, and stomach irritation or bleeding. Contact your doctor if you experience anything unusual while taking any medication.

Vemurafenib

Women taking this drug experienced more severe rashes, joint pain, sun sensitivity, and changes in creatinine levels, a measure of kidney function. Men experienced more keratoacanthoma, a low-grade skin tumor originating in hair follicles, and some liver lab test changes.

- ▼ Most common: fatigue, joint and muscle pain, arm or leg swelling and/or pain, hair loss, nausea, diarrhea, vomiting, constipation, sun sensitivity reactions, skin rash, dry skin, itching, small skin projections known as tags or papillomas, fever, weakness, headache, taste changes, and appetite loss.

Possible Side Effects *(continued)*

- ▼ Common: actinic keratosis (dry, rough, precancerous patches of skin), sunburn, back pain, and cough.
- ▼ Rare: Other vemurafenib side effects can affect almost any area of the body and can include skin peeling, arthritis, dizziness, nerve damage, and weight gain. Contact your doctor if you experience anything unusual while taking any medication.

Drug Interactions

- Aprepitant, atazanavir, clarithromycin, diltiazem, erythromycin, fluconazole, fosamprenavir, indinavir, itraconazole, ketoconazole, nefazodone, nelfinavir, ritonavir, saquinavir, simvastatin, telithromycin, verapamil, and voriconazole increase blood levels of multiple kinase inhibitors by slowing down their breakdown by liver enzymes. They should be avoided if possible. If they must be taken together, dose modification is necessary.
- Carbamazepine, dexamethasone, efavirenz, modafinil, nevirapine, phenobarbital and other barbiturates, phenytoin, pioglitazone, rifabutin, rifampin, and rifapentine can substantially lower blood levels of multiple kinase inhibitors by stimulating the production of enzymes that break them down in the blood. They should be avoided if possible.
- Imatinib stimulates enzymes in the liver that break down phenytoin. Patients taking this combination may need to increase their phenytoin dosage to maintain seizure control.
- Do not mix St. John's wort with any of these medications.
- Long-term use of antacids or drugs that reduce stomach acid production (esomeprazole, lansoprazole, omeprazole, pantoprazole, rabeprazole, ranitidine, famotidine, and cimetidine) can make crizotinib, dasatinib, erlotinib, and gefitinib less soluble in the GI tract, cutting blood levels in ½. Do not take proton-pump inhibitors because their action is very long. H_2 blockers such as cimetidine have a shorter action and should be avoided for 2 hours before or after a dose of dasatinib. Do not mix cimetidine with erlotinib. It affects both stomach acidity and liver enzymes.
- People taking warfarin or another anticoagulant should be cautious when dasatinib, imatinib, sorafenib, or vemurafenib is started because of the increased chance of bleeding. You

may be switched to a heparin (injectable) blood thinner to avoid this interaction. Gefitinib can increase the effect of warfarin, causing bleeding episodes. Your doctor must check your blood regularly and may need to adjust your warfarin dose while you are taking gefitinib.

- Crizotinib, dasatinib, and imatinib may increase blood levels of alfentanil, astemizole, cisapride, cyclosporine, fentanyl, pimozide, quinidine, sirolimus, tacrolimus, terfenadine, some calcium channel blockers, and ergot-based migraine medicines. These drugs should be mixed with caution.
- Imatinib increases the amount of simvastatin in the blood by 3.5 times. Other statin drugs may be similarly affected.
- Nilotinib and sorafenib may increase blood levels of the following drugs by interfering with their breakdown in the liver: amodiaquine, bupropion, cerivastatin, cyclophosphamide, efavirenz, ifosfamide, methadone, paclitaxel, repaglinide, and torsemide.
- Nilotinib may increase blood levels of nonsteroidal anti-inflammatory drug (NSAID) pain relievers, tolbutamide, and glipizide.
- Pazopanib weakly inhibits some liver enzymes responsible for drug breakdown. It can raise blood levels of some medicines, including paclitaxel (Taxol), but for other important medicines usually affected by these enzymes, such as warfarin, this interaction is not clinically important. More research will clarify this.
- Sorafenib also inhibits the liver's ability to break down toxic chemicals and drugs, including acetaminophen. The importance of this effect is not yet known.
- Sorafenib causes a 21% increase in blood levels of the anticancer drug doxorubicin and a 26–42% increase in blood levels of the drug irinotecan. The clinical importance of these interactions is not known but these combinations should be used with caution. Sorafenib has been used safely together with a variety of other anticancer drugs.
- Vandetanib should not be taken with medicines that are used to treat heart arrhythmias, including amiodarone, disopyramide, dofetilide, and sotalol.
- Do not mix vandetanib with other drugs that can affect the heart's electrical system, including chloroquin, clarithromycin, dolasetron, granisetron, haloperidol, methadone, norfloxacin, and pimozide.

Food Interactions

Crizotinib, dasatinib, everolimus, gefitinib, pazopanib, ruxolitinib, sunitinib, vandetanib, and vermurafenib can be taken without regard to food or meals. Imatinib can cause stomach and intestinal irritation. Take each dose with food and a glass of water to minimize this side effect. Erlotinib, lapatinib, nilotinib, and sorafenib should be taken on an empty stomach, at least 1 hour before or 2 hours after a meal. Do not drink or eat any grapefruit or starfruit product while you are taking crizotinib, erlotinib, everolimus, imatinib, nilotinib, pazopanib, ruxolitinib, or sunitinib. These foods reduce the amount of drug absorbed into the bloodstream. Broccoli, brussels sprouts, and char-grilled meats speed the breakdown of erlotinib in the liver, reducing its effectiveness.

Usual Dose

Crizotinib

Adult: 250 mg twice a day to start. Dose may be reduced to 200 mg twice a day for those who are less able to tolerate the medicine or experience severe drug side effects.

Child: not recommended.

Dasatinib

Adult: 100–140 mg a day in 1 or 2 doses. Always take this medication at the same time every day. Modifications of 20 mg a day may be based on response or toxicity assessments. To deal with drug interactions, other medications with the same effect may be substituted for the interacting drugs or the dasatinib dose may be altered.

Child: not recommended.

Erlotinib

Adult: 150 mg a day for NSCLC; 100 mg a day for pancreatic cancer.

Child: not recommended.

Everolimus

Adult: 10 mg at the same time every day; 5 mg a day for people with moderate liver disease.

Child: not recommended.

Gefitinib

Adult: 250 mg once a day.

Child: not recommended.

Imatinib

Adult and Child (age 3 and over): 400–800 mg a day. Treatment should be continued for as long as the patient continues to benefit. If severe liver or other problems develop, drug dosage should be reduced or stopped until they resolve. Children 3 years of age and older can take imatinib in either 1 or 2 daily doses.

Child (under age 3): not recommended.

Lapatinib

Adult: five 250-mg tablets once a day for 3 weeks plus capecitabine twice a day for 2 weeks.

Child: not recommended.

Nilotinib

Adult: two 200-mg capsules every 12 hours. This dose may be modified based on certain lab tests and your heart function.

Child: not recommended.

Pazopanib

Adult: two 200-mg tablets once a day at least 1 hour before or 2 hours after a meal. Adults with moderate liver disease should take only 200 mg a day, and those with a severe liver disease should not take pazopanib.

Child: not recommended.

Ruxolitinib

Adult: 15–25 mg twice a day, depending on blood count; 10 mg twice a day for people with any degree of liver failure. Your doctor will take blood tests every 2–4 weeks. Treatment may be discontinued if no improvement is seen within 6 months.

Child: not recommended.

Sorafenib

Adult: two 200-mg tablets twice a day at least 1 hour before or 2 hours after a meal. Drug dosage may be reduced if you experience a serious side effect.

Child: not recommended.

Sunitinib

Adult: 50 mg once a day for 4 weeks. Then stop for 2 weeks and repeat the 4-week treatment as prescribed. Daily dose may be adjusted in 12.5-mg steps.

Child: not recommended.

Vandetanib

Adult: 300 mg once a day. Dose may be reduced to 100 mg to account for side effects or severe kidney failure. Treatment should be continued until there is no more benefit or side effects are unacceptable. Doctors and pharmacies must be specially certified to prescribe and dispense this drug.

Child: not recommended.

Vemurafenib

Adult: 960 mg (4 tablets) every 12 hours. Dosage may be reduced in people who experience drug side effects but must continue on the medicine. Dose reduction below 480 mg every 12 hours is not recommended.

Child: not recommended.

Overdosage

Take the overdose victim to your doctor or a hospital emergency room. There are no known cases of crizotinib overdose. Animal overdose studies of dasatinib showed cardiac toxicity, bleeding, and high blood pressure. Single doses of 1000 mg of erlotinib and weekly doses of 1600 mg of everolimus were well tolerated in clinical studies. Likely overdose symptoms include diarrhea, rash, liver irritation, and other side effects. Everolimus was reasonably safe in animal studies, and people taking as much as 70 mg per dose had no more reaction than those taking 10 mg. Likely gefitinib and sorafenib overdose symptoms include diarrhea and skin rash. Symptoms should be treated individually but it is particularly important to pay attention to severe diarrhea. There is little experience with imatinib doses larger than 800 mg a day, the maximum human dose. Some overdose effects are muscle cramps and elevated liver enzymes. Lapatinib overdose can cause diarrhea, vomiting, and other drug side effects. Nilotinib overdose has not been reported. In pazopanib clinical studies, people given 1000- and 2000-mg doses developed extreme fatigue and high blood pressure. Ruxolitinib overdose is likely to result in drug side effects, though individual doses of 200 mg have been taken with no severe effects. Sunitinib overdose can cause loss of muscle coordination; head shakes; slowing of thought, speech, and movement; eye discharge; upset stomach; and standing of small hairs on the arm or back of the neck. Vandetanib overdose is likely to lead to drug side effects such as rash, diarrhea, and high blood pressure. In the event of a vandetanib overdose, stop taking the medicine until your doctor has completely evaluated the situation. The risk associated with these side effects is greater because vandetanib stays in the body for weeks after it is taken. In the event of an overdose with vemurafenib, stop treatment and contact your doctor at once. If you seek treatment, ALWAYS bring the prescription bottle or container.

Special Information

You must report any severe side effect or anything unusual to your doctor, especially shortness of breath, feeling like your throat is closing or your tongue is swelling, fatigue, or heart palpitations. These may be signs of heart failure. Treatment may have to be stopped until the side effect improves or resolves. Then, treatment may be resumed.

Contact your doctor if you become confused or have trouble talking or understanding what is said; have sudden blindness in one or both eyes; experience a numb feeling in your face, arms, or legs (especially on one side of your body); have a sudden and severe headache; become dizzy; lose your balance or coordination; or have trouble walking. These are stroke symptoms and require emergency treatment.

Contact your doctor if you become feverish or develop any other sign of infection.

These drugs can cause liver toxicity. Symptoms to watch for and report to your doctor include yellowing of the skin or whites of the eyes, unusually dark-colored urine, appetite loss, unusual tiredness, easy bleeding or bruising, and pain in the upper right stomach area.

Contact your doctor if you experience blurred vision, see halos, or have any other effect on your eyesight while taking vandetanib. You may be told to see an eye doctor.

There are no driving restrictions associated with these medicines. However, some can affect your eyesight, and therefore your ability to drive properly.

Dasatinib contains lactose and may cause GI distress in people who are lactose intolerant.

Crushing dasatinib or everolimus tablets is not recommended. If you cannot swallow a whole pill, the crushed pill must be taken immediately.

If you cannot swallow a vandetanib tablet, place the pill in a glass with about 2 ounces of plain water, stir for 10 minutes, and then drink the entire contents of the glass right away. The pill will not completely dissolve; it will break into tiny pieces. Then, to make sure you get the full dose of medicine and the entire pill, add another 4 ounces of plain water to the glass, stir, and drink that mixture. Vandetanib pill pieces irritate your skin and mucous membranes. Thoroughly wash the area if the medicine comes into contact with skin or mucous membranes.

These drugs commonly increase sun sensitivity and make it easier for your skin to burn. Since vandetanib stays in the body for a long time, people taking it must protect their skin by using sunscreen and wearing long sleeves and pants when they go outside. Continue this practice for 4 months after you stop taking vandetanib.

Women who are or who may be pregnant must avoid contact with the crushed tablets because of risk to the developing fetus. The medication is coated to protect people from unnecessary exposure to dasatinib.

If you are taking erlotinib, contact your doctor immediately if you develop any rash or eye trouble or have severe or persistent diarrhea, nausea, vomiting, appetite loss, difficulty breathing, cough, or fever.

Japanese, Chinese, and black patients taking the same doses of some of these medicines had higher amounts of drug in their blood than patients of other races, but the exact importance of this information is not yet known.

If you are taking gefitinib, contact your doctor at once if you develop cough, wheezing, or fever, or have difficulty breathing. You may have to stop taking gefitinib until the reason for your symptoms is discovered. These symptoms are fatal in ⅓ of people who develop them. Other reasons to contact your doctor right away are severe or persistent diarrhea, nausea, appetite loss, vomiting, eye irritation, or any other new symptom. If your diarrhea is severe, your doctor may have you discontinue the drug for 2 weeks to rest your GI system and manage your symptoms with over-the-counter medicines and electrolyte-replacement solution.

Sorafenib can pass into male ejaculate. Men must use a condom while taking this drug and for 2 weeks after stopping it.

Do not stop or change the dose of these medications unless instructed to do so by your doctor. You should make a special effort to take these medications at the same time every day.

If you forget a dose of crizotinib, take it as soon as you remember, unless less than 6 hours remain until your next scheduled dose. If that is the case, skip the forgotten dose and continue with your regular schedule. Do not take a double dose.

Do not take a double dose of dasatinib. If you take dasatinib twice a day and forget a dose, take it if you remember within an hour of your regular time, and then continue with your regular schedule. Otherwise, skip the forgotten dose. If you take dasatinib once a day and forget a dose, take it if you remember within 12 hours of your regular time. Otherwise, skip the forgotten dose and continue with your regular schedule.

If you forget a dose of erlotinib or everolimus and remember within the next 6 hours, take it as usual and continue with your regular schedule. If you do not remember until more than 6 hours have passed since your regular time, skip the forgotten dose and continue with your regular schedule the next morning. Contact your doctor if you forget your erlotinib or everolimus 2 or more days in a row.

If you forget a dose of imatinib or sorafenib, take it as soon as you remember. If it is almost time for your next dose, space out the remaining doses for the day to allow you to take your total prescribed dosage for the day. Contact your doctor if you forget more than 1 dose in a row or if you take too much medication.

If you forget a dose of pazopanib, take it if you remember within 12 hours of your regular time. Otherwise, skip the forgotten dose and continue with your regular schedule. Contact your doctor if you forget your medicine 2 or more days in a row. Do not crush pazopanib tablets because this increases the speed at which the drug is absorbed into your blood, which raises blood levels and the risk of side effects.

If you forget your daily dose of gefitinib, lapatinib, nilotinib, or sunitinib, skip the forgotten dose and continue with your regular schedule. Tell your doctor if you forget to take any doses of these drugs. Do not take a double dose.

Dialysis patients taking ruxolitinib should take it after treatment, not before. Do not stop taking ruxolitinib unless your doctor tells you to do so. Myelofibrosis will return once you stop.

If you forget to take a dose of vandetanib, take it as soon as you remember unless it is less than 12 hours before your next scheduled dose. If you don't remember until then, skip the dose you forgot. Do not take a double dose.

If you forget to take a dose of vemurafenib, take it as soon as you remember, up until 4 hours before your next regular dose. If you don't remember until after the 4-hour limit, skip the forgotten dose and continue with your regular schedule. Do not take a double dose of vemurafenib.

Special Populations

Pregnancy/Breast-feeding: These drugs are not recommended during pregnancy, as they are known to enter the blood circulation of the developing fetus and can damage the fetus and cause birth defects. Women who are pregnant or may become pregnant should discuss continuing these drugs with their doctor. Women of childbearing age must use effective contraception to avoid pregnancy while taking these drugs and for 2 weeks after stopping them. Women taking vandetanib must avoid pregnancy for 4 months after stopping treatment. If you become pregnant while taking one of these drugs, contact your doctor at once.

Imatinib and vandetanib pass into breast milk. It is not known if dasatinib, erlotinib, gefitinib, or sunitinib pass into breast milk. Nursing mothers taking one of these medicines should use infant formula because of the risk of severe drug side effects for the nursing infant.

Seniors: Seniors have been able to take crizotinib, dasatinib, everolimus, ruxolitinib, vandetanib, and vemurafenib without special precaution, though they may be more sensitive to some side effects, especially fluid retention. No differences in side effect sensitivity have been noted with erlotinib, gefitinib, lapatinib, or sunitinib.

Generic Name

Muromonab-CD3 (muh-ROE-moe-nab)

Brand Names

Orthoclone OKT3 Sterile Solution

Type of Drug

Immunosuppressant.

Prescribed For

Kidney, heart, and liver transplantation.

General Information

Muromonab-CD3 is an important alternative to cyclosporine in treating acute organ transplant rejection. By blocking the activity of T-cells, which protect the body against invading microorganisms or foreign substances, this drug suppresses the immune system and reverses organ rejection. The drug is given as an intravenous (IV) injection by a health care professional in a physician's office or clinic. The drug starts working in minutes and continues working for as long as it is used. T-cells rapidly return to normal within 1 week after the medication is stopped.

Cautions and Warnings

Muromonab-CD3 should be given only by physicians experienced in immunosuppressive therapy and the care of organ-transplant patients.

Do not use muromonab-CD3 if you are **allergic** or **sensitive** to any of its ingredients.

This drug should not be given to people with uncontrolled **hypertension**, untreated **heart failure**, **fluid overload**, or a history of **seizures**. Severe allergic reactions can occur, including arthritis, serum sickness, treatment failure, angioedema (a potentially life-threatening swelling of the lips and throat), and anaphylactic shock.

Muromonab-CD3 is made in cells from mouse tissue and causes the development of anti-mouse antibodies in humans. People who have received other drugs made in this way may already have high levels of this kind of antibody in their blood and, if they do, should not be treated with muromonab-CD3. Your doctor will test for antibody levels.

People who receive this drug usually develop cytokine release syndrome (CRS) from 30 minutes to 2 days after the first dose is given. CRS symptoms range from mild, flu-like symptoms, such as fever, chills, joint aches, weakness, and headaches, to a less common, life-threatening shock-like reaction that involves the heart and nervous system. Some of the more severe symptoms of CRS are shortness of breath, high fever—up to 107°F—wheezing, rapid heartbeat, chest pain, respiratory collapse or failure, heart attack, severe drug reactions, seizures, hallucinations, stiff neck, brain swelling, headache, tremor, altered thinking or mood, lethargy, weakness, and involuntary movements. People who are at risk for more severe forms of CRS include those with a **recent heart attack** or uncontrolled **angina pectoris**, **heart failure**, **fluid in the lungs**, **serious lung disease**, and a history of **seizure** or **shock**. CRS may be prevented or minimized by giving methylprednisolone 1–4 hours before the first dose of muromonab-CD3. CRS symptoms usually become less severe with repeated doses of muromonab-CD3.

Muromonab-CD3 increases the risk of blood clots.

People receiving this drug are more likely to develop infection. Preventive antibiotic therapy is sometimes used to reduce the risk of infection.

Possible Side Effects

More than 90% of people receiving muromonab-CD3 experience some form of CRS, though it is usually mild (see "Cautions and Warnings" for symptoms list).

- ▼ Common: infections, lymphoma, and allergic reactions.
- ▼ Rare: Rare side effects can occur in almost any part of the body. Contact your doctor if you experience anything unusual while taking any medication.

Drug Interactions

- Indomethacin may increase the risk of nervous system side effects of muromonab-CD3.

Usual Dose

Adult: 5 mg by IV injection once a day for 10–14 days.

Child: not recommended.

Overdosage

Little is known about the effects of muromonab-CD3 overdose, although it is unlikely because this drug is usually given in a health care facility. Contact your local poison control center or a hospital emergency room for information.

Special Information

Contact your doctor at the first sign of rash, itching, rapid heartbeat, difficulty swallowing, breathing difficulties, unusual swelling, or allergic reaction, or if you experience any bothersome or persistent side effect. It is essential to maintain close contact with your doctor while taking muromonab-CD3.

Mild reactions due to CRS may be treated by taking acetaminophen or antihistamines. Your body temperature should be no higher than 100°F when each dose is given.

Avoid exposure to bacterial infection and immunizations while you are taking this drug. If an infection develops, your doctor will have to stop muromonab-CD3 therapy and treat the infection.

Maintain good dental hygiene while taking muromonab-CD3 and use extra care when brushing and flossing because this drug increases your risk of oral infection. See your dentist regularly.

This drug may cause confusion or interfere with your alertness, dexterity, or coordination. Be careful when driving or doing any task that requires concentration.

It is essential to complete the full course of treatment. This medication should not be stopped unless an infection or other severe side effect develops. If you miss a dose, contact your doctor to schedule another infusion appointment as soon possible.

Special Populations

Pregnancy/Breast-feeding: Muromonab-CD3 may cross into fetal circulation. Muromonab-CD3 should be taken during pregnancy only if your doctor determines that the potential benefit outweighs the risks.

It is not known if muromonab-CD3 passes into breast milk, but any effect on a nursing infant would be severe. Nursing mothers who must take this drug must use infant formula.

Seniors: Seniors may use this drug without special precaution.

Generic Name

Mycophenolate (mye-coe-FEN-oe-late) G

Brand Names

CellCept

The information in this profile also applies to the following drugs:

Generic Ingredients: Mycophenolic Acid
Myfortic

Type of Drug

Immunosuppressant.

Prescribed For

Kidney, liver, and heart transplantation; also prescribed for kidney damage resulting from lupus and idiopathyic thrombocytopenia purpura (ITP; abnormally low blood platelets), eye inflammation, and Churg-Strauss syndrome.

General Information

Mycophenolate is used with corticosteroids and cyclosporine to prevent the rejection of transplanted organs. In the body, the drug is metabolized into MPA, the active form of mycophenolate. MPA blocks the activity of T- and B-cells, which protect the body against invading microorganisms or foreign substances. MPA also suppresses antibody formation and may act directly on inflammation and organ rejection sites to prevent tissue rejection.

Cautions and Warnings

Mycophenolate should only be prescribed by physicians experienced in immunosuppressive therapy and the care of organ-transplant patients.

Do not take mycophenolate if you are **allergic** or **sensitive** to any of its ingredients or to mycophenolic acid or polisorbate 80.

Also, people with rare hereditary conditions involving the enzyme hypoxanthine-guanine phosphoribosyltransferase, including **Lesch-Nyhan and Kelley-Seegmiller syndromes**, should not take mycophenolate.

As with other immunosuppressants, people taking mycophenolate are at increased risk of infections or developing a lymphoma or other malignancy. The risk increases with the degree of immune suppression and the length of time that the drug is taken.

Out of 100 people taking mycophenolate, 2–5 develop a serious, life-threatening infection known as sepsis.

Several cases of a possibly fatal condition known as progressive multifocal leukoencephalopathy have occurred in people treated with this drug.

About 2 in 100 people receiving mycophenolate develop a severe reduction in white-blood-cell count. Contact your doctor if you develop symptoms of viral infection or other unusual symptoms. A type of anemia known as pure red cell aplasia has also occurred in people taking these drugs.

Because mycophenolate suppresses the immune system, you should not get a live, attenuated vaccine while taking it, or you may become sick with the disease against which you are being vaccinated.

About 3 in 100 people who take this drug develop stomach or intestinal bleeding, though many of these people are also taking other drugs that may affect the gastrointestinal tract. People with **stomach or intestinal disease** should take this drug with caution.

People with **kidney disease** should receive lower dosages.

Mild to moderate hypertension (high blood pressure) is a common side effect of mycophenolate and may be a sign of kidney damage. People taking this drug should measure their blood pressure regularly.

Mycophenolate increases your sensitivity to the sun and susceptibility to skin cancer. Always exercise caution outdoors and wear protective clothing.

People with **phenylketonuria** (PKA disease) should use mycophenolate oral suspension with caution because this mixture contains phenylalanine.

Possible Side Effects

▼ Most common: diarrhea, reduced white-blood-cell counts, sepsis and opportunistic infections, vomiting, and high blood pressure.

▼ Common: kidney damage, general pain, abdominal pain, fever, headache, weakness, chest pain, back pain, anemia, reduced platelet counts, swelling of the arms or legs, anxiety, numbness or tingling, constipation, nausea, upset stomach, cough, breathing difficulties, tremors, urinary tract infections and other problems, high blood cholesterol, low blood-phosphate levels, fluid retention, changes in blood-potassium levels, high blood sugar, sore throat, pneumonia, bronchitis, acne, rash, sleeplessness, and dizziness.

▼ Less common: impotence, heart palpitations and other heart problems, low blood pressure, dizziness when rising from a sitting or lying position, appetite loss, gas, stomach irritation or bleeding, gum irritation or enlargement, liver irritation, mouth ulcer, asthma, lung disorder, stuffy or runny nose, sinus irritation, hair loss, itching, sweating, skin ulcer, depression, stiff muscles, joint or muscle pain, double vision, cataracts, conjunctivitis (pinkeye), abdominal enlargement, facial swelling, cysts, flu-like symptoms, bleeding, hernia, pelvic pain, and black-and-blue marks.

▼ Rare: lymphoma, skin cancer (not melanomas) and other malignancies. Other side effects may occur in almost any part of the body. Contact your doctor if you experience anything unusual while taking any medication.

Children receiving mycophenolate experience similar side effects as adults.

Drug Interactions

- Azathioprine (an immune system suppressant) should not be combined with mycophenolate because of the risk of excess immune system suppression.

- Mycophenolate should not be combined with aluminum/magnesium antacids, charcoal, cholestyramine, iron supplements, metronidazole, norfloxacin, or rifampin, due to excessive reductions in mycophenolate blood levels.
- Combining mycophenolate and antiviral drugs (acyclovir, ganciclovir, and valacyclovir) increases blood levels of both drugs.
- Mycophenolate may moderately increase phenytoin and theophylline blood levels.
- Mycophenolate may reduce the effectiveness of some contraceptive drugs.
- Mycophenolate can make vaccines less effective, although a flu vaccine may be recommended. Do not use live, attenuated vaccines (see "Cautions and Warnings").
- Mycophenolate blood levels may be increased by sirolimus and tacrolimus. Your mycophenolate dosage may need to be changed.
- Probenecid and salicylates (including aspirin) may increase mycophenolate levels.
- Sevelamer may reduce blood levels of mycophenolate. Separate doses by at least 2 hours.
- Amoxicillin + clavulanic acid, ciprofloxacin, cyclosporine, rifabutin, trimethoprim, and sulfamethoxazole may lower mycophenolate blood levels. A dosage adjustment may be necessary.

Food Interactions

These medicines should be taken on an empty stomach at least 1 hour before or 2 hours after meals.

Usual Dose

Do not substitute one of these medicines for another; they are not equivalent to each other.

Mycophenolate

Adult: 1–1.5 g twice a day.

Child (age 3 months and over): capsules—750–1000 mg twice a day; oral suspension—600 mg per m^2 of body surface area twice a day up to a maximum daily dose of 2 g/10 mL.

Mycophenolic Acid

Adult and Child (age 17 and over): 720 mg twice a day.

Child (age 5–16): 400 mg per m^2 of body surface area twice a day up to a maximum daily dose of 1440 mg.

Overdosage

Overdose is likely to cause side effects—especially those relating to the stomach and intestines—and blood abnormalities. Take the victim to a hospital emergency room. If you seek treatment, ALWAYS bring the prescription bottle or container.

Special Information

It is extremely important to take this drug exactly as prescribed. If you forget a dose, take it as soon as you remember. If it is almost time for your next dose, skip the dose you forgot and continue with your regular schedule. Do not take a double dose. Contact your doctor if you forget 2 or more doses in a row.

Because this drug is harmful if not used properly, take extra caution when handling the capsules. Do not open or crush them. Avoid inhaling the powder or allowing it to touch your skin or the inside of your mouth or nose. If such contact does occur, wash thoroughly with soap and water. If the powder gets into your eyes, rinse them thoroughly with plain water.

People taking mycophenolate require regular testing to monitor their progress.

Contact your doctor at the first sign of fever; sore throat; tiredness; weakness; nervousness; unusual bleeding or bruising; tender or swollen gums; convulsions; irregular heartbeat; confusion; numbness or tingling of your hands, feet, or lips; breathing difficulties; severe stomach pain with nausea; blood in the urine; paralysis on one side of your body; apathy; confusion; problems with memory, planning, or judgment; and loss of coordination while doing normal motions. Fatigue, lethargy, and an abnormally pale skin color can be signs of anemia. Other side effects are less serious but should be brought to your doctor's attention, particularly if they are bothersome or persistent.

Maintain good dental hygiene while taking mycophenolate and use extra care when brushing or flossing because this drug increases your risk of oral infection. See your dentist regularly.

This drug should be continued for as long as prescribed by your doctor. Do not stop taking it because of side effects or other issues without your doctor's knowledge.

Special Populations

Pregnancy/Breast-feeding: Pregnant women should not take mycophenolate. Women of childbearing age should have a negative pregnancy test at least 1 week before treatment is started.

They should use 2 effective contraceptive methods beginning 4 weeks before treatment is started and continuing until 6 weeks after mycophenolate is discontinued, or they should practice abstinence during this period. Should you accidentally become pregnant during mycophenolate treatment, discuss with your doctor the advisability of continuing the pregnancy. There are several known cases of serious birth defects in babies born to women treated with this drug after conception, even though the medication was stopped as soon as the pregnancy was discovered.

Mycophenolate passes into breast milk. Nursing mothers who must take this drug should use infant formula.

Seniors: Seniors may require reduced dosage due to loss of kidney and cardiac function.

Generic Name

Naltrexone (nal-TRECK-sohn) G

Brand Names

Depade ReVia

The information in this profile also applies to the following drugs:

Generic Ingredients: Buprenorphine
Subutex

Generic Ingredients: Buprenorphine + Naloxone
Suboxone

Type of Drug

Opioid receptor antagonist.

Prescribed For

Narcotic or alcohol addiction. Also used for multiple sclerosis and other immune system disorders.

General Information

Naltrexone is a pure antagonist of opioid receptors in the brain that are stimulated by narcotic drugs. Buprenorphine is a pure antagonist of one of the opioid receptors and a partial stimulator of another. Buprenorphine satisfies narcotic cravings but seems to have a limit to its effect. Naloxone is an opioid receptor antagonist, added to prevent product abuse. When taken on a regular basis, these drugs block the actions of and physical dependence on narcotic drugs, including methadone, morphine, and heroin. Naltrexone is also beneficial in the treatment of alcoholism and helps reduce alcohol cravings and the number of drinking days. How naltrexone blocks alcohol craving is not known, but it may involve the same brain receptors as narcotic dependence. Naltrexone is a long-acting drug, with effects lasting for 2–3 days.

Low-dose naltrexone (about 1⁄10 of the usual dose) is believed to boost immune system function and has been studied in primary progressive multiple sclerosis, HIV, fibromyalgia, and other immune system disorders. This work is the subject of a growing movement but is controversial and must be confirmed by further larger studies.

Cautions and Warnings

Do not take these medications if you are **allergic** or **sensitive** to any of their ingredients.

Do not take naltrexone if you have taken any narcotic drug within the previous 7–10 days or are **dependent on narcotic drugs**. Taking naltrexone may produce severe drug withdrawal symptoms. People who attempt to overcome the blocking effects of naltrexone by taking large doses of a narcotic drug are at risk for drug overdose. People who have been taking naltrexone are likely to be more sensitive to narcotic drugs.

Naltrexone should be used with caution if you have active **liver disease**, **hepatitis**, or **liver failure**. People with liver disease should receive lower doses of buprenorphine, as hepatitis and jaundice have developed in people taking it.

Naltrexone passes out of the body through the urine. People with **kidney disease** should use it and buprenorphine with caution. The effect of **kidney failure** on naloxone is not known.

People who have a **lung or breathing disorder** should use buprenorphine with caution. It can cause nervous system depression and interfere with your ability to breathe, especially when it is taken with a benzodiazepine drug or other depressant. Caution should also be exercised by people with a **thyroid disorder**, **Addison's disease**, **nervous system depression**, **toxic psychosis**, **prostate enlargement**, **acute alcoholism**, or **delirium tremens (DTs)**.

Buprenorphine produces drug dependence and will lead to withdrawal symptoms if it is suddenly stopped or the dose is not tapered over a long enough time. Buprenorphine and naloxone will cause more intense withdrawal symptoms.

People with **head injuries** or **brain lesions** should use these drugs with caution.

It is not known if naltrexone is safe for use in **rapid detoxification** programs.

The **risk of suicide**, which always accompanies drug abuse, is not reduced by these medications.

Possible Side Effects

Buprenorphine

Side effects increase with drug dosage.

- ▼ Most common: weakness, headache, infections, pain, back pain, drug withdrawal symptoms, constipation, nausea, anxiety, depression, sleeplessness, and sweating.
- ▼ Common: chills, flu-like symptoms, diarrhea, vomiting, dizziness, nervousness, runny eyes, and tiredness.
- ▼ Less common: abscesses, fever, accidental injury, and upset stomach.

Buprenorphine + Naloxone

- ▼ Most common: headache, generalized pain, abdominal pain, drug withdrawal symptoms, flushing, low blood pressure, nausea, sleeplessness, and sweating.
- ▼ Common: weakness, chills, infections, constipation, vomiting, and runny nose.
- ▼ Less common: back pain and diarrhea.

Naltrexone

Most naltrexone side effects appear early in treatment and then improve with time.

- ▼ Common: headache, sleeplessness, nervousness, abdominal cramps, and nausea or vomiting.
- ▼ Less common: dizziness, fatigue, anxiety, tiredness, and weight changes.
- ▼ Rare: Rare side effects can occur in the gastrointestinal tract, heart and blood vessels, respiratory tract, eyes, and ears. Contact your doctor if you experience anything unusual while taking any medication.

Drug Interactions

Buprenorphine and Buprenorphine + Naloxone

- Atazanavir, clarithromycin, darunavir + ritonavir, erythromycin, indinavir, itraconazole, ketoconazole, nefazodone, nelfinavir, ritonavir, simvastatin, and telithromycin may increase buprenorphine blood levels. Dose reduction may be necessary.

- Carbamazepine, dexamethasone, phenobarbital, phenytoin, and rifampin may reduce buprenorphine blood levels. Dose adjustment may be needed.

Naltrexone

- Mixing naltrexone and thioridazine can cause lethargy and tiredness.
- People taking naltrexone will not benefit from narcotic cough suppressants and pain relievers.
- The consequences of mixing naltrexone and disulfiram (for alcohol abuse) are not known.

Food Interactions

None known.

Usual Dose

Buprenorphine and Buprenorphine + Naloxone

Adult and Child (age 16 and over): 8 mg once a day to start, then 12–16 mg once a day. These drugs are interchangeable.

Child (under age 16): not recommended.

Naltrexone

Adult: 25–50 mg once a day to start. Individualization of drug dosage may be needed. Low-dose naltrexone for off-label use of immune system disorders is usually 4.5 mg once a day.

Child: not recommended.

Overdosage

Buprenorphine

Overdose symptoms are those associated with a narcotic overdose: pinpoint pupils, sedation, low blood pressure, and difficulty breathing. Take the victim to a hospital emergency room at once. If you seek treatment, ALWAYS bring the prescription bottle or container.

Naltrexone

There is little experience with naltrexone overdose in humans. However, doses of 50 mg or more can cause liver damage. Take the victim to a hospital emergency room. If you seek treatment, ALWAYS bring the prescription bottle or container.

Special Information

Wear a special identification bracelet or carry an ID card saying you are taking this drug. This may be important if you require emergency medical care.

If you are using heroin, wait at least 4 hours or when early withdrawal signs start to appear before taking buprenorphine. Withdrawal symptoms are possible if you are using methadone, especially if you take more than 30 mg a day.

Buprenorphine and buprenorphine + naloxone sublingual tablets should be placed under the tongue and allowed to dissolve there. If you take more than 2 tablets at a time, either place all the tablets under the tongue at once or 2 at a time.

Take these drugs as directed. If you skip a dose, take it as soon as you remember. If it is almost time for your next dose, skip the forgotten dose and continue with your regular schedule.

Contact your doctor at once and stop taking naltrexone if you develop abdominal pain lasting more than a few days, white bowel movements, dark urine, or yellowing of the whites of the eyes.

Contact your doctor if you are taking buprenorphine and develop a rash, hives, or itching. Do not stop taking buprenorphine without your doctor's permission. Stopping suddenly or too quickly can lead to drug withdrawal symptoms.

Special Populations

Pregnancy/Breast-feeding: These drugs have been found to damage a developing animal fetus, but there is no information on how these drugs affect pregnant women. These drugs should be taken during pregnancy only if your doctor determines that the potential benefit outweighs the risks. Babies born to mothers taking buprenorphine may go through drug withdrawal.

Buprenorphine passes into breast milk but it is not known whether naltrexone does. Nursing mothers who must take these medications should use infant formula.

Seniors: Seniors may be more sensitive to the effects of naltrexone, but dosage adjustments are not needed. Seniors should use buprenorphine with caution.

Namenda *see **Memantine,** page 725*

Type of Drug

Narcotic Analgesics/ Cough Suppressants

Brand Names

Generic Ingredients: Codeine G

Generic Ingredients: Fentanyl

Abstral
Actiq
Duragesic
Fentora
Lasanda
Onsolis
Subsys

Generic Ingredients: Meperidine Hydrochloride G

Demerol

Generic Ingredients: Methadone

Generic Ingredients: Morphine Sulfate

Avinza
Kadian
MS Contin
Oramorph-SR

Generic Ingredients: Oxycodone Hydrochloride

Oxecta
OxyContin
Roxicodone

Generic Ingredients: Tapentadol

Nucynta

Generic Ingredients: Tramadol G

Conzip
Rybix ODT
Ryzolt
Ultram

Combination Products

Generic Ingredients: Acetaminophen + Butalbital + Caffeine + Codeine Phosphate G

Fioricet with Codeine

Generic Ingredients: Acetaminophen + Codeine Phosphate G

Aceta with Codeine
Capital with Codeine
Cocet
Tylenol with Codeine
Vopac

Generic Ingredients: Acetaminophen + Hydrocodone Bitartrate G

Anexsia
Ceta-Plus

Co-Gesic
Hycet
Hydrocet
Hydrogesic
Hy-Phen
Liquicet
Lorcet
Lortab
Maxidone
Norco
Stagesic
T-Gesic
Vicodin
Xodol
Zamicet
Zydone

Generic Ingredients: Acetaminophen + Oxycodone Hydrochloride [G]

Endocet
Magnacet
Percocet
Primlev
Roxicet
Roxilox
Tylox

Generic Ingredients: Acetaminophen + Pentazocine [G]

Generic Ingredients: Aspirin + Butalbital + Caffeine + Codeine Phosphate [G]

Fiorinal with Codeine

Generic Ingredients: Aspirin + Caffeine + Dihydrocodeine Bitartrate [G]

Synalgos-DC

Generic Ingredients: Aspirin + Codeine Phosphate [G]

Ascomp with Codeine
Empirin with Codeine

Generic Ingredients: Aspirin + Oxycodone Hydrochloride + Oxycodone Terephthalate [G]

Percodan
Roxiprin

Generic Ingredients: Codeine Phosphate + Guaifenesin [G]

Brontex
Cheracol with Codeine
Cheratussin AC
Gani-Tuss NR
Glydeine
Guaifen AC
Guaituss AC
Guaitussin with Codeine
Halotussin AC [$] [A]
Mytussin AC
Robitussin AC [$]
Tussi-Organidin NR

Generic Ingredients: Hydrocodone Bitartrate + Chlorpheniramine

Tussionex Pennkinetic

Generic Ingredients: Hydrocodone Bitartrate + Ibuprofen [G]

Ibudone
Reprexain
Vicoprofen

Generic Ingredients: Morphine Sulfate + Naltrexone
Embeda

Generic Ingredients: Naloxone + Pentazocine G

Generic Ingredients: Tramadol + Acetaminophen G
Ultracet

Prescribed For

Mild, moderate, and severe pain, and cough. Long-acting narcotics are meant only for people with chronic pain.

General Information

Codeine and meperidine relieve pain and suppress cough. They may be less effective than aspirin for pain associated with inflammation because aspirin reduces inflammation and they do not. They suppress the cough reflex but do not cure the underlying cause of the cough. Meperidine and other narcotic cough suppressants are stronger pain relievers, but codeine is the best cough medication available. Meperidine is probably the most widely used narcotic in U.S. hospitals as it used before surgery to reduce anxiety and to help bring the patient into early stages of anesthesia.

Fentanyl is a potent pain reliever that can be substituted for other narcotic drugs, generally for people experiencing breakthrough cancer pain. The patch form, which must be replaced about every 3 days, delivers fentanyl to the bloodstream at a steady rate. The lozenge has a shorter length of action than any other narcotic pain reliever, which makes it useful when given to children before surgery because it provides doctors with the flexibility to obtain maximum benefit with minimal side effects. The lozenge on a stick is used for breakthrough cancer pain as a booster for people already taking narcotic pain relievers. Fentanyl nasal spray is intended for people who have become tolerant to other narcotic pain relievers. These forms should only be used under controlled circumstances because of the risk of side effects or overdose. Low dosages of fentanyl relieve pain—larger amounts cause loss of consciousness and breathing difficulties.

Morphine sulfate is a pure narcotic that has been in use for many years. In addition to pain relief, morphine's effects include drowsiness, mood changes, difficulty breathing, slowed movement of the gastrointestinal tract, nausea, vomiting, and changes in the endocrine and autonomic nervous systems. Morphine sulfate liquid, immediate-release tablets, and suppositories must be taken several times a day. The medication they contain is released immediately for absorption into the bloodstream. Extended- and controlled-release morphine products are designed to release some of the narcotic right away and the rest over a 24-hour period, allowing for less-frequent dosage. Embeda is a capsule product containing pellets of naltrexone, a narcotic antagonist coated with morphine. The purpose of giving both drugs together is to minimize the risk of morphine side effects, including drug dependence or addiction, though this has not been conclusively proven. The combination is meant to allow for high-dose around-the-clock morphine treatment for severe pain when narcotic pain relievers have been insufficient. Embeda is not meant for use on an as-needed basis or for pain following surgery.

Oxycodone is a narcotic used to control moderate to severe pain. Most people take it together with aspirin (Percodan) or acetaminophen (Percocet), but it can be used by itself. This is a potent pain reliever that carries a risk of addiction with continued use.

Tapentadol combines the action of a traditional narcotic pain reliever with the ability to work on pain centers in the brain by maintaining levels of the hormone norepinephrine at spaces between nerves, instead of it being absorbed back into nerve endings. Tapentadol is associated with additional cautions and warnings and has increased interactions with other drugs over traditional opioid narcotics like codeine or morphine.

Tramadol is a synthetic compound that works in the central nervous system (CNS) to relieve pain. The exact way in which this drug works is unknown, but it binds to opioid receptors and reduces the uptake of 2 important neurohormones, serotonin and norepinephrine, into nerves. Tramadol is also prescribed with acetaminophen (Ultracet). Pain relief begins about an hour after you take a dose and reaches its maximum effect in 2–3 hours. Like the narcotic pain relievers, tramadol can cause dizziness, tiredness, nausea, constipation, sweating, and itching. Unlike the narcotics, normal doses cause little interference with breathing and do not cause histamine reactions. It has no effect on heart function.

Cautions and Warnings

Do not take narcotics if you are **allergic** or **sensitive** to any of their ingredients. Use narcotics with extreme caution if you suffer from **asthma** or other **breathing problems**.

Long-term use of narcotics may cause drug dependence or addiction and withdrawal symptoms, unless the dose is gradually reduced. Narcotics may make it difficult to monitor the progress of people who have suffered **head injuries** and **acute abdominal conditions**.

These drugs should be used with caution if you have **gallstones** or other **bile tract disease**, including inflammation of the pancreas. They can cause spasm of the bile duct and severe pain.

Meperidine should be used with caution if you have **kidney, heart, or liver disease,** a history of **seizures**, **sickle cell anemia**, **hypothyroidism** (underactive thyroid gland), **Addison's disease**, **pheochromocytoma** (adrenal gland tumor), **inflammatory bowel disease**, **gallstones** or **gallbladder disease**, **enlarged prostate**, or **urinary difficulties**.

Seizures have occurred in people taking oral doses of 700 mg of tramadol or intravenous doses of 300 mg. Other factors may increase the risk of seizures, such as **head trauma**, **metabolic disorder**, and **drug or alcohol withdrawal**.

Actiq contains fentanyl in an amount that can be **fatal to children**. Keep used lozenges, unused lozenges, and lozenges on a stick out of the reach of children.

Mouth sores are more common with fentanyl sublingual spray.

These drugs are broken down in the liver and should be used with caution in people with **liver disease**.

Possible Side Effects

Acetaminophen + Oxycodone

- ▼ Most common: lightheadedness, dizziness, sleepiness, nausea, vomiting, appetite loss, and increased sweating. If any of these effects occur, ask your doctor to consider lowering your dosage. Most of these side effects disappear if you lie down. More serious side effects, including shallow breathing or breathing difficulties, may occur at higher dosages.
- ▼ Less common: euphoria (feeling "high"), weakness, headache, agitation, uncoordinated muscle movements, minor hallucinations, disorientation, visual disturbances, dry mouth, constipation, facial flushing, rapid heartbeat, palpitations, feeling faint, urinary difficulties, reduced sex drive, impotence, rash, itching, depression, abdominal

Possible Side Effects *(continued)*

pain, anemia, low blood sugar, and yellowing of the skin or whites of the eyes.

For more information see Acetaminophen, page 16.

Aspirin + Oxycodone Hydrochloride + Oxycodone Terephthalate

▼ Most common: lightheadedness, dizziness, sleepiness, nausea, vomiting, appetite loss, and increased sweating. If these occur, ask your doctor to consider lowering your dosage. Usually they go away if you lie down. More serious side effects, including shallow breathing or other breathing difficulties, may occur at higher dosages.

▼ Less common: euphoria (feeling "high"), depression, constipation, itching, low blood sugar, and yellowing of the skin or whites of the eyes. These drugs may aggravate convulsions in those who have had them.

For more information, see Aspirin, page 125, and Ibuprofen, page 863.

Codeine, Fentanyl, Hydrocodone, Meperidine, Methadone, Morphine, and Oxycodone

More serious side effects of these drugs include shallow breathing or breathing difficulties.

▼ Most common: lightheadedness, dizziness, drowsiness, nausea, vomiting, appetite loss, and sweating. If these occur, ask your doctor about lowering your dosage. Most of these side effects disappear if you lie down.

▼ Less common: euphoria (feeling "high"), headache, agitation, uncoordinated muscle movement, minor hallucinations, disorientation and visual disturbances, dry mouth, constipation, flushing of the face, rapid heartbeat, palpitations, faintness, urinary difficulties or hesitancy, reduced sex drive or impotence, itching, rash, anemia, lowered or raised blood sugar, and yellowing of the skin or whites of the eyes. Narcotic analgesics may aggravate convulsions in those who have had them.

Tapentadol

▼ Most common: nausea, vomiting, dizziness, and drowsiness.

▼ Common: constipation and itching.

▼ Less common: dry mouth, upset stomach, fatigue, feeling hot, upper-respiratory infection, nose or throat irritation,

Possible Side Effects *(continued)*

urinary infection, appetite reduction, joint pain, tremors, sleeplessness, confusion, unusual dreams, anxiety, excessive sweating, rash, and flushing.

- ▼ Rare: Rare side effects can affect almost any part of the body. Contact your doctor if you experience anything unusual while taking any medication.

Tramadol

- ▼ Most common: constipation, nausea, dizziness, headache, sleepiness.
- ▼ Common: vomiting, upset stomach, itching, weakness, dry mouth, sweating, and diarrhea.
- ▼ Less common: anxiety, confusion, coordination disturbance, euphoria (feeling "high"), nervousness, rash, abdominal pain, weight loss, flatulence, urinary difficulty, urinary frequency, muscle tension, and sleep disorders.
- ▼ Rare: Rare side effects can affect almost any part of the body. Contact your doctor if you experience anything unusual while taking any medication.

Drug Interactions

- Do not mix narcotics with alcohol, sleeping medications, tranquilizers, skeletal muscle relaxants, other depressant drugs, or nonprescription drugs that have alcohol as an ingredient. Alcohol also speeds the release of morphine from Avinza and Embeda. The mixture can result in a deadly narcotic overdose.
- Mixing bupropion with a narcotic can increase the risk of seizures.
- Mixing an anticholinergic medication with a narcotic may lead to difficulty urinating and/or severe constipation.
- Combining a narcotic pain reliever with any other medication that lowers blood pressure can lead to excessive blood-pressure lowering. Avoid this combination.
- Combining cimetidine with any narcotic pain reliever, except tapentadol, may make the narcotic dose more potent and increase the risk of side effects.
- These medicines are broken down mainly by a specific set of liver enzymes. Drugs that interfere with this process can lead to serious narcotic side effects, including difficulty

breathing, sedation, coma, and death. The following drugs strongly inhibit enzyme activity and should be mixed with a narcotic only with extreme caution: aprepitant, clarithromycin, diltiazem, erythromycin, fluconazole, indinavir, itraconazole, ketoconazole, nefazodone, nelfinavir, ritonavir, saquinavir, telithromycin, and verapamil. Meperidine should not be taken with ritonavir.

- Mixing narcotic pain relievers with a monoamine oxidase inhibitor (MAOI) antidepressant can lead to low blood pressure, difficulty breathing, or coma. Some studies have indicated methadone and morphine do not interact in this way, but the combination still should be used with caution. Tapentadol interacts with MAOIs differently from other narcotics, and the mixture can lead to cardiovascular side effects. Do not take an MAOI and a narcotic drug together or within 2 weeks of each other.

Codeine

- Quinidine may decrease the analgesic effects of codeine.

Fentanyl

- Amiodarone, azole antifungals (such as itraconazole, ketoconazole, and voriconazole), droperidol, erythromycin, and protease inhibitors (such as ritonavir and saquinavir) may increase the effects of fentanyl, leading to symptoms that include slowed heart rate, heart conduction disorders, low blood pressure, and breathing difficulties.
- Diazepam and nitrous oxide may produce depressed heart function when given with high doses of fentanyl.

Meperidine

- Acyclovir increases blood levels of meperidine. Use this combination with caution.
- Combining meperidine and the antipsychotic drug chlorpromazine (Thorazine) or thioridazine may lead to serious side effects.
- Hydantoin anticonvulsant drugs (phenytoin) may decrease the effectiveness of meperidine, while enhancing its side effects. Anticonvulsant drugs such as phenytoin increase the breakdown of meperidine in the liver.
- Combining meperidine and a protease inhibitor may increase the risk of breathing and CNS depressant difficulties. These medications should not be used together.

Morphine

- The analgesic effects of morphine may be counteracted if given with rifampin.

Oxycodone

- Combining propofol with oxycodone increases the risk of reduced heart rate.

Tapentadol and Tramadol

- Carbamazepine reduces tramadol's effectiveness. Combining these medications is not recommended.
- Mixing tapentadol or tramadol with a selective serotonin reuptake inhibitor (SSRI) or serotonin-norepinephrine reuptake inhibitor (SNRI-type) antidepressant can lead to a group of symptoms known as serotonin syndrome. Symptoms of this potentially deadly syndrome include changes in mental status (including agitation, hallucinations, or coma), rapid heartbeat, blood-pressure changes, high fever, exaggerated reflexes, poor coordination, nausea, vomiting, and diarrhea. Avoid this combination.
- Tramadol may increase the effects of digoxin or warfarin.
- Serotonin syndrome is also a risk when tricyclic antidepressants (such as amitriptyline, clomipramine, and nortriptyline) are combined with tramadol. These medications should be combined cautiously.

Food Interactions

Codeine may be taken with food to reduce upset stomach. The rest of the drugs in this profile may be used without regard to food or meals. Morphine and naltrexone capsules may be opened and the pellets mixed with applesauce. Other soft foods have not been tested but may also be acceptable. Large amounts of grapefruit or starfruit interfere with the breakdown of these drugs.

Usual Dose

Acetaminophen + Butalbital + Caffeine + Codeine

Adult and Child (age 12 and over): 1–2 capsules every 4 hours. Do not exceed 6 capsules a day.

Child (under age 12): not recommended.

Acetaminophen + Codeine

Elixir

Adult and Child (age 12 and over): 15 mL every 4 hours.

Child (age 7–11): 10 mL 3–4 times a day.

Child (age 3–6): 5 mL 3–4 times a day.
Child (under age 3): not recommended.

Tablets

Adult and Child (age 12 and over): equivalent of 15–60 mg of codeine every 4 hours; do not exceed 360 mg a day.
Child (age 7–11): equivalent of 0.22–0.45 mg of codeine per lb. of body weight every 4–6 hours.

Acetaminophen + Hydrocodone

Adult and Child (age 15 and over): 1–2 tablets every 4 hours; the total daily dose should not exceed 8 tablets.
Child (age 2–14): 0.12 mL per lb. every 4–6 hours.

Acetaminophen + Oxycodone Hydrochloride

Adult: 2.5–10 mg of oxycodone every 6 hours as needed, not to exceed 60 mg of oxycodone per day.
Child: not recommended.

Acetaminophen + Pentazocine

Adult and Child (age 12 and over): 1 tablet every 4 hours; do not exceed 6 tablets a day.
Child (under age 12): not recommended.

Aspirin + Butalbital + Caffeine + Codeine

Adult and Child (age 12 and over): 1–2 capsules every 4 hours. Do not exceed 6 capsules a day.
Child (under age 12): not recommended.

Aspirin + Caffeine + Dihydrocodeine

Adult: 2 capsules every 4 hours.
Child: not recommended.

Aspirin + Codeine

Adult and Child (age 12 and over): 1–2 tablets every 4 hours; not to exceed 6 tablets a day.
Child (under age 12): not recommended.

Aspirin + Oxycodone Hydrochloride + Oxycodone Terephthalate

Adult: 1 tablet every 6 hours as needed for pain; the maximum daily dose of aspirin should not exceed 4 g or 12 tablets.
Child: not recommended.

Codeine

Adult: 15–60 mg every 4–6 hours for relief of pain; 10–20 mg every few hours as needed to suppress cough.
Child: 0.22–0.45 mg per lb. of body weight every 4–6 hours for relief of pain; 2.5–10 mg every 4–6 hours to suppress cough.

Codeine + Guaifenesin

Adult and Child (age 12 and over): 7.5–20 mg of codeine every 4–6 hours; do not exceed 120 mg of codeine in a 24-hour period.

Child (age 6–11): 3.75–10 mg of codeine every 4–6 hours; do not exceed 60 mg of codeine in 24 hours.

Child (age 2–5): 4.5 mg per lb. of body weight of codeine in 4 equal doses per day.

Fentanyl Lozenge and Lozenge on a Stick

Adult: 200–1600 mcg. Dosage may be repeated up to 4 times a day. Allow the lozenge to dissolve in your mouth. DO NOT CHEW.

Child: 2.3–7 mcg per lb. of body weight.

Fentanyl Nasal Spray

Adult: 1 spray (100 mcg) to start. One additional dose may be taken if pain is not relieved within 30 minutes. Wait at least 2 hours before taking more spray for breakthrough pain. Maximum per spray dose is 1600 mcg; final dose should provide maximum pain relief and minimal side effects.

Child: not recommended.

Fentanyl Patch

Apply to a clean and non-irritated patch of skin as directed, usually once every 3 days.

Fentanyl Sub-lingual (under the tongue) Spray

This product is not equal to any other fentanyl product on a mcg per mcg basis; proper daily dosage must be reestablished.

Adult: 1 spray (100 mcg) under the tongue to start, increasing gradually to a maximum of 1600 mcg per spray, 4 sprays per day. Wait at least 4 hours before taking another dose of sublingual spray for breakthrough pain. Final dose should provide maximum pain relief and minimal side effects.

Child: not recommended.

Hydrocodone + Chlorpheniramine Syrup

Adult and Child (age 12 and over): 5 mL twice a day.

Child (age 6–11): 2.5 mL twice a day.

Child (under age 6): not recommended.

Hydrocodone + Ibuprofen

Adult and Child (age 16 and over): 1 tablet every 4–6 hours, up to 5 tablets a day.

Child (under age 16): not recommended.

Meperidine

Adult: 50–150 mg every 3–4 hours as needed.

Child: 0.5–0.8 mg per lb. of body weight every 3–4 hours as needed, up to the adult dosage.

Morphine Extended-Release and Controlled-Release Tablets and Capsules

Adult: 1–3 capsules a day, depending on the specific product and individual need.

Morphine Oral Liquid and Immediate-Release Tablets

Adult: 5–30 mg every 4 hours.

Morphine Suppositories

Adult: 5–30 mg several times a day.

Morphine + Naltrexone

Adult: This product comes in a variety of strengths. When switching to this product from another narcotic, the total daily morphine dose is estimated and given in 2 daily doses. When initiating this medication as a pain reliever, low doses should be used. The highest dose is meant for people who are already tolerant to narcotic medicines.

Naloxone + Pentazocine

Adult: 1 tablet every 3–4 hours; increase to 2 if necessary. Daily dose should not exceed 12 tablets.

Child: not recommended.

Oxycodone

Adult: 10–30 mg every 4 hours as needed. OxyContin should be swallowed whole and not broken.

Child: not recommended.

Tapentadol

Adult: tablet—50–100 mg every 4–6 hours. Dosage should not exceed 700 mg on the first day and 600 mg a day afterward. Extended-release tablet—100–250 mg every 12 hours, not to exceed 500 mg a day.

Child: not recommended.

Tramadol

Adult: 25–100 mg every 4–6 hours; do not exceed 400 mg a day. People with cirrhosis should receive 50 mg every 12 hours. People with severe kidney disease should receive no more than 100 mg every 12 hours.

Child: not recommended.

Senior: Do not exceed 300 mg a day.

Tramadol + Acetaminophen

Adult: 2 tablets every 4–6 hours up to a maximum of 8 tablets for no more than 5 days.

Child: not recommended.

Overdosage

Narcotic overdose can be deadly, especially when mixed with other drugs that slow breathing and the central nervous system. Symptoms include breathing difficulties or slowing of respiration, extreme tiredness progressing to stupor and then coma, pinpoint pupils, no response to pain stimulation, cold and clammy skin, slowing of heartbeat, low blood pressure, convulsions, and cardiac arrest. Children exposed to fentanyl products are at risk of fatal breathing depression, a medical emergency that requires immediate action. The victim should be taken to a hospital emergency room immediately. If you seek treatment, ALWAYS bring the prescription bottle or container.

Special Information

Narcotics are respiratory depressants and slow breathing. They can cause sleepiness, tiredness, and an inability to concentrate. Do not drive or perform any task that requires concentration while taking a narcotic drug. Avoid alcohol.

Contact your doctor if you find it hard to breathe or develop constipation, dry mouth, or any bothersome or persistent side effect.

Apply the fentanyl patch only to non-irritated skin on a flat surface of the upper body. Hair at the application site should be clipped or cut, not shaved, before applying the patch. Do not apply any source of heat directly to the patch, including sunbathing, hot baths, saunas, heat lamps, and heating pads. Do not use any oils, soaps, lotions, alcohol, or anything else that might irritate the skin before applying the patch.

You must discard your fentanyl nasal spray bottle if you no longer need it, if it has been 5 or more days since you last used it, if it has been 2 weeks or more since the bottle was first primed, or after 8 sprays have been used because any remaining sprays will not provide a full dose. You must follow the directions for safe disposal found in the patient information that comes with the product. Spray any remaining spray into the plastic disposal pouch provided with each bottle. Put both the empty spray bottle and pouch into the child-resistant container that comes with the product and throw it away with regular trash. You can get a replacement disposal pouch by calling the manufacturer.

The manufacturer of fentanyl sublingual offers a free child safety kit. The kit consists of a safe interim storage bag, a lock for the bag, and a package of cabinet and drawer child safety latches for securing the storage space at home to help patients store this and other medicines out of the reach of children. Child safety kits are available by calling the manufacturer.

If you forget a dose of your medicine, take it as soon as you remember. If it is almost time for your next dose, skip the one you forgot and continue with your regular schedule. Never take a double dose of a narcotic drug.

Special Populations

Pregnancy/Breast-feeding: Narcotics pass into the fetal blood circulation. Using narcotics during pregnancy, especially in large doses, can make your newborn baby drug dependent. Narcotics may also cause breathing difficulties in infants during delivery. Animal studies show that these drugs may damage the developing fetus. If given to a pregnant woman before cesarean section, fentanyl may cause drowsiness in newborns. A narcotic analgesic should be taken during pregnancy only if your doctor determines that the potential benefit outweighs the risks.

Narcotics pass into breast milk. Methadone and other narcotics may be compatible with nursing, but nursing mothers who must take a narcotic should consider using infant formula.

Seniors: Seniors are more likely to be sensitive to narcotic side effects and should be treated with the lowest effective dosage.

Nasacort AQ *see* ***Corticosteroids, Nasal,*** *page 340*

Nasonex *see* ***Corticosteroids, Nasal,*** *page 340*

Generic Name

Nefazodone (neh-FAZ-oe-doan) G

Brand Names

Only available in generic form.

Type of Drug

Antidepressant.

Prescribed For

Depression.

General Information

A unique compound, nefazodone is chemically unrelated to other antidepressants. It interferes with the ability of nerve endings in the brain to absorb serotonin and norepinephrine, 2 key neurohormones. Nefazodone is broken down in the liver; severe liver disease may increase nefazodone blood levels by 25%. Very little of the drug is released through the kidneys.

Cautions and Warnings

Do not take nefazodone if you are **allergic** or **sensitive** to any of its ingredients.

Nefazodone has been associated with potentially fatal liver failure. People with **liver disease** should use nefazodone with caution.

Antidepressants have been associated with an increased risk of suicide, especially in **teenagers** and **children**. Suicide is always a risk in severely depressed people, who should only be allowed to have minimal quantities of medication in their possession.

Nefazodone may precipitate a manic phase in those with previously undiagnosed bipolar (manic-depressive) disorder. Nefazodone is not used to treat this disorder.

People with a history of **seizure disorders** may experience seizures while taking nefazodone.

People who have recently had a **heart attack** should use this drug with caution because it can substantially reduce heart rate.

Possible Side Effects

- ▼ Most common: weakness, dry mouth, nausea, headache, constipation, blurred or abnormal vision, tiredness, dizziness, insomnia, agitation, lightheadedness, and confusion.
- ▼ Common: upset stomach, increased appetite, cough, memory loss, tingling in the hands or feet, flushing or feelings of warmth, poor muscle coordination, and dizziness when rising from a lying or sitting position.
- ▼ Less common: low blood pressure; fever; chills; flu-like symptoms; joint pain; stiff neck; itching; rash; diarrhea; nausea; vomiting; thirst; sore throat; changes in sense of taste; ringing

Possible Side Effects *(continued)*

or buzzing in the ears; unusual dreams; poor coordination; tremors; muscle stiffness; reduced sex drive; urinary difficulties, including infection; vaginitis; and breast pain.

▼ Rare: Rare side effects can affect your liver, gastrointestinal tract, joints, sexual function, and skin. Severe nefazodone allergy is rare. Contact your doctor if you experience anything unusual while taking any medication.

Drug Interactions

- People who take nefazodone within 2 weeks of taking a monoamine oxidase inhibitor (MAOI) antidepressant may experience severe reactions, including high fever, muscle rigidity or spasm, changes in mental state, and fluctuations in pulse, temperature, and breathing rate. People stopping nefazodone should wait at least 1 week before starting an MAOI.
- Nefazodone should not be taken with astemizole, carbamazepine, cisapride, pimozide, or terfenadine.
- Nefazodone may increase blood levels of alprazolam and triazolam (benzodiazepine antianxiety drugs). Triazolam should not be combined with nefazodone, or only at greatly reduced dosages. Alprazolam and nefazodone should be used together with caution.
- Combining buspirone and nefazodone may lead to increased side effects. Lower buspirone doses should be used.
- When cyclosporine or tacrolimus is given with nefazodone, blood concentrations of these medications should be monitored. Dosage adjustments may be necessary.
- Blood levels of digoxin may be substantially increased by nefazodone. People taking these drugs together should have their digoxin blood levels checked periodically.
- When switching from fluoxetine to nefazodone, a week to several weeks should be allowed between stopping fluoxetine and starting nefazodone to avoid increased side effects.
- The clearance of haloperidol may be reduced by nefazodone; dosage adjustments for haloperidol may be necessary.
- Nefazodone should be used with caution with the blood-pressure-lowering drugs simvastatin, atorvastatin, and lovastatin. Dosages of these drugs may need adjusting.
- Combining nefazodone and propranolol may cause substantial reductions in propranolol blood levels.

- Avoid drinking alcohol or taking St. John's wort while taking nefazodone.

Food Interactions

Take nefazodone on an empty stomach at least 1 hour before or 2 hours after meals.

Usual Dose

Adult: 100 mg twice a day to start. Dosage may be increased by 100–200 mg a week to a maximum daily dose of approximately 600 mg.

Child: not recommended.

Senior: Start at ½ the regular adult dose and increase as needed up to 600 mg a day.

Overdosage

Symptoms of overdose include nausea, vomiting, and sleepiness. Overdose victims should be taken to a hospital emergency room. If you seek treatment, ALWAYS bring the prescription bottle or container.

Special Information

Several weeks of nefazodone treatment may be necessary before you notice any effect. Continue taking the medication during this period. The following symptoms may occur early in treatment or when the dosage is adjusted: anxiety, agitation, panic attacks, sleeplessness, irritability, restlessness, hostility, aggressiveness, acting impulsively, manic reaction, deepening of depression, other unusual changes in behavior, and suicidal thinking. Report any changes to your doctor.

Contact your doctor at once if you develop hives, rash, or other allergic side effects while taking nefazodone.

Nefazodone may make you drowsy. Be careful when driving or doing any task that requires concentration. Avoid alcohol.

Check with your pharmacist or doctor before taking any over-the-counter medication because of the risk of drug interactions.

Special Populations

Pregnancy/Breast-feeding: Animal studies of nefazodone suggest decreased fertility and a risk of fetal damage. Nefazodone should be taken during pregnancy only if your doctor determines that the potential benefit outweighs the risks.

It is not known if nefazodone passes into breast milk. Nursing mothers who must take this drug should use infant formula.

Seniors: Seniors, especially women, should start treatment at ½ the usual dose. Dosage may be gradually increased as needed, up to the maximum recommended dosage.

Brand Names

Neosporin Ophthalmic

Generic Ingredients

Gramicidin + Neomycin Sulfate + Polymyxin B Sulfate G

Type of Drug

Ophthalmic and antibiotic combination.

Prescribed For

Superficial eye infection.

General Information

Neosporin Ophthalmic is a combination of antibiotics that is effective against the most common types of eye infection. It is most useful when the infecting organism is known to be sensitive to any of the 3 antibiotics contained in Neosporin Ophthalmic. It may also be useful when the infecting organism is not known, because of the drug's broad range of coverage. This product is also available as an eye ointment with a minor formula change—bacitracin is substituted for gramicidin. Both the eye drops and eye ointment are used for the same kinds of eye infection.

Cautions and Warnings

Do not use Neosporin Ophthalmic if you are **allergic** or **sensitive** to any of its ingredients.

Prolonged use of any antibiotic product in the eye should be avoided because of the risk of becoming sensitive to it and because other organisms such as fungi may grow. If the infection does not clear up within a few days, contact your doctor.

Possible Side Effects

▼ Less common: occasional eye irritation, itching, swelling, or burning.

Drug Interactions

None known.

Usual Dose

1 or 2 drops in the affected eye every 4 hours for 7–10 days. For severe infections, dosage may be increased to as much as 2 drops every hour.

Overdosage

There is not enough medicine in this product to cause serious problems. Contact your local poison control center or a hospital emergency room for more information. If you seek treatment, ALWAYS bring the prescription bottle or container.

Special Information

To avoid infection, always wash hands first; do not touch the eyedropper tip to your finger, eyelid, or any other surface. Wait at least 5 minutes before using another eye drop or eye ointment.

Contact your doctor if the itching or burning does not go away after a few minutes, or if redness, irritation, swelling, visual disturbance, loss of vision, or eye pain persists.

In general, you should not wear contact lenses if you have an eye infection, but your doctor may determine that the use of lenses is acceptable in your situation.

If you forget to administer a dose, do so as soon as you remember. If it is almost time for your next dose, skip the forgotten dose and continue with your regular schedule. Do not take a double dose.

Special Populations

Pregnancy/Breast-feeding: Neosporin Ophthalmic should be taken during pregnancy only if your doctor determines that the potential benefit outweighs the risks.

This drug has been found to be safe for use during breast-feeding.

Seniors: Seniors may take this drug without special precaution.

Nexium *see **Proton-Pump Inhibitors,** page 956*

Generic Name

Niacin (NYE-uh-sin) G

Brand Names

Endur-Acin	Niacinol

Niacor
Niaspan
Slo-Niacin

Type of Drug

Vitamin.

Prescribed For

Pellagra (niacin deficiency), high blood levels of cholesterol and triglycerides, atherosclerosis (blood vessel disease), and prevention of heart attacks in people who have had a previous heart attack.

General Information

Niacin, also known as vitamin B_3 or nicotinic acid, is essential in maintaining health because of the role it plays in enzyme activity. It is effective in lowering blood-fat levels as part of a comprehensive program including diet and exercise, and it also helps to dilate blood vessels, which can help people with heart disease. However, it is unknown exactly how it works. The effect of niacin on blood fats is seen as early as 1 week after treatment is started.

Cautions and Warnings

Do not take niacin if you are **allergic** or **sensitive** to any of its ingredients or to niacin-related drugs.

Do not take niacin if you have active **liver disease** or a **stomach ulcer**. Those who drink large quantities of **alcohol** or who have **diabetes**, **gallbladder disease**, **glaucoma**, **gout**, or **heart disease**, and people with a past history of **arterial bleeding**, liver disease, or stomach ulcer, should not take niacin unless it is recommended by your doctor and taken under his/her supervision.

When you are taking niacin in therapeutic dosages, your doctor should periodically check your liver function and blood-sugar level. People with **diabetes** may experience an increase in blood sugar. Blood levels of uric acid may rise; people who are prone to **gout** may experience an attack.

Niacin may cause postural low blood pressure (symptoms include dizziness or fainting when rising from a sitting or lying position).

Niacin may affect laboratory tests of your blood or urine.

Possible Side Effects

Most side effects are experienced by people taking niacin in higher doses. Taking a sustained-release form of niacin may reduce the risk of side effects.

Possible Side Effects *(continued)*

- ▼ Most common: flushing, which may occur within 2 hours of taking the first dose of niacin. Flushing may be accompanied by dizziness, rapid heartbeat, heart palpitations, shortness of breath, sweating, chills, swelling, and, rarely, fainting.
- ▼ Common: headache, diarrhea, and itching.
- ▼ Less common: increased blood sugar in people with diabetes, nausea, vomiting, abdominal pain, upset stomach, yellowing of the skin or whites of the eyes, oily or dry skin, aggravation of skin conditions such as acne, high blood levels of uric acid, low blood pressure, runny nose, tingling in the hands or feet, rash, abnormal heartbeat, dizziness, blurred vision, and muscle damage and pain.
- ▼ Rare: Rare side effects can occur in almost any part of the body. Contact your doctor if you experience anything unusual while taking any medication.

Drug Interactions

- Niacin may increase the effect of blood-pressure-lowering drugs, causing dizziness when rising quickly from a sitting or lying position.
- Combining niacin and a statin-type drug such as lovastatin may lead to the destruction of skeletal muscle. Contact your doctor if you experience any unusual muscle pain.
- Aspirin may slow the removal of niacin from the body, but the importance of this interaction is not known.
- Separate any niacin product from a bile acid sequestrant (cholestyramine, colesevelam, or colestipol) by at least 4–6 hours to prevent most of the niacin from being tied up by the other medication.
- Niacin extended-release tablets should be taken with caution with anticoagulants (blood thinners). Blood-platelet counts should be monitored closely.
- Avoid using nutritional supplements or multivitamins that contain niacin, or your niacin-related side effects will be worse.

Food Interactions

Take niacin with or after meals to reduce the risk of upset stomach. Avoid alcohol or hot drinks around the time you take sustained-release niacin to minimize flushing. Sustained-release niacin products should be taken at bedtime with a low-fat snack. Avoid drinking grapefruit juice while taking niacin.

Usual Dose

Do not substitute extended-release tablets for immediate-release tablets, as the dosages and risk of side effects are not the same. If you stop one form of niacin and start another, start with the lowest available dose and increase your dosage slowly.

High Blood-Fat Levels

Immediate-Release

Adult and Child (age 16 and over): 250 mg after the evening meal to start; increase dose slowly (every 4–7 days), to 1500–6000 mg a day, according to your response to the drug.

Child (under age 16): not recommended.

Sustained-Release

Adult (age 21 and over): 500 mg at bedtime for weeks 1–4, then 1000 mg for weeks 5–8. Can then increase dose further if needed (no more than 500-mg increase in a 4-week period). Do not exceed 2000 mg a day.

Child and Adult (under age 21): not recommended.

Pellagra

Adult and Child (age 16 and over): up to 500 mg a day.

Child (under age 16): not recommended.

Overdosage

Symptoms may include drug side effects. Take the victim to a hospital emergency room. If you seek treatment, ALWAYS bring the prescription bottle or container.

Special Information

Skin reactions may occur within 2 hours of the first dose and include flushing and warmth, especially in the face, ears, or neck; tingling; itching; and headache. Contact your doctor if these effects do not disappear as you continue taking niacin.

You can minimize flushing by taking aspirin or a nonsteroidal anti-inflammatory drug (NSAID) such as ibuprofen 30 minutes before your sustained-release niacin tablets. Sustained-release niacin tablets should be swallowed whole, not broken, crushed, or chewed.

Stop taking this drug and contact your doctor immediately if you experience irregular heartbeat, blurred vision, loss of appetite, flu-like symptoms, nausea, vomiting, dark-colored urine, or reduced urination.

Contact your doctor if you have diabetes and notice your blood sugars changing.

If you forget a dose, take it as soon as you remember. If it is almost time for your next dose, skip the missed dose and continue with your regular schedule. Do not take a double dose.

Special Populations

Pregnancy/Breast-feeding: When used in normal doses, niacin may and should be taken during pregnancy as part of a prenatal vitamin formulation (see "Usual Dose"). Doses larger than 20 mg a day are not recommended during pregnancy because their effect on the fetus is unknown.

Niacin passes into human breast milk. Usual doses (up to 17 mg a day; see "Usual Dose") will not affect a nursing infant. Nursing mothers who must take larger doses of niacin should use infant formula.

Seniors: Seniors may be more sensitive to drug side effects than younger adults.

Niaspan *see **Niacin,** page 841*

Generic Name

Nicotine (NIK-uh-teen) G

Brand Names

Commit
Habitrol
Nicoderm
Nicoderm CQ
Nicorelief
Nicorette
Nicorette DS
Nicotrol
Nicotrol Inhaler
Nicotrol NS
Thrive

Type of Drug

Smoking deterrent.

Prescribed For

Addiction to cigarettes. Nicotine gum has also been prescribed with haloperidol for children with Tourette syndrome.

General Information

Nicotine replacement products are prescribed for short-term treatment and make cigarette withdrawal easier for many people. Because nicotine addiction also has a psychological component, counseling or other psychological support is necessary in order for a smoking cessation program to be successful. Patches, inhalers, chewing gum, lozenges, and nasal sprays are available.

Cautions and Warnings

Do not use nicotine if you are **allergic** or **sensitive** to any of its ingredients.

Nicotine should be used only by people addicted to nicotine. It should not be used during the period immediately following a **heart attack** or if you have severe **abnormal heart rhythms** or **angina**.

People with **heart conditions** must be evaluated by a cardiologist before starting treatment.

People with severe **temporomandibular joint (TMJ) disease** should not chew nicotine gum.

Nicotine should be used with caution by people with **diabetes** who take insulin and by people with an **overactive thyroid**, **kidney or liver disease**, **pheochromocytoma** (adrenal gland tumor), **hypertension** (high blood pressure), **stomach ulcer**, or chronic **dental problems** that might be worsened by nicotine chewing gum.

The nasal spray should not be used by people with **asthma**, **bronchospasm**, **allergic rhinitis**, **sinusitis**, or **nasal polyps**.

The inhaler should not be used by people with **asthma** or **chronic pulmonary disease**. It should be used with caution in people with **lung problems** or **bronchospasm**.

It is possible to become addicted to nicotine replacement products. Your nicotine addiction may worsen while using this product.

Possible Side Effects

Chewing Gum and Lozenges

▼ Most common: injury to the gums, jaw, or teeth; sore mouth or throat; and stomach growling due to swallowing air while chewing.

Possible Side Effects *(continued)*

- ▼ Common: nausea, vomiting, upset stomach, and hiccups.
- ▼ Less common: excessive salivation, dizziness, lightheadedness, irritability, headache, more frequent bowel movements, diarrhea, constipation, gas pain, dry mouth, hoarseness, flushing, sneezing, coughing, sleeplessness, swelling of the arms or legs, high blood pressure, heart palpitations, rapid and abnormal heartbeat, confusion, convulsions, depression, euphoria (feeling "high"), numbness, tingling in the hands or feet, ringing or buzzing in the ears, fainting, weakness, redness, itching, and rash.

Inhaler

- ▼ Most common: irritation of the mouth or throat, cough, runny nose, upset stomach, and headache.
- ▼ Common: changes in taste, flu-like symptoms, nausea, and diarrhea.
- ▼ Less common: pain in the neck or jaw, dental problems, sinus inflammation, back pain, numbness or tingling, gas, and fever.

Nasal Spray

- ▼ Most common: headache, chest tightness, tingling in the hands or feet, constipation, inflammation of the mucous membranes of the mouth, and irritation of the nose, throat, or eyes.
- ▼ Common: back pain, difficulty breathing, nausea, and joint pain.
- ▼ Less common: menstrual disorder, heart palpitations, gas, tooth and gum problems, muscle aches, abdominal pains, confusion, acne, and itching.

Transdermal Patch

- ▼ Most common: feeling tired and irritation at the patch site. Transdermal systems may be more irritating to people with eczema or other skin conditions.
- ▼ Common: weakness, back pain, body ache, diarrhea, upset stomach, headache, sleeplessness, dizziness, nervousness, unusual dreams, increased cough or sore throat, muscle and joint pain, changes in the sense of taste, and painful menstruation.

Possible Side Effects *(continued)*

▼ Less common: chest pain, allergic reaction (symptoms include hives, breathing difficulties, and peeling skin), dry mouth, abdominal pain, vomiting, poor concentration, tingling in the hands or feet, sinus irritation or inflammation, increased sweating, and high blood pressure.

Drug Interactions

- Nicotine—and cigarette smoking—may reduce the effects of alcohol, benzodiazepine sedatives, beta blockers, caffeine, clorazepate, clozapine, estradiol, flecainide, fluvoxamine, heparin, imipramine, insulin, mexiletine, olanzapine, opioids, oral lidocaine, propranolol, sleeping pills, and theophylline.

Food Interactions

Do not eat or drink anything while or immediately after you chew nicotine gum. Caffeine, juice, wine, and soft drinks may interfere with its effects.

Usual Dose

Chewing Gum: 1 piece of gum whenever you feel the urge for a cigarette; do not use more than 30 pieces a day. Gradually reduce the number of pieces you chew and the time you chew each piece every 4–7 days. Substituting sugarless gum for nicotine gum may help in the process of gradual dosage reduction. Each piece contains 2–4 mg of nicotine.

Inhaler: Use as needed, generally 3–6 cartridges a day for the first 3–6 weeks; some people use up to 16 cartridges a day. Dosage should be gradually reduced after 12 weeks until you are able to stop. The inhaler should not be used for longer than 6 months.

Lozenge: 1 lozenge every 1–2 hours for the first 6 weeks, gradually reduced over 12 weeks to 1 lozenge every 4–8 hours. Do not use more than 20 lozenges a day. Each lozenge contains 2 or 4 mg of nicotine.

Nasal Spray: 1–2 sprays in each nostril up to 5 times an hour. The spray should be used at least 8 times a day to ease symptoms of nicotine withdrawal. Do not use more than 40 doses a day.

Transdermal Patch: Apply the patch to the skin as soon as you remove it from the package. Nicotrol patches should be applied when you get up in the morning and removed at bedtime. Prescription nicotine patches should be left on for 16–24 hours, depending on the brand. The dosage of the patch will be gradually reduced by your doctor. Do not use the patch for longer than 10 weeks.

Overdosage

Nicotine overdose may be deadly. Symptoms include excessive salivation, nausea, vomiting, diarrhea, abdominal pain, headache, cold sweats, dizziness, hearing and visual disturbances, weakness, and confusion. These symptoms may be followed by fainting; very low blood pressure; a pulse that is weak, rapid, and irregular; convulsions; and death by paralysis of the muscles that control breathing.

Nicotine stimulates the brain's vomiting center, making this reaction common but not automatic; spontaneous vomiting may be sufficient to remove the poison from the victim's system. In case of overdose, contact your local poison control center or a hospital emergency room. If the victim has not already vomited, you may be told to induce vomiting with ipecac syrup—available at any pharmacy—before taking the victim to an emergency room. If you seek treatment, ALWAYS bring the nicotine package.

Special Information

When using the gum, follow the product instructions. Chew each piece slowly and intermittently for about 30 minutes. Rapid chewing releases the nicotine too quickly and may lead to side effects including nausea, hiccups, and throat irritation. Do not chew more than 30 pieces a day. The amount of gum chewed should be gradually reduced and stopped after 3 months of successful treatment.

When using lozenges, place the lozenge in your mouth and let it dissolve, moving it back and forth from time to time. Each lozenge will last 20–30 minutes. Since lozenges come in the form of hard candy, be sure to keep them away from children.

When administering the nasal spray, tilt your head back slightly and do not sniff or inhale through your nose. A dose consists of 1 spray in each nostril. Administering fewer than 8 doses a day may not be effective. Do not exceed 40 doses a day. The spray should not be used for longer than 6 months.

Do not store nicotine patches in an area that is warmer than 86°F. Slight discoloration is not a sign of loss of potency, but do not store a patch after you have removed it from its pouch. Use a different skin site when applying a new patch. Do not wear the same patch for more than 24 hours and do not wear more than 1 patch at a time.

Stop smoking completely when using the nicotine inhaler. When using the inhaler, inhale deeply into the back of your throat or puff in short breaths. Use often and longer at first to control cravings. Nicotine in cartridges is used up after about 20 minutes of active puffing. Do not use more than 16 cartridges a day.

Keep nicotine patches, inhalers, and nasal spray containers—used or unused—out of the reach of children and pets to avoid accidental poisoning.

Consult with your doctor if you continue to smoke while using nicotine products, as you may experience potentially dangerous adverse effects. You dosage may need to be adjusted.

Special Populations

Pregnancy/Breast-feeding: Nicotine is not safe for use during pregnancy. It is known to cause fetal harm when used during the last 3 months of pregnancy and is associated with breathing difficulties in newborns and miscarriage.

Nicotine passes into breast milk. Nursing mothers who use it should use infant formula.

Seniors: Seniors may be more sensitive to side effects, including weakness, dizziness, and body aches.

Generic Name

Nitazoxanide (neye-taz-OX-ah-nyde)

Brand Names

Alinia

Type of Drug

Antiprotozoal.

Prescribed For

Diarrhea caused by the parasites *Giardia lamblia* and *Cryptosporidium parvum*.

General Information

Specific enzyme reactions that occur in the body are used by the *Giardia lamblia* and *Cryptosporidium parvum* microorganisms for energy production, allowing them to thrive inside the body. Nitazoxanide works by blocking these specific enzyme reactions, preventing them from thriving inside humans. It is broken down in the liver.

Cautions and Warnings

Do not take nitazoxanide if you are **allergic** or **sensitive** to any of its ingredients.

People with **liver or kidney disease** should take this drug with caution because it has not been studied in people with these conditions.

This drug has not been shown to be effective in treating diarrhea in people who are HIV-infected or have a **compromised immune system**.

Possible Side Effects

Most side effects are mild and pass with time.

- ▼ Most common: abdominal pain.
- ▼ Less common: headache, diarrhea, nausea, and vomiting.
- ▼ Rare: Other side effects of nitazoxanide can affect almost any part of the body. Contact your doctor if you experience anything unusual while taking any medication.

Drug Interactions

- Nitazoxanide may interact with warfarin and digoxin; however, no specific interactions have been reported.

Food Interactions

Take nitazoxanide with food or meals for maximum effect.

Usual Dose

Adult and Child (age 12 and over): one 500-mg tablet or 5 tsp. every 12 hours with food for 3 days.

Child (age 4–11): 2 tsp. every 12 hours for 3 days.

Child (age 1–3): 1 tsp. every 12 hours for 3 days.

Child (under 1 year): not recommended.

Overdosage

Single doses of nitazoxanide up to 4000 mg have been taken by adults without significant side effects. Overdose victims should be taken to a hospital emergency room for evaluation. If you seek treatment, ALWAYS bring the prescription bottle or container.

Special Information

This product contains 1.48 g of sugar in each teaspoonful of the suspension. This information may be of importance for people with diabetes and others who must manage their sugar intake.

Special Populations

Pregnancy/Breast-feeding: Animal studies using doses about 48 times the usual dose have revealed no adverse reproductive effects. The safety of nitazoxanide during pregnancy is not known. Although animal studies reveal no damage to the fetus, nitazoxanide should be taken during pregnancy only if your doctor determines that the potential benefit outweighs the risks.

It is not known if nitazoxanide passes into breast milk. Nursing mothers who must take it should use infant formula.

Seniors: This drug has been studied in too few seniors to draw definite conclusions about its safety. However, seniors with reduced kidney, liver, or heart function; other diseases; and those taking other medications may respond differently to this medication.

Generic Name

Nitrofurantoin (NYE-troe-few-RAN-toe-in) G

Brand Names

Furadantin
Macrobid
Macrodantin

Type of Drug

Urinary anti-infective.

Prescribed For

Treatment or prevention of acute, uncomplicated urinary tract infections (UTIs), also known as acute cystitis.

General Information

Nitrofurantoin is helpful in treating UTIs because large amounts of it pass into the urine. It works by interfering with the metabolism of carbohydrates, or sugars, in the infecting bacteria. It may also interfere with the formation of the bacterial cell wall.

Cautions and Warnings

Do not take nitrofurantoin if you are **allergic** or **sensitive** to any of its ingredients or if you have **kidney disease**.

Rarely, severe chest pain, breathing difficulties, cough, fever, and chills may develop within a few hours to 3 weeks after taking nitrofurantoin. These symptoms usually go away within 1–2 days after you stop taking it. Nitrofurantoin therapy may cause cough, breathing difficulties, and feelings of ill health after 1–6 months. Respiratory failure and death have occurred in a few cases. Chronic respiratory reactions generally occur in patients receiving continuous treatment for 6 months or longer. These chronic reactions due to longer-term therapy may remain even after treatment has stopped.

Diarrhea caused by antibiotics is a common problem that is usually mild and ends when the antibiotic is discontinued, but it can be serious or even fatal. People can develop watery and bloody stools without stomach cramps and fever as long as 2 months or more after taking the last antibiotic dose. If this happens, contact your doctor right away.

Rarely, nitrofurantoin causes hemolytic anemia. People with a **deficiency of the enzyme G-6-PD** are most susceptible to this reaction and should not take nitrofurantoin.

Rarely, nitrofurantoin causes hepatitis, which may be deadly. It is most likely to develop during long-term treatment. People with **liver disease** and those who have had **jaundice** while on nitrofurantoin should not take this drug.

This drug may cause serious or irreversible peripheral neuropathy (damage to the nerves in the arms and legs). People with **kidney disease**, **anemia**, **diabetes**, **electrolyte imbalance**, or **vitamin B deficiency** are at increased risk.

This drug is only used to treat UTIs caused by organisms susceptible to nitrofurantoin. It should not be used to treat **infections in other parts of the body**. Long-term or chronic use of nitrofurantoin may lead to secondary infection caused by drug-resistant bacteria or fungi.

This drug may cause a false-positive result in urine sugar tests.

Possible Side Effects

Side effects are less prominent with Macrodantin than with Furadantin.

- ▼ Most common: loss of appetite, nausea, vomiting, stomach pain, gas, and diarrhea. Some people develop hepatitis-like symptoms.
- ▼ Less common: fever, chills, cough, chest pain, breathing difficulties, and development of fluid in the lungs. If these reactions occur in the first week of therapy, they can

Possible Side Effects *(continued)*

generally be resolved by stopping the medication. If they develop after taking nitrofurantoin for a longer period, they are considered chronic and may be more serious.

▼ Rare: rash, itching, asthmatic attacks in people with a history of asthma, drug fever, symptoms similar to arthritis, jaundice (yellowing of the skin or whites of the eyes), effects on components of the blood, headache, dizziness, drowsiness, and temporary hair loss. Contact your doctor if you experience anything unusual while taking any medication.

This drug is known to cause changes in white and red blood cells. It should be used only under the strict supervision of your doctor.

Drug Interactions

- Nitrofurantoin may increase other drugs' toxic effects on the liver and the risk of hemolytic anemia if you are taking another drug associated with that condition, including oral antidiabetes drugs, methyldopa, primaquine, quinidine, quinine, and sulfa drugs.
- Nitrofurantoin may interfere with nalidixic acid, norfloxacin, and other fluoroquinolones. Do not combine these drugs.
- Sulfinpyrazone and probenecid may reduce this drug's effectiveness and increase side effects.
- Anticholinergic drugs, including propantheline, may increase the risk of nitrofurantoin side effects.
- Magnesium, found most commonly in antacids, delays the absorption of nitrofurantoin or reduces the amount absorbed. Avoid taking antacids with magnesium when taking nitrofurantoin.
- Combining nitrofurantoin and ethambutol, isoniazid, lincomycin, lindane, lithium, metronidazole, mexiletine, pemoline, long-term high-dose pyridoxine (vitamin B_6), or quinacrine may increase the risk of nervous system effects. Do not combine nitrofurantoin and any of these drugs.

Food Interactions

Nitrofurantoin should be taken with food to minimize upset stomach, loss of appetite, nausea, or other gastrointestinal symptoms. For optimal effectiveness, avoid citrus fruits while taking nitrofurantoin.

Usual Dose

Adult: 50–100 mg 4 times a day, with meals and at bedtime; for long-term therapy, 50–100 mg only at bedtime.

Child (age 1 month and over): 2–3 mg per lb. of body weight in 4 doses.

Child (under age 1 month): not recommended.

People with chronic urinary infections may require lower-dosage, longer-term therapy for up to 6 months. Therapy for longer than 6 months should only be continued when the benefits outweigh the risks.

Overdosage

Induce vomiting with ipecac syrup—available at any pharmacy—and take the victim to a hospital emergency room for treatment. If you seek treatment, ALWAYS bring the prescription bottle or container.

Special Information

Contact your doctor if you develop chest pain or breathing difficulties; cough; sore throat; pale skin; unusual tiredness or weakness; dizziness; drowsiness; headache; rash and itching; yellow skin; achy joints; fever and chills; numbness, tingling, or burning of the fingers or toes; severe diarrhea; abdominal pain; bloody stool; or any persistent or bothersome side effect.

Continue taking this drug until your prescription is finished, even if you stop experiencing symptoms of a UTI.

Nitrofurantoin may give your urine a brownish color. This is not a cause for concern.

The liquid form can stain your teeth if you do not swallow it rapidly.

If you miss a dose, take it as soon as possible. If it is almost time for your next dose and you take it 3 or more times a day, space the missed dose and your next dose by 2–4 hours.

Special Populations

Pregnancy/Breast-feeding: Nitrofurantoin should never be taken by pregnant women with G-6-PD deficiency or those who are near term because it can interfere with the immature enzyme systems of the fetus and cause hemolytic anemia. Otherwise, nitrofurantoin should be taken during pregnancy only if your doctor determines that the potential benefit outweighs the risks.

This drug passes into breast milk. Nursing mothers who must take nitrofurantoin should use infant formula, especially if the baby is G-6-PD deficient.

Seniors: Seniors with kidney disease may be more sensitive to nervous system and lung effects. Seniors may also require reduced dosage due to reduction of kidney function.

Generic Name

Nitroglycerin (nye-troe-GLIH-ser-in) G

Brand Names

Minitran
Nitro-Bid
Nitro-Dur
Nitrolingual
NitroMist
Nitrostat
Nitro-Time

Type of Drug

Antianginal agent.

Prescribed For

Chest pain associated with angina pectoris; prevention and management of angina; nitroglycerin injection is also used as a treatment after a heart attack, for congestive heart failure, and for high blood pressure.

General Information

Nitroglycerin and other nitrates are used to treat pain associated with heart problems. Although the exact nature of their action is not fully understood, they relax vascular smooth muscle. Nitroglycerin is available in several forms: sublingual tablets, which are taken under the tongue and allowed to dissolve; capsules, which are swallowed; transmucosal tablets, which are placed between the lip or cheek and gum and allowed to dissolve; oral sprays, which are sprayed directly onto or under the tongue; transdermal patches, which deliver nitroglycerin for absorption through the skin over a 24-hour period; and ointment, which is usually spread over the chest or another area of the body. One or more forms of nitroglycerin are often used to prevent or alleviate chest pain associated with angina.

Cautions and Warnings

Do not take nitroglycerin if you are **allergic** or **sensitive** to any of its ingredients or to another nitrate product, such as isosorbide. Do not use the patch form if you are allergic to adhesives.

Nitroglycerin should be taken with great caution if **head trauma** or **bleeding in the head** is present.

This drug may be inappropriate for you if you have had a recent **heart attack** or **stroke**, or have severe **anemia**, **glaucoma**, severe **liver or kidney disease**, **overactive thyroid**, **cardiomyopathy** (loss of blood-pumping ability due to damaged heart muscle), or **low blood pressure**, especially postural low blood pressure (symptoms include dizziness or fainting when rising from a sitting or lying position).

Possible Side Effects

- ▼ Most common: flushing and headache, which may be severe or persistent.
- ▼ Less common: lightheadedness, dizziness, and weakness. Blurred vision and dry mouth may occur; if they do, stop taking the drug and contact your doctor. In some people, the blood-pressure-lowering effect of nitroglycerin causes severe responses, including nausea, vomiting, weakness, restlessness, pallor (loss of facial color), increased perspiration, and collapse. Rash may also occur.

Drug Interactions

- Avoid over-the-counter drugs containing stimulants, such as cough, cold, and allergy remedies and appetite suppressants; they may aggravate heart disease.
- Do not take sildenafil, tadalafil, or vardenafil if you are taking nitroglycerin or another nitrate product. The combination can result in a rapid and potentially fatal drop in blood pressure.
- Interaction with large amounts of alcohol may rapidly lower blood pressure, resulting in weakness, dizziness, and fainting.
- Aspirin and calcium channel blockers may increase nitrate blood levels and the risk of side effects.
- Nitroglycerin may interfere with heparin (an injectable anticoagulant drug).
- Nitrates increase dihydroergotamine blood levels, which may raise blood pressure or block the effects of nitroglycerin.
- Use nitroglycerin with caution with antihypertensives such as beta blockers, phenothiazines, or other nitrates.

Food Interactions

Do not use any oral form of nitroglycerin with food or gum in your mouth. Nitroglycerin pills intended for swallowing are best taken on an empty stomach.

Usual Dose

Use only as much as is necessary to control chest pain; overuse may lead to drug tolerance. Nitroglycerin is not recommended for pediatric use.

Aerosol: 1–2 sprays (0.4–0.8 mg) under or on your tongue; repeat as needed to relieve an angina attack, but use no more than 3 doses in a 15-minute period.

Ointment: 1–2 in. squeezed from the tube onto a specially marked piece of paper—some people may require as much as 4–5 in. The ointment is spread on the skin every 4–8 hours as needed to control chest pain. The medication is absorbed through the skin. The application sites should be rotated to prevent skin inflammation and rash.

Sublingual Tablets: Because this form acts within 10–15 seconds, it should be taken only when necessary. Dissolve 1 tablet under the tongue, or between the cheek and gum at first sign of attack. Do not swallow sublingual tablets. Repeat about every 5 minutes until you get relief; take no more than 3 tablets in 15 minutes. You may also take sublingual tablets as a preventative measure 5–10 minutes before an activity that might precipitate an attack.

Sustained-Release Capsules and Tablets: starting dose—2.5–6.5 mg 2–4 times a day. Increase gradually, if needed, to a maximum of 26 mg 4 times a day. Swallow capsules or tablets whole.

Transdermal Patch: The patch is placed on a hairless site on the body that is not associated with excess movement. It is applied once a day and removed after 12–14 hours. Doses start at 0.2–0.4 mg per hour and may increase to 0.8 mg. Higher doses are preferable for once-daily patch applications.

Transmucosal Tablets: The tablets are placed between the upper lip and gum or between the cheek and gum and allowed to dissolve over a 3- to 5-hour period. The tablet releases the drug faster when touched with the tongue or when you drink a hot liquid. Insert another tablet after the previous one is dissolved. Do not sleep with a tablet in your mouth.

Overdosage

Overdose can result in low blood pressure; very rapid heartbeat; flushing; increased perspiration followed by cold, bluish, and clammy skin; headache; heart palpitations; blurred vision and other visual disturbances; dizziness; nausea; vomiting; slow and difficult breathing; slow pulse; confusion; moderate fever; and paralysis. Take the victim to a hospital emergency room immediately. If you seek treatment, ALWAYS bring the prescription bottle or container.

Special Information

Do not change brands of nitroglycerin without your doctor's and pharmacist's knowledge—they may not be equivalent.

Sublingual nitroglycerin should be acquired from your pharmacist only in the original, unopened bottle; the tablets must not be transferred to another bottle or container because they may lose potency. Close the bottle tightly after each use or the drug may evaporate from the tablets. Sublingual nitroglycerin should be taken while you are sitting down, and should not be chewed, crushed, or swallowed. This form of nitroglycerin frequently produces a burning sensation under the tongue, but this sensation does not necessarily indicate that the drug is working for you. If 1 tablet does not relieve your symptoms in 5 minutes, take another. If the second one does not work, take a third. If the pain continues or worsens, contact your doctor or go to an emergency room at once.

When applying nitroglycerin ointment, do not rub or massage it into the skin. Any excess ointment should be washed from the hands after application.

People who use transdermal patches for more than 12 hours a day for an extended period can build up a tolerance to the patch and may have to use another form of nitroglycerin.

Nitroglycerin patches contain a significant amount of medication even after they have been used. They can be a hazard to children and small pets; be certain to dispose of them properly.

Orthostatic hypotension may become a problem if you take nitroglycerin over a long period of time. More blood stays in the extremities and less becomes available to the brain, resulting in lightheadedness or faintness if you stand up suddenly. Avoid prolonged standing and always stand up slowly.

If you take nitroglycerin on a regular schedule and forget a dose, take it as soon as you remember. If you use immediate-release tablets and it is within 2 hours of your next dose, skip the dose you forgot and continue with your regular schedule. If you take sustained-release tablets or capsules and it is within 6 hours of your next dose, skip the dose you forgot and continue with your regular schedule. Do not take a double dose.

Special Populations

Pregnancy/Breast-feeding: Nitroglycerin crosses into the fetal circulation. It should be taken during pregnancy only if your doctor determines that the potential benefit outweighs the risks.

Nitroglycerin passes into breast milk. Nursing mothers who must take it should use infant formula.

Seniors: Seniors may take nitroglycerin without special restriction. Because saliva is necessary for the absorption of sublingual nitroglycerin, seniors with reduced saliva secretion may need to use another form of nitroglycerin or add a saliva substitute; this also applies to younger people with dry mouth.

Type of Drug

Nonsteroidal Anti-inflammatory Drug (NSAID) Eye Drops

Brand Names

Generic Ingredients: Bromfenac G
Bromday

Generic Ingredients: Diclofenac G
Voltaren

Generic Ingredients: Flurbiprofen Sodium G
Ocufen

Generic Ingredients: Ketorolac G
Acular
Acular LS
Acuvail

Generic Ingredients: Nepafenac
Nevanac

Prescribed For

Eye redness and inflammation caused by seasonal allergies; inflammation during and after eye surgery.

General Information

Nonsteroidal anti-inflammatory drug (NSAID) eye drops are used during eye surgery to prevent movement of the eye muscles and are used after surgery to relieve inflammation, pain, and aversion to light. They are also used to treat itching and redness due to seasonal allergies. After cataract surgery, they are used to prevent inflammation.

Cautions and Warnings

Do not use NSAID eye drops if you are **allergic** or **sensitive** to any of their ingredients. Those with a history of **asthma** attacks brought on by an NSAID, iodides, or aspirin should not use these medicines.

Small amounts of these eye drops are absorbed into the bloodstream. NSAIDs may cause gastrointestinal tract bleeding, ulcers, or stomach perforation. They should be used with caution in people with known **bleeding disorders** or those taking other medications that prolong bleeding time.

NSAIDs may increase the risk of high blood pressure, heart disease, and stroke.

They can cause severe toxic effects to the kidney. Report anything to your doctor, who might need to periodically test your kidney function. People taking NSAIDs on a regular basis should also have their liver function tested regularly.

NSAIDs may make you unusually sensitive to the effects of the sun.

Possible Side Effects

- ▼ Most common: temporary burning, stinging, or other minor eye irritation.
- ▼ Less common: nausea; vomiting; viral infections; and eye reactions, including persistent redness, burning, itching, or tearing. The risk of developing bleeding problems or other systemic (whole body) side effects with NSAID eye drops is low because only a small amount of the drug is absorbed into the blood.

Drug Interactions

None known.

Usual Dose

Bromfenac: 1 drop twice a day, beginning 24 hours after cataract surgery and continuing for 2 weeks.

Diclofenac: 1 drop 4 times a day for 2 weeks, beginning 24 hours after cataract surgery.

Flurbiprofen: 1 drop every 30 minutes, beginning 2 hours before surgery (total of 4 drops).

Ketorolac: 1 drop 4 times a day for itching and irritation due to seasonal allergies.

Nepafenac: 1 drop 3 times a day for 2 weeks, beginning 1 day before cataract surgery. Shake this product before using it.

Overdosage

People have died from overdoses of NSAID pills but there is not enough medicine in a bottle of eye drops to cause a severe effect. Contact a hospital emergency room or local poison control center for more information. If you seek treatment, ALWAYS bring the prescription bottle or container.

Special Information

To prevent possible infection, do not allow the dropper to touch your fingers, eyelids, or any surface. Wait at least 5 minutes before using any other eye drops.

Take out contact lenses before using these eye drops.

These medicines may cause blurred vision. Use caution while driving or performing other tasks requiring alertness, coordination, or physical dexterity.

If you forget to administer a dose of NSAID eye drops, do so as soon as you remember. If it is almost time for your next dose, skip the dose you forgot and continue with your regular schedule. Do not take a double dose.

Special Populations

Pregnancy/Breast-feeding: NSAID eye drops should not be used by pregnant women because they may affect the fetal blood circulation and prevent normal labor.

NSAID eye drops may pass into breast milk. There is a possibility that a nursing mother taking NSAIDs could affect her baby's heart or cardiovascular system. Nursing mothers who must use these drugs should use infant formula.

Seniors: Seniors may be more susceptible to side effects, especially ulcer disease.

Type of Drug

Nonsteroidal Anti-inflammatory Drugs (NSAIDs)

Brand Names

Generic Ingredients: Diclofenac Potassium G

Cambia
Cataflam
Zipsor

Generic Ingredients: Diclofenac Sodium G

Flector
Pennsaid
Solaraze
Voltaren

Generic Ingredients: Diflunisal G

Generic Ingredients: Etodolac G

Generic Ingredients: Fenoprofen Calcium G

Nalfon

Generic Ingredients: Flurbiprofen G

Ansaid

Generic Ingredients: Ibuprofen G

Advil*
Bayer Select Pain Relief Formula
Cap-Profen
Children's Elixsure*
Ibuprohm
Ibu-Tab
Medipren
Menadol
Midol Liquid Gels
Motrin*
Pediacare Fever
Profen
Tab-Profen

**Some formulations in this brand-name group are suitable for children and some are alcohol- or sugar-free. Consult your pharmacist.*

Generic Ingredients: Ibuprofen Lysine Injection

Neoprofen

Generic Ingredients: Ketoprofen G

Generic Ingredients: Meclofenamate Sodium G

Generic Ingredients: Mefenamic Acid G

Ponstel

Generic Ingredients: Meloxicam G
Mobic

Generic Ingredients: Nabumetone G

Generic Ingredients: Naproxen/Naproxen Sodium G
Aleve
Anaprox
EC-Naprosyn
Midol Extended Relief
Naprelan
Naprosyn

Generic Ingredients: Oxaprozin G
Daypro

Generic Ingredients: Piroxicam G
Feldene

Generic Ingredients: Sulindac G
Clinoril

Generic Ingredients: Tolmetin Sodium G

Combination Products
Generic Ingredients: Diclofenac Sodium + Misoprostol
Arthrotec

Generic Ingredients: Famotidine + Ibuprofen
Duexis

Prescribed For

Rheumatoid arthritis, osteoarthritis, fever, mild to moderate pain, migraine, juvenile rheumatoid arthritis, sunburn, menstrual pain, acute shoulder pain, ankylosing spondylitis, tendonitis, bursitis, acute gout, and other inflammatory conditions. Ibuprofen lysine injection is used to heal infants with patent ductus arteriosus, a blood vessel that is normal while a baby is in the womb but fails to close after the baby is born, resulting in unwanted additional blood flow to the baby's lungs.

General Information

NSAIDs are used to relieve pain and inflammation. We do not know exactly how NSAIDs work, but they may achieve their effects by blocking the body's production of a hormone called prostaglandin and the action of other body chemicals known as COX-1 and COX-2 enzymes. Pain relief comes within 1 hour after taking the first dose of these medicines, but their anti-inflammatory effects take several days to 2 weeks to become apparent and may take a month or more to reach their maximum effect.

Cataflam, a newer version of diclofenac, has no sodium and is preferred for menstrual pain and cramps. Voltaren, the older version of diclofenac, has sodium. Women taking Cataflam for menstrual problems should not switch to Voltaren. The combination of diclofenac and misoprostol is used to protect against stomach and intestinal irritation and ulcer.

Cautions and Warnings

These cautions and warnings apply to all NSAID products, including those applied directly to the skin.

Do not take ibuprofen or any other NSAID if you are **allergic** or **sensitive** to any of their ingredients. Those with a history of **asthma** attacks brought on by an NSAID, iodides, or aspirin should not take these medicines.

These drugs may cause gastrointestinal (GI) tract bleeding, ulcers, and perforation. This can occur at any time, with or without warning, in people who take ibuprofen regularly. People with a history of active **GI bleeding** should be cautious about taking any NSAID. **Alcoholism** may increase the risk of bleeding. People who develop these symptoms and continue NSAID treatment should be aware of the possibility of developing more serious side effects.

Anemia can develop in people taking an NSAID.

Children taking these medicines may be more likely to vomit blood, suffer acute kidney failure, and develop rashes.

NSAIDs can affect platelets and blood clotting at high doses and should be avoided by people with **clotting problems** and those taking **warfarin**.

People with **heart failure** who use NSAIDs may experience swelling in their arms, legs, or feet.

All NSAIDs may increase the risk of high blood pressure, heart attacks, and stroke. This risk increases with the length of time you are taking the drug. People taking these drugs, especially those with a collagen disease such as **systemic lupus erythematosus** (a chronic autoimmune disease), may experience an unusually severe drug-sensitivity reaction. Report any unusual symptoms to your doctor at once.

Long-term NSAID use may lead to severe kidney toxicity. Report any unusual side effects to your doctor, who might need to periodically test your kidney function. People with advanced **kidney disease** should avoid these medicines.

Diflunisal is a chemical similar to aspirin and should not be given to **children** or **teens**. It may cause a serious complication called Reye's syndrome.

NSAIDs may make you unusually sensitive to the effects of the sun.

NSAIDs may affect your liver, in rare cases with serious or fatal results.

NSAIDs can cause blurred or impaired vision, including changes in color vision. People experiencing these symptoms should stop using the drug and get a vision test, including a test of color vision.

Possible Side Effects

▼ Common: diarrhea, nausea, vomiting, constipation, dizziness, rash, and minor stomach upset, distress, or gas, especially during the first few days of treatment.

▼ Less common: stomach ulcers, GI bleeding, appetite loss, hepatitis, gallbladder attacks, painful urination, poor kidney function, kidney inflammation, blood and protein in the urine, fainting, nervousness, mood elevation, depression, confusion, disorientation, tingling in the hands or feet, lightheadedness, itching, sweating, dry nose and mouth, heart palpitations, chest pain, breathing difficulties, and muscle cramps.

▼ Rare: severe allergic reactions, including closing of the throat; fever and chills; changes in liver function; hallucinations; jaundice (yellowing of the skin and whites of the eyes); and kidney failure. These must be treated in a hospital emergency room or doctor's office. NSAIDs have caused severe skin reactions; see your doctor immediately if this happens to you. Contact your doctor if you experience anything unusual while taking any medication.

Drug Interactions

- These drugs may increase the effects of oral anticoagulant (blood thinning) drugs such as warfarin. Your anticoagulant dose may need to be reduced.
- These drugs may reduce the blood-pressure-lowering effect of beta blockers, ACE inhibitors, and diuretics.

- Combining these drugs with cyclosporine may increase the kidney-related side effects of both drugs.
- Ibuprofen may increase digoxin blood levels and toxicity.
- Ibuprofen may increase phenytoin side effects.
- Lithium blood levels and side effects may be increased by ibuprofen.
- Methotrexate side effects may be increased in people also taking ibuprofen.
- Blood levels of these drugs may be affected by cimetidine.
- Probenecid may increase the risk of NSAID side effects.
- Aspirin and other salicylates should never be combined with an NSAID in the treatment of arthritis.

Food Interactions

Take NSAIDs with food or a magnesium/aluminum antacid if they upset your stomach.

Usual Dose

Diclofenac Gel

Adult: Apply 2–4 g to affected joints 4 times a day. Each tube of diclofenac comes with a dosing card to allow accurate dose measurement. Use the dosing card every time you measure your dose. Your total daily dose must not be more than 32 g a day applied to all affected joints.

Senior: starting dose—⅓–½ the usual dose.

Diclofenac Tablets

Adult: 100–200 mg a day.

Senior: starting dose—⅓–½ the usual dose.

Diclofenac + Misoprostol

Adult: one 50/200-mg tablet 3 or 4 times a day, or one 75/200-mg tablet 3 times a day. For seniors, taking the combination product 4 times a day provides better ulcer protection, but arthritis relief does not improve.

Diflunisal: starting dose—500–1000 mg; maintenance dose—250–500 mg every 8–12 hours. Do not take more than 1500 mg a day. Do not crush or chew diflunisal tablets.

Etodolac

Adult: 200–400 mg every 6–12 hours, not to exceed 1200 mg a day. People weighing 132 lbs. or less should not take more than 20 mg for every 2.2 lbs. of body weight.

Fenoprofen

Adult: mild to moderate pain—200 mg every 4–6 hours. Arthritis—300–600 mg 3–4 times a day to start, individualized to your needs. Total daily dose should not exceed 3200 mg.

Child: not recommended.

Flurbiprofen: 200–300 mg a day in divided doses.

Ibuprofen

Adult and Child (age 12 and over): 200–800 mg 4 times a day depending on the condition being treated; follow your doctor's directions. 200 mg every 4–6 hours is appropriate for mild to moderate pain.

Child (age 6 months–11 years): juvenile arthritis—9–18 mg per lb. of body weight a day, divided into several doses.

Ketoprofen: 50–75 mg 3–4 times a day. Do not exceed 300 mg a day. Seniors and people with kidney problems should start with ⅓–½ of the usual dose.

Ketoprofen Extended-Release: 150–200 mg once a day.

Meclofenamate

Adult and Child (age 14 and over): 200–400 mg a day in divided doses.

Child (under age 14): not recommended.

Mefenamic Acid

Adult and Child (age 14 and over): 500 mg to start, then 250 mg every 6 hours in divided doses.

Child (under age 14): not recommended.

Meloxicam: 7.5–15 mg once a day.

Nabumetone: 1000–2000 mg a day, taken in 1 or 2 doses.

Naproxen

Adult: starting dose—250–500 mg morning and evening; up to 1500 mg a day if needed. Mild to moderate pain—250–275 mg every 6–8 hours.

Child (age 2 and over): 4.5 mg per lb. of body weight divided into 2 doses a day.

Child (under age 2): not recommended.

Oxaprozin: 600–1200 mg once a day. May be increased to up to 1800 mg a day in divided doses. Do not exceed 12 mg per lb. of body weight a day.

Piroxicam

Adult: 20 mg a day.

Child: not recommended.

Sulindac

Adult: 150–200 mg twice a day.

Child: not recommended.

Tolmetin

Adult: 400 mg 3 times a day.

Child (age 2 and over): 9 mg per lb. of body weight divided into 3 or 4 doses a day.

Child (under age 2): not recommended.

Overdosage

People have died from NSAID overdose. Common signs of overdose are drowsiness, nausea, vomiting, diarrhea, abdominal pain, rapid breathing, rapid heartbeat, sweating, ringing or buzzing in the ears, confusion, disorientation, stupor, and coma. Take the victim to a hospital emergency room at once. If you seek treatment, ALWAYS bring the prescription bottle or container.

Special Information

Take each tablet or capsule with a full glass of water and do not lie down for 15–30 minutes afterward.

Do not wash, shower, or bathe the affected joint for at least 1 hour after you apply diclofenac gel. Do not apply diclofenac gel to open wounds or broken skin and do not apply heat to joints that have been treated with diclofenac gel or expose them to sunlight. Do not let diclofenac gel come into contact with your eyes or mucous membranes. This will result in extreme irritation.

After applying diclofenac gel, leave the treated joint exposed for at least 10 minutes before putting on clothing or gloves. Do not apply diclofenac gel at the same time as any other topical medicine, including another NSAID cream or gel, sunscreen, insect repellants, or moisturizer.

NSAIDs may make you drowsy or tired: Be careful when driving or operating hazardous equipment. Do not take over-the-counter products containing aspirin while taking ibuprofen. Avoid alcohol.

Contact your doctor if you develop rash, itching, visual disturbances, weight gain, breathing difficulties, fluid retention, hallucinations, black stools, persistent headache, or any unusual or intolerable side effect.

If you forget a dose of any of these drugs, take it as soon as you remember. If you take several doses a day and it is within 4 hours of your next dose, skip the dose you forgot and continue with your regular schedule. Do not take a double dose.

Special Populations

Pregnancy/Breast-feeding: NSAIDs may affect the developing fetal heart during the last ½ of pregnancy. NSAIDs should be taken during pregnancy only if your doctor determines that the potential benefit outweighs the risks.

Arthrotec, a combination product, contains an ingredient called misoprostol that can induce labor. Pregnant women should never take this product.

NSAIDs may pass into breast milk. There is a possibility that a nursing mother taking ibuprofen could affect her baby's heart or cardiovascular system. Nursing mothers who must take an NSAID should use infant formula.

Seniors: Seniors, especially those with poor kidney or liver function, may be more susceptible to side effects.

NovoLog *see **Insulin,** page 628*

NuvaRing *see **Contraceptives,** page 316*

Generic Name

Nystatin (nye-STAH-tin) G

Brand Names

Nilstat
Nystop

The information in this profile also applies to the following drugs:

Generic Ingredients: Nystatin + Triamcinolone Acetonide G

Type of Drug

Antifungal.

Prescribed For

Fungal infections of the skin, mouth, vagina, and gastrointestinal tract.

General Information

Nystatin comes in a number of dosage forms and can be prescribed when fungal infection is a possible complication of a disease or treatment. Very little nystatin is absorbed into the blood when the product is swallowed. In most cases, nystatin relieves symptoms in 1–3 days. Nystatin vaginal tablets effectively control symptoms such as itching, inflammation, and discharge. Generally, 2 weeks of therapy is sufficient, but prolonged treatment may be necessary. It is important that you continue using this drug during menstruation. This drug has been used to prevent thrush or *Candida* in newborns by treating the mother for 3–6 weeks before her due date. Triamcinolone is a corticosteroid added to nystatin to relieve the discomfort and inflammation associated with a fungal skin infection.

Cautions and Warnings

Do not take this drug if you are **allergic** or **sensitive** to any of its ingredients.

Proper diagnosis is essential for effective treatment. Do not use nystatin without first consulting your doctor.

If large amounts of nystatin + triamcinolone are applied for prolonged periods, the corticosteroid may enter the bloodstream and in rare cases may cause serious side effects, especially in children.

Possible Side Effects

Nystatin is generally well tolerated.

Oral Form

▼ Less common: nausea, upset stomach, and diarrhea may occur with large doses.

Topical Form

Nystatin

▼ Less common: skin irritation.

Nystatin + Triamcinolone

▼ Less common: skin irritation, burning, and dryness.

Vaginal Form

▼ Less common: vaginal irritation; if this occurs, discontinue the drug and contact your doctor.

Drug Interactions

None known.

Usual Dose

Lozenges

Adult and Child: 1 or 2 lozenges (200,000–400,000 units) 4–5 times a day for as long as 14 days if necessary. Allow the lozenges to dissolve slowly on your tongue.

Oral Suspension

Adult and Child (over age 1): 400,000–600,000 units 4 times a day. Shake the bottle well before using. Hold ½ dose in each side of your mouth for as long as possible before swallowing.

Child (under age 1): 200,000 units 4 times a day.

Oral Tablets

Adult and Child: 1–2 tablets (500,000–1,000,000 units) 3 times a day.

Topical Form

Adult and Child: Apply twice a day for as long as your doctor recommends.

Vaginal Tablets

Adult: 1 tablet inserted high in the vagina daily for 2 weeks, or 3–6 weeks before delivery in pregnant women.

Child: not recommended.

Overdosage

Nystatin overdose may cause stomach irritation or upset. Contact your local poison control center for more information. If you seek treatment, ALWAYS bring the prescription bottle or container.

Special Information

If you are taking nystatin + triamcinolone and you notice stretch marks, skin thinning or discoloration, acne, hair growth, or signs of an allergic reaction (which include rash, swelling, dizziness, and trouble breathing), contact your doctor immediately.

Contact your doctor if you develop diarrhea, upset stomach, stomach pain, or skin rash.

Do not stop taking nystatin just because you begin to feel better. You must continue taking the medication as prescribed for at least 2 days after the relief of symptoms.

Insert the vaginal tablets or cream high into the vagina. They each come with a special applicator and directions. Be sure to unwrap the vaginal tablets just before inserting them. Read the directions provided with the tablets or cream and follow these steps:

—Fill the special applicator to the level indicated.

—Lie on your back with your knees drawn upward and spread apart.

—Gently insert the applicator into your vagina and push the plunger to release the medication.

—Withdraw the applicator and wash it with soap and warm water.

—Wash your hands promptly to avoid spreading the infection.

You may want to wear a sanitary pad while using the vaginal cream to protect your clothing against stains. Do not use a tampon because it will absorb the drug. Do not douche unless your doctor tells you to do so. Continue using nystatin vaginal cream or tablets even if you get your period during treatment. Some nystatin brands require storage in the refrigerator. Ask your pharmacist for specific instructions.

If you forget to administer a dose, do so as soon as you remember. If it is almost time for your next dose, skip the one you forgot and continue with your regular schedule. Do not take a double dose.

Special Populations

Pregnancy/Breast-feeding: Pregnant and breast-feeding women may use nystatin with no restrictions. Nystatin + triamcinolone should be used during pregnancy only if your doctor determines that the potential benefit outweighs the risks.

Women who are using nystatin + triamcinolone and breast-feeding should consider using infant formula.

Seniors: Seniors may use nystatin without special precaution.

Generic Name

Omalizumab (oh-ma-LIZ-u-mab)

Brand Names

Xolair

Type of Drug

Anti-IgE.

Prescribed For

Moderate to severe allergic asthma.

General Information

Omalizumab is prescribed only after all other treatment options have been tried. It is the first asthma drug designed specifically for people with allergic asthma. It works by combining with IgE molecules and preventing them from binding to specific cells involved in the allergic response. IgE-binding activates these cells, allowing them to release chemicals that start the actual allergic symptoms and is a key part of how we produce an allergic response. Typically it takes 3–6 months of treatment to see improvement in your asthma symptoms.

Cautions and Warnings

Do not take this drug if you are **allergic** or **sensitive** to any of its ingredients. Severe allergic reactions to omalizumab can develop within the first 3 doses; however, it is possible to experience this reaction as long as a year after treatment has started.

A small percentage of people taking this drug have developed cancer of the breast, skin, prostate, and parotid gland. The exact relationship between omalizumab and cancer is not known.

Heart, brain, and blood-clotting side effects are more likely in people taking omalizumab, including chest pain, heart attack, enlarged heart, heart failure, abnormal heart rhythms, stroke, and pulmonary hypertension (high blood pressure in the arteries of the lungs). Pulmonary hypertension can cause shortness of breath, weakness, chest pain, rapid heartbeat, and increased risk of heart enlargement and failure.

In 1 study, people taking omalizumab were more likely to have a parasitic infection (such as roundworm, hookworm, whipworm, or threadworm) than those not on it. Be cautious if you live in an area where parasitic infections are more likely.

Possible Side Effects

- ▼ Most common: redness, bruising, warmth, burning, stinging, itching, hives, soft or hard lumps, swelling or pain at injection site, viral infection, upper-respiratory infection, sinus irritation, headache, and sore throat.
- ▼ Common: joint and other pain.
- ▼ Less common: tiredness, bone fractures, leg or arm pain, dizziness, itching, rash, and earache.
- ▼ Rare: Contact your doctor if you experience anything unusual while taking any medication.

Drug and Food Interactions

None known.

Usual Dose

Adult and Child (age 12 and over): 150–375 mg once every 2–4 weeks.

Child (under age 12): not recommended.

Overdosage

The chances of an omalizumab overdose are remote because the drug is given only by a health care professional. However, single intravenous doses of 4000 mg have been given with no evidence of a severe response.

Special Information

This medicine is always given at your doctor's office because regular blood tests are necessary and you must be observed to make sure you are not reacting to the shot.

You can be allergic to omalizumab. If so, you can develop many of the same reactions as before you started on this medicine. Contact your doctor immediately if you develop wheezing, difficulty breathing, chest tightness, low blood pressure, dizziness, fainting, fast or slow heartbeat, anxiety, facial flushing or redness, itching, hives, feeling unusually warm, swollen throat or tongue that makes it hard to breathe or swallow, or a hoarse voice.

Contact your doctor if you develop a rash, worsening of your asthma, muscle weakness, cramps, spasms, blood pressure and heart rate changes, reduced perspiration, constipation, bladder incontinence, and sexual dysfunction or nervous system reactions such as loss of balance or coordination, tingling, numbness, feeling of wearing an invisible "glove" or "sock," burning, freezing, electric-like pain, or extreme sensitivity to touch.

Chest pain, unexplained shooting pain in your arm, feeling weak, shortness of breath, heart palpitations, slurring of words or difficulty talking, and sudden numbness or loss of muscle control can be signs of a heart, brain, or blood-clotting side effect.

Report anything unusual to your doctor, especially if you are taking another medicine.

Special Populations

Pregnancy/Breast-feeding: This drug has not been shown to damage the developing fetus in animal studies. Omalizumab should be taken during pregnancy only if your doctor determines that the potential benefit outweighs the risks. The drug's manufacturer has established a pregnancy registry to collect information.

Omalizumab is likely to pass into breast milk, but its effect on infants is not known. Nursing mothers who must take it should consider using infant formula. If you decide to breast-feed, you must coordinate treatment with your pediatrician and observe for possible drug side effects.

Seniors: Seniors may take this drug with no special precaution.

Generic Name

Omega-3-Acid Ethyl Esters

(oh-MAY-gah 3 ASS-id ETH-ill ESS-ters)

Brand Names

Lovaza

Type of Drug

Triglyceride-lowering agent.

Prescribed For

Extremely high blood-triglyceride levels (500 or more).

General Information

This product is a highly concentrated form of 2 omega-3 fatty acids known as EPA and DHA, the identical ingredients contained in over-the-counter fish oil supplements and foods, including fatty seafood such as salmon, halibut, tuna, and scallops, as well as flax seeds, walnuts, soybeans, navy beans, kidney beans, winter squash, and olive oil. The exact way that omega-3 fatty acids lower blood-triglyceride levels is not known, but several possible mechanisms exist and may result in reducing the manufacture of triglycerides in the liver. Large doses of omega-3 fatty acids have been found to help manage blood triglycerides, but research has not established a direct benefit to heart health in people with elevated triglycerides.

Cautions and Warnings

Do not take this drug if you are **allergic** or **sensitive** to fish, shellfish, or any of the drug's ingredients, including soy.

People with **liver disease** who take this product should have their liver enzymes checked regularly.

This product can increase low-density lipoprotein (LDL) levels, which are primarily controlled by statin cholesterol-lowering agents.

Possible Side Effects

- ▼ Less common: belching or stomach gas, upset stomach, infection, flu-like symptoms, back pain, chest pain, skin rash, and taste changes.
- ▼ Rare: Other side effects reported by at least 1 patient include weakness, abdomen enlargement, chills, fever, suicide, body swelling, fungal infections, feeling sick, neck pain, rheumatoid arthritis, cancer, and sudden death. Rare side effects affect almost every part of the body. Contact your doctor if you experience anything unusual while taking any medication.

Drug Interactions

- Omega-3 fatty acids can make it harder for blood clots to form. People taking any anticoagulant medicine must have their clotting time monitored while taking this product.
- Mixing a statin drug and high-dose omega-3 fatty acid treatment can significantly add to the benefits of statins alone, especially in terms of triglyceride and non-high-density lipoprotein (HDL) cholesterol levels.
- Some medications (beta blockers, estrogens, and thiazide-type diuretics) increase triglyceride levels and can counter the benefit of omega-3 fatty acids. Your doctor may want to stop or change these medications as part of your triglyceride treatment.

Food Interactions

Omega-3 fatty acids can be taken without regard to food or meals. People who are allergic to fish or shellfish should not take this medicine.

Usual Dose

Adult: Four 1-g capsules taken either once a day or 2 capsules twice a day. Each capsule contains approximately 900 mg of omega-3 fatty acids: 465 mg EPA and 375 mg DHA.

Child: not recommended.

Overdosage

Overdose symptoms likely mirror drug side effects. Contact your local poison control center for more details. If you seek treatment, ALWAYS bring the prescription bottle or container.

Special Information

This product should be swallowed whole and not opened, crushed, dissolved, or chewed.

You should also be on a lipid-lowering diet as part of your treatment. Omega-3 fatty acids cannot manage triglycerides by themselves.

Other medical issues that affect blood-fat levels must also be treated, including diabetes, obesity, and underactive thyroid disease.

Special Populations

Pregnancy/Breast-feeding: This product has not been studied in pregnant women. Studies of pregnant animals using very large doses of omega-3 fatty acids showed mixed results. Seven times the maximum human dose seemed to affect pregnancy outcomes. Lower doses did not. Discuss the risks of taking this medicine with your doctor if you are or plan to become pregnant.

It is not known if omega-3 fatty acids pass into breast milk. Nursing mothers who must take this product should consider using infant formula.

Seniors: Seniors may take omega-3 fatty acids with no special precautions.

Generic Name

Orlistat (OR-lih-stat)

Brand Names

Alli Xenical

Type of Drug

Fat blocker.

Prescribed For

Obesity management, including weight reduction and maintenance.

General Information

Orlistat works in the stomach and intestine by interfering with an enzyme that is key to the breakdown and absorption of one kind of fat. The unabsorbed fat, about 30% of that in your diet, passes out of the body in the stool. Because fat is the most concentrated form of calories, blocking fat absorption also reduces the number of calories you take in. People taking orlistat usually begin losing weight in a few weeks and continue to lose it for 6 months to a year. After that, weight loss is maintained. If you increase your exercise level or further reduce your caloric intake, you may lose more weight. More than 50% of people taking orlistat in clinical studies lost at least 5% of their body weight after a year of continuous treatment. About 18% lost more than 10% of body weight.

By losing weight, people taking orlistat achieved improved blood-fat profiles and lower blood pressure and blood sugar. They also reduced their waist and hip measurements—2 in. and 2.5 in., respectively—more than people taking a placebo (sugar pill) and following a weight-loss diet.

Orlistat is indicated for obese people with a body mass index (BMI) of 30 kg/m^2 or more, or for those with a BMI of 27 kg/m^2 or more who also have risk factors such as high blood pressure, diabetes, or high cholesterol levels.

Cautions and Warnings

Do not take orlistat if you are **allergic** or **sensitive** to any of its ingredients.

Orlistat should not be used by those with **gastrointestinal absorption disorders** or **cholestasis** (bile duct obstruction).

People taking orlistat have rarely developed severe liver disease, including possible liver failure. Symptoms include yellowing of the skin or whites of the eyes, weakness, and abdominal pain. Some people may develop **kidney stones** while taking this drug, especially those prone to kidney stones.

Orlistat, like any weight-loss drug, may be abused or misused. Orlistat should never be used by those with eating disorders such as **anorexia** or **bulimia**.

The cause of obesity must be determined before taking orlistat; it is not recommended for people who have **hyperthyroidism** or other organic causes of **obesity**.

A reduction in oral hypoglycemic medication or insulin may be necessary for **diabetic patients taking orlistat**.

Possible Side Effects

Most side effects are mild and temporary and tend to decrease during the second year of treatment.

▼ Most common: oily underwear spotting, gas with discharge, the feeling that you have to move your bowels, an oily or fat-laden stool, releasing an oily liquid during a bowel

Possible Side Effects *(continued)*

movement, more frequent bowel movements, abdominal pain or discomfort, influenza, respiratory infections, back pain, and headache.

- ▼ Common: an inability to control bowel movements, nausea, infectious diarrhea, rectal pain or discomfort, arthritis, dizziness, fatigue, rash, menstrual problems, and urinary infection.
- ▼ Less common: tooth or gum problems; vomiting; ear, nose, or throat problems; muscle pain; joint problems; tendonitis; sleep disturbances; dry skin; vaginal irritation; anxiety; depression; and swollen feet.
- ▼ Rare: Rare side effects can occur in almost any part of the body. Contact your doctor if you experience anything unusual while taking any medication.

Drug Interactions

- Orlistat causes blood levels of cyclosporine to decrease when they are taken together. Orlistat and cyclosporine doses should be separated by at least 2 hours.
- Orlistat interferes with the absorption into your bloodstream of fat-soluble vitamins and drugs, including levothyroxine and other thyroid medicines. Separate these drugs by at least 4 hours.
- The blood-fat-lowering effect of statin cholesterol-lowering drugs is increased by orlistat.
- Orlistat may increase the effect of warfarin by interfering with the absorption of vitamin K. Warfarin dosage reduction may be needed.

Food Interactions

Take a dose with, or within an hour of, a fat-containing meal.

Usual Dose

Alli

Adult: 60 mg taken 3 times a day with, or within an hour of, each main meal containing fat.

Child: not recommended.

Xenical

Adult: 120 mg taken 3 times a day with, or within an hour of, each main meal containing fat.

Child: not recommended.

Overdosage

Symptoms are likely to include side effects, especially those related to the stomach and intestines. Take the victim to a hospital emergency room. If you seek treatment, ALWAYS bring the prescription bottle or container.

Special Information

Orlistat should be taken as part of a program of diet and exercise. Taking more than 1 capsule with each meal does not provide extra benefit.

Contact your doctor if you become weak or develop itching, yellowing of the skin or whites of the eyes, dark urine, loss of appetite, or light-colored stools. These may be signs of liver injury.

Distribute your daily fat intake over 3 meals to reduce the chances of developing a stomach or gastrointestinal problem.

Orlistat can interfere with the absorption of the fat-soluble vitamins A, D, and E. Take a multivitamin supplement while using this drug, separated by at least 2 hours.

If you forget to take an orlistat capsule within an hour of any meal, skip the forgotten dose and take a capsule with your next meal. Do not take a double dose.

Special Populations

Pregnancy/Breast-feeding: Although animal studies of orlistat reveal no damage to the fetus, this drug is not recommended during pregnancy and should be taken only if your doctor determines that the potential benefit outweighs the risks.

It is not known if orlistat passes into breast milk. Nursing mothers who must take this drug should use infant formula.

Seniors: Orlistat has not been studied in older adults, who should use caution.

Ortho Tri-Cyclen Lo *see **Contraceptives**, page 316*

Generic Name

Oseltamivir (oe-sel-TAM-ih-veer)

Brand Names

Tamiflu

Type of Drug

Antiviral.

Prescribed For

Treatment and prevention of influenza type A and B. It should only be used for prevention after you know you have definitely been exposed to a flu virus.

General Information

Oseltamivir is the first pill approved to treat both type A and B influenza. It may also lessen the effects of other types of flu. It is thought to work by interfering with a virus enzyme called neuraminidase; this interference limits the spread of virus particles through the respiratory tract. In studies, people taking the drug for 5 days got better 1.3 days sooner than those taking a placebo (sugar pill). Oseltamivir is only prescribed for adults and children over 1 year who have had flu symptoms for no more than 2 days. It may also be used to prevent the flu in children and adults. Studies have shown that it reduces the chances of catching the flu from 17% down to 3%. This drug is broken down in the liver.

Cautions and Warnings

Do not take oseltamivir if you are **allergic** or **sensitive** to any of its ingredients. Serious skin reactions have occurred in people taking this medication. Report any skin or other allergic reaction to your doctor at once.

The effect of oseltamivir in people with **chronic heart disease**, **lung disease**, **suppressed immune systems**, or any condition requiring hospitalization is not known. The safety and effectiveness of repeated oseltamivir use is not known.

Flu viruses can become resistant to oseltamivir, especially those already resistant to zanamivir (another flu medication). Its use should be limited only to situations in which it is absolutely needed. Taking it for the common cold or other viruses does not work and only increases the chances of creating resistant viruses.

People with moderate to severe **kidney disease** require reduced dosage.

People taking oseltamivir can become delirious or exhibit unusual or abnormal behavior, possibly leading to personal injury.

Possible Side Effects

Adult

▼ Most common: nausea and vomiting.

Possible Side Effects *(continued)*

- ▼ Common: diarrhea.
- ▼ Less common: bronchitis, abdominal pain, dizziness or fainting, headache, cough, sleeplessness, abnormal behavior or confusion leading to possible self-injury, and fatigue.
- ▼ Rare: chest pain, anemia, colitis, bone fracture, pneumonia, fever, abscesses around the tonsils, hepatitis, abnormal heart rhythms, gastrointestinal bleeding, colitis, seizures, worsening of diabetes, altered consciousness, confusion, unusual behavior, delusions, hallucinations, agitation, anxiety, and nightmares. Contact your doctor if you experience anything unusual while taking any medication.

Child

- ▼ Most common: vomiting, diarrhea, and middle ear infection.
- ▼ Common: abdominal pain and new or worsened asthma.
- ▼ Less common: nausea, nosebleeds, pneumonia, ear disorders other than infection, sinus irritation, bronchitis, conjunctivitis (pinkeye), rash, and swollen lymph glands.

Drug Interactions

- There is a possible interference between oseltamivir and live attenuated influenza vaccine (LAIV). For this reason, LAIV should not be administered within 2 weeks before or 48 hours after use of oseltamivir.

Food Interactions

Oseltamivir may be taken with food if it upsets your stomach.

Usual Dose

Prevention of Influenza

Adult and Child (age 13 and over): 75 mg once a day for 10 days. Therapy should begin within 2 days of exposure.

Child (age 1 and over and more than 88 lbs.): 75 mg (1¼ tsp.) once a day.

Child (age 1 and over and 52–88 lbs.): 60 mg (1 tsp.) once a day.

Child (age 1 and over and 34–51 lbs.): 45 mg (¾ tsp.) once a day.

Child (age 1 and over and less than 34 lbs.): 30 mg (½ tsp.) once a day.

Child (under 1 year): not recommended.

Treatment of Influenza

Adult and Child (age 13 and over): 75 mg twice a day for 5 days. Daily dosage may be reduced to a single 75-mg capsule in people with kidney disease.

Child (age 1 and over and more than 88 lbs.): 75 mg (2½ tsp.) twice a day.

Child (age 1 and over and 52–88 lbs.): 60 mg (2 tsp.) twice a day.

Child (age 1 and over and 34–51 lbs.): 45 mg (1½ tsp.) twice a day.

Child (age 1 and over and less than 34 lbs.): 30 mg (1 tsp.) twice a day.

Child (under 1 year): not recommended.

Overdosage

Little is known about the effects of oseltamivir overdose, though symptoms may include nausea and vomiting. Contact your local poison control center or a hospital emergency room for more information. If you seek treatment, ALWAYS bring the prescription bottle or container.

Special Information

Oseltamivir should be taken from the first appearance of flu symptoms. Taking oseltamivir is not a substitute for an annual flu shot.

If you forget a dose, take it as soon as you remember. If it is almost time for your next dose, skip the one you forgot and continue with your regular schedule. Do not take a double dose.

Special Populations

Pregnancy/Breast-feeding: Animal studies indicate that oseltamivir may cause fetal abnormalities. It should be taken during pregnancy only if your doctor determines that the potential benefit outweighs the risks.

This drug may pass into breast milk. Nursing mothers who must take it should use infant formula.

Seniors: Oseltamivir may be less effective in seniors.

Type of Drug

Overactive Bladder Drugs

Brand Names

Generic Ingredients: Darifenacin
Enablex

Generic Ingredients: Fesoterodine Fumarate
Toviaz

Generic Ingredients: Oxybutynin G
Ditropan
Ditropan XL
Gelnique
Oxytrol

Generic Ingredients: Solifenacin
VESIcare

Generic Ingredients: Tolterodine
Detrol
Detrol LA

Generic Ingredients: Trospium Chloride G
Sanctura
Sanctura XR

Prescribed For

Overactive bladder.

General Information

These drugs improve bladder control by interfering with nerve receptors that control bladder muscles. By dulling the response of these receptors to nervous system stimulation, these drugs can prevent bladder muscle contractions and the resulting urgent need to urinate. Tolterodine does not work the same for everyone. Darifenacin, solifenacin, and tolterodine are mostly broken down in the liver. Fesoterodine is broken down in the liver to its active form, tolterodine. Thus, how you respond to treatment and your dosage can depend on your degree of liver function, and some people break down these drugs more slowly than others. Trospium is minimally affected by liver enzymes and is not subject to these limitations.

Cautions and Warnings

Do not take any of these drugs if you are **allergic** or **sensitive** to any of their ingredients.

Caution should be taken with these drugs if you are **retaining urine** or have a **stomach obstruction**, severe **constipation**, **ulcerative colitis**, **myasthenia gravis**, or uncontrolled **narrow-angle glaucoma**. People with controlled narrow-angle glaucoma and **dementia** should also use these drugs with caution.

People with **reduced liver function** should take solifenacin, tolterodine, and trospium with caution. Fesoterodine is not recommended for people with severe **liver disease** but may be used in mild to moderate liver disease. People with **reduced kidney function** should be cautious about using all of these drugs except darifenacin and may require a reduced dose.

All of these drugs, except darifenacin, may affect heart rate and cause abnormal heart rhythms.

Possible Side Effects

Darifenacin

- ▼ Most common: dry mouth and constipation.
- ▼ Common: upset stomach and urinary infection.
- ▼ Less common: dizziness, weakness, dry eyes, abdominal pain, nausea, diarrhea, heart palpitations, accidental injuries, and flu infections.
- ▼ Rare: Other side effects may occur anywhere in the body. Contact your doctor if you experience anything unusual while taking any medication.

Fesoterodine

- ▼ Most common: dry mouth.
- ▼ Common: constipation and urinary infection.
- ▼ Less common: nausea; upset stomach; pain in the upper abdomen; upper-respiratory infection; dry eyes; pain on urination; difficulty urinating; cough; swelling in the legs, ankles, or feet; back pain; and sleeplessness.
- ▼ Rare: rash and liver-enzyme increase. Contact your doctor if you experience any unusual side effects.

Oxybutynin

- ▼ Most common: dry mouth, dizziness with or without falling, drowsiness, decreased sweating, nausea, and constipation. Gel or transdermal patch—itching or irritation where the gel or patch is placed.
- ▼ Common: sleeplessness, urinary infection, headache, blurred vision, difficulty urinating, and upset stomach.
- ▼ Less common: sore throat, nasal irritation, sinusitis or headache, upper-respiratory infection, bronchitis, dry throat, thirst, hoarseness, asthma, stuffy nose, diarrhea, eye irritation, pupil enlargement, worsening of glaucoma, palpitations, sleeplessness, memory loss, confusion, fluid retention, abnormal heart rhythms, taste changes, diarrhea or loose stool, difficulty swallowing, stomach gas, bloating,

Possible Side Effects *(continued)*

weakness, impotence, blood-pressure changes, elevated blood sugar, reduced production of breast milk, rash, and itching.

- ▼ Rare: Contact your doctor if you experience anything unusual while taking any medication.

Solifenacin

- ▼ Most common: dry mouth and constipation.
- ▼ Common: urinary retention.
- ▼ Less common: nausea, upset stomach, upper abdominal pain, flu infections, sore throat, dizziness, blurred vision, and fatigue.
- ▼ Rare: vomiting, headache, dry eyes, leg or ankle swelling, cough, and high blood pressure. Contact your doctor if you experience anything unusual while taking any medication.

Tolterodine

- ▼ Most common: dry mouth and headache.
- ▼ Common: dizziness, fainting, abdominal pain, constipation, diarrhea, upset stomach, nausea, and tiredness.
- ▼ Less common: sleepiness, visual problems, very dry eyes, bronchitis, coughing, sore throat, runny nose, sinus irritation, respiratory infection, painful urination, frequent urination, urinary retention, joint pain, back pain, chest pain, high blood pressure, fungal infections, flu-like symptoms, and weight gain.
- ▼ Rare: tingling in the hands or feet, nervousness, itching, rash, dry skin, gas, and vomiting. Contact your doctor if you experience anything unusual while taking any medication.

Trospium

- ▼ Most common: dry mouth.
- ▼ Common: constipation.
- ▼ Less common: upper abdominal pain, aggravated constipation, upset stomach, stomach gas, headache, fatigue, urinary retention, and dry eyes.
- ▼ Rare: severe drug reaction, dizziness, rapid heartbeat, palpitations, blurred vision, abdominal swelling, taste changes, dry throat, dry skin, muscle aches due to tissue breakdown, hallucinations, and swelling around the eyes. Contact your

Possible Side Effects *(continued)*

doctor if you experience anything unusual while taking any medication.

Drug Interactions

- These drugs increase the effects of one another and other medicines with an anticholinergic effect. Do not take more than one agent for an overactive bladder at one time.
- Fluoxetine may increase fesoterodine and tolterodine blood levels and side effects.
- Tolterodine may cause an increase in blood levels of warfarin, escalating anticoagulant effects.
- Combining oxybutynin and atenolol may increase the effect of atenolol.
- Oxybutynin may affect haloperidol blood levels, which in turn may worsen schizophrenic symptoms.
- Oxybutynin may interfere with carbidopa + levodopa.
- Amantadine may increase oxybutynin side effects.
- Clarithromycin, itraconazole, ketoconazole, miconazole, nefazodone, nelfinavir, and ritonavir can interfere with the breakdown of darifenacin, fesoterodine, solifenacin, and tolterodine in the liver. People taking one of these drugs may need only 7.5 mg of darifenacin, 4 mg of fesoterodine, 5 mg of solifenacin, or 1 mg of tolterodine each day.
- Diltiazem, erythromycin, fluconazole, and verapamil may also interact with these drugs, but there is less chance that a dose adjustment will be needed. This interaction is not likely with trospium, because the liver has only a minimal effect on breaking it down in the body.
- Mixing oxybutynin or trospium with digoxin, metformin, morphine, tenofovir, or vancomycin may increase blood levels of either or both drugs.
- Darifenacin may increase the amount of flecainide, thioridazine, or tricyclic antidepressant in the blood. These combinations should be avoided.
- Darifenacin may increase blood levels of digoxin, and people taking this combination should be monitored regularly.

Food Interactions

Darifenacin, fesoterodine, oxybutynin, solifenacin, and tolterodine can be taken without regard to food or meals. Trospium should be taken on an empty stomach. There is no food restriction with the oxybutynin gel or patch.

Usual Dose

Darifenacin

Adult: 7.5–15 mg once a day. People with severe liver disease should not take more than 7.5 mg a day.

Child: not recommended.

Fesoterodine

Adult: 4–8 mg once a day. This is a long-acting product. Do not crush, chew, or split the pill. People with severe kidney disease and those taking certain medications concurrently are limited to 4 mg a day.

Child: not recommended.

Oxybutynin

Ditropan

Adult: 5–20 mg a day in divided doses.

Child (age 6 and over): 5–15 mg a day in divided doses.

Ditropan XL

Adult: 5–30 mg once a day.

Child (age 6 and over): 5–20 mg once a day.

Gel

Adult: Apply once a day to dry, intact skin on the abdomen, upper arms/shoulders, or thighs.

Transdermal Patch (Oxytrol)

Adult: Apply twice a week to dry, intact skin on the abdomen or buttock.

Solifenacin

Adult: 5–10 mg once a day. People with severe kidney or liver disease should not take more than 5 mg a day.

Child: not recommended.

Tolterodine

Adult: 1–2 mg twice a day. People with liver disease should not take more than 1 mg a day. Extended-release tablets—2–4 mg a day.

Child: not recommended.

Trospium

Adult: 20 mg twice a day at least 1 hour before or 2 hours after meals. Extended-release tablets—one 60-mg tablet a day.

Child: not recommended.

Overdosage

Overdose symptoms are those listed under drug side effects, but are likely to include less common and more severe reactions because of the large dose. Take the victim to a hospital emergency room at once. If you seek treatment, ALWAYS bring the prescription bottle or container.

Special Information

These drugs can blur your vision, or cause dizziness or drowsiness.

Contact your doctor if you develop severe or persistent diarrhea.

Tell your doctor if you have any of the following problems before you start taking one of these drugs: stomach or intestinal problems, constipation, trouble emptying your bladder, a weak urine stream, an eye problem called narrow-angle glaucoma, liver problems, or kidney problems. Tell your doctor if you are pregnant or trying to become pregnant, or are breast-feeding.

Heat prostration (fever and heatstroke) is more likely to occur in hot weather if you are taking one of these medicines because it reduces your ability to cool your body by sweating.

Dry mouth may be relieved with sugarless gum, candy, or ice chips. Excessive mouth dryness may lead to tooth decay and should be brought to your dentist's attention if it lasts for more than 2 weeks.

If you forget a dose, take it as soon as you remember. If it is almost time for your next dose, skip the forgotten dose and continue with your regular schedule. Do not take a double dose.

Special Populations

Pregnancy/Breast-feeding: Large doses of these medicines have caused fetal harm and birth defects in animal studies. These drugs should be taken during pregnancy only if your doctor determines that the potential benefit outweighs the risks.

These drugs may pass into breast milk. Nursing mothers who must take one of them should use infant formula.

Seniors: Seniors may take darifenacin, fesoterodine, and tolterodine without special precaution. However, side effects are more likely in people age 75 and over, and a lower dose may be prescribed. Dosage reduction is definitely required for seniors taking solifenacin and trospium.

OxyContin *see **Narcotic Analgesics,** page 823*

Generic Name

Pancrelipase (pan-creh-LIP-ase)

Brand Names

Creon
Pancreaze
Zenpep

Type of Drug

Enzyme combination.

Prescribed For

Pancreatic insufficiency.

General Information

Pancreatic enzyme products are designed to provide the digestive enzymes needed by people with reduced pancreatic function caused by inflammation. The pancreas secretes digestive enzymes into the small intestine, and these enzymes help digest fats, proteins, and carbohydrates in food. The pancreas also releases the hormones insulin and glucagon into the bloodstream, which help the body use the glucose it takes from food for energy.

Normally, digestive enzymes are not active until they reach the small intestine. If these enzymes become active inside the pancreas, they start "digesting" the pancreas itself. Acute pancreatitis is often a result of gallstones. It generally occurs suddenly, lasts for a short time, and usually resolves on its own. Chronic pancreatitis does not resolve itself and results in slow destruction of the pancreas. Chronic pancreatitis is often associated with cystic fibrosis because the tubes that normally carry digestive enzymes to the small intestine are blocked.

Either acute or chronic pancreatitis can cause serious complications. In its acute form, it usually begins with severe pain in the upper abdomen that may last for a few days. It can remain in the abdomen or it may travel to the back and other areas. It can be sudden and intense or start as a mild pain that gets worse when food is eaten. Severe pancreatitis may cause dehydration and low blood pressure. The heart, lungs, or kidneys may fail. Shock and sometimes even death can result from bleeding inside the pancreas. People with acute pancreatitis often look and feel very sick.

Cautions and Warnings

Do not take this product if you are **allergic** or **sensitive** to any of its ingredients, which consist of enzyme combinations made from various animal or plant sources.

High doses of pancrelipase have been associated with a rare and serious side effect called fibrosing colonopathy, in which excessive amounts of connective tissue replace functioning tissues in the colon.

People with **gout**, **reduced kidney function**, or **high blood levels of uric acid** should use this product with caution.

As with all pancreatic enzyme products made from animal materials, there is the theoretical risk of catching a swine virus while using this drug, although no cases of this have been reported.

Possible Side Effects

- ▼ Common: stomach gas, abdominal pain, headache, dizziness, and cough.
- ▼ Less common: abnormal bowel movement and weight loss.

Drug Interactions

None known.

Food Interactions

Pancrelipase must be taken with food or meals.

Usual Dose

Adult and Child (age 4 and over): 227–1136 lipase units per lb. of body weight with each meal.

Child (age 1–4): 455–1136 lipase units per lb. of body weight with each meal.

Child (under age 1): 2000–4000 lipase units per 4 oz. of formula or per breast-feeding. Do not mix capsule contents directly into formula or breast milk prior to administration.

Overdosage

There are no reports of pancrelipase overdose; however, long-term use of high doses or doses larger than 2727 lipase units per lb. of body weight per meal have been associated with fibrosing colonopathy (see "Cautions and Warnings") and high blood levels of uric acid. Contact your doctor or a poison control center if you suspect an overdose. If you seek treatment, ALWAYS bring the prescription bottle or container.

Special Information

These capsules should be swallowed whole to protect the mouth from irritation. People who cannot swallow capsules should mix the contents with a small amount of soft food such as applesauce and swallow the mixture without crushing or chewing. Then, drink a glass of water, juice, or another liquid to be sure all the medicine has been swallowed.

If you forget a dose of pancrelipase with a meal, skip the forgotten dose and take a regular dose with your next meal. Do not take a double dose of pancrelipase.

Numerous products containing pancreatic enzymes are sold without a prescription. They are derived from animal and plant sources but are not considered equivalent to this product or one another. Do not switch brands of pancrelipase without first contacting your doctor. They may not provide the same benefit.

Special Populations

Pregnancy/Breast-feeding: It is not known if pancrelipase affects a developing fetus, though only very small amounts are absorbed into the bloodstream. This drug should be used during pregnancy only if your doctor determines that it is necessary to maintain calorie and food intake required for a safe pregnancy.

It is not known if pancrelipase passes into breast milk, but very little of any oral dose is absorbed into the blood. Nursing mothers who must take it should consider using infant formula because of possible effects on a nursing infant.

Seniors: Seniors may take this drug with no special precaution.

Patanol *see **Antihistamine Eye Drops,** page 109*

Generic Name

Pegloticase (peg-LOW-tih-kace)

Brand Names

Krystexxa

Type of Drug

Enzyme.

Prescribed For

Symptomatic gout that has not responded to other treatment.

General Information

Pegloticase is a long-acting form of the natural enzyme *uricase.* It stimulates the breakdown of uric acid to allantoin, which is harmless and easily eliminated through the kidney. It is not meant for high blood levels of uric acid without gout symptoms.

Cautions and Warnings

Do not take pegloticase if you are **allergic** or **sensitive** to any of its ingredients. Severe reactions occurred in 6.5% of people in pegloticase studies. People receiving it should be given an antihistamine and a corticosteroid drug to prevent a drug reaction, but this is not always successful. These reactions generally appear within 2 hours of the infusion, but they may also develop later than this. It is advisable to stay at your doctor's office for some time after the infusion to make sure that you do not have a reaction.

You may experience an infusion reaction to pegloticase while it is being administered. Infusion reactions are more likely if you are no longer responding to pegloticase, indicated by a rise in uric acid despite pegloticase infusion. Infusion reactions are sudden. Symptoms can be similar to a drug reaction and can include a sudden blood-pressure drop; rapid heartbeat; dizziness; fainting; headache; weakness; sudden skin reactions; itching; flushing; swelling of the tongue, mouth, or throat; difficulty breathing; abdominal pain; nausea; vomiting; and diarrhea. If the reaction is severe, your treatment may have to be stopped.

Do not take pegloticase if you have an inherited condition called **G-6-PD deficiency** because of the risk of red-blood-cell destruction and a blood condition known as methemoglobinemia. People at risk for this problem, especially those of **African and Mediterranean origin** should be screened, via a blood test, before beginning pegloticase treatments.

Your **gout** may flare up when treatment starts. Your doctor may prescribe, or have you continue taking, other gout medicines for at least the first 6 months of treatment to prevent occasional flares.

Some people taking pegloticase in drug studies experienced worsening of their **congestive heart failure**.

Because pegloticase is a biological product, it is normal for people to develop antibodies, proteins created by the body, to disable it. Almost every person receiving pegloticase in studies developed these antibodies. High antibody levels can neutralize its effect and are associated with a greater chance of an infusion reaction.

Possible Side Effects

- ▼ Most common: gout flare, infusion reactions, nausea, bruising, and black-and-blue marks.
- ▼ Common: stuffy nose and sinuses, constipation, chest pain, severe drug reactions, and vomiting.
- ▼ Rare: Other side effects, including worsening heart failure, may occur. Contact your doctor if you experience anything unusual while taking any medication.

Drug Interactions

None known.

Usual Dose

Adult: 8 mg intravenous infusion given over at least 2 hours once every 2 weeks. Pegloticase must be given in a doctor's office.

Child: not recommended.

Overdosage

There is no information on pegloticase overdose, although it would be unlikely since it is given only by a health care provider. Call your doctor if you experience any change in your usual health.

Special Information

Call your doctor and seek emergency treatment at once if you start wheezing, have difficulty breathing, or experience swelling of the mouth, tongue, or throat. These and blood-pressure changes are symptoms of a severe drug reaction, a medical emergency.

Your doctor will carefully monitor blood levels of uric acid while you are on pegloticase. If you miss your regular pegloticase injection, it should be taken as soon as possible. Schedule your next injection 2 weeks from the actual date when you received your last dose.

There were no race or gender differences in how people responded to pegloticase in clinical studies.

Special Populations

Pregnancy/Breast-feeding: It is not known if pegloticase will harm a developing fetus. It should be taken during pregnancy only if your doctor determines that the potential benefit outweighs the risks.

It is not known if this drug passes into breast milk. Nursing mothers who must take pegloticase should use infant formula.

Seniors: A third of people studied with pegloticase were 65 years or older and responded in the same way as younger adults. Some older adults may be more sensitive to pegloticase.

Generic Name

Pemirolast (peh-MEER-oh-last)

Brand Names

Alamast

Type of Drug

Ophthalmic mast-cell stabilizer.

Prescribed For

Eye allergies and redness.

General Information

Pemirolast helps relieve allergy-related itchy, red eyes by stabilizing the cells in eye tissue that are responsible for releasing a number of different chemicals that cause inflammation when in the presence of an allergen.

Cautions and Warnings

Do not use pemirolast if you are **allergic** or **sensitive** to any of its ingredients.

Do not wear **contact lenses** if your eyes are red, and do not use pemirolast for irritation caused by contact lenses because the preservative in this drug may be absorbed by soft contacts.

Do not use this drug if you have an **eye infection**, unless you are also being treated for it.

Possible Side Effects

Serious side effects are not expected with pemirolast.

- ▼ Most common: burning, irritation, or dryness of the eyes and a sensation of something in the eye.
- ▼ Common: headache, inflammation of the mucous membranes of the nose, and flu-like symptoms.

Drug Interactions

None known.

Usual Dose

Adult and Child (age 3 and over): 1–2 drops in each affected eye 4 times a day.

Child (under age 3): not recommended.

Overdosage

The amount absorbed into the blood from a dose is very small but overdose might be expected to produce ordinary drug side effects. Contact your local poison control center for more information. If you seek treatment, ALWAYS bring the prescription bottle or container.

Special Information

To avoid infection, do not touch the dropper tip to your finger, eyelid, or any other surface. Keep the bottle cap tightly closed when it is not being used.

Do not wear contact lenses if your eyes are red. If you wear soft contact lenses and your eyes are not red, remove them before each dose and wait at least 10 minutes after using pemirolast before putting in your lenses.

If you forget a dose of pemirolast, administer it as soon as you remember. If it is almost time for your next dose, skip the dose you forgot and continue with your regular schedule. Do not take a double dose.

Special Populations

Pregnancy/Breast-feeding: Pemirolast, given orally, causes birth defects and miscarriage in animals. It should be taken during pregnancy only if your doctor determines that the potential benefit outweighs the risks.

Pemirolast passes into the breast milk of animals, but no information is available for humans. Nursing mothers should consider using infant formula.

Seniors: Seniors may use pemirolast without special precaution.

Generic Name

Penciclovir (pen-SYE-kloe-veer)

Brand Names

Denavir

Type of Drug

Antiviral.

Prescribed For

Cold sores.

General Information

Penciclovir works against the different types of herpes viruses responsible for common cold sores. Cold sores treated with penciclovir cream go away sooner and are less painful than those that are not treated. Once applied to the skin, penciclovir is converted to its active form and interferes with DNA production inside the viral particle; this inhibits the reproduction process of the herpes virus.

Cautions and Warnings

Do not use penciclovir if you are **allergic** or **sensitive** to any of its ingredients.

Penciclovir should be applied only to the face or lips. Avoid applying it near your eyes because it may be irritating. The effectiveness of penciclovir in people with **compromised immune systems** is not known.

Male animals given massive doses of penciclovir intravenously suffered damage to the testicles. This effect appears to be related to the dose of penciclovir. Men using famciclovir—the oral form of penciclovir—for 8–13 weeks experienced no changes in sperm count.

Drug resistance may develop with repeated use.

Possible Side Effects

Side effects are generally mild and infrequent. In studies, side effects were similar in type and frequency among people who used penciclovir and those who used an inactive cream.

- ▼ Common: headache, redness, and swelling.
- ▼ Less common: skin reactions to the cream.
- ▼ Rare: loss of skin sensation where the cream has been applied, changes in the sense of taste, and rash. Contact your doctor if you experience anything unusual while taking any medication.

Drug Interactions

None known.

Usual Dose

Adult and Child (age 12 and over): Apply to affected areas every 2 hours, during waking hours, for 4 days.

Child (under age 12): not recommended.

Overdosage

Little is known about the effects of penciclovir overdose or accidental ingestion. Contact your poison control center or a hospital emergency room for more information. If you seek treatment, ALWAYS bring the prescription bottle or container.

Special Information

Begin cold sore treatment as early as possible. Early application of penciclovir cream will help prevent cold sores from appearing and reduce accompanying pain.

It is very important to apply penciclovir cream every 2 hours during the day for the drug to work. If you forget to apply a dose of penciclovir, apply it as soon as you remember. If you realize you forgot a dose within 30–45 minutes of your next dose, skip the dose you forgot and continue with your regular schedule.

Special Populations

Pregnancy/Breast-feeding: In animal studies, penciclovir had no effect on the fetus. There is no information on the effect of penciclovir in pregnant women. It should be used during pregnancy only if your doctor determines that the potential benefit outweighs the risks.

It is not known if penciclovir passes into breast milk, though famciclovir—the oral form of penciclovir—passes into breast milk in concentrations larger than those found in the mother's blood. Nursing mothers who must use penciclovir should use infant formula.

Seniors: Seniors may use this drug without special precaution.

Type of Drug

Penicillin Antibiotics (pen-ih-SIL-in)

Brand Names

Generic Ingredients: Amoxicillin G

Amoxil
DisperMox
Larotid
Moxatag

Generic Ingredients: Amoxicillin + Potassium Clavulanate G
Augmentin
Augmentin XR
Augmentin ES-600

Generic Ingredients: Ampicillin G

Generic Ingredients: Dicloxacillin G

Generic Ingredients: Penicillin V Potassium G
Penicillin VK

Prescribed For

Bacterial and other infections.

General Information

Penicillin antibiotics kill bacteria and other microorganisms by destroying the cell wall of the invading organisms. Many infections respond to almost any kind of penicillin; some respond only to a specific penicillin antibiotic. Penicillin cannot cure a cold, the flu, or any other viral infection and should never be taken unless prescribed by a doctor for a specific condition. Always take penicillin exactly as prescribed, including the number of pills to take every day and number of days to take the drug, otherwise you will not get the drug's full effect.

Cautions and Warnings

Do not take penicillin antibiotics if you are **allergic** or **sensitive** to any of their ingredients. Some of these medications contain tartrazine dyes or sulfites, which may cause allergic reactions in certain people. Chewable forms of amoxicillin contain phenylalanine and should not be used by people with **phenylketonuria**.

Do not take amoxicillin or ampicillin if you have **mononucleosis**, as a serious skin rash may develop.

Do not take amoxicillin + potassium clavulanate if you have had a reaction to any penicillin product or if you have severe **kidney disease**. Use this drug with caution if you have had **jaundice** or **liver disease**.

Serious and sometimes fatal allergic reactions have occurred with penicillin. Though more common following penicillin injections, these reactions have also occurred with oral penicillin. Reactions are more common among people who have had a previous penicillin reaction and those who have had **asthma**, **hay fever**, or other **allergies**. Allergic symptoms include itching, rash, swelling, breathing difficulties, very low blood pressure, blood-vessel collapse, peeling skin, chills, fever, muscle aches, arthritis-like pain, and feeling unwell. Sometimes, when an infection is life-threatening and can only be treated with penicillin, minor reactions may be treated with another drug while the penicillin is continued. About 1 in 20 people allergic to a penicillin antibiotic are also allergic to the cephalosporin antibiotics.

Cystic fibrosis patients are more likely to suffer from side effects of certain penicillins.

Prolonged or repeated use of penicillin may lead to a secondary infection that cannot be treated by the penicillin being used. **Women** may be more susceptible to vaginal yeast infections. Contact your doctor if you develop symptoms such as vaginal itching, irritation, or discharge.

Colitis is possible with any broad-spectrum antibiotic; contact your doctor if you have severe cramps or bloody diarrhea while taking penicillin.

Possible Side Effects

The most common penicillin side effect, seen in up to 10% of people, is allergy. About 9% of ampicillin users develop an itchy rash, which is not a true allergic reaction.

- ▼ Common: upset stomach, abdominal pain, nausea, vomiting, diarrhea, colitis (symptoms include severe abdominal cramps and severe, persistent, and possibly bloody diarrhea), sore mouth, coated tongue, anemia, bleeding abnormalities, low platelet and white-blood-cell counts, and oral or rectal fungal infections.
- ▼ Less common: vaginal irritation, appetite loss, itchy eyes, and feelings of body warmth.
- ▼ Rare: yellowing of the skin or whites of the eyes. Contact your doctor if you experience anything unusual while taking any medication.

Drug Interactions

- Penicillin should not be combined with a bacteriostatic antibiotic such as tetracycline. These drugs can interfere with each other.
- Penicillin can interfere with contraceptive drugs. Use additional contraception while taking a penicillin drug. Breakthrough bleeding may occur.

- Penicillins may increase blood levels and side effects of methotrexate.
- Neomycin may decrease blood levels of penicillin and may reduce its effectiveness.
- Penicillin allergies may be intensified by beta blockers, and blood levels of beta blockers may be reduced by penicillins.
- Combining some penicillins and allopurinol may increase the risk of rash and itching.
- Combining penicillins and probenecid may increase blood levels of penicillin.
- Dicloxacillin may interfere with the effects of anticoagulant (blood thinning) drugs such as warfarin.

Food Interactions

Do not take penicillin with fruit juice or carbonated beverages. The acid in these beverages may destroy the drug.

Amoxicillin, amoxicillin + potassium clavulanate, and penicillin V can be taken without regard to food. Other penicillins are best absorbed on an empty stomach and should be taken 1 hour before or 2 hours after meals, or first thing in the morning and last thing at night with the other doses spaced evenly throughout the day.

Usual Dose

Amoxicillin

Adult: *Helicobacter pylori* ulcers—1 g 3 times a day with clarithromycin and/or lansoprazole; infections of the ear, nose, throat, skin, and respiratory and urinary tracts—250–875 mg every 8–12 hours; sexually transmitted diseases—3 g as a single dose; tonsillitis and sinus infection—775 mg once a day.

Child (age 12 weeks and over): 11–20 mg per lb. of body weight a day in 2–3 divided doses.

Amoxicillin + Potassium Clavulanate

Adult and Child (88 lbs. and over): 250–2000 mg every 8–12 hours, depending on infection. Different strengths of this product are not interchangeable. Take only the exact strength and product your doctor has prescribed.

Child (age 3 months and over, less than 88 lbs.): 11–41 mg per lb. of body weight a day divided into 2–3 doses. Use only the exact strength and product your doctor has prescribed.

Dicloxacillin

Adult and Child (88 lbs. and over): 125–250 mg every 6 hours.
Child (under 88 lbs.): 6–11 mg per lb. a day divided into 4 doses.

Penicillin V Potassium

Adult and Child (age 12 and over): 125–500 mg every 6–12 hours.

Child (under age 12): 11–23 mg per lb. of body weight a day divided into 3–4 doses.

Overdosage

Overdose is unlikely, but diarrhea or upset stomach is the primary symptom. Massive overdose may result in seizure. Contact your local poison control center or a hospital emergency room for more information. If you seek treatment, ALWAYS bring the prescription bottle or container.

Special Information

Liquid penicillin should be refrigerated and must be thrown out after 14 days in the refrigerator or 7 days at room temperature.

Contact your doctor if you develop black tongue, rash, itching, hives, diarrhea, breathing difficulties, sore throat, nausea, vomiting, fever, swollen joints, unusual bleeding or bruising, yellowing of the skin or whites of the eyes, or if you are feeling unwell.

Penicillin eradicates most susceptible organisms in 7–10 days; be sure to take all the medication prescribed for the full period of the prescription. It is best taken at evenly spaced intervals throughout the day.

If you miss a dose, take it as soon as possible. If it is almost time for your next dose, space the missed dose and your next dose by 2–4 hours and then continue with your regular schedule.

Special Populations

Pregnancy/Breast-feeding: Penicillin crosses into the fetal circulation but has not been known to cause birth defects and is often prescribed for pregnant women. Penicillin should be taken during pregnancy only if your doctor determines that the potential benefit outweighs the risks.

Penicillin is generally safe during breast-feeding; however, small amounts may pass into breast milk and cause upset stomach, diarrhea, allergic reaction, or other problems in the nursing infant. Nursing women who must take this drug should consider using infant formula.

Seniors: Seniors may take penicillin without special precaution.

Generic Name

Pentosan Polysulfate Sodium

(PEN-toe-san pol-ee-SUL-fate)

Brand Names

Elmiron

Type of Drug

Kidney analgesic (pain reliever).

Prescribed For

Bladder pain or discomfort due to cystitis.

General Information

Interstitial cystitis is a painful, long-term infection of the bladder. Pentosan does not affect the infectious process, but it may stick to the membranes of the bladder wall, preventing irritating substances from reaching bladder cells. About ⅓ of people who take this drug for 3 months or more have less cystitis pain.

Cautions and Warnings

Do not take pentosan if you are **allergic** or **sensitive** to any of its ingredients.

Pentosan is a weak anticoagulant and can cause black-and-blue marks, nosebleeds, and bleeding gums. People with **aneurysms**, **thrombocytopenia**, **hemophilia**, or **gastrointestinal ulcerations**, **polyps**, **or diverticula** should be carefully evaluated before beginning therapy. People having **surgery** must be screened for internal bleeding by their doctor.

People with **liver disease** should use this drug with caution because its breakdown can be reduced in people with liver problems. Pentosan may also cause mild liver toxicity.

Possible Side Effects

- ▼ Most common: patchy hair loss beginning within 4 weeks of treatment, diarrhea, and nausea.
- ▼ Common: headache, emotional upset or depression, dizziness, abdominal pain, upset stomach, and rash.
- ▼ Rare: Rare side effects can include sleeplessness, bleeding, and effects on your blood, eyes, breathing, stomach and intestines, ears, and liver. Contact your doctor if you experience anything unusual while taking any medication.

Drug Interactions

- Aspirin, clopidogrel, warfarin, and other anticoagulant (blood thinning) drugs should be taken with caution if you are already taking pentosan. Pentosan may increase the blood-thinning effect of these drugs.

Food Interactions

Take pentosan with water on an empty stomach, at least 1 hour before or 2 hours after a meal.

Usual Dose

Adult and Child (age 16 and over): 100 mg 3 times a day.
Child (under age 16): not recommended.

Overdosage

Symptoms may include bleeding, liver problems, and upset stomach. Overdose victims should be taken to a hospital emergency room at once. If you seek treatment, ALWAYS bring the prescription bottle or container.

Special Information

Pentosan has a mild anticoagulant effect. Make sure that your pharmacist, dentist, and all of your doctors know you are taking pentosan. Check with your doctor before combining aspirin or other drugs with pentosan.

Patchy hair loss, usually starting within the first 4 weeks of taking pentosan, occurs in about 4% of people who take this medication.

Pentosan should be taken exactly as directed. If you forget to take a dose of pentosan, take it as soon as you remember. If it is almost time for your next dose, skip the dose you forgot and continue with your regular schedule. Do not take a double dose.

Special Populations

Pregnancy/Breast-feeding: Although animal studies of pentosan reveal no damage to the fetus, pentosan should be taken during pregnancy only if your doctor determines that the potential benefit outweighs the risks.

It is not known if pentosan passes into breast milk. Nursing mothers who must take it should use infant formula.

Seniors: Seniors may use this medication without special precaution.

Generic Name

Phenobarbital (FEEN-oe-BAR-bih-tol) G

Brand Names

Solfoton

Type of Drug

Hypnotic, sedative, and anticonvulsant.

Prescribed For

Epileptic and other seizures, convulsions, daytime sedation, and sleeplessness in the short term.

General Information

Phenobarbital is a sustained-release barbiturate. It takes 30–60 minutes to start working and its effect lasts for 10–16 hours. Like other barbiturates, phenobarbital appears to act by interfering with nerve impulses to the brain. When used as an anticonvulsant, phenobarbital is not very effective by itself; when used with anticonvulsant agents such as phenytoin, the combined action is dramatic. This combination has been used very successfully to control epileptic seizures. When used to treat insomnia, phenobarbital loses its effectiveness after 2 weeks.

Cautions and Warnings

Do not take phenobarbital if you are **allergic** or **sensitive** to any of its ingredients or to any barbiturate; have been **addicted to sedatives or hypnotics**; or have a **respiratory condition**, **porphyria**, or severe **liver disease**.

Phenobarbital may dull your physical and mental reflexes. Be extremely careful when driving or performing any task that requires concentration.

Phenobarbital is a Schedule IV drug and is considered a controlled substance. It may be addictive if taken for an extended period of time. It may also cause signs of intoxication, including slurred speech, a wobbly walk, rolling of the eyes, confusion, poor judgment, irritability, and sleeplessness. Combining this drug with alcohol or any other central-nervous-system (CNS) depressant worsens these effects. People who have **depression** or **suicidal tendencies** should use barbiturates with caution. **Children** may experience excitement instead of sedation.

Barbiturates are broken down in the liver and eliminated through the kidneys; people with mild to moderate **liver or kidney disease** should be cautious about taking phenobarbital.

People with **chronic pain** should be careful about taking this drug because it may mask symptoms or cause stimulation rather than sedation, though using phenobarbital after surgery and in people with cancer has proven effective.

People abruptly stopping this drug may develop delirium or seizures. Dosage should be reduced gradually. The symptoms of barbiturate withdrawal may be severe and can be fatal.

Barbiturates may increase your need for vitamin D; take a vitamin supplement while using this drug.

Possible Side Effects

- ▼ Most common: drowsiness, lethargy, headache, dizziness, drug "hangover," breathing difficulties, rash, and general allergic reaction (symptoms include runny nose, watery eyes, sneezing, scratchy throat, and cough).
- ▼ Less common: excitement, nausea, vomiting, constipation, diarrhea, slow heartbeat, low blood pressure, and fainting. Severe adverse reactions may include anemia and yellowing of the skin or whites of the eyes.

Drug Interactions

- Alcohol and other CNS depressants and monoamine oxidase inhibitors (MAOI) increase the effects of phenobarbital.
- Charcoal may counteract the effects of phenobarbital.
- Phenobarbital interferes with the effects of anticoagulant (blood thinning) drugs, contraceptive drugs, corticosteroids, doxycycline, and griseofulvin.
- Phenobarbital enhances the toxic effects of acetaminophen.
- Phenobarbital has a variable effect on phenytoin and other antiseizure medications and on narcotic drugs. Dosage adjustments are necessary.

Food Interactions

Phenobarbital is best taken on an empty stomach but can be taken with food if it upsets your stomach.

Usual Dose

Anticonvulsant

Adult: 60–300 mg a day.

Child: 1.4–2.7 mg per lb. of body weight in 2–3 divided doses a day.

Daytime Sedation

Adult: 30–120 mg in 2–3 divided doses.

Child: 2.7 mg per lb. of body weight in 3 divided doses.

Hypnosis: 100–320 mg.

Overdosage

Severe barbiturate overdose may be fatal. Overdose symptoms include breathing difficulties, moderate reduction in pupil size, lowered body temperature progressing to fever, fluid in the lungs, and eventually coma. These symptoms may not appear for several hours after the overdose. Take the victim to a hospital emergency room immediately. If you seek treatment, ALWAYS bring the prescription bottle or container.

Special Information

Avoid alcohol and other drugs that depress the nervous system, such as other sedatives, hypnotics, or antihistamines.

Take this medication exactly as prescribed.

Contact your doctor at once if you develop fever, sore throat, nosebleeds, mouth sores, unexplainable black-and-blue marks, or easy bruising or bleeding.

If you forget a dose, take it as soon as you remember. If it is almost time for your next dose, skip the one you forgot and continue with your regular schedule. Do not take a double dose.

Special Populations

Pregnancy/Breast-feeding: Barbiturate use during pregnancy may increase the risk of birth defects and cause bleeding problems, brain tumors, and breathing difficulties in newborns. Regular use of a barbiturate during the last 3 months of pregnancy may cause drug dependency in newborns. However, phenobarbital may be necessary to control major episodes of seizure during pregnancy. Phenobarbital should be taken during pregnancy only if your doctor determines that the potential benefit outweighs the risks.

Barbiturates pass into breast milk. They may cause drowsiness, slow heartbeat, and breathing difficulties in infants. Nursing mothers who must take phenobarbital should use infant formula.

Seniors: Seniors are more sensitive to the effects of barbiturates and often need less medication; phenobarbital should be used with caution in seniors.

Generic Name

Phentermine (FEN-tur-meen) G

Brand Names

Adipex P
Suprenza

Type of Drug

Non-amphetamine appetite suppressant.

Prescribed For

Appetite reduction; weight loss.

General Information

This medication is prescribed as a short-term (several weeks) adjunct in a regimen of diet and exercise for weight reduction in those with obesity. Phentermine may reduce your appetite by working on specific areas of the brain or by increasing the amount of energy your body uses, but is always most effective when combined with behavior modification therapy.

Cautions and Warnings

Do not take this product if you are **allergic** or **sensitive** to phentermine or any of its ingredients.

If you notice any of the following unlikely but very serious side effects, stop taking this medication and consult your doctor or pharmacist immediately: chest pain; difficulty breathing with exercise; decreased ability to exercise; fainting; and swelling of the legs, ankles, or feet.

Phentermine should not be used if you have advanced **heart disease**, moderate to severe **high blood pressure**, **thyroid disease**, or **glaucoma**. Phentermine should also not be used by those in a **manic state** or those with a history of **drug abuse**.

The safety and effectiveness of phentermine in combination with other medications for weight loss, including selective serotonin reuptake inhibitors (SSRIs), has not been established and should be avoided.

Phentermine and other stimulant medicines can worsen problems related to emotional issues, including severe **anxiety**, **bipolar disorder**, **psychosis**, **schizophrenia**, and **substance abuse**. Appetite suppressants can be habit forming.

Phentermine is released from the body through the kidneys. People with **reduced kidney function** are at greater risk for drug side effects.

Phentermine can begin to lose its effect after it is taken for several weeks. If this happens, do not increase your dose without first consulting with your doctor. Taking more can increase side effects and not produce any additional appetite suppression.

Possible Side Effects

- ▼ Common: a false sense of well-being, nervousness, euphoria (feeling "high"), overstimulation, restlessness, and trouble sleeping.
- ▼ Less common: heart palpitations, high blood pressure, weakness, dizziness, tremors, headache, dry mouth, nausea, vomiting, diarrhea and other intestinal disturbances, rash, itching, changes in sex drive, hair loss, muscle pain, difficulty urinating, sweating, chills, blurred vision, and fever.
- ▼ Rare: allergic reactions (rash; itching/swelling of the face, tongue, or throat), drowsiness or sedation, severe dizziness, trouble breathing, severe headache, slurred speech, seizure, weakness on one side of the body, and vision changes. Contact your doctor if you experience anything unusual while taking any medication.

Drug Interactions

- Mixing phentermine with any other appetite suppressant or stimulant, including some herbal products, asthma remedies, and nonprescription decongestant products, can lead to excessive stimulation, nervousness, and elevated blood pressure.
- Do not take phentermine within 2 weeks of taking any monoamine oxidase inhibitor (MAOI) medication. This combination can lead to dangerously high blood pressure.
- Appetite suppressants can work against the effects of some blood-pressure-lowering medications and insulin or oral diabetes medicines.
- When phentermine is combined with an SSRI such as fluoxetine, the risk of serotonin syndrome (symptoms include changes in thinking or behavior, fever, high blood pressure, rapid heart rate, and tremor) are increased.
- You should avoid alcohol while taking phentermine.

Food Interactions

Phentermine should be taken on an empty stomach, before breakfast or 2 hours after. Foods containing caffeine can worsen the stimulating effects of phentermine.

Usual Dose

Adult and Child (age 16 and over): 15–37.5 mg a day taken before breakfast or 2 hours after.

Child (under age 16): not recommended.

Overdosage

Overdose symptoms are restlessness, tremors, shallow breathing, confusion, hallucinations, and fever. Fatigue and depression may follow these symptoms. Other symptoms that can develop after phentermine overdose are blood-pressure changes, cold and clammy skin, nausea, vomiting, diarrhea, and stomach cramps. Take the victim to a hospital emergency room for treatment. If you seek treatment, ALWAYS bring the prescription bottle or container.

Special Information

Do not crush or chew the once-daily version of phentermine.

Phentermine and other appetite suppressants should be taken for no more than 12 weeks and always as part of a total weight-loss program that includes diet, exercise, and counseling. Phentermine does not reduce body weight by itself. You must modify and limit your food intake to lose weight.

Contact your doctor right away if you develop fast, irregular, or pounding heartbeat; mood changes such as agitation, uncontrolled anger, hallucinations, or nervousness; uncontrolled muscle movements; or changes in sexual ability/interest.

Seek immediate medical attention and stop taking phentermine if any of these very serious side effects occur: severe headache, slurred speech, seizure, weakness on one side of the body, or vision changes.

Taking phentermine early in the day will help avoid possible interference with your ability to get a good night's sleep.

Appetite suppressants often cause dry mouth, which increases the chance of cavities and gum disease. Pay special attention to oral hygiene. Dry mouth can be avoided with sugarless candy or gum and ice chips.

Phentermine can interfere with your ability to concentrate. Do not drive or use machinery or perform complicated tasks until you are sure the drug is not affecting your judgment.

If you forget a dose of phentermine, take it as soon as you remember, unless it is almost time for your next dose or it is late in the evening. Then continue with your regular schedule. Do not take a double dose.

Special Populations

Pregnancy/Breast-feeding: Appetite suppressants should not be taken by pregnant women, as large doses have been shown to affect the development of animal fetuses.

Phentermine may pass into breast milk. Nursing mothers who must take this medication should use infant formula.

Seniors: Seniors taking phentermine must be closely supervised by their doctor. Phentermine is released from the body through the kidneys. Seniors may be at greater risk for dizziness and high blood pressure because of normal declines in kidney function. Phentermine and other appetite suppressants can interfere with the management of high blood pressure and diabetes, though weight loss is very desirable in both conditions.

Generic Name

Phenytoin (FEN-it-oh-in) G

Brand Names

Dilantin
Dilantin-125
Dilantin Infatab
Phenytek

The information in this profile also applies to the following drugs:

Generic Ingredients: Ethotoin
Peganone

Generic Ingredients: Fosphenytoin G

Type of Drug

Hydantoin anticonvulsant.

Prescribed For

Epileptic seizure; also prescribed for prevention of seizure following neurosurgery and for abnormal heart rhythm.

General Information

Phenytoin is the most widely prescribed of several hydantoin antiseizure drugs. These drugs all inhibit activity in that area of the brain responsible for grand mal seizures. People may respond to some hydantoins and not others.

Immediate-release phenytoin must be taken several times a day; the sustained-release form can be taken either once or several times a day. Many people find the latter more convenient, but the immediate-release form allows your doctor more flexibility in designing an effective dosage schedule. Phenytoin may be used together with other anticonvulsants, such as phenobarbital.

Drugs that control grand mal seizures do not affect petit mal seizures. Combined drug therapy is needed if both conditions are to be treated.

Cautions and Warnings

Do not take phenytoin if you are **allergic** or **sensitive** to any of its ingredients or to any hydantoin anticonvulsant.

When discontinuing phenytoin, dosage should be gradually reduced over a period of about a week—otherwise, severe seizures may occur.

Antiepileptic drugs, including phenytoin, increase the risk of suicidal thoughts or behavior. Patients and caregivers should be alert for worsening of depression, suicidal thoughts or behavior, and/or any unusual changes in mood or behavior.

Phenytoin may exacerbate symptoms of **porphyria**.

People with **liver disease**, the **elderly**, and those who are **gravely ill** are more likely to experience phenytoin side effects.

Elevated blood sugar has been reported by those taking phenytoin. People with **diabetes** should carefully monitor their blood-sugar levels.

Rash may be a sign of a serious reaction and cause for stopping this medication. The risk of severe skin reactions is greatest in people of Asian heritage. Tell your doctor at once if you notice symptoms such as skin rash and blisters, fever, or itching.

If lymph node enlargement occurs, contact your doctor; you may be advised to substitute another anticonvulsant drug or drug combination.

Possible Side Effects

▼ Most common: drowsiness, rapid or unusual growth of the gums, slurred speech, mental confusion, nystagmus (rhythmic, uncontrolled movement of the eye), dizziness, insomnia, nervousness, uncontrollable twitching, double vision, tiredness, irritability, depression, tremors, and headache. These side effects generally disappear as therapy continues and dosage is reduced.

Possible Side Effects *(continued)*

▼ Less common: nausea, vomiting, diarrhea, constipation, fever, rash, balding, weight gain, numbness in the hands or feet, chest pain, bronchitis, cough, water retention, sensitivity to bright light (especially sunlight), conjunctivitis (pinkeye), joint pain and inflammation, and high blood sugar. Phenytoin may cause coarse facial features, lip enlargement, and Peyronie's disease (in which the penis is permanently deformed or misshapen). Phenytoin rash may be accompanied by fever and may be serious or fatal. Some fatal blood-system side effects have occurred with phenytoin.

▼ Rare: liver damage (including hepatitis and jaundice) and unusual body-hair growth. Contact your doctor if you experience anything unusual while taking any medication.

Drug Interactions

- The following drugs may increase the effects of phenytoin, possibly necessitating a decrease in phenytoin dosage: alcohol in small amounts, amiodarone, anticoagulants, aspirin and other salicylate drugs, azole antifungal medications, benzodiazepine drugs, chloramphenicol, cimetidine, contraceptive drugs, disulfiram, efavirenz, erlotinib, estrogens, felbamate, fluorouracil, halothane, isoniazid, methylphenidate, omeprazole, phenacemide, phenothiazine antipsychotic drugs, phenylbutazone, selective serotonin reuptake inhibitor (SSRI) antidepressants, succinimide antiseizure drugs, sulfa drugs, tacrolimus, ticlopidine, tolbutamide, topiramate, trazodone, tricyclic antidepressants, trimethoprim, and valproic acid.
- The following drugs may interfere with the effects of phenytoin, possibly necessitating an increase in phenytoin dosage: alcohol (chronic use), antacids, anticancer drugs, chloral hydrate, colesevelam, diazoxide, folic acid, protease inhibitors, reserpine, rifabutin, rifampin, sucralfate, theophylline drugs, and vigabatrin.
- Phenytoin may reduce the effectiveness of amiodarone, benzodiazepines, contraceptives, corticosteroids, cyclosporine, deferasirox, digoxin, dopamine, doxycycline, dronedarone, efavirenz, erlotinib, estrogen drugs, etravirine, everolimus,

exemestane, felbamate, felodipine, gefitinib, haloperidol, imatinib, irinotecan, itraconazole, ixabepilone, ketoconazole, levodopa + carbidopa, loop diuretics, maraviroc, methadone, metyrapone, mexiletine, mirtazapine, nisoldipine, non-depolarizing muscle relaxants, paroxetine, phenothiazine antipsychotic drugs, posaconazole, praziquantel, protease inhibitors, quetiapine, quinidine, ranolazine, rifampin, SSRIs, statin drugs, tacrolimus, temsirolimus, teniposide, theophylline drugs, tolbutamide, tolvaptan, topiramate, tyrosine kinase receptor inhibitors, valproic acid, vitamin D, and voriconazole. Dosage increases of these drugs may be necessary.

- Phenytoin may increase the effects of primidone.
- The effect of barbiturate sedatives on phenytoin is unpredictable, and phenytoin may increase barbiturate levels. Blood levels of both drugs as well as seizure activity and side effects should be carefully monitored.
- Phenytoin may increase the risk of liver toxicity caused by acetaminophen, especially if phenytoin is taken regularly. The therapeutic effects of acetaminophen may be reduced.
- Combining carbamazepine and phenytoin yields unpredictable results: The effect of either drug may be reduced or phenytoin side effects may occur.
- Chloramphenical, disopyramide, and warfarin concentrations may be increased or decreased when combined with phenytoin.
- Long-term phenytoin therapy may result in extreme folic acid deficiency, or megaloblastic anemia. This imbalance may be corrected with folic acid supplements.

Food Interactions

Take phenytoin with food to avoid stomach upset. Calcium can slow phenytoin absorption. Separate your phenytoin dose from high-calcium foods, such as milk, cheese, almonds, hazelnuts, and sesame seeds, and calcium supplements by 1–2 hours.

Usual Dose

Adult: starting dose—300 mg a day; maintenance dose—300–400 mg a day. Dosage can be raised gradually to 600 mg a day. Sustained-release phenytoin is taken once a day; the immediate-release form must be taken throughout the day.

Child: starting dose—2.5 mg per lb. of body weight a day, divided into 2 or 3 equal doses; maintenance dose—2–4 mg per lb. of body weight a day. Dosage should be adjusted according to the child's needs. Children age 6 and over may take the adult dosage, but no child should take more than 300 mg a day.

Overdosage

Initial symptoms include drug side effects. At lethal doses, the victim may become comatose with unresponsive pupils. Take the victim to a hospital emergency room at once. If you seek treatment, ALWAYS bring the prescription bottle or container.

Special Information

Contact your doctor at once if you feel unwell or develop a rash, severe nausea or vomiting, swollen glands, swollen or tender gums, yellowing of the skin or whites of the eyes, joint pain, sore throat, fever, unusual bleeding or bruising, persistent headache, infection, slurred speech, or poor coordination.

Always carry a medic alert identification that indicates your medication usage and epilepsy status.

Do not stop taking phenytoin or change dosage without your doctor's knowledge.

Phenytoin may cause drowsiness, dizziness, or blurred vision, effects that are increased by alcoholic beverages. Be careful when driving or doing any task that requires concentration.

Phenytoin may reduce the effectiveness of contraceptive drugs. A non-hormonal or alternative method of birth control should be used during treatment.

Phenytoin sometimes produces a pink-brown color in the urine, which is normal and not a cause for concern.

Good oral hygiene—including gum massage, frequent brushing, and flossing—is very important because phenytoin can cause abnormal growth of your gums.

Do not switch phenytoin brands without notifying your doctor. Different brands may not be equivalent.

If you use phenytoin suspension, be sure to shake the bottle vigorously just before a dose.

Do not use phenytoin capsules that have become discolored. Throw them away.

If you forget a dose, take it as soon as you remember. If you take phenytoin once a day and it is almost time for your next dose, skip the one you forgot and continue with your regular schedule. If you take phenytoin several times a day and do not remember it within 4 hours of your regular time, skip the forgotten dose and go back to your regular schedule. Never take a double dose.

Special Populations

Pregnancy/Breast-feeding: Phenytoin crosses into the fetal circulation. The great majority of mothers who take phenytoin deliver healthy babies, but some are born with fetal hydantoin syndrome though the drug has not been definitively established as the cause. This syndrome consists of skull and face abnormalities, reduced brain size, growth deficiency, deformed fingernails, and mental deficiency. Phenytoin also increases the risk of vitamin K deficiency in newborns, which can lead to serious, life-threatening bleeding during the first 24 hours of life. Also, mothers taking phenytoin may be deficient in vitamin K, increasing the risk of bleeding during delivery. Phenytoin should be taken during pregnancy only if your doctor determines that the potential benefit outweighs the risks.

Phenytoin passes into breast milk. Nursing mothers who must take it should use infant formula.

Seniors: Seniors are more sensitive to phenytoin side effects.

Generic Name

Pimecrolimus (pih-meh-CRO-lim-us)

Brand Names

Elidel Cream

Type of Drug

Immune system modulator.

Prescribed For

Mild to moderate eczema.

General Information

The exact way that pimecrolimus works in the management of mild to moderate dermatitis is unknown. However, it is related to drugs that are used to prevent organ rejection in transplant patients. Extremely small amounts of pimecrolimus are absorbed into the blood after application to the skin. Even after long-term use on more than ½ of the body, blood levels of pimecrolimus cannot be detected.

Cautions and Warnings

Do not use pimecrolimus if you are **allergic** or **sensitive** to any of its ingredients or to other related drugs.

Pimecrolimus has been linked to an increased risk of cancer. Pimecrolimus should not be used in those with **compromised immune systems**. Long-term (over 1 year), continuous use of pimecrolimus should be avoided.

Do not apply pimecrolimus cream to infected skin.

Pimecrolimus may cause a mild warmth or burning sensation. Contact your doctor if this reaction persists for more than 1 week.

Pimecrolimus should not be used on children under age 2.

Possible Side Effects

- ▼ Most common: skin burning, headache, sore throat (with or without nasal pain), infections, fever, and cough.
- ▼ Less common: tonsillitis, chickenpox, runny nose, worsening asthma, wheezing, nosebleeds, painful menstruation, conjunctivitis (pinkeye), eye irritation after application near eyes or lids, skin irritation, back pain, joint pain, and earache.
- ▼ Rare: herpes infection; itching; allergic reactions; swelling of the face, lips, or other application site; toothache; constipation or loose stool; and abdominal pain. Contact your doctor if you experience anything unusual while taking any medication.

Drug Interactions

Potential interactions between pimecrolimus cream and other drugs, including immunizations, have not been studied. Interactions are not expected but may still occur.

- People with widespread skin disease should be cautious about taking atazanavir, calcium channel blockers, cimetidine, clarithromycin, erythromycin, fluconazole, indinavir, itraconazole, ketoconazole, nefazodone, nelfinavir, ritonavir, saquinavir, telithromycin, and voriconazole while using large quantities of pimecrolimus cream.

Usual Dose

Adult and Child (age 2 and over): Apply a thin layer of pimecrolimus to the affected skin twice a day. Rub in gently and completely.

Child (under age 2): not recommended.

Overdosage

There have been no cases of pimecrolimus accidental ingestion. Contact your local poison control center or emergency room for more information. If you seek treatment, ALWAYS bring the prescription bottle or container.

Special Information

Contact your doctor if your condition does not improve after 6 weeks of using pimecrolimus cream.

Notify your doctor if you develop swollen lymph glands, or if warts, blemishes, or any other side effect worsen while using pimecrolimus.

Drinking alcohol while using pimecrolimus may cause adverse effects such as skin flushing or redness.

Avoid exposure to the sun or to artificial sun lamps while using pimecrolimus.

Use pimecrolimus cream only as directed by your doctor. It is only for external application to the skin.

Wash your hands after applying pimecrolimus cream, unless your hands are the area being treated.

Do not bathe, shower, or swim immediately after applying pimecrolimus cream. This could wash off the cream.

Stop using pimecrolimus after your eczema has healed. You can begin using pimecrolimus cream again if the condition recurs.

Do not cover the skin being treated with bandages, dressings, or wraps.

Special Populations

Pregnancy/Breast-feeding: Although animal studies of pimecrolimus reveal no damage to the fetus, pimecrolimus should be used during pregnancy only if your doctor determines that the potential benefit outweighs the risks.

It is not known if pimecrolimus passes into breast milk. Nursing mothers who must use it should use infant formula.

Seniors: The effect of pimecrolimus on seniors is not known.

Type of Drug

Platelet Inhibitors

Brand Names

Generic Ingredients: Clopidogrel
Plavix

Generic Ingredients: Prasugrel
Effient

Generic Ingredients: Ticagrelor
Brilinta

Generic Ingredients: Ticlopidine
Ticlid

Prescribed For

Heart attack and stroke prevention; also used for blood thinning after placement of a vascular stent.

General Information

Artery-clogging blood clots are often the cause of heart attacks and strokes. These drugs reduce the risk of both by helping prevent blood-clot formation. They thin the blood by making platelets—the cells that aggregate to begin the process of clot formation—less "sticky." They start working in as little as 2 hours after taking a single tablet. The drug's blood-thinning effect lasts until the body replaces inactivated platelets. Studies suggest that these medicines are more effective than aspirin in preventing heart attack and stroke in people at risk. People taking 1 of these medicines after stent surgery usually take it for a relatively short period. Those taking them to prevent a heart attack or stroke must take the medication for life.

Clopidogrel must be converted by a liver enzyme system before it can do its work. People who do not respond very well to clopidogrel may have a relatively low level of enzyme activity and are more likely to have a heart attack, stroke, or other event related to blood-clot formation while taking it. Your enzyme activity level may be determined by genetic testing. Some medicines can also affect this enzyme system and therefore affect the activity of this drug (see "Drug Interactions").

Prasugrel was found to be more effective than clopidogrel in preventing clot formation around a stent, but it also causes more bleeding. Ticagrelor has been found to be more effective than clopidogrel in lowering the overall risk of heart attack and death due to heart disease. There is no difference in stroke reduction.

Cautions and Warnings

Do not take platelet inhibitors if you are **allergic** or **sensitive** to any of their ingredients or to ticlopidine, a related antiplatelet. These drugs can rarely cause a rapid drop in white-blood-cell count.

People with **bleeding ulcers**, **brain hemorrhages**, or **other bleeding problems** should use these drugs with caution. Those who are **actively bleeding** should not take them. Prasugrel is more likely to cause major, minor, or life-threatening bleeding than clopidogrel.

Other factors that make you more likely to bleed when taking these drugs include **weight less than 122 lbs.**, having a **tendency to bleed**, and taking other medicines that also increase bleeding risk (see "Drug Interactions").

People who have had a **stroke** or **transient ischemic attack** should not take these medicines.

Thrombotic thrombocytopenic purpura (TTP) is a rare but serious complication of clopidogrel and ticlopidine, sometimes reported after less than 2 weeks of treatment. See your doctor right away if you develop a sudden fever, unusual bruising, nosebleeds, bleeding gums, or any other unusual symptoms. TTP reduces your platelet count, interfering with blood clotting, and affects white-blood-cell count.

People with **liver problems** should use clopidogrel with caution because clopidogrel must be acted on in the liver before it can start working. People with reduced liver function will not respond as well to clopidogrel at first, but tend to reach the same response as other individuals within 10 days. Ticagrelor is broken down in the liver. People with moderate liver disease may not be able to break it down as effectively, possibly raising the amount of ticagrelor in the bloodstream. Dose adjustment is not needed if you have mild liver disease. Those with severe liver disease should not take ticagrelor.

People taking prasugrel should also be taking aspirin every day. Clopidogrel may be taken with aspirin as well. The choice of aspirin dose (75–325 mg) is up to your doctor. Daily doses of aspirin larger than 100 mg counter the blood-thinning effect of ticagrelor.

People taking ticagrelor may be more likely to have breathing problems.

Possible Side Effects

Clopidogrel

- ▼ Most common: rash and other skin problems.
- ▼ Common: chest pain, accidents, flu-like symptoms, pain, headache, dizziness, abdominal pain, upset stomach, joint pain, back pain, black-and-blue marks, and respiratory infection.
- ▼ Less common: tiredness, swollen arms or legs, high blood pressure, diarrhea, nausea, bleeding, nosebleeds, breathing difficulties, runny nose, coughing, bronchitis, high blood cholesterol, urinary infection, and depression.
- ▼ Rare: bleeding in the brain and stomach ulcer. Contact your doctor if you experience anything unusual while taking any medication.

Prasugrel

- ▼ Most common: bleeding.
- ▼ Common: high blood pressure, high blood-lipid levels, headache, back pain, dizziness, abdominal pain, and upset stomach.
- ▼ Less common: difficulty breathing; nausea; cough; low blood pressure; fatigue; chest pain (not related to heart attack); heartbeat changes (fast or slow); low white-blood-cell count; rash; fever; swelling in the hands, feet, or ankles; arm or leg pain; and diarrhea.
- ▼ Rare: bleeding in the brain and stomach ulcer. Contact your doctor if you experience anything unusual while taking any medication.

Ticagrelor

- ▼ Most common: difficulty breathing.
- ▼ Common: headache and bleeding (rarely fatal).
- ▼ Less common: cough, dizziness, nausea, abnormal heart rhythm, blood-pressure changes, chest pain, diarrhea, back pain, and fatigue.
- ▼ Rare: fainting and painful, enlarged male breasts. Contact your doctor if you experience anything unusual while taking any medication

Ticlopidine

- ▼ Most common: diarrhea, nausea, upset stomach, rash, and stomach pain.

Possible Side Effects *(continued)*

▼ Less common: reduced white-blood-cell counts, vomiting, bruising, gas, itching, dizziness, appetite loss, and liver function changes.

Drug Interactions

- Clopidogrel may interfere with the body's ability to break down fluvastatin, nonsteroidal anti-inflammatory drugs (NSAIDs), phenytoin, tamoxifen, tolbutamide, torsemide, and warfarin.
- Combining these drugs with NSAIDs may increase blood loss and bleeding in the stomach and intestines.
- Do not combine these drugs with other antiplatelet drugs, direct thrombin inhibitors, or the anticoagulant (blood thinner) warfarin unless you are under your doctor's direct supervision. This interaction may prevent normal blood clotting and lead to severe bleeding problems.
- Calcium channel blockers block the antiplatelet effects of clopidogrel. Avoid this combination.
- Carbamazepine, norethindrone, prednisone, and rifampicin stimulate the enzyme system responsible for converting clopidogrel to its active form, increasing the amount of clopidogrel in the body. Prasugrel is a weak inhibitor of 1 liver enzyme system but is not expected to have an important effect on drugs broken down by it, including bupropion, halothane, nevirapine, and cyclophosphamide.
- The acid reducer omeprazole inhibits the enzyme that breaks down clopidogrel and reduces its effect. Other medicines that have a similar effect on clopidogrel and should be avoided are chloramphenicol, cimetidine, etravirine, felbamate, fluconazole, fluoxetine, fluvoxamine, indomethacin, ketoconazole, lansoprazole, modafinil, oxcarbazepine, pantoprazole, probenecid, rabeprazole, ticlopidine, and topiramate. These drugs also affect blood levels of prasugrel, but not to the extent that drug dose may have to be altered. Acid reducers may be prescribed to combat the upset stomach associated with clopidogrel.
- Do not mix ticagrelor with amiodarone, atazanavir, calcium channel blockers, clarithromycin, cyclosporine, erythromycin, indinavir, itraconazole, ketoconazole, nefazodone, nelfinavir, quinidine, ritonavir, saquinavir, sirolimus, tacrolimus, telithromycin, or voriconazole. These drugs increase the speed with

which ticagrelor is broken down in the body by slowing the release of metabolizing enzymes from the liver.

- Carbamazepine, dexamethasone, efavirenz, modafinil, nevirapine, oxcarbezine, phenobarbital, phenytoin, pioglitazone, rifabutin, rifampin, and St. John's wort can increase the speed at which ticagrelor is broken down, raising the risk of bleeding. Do not mix them.
- Do not take more than 40 mg daily of the statin cholesterol-lowering drugs pravastatin or simvastatin with ticagrelor. This combination carries a greater risk of statin side effects because of interference with statin metabolism. Atorvastatin is not affected to the same extent.
- Digoxin levels may be affected by ticagrelor. Your doctor should check digoxin blood levels when you start ticagrelor.
- Aspirin interacts with these medicines in different ways. Aspirin can be taken with ticagrelor, but you should not take more than 100 mg a day. Prasugrel should be taken with aspirin every day. Clopidogrel may be taken with aspirin.
- Antacids reduce the absorption of ticlopidine. Separate doses by at least 1 hour.
- Taking cimetidine on a regular basis can reduce the clearance of ticlopidine from the body by 50%, increasing the risk of drug toxicity and side effects.
- Ticlopidine reduces the body's clearance of theophylline; your doctor may need to reduce your theophylline dosage.
- Ticlopidine increases the effects of phenytoin and tizanidine. Use caution if taking these drugs simultaneously

Food Interactions

Ticlopidine should be taken at the same meal times every day to reduce stomach upset and gain maximum benefit. The other medicines can be taken without regard to food or meals.

Usual Dose

Clopidogrel

Adult: 75 mg a day.

Prasugrel

Adult: 60 mg to start, then 5–10 mg once a day.

Ticagrelor

Adult: Two 90-mg tablets to start, then 1 tablet twice a day; maintenance dose of 90 mg a day. You may take 1 dose of aspirin (usually 1 regular tablet or 325 mg) when you start ticagrelor and then continue with a daily dose of 75–100 mg of aspirin.

Ticlopidine

Adult: 250 mg taken twice a day with food.

Overdosage

The action of these drugs on platelets cannot be immediately reversed. Their effect is only reversed when the inactive platelet is replaced, usually in 8–12 days. Overdose symptoms can include bleeding, nausea, vomiting, abnormal heart rhythms, tear formation, staggering, sluggishness, and uneven breathing. For ticlopidine, other possible effects include stomach bleeding, convulsions, breathing difficulties, and low body temperature. Overdose victims should be taken to a hospital emergency room. If you seek treatment, ALWAYS bring the prescription bottle or container.

Special Information

You will bruise more easily while taking these medicines and minor cuts may take longer to stop bleeding. If you are having surgery, make sure your doctor knows you are taking clopidogrel or prasugrel. You may have to stop taking the drug 1 week before surgery.

Besides surgery, make sure your doctor knows if you have a history of stroke, stomach ulcer, colon polyps or bleeding, liver problems, or breathing problems, or if you have had a recent serious injury or are planning a dental procedure.

Make sure your doctor knows all the medicines and supplements you take, especially those for HIV/AIDS, heart problems or blood pressure, high cholesterol, seizures, fungal infection, or if you are taking a blood thinner.

Contact your doctor if you develop a rash, swelling under the skin, a sudden fever, difficulty urinating, bleeding, vomiting, diarrhea, weakness or feeling ill, high blood pressure, headache, stroke-like loss of body control, difficulty swallowing, confusion, stupor, coma, or seizures. These may be symptoms of a rare complication of clopidogrel and ticlopidine known as TTP (see "Cautions and Warnings").

It is best to take these medicines exactly as directed. Stopping them too soon increases the risk of clot formation around a new stent, heart attack, and death.

If you forget a dose, take it as soon as you remember. If it is almost time for your next dose, skip the forgotten dose and continue with your regular schedule. Contact your doctor if you forget 2 or more doses in a row.

Special Populations

Pregnancy/Breast-feeding: The safety of using these drugs during pregnancy is not known. Other antiplatelet drugs, such as aspirin, are avoided during pregnancy due to their possible effects on mother and fetus. An antiplatelet should be taken during pregnancy only if your doctor determines that the potential benefit outweighs the risks.

These drugs may pass into breast milk. Nursing mothers who must take this drug should use infant formula.

Seniors: Seniors may take clopidogrel without special precaution. However, in seniors age 75 and over, prasugrel is better for high-risk patients who have diabetes or those who have already had a heart attack. Others in that age group should generally not take prasugrel because of the increased stroke risk and its questionable benefit. There are no restrictions for seniors taking ticagrelor.

Plavix *see **Platelet Inhibitors,** page 920*

Generic Name

Podofilox (poe-DUH-fil-ox) G

Brand Names

Condylox

Type of Drug

Antimitotic drug.

Prescribed For

External genital and perianal warts.

General Information

Podofilox, which can be either manufactured from chemicals or purified from natural sources, kills visible wart tissues. Exactly how it works is not known. Condyloma or genital warts are caused by the human papillomavirus and can appear in various places, including the sex organs, anus, and abdomen. Podofilox is not recommended for treatment of mucous membrane warts. The risk of developing warts increases if your immune system is suppressed.

Cautions and Warnings

Do not use podofilox if you are **allergic** or **sensitive** to any of its ingredients.

Proper diagnosis of genital warts is necessary before you use this product. See your doctor before you start using podofilox. Podofilox is for external use only. Do not use podofilox for any other purpose.

If you get podofilox in your eyes, wash it out at once with cool water and seek medical attention.

Podofilox is flammable. Keep away from any open flame.

Possible Side Effects

- ▼ Most common: burning, pain, inflammation, skin erosion, itching, and bleeding.
- ▼ Common: pain during intercourse, sleeplessness, tingling, tenderness, chafing, bad odor, dizziness, scarring, small sores or ulcers, dryness, difficulty retracting the foreskin, blood in the urine, vomiting, headache, stinging, and redness.
- ▼ Less common: skin peeling, scabbing, skin discoloration, tenderness, crusting, skin cracks, soreness, swelling, rash, and blisters.

Drug Interactions

None known.

Usual Dose

Adult: Apply the solution or gel, morning and night—every 12 hours—for 3 consecutive days, and then apply nothing for 4 days. Repeat this cycle for up to 4 weeks in a row. Use the cotton-tipped applicator supplied with the solution, or your finger if you are using the gel. Try to limit the amount of podofilox that gets on intact skin. Thoroughly wash your hands before and after each application.

Child: not recommended.

Overdosage

Swallowing podofilox may lead to nausea, vomiting, fever, diarrhea, mouth sores, tingling in the hands or feet, changes in mental state, lethargy, coma, rapid breathing, respiratory failure, blood in the urine, kidney failure, and seizures. Excess podofilox should be washed off the skin as soon as possible. In case of overdose or accidental ingestion, take the victim to a hospital emergency room. If you seek treatment, ALWAYS bring the prescription bottle or container.

Special Information

Contact your doctor if you develop any bothersome or persistent side effect. If you do not see any improvement in 4 weeks, stop using the drug and contact your doctor.

Data is not available on the use of podofilox solution for the treatment of warts in the mucous membranes of the genital area including the urethra, rectum, and vagina. Use podofilox exactly as directed by your doctor.

If you forget a dose, apply it as soon as you remember. If it is within 4 hours of your next dose, skip the dose you forgot and continue with your regular schedule.

Special Populations

Pregnancy/Breast-feeding: Podofilox is toxic to animal fetuses at very high dosages. Podofilox should be used during pregnancy only if your doctor determines that the potential benefit outweighs the risks.

It is not known if podofilox passes into breast milk. Nursing mothers who must use it should use infant formula.

Seniors: Seniors may use podofilox without special precaution.

Generic Name

Polyethylene Glycol 3350

(pah-lee-ETH-ih-leen GLYE-cohl) G

Brand Names

GlycoLax MiraLax

Type of Drug

Osmotic laxative.

Prescribed For

Occasional constipation.

General Information

Polyethylene glycol (PEG) laxatives work by preventing water in the stool from being reabsorbed into the body. Other osmotic laxatives such as lactulose, phosphates, citrate of magnesia, and milk of magnesia work by this same mechanism. However, they are not always interchangeable. PEG laxatives soften the stool and help it to pass out of the body. PEG laxatives usually take 2–4 days to produce a bowel movement. Regularity may take a week or more. PEG is also an ingredient in other laxative products, which can contain a stimulant laxative, vitamin C, sodium, and potassium.

Cautions and Warnings

Do not use a PEG laxative if you are **allergic** or **sensitive** to any of its ingredients. The chances of having a PEG allergy are very rare.

Excess use of a PEG laxative can lead to diarrhea and dehydration.

PEG laxatives should be used with caution if you have appendicitis or signs of **appendicitis** (**rectal bleeding**, **colostomy**, **ileostomy**) or signs of **intestinal blockage** (**nausea**, **vomiting**, **abdominal pain**, or **distention**).

PEG laxatives may be preferable over other laxative types for people with **high blood pressure**, **heart or kidney disease**, or some **gastrointestinal (GI) diseases**.

People with **eating disorders** should not use these products without consulting a doctor.

Overuse of this or any other laxative product can lead to laxative dependence and chronic constipation.

Possible Side Effects

- ▼ Common: nausea, cramps, and stomach gas.
- ▼ Less common: confusion, dizziness or lightheadedness, bloating, thirst, and diarrhea.
- ▼ Rare: sweating, irregular heartbeat, unusual tiredness or weakness, and blood in the stool. Contact your doctor if you experience anything unusual while taking any medication.

Drug Interactions

- Laxatives can interfere with the absorption of drugs in the GI tract. Other oral medicines must be taken at least 1 hour before or 2 hours after your laxative dose.

Food Interactions

These products can be taken without regard to food or meals.

Usual Dose

Adult and Child (age 7 and over): 17 g (about 1 heaping tbsp.) once a day for up to 14 days.

Child (under age 6): 1 mg per lb. of body weight once a day, up to a maximum dose of 17 g.

Overdosage

Overdose of PEG laxatives can lead to dehydration and sodium and potassium imbalance, which can cause abnormal heart rhythms and other heart problems. Overdose victims should be taken to a hospital emergency room. If you seek treatment, ALWAYS bring the prescription bottle or container.

Special Information

Contact your doctor if you have had no bowel movement or are still irregular after taking a PEG laxative for 7 days in a row, or if you develop bloody diarrhea, blood in the stool, severe cramping, or signs of a drug reaction or allergy (rash, itching, swelling, or dizziness).

Tell your doctor if you have nausea, vomiting, severe stomach pain, ulcerative colitis, irritable bowel syndrome, kidney disease, or if you have had a sudden change in bowel habits that has lasted 2 weeks or longer.

Mix the powder with a full glass of water, juice, soda, coffee, or tea. Stir well until the powder is completely dissolved before swallowing the mixture.

If you forget a dose of your PEG laxative, take it as soon as you remember. If you do not remember until it is almost time for your next dose, skip the one you forgot and continue with your regular schedule. Do not take a double dose of this medicine.

Special Populations

Pregnancy/Breast-feeding: PEG laxatives may be used during pregnancy if needed but can be harmful to the developing fetus if they are overused. Other laxative types, such as stool softeners or bulk-forming laxatives, are used more commonly. Tell your doctor if you are pregnant or become pregnant while using a PEG laxative. It should be taken during pregnancy only if your doctor determines that the potential benefit outweighs the risks.

It is unlikely that this drug will directly affect a nursing infant. Nursing mothers may occasionally use PEG laxative products if needed.

Seniors: Seniors may be more sensitive to the laxative effects of PEG laxatives; diarrhea is more likely.

Type of Drug

Potassium Replacements

Brand Names

There are many brand-name potassium replacement products, the most common of which are listed here. Many are available over the counter.

K-Dur 20 Klor-Con K-Tab

Generic Ingredients: Potassium G

Generic Ingredients: Potassium Chloride G

Generic Ingredients: Potassium Gluconate G

Generic Ingredients: Potassium Salt Combination G

Prescribed For

Hypokalemia (low blood-potassium levels) and mild hypertension (high blood pressure).

General Information

A major component of body fluids, potassium helps to maintain electrolyte balance, kidney function, and blood pressure. Low potassium levels, which can affect the central nervous system and heart functions, are usually caused by extended diuretic treatment, severe diarrhea, vomiting, complications of diabetes, or other medical conditions.

Potassium supplements are available in different types and forms. Potassium chloride is most often prescribed because it contains the most potassium per unit weight. Another advantage of potassium chloride is that it provides chloride ion, an important body-fluid component. Potassium gluconate provides about ⅓ as much potassium as the chloride, so you have to take 3 times as much to get an equal dose of potassium. However, it is preferable to potassium chloride in circumstances where chloride is undesirable.

Cautions and Warnings

Do not take potassium if you are **allergic** or **sensitive** to any of its ingredients. Potassium replacement therapy should always be monitored and controlled by your doctor.

Do not take potassium if you have severe **kidney disease**, **untreated Addison's disease**, or **high blood-potassium levels** due to dehydration, excessive sun or heat exposure, or other medications that elevate potassium levels.

Anyone with a condition that causes **obstruction or delay of passage through the gastrointestinal (GI) tract**, such as diabetic gastroparesis, should use the liquid form of potassium. People taking medications that slow GI movement, such as anticholinergic drugs, should also use the liquid form.

Potassium tablets have caused ulcers of the esophagus in some people with **compression of the esophagus**, who should use the liquid form. Potassium tablets have been reported to cause small-bowel ulcer, leading to obstruction or perforation (formation of a hole through the bowel into the abdomen). Symptoms of bowel obstruction or perforation are severe vomiting, abdominal pain or distention, and GI bleeding (indicated by black or tarry stools). **Seniors**, people with **diabetes** or **scleroderma**, and people who have had **mitral valve replacement** may be at higher risk for ulcers.People who take potassium may develop hyperkalemia (high blood-potassium levels). Hyperkalemia can develop rapidly, without warning or symptoms, and is potentially fatal. It is often discovered through an electrocardiogram (ECG), but the following symptoms may also occur: tingling in the hands and feet, a feeling of heaviness or weakness in the muscles, listlessness, confusion, low blood pressure, extreme difficulty moving the arms and legs, abnormal heart rhythms, weak pulse, loss of consciousness, pallor, restlessness, and low urine output.

Possible Side Effects

- ▼ Most common: nausea, vomiting, diarrhea, gas, and abdominal discomfort.
- ▼ Rare: skin rash. Contact your doctor immediately if you experience tingling in the hands or feet, weakness and heaviness in the legs, listlessness, mental confusion, decreased blood pressure, and heart-rhythm changes. Contact your doctor if you experience anything unusual while taking any medication.

Drug Interactions

- Potassium supplements should not be taken with the potassium-sparing diuretics spironolactone, triamterene, or amiloride. Severe hyperkalemia may occur.
- Anticholinergic agents may stop or delay the passage of potassium supplements through the GI tract. They should not be taken together.
- Combining supplements with an angiotensin-converting enzyme (ACE) inhibitor may result in hyperkalemia.
- People taking digitalis drugs must keep their blood-potassium levels within acceptable limits. Too little potassium in the blood may increase digitalis side effects and toxic reactions.

Food Interactions

Eating excess salt contributes to the problem of potassium depletion. Salt substitutes contain large amounts of potassium; do not use them while taking a potassium supplement unless directed by your doctor. If stomach upset occurs, take potassium supplements after meals or with food.

Usual Dose

Hypokalemia: prevention—16–24 milliequivalents (mEq) a day; treatment—40–100 mEq a day.

Potassium Depletion: 40–100 mEq a day.

Overdosage

Symptoms include muscle weakness, tingling in the hands or feet, a feeling of heaviness in the legs, listlessness, confusion, breathing difficulties, low blood pressure, shock, abnormal heart rhythms, and heart attack. Contact your local poison control center or a hospital emergency room for more information. If you seek treatment, ALWAYS bring the prescription bottle or container.

Special Information

Directions for taking and using any potassium supplement must be followed closely. Effervescent tablets, powders, and liquids should be properly and completely dissolved, or diluted in 3–8 oz. of cold water or juice and drunk slowly. Noneffervescent tablets or capsules should never be chewed or crushed; they must be swallowed whole, preferably after a meal and with a full glass of water.

Many of the controlled-release potassium supplements contain potassium distributed throughout an indigestible wax core or matrix; you may notice the depleted wax matrix in your stool several hours after swallowing a tablet. This is normal and not a cause for alarm.

Contact your doctor at once if you experience tingling in your hands or feet, a feeling of heaviness in the legs, unusual tiredness or weakness, nausea, vomiting, continued abdominal pain, black stool, if you have trouble swallowing the tablets, or if the tablets seem to stick in your throat.

If you forget a dose, take it right away if you remember within 2 hours of your regular time. If you do not remember until later, skip the dose you forgot and go back to your regular schedule. Do not take a double dose.

Special Populations

Pregnancy/Breast-feeding: The safety of using potassium salts during pregnancy is not known. A potassium supplement should only be taken during pregnancy if your doctor determines that the potential benefit outweighs the risks.

Normal doses of potassium supplements add little to the potassium already in breast milk. Exercise caution and do not take higher doses without consulting your doctor.

Seniors: Seniors may be at higher risk for ulcers caused by potassium supplements.

Generic Name

Pramipexole (pram-ih-PEX-ole) G

Brand Names

Mirapex

Type of Drug

Antiparkinsonian.

Prescribed For

Parkinson's disease and moderate to severe restless legs syndrome.

General Information

Pramipexole is thought to relieve symptoms of Parkinson's disease and restless legs syndrome by stimulating dopamine receptors in the brain. Studies of pramipexole in people with early Parkinson's disease showed improvement after 4 weeks of treatment.

People with advanced Parkinson's disease showed improvement after 6 months.

Restless legs syndrome is a condition that affects about 1 out of every 10 people. Symptoms include an urge to move the legs, usually accompanied by, or caused by, uncomfortable leg sensations. Symptoms begin or worsen during periods of rest or inactivity for most people and are partly or totally relieved by movement. Symptoms usually worsen or occur only in the evening or at night and can disturb sleep. People with restless legs syndrome taking pramipexole may show improvement in symptoms as early as 3 weeks.

Cautions and Warnings

Do not take pramipexole if you are **allergic** or **sensitive** to any of its ingredients.

Pramipexole may make you fall asleep, sometimes suddenly, during the day. Avoid alcohol and use extreme caution when driving or engaging in a potentially hazardous activity.

Pramipexole may cause low blood pressure and make you dizzy or faint when rising from a sitting or lying position, especially during the early stages of treatment.

Pramipexole, like other dopamine stimulants, may worsen pathological gambling, hypersexuality, or overeating, or other **impulsive/compulsive behaviors**, which are generally reversible if the dose is reduced or the drug stopped.

About 1 in 10–15 people who take pramipexole experience hallucinations that may be serious enough to require stopping drug therapy.

One person taking pramipexole developed rhabdomyolysis, a disease in which skeletal muscle tissue is broken down and released into the bloodstream. This condition was resolved when pramipexole therapy was stopped.

Twenty percent of people taking pramipexole for restless legs syndrome experienced their symptoms 2 hours earlier than usual; the reason is unknown.

Those with **kidney disease** should use pramipexole with caution.

People with **Parkinson's disease** have 2–6 times the risk of developing skin cancer (melanoma). It is not known if the increased risk is due to the condition or the drugs used to manage it. People taking this medication should frequently check themselves for skin cancers and see a dermatologist regularly.

Possible Side Effects

Advanced Parkinson's Disease

- Most common: dizziness or fainting when rising from a sitting or lying position, abnormal movements, tremors, muscle rigidity, and hallucinations.
- Common: insomnia.
- Less common: accidental injury, weakness, generalized swelling, chest pain, feeling unwell, abnormal dreaming, confusion, sleepiness, unusual muscle spasms, unusual walking, muscle stiffness, memory loss, a tendency to frequently change positions or pace the floor, odd thoughts, paranoid reactions, delusions, sleeping problems, urinary problems, swelling in the arms or legs, arthritis, twitching, bursitis, muscle weakness, breathing difficulties, runny nose, pneumonia, visual difficulties, constipation, dry mouth, and rash.

Early Parkinson's Disease

- Most common: sleepiness or tiredness and nausea.
- Common: insomnia, hallucinations, and constipation.
- Less common: dizziness, confusion, memory loss, reduced touch sensation, loss of muscle tone, a tendency to frequently change positions or pace the floor, odd thoughts, loss of sex drive, impotence, unusual muscle spasms, swelling in the arms or legs, generalized swelling, appetite loss, difficulty swallowing, weight loss, weakness, feeling unwell, fever, and abnormal vision.

Restless Legs Syndrome

- Most common: nausea, tiredness, and sleepiness.
- Common: constipation.
- Less common: diarrhea, dry mouth, fatigue, insomnia, and abnormal dreaming.

Drug Interactions

- Pramipexole increases levodopa + carbidopa blood levels and may worsen the uncontrolled muscle spasms that occur with levodopa + carbidopa. Your doctor may reduce your dosage of levodopa + carbidopa.
- Drugs that increase the effects of pramipexole include amantadine, cimetidine, diltiazem, quinidine, quinine, ranitidine, triamterene, and verapamil. Dosage adjustment may be required.

- Haloperidol and other antipsychotics, metoclopramide, phenothiazine sedatives, thioxanthene sedatives, and other drugs that antagonize the effects of dopamine can reduce the effect of pramipexole.
- Pramipexole increases the sedative effect of benzodiazepines, sleeping pills, and other nervous system depressants.

Food Interactions

You may take pramipexole with food to prevent nausea.

Usual Dose

Parkinson's Disease

Adult: 0.125 mg 3 times a day to start, gradually increasing to a maximum of 4.5 mg a day. Dosage is reduced for people with kidney disease.

Child: not recommended.

Restless Legs Syndrome

Adult: 0.125 mg taken once a day 2–3 hours before bedtime to start, gradually increasing to a maximum of 0.5 mg a day.

Child: not recommended.

Overdosage

Little is known about the effects of pramipexole overdose. Symptoms are likely to include the most common side effects. Take the victim to a hospital emergency room. If you seek treatment, ALWAYS bring the prescription bottle or container.

Special Information

Take this drug exactly as prescribed.

Pramipexole causes sedation. Be careful when driving or performing any task that requires concentration. Avoid alcohol and other nervous system depressants.

Contact your doctor if you develop hallucinations or any bothersome or persistent side effect.

If you forget a dose, take it as soon as you remember. For Parkinson's disease, space the remaining daily dosage evenly throughout the day. Continue with your regular schedule on the next day. Do not take a double dose.

Special Populations

Pregnancy/Breast-feeding: The safety of using pramipexole during pregnancy is not known. Pramipexole should be taken during pregnancy only if your doctor determines that the potential benefit outweighs the risks.

It is not known if pramipexole passes into breast milk, but this drug can interfere with milk production. Nursing mothers who must take this drug should use infant formula.

Seniors: Seniors are more likely to experience side effects.

Generic Name

Pramlintide (PRAM-lin-tide)

Brand Names

Symlin

Type of Drug

Amylinomimetic.

Prescribed For

Type 1 and 2 diabetes treated with mealtime insulin therapy without satisfactory control.

General Information

Pramlintide is a synthetic form of amylin, a natural hormone that helps control blood sugar. Natural amylin is found in the same part of the pancreas as insulin and it is released into the blood at the same time as insulin. Amylin is also deficient when inadequate amounts of insulin are released by the pancreas. Amylin affects blood-sugar levels in 3 ways. First, it slows the movement of food from the stomach to the small intestine without reducing the overall type and amount of nutrient absorbed from the food. Slowing the movement of food helps because it spreads out the absorption of sugar, avoiding dangerous sugar spikes. Second, amylin also reduces the amount of glucagon released into the bloodstream. Glucagon is a hormone that raises blood sugar released from storage sites in the liver. Third, amylin helps to control your appetite, reducing overall food intake. Pramlintide exerts all the same effects as natural amylin.

Cautions and Warnings

Do not take pramlintide if you are **allergic** or **sensitive** to it or any of its ingredients, including metacresol.

Do not take this drug if you have **gastroparesis**, a diabetes-related condition in which stomach emptying is delayed.

The combination of insulin and pramlintide has been associated with an increased risk of very low blood sugar, especially in people with **type 1 diabetes**. People who have **hypoglycemia unawareness**, or difficulty detecting if or when they have low blood sugar should not use pramlintide. If very low blood sugar is going to occur, it will be within the 3 hours after pramlintide injection.

Do not take pramlintide if you have trouble following your current insulin regimen, have trouble doing regular blood-sugar testing, have a **hemoglobin A1C level above 9%**, or have had several bouts of low blood sugar in which you needed help from another person in the past 6 months.

Antibodies to pramlintide may develop, but antibody levels generally go down with time. Most patients who develop antibodies still have good sugar control and similar types of side effects as people who do not develop pramlintide antibodies.

Possible Side Effects

- ▼ Most common: nausea (usually clears up on its own), appetite loss, headache, vomiting, and very low blood sugar (type 1 diabetes).
- ▼ Common: abdominal pain, dizziness, coughing, sore throat, joint pain, fatigue, and allergic reaction.
- ▼ Less common: very low blood sugar (type 2 diabetes).
- ▼ Rare: reactions where you inject the medication. Other rare side effects can occur in almost any part of the body. Contact your doctor if you experience anything unusual while taking any medication.

Drug Interactions

- Do not take pramlintide if you take drugs that affect stomach emptying, including atropine, or medications that slow nutrient absorption from your intestines, such as alpha-glucosidase inhibitors (e.g., miglitol).
- Pramlintide will slow the rate, but not the total amount, at which some drugs are absorbed into the bloodstream. Take all your pills at least 1 hour before or 2 hours after you inject pramlintide to avoid this interaction.
- Beta blockers, clonidine, guanethidine, and reserpine can mask signs of low blood sugar.
- Doses of other blood-sugar-lowering drugs may need to be modified when you start taking pramlintide. Other drugs that

can increase the blood-sugar-lowering effect of this drug include ACE inhibitors, disopyramide, fibrates, fluoxetine, monoamine oxidase inhibitor (MAOI) antidepressants, pentoxifylline, salicylates, and sulfa antibiotics.

Usual Dose

Adult: 15–60 mcg (type 1 diabetes) or 60–120 mcg (type 2 diabetes) by subcutaneous injection immediately before all major meals (250 or more calories; 30 or more grams of carbohydrate).

Child: not recommended.

Overdosage

The effects of pramlintide overdose are severe nausea, vomiting, diarrhea, dizziness, flushing, and drops in blood pressure. Overdose victims should be taken to a hospital emergency room for evaluation and treatment. If you seek treatment, ALWAYS bring the prescription bottle or container.

Special Information

Pramlintide injections must be given separately from insulin. These drugs cannot be mixed in the same syringe. Always use a new needle and syringe for each insulin and pramlintide injection.

Each dose of pramlintide must be given as an injection under the skin of the thigh or abdomen immediately before all your meals. Do not inject pramlintide into the arm. For more information on injections, see page 1242.

If you forget a dose of pramlintide, skip the forgotten dose and continue with your regular injection just before your next meal. Do not take a double dose.

Unopened pramlintide should be kept in a refrigerator. Never freeze it. Opened vials of pramlintide may be stored for 28 days in a refrigerator or at room temperature no greater than 86°F. Frozen, overheated, or opened vials older than 28 days must be thrown away.

Pramlintide injection is a clear solution. Do not use it if there is any discoloration or cloudiness, or if there are any particles floating in it.

Make sure you know the signs and symptoms of low blood sugar (hunger, headache, sweating, tremor, or irritability; severe symptoms include difficulty concentrating, loss of consciousness, coma, or seizure) and are aware of how your body reacts. Serious injuries can occur if very low blood sugar develops while you are driving, operating heavy machinery, or engaging in other high-risk activities. Your doctor may cut your pre-meal short-acting insulin dose in ½ when you start taking pramlintide.

Do frequent pre- and post-meal blood-sugar testing, and keep a source of sugar on hand.

This drug can cause appetite loss and weight reduction. Do not change your regular dosage if this happens to you.

Special Populations

Pregnancy/Breast-feeding: In animal studies of up to 47 times the usual human dose, pramlintide was associated with some birth defects. Pramlintide should be taken during pregnancy only if your doctor determines that the potential benefit outweighs the risks.

It is not known if this drug passes into breast milk. Nursing mothers taking pramlintide should use infant formula.

Seniors: Seniors may take this drug without special restriction, although careful monitoring and management to avoid very low blood sugar is important.

Generic Name

Pregabalin (pre-GAB-ah-lin)

Brand Names

Lyrica

Type of Drug

Anticonvulsant, pain reliever.

Prescribed For

Fibromyalgia, nerve pain associated with diabetes, pain after herpes zoster (shingles) infection, and partial onset seizures.

General Information

The exact mechanism of pregabalin is not known, but it does bind to tissues in the central nervous system where there is a high flow of calcium. Limiting calcium flow may be the key to its pain-relieving and antiseizure effects. For fibromyalgia, it relieves pain and helps improve daily functioning, but it may not work for everyone. This drug is unique because, unlike others prescribed for partial onset seizures, it does not bind to or affect gamma-aminobutyric acid (GABA) receptors or GABA itself in the brain. It does not affect the flow of sodium in the brain or stimulate opiate receptors. It also does not affect dopamine, serotonin, or norepinephrine, common areas of action for other central-nervous-system drugs.

Cautions and Warnings

Do not take pregabalin if you are **allergic** or **sensitive** to any of its ingredients. Potentially serious reactions include swelling of the face, mouth, lips, gums, tongue, or neck and trouble breathing. People who have had previous episodes of **swelling** and those taking medications associated with increased risk of swelling should take pregabalin with caution. Other reactions include rash, hives, and blisters.

As with other medications to control seizures, increased seizures and symptoms of diarrhea, headache, insomnia, and nausea may occur if pregabalin is abruptly stopped or greatly reduced.

People taking this drug are more likely to have suicidal thoughts or attempt suicide.

People taking pregabalin may accumulate fluid in their legs or arms. People with **congestive heart failure** should take this medication with caution.

Pregabalin may make you dizzy or tired, or interfere with your concentration. People taking this drug may gain weight. In one study of more than 325 people, they gained an average of more than 11 lbs. over 2 years.

Pregabalin may cause blurred vision.

Pregabalin passes out of the body through the kidneys. People with **kidney disease** require lower doses or an extended time between doses.

People with a history of **drug abuse** may be more likely to become dependent on this medicine.

In animal studies, pregabalin reduced sperm counts, increased the numbers of abnormal sperm, and interfered with the ability to reproduce. There were also birth defects. These effects have been studied in humans but are not confirmed.

Possible Side Effects

- ▼ Common: dizziness, tiredness, dry mouth, loss of muscular coordination, swelling in the arms or legs, blurred or double vision, weight gain, and loss of concentration.
- ▼ Less common: accidental injury, increased appetite, constipation, tremors, headache, memory loss, speech disorders, unusual walk, and urinary problems.

Possible Side Effects *(continued)*

▼ Rare: Rare side effects can occur in almost any part of the body, but may not depend on the amount of pregabalin you are taking. Contact your doctor if you experience anything unusual while taking any medication.

Drug Interactions

- Taking pregabalin with an angiotensin-converting enzyme (ACE) inhibitor such as captopril may increase your chance of developing swelling or hives.
- Alcohol, sedatives, lorazepam, opiates, and other nervous system depressants may increase the depressant effects of pregabalin.
- Because of an increased risk of heart failure, pregabalin should be used with caution with thiazolidinedione antidiabetes medication such as pioglitazone or rosiglitazone.

Food Interactions

Pregabalin can be taken without regard to food or meals.

Usual Dose

Adult: 150–450 mg a day in divided doses, depending on the condition being treated. People with reduced kidney function must receive lower doses of pregabalin.

Child: not recommended.

Overdosage

Accidental overdoses as high as 8000 mg have been taken with no symptoms other than side effects. Take the victim to a hospital emergency room for treatment and evaluation. If you seek treatment, ALWAYS bring the prescription bottle or container.

Special Information

Pregabalin can make you dizzy or tired, or interfere with your concentration. Be extremely careful when driving or performing any task that requires concentration. Sedatives, alcohol, and other nervous system depressants will worsen these effects.

Take this medicine exactly as prescribed by your doctor. Suddenly stopping it may lead to seizures, sleeplessness, nausea, headache, and diarrhea. The dose of pregabalin should be reduced gradually over at least 1 week rather than discontinued abruptly.

Tell your doctor if you experience unexplained muscle pain, changes in vision, weight gain, swollen feet or hands, or any bothersome or persistent side effect.

Diabetic patients may develop skin lesions while taking pregabalin.

If you forget a dose, take it as soon as you remember. If it is almost time for your next dose, take the dose you forgot and space the remaining doses evenly throughout the rest of the day. Do not take a double dose.

Special Populations

Pregnancy/Breast-feeding: This medication causes birth defects in laboratory animals given 5 or more times the usual human dose. Also, seizure disorders have been associated with an increased risk of birth defects. Pregabalin should be taken during pregnancy only if your doctor determines that the potential benefit outweighs the risks.

Pregabalin passes into the breast milk of test animals, but it is not known if this also happens in humans. Nursing mothers who must take pregabalin should use infant formula.

Seniors: Seniors may take pregabalin without special precaution, but may require reduced drug dosage because of normal age-related decline in kidney function.

Premarin *see **Estrogens,** page 466*

Prempro *see **Estrogens,** page 466*

Pristiq *see **Venlafaxine,** page 1204*

ProAir HFA *see **Platelet Inhibitors,** page 920*

Generic Name

Prochlorperazine (proe-klor-PER-uh-zeen) G

Brand Names

Compro

Type of Drug

Antinauseant and phenothiazine antipsychotic.

Prescribed For

Severe nausea and vomiting; also used for psychotic disorders.

General Information

Prochlorperazine and other phenothiazine drugs act on a portion of the brain called the hypothalamus. They affect areas of the hypothalamus that control metabolism, body temperature, alertness, muscle tone, hormone balance, and vomiting. How phenothiazines work is not completely understood.

Cautions and Warnings

Do not take prochlorperazine if you are **allergic** or **sensitive** to any of its ingredients or to any phenothiazine drug.

Antipsychotic medications have been associated with increased mortality in **seniors with dementia-related psychosis** and should not be used in this population. The specific causes of death were either due to a heart-related event or infection, mostly pneumonia.

Prochlorperazine should not be used in those who have taken large amounts of sedative drugs, including alcohol, barbiturates, or narcotic medications. It should not be used during **pediatric surgery** or given to **children** under age 2.

Some people taking prochlorperazine develop tardive dyskinesia (symptoms include lip smacking or puckering, puffing of the cheeks, rapid or wormlike tongue movements, uncontrolled chewing motions, and uncontrolled arm and leg movements). This risk increases with long-term use of the medication.

A potentially fatal condition called neuroleptic malignant syndrome (NMS) has been linked to the use of phenothiazine drugs. Symptoms include elevated body temperature, muscle stiffness, altered mental states, and irregularities in pulse or blood pressure.

If you have **heart disease**, **glaucoma**, **epilepsy**, **ulcers**, **intestinal obstruction**, or **difficulty passing urine**, prochlorperazine should be used with caution and under the strict supervision of your doctor.

Prochlorperazine may depress the gag (cough) reflex. Some people who have taken this drug have accidentally choked to death because the gag reflex failed to respond. Because it can prevent vomiting, prochlorperazine may obscure symptoms of disease or drug toxicity.

Because this drug may both increase the risk of Reye's syndrome and mask its symptoms, it should not be used to treat vomiting in children when the underlying cause is unknown. It should be used with caution in children with acute illnesses such as **chickenpox**, **measles**, **central-nervous-system (CNS) infections**, **gastroenteritis**, or any illness that causes **dehydration**.

Women taking this drug develop chronic elevations of the hormone prolactin. About 33% of breast tumors are prolactin-dependent, a factor that you should consider before taking prochlorperazine, especially if you have a history of **breast cancer**.

Avoid extreme heat because prochlorperazine can upset your body's temperature-control mechanism.

Possible Side Effects

▼ Most common: drowsiness, especially during the first or second week of therapy. If the drowsiness becomes troublesome, contact your doctor. Prochlorperazine can cause jaundice (symptoms include yellowing of the skin or whites of the eyes), typically within the first 4 weeks of treatment. It usually goes away when the drug is discontinued. If you notice this effect or feel feverish or unwell, contact your doctor immediately.

▼ Less common: changes in blood components, including anemia (condition characterized by a reduction in the number of red blood cells, amount of hemoglobin, or blood); raised or lowered blood pressure; abnormal heart rate; heart attack; feeling faint; and dizziness. Phenothiazines may produce extrapyramidal effects such as spasm of the neck muscles, rolling back of the eyes, convulsions, difficulty swallowing, and symptoms associated with Parkinson's disease. These effects look very serious but disappear after the drug is withdrawn; however, face, tongue, and jaw symptoms may persist for several years, especially in

Possible Side Effects *(continued)*

seniors with a history of brain damage. If you experience extrapyramidal effects, contact your doctor immediately.

▼ Rare: Prochlorperazine may cause an increase in psychotic symptoms or cause paranoid reactions. Other rare side effects can occur in almost any part of the body. Contact your doctor if you experience anything unusual while taking any medication.

Drug Interactions

- Be cautious about combining prochlorperazine and barbiturates, sleeping pills, narcotics, sedatives, other phenothiazines, or other drugs that produce a depressive effect. Avoid alcohol.
- Prochlorperazine may diminish the effects of oral anticoagulant medications.
- Aluminum antacids may reduce the effectiveness of prochlorperazine. Anticholinergic drugs may reduce the effectiveness of prochlorperazine and increase the risk of side effects.
- The blood-pressure-lowering effect of guanethidine may be counteracted by this drug.
- Combining lithium and prochlorperazine may lead to disorientation, loss of consciousness, and uncontrolled muscle movements.
- Combining propranolol or thiazide diuretics and prochlorperazine may lead to unusually low blood pressure.
- Combining phenytoin and prochlorperazine may increase phenytoin levels in the blood. Prochlorperazine should be combined cautiously with antiseizure medications.

Food Interactions

Prochlorperazine's effectiveness as an antipsychotic may be counteracted by beverages or foods containing caffeine.

Usual Dose

Nausea and Vomiting

Adult: 5–10 mg 3–4 times a day to a maximum of 40 mg a day.

Child (40–85 lbs.): 2.5 mg 3 times a day or 5 mg twice a day. The syrup form contains 5 mg of prochlorperazine per tsp.

Child (30–39 lbs.): 2.5 mg 2–3 times a day.

Child (20–29 lbs.): 2.5 mg 1–2 times a day.

Child (under age 2 or under 20 lbs.): not recommended unless considered to be life-saving. Usually only 1–2 days of therapy are needed to relieve nausea and vomiting.

Schizophrenia

Adult and Child (age 13 and over): 5–10 mg 3–4 times a day. Severe conditions may require 100–150 mg a day.

Child (age 6–12): 2.5 mg 2–3 times a day to a maximum of 25 mg a day.

Child (age 2–5): 2.5 mg 2–3 times a day to a maximum of 20 mg a day.

Child (under age 2): not recommended.

Overdosage

Symptoms include depression, extreme weakness, tiredness or a desire to sleep, lowered blood pressure, uncontrolled muscle spasms, agitation, restlessness, convulsions, fever, dry mouth, abnormal heart rhythms, deep sleep, and coma. Take the victim to a hospital emergency room immediately. If you seek treatment, ALWAYS bring the prescription bottle or container.

Special Information

Prochlorperazine is a sedative and may have a depressive effect, especially during the first few days of therapy. Be careful when driving or performing any task that requires concentration.

Contact your doctor if you develop symptoms of tardive dyskinesia or NMS (see “Cautions and Warnings”) or sore throat, fever, rash, weakness, tremors, visual disturbances, or yellowing of the skin or whites of the eyes.

Do not take any over-the-counter medications without first consulting your doctor.

Prochlorperazine may cause increased sensitivity to the sun. It may also turn your urine reddish-brown to pink; this is not a cause for concern.

If dizziness occurs, avoid sudden changes in posture and climbing stairs. Use caution in hot weather because this medication may make you more prone to heatstroke.

The liquid form of prochlorperazine may cause skin irritation or rash; do not get it on your skin. Liquid prochlorperazine must be protected from light. Do not remove it from its opaque bottle.

If you miss a dose, take it as soon as you remember. If it is almost time for your next dose, skip the dose you forgot and go back to your regular schedule. Do not take a double dose.

Special Populations

Pregnancy/Breast-feeding: Taking prochlorperazine during pregnancy may cause jaundice and CNS effects in newborns. Prochlorperazine should be taken during pregnancy only if your doctor determines the potential benefit outweighs the risks.

Prochlorperazine may pass into breast milk. Nursing mothers who must take it should use infant formula.

Seniors: Seniors with dementia-related psychosis are at a greater risk of dying while taking this and other antipsychotic medicines. Seniors are more sensitive to prochlorperazine's effects and usually require lower dosages to achieve desired results. Some experts feel that they should be treated with 25–50% of the usual adult dosage.

Generic Name

Promethazine (proe-METH-uh-zeen) G

Brand Names

Phenadoz
Phenergan
Promethegan

Combination Products

Generic Ingredients: Promethazine + Codeine Phosphate G

Generic Ingredients: Promethazine + Codeine Phosphate + Phenylephrine Hydrochloride G
Prometh VC with Codeine A

Generic Ingredients: Promethazine + Dextromethorphan Hydrobromide G
Phenergan with Dextromethorphan
Prometh with Dextromethorphan

Generic Ingredients: Promethazine + Phenylephrine Hydrochloride G
Prometh VC Plain A

Type of Drug

Antihistamine.

Prescribed For

Allergy, motion sickness, nausea, vomiting, nighttime sedation, and pain relief following surgery. Combination products are used to treat cough and stuffy/runny nose due to allergy or cold.

General Information

Promethazine hydrochloride, one of the older members of the phenothiazine antihistamine group, is used alone and in combination with cough suppressants and decongestants.

Cautions and Warnings

Do not use promethazine if you are **allergic** or **sensitive** to any of its ingredients or if you cannot tolerate any other phenothiazine drug such as chlorpromazine and prochlorperazine.

This medication is not to be used by **children** under age 2 because of potentially fatal slowing of breathing. Use caution when using this drug in a child over age 2. The lowest effective dose should be used. Children under age 6 should not take promethazine with codeine. Children with **liver disease**, any illness that causes **dehydration**, a history of **sleep apnea**, a family history of **sudden infant death syndrome** (SIDS), or **Reye's syndrome** should not take promethazine.

Promethazine should not be used to treat lower-respiratory tract symptoms, including **asthma**.

Promethazine should be used with caution if you have **heart or liver disease**. This drug should be used under your doctor's strict supervision if you have an **ulcer**, a **seizure disorder**, **bone-marrow depression**, **glaucoma**, or **urinary difficulties**, including an enlarged prostate.

A potentially fatal condition called neuroleptic malignant syndrome (NMS) has been linked to the use of phenothiazine drugs. Symptoms include elevated body temperature, muscle stiffness, altered mental states, and irregularities in pulse or blood pressure.

Possible Side Effects

Suppositories can cause rectal burning or stinging.

- ▼ Most common: drowsiness, thick mucous, and sedation.
- ▼ Less common: sore throat and fever; unusual bleeding or bruising; tiredness; weakness; dizziness; feeling faint; clumsiness; unsteadiness; dry mouth, nose, or throat; facial redness; breathing difficulties; hallucinations; confusion; seizure; muscle spasm, especially in the back and neck; restlessness; a shuffling walk; jerky movements of the head and face; shaking and trembling of the hands; blurred

Possible Side Effects *(continued)*

vision or other changes in vision; urinary difficulties; rapid heartbeat; sensitivity to the sun; increased sweating; and appetite loss. Children and older adults are more likely to develop difficulty sleeping, excitability, nervousness, restlessness, or irritability.

Drug Interactions

- Promethazine may increase the toxic effects of acitretin.
- The effects of promethazine may be decreased by anticholinergic medications.
- If antipsychotic medications are used with promethazine, the risk of NMS (see "Cautions and Warnings") is increased.
- Promethazine may decrease the effects of cabergoline, levodopa + carbidopa, and pergolide. These combinations should be avoided if possible.
- The combination of promethazine with cefotetan, disulfiram, furazolidone, or metronidazole should be avoided.
- Promethazine should be combined cautiously with cisapride; the risk of dangerous heart rhythm abnormalities is increased.
- The sedating effects of promethazine are increased by central-nervous-system (CNS) depressants, including alcohol, hypnotics, sedatives, antianxiety drugs, and narcotics. These combinations should be used with extreme caution.
- Promethazine may increase the risk of seizures and should be taken cautiously with other drugs that have this effect, such as local anesthetics, narcotics, or tramadol.
- Promethazine should be combined cautiously with a monoamine oxidase inhibitor (MAOI) antidepressant. This combination may produce additional unwanted effects.
- Paroxetine may increase blood levels of promethazine, increasing the risk of adverse effects.
- The combination of promethazine and tretinoin increases sun sensitivity and should be avoided.
- Promethazine may interfere with blood-sugar tests and home pregnancy tests.

Food Interactions

Take promethazine with food if it upsets your stomach.

Usual Dose

Allergy

Adult and Child (age 2 and over): 25 mg at bedtime or 6.25–12.5 mg 3 times a day before meals.

Child (under age 2): not recommended.

Motion Sickness

Adult and Child (age 2 and over): 12.5–25 mg ½–1 hour before travel; repeat in 8–12 hours if needed. Then take 1 dose after waking and another before dinner.

Child (under age 2): not recommended.

Nausea and Vomiting

Adult: 12.5–25 mg when needed, up to 6 times a day if necessary.

Child (age 2 and over): 0.5 mg per lb. of body weight; 25 mg every 4–6 hours during and just following surgery.

Child (under age 2): not recommended.

Nighttime Sedation

Adult: 25–50 mg at bedtime.

Child (age 2 and over): 12.5–25 mg at bedtime.

Child (under age 2): not recommended.

Overdosage

Symptoms include drowsiness; confusion; clumsiness; dry mouth, nose, or throat; hallucinations; seizure; and other promethazine side effects. Overdose victims should be taken to a hospital emergency room for treatment. If you seek treatment, ALWAYS bring the prescription bottle or container.

Special Information

Be careful when performing tasks requiring concentration and coordination, such as driving, because promethazine may cause tiredness, dizziness, or lightheadedness. Avoid alcohol.

Contact your doctor if you develop sore throat; dry mouth, nose, or throat; fever; chills; unusual bleeding or bruising; tiredness; weakness; clumsiness; unsteadiness; hallucinations; seizures; sleeping problems; feeling faint; flushing; breathing difficulties; or any bothersome or persistent side effect.

When taking promethazine plus codeine or giving it to a child, you must use an accurate measuring device, such as an oral syringe—available at most pharmacies—to get the correct dose.

Maintain good dental hygiene while taking promethazine because dry mouth may cause you to be more susceptible to oral infections. If the dry mouth caused by promethazine is not eased by gum or hard candy or lasts more than 2 weeks, contact your doctor or dentist. Any dental work should be completed prior to starting this drug.

If you forget a dose of promethazine, take it as soon as you remember. If you take it twice a day and it is almost time for your next dose, take 1 dose right away and another in 5 or 6 hours, then continue with your regular schedule. If you take promethazine 3 or more times a day and forget a dose, take it as soon as you remember. If it is almost time for your next dose, take 1 dose right away and another in 3 or 4 hours, then continue with your regular schedule. Never take a double dose.

Special Populations

Pregnancy/Breast-feeding: Babies born to women who took phenothiazines have suffered side effects at birth such as yellowing of the skin and whites of the eyes, CNS effects, and blood-clotting problems. Do not take any antihistamine without your doctor's knowledge if you are or might be pregnant—especially during the last 3 months of pregnancy—because newborns may have severe reactions to antihistamines.

Nursing mothers who must take promethazine should use infant formula.

Seniors: Seniors are more sensitive to side effects and may require lower dosages.

Prometrium *see **Medroxyprogesterone,** page 720*

Type of Drug

Prostaglandin Agonists

Brand Names

Generic Ingredients: Bimatoprost

Latisse

Lumigan

Generic Ingredients: Latanoprost

Xalatan

Generic Ingredients: Travoprost

Travatan

Travatan Z

Prescribed For

Open-angle glaucoma and ocular hypertension (high pressure inside the eye). May also be prescribed for angle-closure, inflammatory, or neovascular glaucoma. Bimatoprost is prescribed to grow and thicken eyelashes.

General Information

Prostaglandin agonists are believed to reduce pressure inside the eye by combining with prostaglandin receptors to increase the outflow of eye fluid. They are absorbed through the cornea, where all but bimatoprost are transformed into their active forms. Pressure is lowered within 2 hours and lasts up to 12 hours.

Cautions and Warnings

Do not use prostaglandin agonists if you are **allergic** or **sensitive** to any of their ingredients. Sensitivity to one member of this group may not indicate sensitivity to all.

Prostaglandin agonists may change your eye color because they increase the number of pigment granules in the cornea, which in turn increases brown pigment in the iris. This color change occurs gradually over a period of months or years. Typically, the brown color around the pupil spreads slowly to the outer part of the iris. This change is more noticeable in people with green-brown, blue/gray-brown, or yellow-brown eye color. The long-term effect of these medicines on eye pigment granules is not known; your doctor may tell you to stop using these eye drops if the color change persists or is especially noticeable. They can also darken eyelid color and increase eyelash color and length, as well as the number of eyelashes.

The effect of prostaglandin agonists on the cornea is not known.

Possible Side Effects

- ▼ Most common: blurred vision; stinging, burning, itching, and redness of the eyes; and brownish eye coloration.
- ▼ Common: abnormal vision, eyelid problems, excessive tearing, and a sensation of something in the eye.
- ▼ Less common: dry eye; swelling or redness of the eyelid; eyelid discomfort, itching, inflammation, rash, burning, or pain; eyelid changes; temporary loss of lashes or sections of lashes; eyelash breakage; and increased sensitivity to bright light.

Possible Side Effects *(continued)*

- ▼ Rare: blood clot in the artery supplying the retina, bleeding inside the eye, detachment of the retina, increased eye pressure, color blindness, corneal deposits, corneal swelling, droopy eyelid, and irritation of the iris. Contact your doctor if you experience anything unusual while taking any medication.

Systemic side effects from traces of these drugs passing into the blood

- ▼ Common: cold, influenza, or other respiratory infections.
- ▼ Less common: muscle, joint, or back pain; accidental injury; chest pain; bronchitis; cough; diabetes; dizziness; headache; high blood pressure; sleeplessness; sore throat; runny nose; sinus irritation; and rash or allergic reactions.

Drug Interactions

- If you use other eye drops that contain a thimerosal preservative, separate the administration of each eye drop by at least 5 minutes.

Usual Dose

Adult: 1 drop in the affected eye every evening.

Child: not recommended.

Overdosage

Overdose symptoms include eye irritation and redness. Severe overdosage may also cause abdominal pain, dizziness, fatigue, flushing, nausea, and sweating. Contact your doctor, local poison control center, or a hospital emergency room for more information. If you seek treatment, ALWAYS bring the prescription bottle or container.

Special Information

Contact your doctor if you develop eye irritation or any other side effect.

If you use any other eye medication, wait 5 minutes between each application.

To prevent infection, keep the eyedropper from touching your fingers, eyelids, or any surface.

Contact your doctor immediately if you are having eye surgery, experience an eye injury, develop an eye infection such as conjunctivitis (pinkeye), or develop an eyelid reaction to determine if you should continue to use the eye drops.

If you wear contact lenses, take them out before using these eye drops and wait 15 minutes before reinserting them. These drugs contain a benzalkonium preservative that can be absorbed by the contacts.

Store unopened bottles of latanoprost in the refrigerator. Once opened, the eye drops can be kept at room temperature—up to 77°F—for 6 weeks. All other products can be stored at room temperature and should be discarded 6–8 weeks after opening.

Do not take more medication than your doctor has prescribed. Taking it more often may actually reduce its effectiveness. If you forget to administer a dose, do so as soon as you remember. If it is almost time for your next dose, skip the one you forgot and continue with your regular schedule. Do not take a double dose.

Special Populations

Pregnancy/Breast-feeding: Animal studies have shown that prostaglandin agonists may be harmful to the fetus at extremely high dosages. They should be used during pregnancy only if your doctor determines that the potential benefit outweighs the risks.

It is not known if these medications pass into breast milk. Nursing mothers who must use a prostaglandin agonist should use infant formula.

Seniors: Seniors may use these medicines without special precaution.

Protonix *see **Proton-Pump Inhibitors,** below*

Type of Drug

Proton-Pump Inhibitors

Brand Names

Generic Ingredients: Dexlansoprazole
Dexilant

Generic Ingredients: Esomeprazole Magnesium
Nexium

Generic Ingredients: Lansoprazole G
Prevacid

Generic Ingredients: Lansoprazole + Naproxen
NapraPAC

Generic Ingredients: Omeprazole G
Prilosec

Generic Ingredients: Omeprazole + Sodium Bicarbonate
Zegerid

Generic Ingredients: Pantoprazole Sodium G
Protonix

Generic Ingredients: Rabeprazole Sodium
Aciphex

Prescribed For

Stomach or duodenal (upper intestinal) ulcers, gastroesophageal reflux disease (GERD), and conditions in which there is an excess of stomach acid; also used to treat and maintain healing of ulcers of the esophagus.

General Information

Proton-pump inhibitors (PPIs) stop the production of stomach acid by interfering with the "proton pump" in the mucous lining of the stomach at the last stage of acid production. PPIs can turn off stomach acid production within 1 hour. These drugs are useful in treating conditions in which stomach acid plays a key role, as with ulcers and GERD. It is prescribed together with amoxicillin and clarithromycin for people with ulcers caused by *Heliobacter pylori* infections. For more information on this combination, see Erythromycin, page 460.

Cautions and Warnings

Do not take PPIs if you are **allergic** or **sensitive** to any of their ingredients.

PPIs should not be taken as maintenance treatment for **duodenal ulcers** and are not recommended for treatment of **GERD** beyond 8–16 weeks.

People taking a PPI for more than 3 months can develop low blood levels of magnesium, leading to muscle stiffness, abnormal heart rhythms, and seizures.

PPI use has been associated with an increased risk of osteoporosis-related fractures. This risk goes up if multiple daily doses are taken over 1 year.

People with **liver disease** may need to take a lower dose of PPIs.

Possible Side Effects

Generally, PPIs cause few side effects.

- ▼ Common: headache, diarrhea, nausea, gas, abdominal pain, constipation, and dry mouth.
- ▼ Less common: sore throat, upper-respiratory infection, fever, vomiting, dizziness, rash, constipation, muscle pain, unusual tiredness, cough, and back pain.
- ▼ Rare: Drug-sensitivity reactions, including severe skin reactions, may occur. Other rare side effects can affect almost any part of the body. Contact your doctor if you experience anything unusual while taking any medication.

Drug Interactions

- PPIs may interfere with the absorption of azole antifungals such as ketoconazole and itraconazole. These combinations should be avoided. Voriconazole may increase levels of PPIs in the blood.
- PPIs may increase the effects of benzodiazepines such as diazepam and triazolam, digoxin, methotrexate, salicylates such as aspirin, tolterodine (extended release), and warfarin. They may also interact with other drugs broken down by the liver.
- Combining PPIs and clarithromycin may increase blood levels of both drugs.
- PPIs may decrease the blood-thinning effect of clopidogrel. If they must be given together, blood levels should be monitored for dosage adjustments. Clopidogrel should not be taken with omeprazole.
- Fluvoxamine may increase the effects of PPIs.
- PPIs may reduce the effectiveness of dasatinib, erlotinib, nilotinib, and mycophenolate.
- Dexlansoprazole and esomeprazole may decrease the effectiveness of protease inhibitors (HIV drugs). Do not combine PPIs with atazanavir or nelfinavir in particular.

- Dexlansoprazole, lansoprazole, and omeprazole may increase the effects of tacrolimus.
- Sucralfate may interfere with the absorption of lansoprazole into the blood.

Food Interactions

PPIs can be taken without regard to food or meals but are best taken immediately before a meal, preferably breakfast. Capsules may be opened and mixed with 1 tbsp. of cool applesauce for people having difficulty swallowing. Esomeprazole and Zegerid must be taken at least 1 hour before a meal.

Usual Dose

Dexlansoprazole

Adult and Child (age 1 and over): 30–60 mg a day. People with liver disease need a lower dosage.

Esomeprazole

Adult and Child (age 12 and over): 20–40 mg a day, 1 hour before a meal.

Child (age 1–11): 10–20 mg once a day for up to 8 weeks.

Child (age 1–11 months): 2.5–10 mg (exact dosage calculated by weight) once a day for up to 6 weeks.

Lansoprazole

Adult and Child (age 1 and over): 15–30 mg a day. People with liver disease need a lower dosage.

NapraPAC

Adult: 15 mg lansoprazole/1000 mg naproxen a day. One lansoprazole tablet and one 500-mg naproxen tablet are taken in the morning before eating. The second 500-mg naproxen tablet is taken in the evening.

Omeprazole

Adult and Child (age 17 and over): 20–40 mg a day before eating.

Child (age 1–16): 5–20 mg a day based on weight.

Pantoprazole

Adult: 40 mg once or twice a day, preferably in the morning.

Child (age 6 and over): 20–40 mg a day based on weight.

Rabeprazole

Adult and Child (age 12 and over): 20–60 mg a day.

Child (under age 12): not recommended.

Zegerid

Adult: 1 capsule (20 or 40 mg) or 1 powder packet (20 or 40 mg) a day with water. Do not use other liquids or foods. Take at least 1 hour before a meal, on an empty stomach.

Child: not recommended.

Overdosage

Little is known about the effects of PPI overdose. Symptoms are likely to resemble side effects. Contact your local poison control center or a hospital emergency room for more information. If you seek treatment, ALWAYS bring the prescription bottle or container.

Special Information

Contact your doctor if you are unusually tired or weak, or if you develop a sore throat, fever, sores in the mouth that do not heal, unusual bleeding or bruising, bloody or cloudy urine, urinary difficulties, or any persistent or bothersome side effect.

Call your doctor if you develop seizures, dizziness, abnormally fast or skipped heartbeats, jitteriness, shaking or jerking movements, muscle weakness, cramps or muscle aches, or spasms of the hand, foot, or voice box while taking one of these medicines. These can be signs of low blood magnesium.

Take the full course of treatment prescribed, even if your symptoms improve after 1 or 2 weeks.

If you forget a dose, take it as soon as you remember. If it is almost time for your next dose, skip the one you forgot and continue with your regular schedule. Do not take a double dose.

Special Populations

Pregnancy/Breast-feeding: PPIs may be toxic to pregnant animals. A PPI should be taken during pregnancy only if your doctor determines that the potential benefit outweighs the risks.

It is not known if PPIs pass into breast milk. Nursing mothers who use this drug should use infant formula.

Seniors: Seniors report the same side effects as younger adults.

Proventil HFA

see ***Albuterol,*** *page 51*

Generic Name

Quetiapine (kwe-TYE-uh-pene)

Brand Names

Seroquel
Seroquel XR

The information in this profile also applies to the following drugs:

Generic Ingredients: Asenapine
Saphris

Generic Ingredients: Clozapine G
Clozaril
FazaClo Orally Disintegrating Tablets

Generic Ingredients: Loxapine G
Loxitane

Generic Ingredients: Olanzapine G
Zyprexa
Zyprexa Zydis
Zyprexa Relprevv

Combination Products
Generic Ingredients: Olanzapine + Fluoxetine
Symbyax

Type of Drug

Atypical antipsychotic.

Prescribed For

Bipolar disorder, major depression, and schizophrenia. May also be prescribed for obsessive-compulsive disorder, post-traumatic stress disorder, alcohol dependence, and Tourette syndrome.

General Information

These drugs are used for a wide variety of symptoms and each drug has a unique profile. They work by antagonizing a number of different types of brain receptors. This means that the drug decreases levels of certain neurotransmitters, including serotonin, dopamine, and histamine, by preventing them from binding to cell receptors, but dopamine is thought to be the most important of these. People taking an atypical antipsychotic benefit with reduced psychiatric symptoms, better functioning in society, and an improved quality of life. Clozapine was the first atypical antipsychotic to be developed but has been used on a limited basis because of its toxicities. Clozapine is a unique antipsychotic that has the capacity to treat people who do not respond to or cannot tolerate other drugs. It works by a mechanism that differs from that of other antipsychotic drugs.

These drugs are mainly broken down by enzymes produced in the liver. See Fluoxetine, page 1045, for more information on olanzapine + fluoxetine.

Cautions and Warnings

Do not take these drugs if you are **allergic** or **sensitive** to any of their ingredients. Severe reactions include swelling of the lips, tongue, face, arms, or legs; closing of the throat; and intestinal reactions.

A very small number of people who take these medicines develop a rapid drop in their white-blood-cell count called agranulocytosis. This effect, which is most common with clozapine, usually reverses itself when the drug is stopped, but the drug must be stopped as soon as it is discovered. Most cases of agranulocytosis occur between week 4 and week 10 of treatment. It is essential that blood samples be taken approximately every week and for 4 weeks after the drug is stopped to watch for this effect. Because of the risk of agranulocytosis, clozapine should not be tried until at least 2 other antipsychotic medicines have failed. People with **bone marrow diseases** involving an overproduction of cells, uncontrolled **epilepsy**, **intestinal obstruction**, a history of **clozapine-induced agranulocytosis**, **severe granulocytopenia** (a disease of the white blood cells), or severe **central-nervous-system depression** or those in a **coma** should not use clozapine.

Atypical antipsychotics have been associated with increased mortality in seniors with **dementia or Alzheimer's disease**. The causes of death were due to a heart-related event or infection, mainly pneumonia. These medications are not approved for use in people with dementia-related psychosis.

Antidepressants and antipsychotics have been linked to an increase in suicidal behavior among teens and adolescents. All patients started on these drugs should be closely monitored, especially in the first few months of treatment, for changes in behavior, worsening of symptoms, or suicidal tendencies.

A potentially fatal condition called neuroleptic malignant syndrome (NMS) may occur with some antipsychotic drugs. Symptoms include convulsions, breathing difficulties, and back, neck, or leg pain. People who have experienced this syndrome with another antipsychotic drug should be cautious when taking these medications.

Some people taking antipsychotic drugs develop tardive dyskinesia, a potentially irreversible condition marked by uncontrollable movements. Tardive dyskinesia has not been seen in patients taking clozapine, a major advantage of this drug over other antipsychotic medicines. However, there is still a risk that this set of symptoms could occur with clozapine.

These medicines should be used with caution if you have had a **seizure**, or have a seizure disorder or other condition that may make you more susceptible to seizures.

These medicines can make you dizzy or cause you to faint if you rise suddenly from a sitting or lying position. They should be used with caution if you have a history of **heart disease**, including **heart attack**, **angina**, **abnormal heart rhythms**, or **stroke or TIA** ("mini-stroke"). Take these drugs with caution if you have a condition or take any drug that can cause **low blood pressure**.

People taking quetiapine for a long period have developed cataracts, but they have not been directly related to the drug. You should have an eye exam when you start the drug and every 6 months thereafter to detect any cataract formation.

Quetiapine treatment has been associated with low levels of thyroid hormone in the blood. This is usually not a problem, although a small percentage of people taking this drug may need a thyroid supplement.

These medicines may cause significant weight gain, increases in cholesterol and triglyceride levels, high blood sugar, and diabetes. Asenapine patients may experience less weight gain and blood-fat increases. People with **diabetes** or those who are at risk for diabetes should have their blood-glucose levels monitored while taking these drugs.

People with **liver disease** may require dosage adjustments when taking olanzapine. Those with severe liver disease should not take asenapine. Quetiapine has caused liver inflammation without any symptoms, as measured by increases in enzymes produced by the liver. These enzymes generally return to normal with continued treatment.

Antipsychotic medicines can upset the body's temperature-regulating mechanism, creating the risk for heat stroke or dehydration.

Swallowing problems and inhaling food have been experienced by people taking other antipsychotics and may present problems for those taking these medications.

Antipsychotic medicines can raise levels of a hormone called prolactin in men and women, possibly causing infertility, impotence, skipped menstrual periods, breast pain, and abnormal breast milk formation. Left untreated, raised prolactin levels can lead to reduced bone density and may put you at higher risk for breast cancer.

Women eliminate olanzapine about 30% more slowly than men, but this effect is not considered a problem. Women may respond to lower olanzapine doses than men.

Possible Side Effects

Asenapine

▼ Most common: tiredness; sleeplessness; headache; restlessness; inability to sit still; involuntary movements; uncontrollable speech; unusual hand or finger movements; shuffling walk; and eyelid twitching.

▼ Common: constipation, dry mouth, loss of sensation around the mouth, vomiting, and dizziness.

▼ Less common: stomach upset, extra saliva production, fatigue, irritability, weight gain, increased appetite, high blood pressure, anxiety, dry mouth, toothache, upset stomach, joint pain, arm or leg pain, taste changes, anxiety, and depression.

▼ Rare: Rare side effects can affect your heart, blood, eyes, stomach and intestines, and nervous system. Contact your doctor if you experience anything unusual while taking any medication.

Clozapine

▼ Most common: rapid heartbeat, low blood pressure, dizziness, fainting, drowsiness or sedation, salivation, and constipation.

▼ Less common: headache, tremor, sleep disturbance, restlessness, slow muscle motions, absence of movement, agitation, convulsions, rigidity, restlessness, confusion, sweating, dry mouth, visual disturbances, high blood pressure, high cholesterol, high blood triglycerides, nausea, vomiting, heartburn or abdominal discomfort, fever, and weight gain.

Possible Side Effects *(continued)*

▼ Rare: agranulocytosis (symptoms include fever with or without chills, sore throat, and sores or white spots on the lips or mouth), tardive dyskinesia (symptoms include lip smacking or puckering, puffing of the cheeks, rapid or wormlike tongue movement, uncontrolled chewing motions, and uncontrolled arm and leg movements), and NMS (see "Cautions and Warnings"). Other rare side effects can occur in almost any part of the body. Contact your doctor if you experience anything unusual while taking any medication.

Loxapine

▼ Common: blurred vision, confusion, dizziness, lightheadedness or fainting, drowsiness, and dry mouth.

▼ Less common: constipation (mild), decreased sexual ability, breast enlargement or milk secretion in men and women, headache, increased sun sensitivity, missed menstrual periods, nausea or vomiting, trouble sleeping, weight gain. Tardive dyskinesia (symptoms include lip smacking or puckering, puffing of the cheeks, rapid or wormlike tongue movement, uncontrolled chewing motions, and uncontrolled arm and leg movements) can occur and may be permanent.

▼ Rare: seizures, difficult or fast breathing, fast heartbeat or irregular pulse, high fever, blood-pressure changes, sweating, loss of bladder control, muscle stiffness (severe), unusually pale skin, and unusual tiredness or weakness.

Olanzapine

▼ Most common: headache, tiredness, agitation, sleeplessness, nervousness, hostility, dizziness, and runny nose.

▼ Less common: fever; abdominal, back, or chest pain; a rigid neck; dizziness or fainting when rising from a sitting or lying position; rapid heartbeat; low blood pressure; constipation; dry mouth; increased appetite; weight gain; swelling in the arms or legs; joint pain; arm or leg pain; twitching; anxiety; personality changes; restlessness or a feeling that you need to keep moving; muscle stiffness; tremors; memory loss; difficulty speaking or expressing thoughts; euphoria (feeling "high"); stuttering; cough; sore throat; double vision or other eye problems; and symptoms of premenstrual syndrome.

Possible Side Effects *(continued)*

▼ Rare: Other rare side effects can occur in almost any part of the body. Contact your doctor if you experience anything unusual while taking any medication.

Quetiapine

▼ Most common: dizziness, headache, agitation, upset stomach, tiredness, sleepiness, dizziness or fainting when rising from a sitting or lying position, abdominal pain, weight gain, and dry mouth.

▼ Common: swelling in the arms or legs, heart palpitations, spastic movements, difficulty talking, sore throat, runny nose, increased coughing, breathing difficulties, flu-like symptoms, appetite loss, sweating, and low white-blood-cell counts.

▼ Less common: Other side effects can occur in almost any part of the body. Contact your doctor if you experience anything unusual while taking any medication.

Drug Interactions

- These drugs can increase the effects of central-nervous-system depressants. Dosage adjustments may be needed.
- These medications may increase the sedative effects of benzodiazepine drugs such as diazepam and lorazepam, causing symtoms of dizziness, fainting, or even cardiac arrest. At least 1 person has died as a result of combining diazepam and clozapine. These medications should be taken together with caution.
- These drugs may increase the effects of medications to lower blood pressure. Dosage adjustments may be necessary.
- Do not drink alcohol while taking these medications.

Asenapine

- The risk of dangerous heart rhythm disorders is possible if asenapine is combined with amiodarone, arsenic trioxide, bretylium, chlorpromazine, cisapride, disopyramide, dofetilide, dolasetron, droperidol, gatifloxacin, mefloquine, mesoridazine, moxifloxacin, pentamidine, pimozide, quinidine, sotalol, tacrolimus, thioridazine, and ziprasidone.
- Asenapine increases paroxetine levels in the bloodstream. Mix these drugs with caution.

- Asenapine may affect the breakdown of the following medications, causing additional side effects: amitriptyline, amphetamine, aripiprazole, atomoxetine, bupropion, carvedilol, celecoxib, chlorpheniramine, chlorpromazine, cimetidine, cinacalcet, citalopram, clemastine, clomipramine, cocaine, codeine, debrisoquine, desipramine, dextromethorphan, diphenhydramine, donepezil, doxepin, doxorubicin, duloxetine, encainide, escitalopram, flecainide, fluoxetine, halofantrine, haloperidol, hydroxyzine, imipramine, lidocaine, methadone, methoxyamphetamine, metoclopramide, metoprolol, mexiletine, midodrine, moclobemide, nebivolol, nortriptyline, oxycodone, paroxetine, perhexiline, perphenazine, phenacetin, promethazine, propafenone, propranolol, quinidine, ranitidine, risperidone, ritonavir, sertraline, tamoxifen, terbinafine, thioridazine, ticlopidine, timolol, tramadol, tripelennamine, and venlafaxine.

Clozapine

- Clozapine's anticholinergic effects—blurred vision, dry mouth, and confusion—may be enhanced by interaction with other anticholinergics.
- Use of clozapine with carbamazepine, phenobarbital, phenytoin, nicotine, and rifampin may cause decreases in blood levels of clozapine, reducing its effectiveness. The combination of clozapine and carbamazepine is not recommended.
- Caffeine, cimetidine, ciprofloxacin, erythromycin, ketoconazole, and risperidone may increase blood levels of clozapine, resulting in increased side effects.
- Clozapine should be combined cautiously with psychotropic medications such as haloperidol. Dizziness, fainting, and respiratory and cardiac arrest have been reported.
- Clozapine should not be used with ritonavir.
- Selective serotonin reuptake inhibitor (SSRI) antidepressants (such as fluoxetine, fluvoxamine, paroxetine, or sertraline) increase the effects of clozapine. Dosage adjustments may be necessary whenever starting, stopping, or changing the dosage of an SSRI.

Loxapine

- The effects of both drugs are increased if loxapine is combined with metoclopramide, sodium oxybate, and tramadol. These combinations are not recommended.

Olanzapine

- The dosage of olanzapine must be adjusted when the drug is combined with carbamazepine.
- Combining olanzapine with fluvoxamine may cause elevations in olanzapine blood levels and added side effects.
- Combining olanzapine with ritonavir may decrease the effectiveness of olanzapine.
- Olanzapine may antagonize the effects of levodopa + carbidopa. Patients being treated for Parkinson's disease may need dosage adjustments or discontinuation of olanzapine.
- The risk of seizures is increased when olanzapine is given with tramadol.

See Fluoxetine, page 1045, for more information on olanzapine + fluoxetine.

Quetiapine

- The risk of dangerous heart rhythm disorders is possible if quetiapine is combined with amiodarone, arsenic trioxide, bretylium, chlorpromazine, cisapride, disopyramide, dofetilide, dolasetron, droperidol, gatifloxacin, mefloquine, mesoridazine, moxifloxacin, pentamidine, pimozide, quinidine, sotalol, tacrolimus, thioridazine, and ziprasidone.
- Quetiapine decreases the effects of carbamazepine.
- Cimetidine may cause elevations in quetiapine levels in the blood.
- Erythromycin, fluconazole, fluvoxamine, itraconazole, ketoconazole, and protease inhibitors (HIV drugs) such as ritonavir may increase quetiapine blood levels. Caution should be exercised when combining these drugs with quetiapine.
- Combining quetiapine with carbamazepine, glucocorticoids, phenobarbital, phenytoin, or rifampin increases the rate at which quetiapine is released from the body. You may require an increase in quetiapine dosage to achieve the same effect.
- Quetiapine may antagonize the effects of levodopa + carbidopa.
- Thioridazine decreases quetiapine levels by over ½. Dosage adjustments are necessary with this combination.
- Valproic acid may increase the effects of quetiapine.

Food Interactions

There are no food interactions with clozapine or olanzapine. Do not eat or drink immediately before or for 10 minutes after you take asenapine. Broccoli, brussels sprouts, and char-grilled meat may increase the breakdown of asenapine. Avoid these foods. Taking quetiapine with food increases the amount of drug absorbed by a small amount. This is not likely to change its effect on your body.

Usual Dose

Asenapine

Adult: Completely dissolve one 5- or 10-mg tablet twice a day under the tongue. Do not chew or swallow the tablet whole.

Child: not recommended.

Clozapine

Adult: starting dose—12.5 mg twice a day; maintenance dose—generally, 300–450 mg a day in divided doses. Dosage may be increased gradually to a daily maximum of 900 mg in divided doses if required.

Child: not recommended.

Loxapine

Adult: 10–50 mg twice a day to start. Dose is increased to 60–100 mg a day according to response. The lowest effective dose should be used.

Child: not recommended.

Olanzapine

Adult and Child (age 13–17): 5–10 mg a day to start; maintenance dose increases gradually up to 20 mg a day if needed.

Child (under age 13): not recommended.

Olanzapine Long-Acting Injection

Adult: 150–405 mg every 2–4 weeks by deep intramuscular injection.

Olanzapine + Fluoxetine

Adult: one 6/25 (olanzapine/fluoxetine) capsule every evening to start. Dose may be increased gradually to one 12/50 capsule in the evening. Maximum dose is 18/75. Lower doses may be needed by women, seniors, people with liver disease, and those with low blood pressure or those who are inclined to dizziness or fainting.

Quetiapine

Bipolar Disorder

Adult: starting dose—50–100 mg, increased gradually to a maintenance dose of 400–800 mg a day.

Child (age 10 and over): starting dose—50 mg, increased gradually to a maintenance dose of 400–800 mg a day.

Child (under age 10): not recommended.

Schizophrenia

Adult: starting dose—50 mg, increased gradually to a maintenance dose of 150–800 mg a day.

Child (age 13–17): starting dose—50 mg, increased gradually to a maintenance dose of 400–800 mg a day.

Child (under age 13): not recommended.

Quetiapine XR

Major Depressive Disorder

Adult: starting dose—50 mg a day, increased as needed to 150–300 mg a day.

Child: not recommended.

Schizophrenia and Bipolar Disorder

Adult: starting dose—300 mg a day, increased to a maintenance dose of 400–800 mg a day.

Child: not recommended.

Overdosage

Symptoms of overdose depend on the drug but can include delirium, drowsiness, slurred speech, changes in heart rhythm, unusual excitement, nervousness, restlessness, hallucinations, excessive salivation, dizziness or fainting, slow or irregular breathing, and coma. Overdose victims should be taken to a hospital emergency room at once. If you seek treatment, ALWAYS bring the prescription bottle or container.

Special Information

Avoid alcohol or any other nervous system depressants while taking these medications. Smoking can speed the breakdown of these drugs.

Regular blood tests are necessary to monitor blood composition for any changes that might be caused by clozapine.

These drugs may make you drowsy, especially in the first few weeks of treatment and with larger doses. Take care while driving or performing any task that requires concentration.

Contact your doctor at once if you develop lethargy or weakness, a flu-like infection, sore throat, feelings of ill health, fever, sweating, muscle rigidity, mental changes, irregular pulse or blood pressure, mouth ulcers, or dry mouth that lasts for more than 2 weeks.

Dry mouth, a common side effect of these medicines, may be countered by using gum, hard candy, ice, or a saliva substitute such as Orex or Moi-Stir. See your dentist regularly while you are taking these medications, because dental problems are more likely with chronic dry mouth.

Antipsychotic drugs may increase your sensitivity to hot weather and your susceptibility to dehydration by interfering with temperature-control mechanisms.

Do not stop taking these drugs without your doctor's knowledge and approval, because a gradual dosage reduction may be necessary to prevent side effects.

Some of the side effects of these drugs—drowsiness, blurred vision, and seizures—may interfere with the performance of complex tasks such as driving or operating hazardous equipment. While taking these medications, rapidly rising from a sitting or lying position may cause you to become dizzy or faint.

If you take clozapine twice a day and forget a dose, take it as soon as you remember. If it is almost time for your next dose, take 1 dose as soon as you remember and another in 5–6 hours, then go back to your regular schedule. If you take clozapine 3 times a day and forget a dose, take it as soon as you remember. If it is almost time for your next dose, take 1 dose as soon as you remember and another in 3–4 hours, then go back to your regular schedule. Never take a double dose.

If you forget to take a dose of olanzapine or quetiapine, take it as soon as you remember. If it is almost time for your next dose, skip the dose you forgot and continue with your regular schedule. Do not take a double dose.

If you forget a dose of asenapine or loxapine, take it as soon as you remember. If it is almost time for your next dose, take 1 dose as soon as you remember and another in 5–6 hours, then go back to your regular schedule. Do not take a double dose.

Orally disintegrating tablets should be left in the unopened blister until time of use. They should not be pushed through the foil. Just prior to use, peel the foil from the blister and gently remove the orally disintegrating tablet with clean and dry hands. Immediately place the tablet in the mouth, allow it to disintegrate, and then swallow with saliva. No water is needed.

Special Populations

Pregnancy/Breast-feeding: Talk to your doctor if you become pregnant or are trying to become pregnant while taking these drugs. Newborns whose mothers are taking any antipsychotic medicine are more likely to experience agitation, abnormally increased or decreased muscle tone, tremor, sleepiness, severe difficulty breathing, and difficulty in feeding. In some newborns, the symptoms subside within hours or days and do not require specific treatment; other newborns may require longer hospital stays. Do not stop taking your medication without talking to your doctor, because suddenly stopping antipsychotic medications can cause significant treatment complications. These drugs should be taken during pregnancy only if your doctor determines that the possible benefit outweighs the risks.

These drugs may pass into breast milk. Nursing mothers who must take an atypical antipsychotic medicine should use infant formula.

Seniors: Seniors may be more sensitive to side effects, especially dizziness, fainting, and tiredness. Seniors taking olanzapine are at greater risk of having a stroke. Older men are more likely to have prostate problems, a reason to be cautious with clozapine. Seniors with psychosis due to dementia should not take these medications.

Generic Name

Quinidine (QUIN-ih-dene) G

Brand Names

Only available in generic form.

Type of Drug

Antiarrhythmic.

Prescribed For

Abnormal heart rhythms.

General Information

Derived from the bark of the cinchona tree, which also gives us quinine, quinidine works by affecting the flow of potassium into and out of heart muscle cells. This helps quinidine slow the flow of nerve impulses throughout the heart muscle, which allows control mechanisms in the heart to take over and keep the heart beating at a normal, even rate. The 3 kinds of quinidine—gluconate, polygalacturonate, and sulfate—provide different amounts of active drug and cannot be interchanged without dosage adjustments.

Cautions and Warnings

Do not take quinidine if you are **allergic** or **sensitive** to any of its ingredients or to quinine or a related drug. Quinidine sensitivity may be masked if you have **asthma**, **muscle weakness**, or an **infection** when you start taking the drug.

Liver toxicity related to quinidine sensitivity occurs rarely. Unexplained fever or liver inflammation may indicate this effect. Your doctor should monitor your liver function during the first 4–8 weeks of therapy. People with **kidney or liver disease** may require lower dosages.

People taking quinidine for long periods may experience sudden fainting or abnormal heart rhythms. Occasionally, these episodes may be fatal.

Possible Side Effects

▼ Most common: nausea, vomiting, abdominal pain, diarrhea, and appetite loss. These may be accompanied by fever.

▼ Less common: unusual heart rhythms, altering of blood components, irritation of the esophagus, headache, dizziness, feelings of apprehension or excitement, confusion, delirium, muscle ache or joint pain, ringing or buzzing in the ears, mild hearing loss, blurred vision, changes in color perception, sensitivity to bright light, double vision, difficulty seeing at night, flushing of the skin, itching, sensitivity to the sun, cramps, an unusual urge to defecate or urinate, and cold sweat.

▼ Rare: collapse of blood vessels; asthma; swelling of the face, hands, and feet; respiratory collapse; and liver problems.

High dosages of quinidine may cause rash, hearing loss, dizziness, ringing in the ears, headache, nausea, or disturbed vision. This group of symptoms, called cinchonism, is usually related to taking a large amount of quinidine but may appear after a single dose of the medication. Cinchonism is not necessarily a toxic reaction, but you should immediately report any sign of it to your doctor. Do not stop taking this drug unless instructed to do so by your doctor. Contact your doctor if you experience anything unusual while taking any medication.

Drug Interactions

- Quinidine increases the effect of warfarin and other oral anticoagulants (blood thinners).
- Quinidine may increase the effects of metoprolol, propranolol, and other beta blockers; propafenone; succinylcholine; atropine, benztropine, oxybutynin, trihexyphenidyl, and other anticholinergic drugs; and tricyclic antidepressants.
- The effect of quinidine may be decreased by the following medicines: cholinergic drugs such as bethanechol, nifedipine, phenobarbital and other barbiturates, phenytoin and other hydantoins, rifampin, and sucralfate.
- The effectiveness and side effects of quinidine may be increased by taking amiodarone, some antacids, cimetidine, clarithromycin, diltiazem, erythromycin, fluvoxamine, indinavir, itraconazole, ketoconazole, mibefradil, nefazodone, nelfinavir, ritonavir, verapamil, or anything that decreases uric-acid levels.
- Quinidine may dramatically increase the amount of digoxin in the blood, causing possible digoxin toxicity. This combination should be monitored closely by your doctor.
- The combination of disopyramide and quinidine may result in increased disopyramide levels and possible side effects; reduced quinidine activity may also result.
- Avoid over-the-counter cough, cold, allergy, and diet preparations. These medications may contain drugs that stimulate the heart and may be dangerous in combination with quinidine.
- St. John's wort may decrease quinidine levels.
- Avoid taking megadoses of vitamin C while taking this drug.

Food Interactions

You can take quinidine with food if it upsets your stomach. Some forms of quinidine may be less irritating to the stomach. Avoid drinking grapefruit juice.

Usual Dose

Immediate-Release

Adult: extremely variable; generally, 600–1200 mg a day.
Child: not recommended.

Sustained-Release

Adult: generally, 600–1800 mg a day.
Child: not recommended.

Overdosage

Overdose produces depressed mental function, including lethargy, decreased breathing, seizures, and coma. Other symptoms are abdominal pain and diarrhea, abnormal heart rhythms, and symptoms of cinchonism (see "Possible Side Effects"). The victim should be taken to a hospital emergency room. If you seek treatment, ALWAYS bring the prescription bottle or container.

Special Information

Contact your doctor if you develop ringing or buzzing in the ears, hearing or visual disturbances, dizziness, headache, nausea, rash, breathing difficulties, or any intolerable side effect.

Do not crush or chew the sustained-release products.

Some side effects of quinidine may lead to oral discomfort, including dry mouth, cavities, periodontal disease, and oral *Candida* infections. See your dentist regularly while taking this drug.

If you forget to take a dose of quinidine and you remember within 2 hours of your regular time, take it right away. If you do not remember until later, skip the dose you forgot and continue your regular schedule. Do not take a double dose.

Special Populations

Pregnancy/Breast-feeding: Quinidine may cause birth defects. It should be taken during pregnancy only if your doctor determines that the potential benefit outweighs the risks.

Quinidine passes into breast milk but is considered acceptable for use while breast-feeding. Consult your doctor.

Seniors: Seniors may be more sensitive to the effects of this medication due to decreased kidney function.

Generic Name

Raloxifene (rah-LOX-ih-feen)

Brand Names

Evista

Type of Drug

Selective estrogen receptor modulator (SERM).

Prescribed For

Osteoporosis prevention and treatment and breast cancer prevention.

General Information

The female hormone estrogen plays an important role in maintaining bone strength in women by regulating the body's use of calcium. When the ovaries stop producing estrogen after menopause, a woman's risk of developing osteoporosis increases significantly. Raloxifene hydrochloride, which belongs to the SERM class of drugs, is used to increase bone density and prevent broken bones in postmenopausal women by mimicking the protective effect that estrogen has on bone. This drug also lowers cholesterol levels by acting like estrogen therapy in the cardiovascular system. Raloxifene has a potential advantage over estrogen therapy in the treatment of osteoporosis because it does not appear to have an estrogen-like effect in the breast or uterus, where the hormone may increase cancer risk. Raloxifene is broken down in the liver.

Cautions and Warnings

Do not take raloxifene if you are **allergic** or **sensitive** to any of its ingredients, or you are **pregnant** or **nursing**.

There is an increased risk of **venous thromboembolism** with raloxifene; women with a history of this disorder or other **blood-clotting problems** should not take this drug.

Only **postmenopausal women** should use raloxifene. There is no information on the use of this drug by **men**.

People with moderate to severe **kidney or liver disease** should use this drug with caution.

Raloxifene should not be used to prevent **heart disease**. Women with heart disease taking raloxifene have a greater risk of dying of a stroke. Triglycerides should be closely monitored in women with **high blood-triglyceride levels**, as this drug can further increase triglycerides, a risk factor for heart disease.

Possible Side Effects

- ▼ Most common: hot flashes, leg cramps, infections, flu-like symptoms, joint pain, runny nose, and sinus irritation.
- ▼ Common: depression, sleeplessness, headaches, dizziness, rash, nausea, diarrhea, upset stomach, weight gain, muscle aches, sore throat, and cough.
- ▼ Less common: chest pain, fever, migraine, tingling in the hands or feet, sweating, vomiting, gas, stomach and intestinal problems, vaginal irritation, vaginal discharge, urinary

Possible Side Effects *(continued)*

infection, cystitis, endometrial problems, swelling in the arms or legs, arthritis, pneumonia, and laryngitis.

▼ Rare: loss of or changes in speech, coordination, or vision; pain or numbness in the chest, arms, or legs; and shortness of breath. Rare side effects can occur in almost any part of the body. Contact your doctor if you experience anything unusual while taking any medication.

Drug Interactions

- Taking raloxifene and estrogen therapy is not recommended because the effects of this combination are unknown.
- The blood levels of raloxifene may be increased by diazepam, diazoxide, and lidocaine.
- Cholestyramine can reduce the amount of raloxifene absorbed by 60%. Separate doses of these drugs by 2 hours or more.
- Raloxifene can reduce the effect of warfarin (a blood thinner). Your warfarin dosage may need adjustment.

Food Interactions

Raloxifene can be taken without regard to food or meals.

Usual Dose

Adult: 60 mg once a day.

Child: not recommended.

Overdosage

Little is known about the effects of raloxifene overdose. Contact your local poison control center or a hospital emergency room for information. If you seek treatment, ALWAYS bring the prescription bottle or container.

Special Information

Raloxifene can increase your risk of developing a blood clot in the lungs, legs, or another part of the body during any extended period of inactivity. Stop taking raloxifene 3 days before surgery, a long period of bed rest, or lengthy plane or car trips.

It is very important for all postmenopausal women to get 1200 mg of calcium and 10 mcg (400 IU) of vitamin D every day, either from food or a dietary supplement. Women age 70 and over require 1200 mg of calcium and 15 mcg (600 IU) of vitamin D daily.

Regular exercise is recommended for all postmenopausal women because it helps build strong bones.

Raloxifene does not reduce the hot flashes or flushes associated with menopause. Contact your doctor if you experience hot flashes or flushes, uterine bleeding, or breast changes while taking raloxifene.

If you forget a dose, take it as soon as you remember. If it is almost time for your next dose, skip the one you forgot and continue with your regular schedule. Do not take a double dose.

Special Populations

Pregnancy/Breast-feeding: Raloxifene should be used only by women who have undergone menopause. It can harm a fetus or a nursing infant and should not be used by women who are pregnant or nursing.

Seniors: Seniors can use raloxifene without special precaution.

Generic Name

Raltegravir (rahl-TEG-rah-veer)

Brand Names

Isentress

Type of Drug

HIV integrase inhibitor.

Prescribed For

Human immunodeficiency virus (HIV).

General Information

Raltegravir is the first HIV integrase strand transfer inhibitor. HIV integrase is an enzyme required for the HIV virus to reproduce. It is responsible for the integration of HIV-1 DNA into an infected cell. Once introduced into a cell, the DNA forms the provirus that is required to create new HIV virus. Raltegravir's unique mechanism of action makes it a valuable addition to other HIV drug treatments that attack different aspects of HIV reproduction. It is recommended only for adults who have been unsuccessfully treated with other HIV antiviral medicines. It is broken down in the liver. Resistance to the effects of raltegravir can develop in a number of different ways.

Cautions and Warnings

Do not take raltegravir if you are **allergic** or **sensitive** to any of its ingredients.

When beginning treatment with antivirals such as raltegravir, some patients who respond to therapy sometimes develop what is known as immune reconstitution syndrome. This is an inflammatory response to infectious organisms already in the body but in an inactive state, such as *Mycobacterium,* cytomegalovirus, *Pneumocystis carinii* pneumonia, or tuberculosis, or they may experience a reactivation of varicella zoster virus, which may require further evaluation and treatment.

Raltegravir can cause muscle aches and destruction of muscle tissue.

Possible Side Effects

- ▼ Most common: diarrhea.
- ▼ Common: nausea, headache, and fever.
- ▼ Less common: abdominal pain, vomiting, weakness, fatigue, dizziness, selective loss of body fat, anemia, heart attack, reduced white-blood-cell count, hepatitis, herpes simplex infection, shingles, gastritis (a burning pain in your upper abdomen, bloating, belching, nausea, or vomiting), paranoia, anxiety, depression, suicidal thoughts or attempts, and kidney disease.
- ▼ Rare: Skin rash or severe skin reactions (including skin peeling and blisters) and cancers have been reported in people taking this drug. The type and frequency of cancer is consistent with those found in people with poorly functioning immune systems, but their specific relationship to raltegravir is not known. Contact your doctor if you experience anything unusual while taking any medication.

Drug Interactions

- Phenobarbital, phenytoin, and rifampin reduce the amount of raltegravir in the blood; dose adjustment may be needed.
- Efavirenz, nevirapine, rifabutin, St. John's wort, and tipranavir + ritonavir may reduce raltegravir blood concentrations, but dose adjustment is not needed.
- Atazanavir and atazanavir + ritonavir increase the amount of raltegravir in the blood, but dose adjustment is not needed.

Food Interactions

Raltegravir can be taken without regard to food or meals.

Usual Dose

Adult and Child (age 12 and over): 400 mg twice a day; 800 mg twice a day if you are also taking rifampin. Dosage range is 100–1600 mg a day.

Child (age 2–11, 55 lbs. and over): 400 mg twice a day.

Child (age 2–11, under 55 lbs.): 75–300 mg twice a day, based on body weight (2.7 mg per lb. twice a day).

Child (under age 2): not recommended.

Overdosage

No specific information is available on raltegravir overdose. Take the victim to a hospital emergency room at once. If you seek treatment, ALWAYS bring the prescription bottle or container.

Special Information

This drug is not a cure for HIV. It will not prevent you from transmitting the HIV virus to another person; you must still practice safe sex. People taking this drug may still develop opportunistic infections and other complications of advanced HIV infection. It is very important to take these drugs exactly as prescribed. Every dose of HIV medication you forget or skip can make it more difficult for the drugs to do their job and can lead to the development of HIV resistance.

People infected with HIV must take especially good care of their teeth and gums to minimize the risk of developing oral infections.

If you forget a dose of raltegravir, take it as soon as you remember. If you do not remember until it is almost time for your next dose, skip the one you forgot and continue with your regular schedule. Do not take a double dose of this medicine. Contact your doctor if you forget 2 or more doses in a row.

Special Populations

Pregnancy/Breast-feeding: Animal studies of raltegravir have not shown it to be toxic to the developing fetus. It should be taken during pregnancy only if your doctor determines that the potential benefit outweighs the risks.

It is not known if raltegravir passes into breast milk. Mothers with HIV should always use infant formula, regardless of whether they take this drug, to avoid transmitting the virus to their child.

Seniors: Studies have not revealed any differences in response between seniors and younger adults. Caution is recommended because of the likelihood of other concurrent diseases and drug therapy, and reduced liver, kidney, and heart function in seniors.

Generic Name

Ramelteon (RAM-el-tee-on)

Brand Names

Rozerem

Type of Drug

Hypnotic.

Prescribed For

Insomnia characterized by difficulty falling asleep.

General Information

Ramelteon is a unique hypnotic that activates the same nerve endings in the brain that are acted on by melatonin, a hormone essential to natural sleep and our normal circadian rhythms, which dictate sleep-wake patterns. Some have called this drug "super-melatonin." It does not act on brain receptors targeted by other widely used sedatives and hypnotics.

Ramelteon studies have shown it has no potential for abuse, and it is not considered a controlled substance under federal laws. There is also no evidence of memory loss or hangover after 2 days of taking ramelteon. But in a study in which adults with chronic trouble sleeping took ramelteon for 35 consecutive nights, there was some morning-after fatigue and sluggishness as well as short-term memory difficulties. Information from this study also showed no risk for drug withdrawal symptoms or sleeplessness after stopping ramelteon.

Ramelteon passes rapidly into the blood and starts working in a few minutes. It is broken down in the liver and mostly passes out of the body in the urine.

Cautions and Warnings

Do not take ramelteon if you are **allergic** or **sensitive** to any of its ingredients. Allergic reactions may include breathing difficulties;

swelling of the lips, tongue, and throat; and nausea and vomiting. Stop using ramelteon and contact your doctor if you experience any of these symptoms.

People with severe **sleep apnea** should not use ramelteon because it has not been studied in this group. Ramelteon does not worsen mild to moderate sleep apnea.

People with severe **liver disease** should not take this drug. Even those with mild liver disease can have up to 4 times as much ramelteon in their blood as those with normal liver function.

Studies of ramelteon show a single dose does not cause difficulty breathing in people with **chronic obstructive pulmonary disease** (COPD). However, the long-term effects of ramelteon on people with COPD and other respiratory conditions have not yet been studied. People with breathing disorders should use this drug with caution.

Complex sleep-related behaviors, including driving, eating, and walking while asleep, with no memory of the event afterward, can occur with ramelteon and other sleep medications. These activities happen after taking a sedative-hypnotic product while you are not fully awake.

Ramelteon may also cause hallucinations, amnesia, anxiety, and behavioral changes in some people.

Difficulty sleeping may be a sign of another physical or psychiatric problem. If ramelteon does not help you, ask your doctor to look for other issues that might be interfering with your sleep and have not yet been discovered.

In depressed patients taking any hypnotic drug, worsening depression, including suicidal thoughts, is possible.

Ramelteon can affect hormone levels in adults, decreasing testosterone and increasing prolactin.

Possible Side Effects

- ▼ Most common: dizziness.
- ▼ Less common: fatigue, nausea, worsening sleeplessness, and headache.

Report any other side effects, particularly changes in behavior, to your doctor.

Drug Interactions

- Fluvoxamine can dramatically increase the amount of ramelteon in the blood by interfering with enzymes in the liver that break it down. Do not take ramelteon if you are also taking fluvoxamine.

- Ketoconazole and fluconazole increase the amount of ramelteon in the blood by affecting its breakdown in the liver. This combination should be used with caution.
- Rifampin increases the rate at which the liver breaks down ramelteon and can reduce its effectiveness.
- Alcohol can increase ramelteon's effects. Avoid alcoholic beverages before you take ramelteon or during the 30 minutes between taking ramelteon and going to sleep.

Food Interactions

This drug is best taken on an empty stomach. Taking it with or immediately after a high-fat meal will delay the absorption of ramelteon into the bloodstream.

Usual Dose

Adult: 8 mg taken 30 minutes before sleep.
Child: not recommended.

Overdosage

There have been no reports of ramelteon overdose, although symptoms are likely to be sleepiness and some of its side effects. Overdose victims should be taken to a hospital emergency room at once. If you seek treatment, ALWAYS bring the prescription bottle or container.

Special Information

Avoid engaging in activities that require concentration (such as operating a motor vehicle or heavy machinery) after taking ramelteon. Avoid alcohol.

Take ramelteon within 30 minutes of going to bed. After taking this drug, you should restrict your activities, since you are likely to become sleepy within a few minutes.

Contact your doctor if your insomnia gets worse while taking ramelteon or if you develop any behavioral changes, reduced sex drive (men or women), skipped periods, release of breast milk (women), or fertility problems (men or women).

Swallow ramelteon tablets whole; do not break them. Also, do not take more than 1 dose a day.

Special Populations

Pregnancy/Breast-feeding: In animal studies, ramelteon affected the development of a growing fetus, but its effects on the human fetus are unknown. Ramelteon should be taken during pregnancy only if your doctor determines that the potential benefit outweighs the risks.

In animal studies, ramelteon passed into the breast milk of nursing animals, but it is not known if this drug passes into human milk. Nursing mothers who must take this drug should use infant formula.

Seniors: Seniors may use this medication without restriction.

Generic Name

Ranolazine (rah-NO-la-zeen)

Brand Names

Ranexa

Type of Drug

Antianginal agent.

Prescribed For

Treatment of chronic angina that has not responded to other treatments.

General Information

Ranolazine has been studied in people with angina who had not responded to maximum doses of other antianginal drugs. These studies showed significant reductions in the number of angina attacks in people taking ranolazine. It is intended to reduce the number of angina attacks, not to treat an acute attack. It is broken down in the gut and the liver, so its absorption into the bloodstream can be very variable. It takes about 3 days of medicine to produce a steady blood level in your body. About ¾ of each dose passes out of the body via the urine. Ranolazine is prescribed in combination with other antianginal drugs, including some calcium channel blockers, beta blockers, and nitrates. Men appear to benefit more from ranolazine than women.

Cautions and Warnings

Do not take ranolazine if you are **allergic** or **sensitive** to any of its ingredients.

Ranolazine should be used with caution if you have moderate to severe **liver disease**. People with severe **kidney disease** may experience significant blood pressure increases. Check your blood pressure regularly. Ranolazine can affect your heart. People with an **abnormal electrocardiogram** (ECG) should not take this medicine.

Possible Side Effects

- ▼ Common: headache, dizziness, constipation, and nausea.
- ▼ Less common: ringing in the ears, fainting, dry mouth, abdominal pain, vomiting, swelling in the arms or legs, difficulty breathing, slow heartbeat, heart palpitations, blood in the urine, low blood pressure, dizziness when rising from a sitting or lying position, and tremors.
- ▼ Rare: swollen lip or face, choking, kidney failure, blurred vision, confusion, reduced sense of touch, tingling in the hands or feet, tremor, lung disease, and reduced white-blood-cell and platelet counts. Contact your doctor if you experience anything unusual while taking any medication.

Drug Interactions

There are many ranolazine drug interactions that are not listed below because they do not require any action.

- Clarithromycin, indinavir, itraconazole, ketoconazole, nefazodone, nelfinavir, ritonavir, saquinavir, and voriconazole interfere with one of the enzyme systems that break down ranolazine. Do not mix these drugs with ranolazine because they will raise the amount of ranolazine in the blood, leading to drug side effects.
- Other drugs that mildly slow the enzymes that break down ranolazine are aprepitant, diltiazem, erythromycin, fluconazole, and verapamil. These drugs may be mixed with ranolazine but your daily ranolazine dose must be limited to no more than 500 mg twice a day.
- Do not mix ranolazine with carbamazepine, phenobarbital, phenytoin, rifabutin, rifampin, rifapentine, or St. John's wort, drugs that strongly stimulate enzymes responsible for breaking down ranolazine.
- Caution should be exercised if you are taking ranolazine with cyclosporine. Your ranolazine dose may need to be reduced.
- Ranolazine may raise blood levels of antipsychotic drugs, digoxin (by 50%), and tricyclic antidepressants. Dosage adjustments may be needed.
- Like ranolazine, many drugs can affect your heart, including amiodarone, bepridil, cisapride, dofetilide, dolasetron,

droperidol, erythromycin, fluoxetine, halofantrine, haloperidol, mesoridazine, moexipril, quinidine, sotalol, thioridazine, ziprasidone, and others. These drugs should not be taken with ranolazine.

Food Interactions

Ranolazine can be taken without regard to food or meals. Do not drink grapefruit juice or eat any grapefruit- or starfruit-containing products while taking this medicine.

Usual Dose

Adult: 500–1000 mg twice a day. Do not chew, crush, or break the tablets.

Child: not recommended.

Overdosage

There are no cases of ranolazine overdose. Overdose symptoms may include drug side effects. Overdose patients should be taken to a hospital emergency room for treatment because of the possibility of an impact on the heart. If you seek treatment, ALWAYS bring the prescription bottle or container.

Special Information

Ranolazine should only be taken when other antianginal drugs have not worked.

Do not take more than 1000 mg twice a day. Larger doses are likely to affect your heart without producing a greater benefit.

Contact your doctor at once if you faint or have heart palpitations.

Ranolazine can make you dizzy or lightheaded. Take extreme care while driving or operating any complex equipment or machinery.

If you forget a dose, take it as soon as you remember. If it is almost time for the next dose, skip the one you forgot and continue with your regular schedule. Do not take a double dose.

Special Populations

Pregnancy/Breast-feeding: Animal studies show this drug may cause birth defects. Ranolazine should be taken during pregnancy only if your doctor determines that the potential benefit outweighs the risks.

It is not known if ranolazine passes into breast milk. Nursing mothers who must take it should use infant formula.

Seniors: Seniors age 75 and over may experience more ranolazine side effects than younger adults. Seniors should be started on the lowest effective dose of ranolazine.

Brand Names

Rebetron

Generic Ingredients

Interferon Alpha-2b + Ribavirin

Type of Drug

Antiviral combination.

Prescribed For

Hepatitis C virus (HCV) infection.

General Information

This combination should be used only when interferon alpha has failed. Ribavirin is not effective against HCV by itself. The way that this combination works against HCV is not known.

HCV infection can be especially serious in people with HIV. Interferon alpha or a long-acting (pegylated) interferon alpha called Pegasys, taken either alone or in combination with the antiviral pill ribavirin, can be given to people coinfected with chronic HCV and HIV, who are at greatest risk for progression to serious disease. Treatment does not always work, but HIV-infected patients may benefit from treatment with this combination.

For more information on both of these drugs, see also their individual drug profiles, Interferon Alpha, page 634, and Ribavirin, page 997.

Cautions and Warnings

Do not take Rebetron if you are **allergic** or **sensitive** to any of its ingredients.

All people taking this combination must be closely monitored by their doctors, including having periodic blood, liver, and thyroid function tests.

People with **kidney disease**, **heart disease**, **sickle-cell anemia**, or **thalassemia** (a genetic blood disorder) should use this medication with caution. If heart disease worsens during treatment, the drug should be discontinued.

Hearing disorders and fainting have occurred in people taking this medication.

Rebetron can affect both sperm and egg. Men and women taking Rebetron must use effective contraception during treatment and for 6 months after treatment is completed. Contact your doctor if pregnancy occurs.

People with **autoimmune hepatitis** should not use Rebetron.

People who develop severe side effects or become depressed while taking this medication should have their interferon dosage temporarily lowered. The medication should be stopped if severe depression develops.

Children as young as age 1 have been treated with interferon alpha, but the combination product has not been studied in children of any age.

Possible Side Effects

Some people experience no side effects while taking Rebetron, and most feel well enough to work and travel during treatment.

▼ Most common: depression, fever, tiredness, headache, muscle aches, chills, flu-like symptoms, irritability, nausea, diarrhea, appetite loss, abdominal pain, weakness, joint and muscle pain, and feeling unwell.

▼ Common: dry mouth, thirst, dizziness, tingling in the hands or feet, sleep disturbances, vomiting, upset stomach, weight loss, and hemolytic anemia (red-blood-cell destruction).

▼ Less common: loss of concentration, nervousness, constipation, loose stools, changes in sense of taste, sore throat, breathing difficulties, sinus irritation, inflamed injection site (interferon alpha only), chest pain, and sweating.

▼ Rare: confusion, loss of sex drive, stuffy nose, coughing, facial swelling, and cold sores. Other rare side effects can occur in almost any part of the body. Contact your doctor if you experience anything unusual while taking any medication.

Drug Interactions

- Antacids may reduce the amount of ribavirin absorbed.
- Interferon alpha-2b can significantly increase the level of theophylline in the blood.
- Combining interferon alpha-2b with zidovudine (AZT) may result in serious side effects. If taking this combination, your white-blood-cell count must be monitored carefully.

Food Interactions

High-fat meals can increase the amount of ribavirin absorbed, though the importance of this is not known. These drugs can be taken without regard to food or meals.

Usual Dose

Adult (166 lbs. and over): ribavirin—600 mg in the morning and at night; interferon alpha—3 million units 3 times a week by injection under the skin.

Adult (under 166 lbs.): ribavirin—400 mg in the morning and 600 mg at night; interferon alpha—3 million units 3 times a week by injection under the skin.

Child (110–134 lbs.): ribavirin—400 mg morning and night; interferon alpha—3 million units 3 times a week by injection under skin.

Child (81–109 lbs.): ribavirin—200 mg in the morning and 400 mg at night; interferon alpha—3 million units 3 times a week by injection under the skin.

Child (55–80 lbs.): ribavirin—200 mg morning and night; interferon alpha—3 million units 3 times a week by injection under skin.

Child (under 55 lbs.): not recommended.

Overdosage

Little is known about the effects of Rebetron overdose. Take the victim to a hospital emergency room. If you seek treatment, ALWAYS bring the prescription bottle or container.

Special Information

Rebetron is administered in 2 forms—capsule (ribavirin) and injection (interferon alpha-2b). For information on how to properly administer injections, see page 1242.

This medication can make you drowsy. Be careful when driving or performing any task that requires concentration.

Drink lots of water while using Rebetron to make sure you are well hydrated.

Contact your doctor at once if hives, itching, chest tightness, coughing, breathing difficulties, visual difficulties, wheezing, low blood pressure, or lightheadedness develop. These can be signs of drug allergy.

Rebetron can make you more sensitive to the sun. Avoid spending a lot of time in the sun while taking it.

If you forget to take a dose of interferon alpha, take it as soon as you remember. If it is almost time for your next dose, space your remaining weekly doses throughout the rest of the week. If you forget a dose of ribavirin, take it as soon as you remember. If it is almost time for your next dose, skip the dose you forgot and continue with your regular schedule. Do not take a double dose. Contact your doctor if you forget 2 or more doses in a row.

Do not change brands of interferon alpha without your doctor's knowledge—they may not be equivalent.

Special Populations

Pregnancy/Breast-feeding: Rebetron should not be taken by pregnant women or their male partners because of its effect on the sperm, egg, and fetus. Women must be tested monthly to be sure they are not pregnant.

It is not known if the ingredients in Rebetron pass into breast milk. Nursing mothers who must take this medication should use infant formula.

Seniors: Rebetron is partially passed out of the body through the kidneys. Seniors should use this drug with caution because of the risk of kidney damage.

Generic Name

Repaglinide (reh-PAG-lih-nide)

Brand Names

Prandin

The information in this profile also applies to the following drugs:

Generic Ingredients: Nateglinide G
Starlix

Combination Products
Generic Ingredients: Repaglinide + Metformin Hydrochloride
PrandiMet

Type of Drug

Antidiabetic.

Prescribed For

Type 2 diabetes.

General Information

In people with type 2 diabetes, the pancreas does not make enough insulin and the hormone does not work as well as in normal people. Because insulin regulates the amount of sugar in the blood, lack of this hormone causes blood sugar to rise to unhealthy levels. When taken with meals, repaglinide temporarily stimulates the pancreas to release more insulin when it is needed to help process dietary sugar. This helps to stabilize blood sugar. Repaglinide may be used alone or with metformin or other antidiabetes drugs. Repaglinide works only if beta cells in the pancreas are functioning.

Cautions and Warnings

Do not use repaglinide if you are **allergic** or **sensitive** to its ingredients.

Because repaglinide is broken down in the liver, people with **liver problems** may require reduced dosage or more time between doses.

People with severe **kidney disease** must start with the lowest effective dose of repaglinide.

People with **liver disease** should use nateglinide and repaglinide with caution.

Any antidiabetes drug can excessively **lower blood sugar**. Do not use **NPH insulin** while taking one of these drugs. Low blood sugar can develop when you do not consume enough calories, overexert yourself physically, drink alcohol, or combine blood-sugar-lowering drugs (see "Overdosage" for low blood-sugar symptoms).

You may need to temporarily switch to insulin therapy if you have **surgery** or experience **fever**, **infection**, or **trauma**.

Possible Side Effects

Nateglinide

- ▼ Most common: respiratory infection.
- ▼ Less common: bronchitis, cough, back pain, flu-like symptoms, dizziness, joint disease, diarrhea, accidents, and low blood sugar.
- ▼ Rare: allergy. Contact your doctor if you experience anything unusual while taking any medication.

Repaglinide

- ▼ Most common: low blood sugar, headache, and respiratory infection.
- ▼ Common: sinus irritation, runny nose, bronchitis, nausea, diarrhea, and back or joint pain.
- ▼ Less common: constipation, vomiting, upset stomach, tingling in the hands or feet, chest pain, urinary infection, and tooth problems.

Possible Side Effects *(continued)*

▼ Rare: allergy. Contact your doctor if you experience anything unusual while taking any medication.

For more information about PrandiMet, see Metformin, page 731.

Drug Interactions

- Avoid using repaglinide with gemfibrozil and/or itraconazole because of the risk of extremely low blood sugar.
- Combining repaglinide with clarithromycin, erythromycin, ketoconazole, miconazole, and simvastatin may increase repaglinide blood levels and result in low blood sugar. Your repaglinide dose may need to be adjusted.
- Rifampin may decrease blood levels of nateglinide and repaglinide and reduce their effectiveness. Repaglinide effectiveness may also be decreased by barbiturates and carbamazepine. Dose adjustments may be necessary.
- The blood-sugar-lowering effect of all antidiabetes drugs may be increased by aspirin and other salicylates, beta blockers, chloramphenicol, cyclosporine, monoamine oxidase inhibitor (MAOI) antidepressants, nonsteroidal anti-inflammatory drugs (NSAIDs), probenecid, sulfa drugs, and warfarin-type anticoagulants (blood thinners).
- Calcium channel blockers, contraceptive drugs, corticosteroids, estrogens, isoniazid, nicotinic acid, phenothiazines, phenytoin, stimulants, thiazides and other diuretics, and thyroid drugs may increase blood-sugar levels. Your dosage of nateglinide or repaglinide may need to be increased if you combine it with any of these drugs.

For more information about PrandiMet, see Metformin, page 731.

Food Interactions

Repaglinide should be taken before meals because food interferes with its absorption in the blood.

Usual Dose

Nateglinide

Adult: 60–120 mg 1–30 minutes before each meal, 3 times a day.

Child: not recommended.

Repaglinide

Adult: 0.5–4 mg 15–30 minutes before each meal, up to 4 times a day. Adults with severe kidney disease should start at 0.5 mg before each meal.

Child: not recommended.

Repaglinide + Metformin

Adult: 1/500–4/1000 mg, taken as 1–2 tablets 15–30 minutes before a meal twice a day.

Child: not recommended.

Overdosage

Low blood sugar may occur. Symptoms of low blood sugar are cold sweats, anxiety, cool and pale skin, difficulty concentrating, drowsiness, excessive hunger, headache, nausea, nervousness, rapid pulse, shakiness, unusual tiredness or weakness, and vision changes. Take the overdose victim to a hospital emergency room. If you seek treatment, ALWAYS bring the prescription bottle or container.

Special Information

Measurements of blood sugar and glycosylated hemoglobin (A1C) are essential to your doctor's evaluation of your progress. See your doctor regularly.

Repaglinide must be taken 15–30 minutes before you eat. If you skip a meal, do not take this drug. If you have an extra meal, take an extra dose before that meal.

The timing of each repaglinide dose is key to its effectiveness. If you forget to take repaglinide before a meal, take it during the meal. If you have already eaten and forgotten your medication, skip the forgotten dose. If you cannot remember to take repaglinide before each meal, talk to your doctor about changing drugs.

Special Populations

Pregnancy/Breast-feeding: Repaglinide should not be taken during pregnancy. Animal studies indicate that it may affect the skeletal development of the fetus. Most experts recommend that diabetes be controlled with insulin during pregnancy.

It is not known if repaglinide passes into breast milk. Nursing mothers who must take it should use infant formula.

Seniors: Some seniors may be more sensitive to the effects of this drug.

Restasis *see* ***Cyclosporine,*** *page 369*

Generic Name

Retapamulin (reh-tah-PAM-u-lin)

Brand Names

Altabax

The information in this profile also applies to the following drugs:

Generic Ingredients: Mupirocin G
Bactroban Centany

Type of Drug

Antibacterial.

Prescribed For

Impetigo (staphylococcal and streptococcal skin infections) and other minor bacterial skin infections. Mupirocin nasal is used to prevent resistant *Staphylococcus aureus* infections from spreading during outbreaks of the infection. Mupirocin can also be used to treat diaper rash.

General Information

Retapamulin is an antibiotic ointment that is applied directly to the impetigo blisters, especially those that have burst and are leaking pus. Mupirocin is used to supplement other treatments for impetigo, although many doctors prefer oral medication. Mupirocin works by interfering with bacteria's ability to make the proteins it needs for survival. Large amounts of mupirocin kill bacteria and smaller amounts stop the bacteria from growing. It may be effective against antibiotic-resistant bacteria. Impetigo is a skin infection caused by *S. aureus* or *Streptococcus pyogenes.* It is most common in children age 2–6, but it can affect people of all ages. Impetigo usually begins when bacteria enter a break in the skin, such as a cut, scratch, or insect bite. Early symptoms include red or pimple-like sores surrounded by red skin. These sores can be anywhere, but usually they occur on the face, arms, and legs. The sores fill with pus, then break open after a few days and form a thick crust. They are often itchy, but scratching them can spread the sores. Impetigo can spread by contact with sores or nasal discharge from an infected person.

Cautions and Warnings

Do not use these products if you are **allergic** or **sensitive** to any of their ingredients. Stop using them if you experience a severe skin irritation.

Mupirocin nasal should be used only to treat *S. aureus* infections, not to prevent them. Large quantities of mupirocin ointment should not be applied to an open wound because polyethylene glycol—used as a base in mupirocin ointment—may be absorbed through the wound and damage the kidneys.

Long-term or chronic use of mupirocin may lead to secondary infection caused by drug-resistant bacteria or fungi.

Do not swallow this ointment or apply it directly to the eye or to the inside of the mouth, nose, or vagina.

Possible Side Effects

Mupirocin

Cream

- ▼ Less common: headache, rash, and nausea.
- ▼ Rare: abdominal pain, burning, irritation, inflammation, dizziness, itching, secondary infection, and mouth ulcer. Contact your doctor if you experience anything unusual when taking any medication.

Nasal Ointment

- ▼ Most common: headache and runny nose.
- ▼ Less common: respiratory congestion, sore throat, changes in sense of taste, burning or stinging, cough, and itching.
- ▼ Rare: eyelid inflammation, diarrhea, dry mouth, ear pain, nosebleeds, nausea, and rash. Contact your doctor if you experience anything unusual when taking any medication.

Ointment

- ▼ Less common: burning, pain, and itching.
- ▼ Rare: rash, stinging, or pain where the ointment is applied; nausea; skin redness; dry skin; tenderness; swelling; and increased oozing from impetigo lesions. Contact your doctor if you experience anything unusual when taking any medication.

Possible Side Effects *(continued)*

Retapamulin

- ▼ Most common: skin irritation at the application site and itching.
- ▼ Less common: irritation of the nose and throat, headache, nausea, diarrhea, eczema, and fever.
- ▼ Rare: pain at the application site, local swelling, and contact dermatitis. Contact your doctor if you experience anything unusual while taking any medication.

Drug Interactions

None known.

Usual Dose

Mupirocin

Nasal Ointment: Put ½ the ointment from a single-use tube in each nostril morning and evening for 5 days. After the ointment is applied, gently squeeze your nostrils closed and allow them to open again. Repeat this continuously for about 1 minute.

Ointment and Cream: Apply a small amount to the affected area 3 times a day. Cover with sterile gauze if desired.

Retapamulin

Adult and Child (9 months and over): Apply a thin layer of ointment to the affected areas twice a day for 5 days. You should not cover an area of more than 4 in. by 4 in. on any day because of the possibility of absorbing too much antibiotic into the blood. Cover with sterile gauze if desired.

Overdosage

Little is known about overdose with these medications. Contact your local poison control center or a hospital emergency room for more information. If you seek treatment, ALWAYS bring the prescription container.

Special Information

Contact your doctor if this medication does not work within 3–5 days or if any of the following symptoms develop: dry skin or redness, rash, itching, stinging, pain, or other possible drug reactions. Do not use this ointment more often than prescribed or for longer than 5 days. Excessive use can lead to the development of resistant bacteria, making this and other infections harder to treat.

Clean and dry the affected area before applying the cream or ointment.

If you forget a dose, apply it as soon as you remember. If it is almost time for the next dose, skip the one you forgot and continue with your regular schedule. Do not apply a double dose.

Special Populations

Pregnancy/Breast-feeding: There are no studies of these drugs in pregnant women. They should be used during pregnancy only if your doctor determines that the potential benefit outweighs the risks.

It is not known if these drugs pass into breast milk. Nursing mothers should use infant formula.

Seniors: Seniors may use this drug without special precaution.

Generic Name

Ribavirin (ry-bah-VY-rin) G

Brand Names

Copegus
Rebetol
Ribasphere

Type of Drug

Antiviral.

Prescribed For

Hepatitis C virus (HCV) infection.

General Information

Ribavirin is part of a 2-drug combination (with peginterferon injection) that has become a primary treatment for active HCV infection in adults with some liver disease. The exact way that it works against HCV is not known. Ribavirin is not effective for chronic HCV infections without interferon injections or for any other type of virus infection. It does not work against any other form of hepatitis.

HCV infection can be especially serious in people with HIV. Interferon alpha or a long-acting (pegylated) interferon called Pegasys, either alone or taken in combination with the ribavirin drug Copegus, can be given to people co-infected with chronic HCV and HIV, who are at greatest risk for progression to serious disease. Treatment does not always work, but HIV-infected patients may benefit from treatment with this combination.

Because this drug is always taken in combination with injectable interferon alpha, see Interferon Alpha, page 634, for further information.

Cautions and Warnings

Do not take ribavirin if you are **allergic** or **sensitive** to any of its ingredients.

People with **kidney damage** and those with moderate to severe **liver disease** or liver disease caused by an autoimmune reaction (in which the liver is attacked by the body's own defense system) should not take this medicine.

People with **cancer** and those taking antirejection drugs because they have had an **organ transplant** should not take ribavirin.

Ribavirin may worsen **heart disease**, causing high blood pressure, increased heart rate, and chest pain.

People with **sickle-cell disease**, **thalassemia** (a genetic blood disorder), and other **hemoglobin abnormalities** should not take ribavirin.

Serious side effects of combination therapy include severe depression, hemolytic anemia, suppression of bone marrow function, autoimmune and infectious disorders, pulmonary dysfunction, pancreatitis, and diabetes. Ribavirin should not be used by **pregnant** women or by men whose female partners are pregnant.

Possible Side Effects

Virtually every person who takes ribavirin + interferon for HCV will develop a drug side effect.

▼ Most common: nausea; vomiting; diarrhea; depression; insomnia; irritability; anxiety; inability to concentrate; flu-like symptoms such as fatigue, fever, chills, joint pain, and muscle aches; headache; bacterial infections; severe anemia (usually within the first 2 weeks of ribavirin therapy) and reductions in white-blood-cell counts; difficulty breathing; fluid in the lungs; pneumonia; inflammation of the pancreas; hair loss; itching; and rashes.

▼ Common: loss of appetite, diarrhea, abdominal pain, injection-site reactions, liver failure, dizziness, confusion, back pain, mood changes, tiredness or fatigue, dry mouth, coughing, unusual shortness of breath after exertion, upset

Possible Side Effects *(continued)*

stomach, reduced thyroid gland activity, reduced blood-platelet count, blurred vision, sweating, and eczema.

▼ Rare: Rare side effects can occur in almost any part of the body. Some rare side effects include suicidal thoughts, psychosis, aggression, anxiety, drug abuse and overdose, detachment of the retina, heart pain, liver damage, abnormal heart rhythms, worsening diabetes, overactive thyroid, systemic lupus erythematosus (a chronic autoimmune disease), rheumatoid arthritis, nerve damage, aplastic anemia, stomach ulcers, gastrointestinal bleeding, colitis, corneal ulcer, pulmonary embolism, coma, myositis, and stroke. Contact your doctor if you experience anything unusual while taking any medication.

For further side effects for combination treatments, see Interferon Alpha, page 634.

Drug Interactions

- Ribavirin increases blood levels of didanosine and can increase the risk of drug side effects, including fatal liver failure, pancreas inflammation, and nervous system problems. This combination should be avoided.
- Ribavirin should be used with caution with nucleoside analogues.
- Ribavirin slows the metabolism of several HIV antivirals (lamivudine, stavudine, and zidovudine). This may increase the risk of drug side effects, including anemia.
- Treatment with interferon, typically prescribed with ribavirin, increases blood levels of theophylline by 25%, increasing the risk of drug side effects.

For further drug interactions for combination treatments, see Interferon Alpha, page 634.

Food Interactions

Take ribavirin with food.

Usual Dose

Copegus

Adult: chronic HCV infection—800–1200 mg a day, divided into 2 doses, depending on body weight and the type of HCV infection; chronic HCV with HIV co-infection—800 mg a day. Dosage adjustments may be required if severe side effects occur.

Child (age 5 and over): 400–1200 mg a day, divided into 2 doses, depending on body weight.

Child (under age 5): not recommended.

Rebetol and Ribasphere

Adult: 800–1400 mg a day, divided into 2 doses, depending on body weight.

Child (age 3 and over; 103 lbs. and over): 800–1200 mg a day, divided into 2 doses, depending on body weight.

Child (age 3 and over; less than 103 lbs.): 6.8 mg per lb. of body weight a day, divided into 2 doses.

Child (severe respiratory syncytial virus): 20 mg/mL solution once a day via aerosol over 12–18 hours for 3–7 days.

Overdosage

Take the overdose victim to a hospital emergency room at once. If you seek treatment, ALWAYS bring the prescription bottle or container.

Special Information

Contact your doctor at once if you begin to have trouble breathing or develop pneumonia or abdominal pain.

Contact your doctor if you become severely depressed or suicidal or develop flu-like symptoms, fever, chills, muscle pain, headache, hives or swelling, severe stomach pain, lower back pain, bruising or unusual bleeding, worsening psoriasis, changes in your vision, tiredness or weakness, appetite loss, nausea, vomiting, sore throat, unusual bleeding or bruising, yellowing of the skin or whites of the eyes, rash, or itching.

This drug can cause dizziness, confusion, tiredness, or fatigue. Avoid driving or operating machinery until you know how this drug affects you.

Alcoholic beverages can worsen liver disease and should be avoided if you have any form of hepatitis.

If you forget a dose of ribavirin, take it as soon as you remember. If it is almost time for your next dose, skip the forgotten dose and continue with your regular schedule. Do not take a double dose. Regularly missing doses of this medicine will reduce the ability of this drug to fight HCV.

Special Populations

Pregnancy/Breast-feeding: Ribavirin is toxic to a developing fetus and causes birth defects, and it remains in the body for up to 6 months after a course of treatment is finished. Pregnant women and their male partners and women who may be pregnant must avoid this drug.

Use at least 2 reliable forms of contraception to avoid becoming pregnant during treatment and for at least 6 months after a course of ribavirin therapy has been completed. The female partners of men taking ribavirin should also practice this form of contraception.

This drug may pass into breast milk. Nursing mothers who take ribavirin should use infant formula.

Seniors: Seniors should use this drug with caution because of the risk of kidney damage.

Generic Name

Rifampin (rih-FAM-pin) G

Brand Names

Rifadin

Combination Products

Generic Ingredients: Rifampin + Isoniazid G
Rifamate

Generic Ingredients: Rifampin + Isoniazid + Pyrazinamide
Rifater

Type of Drug

Antitubercular.

Prescribed For

Tuberculosis, meningitis carriers, and other infections.

General Information

Rifampin, an important agent in the treatment of tuberculosis, is always used with at least 1 other tuberculosis drug. It is also prescribed to eradicate the organism that causes meningitis in carriers—people who are not infected themselves but carry the organism and can spread it to others. Rifampin can be used to treat strep throat; staphylococcal infections of the skin, bones, or prostate; cat scratch disease; Legionnaires' disease; leprosy; and to prevent meningitis caused by *Haemophilus influenzae.*

Cautions and Warnings

Do not take rifampin if you are **allergic** or **sensitive** to any of its ingredients, or to rifabutin, prescribed for *Mycobacterium avium* complex (an infection associated with advanced cases of AIDS).

Liver damage and death have been reported in people taking rifabutin, a drug that is very similar to rifampin. It is also the principal side effect of pyrazinamide, an ingredient in Rifater. People taking other drugs that may cause liver damage should avoid rifampin. If you have **liver disease**, your doctor should monitor your liver function.

Reduced white-blood-cell and platelet counts that may be severe can occur with high doses of rifampin.

Bacterial resistance develops very quickly if rifampin is used for active **meningococcus infection**. It should not be used for this purpose.

Rifampin should not be used in people with **porphyria**.

It is very important that you comply with the full course of therapy and not miss any doses; otherwise, the drug may not work and may cause increased side effects.

Possible Side Effects

▼ Most common: flu-like symptoms; heartburn; upset stomach; appetite loss; nausea; vomiting; gas; cramps; diarrhea; headache; drowsiness; tiredness; menstrual disturbances; dizziness; fever; pain in the joints, arms, and legs; confusion; visual disturbances; numbness; and hypersensitivity to the drug.

▼ Less common: effects on the blood, kidneys, or liver.

▼ Rare: Rare side effects can occur in almost any part of the body. Contact your doctor if you experience anything unusual while taking any medication.

Drug Interactions

- Severe and sometimes fatal hepatitis has also occurred in people taking isoniazid, another antitubercular drug often combined with rifampin. This combination produces more liver damage than either drug taken alone. People with liver disease should be carefully monitored by their doctors and receive reduced dosage.
- Severe liver damage, including hepatitis, may develop when rifampin is combined with other drugs that may cause liver

toxicity, such as the protease inhibitors ritonavir and saquinavir. Do not use rifampin with any protease inhibitor; their effectiveness may also be affected.

- Rifampin may increase your need for oral anticoagulant (blood thinning) drugs and may also affect angiotensin-converting enzyme (ACE) inhibitors, especially enalapril.
- Rifampin may reduce the effectiveness of acetaminophen; anticonvulsants; oral antidiabetes drugs; barbiturates; benzodiazepines; beta blockers; buspirone; chloramphenicol; clarithromycin, erythromycin, and other macrolide antibiotics; corticosteroids; cyclosporine; digoxin; disopyramide; doxycycline; estrogens; fluoroquinolone anti-infectives; haloperidol; inamrinone; itraconazole; ketoconazole; losartan; methadone; mexiletine; narcotics; ondansetron; phenytoin; quinidine; quinine drugs; sulfa drugs; tacrolimus; theophylline drugs; thyroid hormones; tocainide; tricyclic antidepressants; verapamil; zidovudine (AZT); and zolpidem.
- Drugs that can interfere with rifampin include aminosalicylic acid, itraconazole, and ketoconazole.
- Women taking contraceptive drugs should use another contraceptive method while taking rifampin.
- Liver toxicity has developed when people taking rifampin were given halothane, a general anesthetic, prior to surgery.

Food Interactions

Take rifampin and all rifampin combinations 1 hour before or 2 hours after a meal, at the same time every day.

Usual Dose

Rifamate

Adult: 2 capsules once a day.

Rifampin

Adult: 4.5 mg per lb. of body weight, up to 600 mg a day.
Child: 4.5–9 mg per lb. of body weight, up to 600 mg a day.

Rifater

Adult and Child (age 15 and over): This drug is dosed according to body weight. The following dose should be taken once a day on an empty stomach, either 1 hour before or 2 hours after a meal, with a full glass of water.

120 lbs. or more—6 tablets

100–120 lbs.—5 tablets
97 lbs. or less—4 tablets
Child (under age 15): not recommended.

Overdosage

Take the overdose victim to a hospital emergency room at once. If you seek treatment, ALWAYS bring the prescription bottle or container.

Symptoms of rifampin overdose include nausea, vomiting, and tiredness. Unconsciousness is possible in cases of severe liver damage. Brown-red or orange skin discoloration may also develop.

Early manifestations of an overdose of isoniazid, an ingredient in Rifamate and Rifater, include nausea, vomiting, dizziness, slurring of speech, blurring of vision, and visual hallucinations. Respiratory distress and central-nervous-system depression, moving rapidly from stupor to profound coma, are to be expected with marked overdosage, along with severe, intractable seizures.

Pyrazinamide overdose is likely to cause liver problems.

Special Information

Rifampin may cause a red-brown or orange discoloration of the urine, stool, saliva, sweat, or tears; this is not harmful. Soft contact lenses and dentures may become permanently stained.

Contact your doctor if you develop flu-like symptoms, fever, chills, muscle pain, headache, tiredness or weakness, appetite loss, nausea, vomiting, sore throat, unusual bleeding or bruising, yellowing of the skin or whites of the eyes, rash, or itching.

If you take rifampin once a day and miss a dose, take it as soon as you remember. If it is almost time for your next dose, skip the dose you forgot and continue with your regular schedule. Do not take a double dose. Regularly missing doses of rifampin increases the risk of side effects.

Special Populations

Pregnancy/Breast-feeding: Animal studies indicate that rifampin may cause cleft palate and spina bifida (birth defect in which bones of the lower spinal column do not form properly, leaving the spinal canal partially exposed) in the fetus. Pregnant women should use this drug only if absolutely necessary.

This drug may pass into breast milk. Nursing mothers who must take it should use infant formula.

Seniors: Seniors with liver disease may be more sensitive to the effects of this drug.

Generic Name

Rifaximin (rih-FAX-ih-min)

Brand Names

Xifaxan

Type of Drug

Antibiotic.

Prescribed For

Traveler's diarrhea caused by *Escherichia coli* and prevention of hepatic encephalopathy (HE); also used for *Clostridium difficile* infection and irritable bowel syndrome.

General Information

Many people who travel outside of the United States develop "traveler's diarrhea" because their food and water is contaminated with the bacterium *E. coli.* This bacterium is also responsible for the majority of food poisoning cases in the United States, and some have said that the common "stomach flu" is really just a minor case of food poisoning. Other antibiotics have been successful in treating *E. coli* bacteria, but the advantage of rifaximin is that only a very small amount of it is absorbed into the blood. It stays in the intestines where the offending bacteria are located.

HE occurs in people with cirrhosis and other forms of liver disease. Normally the liver cleans toxins out of the blood, but when the liver is damaged, these toxins continue circulating throughout the body and can damage the brain, resulting in confusion, behavioral changes, and other mental impairments.

Cautions and Warnings

Do not take rifaximin if you are **allergic** or **sensitive** to any of its ingredients or to any of the group of antibiotics known as rifamycins. The best-known member of the group is rifampin. Reported allergic reactions include severe rash, swelling of the face and tongue, difficulty swallowing, hives, flushing, and itching. Some of these reactions have occurred as soon as 15 minutes after taking this medicine.

Do not take rifaximin if you have **fever** and/or **bloody stool** unless you consult your doctor.

Rifaximin should not be used to treat the form of diarrhea known as **dysentery**. Dysentery symptoms are often mild and vague. Usually there is persistent discomfort, nausea, and mild diarrhea with blood and mucus. Occasionally there is also tenderness over the area of the liver.

Treatment with antibiotics can cause diarrhea or, more seriously, colitis. Contact your doctor if diarrhea symptoms worsen while taking rifaximin.

Possible Side Effects

- ▼ Most common: dizziness, swelling of the hands and feet, intestinal gas, headache, abdominal pain, urgent bowel movements, nausea, and constipation.
- ▼ Common: fatigue, itching, fever, and vomiting.
- ▼ Less common: hives and skin rash.
- ▼ Rare: Rare side effects can occur in almost any part of the body. Contact your doctor if you experience anything unusual while taking any medication.

Drug and Food Interactions

None known.

Usual Dose

Hepatic Encephalopathy

Adult: 550 mg twice a day.

Child: not recommended.

Traveler's Diarrhea

Adult and Child (age 12 and over): 200 mg 3 times a day for 3 days.

Child (under age 12): not recommended.

Overdosage

There is no experience with rifaximin overdose, although people in studies using doses larger than the usual dose of 600 mg a day have experienced the same side effects as those taking the usual dose. Contact your local poison control center or a hospital emergency room for more information. If you do seek treatment, ALWAYS bring the prescription bottle or container.

Special Information

You should contact your doctor if you think your condition is getting worse, if diarrhea develops, or if you are not improving after 24–48 hours (1–2 days) while taking rifaximin for traveler's diarrhea.

If you forget a dose, take it as soon as you remember. If it is almost time for your next dose, skip the dose you forgot and continue with your regular schedule. Do not take a double dose.

Special Populations

Pregnancy/Breast-feeding: Animal studies of rifaximin show that it causes birth defects. It should be taken during pregnancy only if your doctor determines that the potential benefit outweighs the risks.

It is not known if rifaximin passes into breast milk. Nursing mothers who must take this drug should use infant formula.

Seniors: Seniors may be more sensitive than younger adults to this medication.

Generic Name

Riluzole (RIL-ue-zole) G

Brand Names

Rilutek

Type of Drug

Glutamate-release blocker.

Prescribed For

Amyotrophic lateral sclerosis (ALS), also known as Lou Gehrig's disease.

General Information

ALS is a chronic disease of the nervous system. Riluzole, the only drug proven to affect ALS, has a number of different actions, although exactly how it works is unknown. The drug slows the release of glutamate, which is thought to damage important nerve centers in the brain of those with ALS, and protects other aspects of nerve function. Riluzole extended survival in people with ALS during 18 months of treatment, though muscle strength and nerve function did not improve. Overall, death rates at the end of the studies were the same whether people took riluzole or not. In one study, the average life extension for people taking riluzole was 60 days. Riluzole is broken down in the liver.

Cautions and Warnings

Do not take riluzole if you are **allergic** or **sensitive** to any of its ingredients.

Riluzole causes liver inflammation; people with severe **liver disease** should use this drug with caution. Liver function should be evaluated regularly. People with **kidney disease** should also use riluzole with caution.

Rarely, there have been cases of neutropenia (low white-blood-cell count) and anemia in people taking riluzole. Report any sign of fever to your doctor, who should check your levels of white blood cells.

Women and **people of Japanese descent** may eliminate riluzole from their bodies twice as slowly as do male Caucasians. The drug may be eliminated more slowly due to genetic factors or because of differences in diet such as decreased use of alcohol, nicotine, and caffeine.

Cigarette smoking is likely to increase the rate at which riluzole is broken down by the liver. The drug may break down more quickly in women than in men. There is no indication that either of these factors is important in determining riluzole dosage.

Taking more than 100 mg a day of riluzole increases side effects and is not more effective.

Possible Side Effects

About 14% of people stop taking riluzole because of side effects.

- ▼ Most common: weakness, nausea, dizziness (twice as common in women), diarrhea, a tingling sensation around the mouth, appetite loss, fainting, and tiredness. These effects increase with dosage.
- ▼ Common: poor lung function, abdominal pain, pneumonia, and vomiting.
- ▼ Less common: back pain, headache, upset stomach at high dosages, gas, stuffy nose, runny nose, cough, high blood pressure, joint aches, and swelling in the arms and legs. At high dosages, side effects can include urinary infection and painful urination, and dizziness when rising from a lying or sitting position.
- ▼ Rare: aggravation, feeling unwell, mouth infection, eczema, rapid heartbeat, and vein irritation. Other rare side effects can occur in almost any part of the body. Contact your doctor if you experience anything unusual while taking any medication.

Drug Interactions

- Allopurinol, methyldopa, sulfasalazine, and other drugs that are toxic to the liver may interact with riluzole. Combinations of liver-toxic drugs should be taken with caution.
- Amitriptyline, caffeine, phenacetin, quinolone antibacterials, and theophylline may slow the elimination of riluzole, increasing the risk of drug side effects.
- Rifampin and omeprazole may quicken the elimination of riluzole.

Food Interactions

Take riluzole on an empty stomach, at least 1 hour before or 2 hours after meals, with a full glass of water. Avoid char-grilled foods, which may speed the elimination of riluzole. Avoid high-fat meals, which decrease the absorption of riluzole.

Usual Dose

Adult: 50 mg every 12 hours.
Child: not recommended.

Overdosage

Little is known about the effects of riluzole overdose. Take the victim to a hospital emergency room at once. If you seek treatment, ALWAYS bring the prescription bottle or container.

Special Information

Taking more than 50 mg twice a day will not improve your condition and may increase drug side effects.

Contact your doctor at once if you become feverish or ill. This could be a sign of a very low white-blood-cell count.

Riluzole should be taken at the same time each day—morning and evening—to achieve maximum benefit.

Riluzole can make you dizzy, tired, or faint. Be careful when driving or doing any task that requires concentration.

People taking riluzole should not drink excessive amounts of alcohol.

Store riluzole tablets at between 68°–77°F and protect them from bright light.

If you forget a dose, take it as soon as you remember. If it is almost time for your next dose, skip the dose you forgot and continue with your regular schedule. Do not take a double dose.

Special Populations

Pregnancy/Breast-feeding: Riluzole is toxic to pregnant lab animals at high dosages. It should be taken during pregnancy only if your doctor determines that the potential benefit outweighs the risks.

It is not known if riluzole passes into breast milk. Nursing mothers who must take it should use infant formula.

Seniors: Seniors with kidney or liver disease should use riluzole with caution.

Generic Name

Rimantadine (rih-MAN-tuh-dene) G

Brand Names

Flumadine

Type of Drug

Antiviral.

Prescribed For

Influenza A viral infection (type A flu).

General Information

Rimantadine is a synthetic antiviral agent that appears to interfere with the reproduction of various strains of the influenza A virus, a common cause of viral infection. Rimantadine is used both to treat and to prevent type A flu; however, it is indicated only for influenza A prevention in children. Annual vaccination against the virus is the best way of preventing the flu, but immunity takes 2–4 weeks to develop. In the meantime, rimantadine may be taken to prevent viral infection in high-risk people or people who may experience greater exposure to the virus.

Cautions and Warnings

Do not take rimantadine if you are **allergic** or **sensitive** to any of its ingredients or to amantadine.

People with severe **liver or kidney disease** clear this drug from their bodies only ½ as fast as those with normal organ function; they will need to have their dosage adjusted appropriately.

People with a history of **seizures** are likely to suffer another one while taking rimantadine. Contact your doctor if this happens to you.

The influenza virus may become resistant to rimantadine in up to 30% of people taking the drug. When this happens, the resistant virus can infect people who are not protected by the vaccine.

Possible Side Effects

- ▼ Most common: sleeplessness, nervousness, loss of concentration, headache, fatigue, weakness, nausea, vomiting, appetite loss, dry mouth, and abdominal pain.
- ▼ Less common: diarrhea, upset stomach, dizziness, depression, euphoria (feeling "high"), changes in gait or walk, tremors, hallucinations, convulsions, fainting, ringing or buzzing in the ears, changes in or loss of the senses of taste or smell, breathing difficulties, pallor, rash, heart palpitations, rapid heartbeat, high blood pressure, heart failure, swelling of the ankles or feet, and heart block.
- ▼ Rare: constipation, swallowing difficulties, mouth sores, agitation, sweating, diminished sense of touch, eye pain or tearing, cough, bronchospasm, increased urination, fever, and fluid oozing from the nipples in women. Contact your doctor if you experience anything unusual while taking any medication.

Drug Interactions

The importance of rimantadine's drug interactions is not known because there is no established relationship between the amount of drug in the blood and its antiviral effect.

- Aspirin and acetaminophen may reduce the amount of rimantadine in the blood by about 10%.
- Cimetidine decreases the rate at which rimantadine is broken down by the liver.
- Do not use rimantadine concurrently with live intranasal influenza virus vaccine, such as FluMist. Wait at least 48 hours between uses of either medicine.

Food Interactions

Rimantadine is best taken on an empty stomach, or at least 1 hour before or 2 hours after meals. You may take it with food if it upsets your stomach.

Usual Dose

Adult and Child (age 10 and over): 100 mg twice a day. People with severe liver or kidney disease—no more than 100 mg a day.

Child (age 1–9): 2.25 mg per lb. of body weight, up to 150 mg, taken once a day.

Child (under 1 year): not recommended.

Overdosage

Symptoms include agitation, hallucination, and abnormal heart rhythm. Overdose victims should be made to vomit with ipecac syrup—available at any pharmacy—as soon as possible. Contact your local poison control center or a hospital emergency room before giving ipecac. Take overdose victims to a hospital emergency room. If you seek treatment, ALWAYS bring the prescription bottle or container.

Special Information

Rimantadine may be given to children age 16 and under to prevent influenza infection, but it is not recommended for treatment of their flu symptoms.

Contact your doctor if you develop seizures, convulsions, or any other serious or unusual side effects.

If you forget a dose, take it as soon as you remember. If it is almost time for your next dose, skip the dose you forgot and continue with your regular schedule. Do not take a double dose.

Special Populations

Pregnancy/Breast-feeding: In animal studies, rimantadine is toxic to fetuses. It should be taken during pregnancy only if your doctor determines that the potential benefit outweighs the risks.

Rimantadine passes into breast milk. Nursing mothers who must take it should use infant formula.

Seniors: Seniors are more likely to suffer from rimantadine side effects of the nervous system, stomach, and intestine and may require reduced dosage due to liver or kidney dysfunction.

Generic Name

Risperidone (ris-PER-ih-done) G

Brand Names

Risperdal
Risperdal M-Tab Orally Disintegrating Tablets

The information in this profile also applies to the following drugs:

Generic Ingredients: Paliperidone
Invega Invega Sustenna

Generic Ingredients: Ziprasidone G
Geodon

Type of Drug

Atypical antipsychotic.

Prescribed For

Psychotic disorders, schizophrenia, bipolar disorder, and irritability associated with autism.

General Information

Paliperidone is a major product of the breakdown of risperidone, so these medications work in exactly the same way and have the same safety profile. They affect brain receptors for serotonin and dopamine, 2 important neurohormones. They are broken down in the liver. Between 6% and 8% of Caucasians and a very small number of Asians have little of the liver enzyme that breaks down these medications and are considered to be "poor metabolizers" of the drug. Because these people break down these medications very slowly, it takes about 5 days for the drug to reach a steady level in their blood. People with normal amounts of the enzyme reach a steady level in about 1 day. People with kidney or liver disease require reduced dosage.

Ziprasidone may be prescribed for people who have not been helped by other antipsychotics or for whom other antipsychotics have stopped working. Ziprasidone affects serotonin and dopamine, neurotransmitters in the brain, normalizing their chemical balance and relieving symptoms of schizophrenia.

Cautions and Warnings

Do not take these medications if you are **allergic** or **sensitive** to any of their ingredients.

People taking them for longer than 6–8 weeks must be reevaluated at least every 2 months.

These medications have been associated with increased risk of death in seniors with **dementia** or **Alzheimer's disease**. The specific causes of death related to atypical antipsychotic drugs were either due to a heart-related event or infection, mostly pneumonia. The drugs should not be used to treat people with dementia-related psychosis.

A serious set of side effects known as neuroleptic malignant syndrome (NMS) has been associated with some antipsychotic drugs. The symptoms that constitute NMS include high fever, muscle rigidity, mental changes, irregular pulse or blood pressure, sweating, and abnormal heart rhythm. NMS is potentially fatal and requires immediate medical attention.

These medicines can cause a life-threatening abnormal heart rhythm called torsade de pointes. These drugs should therefore be used with caution in people with **heart or blood vessel disease. Slow heart rate**, **electrolyte imbalance**, and taking other drugs that carry a risk of torsade de pointes may increase the chances of developing this abnormality. Dizziness and fainting can also occur.

Some people taking antipsychotic medications have developed tardive dyskinesia (symptoms include lip smacking or puckering, puffing of the cheeks, rapid or wormlike tongue movements, uncontrolled chewing motions, and uncontrolled arm and leg movements). This risk increases with long-term use of the medication.

These drugs have been associated with obesity, high cholesterol, high blood sugar, and diabetes. People with **diabetes or prediabetes** and those who are at risk for diabetes should have their blood-glucose levels checked regularly while taking these drugs.

Atypical antipsychotic medicines raise levels of a hormone called prolactin. Increased prolactin has been associated with tumors of the pituitary gland, breast, and pancreas.

Seizures have occurred in people taking antipsychotic medications. People with a history of seizures or those who are taking medications or have conditions that put them at higher risk for seizures should take this medication with caution.

Swallowing problems and inhaling food have been experienced by people taking other antipsychotics and may present problems for those taking these drugs.

Levels of some white blood cells can drop drastically in people taking these medicines, making it harder to fight infection. Your doctor will monitor your blood count.

Avoid extreme heat because these medications can upset your body's temperature-control mechanism.

Lower dosages should be used for people with **kidney or liver disease**.

Possible Side Effects

Paliperidone

- ▼ Most common: rapid heartbeat, headache, and tiredness.
- ▼ Common: nausea, anxiety, inability to sit still or remain motionless, dizziness, extrapyramidal syndrome (involuntary movements, muscle tremors or rigidity, body restlessness, muscle contractions, and changes in breathing and heart rate), and weight gain.
- ▼ Less common: other heart disorders, electrocardiogram (ECG) changes, blurred vision, upper abdominal pain, dry mouth, upset stomach, excess saliva, weakness, fatigue, fever, high blood pressure, back pain, pain in the arms or legs, twisting and repetitive movement or abnormal postures, muscle tightness that can lead to deformity and functional loss, Parkinson's-like symptoms, tremors, coughing, and dizziness or fainting when rising from a sitting or lying position.
- ▼ Rare: Rare side effects can occur in almost any part of the body. Contact your doctor if you experience anything unusual while taking any medication.

Risperidone

- ▼ Most common: Parkinson's-like symptoms, sleepiness, sleeplessness, agitation, anxiety, uncontrolled movements, headache, and nasal stuffiness and irritation.
- ▼ Less common: dizziness, constipation, nausea, vomiting, upset stomach, abdominal pain, weight gain, absence of menstrual periods, increased sleep duration, coughing, upper-respiratory infection, sinus infection, sore throat, breathing difficulties, rapid heartbeat, joint or back pain, chest pain, fever, abnormal vision, rash, dry skin, and dandruff.
- ▼ Rare: Rare side effects can occur in almost any part of the body. Contact your doctor if you experience anything unusual while taking any medication.

Ziprasidone

- ▼ Most common: sleepiness and nausea.
- ▼ Common: itching, weakness, headache, rapid heartbeat, dizziness, constipation, nausea, upset stomach, diarrhea, inability to remain in a sitting position, restlessness and a

Possible Side Effects *(continued)*

feeling of muscular quivering, extrapyramidal symptoms (see "Cautions and Warnings"), and respiratory conditions.

- ▼ Less common: accidental injury, rash, fungal infection of the skin, dry mouth, appetite loss, muscle aches, abnormal muscle tone, rigid muscles, runny nose, coughing, and abnormal vision.
- ▼ Rare: fainting and seizures. Other rare side effects can occur in almost any part of the body. Contact your doctor if you experience anything unusual while taking any medication.

Drug Interactions

- Do not mix these drugs with amiodarone, arsenic trioxide, bretylium, chlorpromazine, disopyramide, dofetilide, dolasetron, droperidol, gatifloxacin, halofantrine, levomethadyl, mefloquine, mesoridazine, moxifloxacin, pentamidine, pimozide, probucol, quinidine, sotalol, sparfloxacin, tacrolimus, or thioridazine. The risk of life-threatening heart rhythm disorders is increased with these combinations. Chloroquine, haloperidol, maprotiline, methadone, romidepsin, tetrabenazine, toremifene, and vandetanib should not be combined with paliperidone for this reason. In addition, cisapride and levomethadyl should not be taken with ziprasidone.
- These medications increase the effects of blood-pressure-lowering drugs and central-nervous-system depressants, increasing the risk of dizziness when rising from a sitting or lying position.
- Combining alcohol with these drugs may cause weakness and poor coordination.
- Carbamazepine may antagonize the effects of these medications, necessitating dosage adjustments.
- These drugs may decrease the effects of levodopa + carbidopa and other dopamine agonists.
- Paroxetine may increase levels of paliperidone, requiring dosage adjustments.
- Valproic acid may increase the effects of paliperidone.
- Antipsychotics (such as haloperidol, lithium, or thioridazine) may increase the effects of risperidone and ziprasidone.
- Long-term use of clozapine may decrease the effects of risperidone. Dosage adjustments may be needed.

- Abiraterone, fluoxetine, and paroxetine may increase blood concentrations of risperidone. Abiraterone and risperidone should not be combined.
- Risperidone should not be taken with ginkgo biloba.
- Cimetidine, ranitidine, protease inhibitors (such as indinavir and ritonavir), and verapamil may increase the effect of risperidone and its side effects.
- Risperidone may increase levels of maprotiline and valproate, requiring additional monitoring and possible dose adjustments.
- Phenobarbital, phenytoin, and rifampin may reduce blood levels of risperidone.

Food Interactions

Risperidone and paliperidone can be taken without regard to food or meals. Take ziprasidone with food. Avoid grapefruit juice and starfruit, as they may interfere with the breakdown of ziprasidone.

Usual Dose

Paliperidone

Adult: 6 mg once a day to start. Daily dosage may be increased to 12 mg if needed. Do not crush or chew these tablets.

Child (age 12–17): 1.5–12 mg a day.

Child (under age 12): not recommended.

Paliperidone Long-Acting Injection: 39–234 mg every 4 weeks by deep intramuscular injection.

Risperidone

Bipolar Disorder

Adult: starting dose—2–3 mg once a day. Dosage may be increased gradually up to 6 mg a day if needed.

Child (age 10–17): starting dose—0.5 mg once a day. Dosage may be increased gradually up to a recommended 2.5 mg a day.

Irritability Associated with Autism

Child (age 5–16): starting dose—0.25 mg a day for children weighing less than 44 lbs. and 0.5 mg a day for those weighing 44 lbs. or more. Dosage may be increased gradually up to 0.5 mg a day for children weighing less than 44 lbs. and 1 mg a day for those weighing 44 lbs. or more.

Child (under age 5): not recommended.

Schizophrenia

Adult: starting dose—1 mg twice a day. Dosage may be increased gradually up to 8 mg a day if needed.

Child (age 13–17): starting dose—0.5 mg once a day. Dosage may be increased gradually up to 3 mg a day if needed.

Ziprasidone

Adult: 20–100 mg twice a day. The lowest effective dose is recommended.

Child: not recommended.

Overdosage

Symptoms include drowsiness, rapid heartbeat, low blood pressure, and abnormal and uncontrolled muscle movements. Overdose victims should be taken to a hospital emergency room. If you seek treatment, ALWAYS bring the prescription bottle or container.

Special Information

These drugs can make you tired and affect your judgment, an effect that increases with dosage. Be careful when driving or performing any task that requires concentration. Avoid alcohol.

Some antipsychotic drugs can interfere with the body's temperature-regulating mechanism. Avoid extreme heat while you are taking these drugs.

Some people develop a rapid heartbeat and become dizzy or faint when first taking these medicines. This risk can be minimized by starting at a low dose.

Be sure to notify your doctor if you have or had heart disease and you become dizzy, faint, or have heart palpitations (signs of torsade de pointes). Contact your doctor if you have very high fever, muscle rigidity, mental changes, irregular pulse or blood pressure, rapid heartbeat, sweating, or abnormal heart rhythms (signs of NMS).

Rash is common with ziprasidone and may be a sign of a more serious illness. Contact your doctor at once if a rash develops.

These drugs can make you unusually sensitive to the sun. Wear protective clothes and use sunscreen.

Because of the controlled-release design of the paliperidone tablet, it should only be taken by people who are able to swallow the tablet whole. It should not be cut or split. You may notice an empty tablet-shaped shell in your stool. This is normal and not a cause for alarm.

If you forget a dose of risperidone or paliperidone, take it as soon as you remember. If it is almost time for your next dose, skip the dose you forgot and continue with your regular schedule. Contact your doctor if you forget 2 doses in a row.

If you forget to take a dose of ziprasidone and it is more than 2 hours until your next dose, take the one you forgot. Otherwise, skip the forgotten dose and continue with your regular schedule. Do not take a double dose.

Special Populations

Pregnancy/Breast-feeding: Studies of risperidone in animals show an increase in birth defects and stillbirth. There is also a report of an infant who was born with an abnormally developed brain after the mother took risperidone. Newborns whose mothers are taking any antipsychotic medicine are more likely to experience agitation, abnormally increased or decreased muscle tone, tremor, sleepiness, severe difficulty breathing, and difficulty in feeding. In some newborns, the symptoms subside within hours or days and do not require specific treatment; other newborns may require longer hospital stays. If you are or might be pregnant, do not stop taking these medications without talking to your doctor, because suddenly stopping antipsychotic medications can cause significant treatment complication.

Both risperidone and paliperidone pass into breast milk. It is not known if ziprasidone passes into breast milk. Nursing mothers who must take these medications should use infant formula.

Seniors: Seniors with reduced kidney function require lower dosages. Seniors may also be more sensitive to side effects.

Generic Name

Roflumilast (row-FLU-mih-last)

Brand Names

Daliresp

Type of Drug

PDE4 inhibitor.

Prescribed For

Chronic obstructive pulmonary disease (COPD).

General Information

Roflumilast is used to reduce the frequency and number of attacks in people with severe COPD associated with chronic bronchitis (long-lasting inflammation of the main air passages to the lungs). It does not ease bronchospasm and should not be used to treat an attack of COPD. It works by interfering with a major metabolizing enzyme, PDE4, in lung tissue, leading to the accumulation of cyclic AMP, a chemical messenger that is important in normal cellular function.

Cautions and Warnings

Do not use roflumilast if you are **allergic** or **sensitive** to any of its ingredients.

People with moderate to severe **liver disease** break down the drug much more slowly and should not take this medication.

People using roflumilast have an increased chance of sleeplessness, depression, anxiety, and other mood changes, including suicidal thoughts or actions. People with a history of **depression** should use roflumilast with caution.

People taking roflumilast can experience unintended or unusually large weight loss.

Possible Side Effects

- ▼ Common: diarrhea and weight loss.
- ▼ Less common: nausea, headache, back pain, flu-like symptoms, sleeplessness, dizziness, and appetite loss.
- ▼ Rare: Other side effects, including mood changes and other psychiatric effects, gastrointestinal (GI) upset, vomiting, upset stomach, muscle spasms, and tremors may occur. Contact your doctor if you experience anything unusual while taking any medication.

Drug Interactions

- Roflumilast's breakdown by enzymes produced in the liver is slowed if you are also taking one of the following medicines, increasing the chance of drug-related side effects: aprepitant, atazanavir, cimetidine, clarithromycin, delavirdine, diltiazem, enoxacin, erythromycin, fluconazole, fluvoxamine, indinavir, itraconazole, ketoconazole, nefazodone, nelfinavir, ritonavir, saquinavir, telithromycin, verapamil, and voriconazole. Do not mix these medicines with roflumilast.

- Taking a contraceptive drug containing the hormones ethinyl estradiol or gestodene may interfere with the breakdown of roflumilast, increasing the risk of drug side effects. Use this combination with caution.
- Barbiturates such as phenobarbital, carbamazepine, corticosteroid drugs, efavirenz, modafanil, nevirapine, oxcarbazepine, phenytoin, pioglitazone, rifabutin, rifampicin, rifampin, and St. John's wort stimulate the production of liver enzymes responsible for the breakdown of roflumilast, reducing its effect on your body. Do not mix these medicines with roflumilast.

Food Interactions

This medicine can be taken without regard to food or meals. Avoid grapefruit products because they slow the breakdown of roflumilast by liver enzymes and can increase the risk of drug side effects.

Usual Dose

Adult: 500 mcg once a day.
Child: not recommended.

Overdosage

Symptoms of roflumilast overdose can include headache, GI problems, dizziness, heart palpitations, lightheadedness, clamminess, and low blood pressure. Overdose victims should be taken to a hospital emergency room for treatment. If you seek treatment, ALWAYS bring the prescription container.

Special Information

Check your weight regularly and contact your doctor if you experience unintended or unusual weight loss.

Contact your doctor if your mood changes, especially if you have trouble sleeping, act on dangerous impulses, or have suicidal thoughts. Make sure your doctor knows all the medicines and supplement products you are taking because of the interaction risk.

Special Populations

Pregnancy/Breast-feeding: Animal studies have shown this drug had some effect on the fetus; however, it is not known how roflumilast affects a human fetus. It should be taken during pregnancy only if your doctor determines that the potential benefit outweighs the risks.

Roflumilast passes into breast milk. Nursing mothers who must take it should use infant formula.

Seniors: More than ½ of people studied with roflumilast were 65 years or older and responded in the same way as younger adults. Seniors can safely take roflumilast with no special precaution.

Generic Name

Ropinirole (roe-PIN-ih-role) G

Brand Names

Requip Requip XL

Type of Drug

Antiparkinsonian.

Prescribed For

Parkinson's disease (PD) and moderate to severe restless legs syndrome (RLS).

General Information

Ropinirole relieves symptoms of PD and RLS by stimulating dopamine receptors in the brain. A study of people with early PD showed improvement in about 70% of people taking the drug for 10–12 weeks, compared to 40% of people taking a placebo (sugar pill). In another study, 28% of people with advanced PD who received ropinirole for 6 months showed improvement, compared to 11% of people in the placebo group. Ropinirole is broken down in the liver.

RLS is a condition that affects about 1 out of every 10 people. Symptoms include an urge to move the legs, usually accompanied by, or caused by, uncomfortable leg sensations. Symptoms begin or worsen during periods of rest or inactivity for most people and are partly or totally relieved by movement. Symptoms usually worsen or occur only in the evening or at night, and can disturb sleep.

Cautions and Warnings

Do not take ropinirole if you are **allergic** or **sensitive** to any of its ingredients.

Ropinirole may cause low blood pressure and make you dizzy or faint when rising from a sitting or lying position, especially during the early stages of treatment.

About 1 in 10–15 people who take ropinirole experience hallucinations that may be serious enough to require stopping drug therapy.

Ropinirole may make you fall asleep, sometimes suddenly, during the day. Avoid alcohol and use extreme caution when driving or engaging in a potentially hazardous activity.

People with severe **cardiovascular disease** should use ropinirole with caution.

Ropinirole, like other dopamine stimulants, may worsen pathological gambling, hypersexuality, or overeating, or other **impulsive/compulsive behaviors**, which are generally reversible if the dose is reduced or the drug is stopped.

People stopping other treatments for PD have developed high fever and confusion. Breathing difficulties caused by lung changes have occurred with the use of other antiparkinsonians. These problems have not been associated with ropinirole, but there is a risk that you may experience similar problems if you stop taking ropinirole.

Ropinirole may cause symptoms of RLS to occur earlier than usual or in other extremities; this has been seen with similar drugs, but has not been studied specifically in ropinirole.

People with PD have 2–6 times the risk of developing skin cancer. It is not known if the increased risk is due to the condition or the drugs used to manage it. People taking this medication should frequently check themselves for skin cancers and see a dermatologist regularly.

Ropinirole should be used cautiously in those with **liver disease**.

Possible Side Effects

Advanced Parkinson's Disease

- ▼ Most common: abnormal movements, tremor, muscle rigidity, hallucinations, and urinary infection.
- ▼ Common: confusion, constipation, pneumonia, sweating, abdominal pain, and twitching.
- ▼ Less common: dizziness or fainting when rising from a sitting or lying position, unusual dreaming, changes in gait or walk, poor muscle coordination, memory loss, nervousness, tingling in the hands or feet, temporary paralysis, diarrhea, difficulty swallowing, gas, increased salivation, poor urinary control, pus in the urine, arthritis, breathing difficulties, dry mouth, anemia, and weight loss.

Possible Side Effects *(continued)*

Early Parkinson's Disease

- ▼ Most common: sleepiness or tiredness, nausea, dizziness, fainting, upset stomach, vomiting, and virus infection.
- ▼ Common: general pain, sweating, weakness, fainting, abdominal pain, sore throat, and changes in vision.
- ▼ Less common: dry mouth; flushing; chest pain; feeling unwell; blood-pressure changes; heart palpitations; rapid heartbeat; hallucinations; confusion; memory loss; very sensitive reflexes; yawning; unusual movements; difficulty concentrating; appetite loss; gas; swollen arms or legs; runny nose; sinus irritation; bronchitis; breathing difficulties; eye problems; urinary infection; impotence; and poor blood supply to the hands, legs, and feet.

Restless Legs Syndrome

- ▼ Most common: nausea, tiredness, sleepiness, vomiting, dizziness, and fatigue.
- ▼ Common: sweating.
- ▼ Less common: dry mouth, diarrhea, nasal congestion, and swelling.

Drug Interactions

- Ropinirole increases levodopa + carbidopa blood levels and may worsen uncontrolled muscle spasm that occurs with levodopa + carbidopa. Your doctor may reduce your dosage.
- Cimetidine, ciprofloxacin, diltiazem, enoxacin, erythromycin, estrogen, fluvoxamine, mexiletine, and norfloxacin increase ropinirole's effects.
- Phenothiazine sedatives, haloperidol and other antipsychotics, thioxanthene sedatives, and metoclopramide and other drugs that antagonize the effects of dopamine may reduce the effect of ropinirole. Phenobarbital, carbamazepine, and cigarette smoking may also cause a decrease in the effect of ropinirole.
- Ropinirole increases the sedative effect of benzodiazepines, sleeping pills, and other nervous system depressants.
- Dosages of ropinirole may need adjusting if estrogen therapy is started or stopped.

- Ropinirole may increase the blood-thinning effects of warfarin. Dosage adjustments may be necessary.

Food Interactions

You may take ropinirole with food to prevent nausea.

Usual Dose

Parkinson's Disease

Adult: 0.25 mg 3 times a day to start, gradually increasing, if needed, in intervals of 0.75 mg a week, to a maximum of 24 mg a day. Dosage is reduced for people with kidney disease. The long-acting version of ropinirole should be taken once a day.

Child: not recommended.

Restless Legs Syndrome

Adult: 0.25–4 mg a day 1–3 hours before bedtime.

Child: not recommended.

Overdosage

Little is known about the effects of ropinirole overdose. Symptoms are likely to include the most common side effects. Take the victim to a hospital emergency room. If you seek treatment, ALWAYS bring the prescription bottle or container.

Special Information

Take this drug exactly as prescribed. If you forget a dose, take it as soon as you remember. If you take the regular ropinirole, space the remaining daily dosage evenly throughout the day. If you take the long-acting version and do not remember until the next day, skip the forgotten dose and go back to your regular schedule the next day. Do not take a double dose.

Special Populations

Pregnancy/Breast-feeding: In animal studies, ropinirole causes birth defects and damages the fetus. Ropinirole should be taken during pregnancy only if your doctor determines that the potential benefit outweighs the risks.

Animal studies show that ropinirole passes into breast milk, but it is not known if this occurs in humans. Ropinirole may interfere with milk production. Nursing mothers who must take this drug should use infant formula.

Seniors: Hallucinations are more likely to occur in seniors.

Generic Name

Rufinamide (roo-FIN-ah-myde)

Brand Names

Banzel

Type of Drug

Anticonvulsant.

Prescribed For

Lennox-Gastaut syndrome.

General Information

Rufinamide is chemically unique from other anticonvulsants and is generally given as part of a combination treatment program. It is broken down in the liver and mainly leaves the body through the kidneys. It is not known exactly how rufinamide produces its effect, but it slows the action of nerve cells, reducing the chances for a seizure.

Cautions and Warnings

Do not take this drug if you are **allergic** or **sensitive** to any of its ingredients. With some anticonvulsant medicines, sensitivity reactions can occur in more than one organ, such as the liver, kidney, heart, and/or lymph glands. This has been reported in **children** under age 12 taking rufinamide. Symptoms include rash, itching, facial swelling, fever, stupor, and liver inflammation. Your doctor may decide to change medicines if multiple reactions develop, as symptoms may go away after the medicine is stopped.

Anticonvulsant medicines increase the risk of depression, suicidal thoughts, and the risk of attempted suicide. Anyone taking rufinamide or any other anticonvulsant medicine should be carefully watched for new or worsening mood changes or behaviors.

Rufinamide can affect heart function. It is associated with a genetic disorder called QT-shortening, in which electrical impulses between heart chambers are affected. People with a family history of **short QT syndrome** should not take rufinamide. Your doctor may take an electrocardiogram (ECG) immediately after you take the medicine to see if it affects your heart's electrical system.

As with all anticonvulsant medicines, do not abruptly stop taking rufinamide. The drug dose should be gradually reduced to reduce the chances of drug-withdrawal seizures.

People with mild to moderate **liver disease** should use rufinamide with caution. People with severe liver disease should not use this medicine at all. People with **kidney disease** generally do not need any dose adjustment. Daily dose may be adjusted during **kidney dialysis**.

Possible Side Effects

- ▼ Most common: dizziness, headache, fatigue, and tiredness.
- ▼ Common: double vision, blurred vision, tremors, and unusual eyeball movements.
- ▼ Less common: poor muscle coordination, upper abdominal pain, anxiety, constipation, upset stomach, back pain, gait changes, and unexpected fainting.
- ▼ Rare: Other drug side effects include appetite changes and can affect the blood, heart, and kidneys. Contact your doctor if you experience anything unusual while taking any medication.

Drug Interactions

- Rufinamide may increase blood levels of the anticonvulsant medicines phenobarbital and phenytoin. These effects may be greater in children.
- Rufinamide may reduce blood levels of the anticonvulsant medicines carbamazepine and lamotrigine. These effects may be greater in children.
- Carbamazepine, phenobarbital, phenytoin, and primidone may reduce blood levels of rufinamide.
- Valproate may increase blood levels of rufinamide. These effects may be greater in children.
- Rufinamide may reduce blood levels of the hormones in contraceptive drugs, possibly reducing their effectiveness. Women using contraceptive drugs for birth control should use non-hormonal contraception while taking rufinamide.
- Rufinamide can reduce blood levels of triazolam, a benzodiazepine-type sedative, possibly reducing its effectiveness.
- Taking this medication causes tiredness, fatigue, and poor coordination. Mixing rufinamide with other medicines that cause similar effects should be avoided.

Food Interactions

Rufinamide should be taken with food because it increases the amount of drug absorbed by ⅓.

Usual Dose

It is not known if doses less than 1600 mg twice a day are effective.

Adult: 200–400 mg twice a day to start, increasing gradually to a maximum dose of 1600 mg twice a day.

Child (age 4 and over): 2.25–4.5 mg per lb. of body weight twice a day to start, increasing gradually to either 10.25 mg per lb. or 1600 mg per dose, whichever is less.

Overdosage

One person took 7200 mg of rufinamide and experienced no major side effects or symptoms. Take the overdose victim to a hospital emergency room at once for evaluation and treatment. If you seek treatment, ALWAYS bring the prescription bottle or container.

Special Information

Your doctor must balance the potential benefits of treatment with rufinamide against the risk of new or worsening irritability, anxiety, depression, or suicidal thoughts or actions. Other symptoms include panic attacks, difficulty sleeping, and unusual mood changes, including new or worsening aggressiveness and an extreme increase in talking and activity. Report anything unusual to your doctor at once.

Report any rash, with or without fever, to your doctor at once. These may be signs of a severe drug reaction.

Rufinamide may cause dizziness and/or poor muscle coordination. Do not drive or do anything requiring coordination and concentration until you see how the medicine affects you.

Rufinamide can affect your heart. Contact your doctor at once if you experience heart palpitations or sudden fainting.

Do not stop taking this drug unless your doctor tells you to do so. If you forget a dose, take it as soon as you remember. If you don't remember until it is almost time for your next dose, skip the forgotten dose and continue with your regular schedule. Contact your doctor if you forget 2 or more doses in a row. Do not take a double dose of this medicine.

Special Populations

Pregnancy/Breast-feeding: In animal studies, rufinamide damaged the developing fetus at doses similar to those taken by people.

There is no information on the effect of rufinamide during pregnancy. Rufinamide should be taken during pregnancy only if your doctor determines that the potential benefit outweighs the risks.

This drug is likely to pass into breast milk. Nursing mothers who must take it should use infant formula.

Seniors: Seniors may take rufinamide with no special precaution.

Generic Name

Salmeterol (sal-METE-er-ol)

Brand Names

Serevent
Serevent Diskus

The information in this profile also applies to the following drugs:

Generic Ingredients: Arformoterol
Brovana

Generic Ingredients: Formoterol
Foradil Aerolizer
Perforomist

Combination Products
Generic Ingredients: Formoterol + Budesonide
Symbicort

Generic Ingredients: Formoterol + Mometasone
Dulera

Type of Drug

Bronchodilator.

Prescribed For

Asthma and bronchospasm.

General Information

These drugs are long-acting beta-2 agonists that work on nervous system receptors that relax the muscle bands surrounding your airways, making it easier to breathe. They should only be used if other asthma control medicines do not work. They differ from some other bronchodilators in that they do not provide immediate symptom relief, but instead are prescribed for long-term prevention. When you start treatment with one of these, you may need to continue your other asthma inhalers for symptom relief.

After a while, however, you should have less need for the other drugs. These drugs are somewhat safer for people with heart conditions than other bronchodilators due to their weaker effect on the heart and blood vessels. Still, very large doses may lead to abnormal heart rhythms. Salmeterol begins working within 20 minutes after a dose and continues for 12 hours. These medicines should be used together with a corticosteroid inhaler. To make it more convenient, these medicines have been combined with a corticosteroid into a single product for inhalation. These fixed-dose combinations are especially useful for teens and children who require these medicines.

Cautions and Warnings

Do not take these medicines if you are **allergic** or **sensitive** to any of their ingredients.

They should be used with caution by people with a history of **angina pectoris** (a condition characterized by brief attacks of chest pain), **heart disease**, **high blood pressure**, **stroke** or **seizure**, **thyroid disease**, **prostate disease**, or **glaucoma**.

Used in excess, these medicines can rarely lead to more severe asthma attacks, rather than asthma relief. In the most extreme cases, people have had heart attacks after using excessive amounts of inhalant bronchodilators such as salmeterol.

A large study comparing the safety of salmeterol to a placebo (sugar pill) showed a small but significant increase in asthma-related deaths among people taking salmeterol—13 deaths out of 13,174 patients treated for 28 weeks versus only 3 deaths among 13,179 taking the placebo. The risk of asthma-related death might be greater in **blacks** than Caucasians.

Long-term use of salmeterol and related drugs can lead to increases in certain ovarian tumors.

Salmeterol should not be used by patients with **acutely deteriorating asthma**, which can lead to serious respiratory events.

People with **lung disease** who use a salmeterol inhaler, with or without a corticosteroid, develop lung infections or pneumonia more often.

Possible Side Effects

Arformoterol and Formoterol

▼ Common: joint pain, back pain, and headache.

Possible Side Effects *(continued)*

- ▼ Less common: common cold symptoms, increased cholesterol or triglycerides, and weight gain.
- ▼ Rare: drug reactions (itching, skin reactions, swollen lips and eyelids, difficulty breathing), low blood sugar, muscle aches, and irritation of the pancreas. Contact your doctor if you experience anything unusual while taking any medication.

Salmeterol

- ▼ Most common: heart palpitations, rapid heartbeat, tremors, cough, dizziness and fainting, shakiness, nervousness, tension headache, diarrhea, heartburn or upset stomach, dry or sore and irritated throat, respiratory infections, and nasal or sinus conditions.
- ▼ Less common: nausea and vomiting, joint or back pain, muscle cramps, muscle soreness, muscle ache or pain, giddiness, viral stomach infections, itching, dental pain, not feeling well, rash, and menstrual irregularity.

Drug Interactions

- Salmeterol breakdown is slowed by aprepitant, clarithromycin, diltiazem, erythromycin, fluconazole, indinavir, itraconazole, ketoconazole, nefazodone, nelfinavir, ritonavir, saquinavir, telithromycin, and verapamil. This interaction can raise salmeterol to the point where it can affect your heart. Do not mix these medicines.
- Monoamine oxidase inhibitor (MAOI) and tricyclic antidepressants, thyroid drugs, other bronchodilator drugs, and some antihistamines may increase the effects of salmeterol.
- The risk of cardiotoxicity may be increased in people taking both salmeterol and theophylline.
- Beta-blocker drugs may reduce the effect of salmeterol, and may also produce severe bronchospasm in people with asthma.
- Salmeterol may exacerbate certain effects of non-potassium-sparing (loop or thiazide) diuretics.
- Salmeterol may decrease the effects of blood-pressure-lowering drugs, especially reserpine, methyldopa, and guanethidine.

Food Interactions

Large amounts of grapefruit or starfruit products can slow the breakdown of salmeterol. Avoid these foods while using this medicine.

Usual Dose

Salmeterol

Aerosol

Adult and Child (age 12 and over): 2 inhalations every 12 hours.
Child (under age 12): not recommended.

Powder

Adult and Child (age 4 and over): 1 inhalation every 12 hours.
Child (under age 4): not recommended.

Overdosage

Overdose of salmeterol inhalation usually results in exaggerated side effects, including chest pain and high blood pressure, although blood pressure may drop to a low level after a short period of elevation. People who inhale too much salmeterol should see a doctor. If you seek treatment, ALWAYS bring the prescription bottle or container.

Special Information

Be sure to follow the inhalation instructions that come with the product. Wait at least 1 minute between puffs. Do not inhale salmeterol if you have food or anything else in your mouth. Rinse mouth with water after each use.

Contact your doctor immediately if you develop chest pain, palpitations, rapid heartbeat, muscle tremors, dizziness, headache, facial flushing, or urinary difficulty, or if you continue to experience difficulty in breathing after using salmeterol.

If you forget a dose of salmeterol, take it as soon as you remember. If it is almost time for your next dose, skip the one you forgot and go back to your regular schedule. Do not take a double dose.

Special Populations

Pregnancy/Breast-feeding: When used during childbirth, salmeterol may slow or delay natural labor. It can cause rapid heartbeat and high blood sugar in the mother and rapid heartbeat and low blood sugar in the baby. It is not known whether salmeterol causes birth defects in humans, but it has caused defects in animals.

Salmeterol should be taken during pregnancy only if your doctor determines that the potential benefit outweighs the risks.

Salmeterol may pass into breast milk. Nursing mothers who must take this drug should use infant formula.

Seniors: Seniors should use the same dosage of salmeterol as younger adults.

Type of Drug

Sedatives (Benzodiazepine Type)

Brand Names

Generic Ingredients: Estazolam G
Prosom

Generic Ingredients: Eszopiclone G
Lunesta

Generic Ingredients: Flurazepam G
Dalmane

Generic Ingredients: Quazepam G
Doral

Generic Ingredients: Temazepam G
Restoril

Generic Ingredients: Triazolam G
Halcion

Generic Ingredients: Zaleplon G
Sonata

Generic Ingredients: Zolpidem G
Ambien
Ambien CR
Intermezzo
Zolpimist Oral Spray

Prescribed For

Insomnia and sleep disturbances.

General Information

Benzodiazepines work by a direct effect on the brain. In addition to being used as sedatives, benzodiazepines are prescribed for their antianxiety, anticonvulsant, and muscle relaxant effects. As sedatives, they make it easier to go to sleep and decrease the number of times you wake up during the night.

Short-acting drugs in this class have the advantage of helping you get to sleep faster. Although this virtually eliminates the "hangover" effect, it may also cause some people to wake up earlier than they would like because the drug has stopped working. Longer-acting drugs have the opposite effect; they take longer to work and keep you asleep all night but also carry a risk of morning "hangover." Intermediate-acting benzodiazepines generally remain in your body long enough to give you a good night's sleep with minimal drug hangover. The following table summarizes important information about benzodiazepine sedatives.

Drug name	**Starts working**	**Half-life (hours)**	**Equivalent sedative dose (approximate)**
Estazolam	1–5 hrs.	10–24	1–2 mg
Eszopiclone	10–18 min.	6	3 mg
Flurazepam	1–1.5 hrs.	40–250	15–30 mg
Quazepam	1–5 hrs.	39–120	20 mg
Temazepam	30 min.–3 hrs.	8–22	20 mg
Triazolam	30 min.–2 hrs.	2	0.25 mg
Zaleplon	30 min.–1 hr.	1	20 mg
Zolpidem	15–30 min.	2.6	20 mg

These drugs are not all equal in their effects because they do not all act on every benzodiazepine receptor. Several are chemically different from the benzodiazepines, but they act on benzodiazepine receptors and so are included in this profile.

Zolpidem causes little or no "hangover," and there are few rebound effects after stopping the drug. The CR (controlled-release) formulation was created to address the problem of people not getting a full night's sleep when taking the older, immediate-release product. It does not act as quickly as the older formulation because the drug enters the bloodstream much more slowly. These drugs are broken down by enzymes produced in the liver.

Cautions and Warnings

Do not take these drugs if you are **allergic** or **sensitive** to any of their ingredients. Severe reactions (including swelling of the lips, face, tongue, or throat that can lead to difficulty swallowing or breathing) have occurred with them. People who react to one benzodiazepine may also react to other members of this group.

People with **respiratory disease** may experience **sleep apnea** (intermittent cessation of breathing during sleep) while taking a benzodiazepine. People who have sleep apnea should not take these medicines.

People with **kidney or liver disease** should be carefully monitored while taking these drugs and may dictate a lower dosage. In general, you should take the lowest possible benzodiazepine dose to help you sleep.

Clinical **depression** may be increased by triazolam, which can depress the nervous system. Intentional overdose is more common among depressed people who take sleeping pills than among those who do not.

All benzodiazepines can be addictive if taken for long periods of time and can cause drug-withdrawal symptoms if suddenly discontinued. Withdrawal symptoms include tremors, muscle cramps, insomnia, agitation, diarrhea, vomiting, sweating, and convulsions. Continued difficulty sleeping may be a sign of another physical or psychiatric problem. If these drugs do not help you, ask your doctor to look for other issues that might be interfering with your sleep but have not yet been discovered.

Tapering the drug when stopping will help prevent withdrawal symptoms. People with a history of **seizures** should be particularly cautious when stopping use of this drug. You may also experience rebound sleeplessness if you stop abruptly, in which sleep is worse during the first 1–3 nights after you stop the drug than it was before you started it.

Benzodiazepines have been associated with unusual behavior while asleep, including making and eating food, making telephone calls, or driving, with no memory of the event. Memory loss is especially possible when higher doses are taken. This effect, known as "traveler's amnesia," is most common among people who take this medication to adjust to **time zone changes** during travel; it may be linked to the use of alcoholic beverages and to attempts at starting daily activity too soon after waking up.

Possible Side Effects

Rare side effects experienced with these medications can occur in almost any part of the body. Contact your doctor if you experience anything unusual while taking any medication.

Possible Side Effects *(continued)*

Estazolam

▼ Common: drowsiness, headache, dizziness, talkativeness, nervousness, apprehension, poor muscle coordination, lightheadedness, daytime tiredness, muscle weakness, slowness of movement, hangover, and euphoria (feeling "high").

▼ Less common: nausea, vomiting, rapid heartbeat, confusion, temporary memory loss, upset stomach, stomach cramps and pain, depression, blurred or double vision and other visual disturbances, constipation, changes in sense of taste, appetite changes, stuffy nose, nosebleeds, common cold symptoms, asthma, sore throat, cough, breathing difficulties, diarrhea, dry mouth, allergic reaction, fainting, abnormal heart rhythm, itching, acne, dry skin, sensitivity to bright light or to the sun, rash, nightmares or strange dreams, sleeplessness, tingling in the hands or feet, ringing or buzzing in the ears, ear or eye pain, menstrual cramps, frequent urination and other urinary difficulties, blood in the urine, discharge from the penis or vagina, lower back and joint pain, muscle spasms and pain, fever, swollen breasts, and weight changes.

Eszopiclone

Adult

Some side effects are more likely with larger doses (viral and other infections, dry mouth, dizziness, hallucinations, rash, and unpleasant taste).

▼ Most common: headache, drowsiness, unpleasant taste, and lung infections.

▼ Common: dry mouth, dizziness, and nausea.

▼ Less common: nervousness, vomiting, viral infections, anxiety, confusion, depression, hallucinations, reduced sex drive, rash, male breast enlargement and/or pain, painful menstruation, chest pain, migraines, and swelling of the arms or legs.

Seniors

Some side effects are more common with larger doses, including dry mouth, pain, and unpleasant taste.

▼ Most common: headache.

Possible Side Effects *(continued)*

- ▼ Common: pain, dry mouth, diarrhea, and upset stomach.
- ▼ Less common: accidental injury, abnormal dreaming, nervousness, nerve pain, itching, and urinary infection.

Flurazepam

- ▼ Common: drowsiness, headache, dizziness, talkativeness, nervousness, apprehension, poor muscle coordination, lightheadedness, daytime tiredness, muscle weakness, slowness of movement, hangover, and euphoria (feeling "high").
- ▼ Less common: nausea, vomiting, rapid heartbeat, confusion, temporary memory loss, upset stomach, stomach cramps and pain, depression, blurred or double vision and other visual disturbances, constipation, changes in sense of taste, appetite changes, stuffy nose, nosebleeds, common cold symptoms, asthma, sore throat, cough, breathing difficulties, diarrhea, dry mouth, allergic reaction, fainting, abnormal heart rhythm, itching, rash, acne, dry skin, sensitivity to the sun, nightmares or strange dreams, sleeplessness, tingling in the hands or feet, ringing or buzzing in the ears, ear or eye pain, menstrual cramps, frequent urination and other urinary difficulties, blood in the urine, discharge from the penis or vagina, lower back and other pain, muscle spasms and pain, fever, swollen breasts, and weight changes.

Quazepam, Temazepam, and Triazolpam

- ▼ Common: drowsiness, headache, dizziness, talkativeness, nervousness, apprehension, poor muscle coordination, lightheadedness, daytime tiredness, muscle weakness, slowness of movement, drug hangover, and euphoria (feeling "high").

Zaleplon

Overall side effects are similar in people taking zaleplon and those taking a placebo (sugar pill).

- ▼ Most common: headache.
- ▼ Common: abdominal pain, weakness, muscle aches, memory loss, dizziness, and tiredness.
- ▼ Less common: fever, difficulty swallowing, tingling in the hands or feet, tremors, eye pain, unusually sensitive

Possible Side Effects *(continued)*

hearing, changes in sense of smell, and painful menstrual periods.

Zolpidem

Short-Term Use (10 Days or Less)

▼ Most common: headache, drowsiness, dizziness, lightheadedness, nausea, and diarrhea.

▼ Less common: chest pain, fatigue, unusual dreams, memory loss, anxiety, nervousness, difficulty sleeping, appetite loss, vomiting, and runny nose.

Long-Term Use

▼ Most common: headache, dizziness, nausea, drowsiness, and a feeling of being drugged.

▼ Common: allergy symptoms, back pain, flu-like symptoms, lethargy, sensitivity to light, depression, upset stomach, constipation, abdominal pain, muscle and joint pain, upper-respiratory infection, sinus irritation, sore throat, rash, urinary infection, heart palpitations, and dry mouth.

Drug Interactions

- The effects of benzodiazepines are enhanced if they are taken with alcohol, anticonvulsants, antihistamines, barbiturates, sedatives, selective serotonin reuptake inhibitors (SSRIs), or tricyclic and monoamine oxidase inhibitor (MAOI) antidepressants.
- Cimetidine, contraceptive drugs, disulfiram, isoniazid, itraconazole, ketoconazole, and nefazodone may increase the effect of triazolam by interfering with the drug's breakdown in the liver. Probenecid may also increase their effect.
- Cigarette smoking, rifampin, and theophylline may reduce the effect of these medicines.
- Benzodiazepines reduce the effectiveness of levodopa + carbidopa.
- Benzodiazepines may increase the amount of digoxin, phenytoin, or zidovudine (an HIV drug also known as AZT) in your blood, increasing the chances of side effects.
- Combining clozapine and a benzodiazepine has led to respiratory collapse in a few people. Benzodiazepine sedatives should be stopped at least 1 week before starting clozapine treatment.

- The effects of the benzodiazepines may be increased by the macrolide antibiotics azithromycin, erythromycin, and clarithromycin.
- Do not combine zaleplon and diphenhydramine (an over-the-counter antihistamine and sleeping pill).
- Zaleplon increases the depressant effects of alcohol and other nervous system depressants, promethazine, imipramine, and thioridazine.
- Barbiturates, carbamazepine, efavirenz, modafinil, nevirapine, oxcarbazepine, phenobarbital, phenytoin, pioglitazone, rifampin, and St. John's wort may reduce these drugs' effect by stimulating a liver enzyme that breaks it down.
- Combining zaleplon and cimetidine can almost double zaleplon blood levels. People taking cimetidine regularly for heartburn, ulcers, or stomach acid reduction should begin with the lowest effective dosage of zaleplon.
- Ketoconazole strongly inhibits the enzyme system responsible for breaking down the benzodiazepines. Other strong inhibitors of the same enzymes likely to interact zolpidem are itraconazole, indinavir, nelfinavir, ritonavir, saquinavir, clarithromycin, telithromycin, and nefazodone. Your zolpidem dose will likely be reduced when mixing these medicines. Aprepitant, diltiazem, erythromycin, fluconazole, and verapamil moderately inhibit the same system. Many other medicines inhibit this system, but the importance of those interactions is not known. Mixing these drugs increases the sedative effect of benzodiazepine drugs.
- The combination of zolpidem and ritonavir may cause severe sedation and respiratory depression.

Food Interactions

Estazolam, flurazepam, quazepam, temazepam, and triazolam can be taken with food if it upsets your stomach. Take eszopiclone, zolpidem, and zaleplon on an empty stomach. High-fat meals can slow their absorption and reduce their effectiveness. Avoid taking large amounts of starfruit, grapefruit juice, or other grapefruit products with benzodiazepines.

Usual Dose

Estazolam

Adult: 1–2 mg at bedtime. Small or frail patients should start with 0.5 mg. Dosage should be increased cautiously.

Child: not recommended.

Senior: 1 mg at bedtime.

Eszopiclone

Adult: 2–3 mg immediately before bedtime or after you are in bed and have trouble falling asleep. Eszopiclone can act very quickly. People with liver disease should take only 1 mg.

Child: not recommended.

Senior: 1–2 mg immediately before bedtime.

Flurazepam

Adult and Child (age 15 and over): 15–30 mg at bedtime. Dosage must be individualized for maximum benefit.

Child (under age 15): not recommended.

Senior: starting dose—15 mg at bedtime.

Quazepam

Adult: 7.5–15 mg at bedtime. The dose must be individualized for maximum benefit. Seniors should take the lowest effective dose.

Child: not recommended.

Temazepam

Adult: 7.5–30 mg at bedtime. The dose must be individualized for maximum benefit.

Child: not recommended.

Senior: starting dose—7.5 mg at bedtime. The dose may be increased if needed.

Triazolam

Adult: 0.125–0.5 mg about 30 minutes before sleep.

Child: not recommended.

Senior: starting dose—0.125 mg, then increase in 0.125-mg steps until the desired effect is achieved.

Zaleplon

Adult: 5–10 mg at bedtime.

Child: not recommended.

Senior: Begin with 5 mg at bedtime and increase if needed.

This medication is usually taken for 7–10 days and rarely longer than 2–3 weeks.

Zolpidem

Controlled-Release

Adult: 12.5 mg immediately before bedtime.

Child: not recommended.

Seniors and People with Liver Disease: 6.25 mg immediately before bedtime.

Immediate-Release

Adult: 10 mg immediately before bedtime. Zolpidem can act very quickly.

Child: not recommended.

Seniors and People with Liver Disease: 5 mg immediately before bedtime.

Oral Spray

Adult: 2 sprays (10 mg) at bedtime.

Child: not recommended.

Seniors and People with Liver Disease: 1 spray (5 mg) immediately before bedtime.

Overdosage

The most common symptoms of benzodiazepine overdose are confusion, sleepiness, depression, loss of muscle coordination, and slurred speech. Coma may also occur. Overdose victims must be made to vomit with ipecac syrup—available at any pharmacy—to remove any remaining drug from the stomach. Contact your doctor or a poison control center before doing this. If 30 minutes have passed since the overdose was taken or if symptoms have begun to develop, the victim must immediately be taken to a hospital emergency room. If you seek treatment, ALWAYS bring the prescription bottle or container.

Special Information

Never take more benzodiazepine sedative than your doctor has prescribed. Do not take a double dose of a benzodiazepine.

Avoid alcohol and other nervous system depressants while taking these drugs.

Exercise caution while performing tasks that require concentration and coordination. These drugs may make you tired, dizzy, or lightheaded.

Contact your doctor if your insomnia worsens or does not improve within 7–10 days. It may be the result of an underlying medical or psychiatric condition.

If you take one of these medicines every day for 3 or more weeks, you may experience some withdrawal symptoms when you stop taking it (see "Cautions and Warnings").

Benzodiazepines can cause a morning-after "hangover." Do not take these drugs unless circumstances will allow for a full night's sleep and some time before you need to be alert and active.

Special Populations

Pregnancy/Breast-feeding: Taking a benzodiazepine in the weeks just before delivery may cause tiredness or listlessness in newborns. Benzodiazepines should absolutely not be used by pregnant women.

These medicines pass into breast milk. Nursing mothers taking a benzodiazepine sedative should use infant formula.

Seniors: Seniors are more susceptible to the effects of these drugs.

Type of Drug

Selective μ-Opioid Receptors

Brand Names

Generic Ingredients: Alvimopan
Entereg

Generic Ingredients: Methylnaltrexone Bromide
Relistor

Prescribed For

Alvimopan is prescribed in the hospital to shorten the recovery time after major bowel surgery. Methylnaltrexone is prescribed to relieve constipation due to narcotic pain relievers that is not relieved by other treatments.

General Information

The ability of the gastrointestinal (GI) tract to move food and waste is often slowed after surgery (postoperative ileus). This can affect individual sections or the entire GI tract and can last 5–6 days or more after surgery. Because you cannot be discharged until bowel function is normal, ileus delays hospital discharge. Symptoms of this condition include bloating, nausea, vomiting, pain, gas, fluids in the bowel, and constipation. Two sources of postoperative ileus are inflammation and the morphine and other narcotic pain relievers that cause constipation. Constipation is also a major problem for people who take large doses of narcotic pain relievers, often because of surgery or a major illness. These drugs work against one of the opioid receptors in the bowel that is responsible for the speed of bowel movement. Antagonizing this receptor makes it possible to regain bowel function without interfering with the pain-relieving effects of narcotic drugs.

Cautions and Warnings

Do not take these drugs if you are **allergic** or **sensitive** to any of their ingredients.

People with severe **liver or kidney disease** should not take alvimopan. People with mild or moderate liver or kidney disease may be more likely to experience drug side effects than those with a healthy kidney and liver. People with severe kidney disease should receive ½ the normal dose of methylnaltrexone. Those with mild to moderate kidney or liver disease may take regular doses of the medicine. There is no experience with methylnaltrexone in severe liver disease.

If severe diarrhea develops while using methylnaltrexone, stop using the medicine and contact your doctor at once.

One study showed an increase in heart attack among people who took low doses of alvimopan for a year. This has not been seen in alvimopan studies where the drug is used at normal dosages for the typically short course of treatment.

People who have recently or are currently taking a narcotic pain reliever may be more sensitive to alvimopan's GI side effects of abdominal pain, nausea, vomiting, and diarrhea.

These drugs should not be used by people who have a **bowel obstruction**.

Possible Side Effects

Alvimopan

▼ Most common: upset stomach and low blood potassium.

▼ Common: anemia.

▼ Less common: constipation, stomach gas, back pain, and urinary difficulty.

Methylnaltrexone

▼ Most common: abdominal pain, gas, nausea, dizziness, and excessive sweating.

▼ Common: diarrhea.

Drug Interactions

None known.

Food Interactions

These drugs can be taken without regard to food or meals.

Usual Dose

Alvimopan

Adult: 12 mg before surgery, then 12 mg twice a day starting on the day after surgery for up to 7 days or until discharge. You should not take a total of more than 15 doses of alvimopan.

Child: not recommended.

Methylnaltrexone

Adult

252 lbs. or more: 0.0034 mL per lb. of body weight injected under the skin every 2 days. Daily injection may be needed.

136–251 lbs.: 0.6 mL (12 mg) injected under the skin every 2 days. Daily injection may be needed.

84–135 lbs.: 0.4 mL (8 mg) injected under the skin every 2 days. Daily injection may be needed.

Under 84 lbs.: 0.0034 mL per lb. of body weight injected under the skin every 2 days. Daily injection may be needed.

Overdosage

Up to 10 alvimopan pills have been taken at once with few side effects. Methylnaltrexone doses more than 100 times the regular dose have been studied with no problems; people taking a single dose about 200 times the regular dose suffered low blood pressure and some fainting. Contact your local poison control center or a hospital emergency room for more information. If you seek treatment, ALWAYS bring the prescription bottle or container.

Special Information

You should receive 2 doses of alvimopan every day after surgery. If 1 is not provided at the regular time, it should be taken when the dose is provided by hospital staff. If it is completely forgotten, continue with your regular schedule. Do not take a double dose of alvimopan.

Methylnaltrexone injection is clear and colorless to pale yellow. Do not use it if it has changed color or has particles floating in it. Inject the solution right after drawing into a syringe. It may be stored at room temperature for up to 24 hours.

Stop using methylnaltrexone when you stop taking narcotic pain relievers.

Be sure you are near a bathroom after injecting methylnaltrexone. About 1 of every 3 people who use methylnaltrexone responds within 30 minutes after being injected.

Special Populations

Pregnancy/Breast-feeding: Animal studies of these drugs revealed no clear effects on a developing fetus. They should be taken during pregnancy only if your doctor determines that the potential benefit outweighs the risks.

These drugs may pass into human breast milk. Nursing mothers who must take them should use infant formula because of possible drug side effects in a nursing infant.

Seniors: This drug has not been studied in seniors.

Type of Drug

Selective Serotonin Reuptake Inhibitors (SSRIs)

Brand Names

Generic Ingredients: Citalopram Hydrobromide G
Celexa

Generic Ingredients: Escitalopram Oxalate G
Lexapro

Generic Ingredients: Fluoxetine Hydrochloride G
Prozac
Prozac Weekly
Sarafem

Generic Ingredients: Fluvoxamine Maleate G
Luvox
Luvox CR

Generic Ingredients: Paroxetine Hydrochloride G
Paxil
Paxil CR

Generic Ingredients: Paroxetine Mesylate
Pexeva

Generic Ingredients: Sertraline Hydrochloride G
Zoloft

Prescribed For

Depression, bulimic binge-eating and vomiting, obsessive-compulsive disorder (OCD), social anxiety disorder, generalized anxiety disorder, panic disorder, migraine, diabetic peripheral neuropathy, hot flashes, post-traumatic stress disorder, premenstrual dysphoric disorder, Raynaud's syndrome, and borderline personality disorder. Also prescribed for alcoholism, anorexia, kleptomania, irritable bowel syndrome, dyskinetic side effects of levodopa + carbidopa, and Tourette syndrome.

Fluoxetine is approved for treating major depressive disorder and OCD in children. Fluvoxamine is also approved for treating OCD in children. Other SSRIs are not approved for use in children for any indication.

General Information

SSRIs, which are chemically unrelated to other antidepressant drugs, prevent the movement of the neurotransmitter serotonin into nerve endings. This forces serotonin to remain in the spaces surrounding nerve endings, increasing its action. Abnormal serotonin function may be involved in depression, and the SSRIs are effective in treating the common symptoms of depression. For example, they can help improve mood and mental alertness, alleviate anxiety, and improve sleep patterns.

Cautions and Warnings

Do not take SSRIs if you are **allergic** or **sensitive** to any of their ingredients. Some people have experienced serious drug reactions to SSRIs.

SSRIs can increase the risk of suicidal thinking and behavior. The risk of suicide is higher in teens and adults up to age 24, about the same in people age 25–64, and reduced in people age 65 and over. Younger people who are started on an antidepressant should be observed closely for clinical worsening of depression, suicidality, or unusual changes in behavior, especially at the beginning of therapy or when the dose is increased or decreased. Suicide risk is especially high in **severely depressed people** and may continue until the condition is significantly improved. Severely depressed people should be allowed to carry only small quantities of SSRIs to limit the risk of overdose.

Serious, potentially fatal reactions may occur if SSRIs and a monoamine oxidase inhibitor (MAOI) antidepressant are taken within 2 weeks of one another (see "Drug Interactions").

About 7% of people taking fluoxetine develop an itching rash, ⅓ of whom have to stop taking the medication.

As many as ⅓ of people taking an SSRI experience anxiety, sleeplessness, and nervousness.

Underweight depressed people who take fluoxetine may lose more weight. About 9% of people taking fluoxetine experience appetite loss, and 13% lose more than 5% of their body weight.

SSRIs may affect blood platelets, although their exact effect is not known. Some people have had abnormal bleeding while taking these drugs, especially if they are taken with other drugs that affect blood-clotting function.

SSRIs are significantly broken down in the liver. People with **liver disease** should use these drugs with caution and may require lower doses than people without liver disease. People with severe **kidney disease** should begin with smaller doses of citalopram, escitalopram, paroxetine, and sertraline.

People taking SSRIs may experience a severe drop in their blood-sodium level, especially if taking diuretics as well. Sodium levels usually return to normal when the medicine is stopped, but medical treatment is often necessary.

SSRIs should be used with caution by people with **seizure disorders** and by people with **glaucoma**.

People with **mania** or **hypomania** may experience an activation or worsening of their condition when taking SSRIs, especially if they are not also taking an antimanic medication.

Fluoxetine may alter blood-sugar control in people with **diabetes**.

SSRIs should be discontinued gradually, as significant side effects from discontinuing too quickly may occur.

Rarely, people taking SSRIs develop a group of symptoms called serotonin syndrome, consisting of 1 or more of the following symptoms: excitement, a mild manic reaction, restlessness, loss of consciousness, confusion, disorientation, anxiety, agitation, muscle weakness, muscle spasms, tremors, involuntary muscle movements on one side of the body, shivering and dilated pupils, sweating, vomiting, and rapid heartbeat. Serotonin syndrome requires immediate medical treatment.

Babies born of mothers who took an SSRI may develop a rare heart and lung condition known as PPHN (persistent pulmonary hypertension of the newborn). PPHN occurs when a newborn baby cannot properly adapt to breathing on his own outside the womb. Newborns with PPHN may need intensive care to increase their blood-oxygen level. Severe PPHN can damage multiple organs, including the brain, and even cause death.

Possible Side Effects

▼ Common: headache, anxiety, nervousness, sleeplessness, drowsiness, tiredness, weakness, sexual dysfunction,

Possible Side Effects *(continued)*

tremors, night sweats, dizziness, lightheadedness, dry mouth, upset or irritated stomach, appetite loss, appetite increase, nausea, vomiting, diarrhea, gas, rash, weight loss or gain, electric-shock sensations, increased sweating, increased yawning, tinnitus, abnormal dreams, difficulty concentrating, acne, hair loss, dry skin, dizziness or fainting when rising suddenly from a sitting or lying position, and itching.

▼ Less common: chest pain, allergy, runny nose, bronchitis, abnormal heart rhythms, blood pressure changes, bone pain, bursitis, twitching, breast pain, cystitis, urinary pain, double vision, eye or ear pain, conjunctivitis (pinkeye), anemia, swelling, low blood sugar, and low thyroid activity.

▼ Rare: Rare side effects can occur in almost any part of the body. Contact your doctor if you experience anything unusual while taking any medication.

Drug Interactions

- Five weeks should elapse between stopping fluoxetine and starting an MAOI antidepressant. At least 2 weeks should elapse between stopping other SSRIs and starting an MAOI. Two weeks should elapse between stopping an MAOI and starting an SSRI. Taking these drugs too close together or at the same time may cause serious, life-threatening reactions.
- Combining an SSRI with linezolid, metoclopramide, St. John's wort, tramadol, or triptan antimigraine drugs may increase the risk of serotonin syndrome (see "Cautions and Warnings"). Avoid combining these medications.
- Combining an SSRI with aspirin or a nonsteroidal anti-inflammatory drug (NSAID) substantially increases the risk of gastrointestinal (GI) side effects. These combinations should be avoided over the long term. The risk of bleeding is increased with these combinations or with an SSRI and warfarin.
- Alcohol may increase tiredness and other depressant effects of SSRIs.
- SSRIs may affect lithium blood levels. Your lithium dosage may need to be adjusted.

- Tricyclic antidepressant blood levels may increase if they are taken with SSRIs. Combine these drugs with caution.
- Cyproheptadine (an antihistamine) may reverse the effects of SSRIs.
- SSRIs can increase blood levels of many drugs, including any other SSRI, amphetamines, some antiarrhythmics (encainide, flecainide, propafenone), codeine, and phenothiazines, leading to an increased risk of side effects.
- People who combine L-tryptophan and an SSRI may become agitated and restless and may experience an upset stomach. This combination is not recommended.
- Combining an SSRI with pimozide can significantly increase the amount of pimozide in the blood. Do not combine these drugs.
- Fluoxetine, fluvoxamine, and paroxetine increase thioridazine levels. Do not combine these drugs.
- Cimetidine can increase citalopram, escitalopram, paroxetine, and sertraline levels in the blood.
- Citalopram, escitalopram, and fluvoxamine may increase the effects of beta blockers.
- Citalopram, fluoxetine, paroxetine, and sertraline can raise the blood levels of cyclosporine (an immune suppressant).
- Citalopram and escitalopram may decrease levels of ketoconazole. The risk of GI side effects may be increased with this combination.
- Hallucinations have occurred after combining fluoxetine with dextromethorphan (the most common cough suppressant in over-the-counter products).
- Combining fluoxetine, fluvoxamine, and sertraline with phenytoin can lead to increased phenytoin side effects.
- Combining paroxetine and phenytoin may reduce blood levels of both drugs.
- Fluoxetine, fluvoxamine, and sertraline can raise the blood level of the antipsychotic drugs clozapine, olanzapine, and risperidone.
- Fluoxetine and fluvoxamine may increase the risk of carbamazepine side effects and increase haloperidol levels.
- Fluoxetine and fluvoxamine may reduce the effectiveness of buspirone, which can lead to a worsening of OCD in people taking this combination to treat OCD.

- Fluoxetine and fluvoxamine may increase the effect of benzodiazepine antianxiety drugs.
- Fluoxetine may affect ritonavir, possibly leading to serotonin syndrome (see "Cautions and Warnings").
- Fluoxetine may raise levels of vinblastine. Dosage adjustments may be needed.
- Quetiapine raises blood levels of fluvoxamine. The risk of neuroleptic malignant syndrome may be increased.
- Fluvoxamine should not be taken with alosetron.
- The antihistamines astemizole and terfenadine should not be taken with fluvoxamine due to the risk of serious heart rhythm abnormalities.
- Fluvoxamine can raise levels of oral antidiabetes drugs, methadone, proton-pump inhibitors, ropivacaine, rosiglitazone, and zolpidem.
- Sildenafil dosage may need to be reduced if combined with fluvoxamine.
- Fluvoxamine and paroxetine may affect theophylline blood levels.
- Smoking increases the metabolism of fluvoxamine.
- Paroxetine increases blood levels of atomoxetine, galantamine, procyclidine, trazodone, and zolpidem. Dosage adjustments may be necessary.
- Paroxetine may affect the effectiveness of digoxin.
- Paroxetine may increase risperidone blood levels, and the combination may lead to serotonin syndrome (see "Cautions and Warnings").
- Tamoxifen must be broken down by the enzyme system slowed by paroxetine. Mixing it with paroxetine reduces its effectiveness.
- Paroxetine blood levels may be reduced by barbiturates, fosamprenavir, and ritonavir.
- Carbamazepine may lower citalopram, escitalopram, and sertraline blood levels.
- Sertraline may increase the effects of tolbutamide and zolpidem.
- Sertraline may decrease the effects of cisapride.
- The oral concentration of sertraline should not be used with disulfiram.

Food Interactions

SSRIs can be taken without regard to food or meals.

Usual Dose

Citalopram

Adult: 20–60 mg a day. Seniors and people with liver disease should take no more than 20 mg a day. People with kidney disease may need a lower dose.

Child: not recommended.

Escitalopram

Adult and Child (age 12 and over): 10–20 mg once a day. Seniors and people with liver disease should take no more than 10 mg.

Child (under age 12): not recommended.

Fluoxetine

Adult: 20–80 mg a day, taken in the morning, or a single 90-mg capsule weekly. Seniors, people with kidney or liver disease, and people taking several different drugs may need a lower dose.

Child (age 7–17): 10–60 mg a day.

Fluvoxamine

Adult: 50–300 mg a day at bedtime. Seniors and people with liver disease may need a lower dose.

Child (age 8–17): 25–200 mg a day. Adolescents may take up to 300 mg a day. Doses larger than 50 mg should be divided in 2 and given morning and night. If the 2 divided doses are not equal, give the larger dose at bedtime.

Child (under age 8): not recommended.

Paroxetine

Adult: 20–60 mg a day, or 25–75 mg a day for the controlled-release form. Seniors and people with liver disease should start at 10 mg a day and take no more than 40 mg a day. People with kidney disease may need a lower dose.

Child: not recommended.

Prozac Weekly

Adult: 90 mg (1 capsule) every 7 days.

Child: not recommended.

Sertraline

Adult and Child (age 6–17): 25–200 mg a day. In adults, lower doses may be used to start, but most adults take at least 50 mg a day. Children age 12 and under should start with 25 mg a day. Seniors and people with liver disease should take a lower dose.

Overdosage

Overdose symptoms may include seizures, nausea, vomiting, agitation, restlessness, and nervous system excitation. Any person suspected of having taken an SSRI overdose should be taken to a hospital emergency room at once. If you seek treatment, ALWAYS bring the prescription bottle or container.

Special Information

SSRIs can make you dizzy or drowsy. Take care when driving or performing other tasks that require alertness and concentration, especially when you first start the drug or increase your dose. Avoid alcohol.

Low blood sodium can cause headache, dizziness, falling, trouble concentrating, confusion, weakness, and memory loss. Contact your doctor if you develop these symptoms. Symptoms of potentially fatal severe sodium loss include hallucinations, fainting, seizures, coma, and inability to breathe.

Be sure your doctor knows if you are pregnant, breast-feeding, or taking other drugs, including over-the-counter drugs, while taking an SSRI.

Contact your doctor if you develop a rash or hives, become excessively nervous or anxious, lose your appetite—especially if you are already underweight—or experience any unusual side effects.

If you forget a dose, take it as soon as you remember. If it is almost time for your next dose, skip the dose you forgot and continue with your regular schedule. Do not take a double dose.

Discontinuing SSRIs suddenly may cause adverse effects such as mood changes, irritability, agitation, dizziness, tingling in the hands or feet, anxiety, confusion, headache, tiredness, and insomnia. These effects can be serious but are usually temporary. A gradual reduction in dose is recommended.

Special Populations

Pregnancy/Breast-feeding: These drugs pass into the circulation of the developing fetus. Studies in animals and people have shown that SSRIs may cause birth defects and premature birth. An SSRI should be taken during pregnancy only if your doctor determines that the potential benefit outweighs the risks.

These drugs pass into breast milk. Nursing mothers who must take an SSRI should use infant formula.

Seniors: These drugs can lower blood levels of sodium in seniors, potentially leading to serious side effects. Seniors generally start with lower doses and may need less of the drug to achieve the desired results.

Seroquel *see **Quetiapine,** page 961*

Generic Name

Sevelamer (seh-VEL-ah-mer)

Brand Names

Renagel (sevelamer hydrochloride)
Renvela (sevelamer carbonate)

Type of Drug

Phosphate binder.

Prescribed For

High blood-phosphate levels in people with end-stage renal disease (ESRD).

General Information

People with ESRD, a form of kidney disease, tend to retain phosphorous. High phosphate levels, in turn, can affect calcium balance in the body and cause deposits of this mineral to build up in the wrong places. Sevelamer hydrochloride helps to reduce phosphate levels by limiting the amount of phosphorous absorbed from food. Sevelamer also lowers levels of total and low-density lipoprotein (LDL) cholesterol.

Cautions and Warnings

Do not take sevelamer if you are **allergic** or **sensitive** to any of its ingredients or you have a **low phosphate level** or a **bowel obstruction**.

Use this drug with caution if you have had **gastrointestinal surgery** or have **difficulty swallowing** or severe **stomach or intestinal problems**.

Possible Side Effects

▼ Most common: diarrhea, nausea, upset stomach, and vomiting.

▼ Common: abdominal pain, stomach gas, constipation, headache, infection, pain, blood-pressure changes, and blood-clotting problems.

▼ Less common: back pain; fever; and bowel impaction, obstruction, and perforation.

▼ Rare: Rare side effects can occur in almost any part of the body. Contact your doctor if you experience anything unusual while taking any medication.

Drug Interactions

- Sevelamer may interfere with other drugs taken at the same time. Take sevelamer either 1 hour before or 3 hours after other medications.
- Sevelamer reduces the amount of ciprofloxacin in the blood by ½.
- Sevelamer can interfere with the absorption of vitamins D, E, K, and folic acid from food.

Food Interactions

Sevelamer should be swallowed whole with meals.

Usual Dose

Renagel

Adult: starting dose—1–4 capsules with each meal for people not taking a phosphate binder. For people switching from calcium acetate to sevelamer, consult your doctor for correct dosing.

Child: not recommended.

Renvela

Adult: starting dose—1–2 800-mg tablets 3 times a day. Dose is adjusted every 2 weeks as needed to obtain target phosphorous level. The highest daily dose studied in trials was 17 tablets a day.

Child: not recommended.

Overdosage

Symptoms may include drug side effects. Contact your local poison control center or a hospital emergency room for more information. If you seek treatment, ALWAYS bring the prescription bottle or container.

Special Information

Sevelamer can interfere with the absorption of vitamins from food. Take a supplemental multivitamin while using this drug.

It is important to take sevelamer with each meal. If you forget a dose, skip it and continue to take the drug with subsequent meals.

Do not chew or break the capsules before swallowing them.

Special Populations

Pregnancy/Breast-feeding: In animal studies, sevelamer interfered with fetal bone development. It also interferes with the absorption of vitamins and nutrients, which are essential for a healthy pregnancy. Sevelamer should be taken during pregnancy only if your doctor determines that the potential benefit outweighs the risks.

It is not known if sevelamer passes into breast milk. Nursing mothers who must take it should use infant formula.

Seniors: Seniors may take this drug without special precaution.

Brand Names

Sinemet

Generic Ingredients

Carbidopa + Levodopa G

Other Brand Names

Parcopa
Sinemet CR

The information in this profile also applies to the following drugs:

Generic Ingredients: Carbidopa
Lodosyn

Generic Ingredients: Carbidopa + Levodopa + Entacapone
Stalevo

Type of Drug

Antiparkinsonian.

Prescribed For

Parkinson's disease (PD) and parkinsonism following nervous system damage.

General Information

In Sinemet, levodopa, which increases dopamine, is the active ingredient that affects PD; carbidopa slows the breakdown of levodopa, making more available to the brain and reducing the side effects from levodopa. Carbidopa is sold under the brand name Lodosyn for people who need individual doses of carbidopa. Entacapone is added to levodopa + carbidopa to help alleviate periods when the levodopa stops working. Other antiparkinsonian drugs are often prescribed with Sinemet.

Cautions and Warnings

Do not take Sinemet if you are **allergic** or **sensitive** to any of its ingredients.

When Sinemet is given to people already taking levodopa, the levodopa must be stopped at least 12 hours before the Sinemet is started to decrease incidents of side effects.

The sustained-release form of Sinemet has a lesser incidence of nervous system side effects; the immediate-release version may produce such effects even at lower dosages.

Sinemet may cause depression and suicidal thoughts. People with current **depression** or a history of **mental disturbances** should be observed for worsening symptoms.

Sinemet should be used with caution in people with an **endocrine disorder**, severe **heart or lung disease**, **kidney or liver disease**, or **asthma**. Care should be used when Sinemet is given to those who have had a **heart attack** and have resulting **heart rhythm disorders**. Heart function should be monitored after initial dose.

A potentially fatal condition called neuroleptic malignant syndrome (NMS) has been linked to the use of Sinemet. Symptoms include elevated body temperature, muscle stiffness, altered mental states, and irregularities in pulse or blood pressure.

Sinemet can worsen **narrow-angle glaucoma**. People with this condition should not use it.

People with PD have 2–6 times the risk of developing skin cancer (melanoma). It is not known if the increased risk is due to the condition or the drugs used to manage it. People taking this medication should frequently check themselves for skin cancers and see a dermatologist regularly. Patients with suspected **melanoma** should not take Sinemet.

Sinemet may increase the risk of bleeding in patients with a history of **ulcer**.

For more information about Stalevo, see Entacapone, page 442.

Possible Side Effects

- ▼ Common: uncontrolled muscle movements, appetite loss, nausea, vomiting, stomach pain, dry mouth, difficulty swallowing, drooling, shaky hands, headache, dizziness, numbness, weakness, feeling faint, grinding of the teeth, confusion, sleeplessness, nightmares, hallucinations, anxiety, agitation, tiredness, feeling unwell, and euphoria (feeling "high").
- ▼ Less common: heart palpitations; chest pain; dizziness when rising quickly from a sitting or lying position; increased sex drive; sudden extreme slowness of movement ("on-off" phenomenon); changes in mental state, including paranoia, psychosis, depression, and a slowdown of mental functioning; difficulty urinating; muscle twitching; eyelid spasms; lockjaw; burning sensation on the tongue; bitter taste; diarrhea; constipation; gas; flushing; rash; sweating; drug allergy (including serious skin reactions); unusual breathing; blurred or double vision; pupil dilation; hot flashes; weight changes; and darkening of urine or sweat.
- ▼ Rare: Rare side effects can occur in almost any part of the body. Contact your doctor if you experience anything unusual while taking any medication.

For more information about Stalevo, see Entacapone, page 442.

Drug Interactions

- Combining Sinemet and a monoamine oxidase inhibitor (MAOI) antidepressant may cause a rapid increase in blood pressure. MAOIs should be stopped 2 weeks before starting on Sinemet. Do not combine these medications.
- Antacids may increase the effects of Sinemet.
- People taking a medication to treat high blood pressure may need less if they start taking Sinemet.
- Antipsychotic drugs, isoniazid, papaverine, and phenytoin may interfere with Sinemet.
- Clonidine, metoclopramide, and vitamin B_6 may interfere with the effects of Sinemet.
- There are rare reports of high blood pressure and dyskinesia (involuntary movements) with a combination of Sinemet and tricyclic antidepressants. These drugs may also inhibit the effectiveness of Sinemet.

For more information about Stalevo, see Entacapone, page 442.

Food Interactions

Immediate-release Sinemet can be taken with food to reduce upset stomach. Sinemet CR, the sustained-release form, should be taken on an empty stomach.

Usual Dose

Sinemet

Three Sinemet strengths are available: 10/100, 25/100, and 25/250. The first number represents carbidopa content, the second the levodopa content, in mg. Dosage must be individualized. Dosage adjustments are made by adding or omitting ½–1 tablet a day. Maximum daily dosage is eight 25/250 tablets. Sinemet CR is started at dosages roughly equal to 10% more levodopa a day than was being taken previously.

If extra carbidopa is needed, your doctor may prescribe Lodosyn to be taken together with Sinemet. Lodosyn is added in steps of no more than 25 mg a day until the desired effect is achieved.

Stalevo

Carbidopa + Levodopa + Entacapone (12.5/50/200; 18.75/75/200; 25/100/200; 31.25/125/200; 37.5/150/200): 1 tablet every 3–8 hours, up to 8 tablets a day.

Carbidopa + Levodopa + Entacapone (50/200/200): 1 tablet every 3–8 hours, up to 6 tablets a day.

Overdosage

Symptoms include exaggerated side effects. Take the victim to a hospital emergency room. If you seek treatment, ALWAYS bring the prescription bottle or container.

Special Information

Sinemet can cause tiredness or an inability to concentrate. Be careful when driving or doing any task that requires concentration. Sinemet may also make you fall asleep, sometimes suddenly, during the day. If you have experienced this, do not drive or operate machinery.

Contact your doctor if you experience dizziness, lightheadedness, or fainting spells; changes in mood or mental state; abnormal heart rhythm or heart palpitations; difficulty urinating; persistent nausea, vomiting, or other stomach complaints; or uncontrollable movements of the face, eyelids, mouth, tongue, neck, arms, hands, or legs.

When stopping or reducing this drug, fever or hot flashes may be a symptom of a very dangerous condition similar to NMS. Contact your doctor immediately.

People taking entacapone and other medicines for PD have experienced intense urges (e.g., sexual activity and gambling) and difficulty controlling these and other urges. This may be due to the increase in brain dopamine produced by PD medicines, as the urges can pass after the medicine is reduced or stopped. Report any changes to your doctor.

This drug may cause darkening of urine or sweat. This effect is not harmful, but may interfere with urine tests for diabetes. Make sure all your doctors know you are taking this medication.

Take Sinemet exactly as prescribed.

If you forget a dose, take it as soon as you remember. If it is within 2 hours of your next dose, skip the one you forgot and continue with your regular schedule. Do not take a double dose.

Do not cut, crush, or chew Sinemet CR or Stalevo tablets.

Special Populations

Pregnancy/Breast-feeding: Both of the ingredients in Sinemet cause birth defects in animals. Sinemet should be taken during pregnancy only if your doctor determines that the potential benefit outweighs the risks.

The ingredients in Sinemet may pass into breast milk and are considered unsafe for infants. Nursing mothers who must take this drug should use infant formula.

Seniors: Seniors may require reduced dosage. They are also more likely to develop abnormal heart rhythms or other cardiac side effects, especially if they have heart disease.

Singulair *see **Leukotriene Antagonists/Inhibitors,** page 679*

Generic Name

Sodium Oxybate (so-DEE-um OX-ee-bate)

Brand Names

Xyrem

Type of Drug

Central-nervous-system (CNS) depressant.

Prescribed For

Narcolepsy, cataplexy, and fibromyalgia.

General Information

Sodium oxybate, also known as GHB, is a CNS depressant that reduces daytime sleepiness in people with narcolepsy, a condition in which people suddenly fall asleep without warning. People can stay asleep for anywhere from a few seconds to a few hours, and may continue to function as if they were completely awake and aware but later have no memory of the event. Some narcoleptic people also have attacks of cataplexy, in which they suddenly lose all muscle tone and strength. Cataplexy symptoms last for up to 30 minutes and can range from minor sagging of the facial muscles to dropping of the jaw or head, weak knees, or a total collapse. Speech is slurred, and double vision and inability to focus the eyes may occur; however, hearing and awareness are unaffected. Cataplexy is often triggered by strong emotions such as exhilaration, anger, fear, surprise, awe, embarrassment, laughter, or orgasm and is often confused with epilepsy. Sodium oxybate has also been used to treat fibromyalgia. This drug is available through a centralized pharmacy and is distributed only to legitimate patients. Ninety-five percent of this drug is broken down in the body to form carbon dioxide, which is then passed out through the lungs. The rest passes out of the body in the urine.

Cautions and Warnings

Do not take this drug if you are **allergic** or **sensitive** to it.

People with a rare genetic disease known as **succinic semialdehyde dehydrogenase (SSD) deficiency** cannot take this drug.

Sodium oxybate (GHB) is a known drug of abuse and has been associated with important CNS events. Because of this, it is a federally controlled substance and should only be used as prescribed. Prescribed sodium oxybate doses are much lower than those used by drug abusers. Confusion, depression, difficulty breathing, and loss of consciousness can occur even at recommended doses.

Sodium oxybate can cause drug dependence and physical withdrawal symptoms if stopped suddenly. Your dosage should always be reduced gradually to prevent drug-withdrawal symptoms.

People with **respiratory illnesses**, including **sleep apnea**, should use this drug with caution. Loss of consciousness in drug abusers taking GHB has led to coma or death.

People with **liver disease** should take only ½ the usual dose of sodium oxybate. Some patients taking larger doses of sodium oxybate can experience nighttime urinary incontinence (bed-wetting). Sleepwalking or confused nighttime behavior can occur.

This drug has large amounts of sodium. People with **heart failure**, **high blood pressure**, or **kidney disease** should avoid salt in their diet.

Possible Side Effects

Side effects increase noticeably as the drug dose increases.

- ▼ Most common: headache, nausea, and dizziness.
- ▼ Common: vomiting, tiredness, inflamed throat and nasal passages, throat pain, sleepiness, lethargy, weakness, loss of urinary control, ringing or buzzing in the ears, blurred vision, gastrointestinal pain, diarrhea, upset stomach, stomach virus, respiratory infections, increased blood pressure, back pain, reduced sense of touch, sleep paralysis, confusion, sleep disorders, and sleepwalking.
- ▼ Less common: sweating, difficulty focusing or paying attention, depression, and nightmares.
- ▼ Rare: Other side effects can occur in almost any part of the body. Contact your doctor if you experience anything unusual while taking any medication.

Drug Interactions

- Sodium oxybate is a CNS depressant. Avoid alcohol, certain antihistamines, barbiturates, narcotics, and other sedatives. Taking sodium oxybate with these drugs may lead to excessive depression, drowsiness, or difficulty breathing.
- Sodium oxybate may be mixed with other drugs often taken by people with narcolepsy, including modafinil, protriptyline, and zolpidem.

Food Interactions

Sodium oxybate must be taken on an empty stomach, at least 2 hours after eating.

Usual Dose

Adult and Child (age 16 and over): 2.25 g at bedtime and again 2.5–4 hours later to start. Your daily dose can be increased to 4.5 g in each of the doses. Most people require 6–9 g a day. People with liver disease should take ½ the regular dose.

Child (under age 16): not recommended.

Overdosage

Two overdoses were reported in clinical studies. Symptoms include drug side effects such as loss of consciousness, loss of urinary and stool control, blurred vision, seizures, and others. One patient died from an overdose of sodium oxybate with alcohol and other drugs. Sodium oxybate overdose victims are intoxicated and can injure themselves or pass out. In the past, people taking 18–250 g of GHB per day have become addicted to GHB. These people experienced withdrawal symptoms for several days to 2 weeks after abruptly stopping GHB. Overdose victims should be taken to a hospital emergency room at once. If you seek treatment, ALWAYS bring the prescription bottle or container with you.

Special Information

Sodium oxybate solution contains 2.5 g per mL. Each evening, measure both doses of sodium oxybate for the night using the oral syringe in the package and place them into the 2 dosing cups supplied in the package. Dilute each dose with 2 oz. of water. Set your alarm clock to wake up 2½–4 hours after the first dose. Then, take your first dose while sitting in bed. When your alarm wakes you, take the second dose also while sitting in bed. Mixed solutions should be used on the same night.

Avoid any activity that requires coordination and alertness for at least 6 hours after you take this medication. Be aware that it can also affect your alertness and coordination during the day. Be careful until you know how it affects you.

Depression, psychosis, paranoia, hallucinations, agitation, or abnormal behavior or thinking should be reported to your doctor as soon as possible. They can be psychiatric side effects of sodium oxybate.

Do not allow children or pets access to your medication.

Special Populations

Pregnancy/Breast-feeding: Animal studies of sodium oxybate have found no effects on the developing fetus. However, there are no sodium oxybate studies in pregnant women. It should be taken during pregnancy only if your doctor determines that the potential benefit outweighs the risks.

It is not known if this drug passes into breast milk. Nursing mothers should use infant formula.

Seniors: This drug has not been studied in seniors.

Generic Name

Spinosad (SPIN-oh-sad)

Brand Names

Natroba

Type of Drug

Pediculocide.

Prescribed For

Head lice.

General Information

Spinosad kills head lice by overexciting the parasite's nervous system. Lice become paralyzed and die after this period of over-excitement. In clinical studies, almost twice as many spinosad users were free of live lice 14 days after treatment compared with traditional scabicides. Spinosad is not absorbed through the skin into the bloodstream but contains benzyl alcohol, which can be absorbed and therefore should not be used for infants.

Cautions and Warnings

Do not use spinosad if you are **allergic** or **sensitive** to any of its ingredients. Stop using spinosad if you develop a reaction to it.

Spinosad should not be used for **infants younger than 6 months** because of the chances of toxicity from benzyl alcohol, an ingredient in this product.

Spinosad is for use only on scalp hair. Do not use it for lice on any other area of the body.

Possible Side Effects

- ▼ Less common: skin or eye redness or irritation.
- ▼ Rare: skin or hair dryness, skin peeling, and hair loss.

Contact your doctor if you experience anything unusual while taking any medication.

Drug Interactions

- Do not apply this product with any other topical medication.

Usual Dose

Adult and Child (age 4 and over): Shake bottle well before using. Do not shampoo or wet your hair and scalp before use. Apply enough spinosad suspension to cover the hair and scalp and leave it in for a full 10 minutes. Rinse off with warm water. Repeat if live lice are seen 7 days after the first treatment. Avoid eye contact.

Child (under age 4): not recommended.

Overdosage

In case of accidental ingestion, take the victim to an emergency room. If you seek treatment, ALWAYS bring the prescription container.

Special Information

Hair and scalp must be dry before applying spinosad suspension. Be sure to apply enough spinosad to completely cover every head louse. Long hair may require using a whole bottle.

This drug should be applied only to scalp hair and skin. It should never be applied to any other area of the body or swallowed.

Do not apply spinosad to areas around the eyes, nose, or mouth. Contact your doctor if anything unusual develops or if irritation continues after you have stopped using the drug. If spinosad gets into your eye, you must immediately flush the eye with water to completely wash it away.

Wash your hands thoroughly after applying spinosad to remove all traces from your skin, to prevent accidentally irritating your eyes later on.

This product should be part of a lice prevention program including warm water washing or dry cleaning of all recently worn clothes and hats, used bedding, and towels. Wash all combs, brushes, and hair clips in warm water. Use a fine-tooth comb or special lice comb to remove dead lice and nits.

Special Populations

Pregnancy/Breast-feeding: Animal studies with spinosad did not damage the developing fetus, but the safety of using spinosad during pregnancy is not known. It should be taken during pregnancy only if your doctor determines that the potential benefit outweighs the risks.

Spinosad is not absorbed into the blood and does not pass into breast milk. However this product contains benzyl alcohol, which can affect a developing fetus and may be found in breast milk. Nursing mothers who use it must pump and throw away their breast milk for 8 hours after using spinosad. New mother's milk produced after 8 hours has passed can be safely fed to an infant. Or you may choose to temporarily use infant formula.

Seniors: This drug may be used without special precaution.

Spiriva *see **Ipratropium,** page 644*

Type of Drug

Statin Cholesterol-Lowering Agents

Brand Names

Generic Ingredients: Atorvastatin G
Lipitor

Generic Ingredients: Atorvastatin + Amlodipine Besylate
Caduet

Generic Ingredients: Fluvastatin
Lescol
Lescol XL

Generic Ingredients: Lovastatin G
Altoprev
Mevacor

Generic Ingredients: Lovastatin + Niacin
Advicor

Generic Ingredients: Pitavastatin
Livalo

Generic Ingredients: Pravastatin G
Pravachol

Generic Ingredients: Rosuvastatin
Crestor

Generic Ingredients: Simvastatin G
Zocor

Generic Ingredients: Simvastatin + Niacin
Simcor

Prescribed For

High blood levels of cholesterol, low-density lipoprotein (LDL) cholesterol, triglycerides, and C-reactive protein; also prescribed for atherosclerosis (hardening of the arteries), diabetes-related blood-fat problems, preventing heart attacks and strokes, and reducing the risk of cardiac bypass surgery. Some of these drugs may also be used for blood-fat disorders related to kidney disease and inherited blood-fat problems.

General Information

High blood-fat levels are believed to play a role in the development of cardiovascular disease. Statin drugs help to lower blood-fat levels by blocking the effects of the enzyme HMG-CoA reductase, which in turn interferes with the production of cholesterol in the body. They also increase levels of high-density lipoprotein (HDL) cholesterol, the "good" cholesterol considered to have a beneficial effect on heart health. Statin drugs are proven to slow the progression of atherosclerosis, help prevent heart attacks, and reduce the risk of dying from heart disease. Other related benefits have been discovered. Atorvastatin, for example, has been found to improve the walking ability of people with intermittent claudication (a blood-vessel disease). Advicor combines lovastatin with niacin, a nutrient that helps raise levels of "good" cholesterol. Simcor combines 2 cholesterol drugs, but no additional benefit on heart health beyond that already known for taking simvastatin alone has been proven for this combination product. Atorvastatin has also been combined in single pills with a blood-pressure-lowering medicine (Caduet).

These drugs begin working quickly. Blood-fat levels are significantly improved after 1–2 weeks of treatment. Maximum effect occurs in 4–6 weeks, persists for the remainder of drug therapy, and continues for 4–6 weeks after you stop taking these drugs. Statins are generally not recommended for people under age

30, although they may be prescribed for teenagers under certain circumstances. Only a small amount of these drugs enters the bloodstream. They are largely broken down in the liver.

Cautions and Warnings

Do not take statins if you are **allergic** or **sensitive** to any of their ingredients. It is possible to be allergic to one of these drugs and tolerate another. Contact your doctor if you develop a rash, itching, or hives.

People with **liver disease**, those who have had it in the past, and those who drink large amounts of **alcohol** should not take a statin because they can worsen or cause liver disease. Liver failure has occurred. About 1 in 100 people who take these drugs develops high liver-enzyme counts. The risk of this effect varies somewhat between statins but generally increases with higher dosages. Your doctor should take a blood sample to test your liver function before you begin a statin drug and every month or so during the first year of treatment.

People taking these drugs may develop severe muscle aches or weakness, which can be a sign of a more serious condition that could lead to kidney damage, confusion, and death. This is usually a rare problem but is more common at higher drug doses. Due to the risk of muscle damage within the first year of treatment, maximum doses of these medicines should be prescribed only after a person has been taking a statin for at least a year without symptoms such as weakness, muscle cramps, stiffness, or spasm.

People with **kidney disease** who take pitavastatin, pravastatin, rosuvastatin, or simvastatin must be closely monitored by their doctors. A reduced drug dosage is recommended.

People in early studies of lovastatin developed cloudy vision due to an effect on the lens of the eye, but this effect has not been seen in further studies. Statins have also been reported to cause degeneration of the optic nerve and cataracts at doses 30–60 times the average dose. Report any changes in vision to your doctor.

Elevated levels of hemoglobin A1C and blood sugar measured on diabetes blood tests, new cases of diabetes, and deterioration in diabetes control have been seen in studies of atorvastatin, pravastatin, rosuvastatin, and simvastatin, but there is no definite link to the statin drugs.

Many studies have found no link between statins and cancer. Others have linked long-term statin use to a higher risk of colorectal, bladder, and lung cancer and a lower risk of blood cancer.

Possible Side Effects

Side effects are usually mild and temporary. Rare side effects associated with these drugs can occur in almost any part of the body. Contact your doctor if you experience anything unusual while taking any medication.

Atorvastatin

▼ Most common: headache, diarrhea, joint pain, muscle aches, sinus irritation, and infection.

▼ Common: back pain, abdominal pain or cramps, flu-like symptoms, and weakness.

▼ Less common: gas, upset stomach, rash, and allergy.

Atorvastatin + Amlodipine

See Calcium Channel Blockers, page 224, for more information.

Fluvastatin

▼ Most common: headache and upset stomach.

▼ Common: muscle aches, abdominal pain or cramps, diarrhea, and flu-like symptoms.

▼ Less common: sleeplessness, nausea, gas, urinary tract infection, joint pain, bronchitis, sinus irritation, allergy, and fatigue.

Lovastatin

▼ Most common: infection, headache, and sinus irritation.

▼ Common: abdominal pain or cramps, gas, constipation, diarrhea, joint pain, back pain, and flu-like symptoms.

▼ Less common: dizziness, heartburn, upset stomach, itching, rash, nausea, vomiting, urinary tract infection, muscle aches, blurred vision, eye irritation, and weakness.

Lovastatin + Niacin

See Niacin, page 841, for more information.

Pitavastatin

▼ Common: back pain, constipation, diarrhea, and muscle aches.

Possible Side Effects *(continued)*

Pravastatin

▼ Most common: muscle aches, pain, or cramps.
▼ Common: nausea, vomiting, upset stomach, fatigue, and abdominal pain or cramps.
▼ Less common: headache, dizziness, constipation, gas, diarrhea, heartburn, pain, breathing difficulties, upper-respiratory infection, chest pain, rash, and urinary difficulties, and visual changes.

Rosuvastatin

▼ Most common: joint pain and muscle aches or pain.
▼ Common: headache and dizziness.
▼ Less common: abdominal pain or cramps, stomach irritation, constipation, nausea, weakness, and pain.

Simvastatin

▼ Common: headache, sleeplessness, vertigo, eczema, nausea, abdominal pain or cramps, constipation, stomach irritation, bronchitis, and respiratory infection.
▼ Less common: urinary tract infection, muscle aches, swelling in the arms and legs, and sinus irritation.

Simvastatin + Niacin

See Niacin, page 841, for more information.

Drug Interactions

- Do not mix atorvastatin, lovastatin, or simvastatin with clarithromycin, erythromycin, HIV protease inhibitors, itraconazole, ketoconazole, nefazodone, posaconazole, or telithromycin.
- Do not use lovastatin extended-release, pitavastatin, or simvastatin if you must take cyclosporine.
- Do not use the following statins with the following drugs: tacrolimus with atorvastatin; lopinavir/ritonavir with pitavastatin; darunavir or nelfinavir with lovastatin or simvastatin; baicalin with rosuvastatin; and conivaptan, danazol, and mibefradil with simvastatin.
- Taking both a statin drug and any fibrate drug—gemfibrozil, fenofibrate, or fenofibric acid—increases the risk of painful muscle damage. A reduced statin dosage may be required.

Gemfibrozil should not be taken together with atorvastatin and simvastatin.

- The risk of painful muscle damage or other statin side effects may be increased if they are used with the following drugs: amiodarone, cilostazol, colchicine, danazol, delavirdine, diltiazem, fluconazole, imatinib, niacin, quinine, and verapamil. In particular, the lowest possible doses of atorvastatin, lovastatin, or simvastatin should be used. Fluvastatin, pitavastatin, pravastatin, or rosuvastatin may be used with caution.
- If simvastatin must be used with amiodarone, amlodipine, or ranolazine, the daily dose should not exceed 20 mg due to an increased risk of muscle damage. Do not use more than 10 mg a day of simvastatin with diltiazem or verapamil.
- Statin blood levels and effectiveness may be reduced by bosentan, carbamazepine, efavirenz, isradipine, nevirapine, phenytoin (except fluvastatin; see below), and St. John's wort. Your statin dose may need to be changed.
- Cimetidine, ranitidine, and omeprazole may increase the effects of statins.
- Adding glyburide to fluvastatin can increase the effects of both drugs.
- The cholesterol-lowering effects of statins and bile acid sequestrants are additive. Take a statin drug 1 hour before or 4 hours after a bile acid sequestrant. Colestipol reduces atorvastatin blood levels, but this combination nevertheless more effectively lowers blood-fat levels than either drug used alone.
- Antacids reduce statin blood levels, although their actual cholesterol lowering may not change. Separate doses of these drugs by at least 2 hours.
- Statins increase blood levels of estrogens and progestins in contraceptive drugs, which can lead to side effects. If you must take both drugs, talk to your doctor about switching to a lower-dose hormonal contraceptive.
- Statins may increase the effects of warfarin. People taking these drugs together should be periodically examined by their doctors. Warfarin dosage adjustment may be necessary.
- Statins may enhance and prolong the effects of benzodiazepine sedatives such as midazolam.
- Statin drugs can increase the amount of diclofenac and digoxin in the blood.

- Drinking alcohol while taking a statin increases the risk of side effects.
- Phenytoin and fluvastatin interact in a way that increases the blood levels of both drugs.
- Rifampin increases blood levels of pitavastatin. People mixing these drugs may take no more than 2 mg a day of pitavastatin. Rifampin may reduce the blood levels of other statins.
- Separate doses of pravastatin and pectin by as much time as possible.
- Rosuvastatin blood levels and side effects may be increased by eltrombopag. Your daily rosuvastatin dose may be reduced if you must take these drugs together.
- A simvastatin dose reduction may be necessary if you must take dronedarone, ticagrelor, or voriconazole.

For more information, see Calcium Channel Blockers, page 224, for Caduet; and Niacin, page 841, for Advicor and Simcor.

Food Interactions

Grapefruit juice can slow the breakdown of statin drugs (except pravastatin) in the liver, increasing the risk of drug side effects. Lovastatin must be taken with meals. Other statin drugs can be taken without regard to food or meals.

Usual Dose

Atorvastatin

Adult: 10–80 mg a day.
Child (age 10–17): 10–20 mg a day.
Child (under age 10): not recommended.

Atorvastatin + Amlodipine

Adult: 2.5/10–10/80 mg a day.
Child: not recommended.

Fluvastatin

Adult and Child (over age 16): 20–80 mg a day, taken in the evening.
Child (age 9–16): 20 mg a day.
Child (under age 9): not recommended.

Lovastatin

Adult: 10–80 mg a day, usually taken with your evening meal.

Child (age 10–17): 10–40 mg a day.
Child (under age 10): not recommended.

Lovastatin + Niacin
Adult: 500/20–2000/40, taken at bedtime with a low-fat snack.
Child: not recommended.

Pitavastatin
Adult: 1–4 mg a day. People with moderate to severe kidney disease should take no more than 2 mg a day.
Child: not recommended.

Pravastatin
Adult: 10–80 mg a day.
Child (age 14–17): 10–40 mg a day.
Child (age 8–13): 10–20 mg a day.
Child (under age 8): not recommended.

Rosuvastatin
Adult: 5–40 mg a day.
Child (age 10–17): 5–20 mg a day.
Child (under age 10): not recommended.

Simvastatin
Adult: 5–40 mg, taken in the evening. Dosage may be increased to a maximum of 80 mg a day.
Child (age 10–17): 10–40 mg a day.
Child (under age 10): not recommended.

Simvastatin + Niacin
Adult: 500/20–2000/40, taken in the evening.
Child: not recommended.

Overdosage

People taking an overdose of these drugs have experienced no specific symptoms and have recovered without a problem after the drug was removed by making them vomit. Overdose victims should be taken to a hospital emergency room for evaluation and treatment. If you seek treatment, ALWAYS bring the prescription bottle or container.

Special Information

Contact your doctor if you develop blurred vision, muscle aches, pain, tenderness, or weakness, especially if you are also feverish or do not feel well.

Statin drugs are prescribed in combination with a low-fat diet. Following your doctor's dietary instructions will help reduce your blood fats and keep them low. Do not take more cholesterol-lowering medication than your doctor has prescribed. Do not stop taking it without your doctor's knowledge.

These drugs may cause increased sensitivity to the sun. Use sunscreen and wear protective clothing.

If you forget a dose, take it as soon as you remember. If it is almost time for your next dose, skip the one you forgot and continue with your regular schedule. Do not take a double dose.

Special Populations

Pregnancy/Breast-feeding: Pregnant women and those who might become pregnant must not take any of these drugs.

Fluvastatin and pravastatin pass into breast milk in humans, and other statins have been shown to do the same in animal studies. Nursing mothers who must take them should use infant formula.

Seniors: Seniors are more sensitive to the effects of some statin drugs and may require reduced dosage.

Strattera *see **Atomoxetine,** page 130*

Suboxone *see **Naltrexone,** page 818*

Generic Name

Sucralfate (sue-KRAL-fate) G

Brand Names

Carafate

Type of Drug

Anti-ulcer.

Prescribed For

Short-term (less than 8 weeks) treatment and maintenance therapy of duodenal (intestinal) ulcer. Also used for stomach ulcer, irritation, and bleeding; gastroesophageal reflux disease (GERD); irritation of the esophagus and mouth; throat ulcer; and prevention of stress ulcer and stomach bleeding.

General Information

Sucralfate works within the gastrointestinal (GI) tract by exerting a soothing local effect on ulcer tissue; very little of the drug is absorbed into the bloodstream. After the drug binds to proteins in the damaged mucous tissue within the ulcer, it forms a barrier to the normal acids and enzymes of the GI tract. This barrier protects ulcer tissue from further damage, allowing it to heal naturally. Sucralfate is not an antacid and works differently than cimetidine, omeprazole, and other anti-ulcer drugs, but it is as effective in treating duodenal ulcer disease as these drugs.

Cautions and Warnings

Do not take sucralfate if you are **allergic** or **sensitive** to any of its ingredients.

Small amounts of aluminum are absorbed while you take sucralfate. This can be a problem for people with chronic **kidney failure** and for those on **dialysis**.

Possible Side Effects

Side effects are usually minimal.

▼ Most common: constipation.

▼ Less common: diarrhea, nausea, upset stomach, indigestion, dry mouth, rash, itching, back pain, dizziness, and sleepiness.

Drug Interactions

- Sucralfate may interfere with the absorption of cimetidine, diclofenac, famotidine, ketoconazole, levothyroxine, nizatidine, penicillamine, phenytoin, quinidine, quinolone antibiotics, ranitidine, tetracycline, theophylline, and warfarin. Separate these drugs and sucralfate by at least 2 hours to avoid this effect.
- Avoid aluminum-containing antacids while you are taking sucralfate, especially if you have reduced kidney function. This combination increases aluminum absorption into the bloodstream and may lead to aluminum poisoning.

Food Interactions

Take each dose on an empty stomach, at least 1 hour before or 2 hours after meals.

Usual Dose

Adult: starting dose—1 g 4 times a day for active ulcers; maintenance dose (tablets only)—1 tablet twice a day.

Child: not recommended.

Overdosage

Little is known about the effects of sucralfate overdose, although the risk associated with it is thought to be minimal. Contact your local poison control center or a hospital emergency room for more information. If you seek treatment, ALWAYS bring the prescription bottle or container.

Special Information

Complete the full course of drug therapy.

Notify your doctor if you develop constipation, diarrhea, or other GI side effects.

If you forget a dose, take it as soon as you remember. If it is almost time for your next dose, skip the one you forgot and continue with your regular schedule. Do not take a double dose.

Special Populations

Pregnancy/Breast-feeding: Although animal studies of sucralfate reveal no damage to the fetus, sucralfate should be taken during pregnancy only if your doctor determines that the potential benefit outweighs the risks.

It is not known if sucralfate passes into breast milk. Nursing mothers who must take it should use infant formula.

Seniors: Seniors should take the lowest effective dose.

Type of Drug

Sulfa Drugs

Brand Names

Generic Ingredients: Sulfadiazine G

Generic Ingredients: Sulfasalazine G

Azulfidine Azulfidine EN-Tabs

Combination Products

Generic Ingredients: Sulfamethoxazole + Trimethoprim G

Bactrim
Bactrim DS
Septra
Septra DS
Sulfamethoprim
Sulfatrim Pediatric

Prescribed For

Sulfadiazine is prescribed for urinary tract and other infections, including malaria, rheumatic fever, and toxoplasmosis encephalitis. Sulfasalazine is prescribed for rheumatoid arthritis and ulcerative and other forms of colitis; also prescribed for psoriasis, Crohn's disease, and ankylosing spondylitis. The combination of trimethoprim + sulfamethoxazole (TMP-SMX) is also prescribed for a wide variety of infections, including urinary tract infection, bronchitis, and ear infection in children; also prescribed for traveler's diarrhea, *Pneumocystis carinii* pneumonia (PCP), prostate infection, cholera, nocardiosis (lung infection), and *Salmonella* infection.

General Information

In use for many years, sulfa drugs are prescribed for infections in various parts of the body but are particularly helpful for urinary tract infections. They kill bacteria and some fungi by interfering with the metabolic processes of these organisms. Some organisms may become resistant to the effects of sulfa drugs. TMP-SMX interferes with the infecting microorganism's normal use of folic acid in 2 ways, making it more efficient than other antibacterial drugs.

Sulfasalazine has specific anti-inflammatory and immune system effects, and is effective against colitis, intestinal irritation, and arthritis and other inflammatory conditions.

Cautions and Warnings

Do not take sulfa drugs if you are **allergic** or **sensitive** to any of their ingredients or to any drug chemically related to the sulfa drugs, including thiazide and loop diuretics, carbonic anhydrase inhibitors, and sulfonylurea-type oral antidiabetes drugs.

Do not use any sulfa drug if you are allergic to **aspirin**, **PABA-containing sunscreens**, **local anesthetics**, or if you have **porphyria**.

Allergic reactions to sulfa drugs are more common in people with severe **allergies**, **bronchial asthma**, or **glucose-6-phosphate dehydrogenase (G-6-PD) deficiency**. Use with caution if you have one of these conditions.

Do not take TMP-SMX if you have a **folic acid deficiency**

Sulfasalazine should not be used by people with **intestinal or urinary obstruction**. Colitis has occurred in people taking TMP-SMX.

Sulfa drugs should be taken by people with severe **kidney or liver disease** only after a doctor has evaluated their condition and need for the drug.

Deaths in people taking sulfasalazine and sulfadiazine have been related to a variety of effects on the blood, kidney and liver damage, and nervous system changes. Symptoms may include sore throat, fever, pale or yellow skin, chills, unusual bleeding or bruising, rash, and drowsiness; these should be reported to your doctor at once. Also contact your doctor if you experience ringing in the ears, blood in the urine, breathing difficulties, or anything unusual while taking a sulfa drug.

Men taking sulfasalazine may have low sperm count or become infertile. This effect reverses when the drug is stopped.

Sulfa drugs can cause increased sensitivity to the sun or bright light. Use sunscreen and wear protective clothing.

People taking TMP-SMX for **PCP** who also have compromised immune function may not respond to the drug as well and are more likely to develop the less common side effects.

Possible Side Effects

- ▼ Most common: appetite loss, headache, itching, rash, skin sensitivity to strong sunlight, nausea, vomiting, abdominal or stomach cramps or pain, hallucinations, diarrhea, dizziness, ringing or buzzing in the ears, and chills.
- ▼ Less common: blood diseases or changes in blood composition, anemia, mouth sores, blue or purple tint to skin, arthritic pain, drowsiness, hearing loss, itchy eyes, fever, hair loss, and yellowing of the skin or whites of the eyes.
- ▼ Rare: goiter, increased urination, and hypoglycemia. Rare side effects can occur in almost any part of the body. Contact your doctor if you experience anything unusual while taking any medication.

Possible Side Effects *(continued)*

Trimethoprim + Sulfamethoxazole (TMP-SMX)

▼ Most common: nausea, vomiting, rash, and itching.

▼ Less common: abdominal pain, diarrhea, upset stomach, fever, chills, cough, sensitivity to sunlight, reduced levels of red and white blood cells and platelets, allergic reaction (symptoms include rash, itching, hives, and breathing difficulties), swelling around the eyes, arthritis-like pain, low blood sugar, coating of the tongue, headache, tingling in the arms or legs, depression, convulsions, hallucinations, ringing in the ears, dizziness, difficulty sleeping, apathy, tiredness, weakness, and nervousness. Septra may also affect your kidneys and cause you to produce less urine.

Drug Interactions

- Sulfa drugs may increase the effects of methotrexate, phenytoin and other hydantoin antiseizure drugs, sulfonylurea-type oral antidiabetes drugs, thiazide diuretics, uricosuric (gout) drugs, and warfarin and other anticoagulant drugs. Dosages of these drugs may need to be reduced by your doctor.
- Cyclosporine blood levels may be reduced by sulfa drugs, possibly increasing kidney toxicity.
- Indomethacin, probenecid, and aspirin and other salicylates may increase blood levels of sulfa drugs, increasing the risk of side effects.
- The effects of folic acid and digoxin may be diminished by sulfasalazine; dosage increases may be needed.
- Taking sulfasalazine and thiopurines (including azathioprine, mercaptopurine) together may reduce your white-blood-cell count.
- Combining TMP-SMX with the following drugs may increase the risk of abnormal heart rhythms: antiarrhythmic agents (including amiodarone, bretylium, disopyramide, dofetilide, quinidine, and sotalol), arsenic trioxide, chlorpromazine, cisapride, dolasetron, droperidol, mefloquine, mesoridazine, moxifloxacin, pentamidine, pimozide, tacrolimus, thioridazine, and ziprasidone. TMP-SMX should not be used at all if you take dofetilide.
- Do not take TMP-SMX if you take methenamine or tretinoin, due to risk of severe side effects.

- Do not drink alcohol while taking TMP-SMX, or a dangerous reaction may occur.
- Live vaccines may be less effective while using TMP-SMX and should be avoided.
- Septra may prolong the effects of anticoagulant (blood thinning) agents, such as warfarin.
- The trimethoprim in TMP-SMX may reduce the effectiveness of cyclosporine and increase its toxic effect on the kidney.
- TMP-SMX may increase blood levels of certain antidiabetes drugs (glitazones, meglitinides, and sulfonylureas), digoxin, methotrexate, and phenytoin, increasing the chance of side effects. Your doctor may reduce the dosage of these medicines or stop TMP-SMX, depending on your reaction.
- People taking a thiazide diuretic with TMP-SMX are more likely to develop reduced levels of blood platelets and an increased chance of bleeding under the skin.
- Caution should be used when combining TMP-SMX with angiotensin-converting enzyme (ACE) inhibitors because potassium levels may be affected. Seniors in particular are prone to dangerously high potassium levels.
- The combination of TMP-SMX with pyrimethamine may increase the risk of anemia. Treatment with folic acid may be necessary, or your doctor may stop 1 or both drugs.
- Taking TMP-SMX with leucovorin for AIDS-related pneumonia increases the risk of overall treatment failure.
- TMP-SMX can decrease blood levels and effectiveness of tricyclic antidepressants (e.g., amitriptyline), and a dosage increase may be necessary while you take Septra.
- Amantadine, dapsone, and indomethacin may increase blood levels of TMP-SMX and increase the risk of side effects. Your doctor may change your dosage or stop TMP-SMX treatment, depending on your reaction.

Food Interactions

Sulfa drugs should be taken on an empty stomach with a full glass of water. Sulfasalazine can be taken with food if it upsets your stomach. Drink plenty of water throughout the day.

Usual Dose

Sulfadiazine

Adult: 2–4 g a day in 3–6 divided doses.

Child (age 2 months and over): 330 mg per lb. of body weight, up to 6 g a day.

Sulfasalazine

Adult: 500 mg–4 g a day in evenly divided doses.

Child (age 6 and over): 3.4–27 mg per lb. of body weight, in evenly divided doses, up to 2 g a day.

Child (under age 6): not recommended.

Trimethoprim + Sulfamethoxazole (TMP-SMX)

Non-PCP Infections

Adult: 2 regular tablets or 1 Septra DS tablet every 6–12 hours for 5–14 days, depending on the condition being treated.

Child (67–88 lbs.): 4 tsp. (or 2 tablets) every 12 hours.

Child (45–66 lbs.): 3 tsp. (or 1½ tablets) every 12 hours.

Child (23–44 lbs.): 2 tsp. (or 1 tablet) every 12 hours.

Child (under 22 lbs.): 1 tsp. every 12 hours.

Child (under age 2 months): not recommended.

PCP Infections

Adult and Child (2 months and over): sulfamethoxazole 34–45 mg per lb. of body weight + trimethoprim 7–9 mg per lb. every 6 hours for 14–21 days.

Child (under age 2 months): not recommended.

Overdosage

Symptoms include appetite loss, nausea, vomiting and colic, dizziness, headache, drowsiness, unconsciousness, high fever, severe bleeding or bruising, and irritation or soreness of the tongue. Take the victim to a hospital emergency room at once. If you seek treatment, ALWAYS take the prescription bottle or container.

Special Information

Be sure to take the full course of medication as prescribed, even if you notice an improvement in your symptoms.

Sulfasalazine may turn your urine orange-yellow. This is a harmless reaction. Skin discoloration has also occurred. This drug may permanently stain soft contact lenses.

Maintain adequate fluid intake to reduce the chance of kidney stone formation when taking sulfasalazine.

Some people may not adequately digest delayed-release sulfasalazine. If you find undigested tablets in your stool, notify your doctor because you will need to take a different drug.

Contact your doctor if you develop a sore throat, rash, unusual bleeding or bruising, or any other persistent or intolerable side effect.

You may develop unusual sensitivity to bright light, particularly sunlight. If you have a history of light sensitivity or if you have sensitive skin, avoid prolonged exposure to sunlight while using TMP-SMX.

Sulfa drugs may interfere with some tests for sugar in the urine.

If you forget a dose, take it as soon as you remember. If you take the drug twice a day and it is almost time for your next dose, take 1 dose right away, another after 5–6 hours, and then go back to your regular schedule. If you take the drug 3 or more times a day and it is almost time for your next dose, take 1 dose right away, another after 2–4 hours, and then go back to your regular schedule. Never take a double dose.

Special Populations

Pregnancy/Breast-feeding: Sulfa drugs pass into the fetal circulation and may affect the fetus. Malformations have been seen in animal studies and so these drugs should not be taken during pregnancy.

Small amounts of sulfa drugs pass into breast milk and may harm the nursing infant. Nursing mothers who must take them should use infant formula.

Seniors: Seniors with kidney or liver problems should take sulfa drugs with caution.

Type of Drug

Sulfonylurea Antidiabetes Drugs

Brand Names

Generic Ingredients: Chlorpropamide G
Diabinese

Generic Ingredients: Glimepiride G
Amaryl

Generic Ingredients: Glipizide G
Glucotrol
Glucotrol XL

Generic Ingredients: Glyburide G
DiaBeta
Glynase

Generic Ingredients: Tolazamide G

Generic Ingredients: Tolbutamide G

Combination Products
Generic Ingredients: Glipizide + Metformin G

Generic Ingredients: Glyburide + Metformin G
Glucovance

Prescribed For

Type 2 diabetes mellitus. Chlorpropamide may also be used to treat diabetes insipidus (a hormonal condition unrelated to blood sugar).

General Information

The sulfonylureas stimulate the production and release of insulin from the pancreas. These drugs are not a form of oral insulin or a substitute for insulin. The pancreas must be functioning for them to work; they are not effective in type 1 diabetes. These drugs differ from each other in how long they take to start working, the duration of their effectiveness, and the amount of each required to produce a roughly equivalent antidiabetic effect.

Some sulfonylureas are available in combination with metformin. Metformin lowers the amount of glucose produced by the liver, reduces the amount of glucose you absorb from food, and helps cells use glucose. Metformin can also moderately lower body fats. Glipizide is also available with pioglitazone (Duetact) and rosiglitazone (Avandaryl); for more information on these medicines, see Glitazone Antidiabetes Drugs, page 529.

These drugs may be used alone or in combination with other antidiabetes drugs to control your blood sugar.

Cautions and Warnings

Do not take a sulfonylurea if you are **allergic** or **sensitive** to any of its ingredients or to sulfa drug antibacterials.

People with acidosis, including those with diabetic ketoacidosis, should not take these drugs.

People with an inherited condition known as **glucose-6-phosphate dehydrogenase (G-6-PD) deficiency** should not take these medicines because they can trigger red-blood-cell destruction.

Do not use Glucovance if you have **heart failure**, **liver disease**, or moderate to severe **kidney disease**. These conditions increase the risk for lactic acidosis, a rare, potentially fatal condition that can occur with metformin treatment.

People with severe **narrowing of the gastrointestinal (GI) tract** should not take the extended-release form of glipizide due to risk of intestinal obstruction. Glipizide extended-release make not work as well in people with other forms of GI disease.

Infection, **fever**, **surgery**, **injury**, or **emotional upset** reduce the effectiveness of these drugs. If you are having surgery or an X-ray that requires the injection of an iodine-based contrast material, you should temporarily stop taking Glucovance because the combination could result in acute kidney problems. You must be under your doctor's continuous care while taking any of these drugs.

Studies have found that people taking tolbutamide are up to 2½ times more likely to have fatal heart trouble than those whose diabetes is controlled with diet and/or other medications.

These drugs can cause low blood sugar (see "Overdosage") that may require medical attention.

These drugs should be used with caution if you have serious **liver or kidney disease**; monitor your blood sugar very closely.

Possible Side Effects

- ▼ Most common: low blood sugar (see "Overdosage" for symptoms), loss of appetite, nausea, vomiting, stomach upset, and weakness or tingling in the hands and feet.
- ▼ Less common: sensitivity to sunlight, itching, dizziness, and headache.
- ▼ Rare: yellowing of the skin or whites of the eyes and rash. Rare side effects can occur in almost any part of the body. Contact your doctor if you experience anything unusual while taking any medication.

For more information about Glucovance, see Metformin, page 731.

Drug Interactions

- Mixing glyburide and bosentan increases the risk of liver damage. Do not mix these drugs.
- The following drugs may increase your need for sulfonylureas: beta blockers, calcium channel blockers, charcoal tablets, cholestyramine, contraceptive drugs, corticosteroids, diazoxide, estrogens, isoniazid, nicotinic acid, phenothiazines, phenytoin and other hydantoin drugs, rifampin, stimulants, thiazide diuretics, thyroid replacement drugs, and anything that makes your urine less acidic.

- The following drugs may increase blood levels of oral sulfonylureas; dosage adjustments may be needed to account for this effect. Some of these drugs can cause drastic drops in blood sugar levels: androgens (male hormones), angiotensin-converting enzyme (ACE) inhibitors, aspirin and other salicylates, azole antifungals, chloramphenicol, fenfluramine, fluoroquinolone antibiotics (ciprofloxacin), fluoxetine, gemfibrozil, histamine H_2 antagonists, magnesium-containing products, methyldopa, monoamine oxidase inhibitor (MAOI) antidepressants, probenecid, sulfa drugs, sulfinpyrazone, tricyclic antidepressants, large doses of vitamin C, and warfarin and other anticoagulants.
- Mixing these drugs with alcohol can cause flushing and breathing difficulties. Other possible effects are throbbing pain in the head and neck, nausea, vomiting, increased sweating, excessive thirst, chest pains, palpitations, lowered blood pressure, weakness, dizziness, blurred vision, and confusion. Alcohol also increases the risk of lactic acidosis while taking Glucovance. If you experience any of these reactions, contact your doctor immediately.
- Sulfonylureas may increase the effects of digitalis drugs.
- Chlorpropamide may increase the effects of barbiturates.
- Glyburide may alter the effectiveness of oral anticoagulant (blood thinning) drugs. Dosage may need to be adjusted by your doctor.

For more information about Glucovance, see Metformin, page 731.

Food Interactions

All the sulfonylureas except glipizide can be taken with food. Glipizide should be taken 30 minutes before a meal for best results. Citrus fruits and other foods that make your urine more acidic may increase blood levels of sulfonylureas and should be eaten in limited quantities. To minimize stomach problems, you should take Glucovance with food.

Usual Dose

Child: None of the sulfonylureas are recommended for children.

Chlorpropamide

Adult: 250–500 mg a day.
Senior: Start with 100 mg a day.

Glimepiride: 1–8 mg once a day.

Glipizide

Adult: 5–20 mg once a day for extended-release tablets; 5–40 mg a day in single or divided doses for immediate-release tablets.

Senior: Start with 2.5 mg a day.

Glipizide + Metformin: 2.5/250 mg–20/2000 mg in single or divided doses.

Glyburide

DiaBeta

Adult: 2.5–20 mg a day in single or divided doses.

Senior: Start with 1.25 mg a day.

Glynase

Adult: 1.5–12 mg a day in single or divided doses.

Senior: Start with 0.75 mg a day.

Glynase is not equivalent to DiaBeta and may not be substituted for it.

Glyburide + Metformin: 1.25/250 mg–20/2000 mg in single or divided doses.

Tolazamide: 100–1000 mg a day.

Tolbutamide: 1–3 g a day.

Overdosage

Sulfonylurea overdose causes low blood sugar. Symptoms may occur suddenly and include weakness, fatigue, nervousness, confusion, headache, double vision, convulsions, dizziness, psychosis, unconsciousness, rapid and shallow breathing, numbness or tingling around the mouth, hunger, nausea, loss of skin color, dry skin, and pulse changes. Overdose victims should eat high-sugar, low-fat foods such as fruit juice or a glucose product for diabetics to raise blood-sugar levels. If victims are unable to eat or drink (due to a seizure, unconsciousness, or other debilitating condition), they should be immediately taken to a hospital emergency room. If you seek treatment, ALWAYS bring the prescription bottle or container.

Special Information

Managing diabetes is your responsibility. Follow your doctor's instructions about diet, exercise, hygiene, and measures to avoid infection. Take all your medicines as prescribed.

Contact your doctor if you develop low blood sugar (see "Overdosage") or high blood sugar (symptoms include excessive thirst or urination and sugar or ketones in the urine), if you are not feeling well, or if you have symptoms such as itching, rash, yellowing of the skin or whites of the eyes, abnormally light-colored stools, a low-grade fever, sore throat, diarrhea, or unusual bruising or bleeding.

Alcohol increases the risk of developing lactic acidosis while taking Glucovance. Lactic acidosis is a medical emergency. If you develop it, immediately contact your doctor and stop taking these drugs. The symptoms of lactic acidosis (not feeling well, muscle aches, difficulty breathing, and slow heartbeat) can develop with more severe acidosis. Regular monitoring of kidney function minimizes the risk of developing lactic acidosis, as does using the smallest effective dosage of Glucovance.

Do not stop taking these drugs, except under your doctor's supervision. If you forget a dose, take it as soon as you remember. If it is almost time for your next dose, skip the one you forgot and continue with your regular schedule. Do not take a double dose.

Special Populations

Pregnancy/Breast-feeding: Animal studies have shown that all these drugs except glyburide cause birth defects or interfere with fetal development. Do not take a sulfonylurea if you are pregnant. Pregnant women with diabetes are usually treated with insulin.

These drugs pass into breast milk and may lower blood-sugar levels in an infant receiving breast milk. Nursing mothers taking one of these medications should use infant formula.

Seniors: Seniors, especially those with reduced kidney function, are very sensitive to the blood-sugar-lowering effects and side effects of these drugs. Low blood sugar, the major sign of drug overdose, may be more difficult to identify in seniors and is more likely to cause nervous system side effects. Seniors taking these drugs must keep in close contact with their doctors and follow their directions. Dosages should usually be lower, especially when first taking sulfonylureas.

Symbicort

see ***Corticosteroids, Inhalers,*** *page 334*

Synthroid

see ***Thyroid Hormone Replacements,*** *page 1136*

Generic Name

Tacrolimus (tak-ROE-lim-us) G

Brand Names

Prograf Protopic Ointment

The information in this profile also applies to the following drugs:

Generic Ingredients: Sirolimus
Rapamune

Type of Drug

Immunosuppressant.

Prescribed For

Organ transplant rejection, autoimmune disease, severe psoriasis, and atopic dermatitis.

General Information

Tacrolimus is derived from a bacterium and is used to prevent the rejection of transplanted organs. The drug is used in liver transplants and has been studied in kidney, bone marrow, heart, pancreas, and small bowel transplants, among others. Tacrolimus works by blocking the activity of T-cells, which protect the body against invading microorganisms or foreign substances, producing immune system suppression. Tacrolimus may be used with corticosteroids and cyclosporine for further transplant protection.

Cautions and Warnings

These drugs should only be prescribed by physicians experienced in immunosuppressive therapy and the care of organ transplant patients.

Do not take these drugs if you are **allergic** or **sensitive** to any of their ingredients. Some people may be allergic to chemically modified castor oil, which is used in tacrolimus injection.

These medicines are not recommended for people undergoing lung transplant procedures. Sirolimus is not recommended for liver transplant patients.

As with other immune suppressants, people taking these drugs have an increased risk of developing infection or lymphoma or another malignancy. The risk increases with the degree of immune suppression and the length of time that the drug is taken.

Do not use tacrolimus ointment if you have **skin cancer**,

Netherton syndrome, or a **skin infection** at the site of application. These drugs increase your sensitivity to the sun and susceptibility to skin cancer. Always wear protective clothing and sunscreen when outdoors.

Sirolimus increases the risk of angioedema, a potentially life-threatening swelling of the lips and throat. Contact your doctor immediately if you experience this effect.

Between 10% and 20% of transplant patients treated with tacrolimus develop post-transplant diabetes mellitus, though the condition is sometimes reversible.

People with **liver disease** should receive lower dosages of sirolimus.

Kidney toxicity has been found in more than 50% of kidney transplant patients and about 40% of liver transplant patients, particularly those who experienced post-transplant reduction in liver function who were taking tacrolimus. People with **kidney disease** should receive lower dosages. Mild to moderate high blood pressure is a common side effect of tacrolimus and may be a sign of kidney damage. People taking this drug should measure their blood pressure regularly.

About 10–45% of patients who take tacrolimus develop mild to severe elevations of blood potassium.

Tremors, headaches, muscle function changes, changes in mental state and sense perception, or other nervous system problems occur in about ½ of the people receiving liver or kidney transplants. Seizure has also occurred. In some cases, these side effects may be associated with large amounts of tacrolimus in the blood.

Tacrolimus may cause a thickening of the heart muscle. This condition is reversible with a dosage reduction.

Sirolimus can cause increases in cholesterol and triglyceride levels that may require treatment with diet or lipid-lowering drugs.

Wounds may not heal as quickly or as well as normal if you take sirolimus.

People taking tacrolimus may develop a disorder related to Epstein-Barr virus infection.

Possible Side Effects

Sirolimus

Drug side effects increase as drug dosage increases. Rare side effects can occur in almost any part of the body. Contact

Possible Side Effects *(continued)*

your doctor if you experience anything unusual while taking any medication.

- ▼ Most common: abdominal pain; fever; headache; joint pain; urinary tract infection; high blood pressure; high blood lipids; acne; rash; constipation; diarrhea; nausea; anemia; low blood-platelet levels; swollen legs, ankles, or arms; and decreased kidney function.
- ▼ Less common: rapid heartbeat, blood clots, skin cancer, blood cell abnormalities, low blood potassium, pneumonia, poor wound healing, bone damage, herpes infection, mouth sores, and nosebleeds.

Protopic

- ▼ Most common: burning or itching skin, redness or infection of the skin, headache, and flu-like symptoms.
- ▼ Less common: herpes simplex, rash, acne, allergic reaction, asthma, sinusitis, sleeplessness, and painful menstruation.

Tacrolimus

- ▼ Most common: headache, tremors, sleeplessness, tingling in the hands or feet, diarrhea, nausea, constipation, vomiting, high blood pressure, urinary tract infection, decreased kidney function, anemia, increased white-blood-cell counts, changes in blood-potassium level, reduced blood magnesium, high blood sugar, high blood fats, breathing difficulties, itching, rash, abdominal pain, generalized pain, fever, infection, weakness, back pain, and retention of fluid.
- ▼ Less common: infrequent urination, fluid in the lungs and other lung problems, abnormal dreaming, anxiety, confusion, depression, dizziness, instability, hallucination, poor coordination, muscle spasms, psychosis, tiredness, unusual thoughts, double vision or other visual disturbances, ringing or buzzing in the ears, appetite loss, upset stomach, liver abnormalities, yellowing of the skin or whites of the eyes, reduced blood-platelet counts, difficulty swallowing, gas, stomach bleeding, fungal infection of the mouth, blood in the urine, chest pain, rapid heartbeat, low blood pressure, black-and-blue marks, muscle and joint aches, leg cramps, muscle weakness, asthma, bronchitis, coughing, sore throat, pneumonia, stuffy and runny nose, sinus irritation, voice changes, sweating, and herpes infection.

Drug Interactions

- Sirolimus and tacrolimus should not be combined due to reduced efficacy and potentially fatal side effects.
- Live vaccines may be less effective while using these drugs and should be avoided.
- Rifampin and rifabutin drastically reduce blood levels of sirolimus in the blood by increasing its metabolism. Do not mix these drugs.
- Blood levels of these drugs and side effects may be increased—in some cases by up to 10 times, by the following drugs: antifungal drugs such as clotrimazole, fluconazole, itraconazole, ketoconazole, and voriconazole; bromocriptine; calcium channel blockers; chloramphenicol; cimetidine; cisapride; clarithromycin; danazol; erythromycin; ethinyl estradiol; lansoprazole; methylprednisolone; metoclopramide; nefazodone; omeprazole; protease inhibitors, and telithromycin. Do not mix clarithromycin, erythromycin, telithromycin, ketoconazole, itraconazole, and voriconazole with sirolimus.
- Do not use sirolimus with disulfiram, furazolidone, or metronidazole to avoid a severe alcohol intolerance reaction. Avoid alcohol while using tacrolimus ointment. Temporary facial flushing may occur.
- Do not mix tacrolimus with ziprasidone as life-threatening abnormal heart rhythms may occur. The risk of abnormal heart rhythms is also increased if tacrolimus is used with any of the following; combine with caution: antiarrhythmic drugs (including amiodarone, bretylium, disopyramide, dofetilide, flecainide, quinidine, sotalol), arsenic trioxide, chlorpromazine, cisapride, dolasetron, droperidol, lapatinib, mefloquine, mesoridazine, methadone, moxifloxacin, nilotinib, paliperidone, pentamidine, perflutren, pimozide, propafenone, quinupristin/dalfopristin, tetrabenazine, and thioridazine.
- Combining tacrolimus with cyclosporine (another organ transplant drug) can worsen kidney disease; avoid this combination. People switching from cyclosporine to tacrolimus should not begin tacrolimus therapy until at least 24 hours after the last cyclosporine dose. Cyclosporine can double the amount of sirolimus in the blood. Take sirolimus at least 4 hours after cyclosporine capsules or solution.
- The risk of angioedema (a potentially life-threatening swelling of the lips and throat) is increased if sirolimus is taken

with an angiotensin-converting enzyme (ACE) inhibitor. Use these drugs together with caution.

- The risk of severe muscle damage is increased when these drugs are combined with fibrates or statins. Fluvastatin and pravastatin may be safer choices.
- These drugs may increase blood levels and side effects of mycophenolate and phenytoin. A dose adjustment may be necessary.
- Sirolimus and tacrolimus blood levels may be reduced by carbamazepine, caspofungin, phenobarbital, phenytoin, rifabutin, rifampin, and St. John's wort.
- Do not use potassium-sparing diuretics or other drugs that can raise potassium levels while taking tacrolimus.
- Tacrolimus may cause more kidney damage when combined with other drugs that also cause kidney problems, including aminoglycoside antibiotics, amphotericin B, and cisplatin. Use with caution.

Food Interactions

Fresh grapefruit juice contains an inhibitory substance that blocks the liver enzyme that breaks down these drugs, increasing their levels in the blood. The same effect does not occur with frozen grapefruit juice because the inhibitory substance has a short shelf life and breaks down when the juice is frozen.

These drugs should be taken consistently either 1 hour before or 2 hours after meals.

Usual Dose

Sirolimus

Adult and Child (age 13 and over): Dosage is individualized based on height and weight, and is usually in the range of 2–40 mg a day. Dosing is usually started at the high end of the recommended amount and then reduced to the lowest effective level. Mix the solution with 2 or more oz. of water or orange juice only (see "Special Information").

Child (under age 13): not recommended.

Tacrolimus

Adult and Child: 0.03–0.09 mg per lb. of body weight a day divided into 2 doses. Children may require more than adults. Dosing is usually started at the high end of the recommended amount and then reduced to the lowest effective level.

Protopic

Adult and Child (age 16 and over): Rub 0.1% ointment into affected areas twice a day and continue until symptoms go away, for up to 6 weeks.

Child (age 2–15): Rub 0.03% ointment into affected areas twice a day for up to 6 weeks.

Contact your doctor if symptoms do not improve within 6 weeks.

Overdosage

Tacrolimus overdose produces expected drug side effects. Sirolimus overdose has produced abnormal heart rhythms. Take the victim to a hospital emergency room. If you seek treatment, ALWAYS bring the prescription bottle or container.

Special Information

It is extremely important to take this drug exactly as prescribed. If you forget a dose, take it as soon as you remember. If it is almost time for your next dose, skip the forgotten dose and continue with your regular schedule. Do not take a double dose. Contact your doctor if you forget 2 or more doses in a row.

Sirolimus solution must be stored in the refrigerator. If the solution becomes cloudy in the refrigerator, let it stand at room temperature until the cloudiness disappears. The cloudiness does not affect the quality of the drug.

If you are taking sirolimus oral solution, use the amber oral-dose syringe that comes in the package to withdraw the prescribed amount of medicine, and place that into a glass or plastic container with at least 2 oz. of water or orange juice. Do not use any other liquids, including grapefruit juice, for dilution. Stir the mixture and drink at once. Then pour another 4 oz. of water or orange juice into the same container, mix, and drink right away.

People taking these medicines require regular testing to monitor their progress.

Contact your doctor at the first sign of fever; sore throat; tiredness; weakness; nervousness; unusual bleeding or bruising; tender or swollen gums; convulsions; irregular heartbeat; confusion; numbness or tingling of your hands, feet, or lips; breathing difficulties; severe stomach pain with nausea; or blood in the urine. Other side effects should be brought to your doctor's attention.

Maintain good dental hygiene while taking these drugs and use extra care when brushing and flossing because the drug increases your risk of oral infection. See your dentist regularly.

These drugs should be continued as long as prescribed by your doctor. Do not stop taking the medication because of side effects or other problems. If you cannot tolerate the oral form, this drug may be given by injection, though the oral capsules are preferable.

Special Populations

Pregnancy/Breast-feeding: These drugs pass into the fetal circulation and cause miscarriage and reduced fertility in animals. In humans, babies born to mothers taking tacrolimus have had high blood potassium and poor kidney function. There is no reliable experience with sirolimus. These drugs should be taken during pregnancy only if your doctor determines that the potential benefit outweighs the risks. Women who might become pregnant while taking these medicines must begin using reliable contraception before starting treatment and continue at least 12 weeks after treatment has stopped.

These medicines pass into breast milk. Nursing mothers who must take one of these drugs should use infant formula.

Seniors: Seniors may require a reduced dosage of these drugs due to reduced heart, liver, or kidney function.

Generic Name

Tamoxifen Citrate

(tuh-MOX-ih-fen SYE-trate) G

Brand Names

Only available in generic form.

The information in this profile also applies to the following drugs:

Generic Ingredients: Toremifene Citrate
Fareston

Type of Drug

Antiestrogen.

Prescribed For

Breast cancer. Tamoxifen is also used for painful breasts, menstrual migraine, and ovulation induction in women; swollen or painful breasts, breast cancer, and low sperm count in men; and pancreatic, endometrial, and liver-cell cancer.

General Information

Tamoxifen is effective in treating estrogen-positive breast cancer in women. It works by blocking the effects of estrogen in breast tissue. When used together with chemotherapy after mastectomy, tamoxifen can prevent or delay the recurrence of breast cancer. It is used to treat metastatic breast cancer (that which has spread) and to prevent breast cancer in women at high risk. Up to 60% of women whose breast cancer has metastasized may benefit from taking tamoxifen. Toremifene is used only to treat breast cancer, not to prevent it.

Cautions and Warnings

Do not take these drugs if you are **allergic** or **sensitive** to any of their ingredients.

Women taking these drugs have an increased risk of serious blood clots such as deep vein thrombosis and pulmonary embolism. Women undergoing **coumarin-based anticoagulant** therapy or those with a history of **heart disease**, **deep vein thrombosis**, or **pulmonary embolism** should not take these drugs.

Do not take toremifene if you have or have had **long QT syndrome** (abnormal heart rhythms), **congestive heart failure**, **liver disease**, or **electrolyte abnormalities**. People with **low blood levels of potassium or magnesium** should not take toremifene until these problems have been corrected.

Women taking tamoxifen for **ductal carcinoma**, or those at **high risk for breast cancer**, have an increased risk of uterine cancer, stroke, or pulmonary embolism. Other women may also be at risk of developing uterine cancer and other noncancerous growths in the uterus, including polyps and fibroids.

These drugs may increase blood-calcium levels and bone growth, sometimes accompanied by pain. These may be a sign of a good response to the drug and usually decline rapidly. However, you should contact your doctor if you feel any bone pain.

Visual difficulties have occurred in people taking tamoxifen for 1 year or more in dosages at least 4 times above the maximum recommended dosage. These include cataracts, loss of color vision, and damage to the retina. A few cases of decreased visual clarity and other vision problems have been reported at normal dosages.

People taking tamoxifen have experienced liver inflammation and, rarely, more serious liver abnormalities. Very high dosages of this drug (15 mg per lb. of body weight) may cause liver cancer.

Possible Side Effects

Side effects are generally mild. Lowering drug dosage can sometimes control severe reactions.

- ▼ Most common: hot flashes, flushing, sweating, weight changes, vaginal discharge, menstrual changes, nausea, elevated liver enzymes, visual changes, and dry eyes.
- ▼ Less common: cough, swelling, fatigue, muscle pain, abdominal cramps, appetite loss, vomiting, vaginal bleeding, and skin changes. In men: impotence and lowered sex drive.
- ▼ Rare: high blood-calcium levels, swelling of the arms or legs, changes in the sense of taste, vaginal itching, depression, dizziness, lightheadedness, visual difficulties, and reduced white-blood-cell or platelet count. Ovarian cysts have occurred in premenopausal women with advanced breast cancer who took tamoxifen. Contact your doctor if you experience anything unusual while taking any medication.

Drug Interactions

- These drugs should not be combined with drugs that cause heart rhythm changes, including amiodarone, arsenic trioxide, bretylium, chlorpromazine, cisapride, disopyramide, dofetilide, dolasetron, droperidol, mefloquine, mesoridazine, moxifloxacin, pentamidine, pimozide, quinidine, sotalol, tacrolimus, thioridazine, and ziprasidone.
- These drugs may increase blood-calcium levels, and the use of thiazide diuretics and other drugs that stimulate calcium release from cells may increase this effect.
- The combination of tamoxifen and cytotoxic agents may increase the risk of blood clots.
- The effects of warfarin and other anticoagulant (blood thinning) drugs may be increased by tamoxifen.
- Bromocriptine may increase tamoxifen blood levels.
- Medroxyprogesterone and rifamycins such as rifampin decrease tamoxifen levels.
- Tamoxifen lowers the level of letrozole in the blood.
- Toremifene blood levels are reduced by carbamazepine, dexamethasone, phenobarbital, phenytoin, rifabutin, rifampin, St. John's wort, and other drugs that enhance its breakdown in the liver.
- Drugs interfering with the breakdown of toremifene, and which may increase its blood levels and side effects, include

azole antifungals, clarithromycin and related antibiotics, nefazodone, and protease inhibitors.
- Toremifene may interfere with the breakdown of phenytoin, tolbutamide, and warfarin in the liver. Dosage adjustments may be necessary.

Food Interactions

Tamoxifen can be taken with food or milk if it upsets your stomach.

Usual Dose

Adult

Tamoxifen: 20–40 mg a day. Doses higher than 20 mg should be divided and taken morning and evening.

Toremifene: 60 mg once a day.

Child: not recommended.

Overdosage

Symptoms may include breathing difficulties, convulsions, tremors, overactive reflexes, dizziness, and unsteadiness. Take the victim to a hospital emergency room. If you seek treatment, ALWAYS bring the prescription bottle or container.

Special Information

Take this medication according to your doctor's directions. Inform your doctor if you become very weak or sleepy or if you experience confusion, pain, swelling of the legs, breathing difficulties, blurred vision, bone pain, hot flashes, nausea or vomiting, weight gain, irregular periods, dizziness, headache, or appetite loss. Contact your doctor if you vomit shortly after taking a dose of tamoxifen. Your doctor may tell you to take another dose immediately or wait until the next dose.

Hormonal birth control may not work while taking tamoxifen. Women taking tamoxifen should use a non-hormonal contraceptive for 2 months after treatment is complete.

If you forget a dose, contact your doctor. If you cannot reach your doctor, skip the forgotten dose and continue your regular schedule. Do not take a double dose.

Special Populations

Pregnancy/Breast-feeding: Tamoxifen can harm the fetus and cause vaginal bleeding and spontaneous abortion. It should not be taken by pregnant women. Women of childbearing age taking tamoxifen must use non-hormonal contraception to prevent pregnancy. Contact your doctor at once if you think you may be pregnant.

It is not known if tamoxifen passes into breast milk. Nursing mothers who must take this drug should use infant formula.

Seniors: Seniors may take tamoxifen without special precaution.

Generic Name

Telavancin (tell-uh-VAN-sin)

Brand Names

Vibativ

Type of Drug

Antibiotic.

Prescribed For

Bacterial infection of the skin.

General Information

Telavancin is meant for specific bacterial infections that cannot be cured by other medications. It will be given to you by intravenous (IV) infusion in your doctor's office or another health care setting. One advantage of telavancin is that it kills methicillin-resistant *Staphylococcus aureus* (MRSA), an increasingly difficult type of bacteria to manage because it has evolved to develop resistance against other antibiotics. Telavancin works by interfering with cell wall creation during growth of this bacterium.

Cautions and Warning

Do not use telavancin if you are **allergic** or **sensitive** to any of its ingredients.

Telavancin may cause or worsen **kidney disease** and it has been found to be less effective in people with kidney disease. The dose of telavancin must be adjusted if you have any degree of kidney disease.

Diarrhea is a frequent by-product of all antibiotic treatment, and side effects of telavancin have included reactions from mild diarrhea to fatal colitis.

Telavancin can cause abnormal heart rhythms. Do not take it if you have uncontrolled **heart failure**, severe **enlargement of the left ventricle** of the heart, or **abnormal heart rhythms**.

Telavancin increases your risk of superinfection with other bacteria or fungi.

Telavancin can affect some laboratory tests used to measure blood clotting. It does not affect blood clotting.

Possible Side Effects

- ▼ Most common: taste changes (metallic or soapy), nausea, vomiting, and foamy urine.
- ▼ Common: diarrhea, itching, dizziness.
- ▼ Less common: chills, rash, abdominal pain, reduced appetite, and swelling and redness at the injection site.
- ▼ Rare: Other side effects may occur. Contact your doctor if you experience anything unusual while taking any medication.

Drug Interactions

- The risk of life-threatening abnormal heart rhythms is increased if tacrolimus is used with any of the following drugs; combine with caution: antiarrhythmic drugs (including amiodarone, bretylium, disopyramide, dofetilide, quinidine), arsenic trioxide, chlorpromazine, cisapride, dolasetron, droperidol, mefloquine, mesoridazine, moxifloxacin, pentamidine, pimozide, tacrolimus, thioridazine, and ziprasidone.
- Tacrolimus should be used cautiously with any the following drugs due to an increased risk of kidney damage: angiotensin-converting enzyme (ACE) inhibitors, loop diuretics, and nonsteroidal anti-inflammatory drugs (NSAIDs).

Food Interactions

This drug can be taken without regard to food or meals.

Usual Dose

Adult: 4.5 mg per lb. of body weight once a day for 1–2 weeks by 60-minute IV infusion; lower doses are given to people with kidney disease.

Child: not recommended.

Overdosage

Overdose is unlikely because telavancin is given only in a health care setting. However, kidney damage may occur in the event of an overdose. The treatment must be stopped at once and emergency room treatment sought.

Special Information

This drug is delivered by IV infusion over the course of 1 hour to minimize infusion reactions including itching, rash, and upper body flushing.

Skipping telavancin doses interferes with your antibiotic treatment. If you must miss an infusion appointment, contact your doctor right away for instructions. Do not stop taking this drug before the full course of therapy is completed, even if you feel well.

Make sure your doctor knows all the medicines you are taking, especially blood thinners and those that can affect kidney function (see "Drug Interactions").

Special Populations

Pregnancy/Breast-feeding: Telavancin causes birth defects in animal studies, but it is unknown how it affects humans. This drug should not be used during pregnancy unless your doctor determines that the potential benefit outweighs the risks. Women of childbearing age should have a pregnancy test before starting on telavancin treatment and should use birth control while they take it. A registry has been created to keep records of women who become pregnant while taking telavancin and to track how their babies progress up to 12 months of age. This will help doctors better understand the actual risks of telavancin. Your doctor may enroll you in this anonymous registry.

It is not known if telavancin passes into breast milk. Nursing mothers who must take this drug should use infant formula.

Seniors: Seniors may be at a greater risk of drug side effects due to declining kidney function. In clinical studies, seniors receiving telavancin experienced side effects no more often than younger adults but were less likely to be cured of the infection.

Generic Name

Telithromycin (tel-ith-row-MY-sin)

Brand Names

Ketek

Type of Drug

Antibiotic.

Prescribed For

Pneumonia that develops outside of the hospital and is resistant to other antibiotics. May also be prescribed for infections in other areas of the body.

General Information

Telithromycin is effective against a variety of common bacteria. When tested against commonly used antibiotics, telithromycin was at least as good as the others and sometimes better. Telithromycin should only be taken for infections that are caused by bacteria it can treat.

Telithromycin is related to erythromycin, another antibiotic that has been in use for many years, but telithromycin has a different chemical structure and is known as a ketolide antibiotic. Bacteria that are resistant to erythromycin may still be treated with telithromycin.

Telithromycin is absorbed into the body within an hour after it is taken, but only about 50% of the drug finds its way into the bloodstream. It is broken down in the liver.

Cautions and Warnings

Do not take telithromycin if you are **allergic** or **sensitive** to any of its ingredients.

Telithromycin can be toxic to the liver—resulting in serious liver injury and some deaths—and should not be taken by people with a history of **jaundice** and/or **hepatitis** when those effects were caused by a macrolide antibiotic. People with **liver disease** may take this drug, but should be closely monitored by their doctors. If you develop signs of liver problems (nausea, fatigue, loss of appetite, light-colored stools, dark urine, yellowing of the skin or whites of the eyes, and pain in the upper right abdomen), stop the treatment and contact your doctor immediately.

People with **myasthenia gravis** must not use telithromycin because it can worsen this condition, sometimes within a few hours of the first dose of telithromycin. The most common symptom is weakness, and some muscles can be completely wasted by myasthenia gravis over time.

Telithromycin may increase the risk for severe abnormal heart rhythms. This drug should be avoided by people with **congenital heart defects**, **abnormal heart rhythms**, **low blood levels of potassium or magnesium**, or certain antiarrhythmic drugs (see "Drug Interactions").

People with severe **kidney failure** must receive a reduced dose of this drug.

Colitis (severe diarrhea) is possible with nearly any antibacterial agent, including telithromycin, and may range from mild to life-threatening.

Telithromycin has been known to cause visual disturbances or a sudden loss of consciousness. When taking telithromycin, you should not drive or engage in any potentially hazardous activities.

Possible Side Effects

- ▼ Most common: diarrhea.
- ▼ Common: nausea and headache.
- ▼ Less common: dizziness, vomiting, loose stools, and loss of taste perception.
- ▼ Rare: visual problems, fungal infection, fatigue, allergic reactions, heart palpitations, liver inflammation, myasthenia gravis, and muscle cramps. Other rare side effects can occur in almost any part of the body. Contact your doctor if you experience anything unusual while taking any medication.

Drug Interactions

- Telithromycin should never be used with the antiarrhythmic drugs amiodarone, bretylium, disopyramide, dofetilide, quinidine, or sotalol; cisapride; or pimozide, due to a significantly increased risk of potentially life-threatening abnormal heart rhythms. Other drugs that may cause heart rhythm changes and should be avoided include arsenic trioxide, chlorpromazine, dolasetron, droperidol, mefloquine, mesoridazine, moxifloxacin, pentamidine, tacrolimus, thioridazine, and ziprasidone.
- Carbamazepine, phenobarbital, phenytoin, and rifampin reduce the amount of telithromycin in the bloodstream, interfering with its antibacterial action. Avoid using telithromycin with rifampin.
- Combining telithromycin with ergot alkaloid derivatives is not recommended.
- Avoid mixing telithromycin with atorvastatin, lovastatin, or simvastatin. Telithromycin increases blood levels and the potential for muscle damage with these drugs.
- Mixing telithromycin with verapamil may increase the risk of heart problems. Your doctor should closely monitor your heart if you must take these drugs together.

- Telithromycin may increase the effects of warfarin and other blood thinners. Patients taking this combination should have their blood-clotting times checked.
- Telithromycin significantly increases the amount of digoxin in the blood. Digoxin levels and side effects should be monitored.
- Telithromycin can increase levels of cyclosporine, hexobarbital, phenytoin, sirolimus, and tacrolimus in the blood, exposing the person taking the combination to drug side effects.
- Telithromycin increases the amount of midazolam absorbed into the blood by several times by slowing its breakdown in the liver. The midazolam dose may have to be reduced to avoid drug side effects. This interaction may also occur with other benzodiazepine drugs.
- Telithromycin increases blood levels and possible side effects of buspirone, cabergoline, colchicine, ranolazine, and repaglinide.
- Telithromycin slows the breakdown of the beta blocker metoprolol and should be used with caution in people with heart failure who must take this drug.
- Telithromycin may increase blood levels of contraceptive drugs.
- Mixing telithromycin and theophylline produces an increase in theophylline blood levels and side effects such as nausea and vomiting. Take these drugs at least 1 hour apart.
- Azole antifungal drugs such as itraconazole and ketoconazole substantially increase the amount of telithromycin absorbed into the blood.

Food Interactions

This drug can be taken without regard to food or meals.

Usual Dose

Adult: 800 mg (two 400-mg tablets) at the same time every day for 5–10 days, depending on the infection. People with severe kidney failure, including dialysis patients, can take 600 mg a day. For patients with both severe kidney and liver disease, the daily dose is 400 mg a day.

Child: not recommended.

Overdosage

Anyone suspected of having taken a telithromycin overdose should be taken to a hospital emergency room. If you seek treatment, ALWAYS bring the prescription bottle or container.

Special Information

Use caution when driving, operating machinery, or performing other hazardous activities.

Contact your doctor if changes in vision caused by telithromycin affect your daily activities. Avoid quickly changing focus between objects in the distance and objects nearby, which may help to decrease the impact of these visual difficulties.

Telithromycin should only be used to treat bacterial infections. It does not treat viral infections such as the common cold.

Report any diarrhea to your doctor because of the chance that it can be drug-related.

If you forget to take a dose of telithromycin, take it as soon as you remember, and then continue with your regular dose on the next day. Do not skip doses or fail to complete the full course of therapy, even if you feel better. This can reduce the effectiveness of this antibiotic and increase the chances that bacteria will become resistant to telithromycin. Tell your doctor or pharmacist if you forget more than 1 dose of telithromycin.

Do not take more than 2 tablets of telithromycin in any 24-hour period.

Be sure to tell your doctor about any other medicines you are taking, including over-the-counter and herbal remedies.

Special Populations

Pregnancy/Breast-feeding: This medication caused birth defects in animal studies. Women who are or might be pregnant should talk with their doctor before taking telithromycin. It should be taken during pregnancy only if your doctor determines that the potential benefit outweighs the risks.

Telithromycin passes into breast milk. Nursing mothers who must take it should use infant formula.

Seniors: Seniors can take telithromycin in the same dosage as younger adults.

Generic Name

Temozolomide (tem-oh-ZOHL-oh-mide)

Brand Names

Temodar

Type of Drug

Antineoplastic.

Prescribed For

Brain cancer; also used for certain kinds of advanced skin cancer.

General Information

Temozolomide is used to treat newly diagnosed glioblastoma together with radiation therapy and then continued as a maintenance treatment. It is also prescribed for astrocytoma, a specific type of cancer of the brain, in adults whose tumors have returned after other treatments have failed. Once absorbed, it seems to interfere with the growth of cancer cells, which are then eventually destroyed by the body.

Cautions and Warnings

Do not take this medicine if you are **allergic** or **sensitive** to any of its ingredients or to dacarbazine, another anticancer drug.

People taking temozolomide may experience reduced white-blood-cell and platelet counts. These generally occur late in the first treatment cycle and may increase your risk of infection.

People with **impaired liver function** should use temozolomide with caution.

Secondary cancers, including leukemia, have occurred in people taking this drug.

People taking temozolomide should receive preventive antibiotic treatment for *Pneumocystis carinii* pneumonia (PCP) during glioblastoma treatment and radiation therapy.

Temozolomide may cause infertility in **men**.

Possible Side Effects

- ▼ Most common: headache, fatigue, general weakness, weakness on one side of the body, convulsions, dizziness, diarrhea, nausea, constipation, vomiting, rash, leg or arm swelling, poor muscle coordination, memory loss, weight gain, sleeplessness, viral infection, and fever.
- ▼ Common: partial paralysis; anxiety; difficulty swallowing; taste changes; jerking movements of the face, trunk, arms, or legs; depression; unusual walk; excessive adrenal gland output; confusion; itching; dry skin; increased urination; loss of urinary control; urinary infection; appetite loss; abdominal pain; double vision and other visual abnormalities; cough; sore throat; runny nose; respiratory tract infection; muscle aches; breast pain (women); and back pain.

Possible Side Effects *(continued)*

▼ Rare: Rare side effects can occur in almost any part of the body. Contact your doctor if you experience anything unusual while taking any medication.

Drug Interactions

- Valproic acid reduces the amount of temozolomide cleared through the kidney. The importance of this interaction is not known.

Food Interactions

Food interferes with the absorption of temozolomide into the blood. Take it on an empty stomach with a full glass of water to reduce nausea and vomiting.

Usual Dose

Adult: 75–500 mg at bedtime. Dosage is adjusted according to body weight and height and white-blood-cell and platelet counts.

Child: not recommended.

Overdosage

Temozolomide overdose causes drastic reductions in platelets and white blood cells. Overdose victims must be taken to a hospital emergency room at once. If you seek treatment, ALWAYS bring the prescription bottle or container.

Special Information

Nausea and vomiting usually decline with time and are readily controlled with antinausea drugs. Antinauseant medication may be taken before or after your temozolomide dose.

Women clear temozolomide from the body more slowly than men and are more likely to experience low white-blood-cell and platelet counts in the first cycle of temozolomide treatment.

Do not open or chew temozolomide capsules. Swallow them whole with a glass of water.

Exposure to temozolomide powder causes malignant tumors in animals. Be sure that you and others do not inhale the contents of any capsule or get any of the drug on your skin or mucous membranes from a capsule that has been damaged or opened and keep this drug away from children and pets.

If you forget to take a dose of temozolomide, be sure to tell your doctor and continue with your regular schedule on the next day. Do not take a double dose.

Special Populations

Pregnancy/Breast-feeding: Temozolomide will damage a developing fetus. Women who must take it should use an effective contraceptive method and wait 6 months after the treatment is finished before becoming pregnant. Men should not father a child up to 6 months after treatment.

Women who must take temozolomide should use infant formula, because temozolomide may pass into breast milk and cause severe reactions in the nursing infant.

Seniors: Seniors are more likely to experience reduced white-blood-cell and platelet counts.

Generic Name

Terbutaline (ter-BUE-tuh-leen) G

Brand Names

Only available in generic form.

Type of Drug

Bronchodilator.

Prescribed For

Asthma and bronchospasm.

General Information

Terbutaline is similar to other bronchodilator drugs, such as metaproterenol and isoetharine, but it has a weaker effect on nerve receptors in the heart and blood vessels. For this reason, it may be safer for people with heart conditions.

Terbutaline tablets begin to work within 30 minutes and continue working for 4–8 hours.

Cautions and Warnings

Do not take terbutaline if you are **allergic** or **sensitive** to any of its ingredients. Terbutaline should not be used to manage or delay labor contractions because of the risk of heart problems and death.

Terbutaline should be used with caution by people with a history of **angina pectoris** (brief attacks of chest pain), **heart disease**, **high blood pressure**, **cardiac arrhythmia**, **stroke**, **seizure**,

liver or kidney disease, **diabetes**, **thyroid disease**, **prostate disease**, or **glaucoma**.

Possible Side Effects

- ▼ Most common: heart palpitations, abnormal heart rhythm, tremors, dizziness and fainting, shakiness, nervousness, tension, drowsiness, headache, nausea and vomiting, and heartburn or upset stomach.
- ▼ Less common: rapid heartbeat, chest pain and discomfort, angina, weakness, sleeplessness, wheezing, bronchial spasms and difficulty breathing, dry or sore throat, flushing, sweating, and changes in the sense of smell and taste.
- ▼ Rare: hallucinations, rash, seizures, and increased liver enzyme levels. Contact your doctor if you experience anything unusual while taking any medication.

Drug Interactions

- Terbutaline's effects may be increased by some antihistamines, other bronchodilator drugs, monoamine oxidase inhibitor (MAOI) or tricyclic antidepressants, and thyroid drugs.
- The risk of cardiac toxicity may be increased in people taking both terbutaline and theophylline.
- Terbutaline's effectiveness is reduced by beta-blocker drugs such as propranolol.
- Terbutaline may reduce the effects of blood-pressure-lowering drugs, especially guanethidine, methyldopa, and reserpine.
- Use caution when combining terbutaline with potassium-sparing diuretics, especially in higher doses.

Food Interactions

Terbutaline tablets are more effective when taken on an empty stomach—1 hour before or 2 hours after meals—but can be taken with food if they upset your stomach.

Usual Dose

Adult and Child (age 15 and over): 2.5–5 mg every 6 hours, 3 times a day. Do not take more than 15 mg within 24 hours.

Child (age 12–14): 2.5 mg 3 times a day. Do not take more than 7.5 mg within 24 hours.

Child (under age 12): not recommended.

Overdosage

Overdose of terbutaline is more likely to trigger changes in heart rate, palpitations, unusual heart rhythms, chest pain, high blood pressure, fever, chills, cold sweats, nausea, vomiting, and dilation of the pupils. Convulsions, sleeplessness, anxiety, and tremors may also develop, and the victim may collapse.

If the overdose was taken within the past 30 minutes, give the victim ipecac syrup—available at any pharmacy—to induce vomiting and to remove any remaining medication from the stomach. Do not give ipecac syrup if the victim is unconscious or convulsing. If symptoms have already begun to develop, the victim should be taken to a hospital emergency room. If you seek treatment, ALWAYS bring the prescription bottle or container.

Special Information

Do not take more terbutaline than your doctor prescribes. Taking more than you need could actually worsen your symptoms. If your condition worsens rather than improves after taking terbutaline, stop taking it and contact your doctor.

Contact your doctor immediately if you develop chest pain, palpitations, rapid heartbeat, muscle tremors, dizziness, headache, facial flushing, or urinary difficulty, or if you continue to experience difficulty in breathing after using the medication.

If you forget a dose of terbutaline, take it as soon as you remember. If it is almost time for your next dose, skip the one you forgot and return to your regular schedule. Do not take a double dose.

Special Populations

Pregnancy/Breast-feeding: When used during childbirth, terbutaline can slow or delay labor. Generally, terbutaline should not be taken after the first 3 months of pregnancy; it can cause rapid heartbeat and high blood sugar in the mother, and rapid heartbeat and low blood sugar in the fetus. It is not known if terbutaline causes birth defects in humans, but it has caused defects in pregnant animals. It should be taken during pregnancy only if your doctor determines that the potential benefit outweighs the risks.

Terbutaline passes into breast milk. Nursing mothers who must take this drug should use infant formula.

Seniors: Seniors are more sensitive to the effects of terbutaline. Follow your doctor's directions closely and report any side effects at once.

Generic Name

Teriparatide (terr-ih-PAR-a-tide)

Brand Names

Forteo

Type of Drug

Parathyroid hormone.

Prescribed For

Osteoporosis in men and women at high risk of bone fracture.

General Information

Teriparatide is a synthetic form of the human parathyroid hormone, which is involved in maintaining calcium balance in the body. Unlike other osteoporosis treatments, which slow the rate of bone loss, this treatment builds new bone and improves bone structure in women suffering from osteoporosis. Studies of teriparatide have shown that people taking it experience significant increases in bone mineral density and suffer fewer bone fractures while they are taking teriparatide as well as after they stop it. Typically, people take teriparatide for 1–2 years to build bone mass, which can help prevent additional fractures.

Cautions and Warnings

Do not take teriparatide if you are **allergic** or **sensitive** to any of its ingredients.

Teriparatide increased the risk of osteosarcoma in animal studies. This rare but very serious cancer of the bone has not appeared in humans taking teriparatide, but the drug should not be used by people with a **bone disease** other than osteoporosis—such as **Paget's disease**. Those with a history or an increased risk of **bone cancer** or those who have had **radiation therapy** or **cancer that has spread to the bone** should not use this drug.

People known to have an underlying **hypercalcemia disorder** (high blood-calcium levels), such as **hyperparathyroidism**, should not use teriparatide.

The long-term safety of teriparatide has not been studied; therefore the drug should not be taken for more than 2 years.

People who have or have had **kidney stones** should use teriparatide with caution because of the risk that it could worsen this condition.

Possible Side Effects

▼ Most common: generalized pain and joint pain.

▼ Common: dizziness, headache, weakness, high blood pressure, nausea, constipation, diarrhea, upset stomach, runny nose, coughing, and sore throat.

▼ Less common: neck pain, angina, fainting, vomiting, stomach problems, dental problems, leg cramps, depression, sleeplessness, vertigo, shortness of breath, pneumonia, rash, and sweating.

▼ Rare: difficulty breathing after injection, swelling of the mouth or face, hives, and chest pain. Other rare side effects can occur in almost any part of the body. Contact your doctor if you experience anything unusual while taking any medication.

Drug Interactions

- Teriparatide increases blood levels of calcium and should be used cautiously when combined with digoxin.

Usual Dose

Adult: 20 mcg a day by subcutaneous injection (under the skin) in the thigh or abdomen (lower stomach area).

Child: not recommended.

Overdosage

Little is known about the effects of teriparatide overdose. Likely symptoms include high blood calcium, dizziness or fainting, low blood pressure, nausea, vomiting, and headache. Take the victim to a hospital emergency room. If you seek treatment, ALWAYS bring the prescription bottle or container.

Special Information

Teriparatide comes in a "pen" containing 28 days' worth of medicine. Read your pen user manual thoroughly before administering this drug, and re-read it each time you renew your prescription. Do not use teriparatide after the expiration date printed on the pen and pen packaging. Throw away your teriparatide pen 28 days after you start using it, even if it still contains medicine. For more information on injections, see page 1242.

Teriparatide must be injected under the skin. If you cannot inject yourself, you must have someone else do it for you every day.

When you first start taking teriparatide, you should be in a place where you can sit or lie down if you get dizzy. Contact your doctor if dizziness continues.

Store this product in the refrigerator. Teriparatide should be injected shortly after you take the pen out of the refrigerator. Replace the cap and put it back into the refrigerator immediately after use.

You must continue taking calcium and/or vitamin D supplements as prescribed by your doctor. Also, regular weight-bearing exercise, reducing alcohol consumption, and stopping smoking will help improve your osteoporosis.

Take teriparatide at the same time every day. If you forget to take a dose, take it as soon as you remember. Do not take a double dose and do not take more than 1 dose a day.

Special Populations

Pregnancy/Breast-feeding: In animal studies, teriparatide entered the fetal circulation and caused changes in bone development. Pregnant women should use this drug only if their doctor determines the potential benefit outweigh the risks.

It is not known if teriparatide passes into breast milk. Nursing mothers who must take it should use infant formula.

Seniors: Seniors may use this drug without special precaution.

Generic Name

Tesamorelin (tess-ah-MOHR-eh-lin)

Brand Names

Egrifta

Type of Drug

Growth-hormone-releasing factor.

Prescribed For

HIV-associated lipodystrophy.

General Information

Tesamorelin is a synthetic growth-hormone-releasing factor that acts on the pituitary gland to stimulate the formation and release of growth hormone. Growth hormone plays an important role in how the body manages muscle mass, lipid metabolism, and glucose. Tesamorelin increases muscle mass and reduces excess fat that has accumulated in the abdominal area and which is thought to be a risk factor for heart disease and type 2 diabetes. It is the first treatment approved for HIV lipodystrophy and produces fewer side effects than growth hormone itself. Tesamorelin is not a weight-loss drug and should not be used for that purpose.

Cautions and Warnings

Do not use tesamorelin if you are **allergic** or **sensitive** to any of its ingredients. Seek emergency treatment if you experience a reaction to tesamorelin (symptoms include itching, redness, flushing, hives or other rash, difficulty breathing, swelling of your face or throat, rapid heartbeat, or fainting).

People with a history of **head trauma**, **underactive pituitary gland**, **pituitary tumor or surgery**, or any other disruption of pituitary gland function should not use tesamorelin. People receiving head irradiation should not use this drug.

If you have or have had any form of **cancer**, do not start using this drug until all treatment has been completed and your cancer is inactive. Growth hormone can stimulate the growth of an active tumor. HIV-positive patients have an increased background risk of malignancy.

Tesamorelin affects blood-sugar metabolism. As a result, type 2 diabetes can develop or become worse. Check your blood sugar regularly while taking tesamorelin. People with **diabetes** who use this medicine may have to alter their antidiabetes therapy.

The long-term cardiovascular (heart and blood vessel) safety of tesamorelin is not known. People who do not show a clear positive response to tesamorelin, as measured by CT scan or a reduced waist size, should not risk the long-term use of this medicine.

Joint pain, carpal tunnel syndrome, and swelling can develop due to fluid retention caused by increased levels of growth hormone. Tesamorelin treatment may be stopped if any acute critical illness develops.

You may develop antibodies to tesamorelin, but this should not affect how the drug works in your body.

Possible Side Effects

Side effects are more likely during the first 6 months of treatment.

Possible Side Effects *(continued)*

▼ Most common: joint pain and injection site reactions, including itching, pain, redness, swelling, irritation, and bleeding.

▼ Common: muscle aches, spasms, and stiffness; joint stiffness; and swelling in the hands, ankles, or feet.

▼ Less common: rash, pain, chest pain, tingling in the hands or feet, carpal tunnel syndrome, reduced sense of touch, nausea, vomiting, upset stomach, upper-abdominal pain, heart palpitations, depression, night sweats, muscle strain, high blood pressure, flushing, sleeplessness, new type 2 diabetes, and increased blood level of creatinine phosphokinase (elevations of this enzyme indicate muscle damage).

▼ Rare: Other side effects may affect almost any part of the body. Contact your doctor if you experience anything unusual while taking any medication.

Drug Interactions

- Tesamorelin may affect the breakdown of some drugs because of the effect of growth hormone release.
- Tesamorelin may reduce the blood levels and effectiveness of anticonvulsant drugs, corticosteroids, cyclosporine, and hormone-based therapies such as contraceptive drugs, estrogen, and testosterone. Caution should be used when combining these drugs, and dosage adjustments may be necessary.
- Do not depend on any oral, injected, or implanted hormone-based contraceptive, including emergency contraceptives, while using this medicine. You must use a non-hormonal contraceptive or remain abstinent while taking it.
- The dose of antidiabetes medicines may need to be adjusted because of tesamorelin's effect on sugar metabolism.

Usual Dose

Adult: 2 mg (2 mL) injected under the skin of your abdomen once a day.

Child: not recommended.

Overdosage

There is no information on tesamorelin overdose. Call your local poison control center or a hospital emergency room for more information. If you seek treatment, ALWAYS bring the prescription bottle or container.

Special Information

Take this medicine at the same time each day to help you get into a regular routine. If you forget a dose, take it as soon as you remember. Do not take a double dose.

Store tesamorelin in the refrigerator before you use it. Do not freeze this drug at any time. This medicine must be mixed just before you inject it. Carefully follow package instructions and throw away any part of the vial that you have not used. After mixing, it cannot be refrigerated, frozen, or saved for use at another time. The final injection must be clear, colorless, and free of any particles floating in it. If not, throw it away and use another vial. Be sure to inject your medicine at different places on your abdomen each day to minimize injection site reactions, which may include redness, itching, irritation, painful rash, bleeding, and swelling.

Do not share needles or syringes with another person.

Special Populations

Pregnancy/Breast-feeding: Pregnant women should not use this medicine because it may harm the developing fetus by interfering with normal fat growth during pregnancy. Animal studies have resulted in damage to the fetus. Stop using tesamorelin if you become pregnant.

It is not known whether tesamorelin passes into breast milk, but HIV-positive mothers must use infant formula to avoid transmitting the virus to their child.

Seniors: There is no information on seniors using this medicine.

Generic Name

Testosterone (tes-TOS-ter-own) G

Brand Names

Androderm
AndroGel
Axiron
Fortesta
Striant
Testim
Testopel

The information in this profile also applies to the following drugs:

Generic Ingredients: Methyltestosterone G
Android
Methitest
Testred

Type of Drug

Hormone replacement.

Prescribed For

Impotence due to hormone deficiency and testosterone replacement in men who have lost their testicle function or have low blood levels of testosterone. Androgen may be prescribed for boys before they reach puberty to maintain secondary sex characteristics if testosterone is lacking or if puberty is delayed. In women, testosterone may be used to treat metastatic cancer (cancer that has spread from one part of the body to another) and breast enlargement or pain in women who have just given birth. It has also been studied for low sex drive in women.

General Information

Testosterone is the principal androgen (male hormone). In men, testosterone is produced in the testicles. Women make small amounts of testosterone in their ovaries and in the adrenal gland. Testosterone is responsible for the growth and development of male sex organs as well as secondary sex characteristics such as beard, pubic, chest, and underarm hair; vocal cord thickening, which lowers the voice; and muscle and fat distribution. Androgens are also responsible for the adolescent growth spurt.

Weekly testosterone injection of 200 mg, for up to 1 year, has been studied as a reversible male contraceptive.

Cautions and Warnings

Do not take testosterone if you are **allergic** or **sensitive** to any of its ingredients.

The following people should avoid testosterone: **pregnant women, men with breast or prostate cancer**, and people with **heart, liver, or kidney disease**, who may respond to the drug by retaining fluid, which may lead to heart failure. **Seniors** taking testosterone may be at an increased risk of prostate cancer.

Sleep apnea may occur in some patients taking testosterone, especially if they are **obese** or have **lung disease**.

Some **athletes** have taken testosterone in order to improve performance, but this is unsafe and ineffective.

Male hormones may cause very high blood-calcium levels in people with **breast cancer**, who should avoid taking testosterone.

Continuous use of high dosages of male hormones may cause life-threatening liver problems. Liver function should be monitored regularly. Hepatitis and jaundice have occurred with androgen use, but may be reversible when treatment is stopped.

Taking male hormones for an extended period of time causes reduced sperm count and semen volume. Men taking testosterone as hormone replacement may develop enlarged breasts.

Testosterone may cause frequent or persistent erections or an excessive sex drive. Report any bothersome symptoms to your doctor. **Seniors** should check with their doctors to be sure that they may safely engage in sexual activity.

A man using a scrotal testosterone patch may transfer some hormone to his sexual partner, which may result in unwanted changes in the partner's secondary sex characteristics.

Testosterone may affect glycemic control in people with **diabetes**.

Testosterone must be used with caution in **children** as it can interfere with bone maturation. Boys should be treated only by specialists who are experienced with testosterone and understand its effects on bone development. Adolescent males should have their bone development checked every 6 months.

Women should inform their doctors of any signs of virilization—a deepening voice, increased hairiness, acne, menstrual problems, and enlarged clitoris—as they may need to stop treatment to prevent irreversible changes.

Testosterone may interfere with laboratory tests of thyroid function; it does not affect the thyroid gland or normal thyroid function.

Possible Side Effects

- ▼ Most common: women—menstrual irregularities, a deepening voice, hairiness, acne, and enlargement of the clitoris. Men—prostate problems, acne, and skin reactions at the site of patch application.
- ▼ Common: men and women—swelling of the feet or lower legs, rapid weight gain, water retention, dizziness, headache, tiredness, flushing or redness, bleeding, nausea, vomiting, yellowing of the skin or whites of the eyes, confusion, depression, increased or decreased libido, thirst, increased urination, and constipation. Men—breast soreness or enlargement, excessive erections, chills, pain in the scrotum or groin, and difficult urination.
- ▼ Less common: men and women—diarrhea, increased pubic hair, and difficulty sleeping. Men—impotence, irritation or

Possible Side Effects *(continued)*

infection of the skin of the scrotum, and decreased testicle size.

▼ Rare: men and women—male-pattern baldness, oily skin, jaundice, and changes in liver function tests. Contact your doctor if you experience anything unusual while taking any medication.

Drug Interactions

- Testosterone may increase the effects of anticoagulants (blood thinners) such as warfarin.
- Using testosterone with a corticosteroid increases the risk of swelling of the hands and feet and fluid retention. These drugs should be used together with caution, particularly in people with heart or liver disease.
- Consult with your doctor if you are taking insulin or other diabetes medications, oxyphenbutazone, or propanolol. You may require dosage adjustment or monitoring.

Food Interactions

You may take this drug with food if it upsets your stomach. Food does not interfere with testosterone skin patches or gel.

Usual Dose

Oral Tablets

Men: 10–50 mg a day.
Women: 50–200 mg a day.
Children:10–50 mg a day.

Transdermal and Buccal

These forms of testosterone should be used by men only, not by women or children.

Skin Patches: 2.5–5 mg a day in 1 or 2 patches. Apply nightly to clean, dry skin on your back, abdomen, upper arm, or thigh, according to your doctor's instructions.

Topical Gels and Solutions: Apply once a day to shoulders, upper arms, thighs and/or abdomen, according to your doctor's instructions. Do not wash site for at least 2 hours after applying.

Striant: Apply to the gums every 12 hours, holding in place for 30 seconds. Do not chew or swallow it. Alternate sides of mouth with each application.

Overdosage

Symptoms resemble drug side effects. Contact your local poison control center or a hospital emergency room for more information. If you seek treatment, ALWAYS bring the prescription package or container.

Special Information

If you develop nausea, vomiting, changes in skin color, or ankle swelling, contact your doctor right away.

If you are using a testosterone skin patch, apply it as directed by your doctor. The site of the patch application should be rotated, with an interval of 7 days between applications to the same site. The patch should not be applied to oily or irritated skin.

Testosterone gels are flammable and should not be used near an open flame or while smoking.

If pregnant women or children come into accidental contact with a testosterone gel, wash the area of contact with soap and water as soon as possible to prevent the testosterone from soaking through the skin.

Take this drug exactly as prescribed. If you forget a dose, take it as soon as possible. If it is almost time for your next dose, skip the dose you forgot and continue with your regular schedule. Do not take a double dose.

Special Populations

Pregnancy/Breast-feeding: Testosterone should not be used during pregnancy. Taking this drug during pregnancy, especially during the first 3 months, results in excessive masculinization of the fetus.

It is not known if testosterone passes into breast milk. Nursing mothers who must take it should use infant formula.

Seniors: Seniors who take testosterone may have an increased risk of developing prostate disease, including cancer. A marked increase in sex drive may also develop.

Generic Name

Tetrabenazine (teh-tra-BEN-ah-zeen)

Brand Names

Xenazine

Type of Drug

Monoamine depletor.

Prescribed For

Involuntary or excessive muscle movements of Huntington's disease.

General Information

Tetrabenazine is the first drug to be approved for Huntington's disease, a devastating genetic neurodegenerative disease and ultimately fatal condition. Excessive, involuntary, and repetitive movements, called chorea, are the most visible and dangerous symptom of Huntington's, because they interfere with the ability to perform normal daily activities. Tetrabenazine helps manage the chorea symptoms of Huntington's disease but does not cure them. It can worsen other aspects of the disease, including mood, understanding, muscle rigidity, and functional capacity. It is not yet known if these effects continue, get better, or worsen with continued drug treatment. Tetrabenazine works by temporarily inhibiting an enzyme that transports monoamines into nerve endings, reducing the ability of nerves to trigger muscle contractions.

Cautions and Warnings

Do not take this drug if you are **allergic** or **sensitive** to any of its ingredients.

Tetrabenazine can increase the risk of depression and suicidal thoughts and behavior. This is a particular problem for people with Huntington's disease because 1 of every 4 Huntington's patients will attempt suicide. People taking this medicine should be monitored for new or **worsening depression**, **suicidal thoughts**, or **unusual behavioral changes**. Report anything unusual to your doctor.

Tetrabenazine can cause Parkinson's disease (PD) symptoms—extremely slow movements and reflexes (bradykinesia) and increased muscle rigidity, tension, and spasticity of the muscles (hypertonia). Muscle rigidity can also develop as part of Huntington's disease, making it difficult to distinguish between the drug side effect and worsening of Huntington's. Drug-related PD symptoms can cause more functional disability than untreated chorea for some patients. Report any of these symptoms to your doctor at once. Dose reduction or stopping tetrabenazine may be necessary.

Tetrabenazine is broken down in the liver. People with **liver disease** should not take this drug because it is not yet known how people with liver disease react to tetrabenazine.

A serious set of side effects, known as neuroleptic malignant syndrome (NMS), has been associated with other drugs that affect nerve transmission and may occur with tetrabenazine. The symptoms that constitute NMS include high fever, muscle rigidity, mental changes, irregular pulse or blood pressure, increased sweating, and abnormal heart rhythm. NMS is potentially fatal and requires immediate medical attention.

Agitation and restlessness that ranges from a feeling of inner distress to an inability to sit still (akathisia) can occur with some drugs that affect the nervous system, including tetrabenazine. These symptoms may be relieved by lowering the drug dose. Some people may require stopping drug therapy to eliminate these symptoms.

Up to 10% of people taking tetrabenazine can develop difficulty swallowing, which has led to accidental inhalation of food or drink (aspiration pneumonia).

About 1 of every 3 patients taking this drug report being sedated by tetrabenazine. Sedation is the most common reason for reducing drug dose or not reaching an effective dose.

People with a history of **abnormal heart rhythms** should not take tetrabenazine.

Tetrabenazine raises levels of the hormone prolactin in the blood. Elevated prolactin has been linked with ⅓ of breast cancers in women and with menstrual changes and other side effects. The risk of these effects with tetrabenazine is unknown.

Possible Side Effects

- ▼ Most common: sedation, fatigue, sleeplessness, depression, and restlessness.
- ▼ Common: anxiety, irritability, loss of balance, PD symptoms, nausea, injuries from falling down, and upper-respiratory infections.
- ▼ Less common: reduced appetite, obsessive reactions, dizziness or fainting when rising from a sitting or lying position, difficulty walking, stammering or stuttering, headache, vomiting, black-and-blue marks, difficulty breathing, bronchitis, and pain while urinating.

Drug Interactions

- Mixing tetrabenazine with reserpine (for high blood pressure) may increase the risk of a severe side effect called tardive dyskinesia. You must stop taking reserpine for 20 days before beginning tetrabenazine.
- Do not mix tetrabenazine with other drugs that are known to affect heart rhythm, including some antiarrhythmic drugs such as amiodarone, and sotalol; some antibiotics such as moxifloxacin; and antipsychotic medications such as chlorpromazine, thioridazine, and ziprasidone.
- Bupropion, fluoxetine, paroxetine, and quinidine strongly inhibit the enzyme that breaks down tetrabenazine, increasing tetrabenazine drug levels. Do not mix these drugs.
- Other, weaker inhibitors of this enzyme are cimetidine, chlorpheniramine, clomipramine, doxepin, duloxetine, haloperidol, methadone, mibefradil, and ritonavir. Caution should be exercised when mixing these medicines with tetrabenazine.
- Mixing this drug with some other drugs that affect the nervous system—such as olanzapine or risperidone—and that have similar side effects may lead to more severe drug side effects. These combinations should be used with caution.
- Alcoholic beverages, sedatives, and other nervous system depressants worsen the sedating effect of tetrabenazine.

Food Interactions

Tetrabenazine can be taken without regard to food or meals.

Usual Dose

Adult: 12.5–100 mg a day. Dosage is gradually increased in 12.5-mg steps until maximum benefit with minimum side effects is reached. If tetrabenazine is stopped for any reason, it should be restarted at 12.5 mg and slowly increased again.

Child: not recommended.

Overdosage

The most common overdose symptoms are loss of muscle tone, rolling eyeballs, nausea and vomiting, sweating, sedation, low blood pressure, confusion, diarrhea, hallucinations, skin redness, and tremors. Take the victim to a hospital emergency room at once. If you seek treatment, ALWAYS bring the prescription bottle or container.

Special Information

If you need to take more than 50 mg a day of tetrabenazine, your doctor should do a special blood test to determine your genetic capacity to break down this drug.

People taking this medicine should be cautious about doing anything that requires mental alertness, such as driving or operating hazardous machinery, until they are on a maintenance dose of tetrabenazine and know how the drug affects them.

Report any changes in mental state, unusual muscle movements, difficulty swallowing, excessive sedation, or other severe side effect to your doctor at once. Dosage adjustment may be necessary.

Chorea symptoms return 12–18 hours after you stop taking tetrabenazine.

If you forget a dose of tetrabenazine, take it as soon as you remember. If you do not remember until it is almost time for your next dose, skip the one you forgot and continue with your regular schedule. Do not take a double dose of this medicine.

Special Populations

Pregnancy/Breast-feeding: Animal studies of tetrabenazine revealed no clear effects on a developing fetus. This drug should be taken during pregnancy only if your doctor determines that the potential benefit outweighs the risks.

It is not known if tetrabenazine passes into breast milk. Nursing mothers who must take tetrabenazine should use infant formula.

Seniors: Tetrabenazine has not been studied in seniors.

Type of Drug

Tetracycline Antibiotics

(teh-tra-SIKE-lene)

Brand Names

Generic Ingredients: Demeclocycline Hydrochloride G
Declomycin

Generic Ingredients: Doxycycline G
Atridox
Doryx
Monodox
Oracea
Periostat
Vibramycin

Generic Ingredients: Minocycline Hydrochloride G

Arestin
Dynacin
Minocin
Solodyn

Generic Ingredients: Tetracycline Hydrochloride G

Prescribed For

Infection, including methicillin-resistant *Staphylococcus aureus* (MRSA); some sexually transmitted diseases; infection of the mouth, gums, and teeth; severe acne; Rocky Mountain spotted fever and other types of fever caused by ticks and lice, including Lyme disease; urinary tract infection; and respiratory infection such as pneumonia or bronchitis. Doxycycline is also prescribed for malaria, rosacea, and to treat and prevent traveler's diarrhea. Tetracycline is also used to treat amebic dysentery. Low-dose tetracycline is the most widely prescribed antibiotic for acne.

General Information

Tetracycline antibiotics are effective against a variety of bacterial infections. They work by interfering with the normal growth cycle of the invading bacteria. This allows the body's normal defenses to fight off the infection. Tetracycline may be substituted for penicillin in people who are allergic to penicillin.

Tetracyclines have been used to treat skin infection but are not considered the first-choice antibiotic. Tetracyclines have been used successfully in the treatment of acne, in low dosages over a long period of time.

Cautions and Warnings

Do not take tetracycline antibiotics if you are **allergic** or **sensitive** to any of their ingredients. If you are allergic to one tetracycline antibiotic, you are probably allergic to them all.

Tetracyclines should not be given to people with **liver or kidney disease** or **certain urinary problems**.

Avoid prolonged exposure to the sun if you are taking high dosages of tetracyclines, especially demeclocycline, because these antibiotics may interfere with your body's normal sun-screening mechanism, making you more prone to severe sunburn.

Tetracyclines should not be used by **children under age 8**, because they have been shown to interfere with the development of the long bones and may retard growth. Permanent tooth discoloration may also result.

People taking demeclocycline may experience diabetes insipidus syndrome (symptoms include excessive thirst, urination, and weakness). The severity of this condition depends on the amount of drug taken and is reversible when the drug is withdrawn.

Minocycline may cause lightheadedness, dizziness, or fainting.

Tetracyclines have been associated with pseudotumor cerebri (increased pressure in the brain). Symptoms include headache and blurred vision.

Treatment with antibiotic medications such as tetracycline may cause diarrhea or, more seriously, colitis. Contact your doctor if you develop diarrhea while taking tetracyclines.

Possible Side Effects

- ▼ Most common: upset stomach, nausea, vomiting, diarrhea, sensitivity of the skin to the sun, and rash.
- ▼ Less common: hairy tongue and itching and irritation of the anal or vaginal region. If these symptoms appear, contact your doctor immediately. Periodic physical examinations and laboratory tests should be given to those who are on long-term tetracycline antibiotic therapy.
- ▼ Rare: appetite loss, peeling skin, fever, chills, anemia, brown spotting of the skin, reduced kidney function, and liver damage. Contact your doctor if you experience anything unusual while taking any medication.

Drug Interactions

- Tetracyclines may interfere with bactericidal (bacteria-killing) agents such as penicillin. You should not take both kinds of antibiotics for the same infection.
- Do not combine tetracyclines with isotretinoin or methoxyflurane.
- Antacids, mineral supplements, and multivitamins containing bismuth, calcium, zinc, magnesium, or iron may reduce the effectiveness of tetracyclines—with the exception of doxycycline and minocycline. Sodium bicarbonate powder may also be a problem if used as an antacid. Separate doses of an antacid, mineral supplement, vitamin with minerals, or sodium bicarbonate and a tetracycline antibiotic by at least 2 hours.
- Tetracyclines increase the effect of anticoagulant (blood thinning) drugs such as warfarin. Your anticoagulant dosage may need an adjustment.

- Barbiturates, carbamazepine, and hydantoin antiseizure drugs may reduce doxycycline's effectiveness. More doxycycline or a different antibiotic may be required.
- Cimetidine, ranitidine, and other H_2 antagonists may reduce the effectiveness of tetracyclines.
- Tetracyclines may increase digoxin side effects in a small number of people. This effect may last for months after the tetracycline has been withdrawn. If you are taking this combination, be vigilant for the appearance of digoxin side effects; contact your doctor if they develop.
- Tetracyclines may reduce insulin requirements for diabetics. If you are using this combination, be sure to carefully monitor your blood-sugar level.
- Tetracyclines may increase or decrease blood-lithium levels.
- These drugs may reduce the effectiveness of contraceptive drugs. Breakthrough bleeding or pregnancy is possible; you should use another method of contraception in addition to a hormonal contraceptive while taking one of these antibiotics.

Food Interactions

Take all tetracycline antibiotics, except for doxycycline and minocycline, on an empty stomach, 1 hour before or 2 hours after meals, and with 8 oz. of water. The antibacterial effect of these antibiotics may be neutralized when they are taken with food, dairy products such as milk or cheese, or antacids. Doxycycline and minocycline can be taken with food or milk. Oracea, a particular brand of doxycycline, should be taken on an empty stomach.

Usual Dose

Demeclocycline

Adult: 600 mg a day.

Child (age 9 and over): 3–6 mg per lb. of body weight a day.

Child (under age 9): not recommended.

Doxycycline

Adult and Child (age 9 and over; over 100 lbs.): starting dose—200 mg in 2 doses of 100 mg given 12 hours apart; maintenance dose—100 mg a day in 1 or 2 doses. Oracea—40 mg once a day in the morning. For gonorrhea, take 300 mg in 1 dose and then a second 300-mg dose in 1 hour, or 100 mg twice a day for at least 7 days; for syphilis, 100–300 mg for 10 days to 4 weeks. For malaria prevention, take 100 mg a day, beginning 1–2 days before you leave home. Take your medicine every day and continue for 4 weeks after leaving the malaria-infested area. Do not take doxycycline for more than 4 consecutive months.

Child (age 9 and over; under 100 lbs.): starting dose—2 mg per lb. of body weight divided into 2 doses; maintenance dose—1 mg per lb. of body weight as a single daily dose. Child's dose for malaria prevention is 1 mg per lb. of body weight as a single daily dose.

Your doctor may double the maintenance dosage for severe infection. An increased incidence of side effects is observed with dosages over 200 mg a day.

Minocycline

Adult: starting dose—200 mg; maintenance dose—100 mg every 12 hours. Alternate dosage: starting dose—100–200 mg; maintenance dose—50 mg 4 times a day. Solodyn—45–135 mg a day.

Child (age 9 and over): starting dose—2 mg per lb. of body weight; maintenance dose—1 mg per lb. of body weight every 12 hours.

Child (under age 9): not recommended.

Tetracycline

Adult: 250–500 mg 4 times a day.

Child (age 9 and over): 10–20 mg per lb. of body weight a day in 4 equal doses.

Child (under age 9): not recommended.

Tetracycline Ointment and Solution: Apply to affected area morning and night.

Overdosage

Overdose is most likely to affect the stomach and digestive system. Contact your local poison control center or a hospital emergency room for more information. If you seek treatment, ALWAYS bring the prescription bottle or container.

Special Information

Do not take any antibiotic after the expiration date on the label. Decomposed tetracycline may cause serious kidney damage.

Because the action of tetracyclines depends on its concentration within the invading bacteria, it is imperative that you completely follow the doctor's directions and complete the full course of treatment prescribed.

Contact your doctor if you develop excessive thirst, urination, and weakness; blue-gray discoloration of the skin or mucous membranes (with minocycline); appetite loss; headache; vomiting; changes in vision; abdominal pain with nausea and vomiting; yellowing of the skin or whites of the eyes; or any persistent or intolerable side effect, including dizziness, lightheadedness, or unsteadiness; burning or cramps in the stomach; diarrhea with nausea and vomiting; or itching of the mouth, rectal, or vaginal areas (may indicate the presence of a superinfection). Contact your doctor if your child develops tooth discoloration.

Avoid excessive exposure to the sun while taking tetracyclines, especially demeclocycline, because these drugs may cause susceptibility to sunburn.

Tetracyclines may cause dizziness, lightheadedness, or fainting. Be careful when driving or performing any task that requires concentration.

If you are using tetracycline antibiotic topical solution for acne, apply the product generously to your skin until the area to be treated is completely wet. Stinging or burning may occur, but this lasts only a few minutes. Tetracycline antibiotic solution may stain your skin yellow, but the stain usually washes away. Do not apply the solution or cream inside your eyes, nose, or mouth.

If you miss a dose of an oral tetracycline, take it as soon as possible. If you take the drug once a day and it is almost time for your next dose, space the missed dose and your next dose 10–12 hours apart, then go back to your regular schedule. If you take tetracycline twice a day and it is almost time for your next dose, space the missed dose and your next dose by 5–6 hours, then go back to your regular schedule. If you take the drug 3 or more times a day and it is almost time for your next dose, space the missed dose and your next dose by 2–4 hours, then go back to your regular schedule. Never take a double dose.

Special Populations

Pregnancy/Breast-feeding: Tetracycline should not be taken if you are pregnant, especially during the last 5 months of pregnancy. It interferes with the formation of skull and bone structures in the fetus.

Tetracycline passes into breast milk. It interferes with the development of a child's skull, bones, and teeth. Nursing mothers who must take tetracycline should use infant formula.

Seniors: Seniors, especially those with poor kidney function, are more likely to experience less common side effects.

Generic Name

Thalidomide (thal-IH-doe-mide)

Brand Names

Thalomid

Type of Drug

Immune system modulator.

Prescribed For

Erythema nodosum leprosum (ENL)—a painful skin condition associated with leprosy—and for multiple myeloma, a blood cancer.

General Information

The U.S. Food and Drug Administration (FDA) approved thalidomide in 1998 for ENL under a very strict distribution system called S.T.E.P.S. (System for Thalidomide Education and Prescribing Safety), as this drug causes serious birth defects. Only doctors who are registered with the S.T.E.P.S. program can prescribe thalidomide. The exact way that thalidomide works is not known, but it appears to suppress excessive amounts of tumor necrosis factor and also affects the movement of white blood cells. Thalidomide is also prescribed for leprosy, scleroderma, and other skin conditions, and is being studied for prostate and other cancers.

Cautions and Warnings

Do not use thalidomide if you are **allergic** or **sensitive** to any of its ingredients. A drug-sensitivity or allergic reaction to thalidomide (symptoms include rash, fever, rapid heartbeat, and low blood pressure) may be cause to temporarily stop your treatment.

As little as 1 dose of thalidomide can cause birth defects. It should not be taken by **pregnant** women under any circumstances. Women must take a pregnancy test before the drug will be prescribed. Women of childbearing age should use contraceptives 4 weeks prior to, during, and 4 weeks following drug therapy, even if they have a history of infertility. Regular pregnancy tests should be administered throughout treatment. Men taking thalidomide can also transmit the drug through semen. These men should use a condom during intercourse with a pregnant partner or a woman of childbearing age, even if they have had a vasectomy. Using 2 methods of non-hormonal contraception is preferred.

The use of thalidomide in treating multiple myeloma has been associated with an increased risk of developing blood clots, especially if dexamethasone and other drugs are also part of the treatment. Symptoms include shortness of breath, chest pain, or swelling of the arms and legs. Aspirin or another blood-thinning treatment can be used to counter this risk.

Thalidomide frequently causes nerve damage (symptoms include numbness, tingling, or pain in the hands or feet) that may be permanent. It generally occurs after a few months of regular treatment but can also develop after taking thalidomide for a short time. Thalidomide should not be used as the sole treatment for ENL by people with **neuritis** (nerve irritation).

Thalidomide can cause a rapid drop in white-blood-cell count, increasing the risk of infection.

Thalidomide can increase the level of human immunodeficiency virus (HIV) RNA in people with **AIDS**, but the importance of this finding is unclear.

Serious, possibly life-threatening skin reactions, including Stevens-Johnson syndrome, have occurred in children and adults taking this medicine. Tell your doctor at once if you develop any type of skin reaction to the drug.

Thalidomide is generally not recommended for **children under age 18**, though a small number of children have been safely treated with the drug.

Possible Side Effects

- ▼ Most common: drowsiness, rash, dizziness, impotence, fainting, headache, and stomach pain.
- ▼ Common: muscle weakness; tingling, burning, numbness, or pain in the hands, arms, feet, or legs; tremors; constipation; diarrhea; nausea; mouth infections; sinus irritation; back pain; fever, alone or with chills and sore throat; infections; and feeling unwell.
- ▼ Less common: dry mouth, liver inflammation, gas, dry skin, mood change, leg swelling, acne, fungal skin infections, nail problems, itching, sweating, loss of appetite, tooth pain, anemia, low white-blood-cell count, swollen lymph glands, runny nose, abdominal pain, accidental injuries, and a rigid or painful neck.
- ▼ Rare: blood in the urine, decreased urination, irregular heartbeat, low blood pressure, and agitation. Other rare

Possible Side Effects *(continued)*

side effects can occur in almost any part of the body. Contact your doctor if you experience anything unusual while taking any medication.

Drug Interactions

- Mixing thalidomide with dexamethasone increases the risk of life-threatening blood clots (see "Cautions and Warnings").
- Combining thalidomide with alcohol, barbiturates, chlorpromazine, reserpine, sedatives, tricyclic antidepressants, or other nervous system depressants can cause extreme tiredness. Avoid these combinations.
- Combining thalidomide and chloramphenicol, cisplatin, didanosine, ethambutol, ethionamide, hydralazine, isoniazid, lithium, metronidazole, nitrofurantoin, nitrous oxide, phenytoin, stavudine, or vincristine may worsen peripheral neuropathy (symptoms include tingling, burning, numbness, or pain in the hands or feet) or increase your risk of developing it.
- Medications that interfere with contraceptive drugs must be avoided if you are taking thalidomide, because they increase the risk of an unwanted pregnancy. These drugs include protease inhibitors, carbamazepine, griseofulvin, modafinil, penicillins, rifampin, rifabutin, phenytoin, and St. John's wort.

Food Interactions

For optimal effectiveness, do not take thalidomide with a high-fat meal.

Usual Dose

Adult: 100–400 mg a day at bedtime.
Child: not recommended.

Overdosage

Symptoms are likely to be common side effects. Take the victim to a hospital emergency room. If you seek treatment, ALWAYS bring the prescription bottle or container.

Special Information

Women of childbearing age who take thalidomide should have weekly pregnancy tests. Women with irregular periods may have to be tested every 2 weeks. Stop taking the drug at once if you are or think you may be pregnant.

Drowsiness is common with thalidomide. Be careful when driving or performing any task that requires concentration.

Thalidomide can make you dizzy or faint if you rise suddenly from a lying position. Sitting up for a few minutes before attempting to stand may help prevent this problem.

Contact your doctor if you experience shortness of breath; chest pain; arm or leg swelling; or numbness, tingling, or burning of the feet or hands.

People taking thalidomide may not donate blood or semen.

Thalidomide can increase your sensitivity to the sun. Use sunscreen and wear protective clothing while taking this drug.

Take this drug exactly as prescribed. Do not stop taking it without your doctor's knowledge. Do not share this medication with anyone else.

If you forget a dose, take it as soon as you remember. If it is almost time for your next dose, skip the one you forgot and continue with your regular schedule. Do not take a double dose.

Special Populations

Pregnancy/Breast-feeding: Women who are or might be pregnant should never take thalidomide, especially during the first 2 months of pregnancy. Women of childbearing age who take thalidomide should use 2 reliable methods of contraception (for example, a contraceptive drug and a condom). Contraception must be used for at least 1 month before treatment is begun, during treatment, and for 1 month after treatment has been completed.

It is not known if thalidomide passes into breast milk, but it could cause serious reactions in a nursing infant. Nursing mothers who must take thalidomide should use infant formula.

Seniors: Seniors may take this drug without special restriction.

Type of Drug

Thiazide Diuretics

(THYE-uh-zide dye-ur-RET-iks)

Brand Names

Generic Ingredients: Chlorothiazide G
Diuril

Generic Ingredients: Chlorthalidone G
Thalitone

Generic Ingredients: Hydrochlorothiazide G
Microzide Oretic

Generic Ingredients: Indapamide G

Generic Ingredients: Methyclothiazide G
Enduron

Generic Ingredients: Metolazone
Zaroxolyn

Prescribed For

Edema associated with congestive heart failure (CHF), cirrhosis of the liver, kidney malfunction, hypertension (high blood pressure), and other conditions where it is necessary to rid the body of excess water.

General Information

Thiazide diuretics increase urine production by affecting the movement of sodium and chloride in the kidney. Thiazide diuretics reduce sodium, magnesium, bicarbonate, chloride, and potassium-ion levels. Calcium elimination is moderated and uric acid is retained as a result of thiazide treatment. Thiazide diuretics may also raise blood sugar. These drugs are used in the treatment of any disease where it is desirable to eliminate large quantities of water. Thiazide diuretics are often taken with other drugs to treat high blood pressure and other conditions. The exact way in which they reduce blood pressure is not known; sodium elimination is of primary importance. These diuretics begin to work within 2 hours and produce their effect in 2–6 hours. The differences between thiazide diuretic drugs lie in duration of effect—6–12 hours for some and as long as 48–72 hours for others—and quantity of drug absorbed.

Cautions and Warnings

Do not take a thiazide diuretic if you are **allergic** or **sensitive** to any of its ingredients, to any drugs in this group, or to sulfa drugs. If you have a history of **allergy** or **bronchial asthma**, you may also have a sensitivity or allergy to thiazide diuretics.

Thiazide diuretics may aggravate **systemic lupus erythematosus** (a chronic autoimmune disease).

These medications reduce levels of potassium, sodium, and magnesium in the body, which can cause serious complications.

People with a history of **gout** should use these medications with caution.

Thiazides may raise total **cholesterol**, low-density lipoprotein

(LDL) cholesterol, and total **triglyceride** levels. They should be used with caution by people with moderate to high blood-cholesterol or triglyceride levels. Indapamide does not appear to raise blood-cholesterol levels.

Thiazides should be used with caution if you have severe **kidney disease**, because they may precipitate kidney failure; only metolazone and indapamide may be safely given in this group. People with severe **liver disease** should be treated carefully with diuretics because minor changes in electrolyte (body fluid) balance may cause hepatic coma.

People with **diabetes** may experience increased blood-sugar levels and will need dosage adjustments of their antidiabetic medication.

Thiazide diuretics can cause temporary near-sightedness or glaucoma. Untreated glaucoma can lead to blindness.

Possible Side Effects

- ▼ Most common: Thiazide diuretics cause loss of body potassium (symptoms include dry mouth, thirst, weakness, lethargy, drowsiness, restlessness, muscle pain or cramp, muscular tiredness, low blood pressure, decreased frequency of urination and decreased urine production, abnormal heart rate, and upset stomach with nausea and vomiting). Potassium supplements are given to prevent this problem—or you can eat high-potassium foods such as bananas, citrus fruits, melons, and tomatoes.
- ▼ Less common: appetite loss, abdominal pain, bloating, diarrhea, constipation, dizziness, yellowing of the skin or whites of the eyes, headache, tingling of the toes and fingers, restlessness, changes in blood composition, increased sensitivity to the sun, rash, itching, fever, breathing difficulties, allergic reaction, dizziness when rising quickly from a sitting or lying position, muscle spasm, impotence and reduced sex drive, and blurred vision.

Drug Interactions

- Thiazide diuretics increase the action of other blood-pressure-lowering drugs. Consequently, people with high blood pressure often take more than 1 drug.
- The risk of developing imbalances in electrolytes is increased if you take medicines such as digitalis drugs, amphotericin B, and adrenal corticosteroids while taking a thiazide diuretic.

- Dosage adjustments of anesthetics may be required while taking thiazide diuretics.
- Thiazide diuretics may increase the risk of allopurinol side effects.
- Anticholinergic medications may increase the effects of thiazide diuretics.
- Thiazide diuretics may decrease the effects of oral anticoagulant (blood thinning) drugs.
- If you begin taking a thiazide diuretic, your insulin or antidiabetic dosage may have to be modified.
- Antigout drug dosage may have to be modified because thiazide diuretics raise blood levels of uric acid.
- Thiazide diuretics may prolong the white-blood-cell-reducing effects of chemotherapy drugs.
- Thiazide diuretics may increase the effects of diazoxide, leading to symptoms of diabetes.
- Combining thiazide diuretics and loop diuretics may lead to an extreme diuretic effect and extreme effect on blood-electrolyte levels.
- Rare occurrences of anemia have occurred when thiazide diuretics were taken with methyldopa.
- Thiazide diuretics increase the risk of lithium side effects.
- Methenamine and other urinary agents may reduce the effect of thiazide diuretics.
- Certain nonsteroidal anti-inflammatory drugs (NSAIDs), particularly indomethacin, may reduce the effectiveness of thiazide diuretics. Sulindac, another NSAID, may increase the effect of thiazide diuretics.
- Thiazide diuretics may increase the action of vitamin D, possibly leading to high blood-calcium levels.

Food Interactions

Thiazide diuretics can be taken with food if they upset your stomach. Your doctor may recommend high-potassium foods such as bananas and orange juice to offset the potassium-lowering effect of these drugs.

Usual Dose

Chlorothiazide

Adult: 0.5–1 g 1–2 times a day. Often, people respond to intermittent therapy—that is, taking the drug on alternate days or 3–5 days a week. This reduces side effects.

Child (age 6 months and over): 5–10 mg per lb. of body weight a day in 2 equal doses.

Child (under age 6 months): not more than 15 mg per lb. of body weight a day in 2 equal doses.

Chlorthalidone

Adult: 25–100 mg a day, or 100 mg on alternate days. Some people may need up to 200 mg a day.

Child (age 1 and over): 0.14 mg per lb. of body weight a day to a maximum of 50 mg a day.

Hydrochlorothiazide

Adult and Child (age 13 and over): 25–200 mg a day, depending on the condition being treated; maintenance dose—25–100 mg a day. Some people may need up to 200 mg a day.

Child (age 3–12): 37.5–100 mg a day in 2 doses.

Child (age 6 months–2 years): 12.5–37.5 mg a day in 2 doses.

Child (under age 6 months): not more than 1.5 mg per lb. of body weight a day in 2 doses.

Indapamide

Adult: 1.25–2.5 mg every morning. Dosage may be increased to 5 mg a day.

Child: not recommended.

Methyclothiazide

Adult: 2.5–10 mg a day.

Child: not recommended.

Metolazone: Dosage is individualized: 0.5–20 mg once a day depending on formulation. Do not switch formulations of metolazone without consulting your doctor.

Overdosage

Symptoms include tingling in the arms or legs, weakness, fatigue, fainting, dizziness, changes in heartbeat, feeling unwell, dry mouth, restlessness, muscle pain or cramp, urinary difficulties, nausea, and vomiting. Take the victim to a hospital emergency room at once. If you seek treatment, ALWAYS bring the prescription bottle or container.

Special Information

Ordinarily, diuretics are prescribed early in the day to prevent excessive nighttime urination from interfering with sleep.

Thiazide diuretics cause excess urination at first, but it subsides after several weeks.

Contact your doctor if you develop eye pain or changes in your vision, muscle pain, sudden joint pain, weakness, cramps, nausea, vomiting, restlessness, excessive thirst, tiredness, drowsiness, increased heart or pulse rate, diarrhea, or dizziness.

Avoid alcohol and other medications while taking a thiazide diuretic, unless directed by your doctor.

Avoid over-the-counter medications for the treatment of coughs, colds, and allergy if you have hypertension or CHF because such medication may contain stimulants.

Thiazide diuretics may cause sensitivity to sunlight. Use sunscreen and wear protective clothing if necessary.

If you forget a dose, take it as soon as you remember. If it is almost time for your next dose, skip the one you forgot and continue with your regular schedule. Do not take a double dose.

Special Populations

Pregnancy/Breast-feeding: Thiazide diuretics enter the fetal circulation and may cause side effects in the newborn such as jaundice, blood problems, and low potassium levels. Diuretics are used to treat specific medical conditions during pregnancy, but their routine use during a normal pregnancy is improper. A thiazide diuretic should be taken during pregnancy only if your doctor determines that the potential benefit outweighs the risks.

Thiazide diuretics pass into breast milk. Nursing mothers who must take diuretics should use infant formula.

Seniors: Seniors are more likely to have reduced kidney function. Because these drugs leave the body through the kidneys, seniors should use the lowest effective dose and be aware of the possibility of increased side effects, especially dizziness.

Type of Drug

Thyroid Hormone Replacements

Brand Names

Generic Ingredients: Levothyroxine G

Levo-T
Levothroid
Levoxyl
Synthroid
Tirosint
Unithroid

Generic Ingredients: Liothyronine G

Cytomel
Triostat

Generic Ingredients: Liotrix
Thyrolar

Generic Ingredients: Thyroid Hormone G
Armour Thyroid
Nature-Throid
NP Throid
Westhroid

Prescribed For

Hypothyroidism (underactive thyroid gland).

General Information

The major differences between these drugs are their sources and hormone content. Thyroid hormone is made from beef and pork thyroid. It is effective but lacks standardization, making it difficult for doctors to control dosage. Synthetic drugs are more desirable because their content is easily standardized, ensuring that you receive the correct amount of hormone.

There are 2 important thyroid hormones: levothyroxine and liothyronine. Levothyroxine is converted to liothyronine in the body. This process slows the absorption of levothyroxine and lowers the risk of side effects. Liothyronine's potency and its potential for side effects make it less desirable for older adults. Liotrix contains both levothyroxine and liothyronine; because levothyroxine is converted naturally to liothyronine, there is usually no advantage in taking both hormones unless there is a problem with the conversion process. These considerations tend to make levothyroxine the treatment of choice for thyroid hormone replacement.

Cautions and Warnings

Do not use a thyroid hormone replacement if you are **allergic** or **sensitive** to any of its ingredients or to pork.

Thyroid hormone replacements should not be used for weight loss in people with a normal thyroid status. Standard dosages of these drugs will not work, whereas larger dosages may produce serious or fatal side effects, especially when taken with appetite-suppressing drugs.

If you have **hyperthyroid disease** (symptoms include headache, nervousness, sweating, rapid heartbeat, chest pain, and other signs of central-nervous-system stimulation) or **high output of thyroid hormone**, you should not use these drugs.

If you have **heart disease** or **hypertension** (high blood pressure), thyroid hormone replacement therapy should not be used unless it is clearly indicated and supervised by your doctor, as it can aggravate the condition. If you develop chest pain or other signs of heart disease while taking this drug, contact your doctor immediately. Do not use levothyroxine if you have recently had a heart attack.

Natural thyroid hormones are not recommended for **seniors** because of an increased risk of adverse effects on the heart.

Women, especially postmenopausal women, on long-term thyroid replacement therapy can develop osteoporosis or break a bone. Regular monitoring and using the lowest effective dose helps avoid this effect.

These drugs should not be used to treat **infertility** unless the person also has hypothyroidism.

Thyroid hormone replacement therapy increases metabolism and may worsen the symptoms of other endocrine system (hormone-related) diseases such as **diabetes** and **Addison's disease**. Adjustments in the levels of treatment for these diseases may be needed when you begin using these drugs. You may also require treatment with glucocorticoids.

People with **myxedema** (a dry, waxy swelling under the skin of the face) are very sensitive to thyroid replacement hormones and should start treatment at a very low dose.

Possible Side Effects

Side effects are rare except during the start of therapy or when dosage is adjusted.

▼ Most common: heart palpitations, rapid heartbeat, abnormal heart rhythms, weight loss, chest pain, hand tremor, headache, diarrhea, nervousness, menstrual irregularity, inability to sleep, sweating, intolerance to heat, and hair loss. These symptoms may be controlled by adjusting dosage.

Drug Interactions

- Avoid taking over-the-counter drugs that contain stimulants—such as many of the products used to treat cough, cold, or allergy—which affect the heart and may cause symptoms of overdose.
- Combining tricyclic or tetracyclic antidepressants with levothyroxine may increase the risk of toxic effects of both drugs.
- Using a thyroid replacement hormone with ketamine may lead to severe high blood pressure and rapid heart rate; these drugs should be used together with caution.

- Antacids; bile acid sequestrants; calcium, iron, and sodium supplements; orlistat; simethicone; and sucralfate may reduce the amount of thyroid product absorbed into the blood and its effectiveness. Take your thyroid hormone replacement and these drugs 4–6 hours apart.
- The following drugs may reduce the natural production of thyroid hormone or interfere with the body's response to thyroid replacement hormones; an increased dosage of the thyroid replacement may be necessary: beta blockers, contraceptive drugs, dexamethasone, estrogen, fluorouracil, heroin and methadone, lithium, methimazole, mitotane, propylthiouracil, sulfa drugs, tamoxifen, and tolbutamide.
- The following drugs may increase the natural production of thyroid hormone in your body; a decreased dosage of the thyroid replacement may be necessary: androgens, anabolic steroids, asparaginase, glucocorticoids, and slow-release nicotinic acid.
- The following drugs may have a variable effect on your body's natural thyroid function and/or your response to thyroid hormone therapy; dosage adjustments may be necessary: aminosalicylate sodium, amiodarone, diazepam, ethionamide, interferon drugs, lovastatin, mercaptopurine, metoclopramide, perphenazine, resorcinol, and thiazide diuretics.
- Use of carbamazepine, phenobarbital, phenytoin, rifamycins, and selective serotonin reuptake inhibitor (SSRI) antidepressants may result in a need for increased dosages of levothyroxine.
- Thyroid hormone replacements increase the effects of anticoagulant drugs; your dose of the anticoagulant may need to be reduced.
- People with diabetes may need to have their doctors increase their antidiabetic drug dosages when they start taking a thyroid hormone replacement.
- These drugs may reduce the effectiveness of beta blockers. Dosage of a beta blocker may need to be increased.
- Blood levels of digoxin and similar drugs, and their effectiveness, may be reduced by thyroid hormone replacements.
- Thyroid hormone replacements may interfere with growth hormones if the thyroid drug dosage is too high or too low. A doctor should closely monitor your condition.

- Thyroid hormones may interfere with radiographic imaging agents (which are used to help doctors see body organs in X-rays).
- Dosage reduction of theophylline may be required if you take a thyroid hormone replacement.

Food Interactions

Thyroid hormone replacements should be taken as a single dose on an empty stomach at least 30 minutes before breakfast with a full glass of water.

Soybean-based foods, dietary fiber, and walnuts may interfere with the absorption of levothyroxine from the intestines. Dosage adjustments may be necessary if you frequently consume these foods.

Usual Dose

Thyroid hormone replacements are usually started at a low dose and increased in steps until an adequate response is achieved. The required dosage will vary depending on the condition being treated, your age, and your response to therapy.

Adult

Levothyroxine: 12.5–300 mcg a day. It is essential to take levothyroxine with a full glass of water at the same time each day.

Liothyronine: 5–100 mcg a day.

Liotrix: ¼–2 tablets a day. Liotrix tablets are rated according to their approximate equivalent to thyroid hormone.

Natural Thyroid Hormone: 30–120 mg a day.

Overdosage

Symptoms include headache; irritability; nervousness; sweating; rapid heartbeat with unusual stomach rumbling, with or without cramps; chest pain; heart failure; and shock. Take the victim to a hospital emergency room immediately. If you seek treatment, ALWAYS bring the prescription bottle or container.

Special Information

Thyroid hormone replacement therapy is usually a lifelong treatment and requires periodic monitoring. Take the drug as prescribed and do not stop taking it unless instructed by your doctor.

Do not switch brands, especially in the case of levothyroxine, without your doctor's or pharmacist's knowledge. Different brands of the same thyroid hormone replacement are not always equivalent.

Many drugs have been reported to affect thyroid hormone levels. Make sure your doctor is aware of every prescription or nonprescription drug and supplement you are taking.

Contact your doctor if you develop nervousness, diarrhea, excessive sweating, chest pain, increased pulse rate, heart palpitations, and intolerance to heat—which are signs you may be taking too high a dose—or any bothersome or persistent side effect.

Children beginning thyroid hormone replacement therapy may lose some hair during the first few months, but this is only temporary and the hair generally grows back.

If you forget a dose, take it as soon as you remember—preferably before a meal when your stomach will be emptiest. If it is almost time for your next dose, skip the one you forgot and continue with your regular schedule. Do not take a double dose. Contact your doctor if you miss 2 or more consecutive doses.

Special Populations

Pregnancy/Breast-feeding: Small amounts of these drugs enter the fetal bloodstream. These medications have not been associated with any problems when used to maintain normal thyroid function in the mother. Pregnant women who have been taking a thyroid hormone replacement should continue their treatment under medical supervision.

Small amounts of these drugs pass into breast milk. Nursing mothers who must take them should use infant formula.

Seniors: Seniors, who may be more sensitive to the effects of these drugs, generally require reduced dosage. Broken bones are more likely in people age 70 and older.

Generic Name

Tiagabine (tye-AG-a-bene)

Brand Names

Gabitril

The information in this profile also applies to the following drugs:

Generic Ingredients: Gabapentin G

Gralise Neurontin

Generic Ingredients: Gabapentin Encarbil

Horizant

Type of Drug

Anticonvulsant and analgesic (pain reliever).

Prescribed For

Partial seizures; gabapentin may also be used for pain after herpes zoster (shingles) infection, tremors associated with multiple sclerosis, nerve pain, chronic pain, fibromyalgia, restless legs syndrome (RLS), hot flashes in women receiving chemotherapy for breast cancer or due to menopause, and prevention and treatment of migraine headaches. Gabapentin encarbil is approved for moderate to severe RLS.

General Information

The exact way in which tiagabine works is not known but may be related to its ability to improve the activity of gamma-aminobutyric acid (GABA), the major inhibitor of nerve transmission in the brain and central nervous system. This means that tiagabine probably slows GABA-related nerve impulses that lead to a seizure. The medication achieves maximum blood levels in 45 minutes. It is broken down in the liver.

Tiagabine is only prescribed as additional therapy for those already taking other antiepileptic drugs.

Gabapentin is related to GABA, but it does not modify GABA in the body. It may bind directly to receptors in the brain, but has no effect on those receptors commonly affected by other drugs that act on the central nervous system.

Gabapentin encarbil is broken down to gabapentin, and its benefit for RLS is attributable to gabapentin.

Cautions and Warnings

Do not take these drugs if you are **allergic** or **sensitive** to any of their ingredients. Several people taking tiagabine have developed a severe rash.

These medications have been associated with seizure development in people without epilepsy. In most cases, those who experienced seizures were also taking other medications such as antidepressants, antipsychotics, stimulants, or narcotics. Seizures may also occur with dose increase. If seizures occur in people taking one of these drugs who have not experienced them prior to treatment, the drug should be stopped and you should be evaluated for an underlying seizure disorder.

Suddenly stopping any antiepileptic drug can increase the chance of seizures. Dosage should be reduced gradually.

People taking these or any other seizure-disorder medications are more likely to have suicidal thoughts or attempt suicide.

In studies of tiagabine, a small percentage of those participating experienced status epilepticus, a life-threatening condition of persistent seizure. Although researchers were unable to determine whether tiagabine therapy was causative, those with a history of status epilepticus should be aware of this possible association.

People with **liver disease** should take these drugs with caution and receive reduced dosages. People with **kidney disease** may require reduced dosages of gabapentin. Gabapentin encarbil tablets should not be taken by people with severe kidney disease and by those who are on **dialysis**. In studies, a small number of people died suddenly while taking gabapentin. It is not known if the drug caused these deaths.

A feeling of severe weakness has developed in a small number of people taking tiagabine. The weakness goes away when the medication is reduced or stopped.

Tiagabine may bind to parts of the eye. There is no evidence that this produces long-term effects. Tell your doctor if you experience any changes in vision.

Possible Side Effects

Gabapentin and Gabapentin Encarbil

▼ Most common: tiredness, dizziness, and headache.

▼ Common: fatigue, double vision, blurred vision, and tremors.

▼ Less common: increased appetite, weight gain, arm or leg swelling, back pain, upset stomach, intestinal gas, dry mouth or throat, constipation, dental problems, muscle aches, runny nose, sore throat, speech problems, memory loss, depression, irritability, abnormal thinking, twitching, itching, abrasions, impotence, and visual disturbances.

▼ Rare: dizziness, depression, reduced sex drive, broken bones, poor coordination, low red- and white-blood-cell counts, and flushing. Contact your doctor if you experience anything unusual while taking any medication.

Tiagabine

▼ Most common: dizziness, sleepiness, confusion, depression, weakness, nervousness, and nausea.

▼ Common: poor concentration, speech or language problems, abdominal or other pain, tremor, sleeplessness, diarrhea, vomiting, sore throat, and rash.

Possible Side Effects *(continued)*

▼ Less common: forgetfulness, tingling in the hands or feet, emotional upset, changes in gait or walk, hostility, visual disturbances, agitation, hunger, mouth sores, cough, itching, and flushing.

Drug Interactions

- Taking tiagabine with other medications for seizure control, including carbamazepine, phenytoin, phenobarbital, primidone, and valproate may decrease the amount of tiagabine in the blood. Dosage adjustments may be necessary.
- The risk of seizures is increased if tiagabine is combined with bupropion or tramodol.
- Gemfibrozil may increase the effects of tiagabine.
- Antacids reduce the absorption of gabapentin; take these drugs at least 2 hours apart.
- Combining gabapentin and hydrocodone may affect the blood levels of both.
- Cimetidine, morphine, and naproxen increase blood levels of gabapentin.

Food Interactions

Take tiagabine with food, but avoid high-fat meals, which slow its absorption. Gabapentin encarbil tablets should be taken with food. Gabapentin can be taken without regard to food or meals.

Usual Dose

Gabapentin

Adult and Child (age 13 and over): 300–600 mg 3 times a day. Dosage must be reduced in people with kidney disease.

Child (age 3–12): 4.5–7 mg per lb. of body weight a day in 3 divided doses to start, increasing gradually over a period of about 3 days to a maximum of 22 mg per lb. a day in divided doses.

Child (under age 3): not recommended.

Gabapentin Encarbil

Adult: 600 mg a day in the evening. Dosage must be reduced in people with kidney disease.

Child: not recommended

Tiagabine

Adult: starting dose—4 mg once a day. Dosage may be increased in steps of 4 or 8 mg to 56 mg a day in divided doses.

Child (age 12 and over): starting dose—4 mg once a day. Dosage may be increased in steps of 4 or 8 mg to 32 mg a day in divided doses.

Overdosage

Gabapentin: Symptoms include double vision, slurred speech, drowsiness, diarrhea, lethargy, weakness, breathing difficulties, sedation, droopy eyelids, and excitation.

Tiagabine: Symptoms include tiredness, loss of consciousness, agitation, confusion, difficulty talking, hostility, depression, weakness, and muscle spasm.

Take the victim to a hospital emergency room. If you seek treatment, ALWAYS bring the prescription bottle or container.

Special Information

This drug may make you dizzy or tired, or interfere with your concentration. Be extremely careful when driving or performing any task that requires concentration. Avoid alcohol or other nervous system depressants, because they increase these effects.

Tell your doctor if you experience worsening depression, suicidal thoughts, a panic attack, anxiety, agitation, new or worsening restlessness, trouble sleeping, acting on dangerous impulses, mood changes (including extreme increase in your activity level), changes in vision, rash, or any bothersome or persistent side effect.

Gabapentin encarbil cannot be interchanged with another gabapentin product because it releases medicine into your blood at a specific rate that is different from other products.

Gabapentin encarbil is not recommended for people who work at night or must sleep during the day.

If you forget a dose of tiagabine or gabapentin, take it as soon as you remember. If it is almost time for your next dose, take the dose you forgot and space the remaining daily dosage evenly throughout the day. Do not take a double dose.

If you forget your dose of gabapentin encarbil or do not take it at the correct time, continue with your next regular dose; do not take a double dose. Extended-release products should be swallowed whole, not crushed or chewed, because the tablet is designed to release the medicine slowly over time. Crushing or chewing would release all of the medicine at once, increasing side effect risks.

Special Populations

Pregnancy/Breast-feeding: These medications cause birth defects in laboratory animals. Seizure disorder itself has been associated with an increased risk of birth defects. Discuss with your doctor the need to control seizures and the potential benefit and risks of taking this medication during pregnancy.

Tiagabine may pass into breast milk. It is not known if gabapentin does. Nursing mothers who must take either drug should consider using infant formula.

Seniors: Seniors may take tiagabine without special precaution but may require reduced dosage of gabapentin due to age-related decline in kidney function.

Generic Name

Tizanidine (tih-ZAN-ih-deen) G

Brand Names

Zanaflex

Type of Drug

Skeletal muscle relaxant.

Prescribed For

Spastic muscle movements.

General Information

Tizanidine is prescribed for people who suffer from uncontrolled muscle spasms usually associated with a nervous system condition. It is presumed to work on the central nervous system by affecting nerves that control major muscle systems; it has no direct effect on skeletal muscles. Tizanidine begins working 1–2 hours after it is taken and lasts for 3–6 hours. Because of its short duration of effect, treatment should be reserved for those times when relief is most important.

Cautions and Warnings

Do not take tizanidine if you are **allergic** or **sensitive** to any of its ingredients.

Tizanidine can cause low blood pressure. This effect usually begins within 1 hour after taking the drug and reaches its height after 2–3 hours. Low blood pressure triggered by tizanidine is associated with slow heart rate, lightheadedness, and dizziness when rising from a sitting or lying position.

About 50% of people taking tizanidine experience some sedation. Sedation usually begins 30 minutes after taking the drug and continues to get worse for about 1 hour. Sedative effects usually start during the first week of treatment or do not occur at all.

Tizanidine may cause liver injury. About 1 in 20 people who take this drug experience some liver inflammation, although most cases resolve once the drug is stopped. Several people have died from liver failure after taking tizanidine; it should be avoided by people with **liver disease**.

Slowed heart rate has occurred in people taking tizanidine.

Do not switch between tizanidine tablets and capsules. They are not equivalent.

Some people taking tizanidine have experienced hallucinations, delusions, and psychotic symptoms.

Tizanidine should be used with caution by people who have **reduced kidney function**. These people need smaller-than-usual doses.

Possible Side Effects

- ▼ Most common: dry mouth, sleepiness, tiredness, and weakness.
- ▼ Common: dizziness.
- ▼ Less common: uncontrolled muscle movement, nervousness, constipation, sore throat, vomiting, frequent urination, urinary infection, liver inflammation, double vision, flu-like symptoms, runny nose, speech disorders, fever, depression, anxiety, tingling in the hands or feet, rash, sweating, skin sores, diarrhea, abdominal pain, and upset stomach.
- ▼ Rare: Rare side effects can occur in almost any part of the body. Contact your doctor if you experience anything unusual while taking any medication.

Drug Interactions

- Tizanidine should never be used with fluvoxamine or ciprofloxacin. These combinations can cause serious adverse effects.
- Avoid combining alcohol or any other central-nervous-system depressant and tizanidine because increased sedation may result.

- The addition of acyclovir; antiarrhythmics such as amiodarone, mexiletine, propafenone, or verapamil; cimetidine; famotidine; fluoroquinolones; ticlopidine; or zileuton may increase the amount of tizanidine in the blood, which can lead to serious adverse effects. These combinations should be avoided.
- Women who combine contraceptive drugs and tizanidine should receive reduced dosages of the latter to avoid increased side effects.
- Tizanidine may increase the effects of blood-pressure-lowering drugs.
- Tizanidine may delay the effects of acetaminophen.

Food Interactions

Tizanidine can be taken without regard to food or meals, though it may work faster with food. It should always be taken at the same times of the day and consistently with or without food.

Usual Dose

Adult: 8 mg every 6–8 hours as needed, up to 3 doses a day. Do not exceed 36 mg a day.

Child: not recommended.

Overdosage

Little is known about the effects of tizanidine overdose, but it may lead to very slow breathing. Overdose victims should be taken to a hospital emergency room. If you seek treatment, ALWAYS bring the prescription bottle or container.

Special Information

People taking tizanidine should be careful not to exceed the prescribed dosage because little is known about using higher dosages over an extended period.

Do not suddenly stop taking tizanidine, especially if you have been taking higher doses. Dosage should be reduced gradually to minimize the occurrence of withdrawal side effects. Rebound high blood pressure, muscle rigidity, and increased heart rate are all possible.

Because of the possibility of sedation, be careful when driving or performing any task that requires concentration.

If you take tizanidine on a regular basis and forget a dose, take it as soon as you remember. If it is almost time for your next dose, skip the one you forgot and continue with your regular schedule. Do not take a double dose.

Special Populations

Pregnancy/Breast-feeding: Tizanidine should be taken during pregnancy only if your doctor determines that the potential benefit outweighs the risks.

Tizanidine may pass into breast milk. Nursing mothers who must take this drug should consider using infant formula.

Seniors: Seniors should use tizanidine with caution.

Type of Drug

TNF Blockers

Brand Names

Generic Ingredients: Adalimumab
Humira

Generic Ingredients: Certolizumab
Cimzia

Generic Ingredients: Etanercept
Enbrel

Generic Ingredients: Golimumab
Simponi

Generic Ingredients: Infliximab
Remicade

Generic Ingredients: Tocilizumab
Actemra

Prescribed For

Crohn's disease, ankylosing spondylitis, and rheumatoid arthritis (RA). Infliximab may also be used for plaque psoriasis, ulcerative colitis, psoriatic arthritis, psoriasis, and juvenile arthritis.

General Information

A TNF blocker binds to a specific protein in the body known as tumor necrosis factor (TNF) and blocks it from interacting with cell surfaces. TNF is involved in normal inflammatory and immune responses as well as the inflammatory processes of RA, juvenile RA, and other conditions. A TNF blocker can also interfere with normal biological activities that are either caused or regulated by TNF. Many of these products are prescribed with methotrexate in the treatment of RA for a better result. Other conditions can be treated with a TNF blocker alone.

People who do not do well on a TNF blocker may be given tocilizumab (Actemra) once every 4 weeks by intravenous injection instead of the TNF blocker. Tocilizumab can be used by itself or with another RA medication such as methotrexate. Tocilizumab has been approved only for RA that has not responded to other treatments, but may be taken with methotrexate or some other drugs used to treat RA.

Cautions and Warnings

Do not take a TNF blocker if you are **allergic** or **sensitive** to any of its ingredients or to any murine proteins. Allergic reactions include itching, breathing difficulties, and low blood pressure (symptoms include dizziness and fainting). These reactions may require emergency treatment. Lupus erythematosus (a chronic autoimmune disease) may develop but goes away once drug treatment is stopped.

Serious and sometimes fatal infections and malignancies are possible in people using a TNF blocker because of its ability to suppress the immune response. Lymphoma, leukemia, and some cancers may be more common in children, teens, and people with conditions that predispose them to infections such as advanced or uncontrolled **diabetes**. These drugs should be avoided if you have a **chronic or recurrent infection**. If a serious infection does occur, treatment should be interrupted until the infection can be cured.

People receiving other biologicals for RA have experienced the reactivation of pre-existing **herpes** and **hepatitis**.

Teens and **young adults** receiving a TNF blocker or other immune system suppressant for Crohn's disease, psoriasis, or another condition may be at risk of developing a rare, aggressive white-blood-cell cancer called HSTC that is usually fatal.

Live virus or attenuated virus vaccines should be avoided by people taking a TNF blocker because these drugs suppress the immune response to the vaccine, making them risky.

Levels of blood platelets and some white blood cells may be reduced in rare cases, leading to persistent fever, bruising, bleeding, and pale skin. Contact your doctor if any of these symptoms develop.

The safety and effectiveness of more than 3 infliximab infusions are not known.

People with **congestive heart failure** should take a TNF blocker with caution because it may worsen heart function.

People with **nervous system disorders** or **seizures** should take a TNF blocker with caution.

TNF blockers have been associated with new or worsening nervous system disorders, including **multiple sclerosis**. People with a history of these conditions should be cautious about using TNF blockers.

Tocilizumab should not be used if you have active **liver disease**. It may lead to higher levels of liver enzymes and high blood cholesterol, triglycerides, and other blood fats.

Possible Side Effects

Adalimumab

- ▼ Most common: upper-respiratory infection, sinusitis, headache, rash, accidental injuries, and pain after injection.
- ▼ Common: flu-like symptoms, nausea, abdominal pain, back pain, high blood pressure, and abnormal lab tests (such as cholesterol or blood in urine).
- ▼ Less common: Adalimumab can affect your heart, gastrointestinal system, bones, skin and connective tissue, blood, muscles and skeleton, nervous system, lungs, eyes, and kidneys.
- ▼ Rare: lymphoma, abnormal vision, lupus-like syndrome, liver failure, blood abnormalities, and seizure. Contact your doctor if you experience anything unusual while taking any medication.

Certolizumab

- ▼ Most common: lung or urinary infections and rash.
- ▼ Common: joint pain and anemia and other blood disorders, including bleeding.
- ▼ Less common: angina; abnormal heart rhythms; heart failure; heart attack; high blood pressure; fluid accumulation in heart muscle and around the heart; stroke and TIA; bleeding in the eye; visual disturbances; liver irritation and hepatitis; hair loss; anxiety; bipolar symptoms; attempted suicide; kidney disease, including kidney failure; menstrual disorders; itching; reddish, painful, or tender lumps most commonly located in the front of the legs; and blood clots.

Possible Side Effects *(continued)*

Etanercept

- ▼ Most common: infection, injection-site reactions, upper-respiratory infection, headache, and runny nose.
- ▼ Common: nausea, dizziness, sore throat, cough, weakness, abdominal pain, rash, and respiratory problems.
- ▼ Less common: upset stomach, sinus irritation, vomiting, swelling in the legs or feet, mouth sores, and hair loss.
- ▼ Rare: malignancy, stroke, seizure, tingling in the hands or feet, nervous system irritation similar to multiple sclerosis, eye inflammation, joint pain, generalized pain, appetite loss, blood-vessel inflammation in the skin, dry eyes, lumps under the skin, fever, flu-like symptoms, weight gain, chest pain, flushing, diarrhea, taste changes, difficulty breathing, worsening of existing lung conditions, itching, and skin reactions. Contact your doctor if you experience anything unusual while taking any medication.

Golimumab

- ▼ Common: upper-respiratory infection, and nose and throat irritation.
- ▼ Less common: liver irritation, injection-site reactions, allergic reactions, high blood pressure, bronchitis, dizziness, runny nose, fever, sore throat, and tingling in the hands or feet.
- ▼ Rare: lymphoma, abnormal vision, lupus-like syndrome, liver failure, blood abnormalities, and seizure. Contact your doctor if you experience anything unusual while taking any medication.

Infliximab

Most people (8 of 10) experience more than 1 side effect. Sixteen percent develop a reaction to the drug within 2 hours. Those reactions include fever, chills, itching, rash, chest pain, changes in blood pressure, and breathing difficulties.

- ▼ Most common: headache, nausea, upper-respiratory infection, abdominal pain, fatigue, and fever.
- ▼ Common: sore throat, vomiting, pain, dizziness, bronchitis, rash, runny nose, chest pain, coughing, itching, sinus inflammation, muscle aches, back pain, and fungal infection.
- ▼ Less common: Less common side effects can occur in almost any part of the body.

Possible Side Effects *(continued)*

Tocilizumab

▼ Common: infection, infusion reactions, upper-respiratory infection, headache, runny nose, elevated liver enzyme measurements, and high blood pressure.

▼ Less common: dizziness, bronchitis, rash or other skin reactions, mouth ulcers, and upper stomach or abdominal pain.

▼ Rare: oral herpes infections, gastrointestinal perforation, stomach ulcers, malignancy, weight gain, cough, difficulty breathing, conjunctivitis (pinkeye), kidney stones, and underactive thyroid. Contact your doctor if you experience anything unusual while taking any medication.

Drug Interactions

- Using these drugs with other biological products (abatacept, anakinra, or another TNF blocker) increases the risk of serious infection.
- Do not mix these drugs in the same syringe as another drug.
- If you take golimumab with a drug that requires close monitoring by your doctor, such as warfarin, cyclosporine, or theophylline, your drug dose may be altered by golimumab.
- Tocilizumab increases the production of drug-metabolizing enzymes by the liver while you are receiving it and for several weeks afterward. Dose adjustments may be needed if you mix this drug with conivaptan, omeprazole and other proton-pump inhibitors, simvastatin and other statin drugs, tolvaptan, and warfarin.
- Other medicines that may be compromised by tocilizumab's effect on liver enzymes include some antiepileptic drugs, antidepressants, benzodiazepines, bupropion, clozapine, colchicine, cyclosporine, eplerenone, erlotinib and other multiple kinase inhibitors, irbesartan, losartan, narcotic pain relievers, nonsteroidal anti-inflammatory drug (NSAID) pain relievers, quinidine and other drugs for abnormal heart rhythms, protease inhibitors, sildenafil and other erectile dysfunction drugs, sulfonylurea and other antidiabetes drugs, and tacrolimus.
- Consider using an alternate form of contraception while you are receiving tocilizumab. Contraceptive drug effectiveness may be compromised.

Usual Dose

Adalimumab

Rheumatoid and Psoriatic Arthritis; Ankylosing Spondylitis

Adult and Child (66 lbs. and over): 40 mg injected under the skin every other week.

Child (33–65 lbs.): 20 mg under the skin every other week.

Crohn's Disease

Adult: 160 mg (4 injections of 40 mg) to start, 80 mg 2 weeks later, then 40 mg every other week.

Child: not recommended.

Plaque Psoriasis

Adult: 80 mg to start, then 40 mg every other week starting 1 week later.

Child: not recommended.

Certolizumab

Adult: 400 mg (2 injections of 200 mg each) under the skin to start. Maintenance dose—Crohn's disease: 400 mg every 4 weeks; rheumatoid arthritis: 400 mg at week 2 and 4, then 200 mg every other week or 400 mg every 4 weeks.

Etanercept

Adult: for rheumatoid arthritis, psoriatic arthritis, and ankylosing spondylitis—50 mg a week.

Child (age 4–17): 0.2 mg per lb. of body weight, up to 25 mg twice a week, injected under the skin 3–4 days apart.

Child (under age 4): not recommended.

Golimumab

Rheumatoid and Psoriatic Arthritis; Ankylosing Spondylitis

Adult: 50 mg under the skin once a month.

Child: not recommended.

Infliximab

Adult and Child (age 6–17): 1.35–2.25 mg per lb. of body weight. Another dose may be given 2 and 6 weeks after the first injection, then every 8 weeks.

Child (under age 6): not recommended.

Tocilizumab

Adult: 1.8 mg per lb. of body weight by intravenous infusion over 1 hour, once every 4 weeks. The dose may be increased to 3.6 mg per lb. if needed.

Child: not recommended.

Overdosage

Overdose symptoms are likely to include drug side effects. However, large doses of these medicines have been used with no serious side effects. There is a risk of lowering your white-blood-cell count. Contact your local poison control center or a hospital emergency room for more information. If you seek treatment, ALWAYS bring the prescription bottle or container.

Special Information

Contact your doctor at once if you develop chest pain; fever; chills; warm, red, or painful skin; itching; hives; facial flushing; open cuts or sores on your body; or trouble breathing within a few hours after receiving your medicine, or if you develop yellowing of the skin or whites of the eyes, dark brown urine, right-sided abdominal pain, fever, or severe tiredness.

Tell your doctor if you experience abdominal pain, persistent fever, night sweats, unexplained weight loss, or if your liver or spleen grow larger. These can be signs of a rare and potentially fatal blood cancer.

Make sure your doctor knows your complete medical and medication history, especially if you have had tuberculosis (TB) or any chronic infection. Tell your doctor if you have recently traveled to an area where TB or fungal infections are common.

Contact your doctor if you have or think you are coming down with an infection. Signs of infection may include, fever, sweating, chills, muscle aches, cough, trouble breathing, coughing up blood, weight loss, painful skin (also warm and red) or sores, diarrhea or stomach pain, burning when you urinate or urinating more than usual, and feeling unusually tired.

Contact your doctor if you develop signs of hepatitis or liver damage, including sudden and severe abdominal pain, yellowing of the skin or whites of the eyes, dark-colored urine, tiredness, appetite loss, vomiting, light-colored stool, fever, muscle aches, stomach discomfort, and skin rash.

These drugs may be stored in a refrigerator, but never frozen. Single-use pre-filled syringes must be refrigerated or cold while traveling. Do not attempt to speed the warming of the product after it is removed from the refrigerator in any way, including in a microwave or hot water bath. Simply allow it to slowly reach room temperature. Do not use after the expiration date.

Each medication has specific directions for preparation. Some must be mixed and others come in a syringe ready to be injected.

Be sure you know exactly how to use the product your doctor has prescribed. Contact your doctor or pharmacist if you have any questions about how to administer these drugs. For more information on injections, see page 1242.

Tocilizumab must be mixed and given by a health professional.

Etanercept is taken by injection under the skin. Be sure you understand how to measure the proper dose of etanercept and how to self-inject it.

To mix and inject etanercept: Withdraw all the water supplied with the medicine into a syringe and slowly inject it into the vial containing the etanercept. Swirl the mixture gently to avoid excess foaming in the vial. *Do not shake the vial.*

If you forget to administer a dose, do so as soon as you remember.

Remember that etanercept doses must be administered at least 3 days apart. Contact your doctor or pharmacist if you have any questions about how to time your etanercept doses.

Special Populations

Pregnancy/Breast-feeding: The safety of TNF blockers used during pregnancy is not known. A TNF blocker should be taken during pregnancy only if your doctor determines that the potential benefit outweighs the risks. TNF blocker manufacturers have established systems to keep track of pregnant women who take their products and what happens to them. Your doctor will enroll you in the appropriate program.

It is not known if TNF blockers pass into breast milk. Nursing mothers who must take it should use infant formula.

Seniors: Seniors are more likely to develop infections while using these medicines.

Generic Name

Tolcapone (TOL-kap-own)

Brand Names

Tasmar

Type of Drug

COMT inhibitor.

Prescribed For

Parkinson's disease (PD).

General Information

Tolcapone is believed to block the effects of an enzyme known as COMT, which is found throughout the body. COMT is an essential part of the process by which natural stimulants or catecholamines are eliminated. This extends levodopa + carbidopa's beneficial effect on PD.

Cautions and Warnings

Do not take tolcapone if you are **allergic** or **sensitive** to any of its ingredients.

Tolcapone can cause liver irritation, injury, and failure, which may be fatal. Liver function should be evaluated every 2 weeks for the first year of therapy, then every 4–8 weeks. People with **liver disease** should not take tolcapone. Due to the risk of serious liver damage, people who do not show a benefit from tolcapone 3 weeks from initiation of treatment should stop taking it.

People with severe **kidney disease** should also use tolcapone with caution.

Tolcapone increases levodopa + carbidopa side effects, including low blood pressure, dizziness or fainting, and uncontrolled muscle movements.

Some people have suffered from hallucinations after initiating therapy with tolcapone.

Diarrhea requiring hospitalization has occurred in people taking tolcapone.

Cases of rhabdomyolysis, a potentially fatal disorder involving destruction of skeletal muscle, have been reported with tolcapone use. It is unclear what role, if any, tolcapone may have had in these cases.

Possible Side Effects

- ▼ Most common: abnormal muscle movements, sleep disturbances, stiffness, vivid dreams, tiredness, confusion, nausea, appetite loss, diarrhea, vomiting, muscle cramps, dizziness, and fainting.
- ▼ Common: hallucinations, constipation, dry mouth, abdominal pain, respiratory infections, sweating, falling, and fatigue.
- ▼ Less common: loss of balance, changes in muscular activity, tingling in the hands or feet, upset stomach, gas, arthritis, neck pain, chest pain, low blood pressure, chest

Possible Side Effects *(continued)*

discomfort, breathing difficulties, sinus congestion, flu-like symptoms, urine discoloration, and difficulty urinating.

▼ Rare: agitation, irritability, hyperactivity, minor skin bleeding, hair loss, a burning sensation, feeling unwell, fever, cataracts, and eye inflammation. Contact your doctor if you experience anything unusual while taking any medication.

Drug Interactions

- Do not combine tolcapone and any monoamine oxidase inhibitor (MAOI) antidepressant except selegiline.
- Dose reductions may be necessary when tolcapone is given with drugs that are metabolized by COMT, such as α-methyldopa, apomorphine, dobutamine, and isoproterenol.
- Blood monitoring should be conducted when tolcapone is given with warfarin.
- Tolcapone increases levodopa + carbidopa side effects.

Food Interactions

Take tolcapone at least 1 hour before or 2 hours after meals.

Usual Dose

Adult: 100–200 mg 3 times a day.

Child: not recommended.

Overdosage

Common symptoms include nausea, vomiting, and dizziness. Take the victim to a hospital emergency room. If you seek treatment, ALWAYS bring the prescription bottle or container.

Special Information

Nausea, dizziness or fainting, hallucinations, and other side effects are more likely when you first start taking this drug.

Tolcapone can make you tired and dizzy. Be careful when driving or performing any task that requires concentration.

Your doctor may reduce your dosage of levodopa + carbidopa when you begin taking tolcapone.

If you forget a dose, take it as soon as you remember. If it is almost time for your next dose, skip the forgotten dose and continue with your regular schedule. Do not take a double dose.

Special Populations

Pregnancy/Breast-feeding: The safety of using tolcapone during pregnancy is not known, though there is a risk that it may be toxic to a pregnant woman. It is always prescribed with levodopa + carbidopa, which is known to cause birth defects. Tolcapone should be taken during pregnancy only if your doctor determines that the potential benefit outweighs the risks.

Tolcapone may pass into breast milk. Nursing mothers who must take it should use infant formula.

Seniors: Seniors may be more sensitive to side effects, especially hallucinations.

Generic Name

Tolvaptan (toll-VAP-tan)

Brand Names

Samsca

Type of Drug

Vasopressin antagonist.

Prescribed For

Very low blood-sodium levels.

General Information

Tolvaptan is used for people whose blood sodium cannot be corrected with traditional treatments when they cannot pass sodium out of their bodies through the kidneys. Tolvaptan works within 2 hours of taking it and produces rapid passing of water and sodium. This helps restore urine to its normal balance of salt and other electrolytes. You must be in the hospital when you start or restart taking it because of the drug's very rapid action.

Cautions and Warnings

Do not use tolvaptan if you are **allergic** or **sensitive** to any of its ingredients.

Do not take this medicine if your blood-sodium level must be raised immediately.

Do not take tolvaptan if your kidneys are not making urine.

Tolvaptan may cause you to lose too much water. People who **cannot sense when they are thirsty** or who are **unable to**

respond to feeling thirsty should not take it. Contact your doctor if you feel dizzy, faint, or your kidneys are not working properly.

People with **cirrhosis** should not take tolvaptan unless their doctor determines that the potential benefit outweighs the risks. People with other forms of liver disease may take tolvaptan without restriction.

Tolvaptan treatment must be started in the hospital because overly fast correction of blood-sodium levels can severely affect muscle control, leading to difficulty speaking and swallowing, seizures, coma, paralysis, and possibly death. Other symptoms may include drowsiness, confusion, or mood changes. This is of particular concern in those who are **alcoholic**, severely **malnourished**, or who have advanced **liver disease**. Notify your doctor immediately if you experience any of these symptoms after returning home while taking tolvaptan.

Possible Side Effects

▼ Most common: dry mouth, thirst, and frequent urination.

▼ Common: constipation, weakness, and high blood sugar.

▼ Less common: fever and appetite loss.

▼ Rare: Other side effects can affect your blood, heart and blood vessels, gastrointestinal tract, muscles, nervous system, and reproductive system. Contact your doctor if you experience anything unusual while taking any medication.

Drug Interactions

- Do not mix tolvaptan with azole antifungal drugs (such as itraconazole or ketoconazole) clarithromycin, nefazodone, protease inhibitors (such as indinavir, nelfinivir, ritonavir, and saquinavir), or telithromycin. They slow the clearance of tolvaptan, increasing the amount of medicine in your system and the risk of dangerous side effects.
- Tolvaptan dose may have to be reduced if it is mixed with aprepitant, calcium channel blockers (such as diltiazem or verapamil), cyclosporine, or erythromycin (use with caution).
- Your tolvaptan dose may need to be increased with barbiturates (such as phenobarbital), carbamazepine, phenytoin, rifamycins (such as rifampin), or St. John's wort, which can speed the breakdown of tolvaptan, making it less effective.
- Using tolvaptan with angiotensin-converting enzyme (ACE) inhibitors, angiotensin receptor blockers, or potassium-sparing diuretics can lead to abnormally elevated blood potassium.

- Digoxin levels may rise by 30% if mixed with tolvaptan. Other drugs can be affected by tolvaptan in this same way but the increase is not enough to require a dose or medicine change.

Food Interactions

This drug can be taken without regard to food or meals at any time of the day. Do not drink grapefruit juice because it slows the clearance of tolvaptan from the body.

Usual Dose

Adult: 15–60 mg once a day.

Child: not recommended.

Overdosage

Tolvaptan overdose is likely to make you extremely thirsty, urinate frequently, and become dehydrated. Victims must be taken to a hospital emergency room immediately. If you seek treatment, ALWAYS bring the prescription bottle or container with you.

Special Information

You must take this medicine exactly as directed by your doctor. Do NOT stop taking tolvaptan or restart it on your own. If you forget a dose, take it as soon as you remember. If it is almost time for your next dose, skip the forgotten dose and continue with your regular schedule. Do not take a double dose.

As your blood-sodium level drops and you pass large volumes of water, you will feel thirsty. Drink water until this feeling is satisfied. Your body is trying to re-establish its normal balance. When you stop taking the medicine, your doctor will advise you to go back to restricting fluid intake and monitoring your blood sodium.

Contact your doctor if you develop anything that can affect your body fluids, including diarrhea or vomiting.

Special Populations

Pregnancy/Breast-feeding: Tolvaptan's effect on the developing fetus is not known. Animal studies have shown changes in skeleton, weight, and survival of the fetus. It should be taken during pregnancy only if your doctor determines that the potential benefit outweighs the risks.

It is not known if tolvaptan passes into breast milk. Nursing mothers who must take it should use infant formula.

Seniors: Seniors may take tolvaptan without special precautions, though older adults may be more sensitive to the effects of this drug.

Generic Name

Topiramate (toe-PI-ruh-mate)

Brand Names

Topamax
Topamax Sprinkle

Type of Drug

Anticonvulsant; antimigraine.

Prescribed For

Partial onset seizures, tonic-clonic seizures, Lennox-Gastaut syndrome, and migraine prevention. Topiramate has also been used for alcohol dependence, cluster headaches, infantile spasms, bipolar disorder, bulimia, and obesity.

General Information

Topiramate has a broad spectrum of antiepileptic activity. It inhibits nerve transmission in the brain and nervous system by blocking sodium channels and the neurotransmitter glutamate, and by increasing the effect of the neurotransmitter gamma-aminobutyric acid (GABA). Topiramate reaches peak blood levels within 2 hours. It passes out of the body through urine.

Cautions and Warnings

Do not take topiramate if you are **allergic** or **sensitive** to any of its ingredients.

People taking topiramate may develop reduced bicarbonate levels in their blood (called metabolic acidosis) because it promotes bicarbonate loss through the kidney by inhibiting an enzyme called carbonic anhydrase. Existing **kidney disease**, severe **respiratory disorders**, **status epilepticus**, **diarrhea**, **surgery**, a **ketogenic diet**, or some other drugs can worsen the degree of acidosis. Common symptoms of metabolic acidosis include rapid breathing, confusion, and lethargy. Other possible symptoms include heart palpitations or chest pain, abnormal heart rhythms, headache, visual changes, difficulty breathing, nausea and vomiting, abdominal pain, diarrhea, appetite changes, weight loss, muscle weakness, bone pain, stupor, and coma.

People who suddenly stop taking topiramate may worsen their seizures. Anticonvulsant drugs should be reduced gradually.

People taking this drug are more likely to have suicidal thoughts or attempt suicide.

Some patients receiving topiramate have experienced acute visual disturbances with symptoms of decreased clarity and eye pain. The treatment to reverse this condition is discontinuation of topiramate, according to the treating physician's judgment as to the necessity of the drug.

Topiramate can cause decreased sweating, which may result in body temperature changes that could be dangerous, especially in children.

People with moderate to severe **kidney disease** should receive ½ the usual dose; other dosage adjustments may be needed. About 1.5% of people taking topiramate develop kidney stones. This effect may be avoided by drinking several glasses of water a day during treatment.

People with **liver disease** may clear topiramate from their bodies more slowly than others do, but the reasons for this are not well understood.

People taking topiramate may experience slowness in response, difficulty with concentration, speech disorders, and language problems. Tiredness and fatigue are also common side effects of topiramate. Adults may also experience depression or mood changes. Stopping topiramate therapy may cause concentration or attention difficulty.

Topiramate exerts long-term effects on calcium levels in bone and bone metabolism, possibly increasing the risk of osteoporosis.

Possible Side Effects

Side effects usually affect the central nervous system and are more likely with increasing drug dose.

- ▼ Most common: tiredness or fatigue; slow reflexes; slow thought processes; difficulty concentrating; speech or language problems, especially word-finding; dizziness; weakness; poor muscle coordination; tingling in the hands or feet; tremors; nervousness; insomnia; depression; nausea; loss of appetite; respiratory infections; sensitivity to the sun; and visual disturbances, including double vision.
- ▼ Less common: back or chest pain, leg pain, flushing, body odor, swelling, abnormal coordination, agitation, mood changes, aggressive reactions, reduced touch sensation, apathy, emotional instability, depersonalization, itching, rash, hair loss (in children), upset stomach, abdominal pain, constipation, dry mouth, breast pain, menstrual disorders,

Possible Side Effects *(continued)*

painful menstruation, sore throat, sinus inflammation, breathing difficulties, eye pain, weight loss, loss of white blood cells, muscle ache, hearing loss, and aggravated convulsions.

▼ Rare: chills, sweating, gum irritation, tongue swelling, blood in the urine, nosebleeds, vision loss, a decrease in sexual desire, severe skin reactions, hepatitis, liver failure, pancreatitis, pemphigus (a chronic autoimmune skin disease), and kidney damage. Other rare side effects can occur in almost any part of the body. Contact your doctor if you experience anything unusual while taking any medication.

Drug Interactions

- Combining topiramate with a carbonic-anhydrase inhibitor drug such as acetazolamide may increase your risk of kidney stones. This combination should be avoided.
- Topiramate increases the depressive effect of alcohol and other nervous system depressants. Avoid these combinations.
- Topiramate increases the amount of amitriptyline in the blood. Reductions in amitriptyline dose may be required to avoid drug side effects.
- Certain other anticonvulsant drugs—phenytoin, carbamazepine, and valproic acid—reduce topiramate levels. Using topiramate with valproic acid may also cause elevated levels of ammonia, resulting in mental symptoms and/or vomiting.
- Hydrochlorothiazide increases the amount of topiramate in the blood.
- Lamotrigine may reduce topiramate blood levels.
- Topiramate may reduce the effect of digoxin, lithium, contraceptive drugs, and risperidone.
- Combining metformin or pioglitazone with topiramate requires careful monitoring of diabetes control.

Food Interactions

None known.

Usual Dose

Adult (age 10 and over): starting dose—25–50 mg a day. Increase gradually to 200 mg twice a day. People with moderate to severe kidney failure should begin with ½ the usual dose. The recommended maintenance dose for migraine is 50 mg twice a day.

Child (age 2–9): Topiramate alone—starting dose is 25 mg once a day at night, increased gradually to a maximum of 400 mg a day; individual dosage is based on weight. Adjunct therapy—starting dose is 0.5–1.4 mg per lb. of body weight, up to 25 mg, at night for 1 week. Increase gradually until an optimal response is achieved (2.3–4 mg per lb. of body weight per day, divided into 2 doses).

Child (under age 2): not recommended.

Overdosage

Overdose is likely to cause convulsions, drowsiness, speech disturbance, blurred or double vision, impaired thinking, lethargy, abnormal coordination, stupor, low blood pressure, abdominal pain, agitation, dizziness, and depression. Overdose victims must be taken to a hospital emergency room immediately. If you seek treatment, ALWAYS bring the prescription bottle or container.

Special Information

Drink several glasses of water or other fluids every day to avoid developing kidney stones.

Sprinkle capsules may be swallowed whole or may be opened and sprinkled onto a teaspoon of soft food. The mixture should be swallowed at once without chewing.

Contact your doctor if you develop heart palpitations or chest pain, headache, visual changes, confusion or other changes in mental status, difficulty breathing, nausea and vomiting, abdominal pain, diarrhea, appetite changes, weight loss, muscle weakness, bone pain, lethargy, stupor, or coma.

Be careful when driving or performing any task that requires concentration.

If you forget a dose, take it as soon as you remember. If it is almost time for your next dose, skip the dose you forgot and continue with your regular schedule. Do not take a double dose.

Special Populations

Pregnancy/Breast-feeding: Topiramate has been linked to cleft lip and palate in newborns whose mothers took the drug. Topiramate should be taken during pregnancy only if your doctor determines that the potential benefit outweighs the risks.

Animal studies show that topiramate passes into breast milk. Nursing mothers who must take it should use infant formula.

Seniors: Lower dosage may be needed because of age-related kidney impairment.

Generic Name

Tranexamic Acid (trah-nex-AM-ik)

Brand Names

Lysteda

Type of Drug

TRPV1 nerve channel stimulator.

Prescribed For

Heavy menstrual bleeding.

General Information

Tranexamic acid interferes with the normal breakdown of fibrin, a component of blood clots. It stabilizes fibrin and the structure it provides for the blood clot. Tranexamic acid injection has been available in the United States since 1986 and is now used for people with hemophilia to prevent bleeding during dental surgery. In clinical studies, oral tranexamic acid reduced the amount of menstrual blood loss and excessive staining and improves the social, leisure, and physical activities of women taking it. It does not affect premenstrual syndrome.

Cautions and Warnings

Do not take this drug if you are **allergic** or **sensitive** to any of its ingredients.

This product passes out of the body through the kidneys. Thus, people with moderate to severe **kidney disease** must take lower doses of tranexamic acid.

Women with a history of conditions associated with **blood-clot** formation should not take tranexamic acid. Women with a clot in a blood vessel in or around their brain who take tranexamic acid may develop swelling of brain tissue or a stroke. Women with a higher risk of blood-clot formation, including those with some abnormal heart rhythms, should not take this medicine, because it increases the risk of further clot formation.

People taking tranexamic acid have experienced blood flow blockage in vessels supplying the eye, affecting vision. If this happens you must stop taking the medicine and contact your doctor at once. Tranexamic acid has also been linked to a form of conjunctivitis (pinkeye).

Possible Side Effects

- ▼ Most common: headache, sinus and nasal symptoms, back pain, abdominal pain, muscle and joint pain, and muscle cramps.
- ▼ Common: migraine, anemia, and fatigue.
- ▼ Less common: nausea, vomiting, diarrhea, dizziness, skin reactions, visual disturbances (including changes in color vision), and abnormal blood-clot formation.
- ▼ Rare: severe allergy. Contact your doctor if you experience anything unusual while taking any medication.

Drug Interactions

- Mixing tranexamic acid with hormonal contraceptives (including pill, patch, vaginal ring, or intrauterine device [IUD]) increases the risk of blood-clot-related conditions, including stroke and heart attack. Non-hormonal birth control should be used instead.
- Mixing tranexamic acid oral with isotretinoin or tretinoin products increases the risk of blood-clot formation.
- Women being treated for hemophilia with factor IX injection complex who also take this medicine increase their risk of forming a dangerous blood clot.

Food Interactions

Tranexamic acid can be taken without regard to food or meals.

Usual Dose

Adult: Two 650-mg tablets 3 times a day (3900 mg a day) for up to 5 days a month during menstruation. Dose is reduced for women with kidney disease.

Overdosage

Overdose symptoms can include nausea, vomiting, diarrhea, dizziness or fainting when rising from a sitting or lying position, blood-clot formation, vision changes, changes in mental state, seizures, and rash. Overdose victims should be taken to a hospital emergency room. If you seek treatment, ALWAYS bring the prescription bottle with you.

Special Information

If you forget a dose of tranexamic acid, take it as soon as you remember. Then take your next dose at least 6 hours later and continue with your regular schedule. Do not take more than 2 pills at a time and do not take more than 6 pills within 24 hours.

This medicine can affect your vision. If this happens, stop taking the medicine and contact your doctor immediately.

Go to a hospital emergency room for treatment if you develop signs of a severe allergic reaction to tranexamic acid. Symptoms include difficulty breathing, closing of the throat, and facial flushing.

Contact your doctor if your heavy periods persist despite taking this medication.

Do not use any birth control (pill, patch, vaginal ring, or IUD) that depends on a hormone for its action.

Special Populations

Pregnancy/Breast-feeding: This drug is not meant for pregnant women because it is only for women who are menstruating. Animal studies indicate that the drug passes into the bloodstream of a developing fetus.

Small amounts of tranexamic acid pass into breast milk. Nursing mothers should use infant formula and should take this medicine only if absolutely necessary.

Seniors: This product is not meant for women who have passed menopause.

Travatan *see **Prostaglandin Agonists,** page 953*

Generic Name

Trazodone (TRAY-zoe-done) G

Brand Names

Oleptro

Type of Drug

Antidepressant.

Prescribed For

Depression with or without anxiety; also used for cocaine withdrawal, alcoholism, insomnia, and aggressive behaviors.

General Information

Trazodone is chemically different from other antidepressants. It is just as effective as other drugs, such as tricyclic antidepressants, in treating the symptoms of depression. Symptoms can often be relieved as early as 2 weeks after starting trazodone, but 4 or more weeks may be required to achieve maximum benefit.

Cautions and Warnings

Do not use trazodone if you are **allergic** or **sensitive** to any of its ingredients.

Antidepressants have been associated with an increased risk of suicide, especially in **teenagers**. Suicide is always a risk in severely depressed people, who should only be allowed to have minimal quantities of medication in their possession.

Trazodone may cause symptoms resembling those of neuroleptic malignant syndrome or serotonin syndrome, including very high fever, muscle rigidity, changes in mental state, irregular pulse or blood pressure, sweating, abnormal heart rhythms, and rapid heartbeat. If these symptoms develop, stop taking your medication at once and contact your doctor. The risk increases if trazodone is combined with other antidepressant medications, triptans, or antipsychotic drugs.

A major depressive episode may be the first sign of bipolar disorder. Trazodone is not approved to treat bipolar disorder. Do not use trazodone if you are recovering from a **heart attack**. People with a previous history of **heart disease** should not use trazodone, because it may cause abnormal heart rhythms.

Rarely, priapism (a persistent, painful erection) has occurred with trazodone. If this happens, stop taking the drug and contact your doctor. One-third of these cases may require surgery or may lead to a permanent inability to achieve erection.

Treatment with antidepressants has been associated with depleted levels of sodium in the body. Symptoms include headache, difficulty concentrating, memory impairment, confusion, weakness, and unsteady walking.

Withdrawal symptoms of anxiety, agitation, and sleep disturbances have been reported with sudden discontinuation of trazodone. Your medication should be tapered off gradually to prevent these symptoms.

Possible Side Effects

- ▼ Common: upset stomach; constipation; abdominal pain; a bad taste in the mouth; nausea; vomiting; diarrhea; palpitations; rapid heartbeat; rash; swelling of the arms or legs; blood-pressure changes; feeling of paralysis of the body; breathing difficulties; dizziness; anger; hostility; nightmares; vivid dreams; confusion; disorientation; loss of memory or concentration; drowsiness; fatigue; lightheadedness; difficulty sleeping; nervousness; excitement; headache; loss of coordination; tingling in the hands or feet; tremor of the hands or arms; ringing or buzzing in the ears; blurred vision; red, tired, and itchy eyes; stuffy nose or sinuses; loss of sex drive; muscle ache and pain; appetite loss; weight gain or loss; increased sweating; clamminess; and feeling unwell.
- ▼ Less common: drug allergy, chest pain, heart attack, gas, delusions, hallucinations, agitation, difficulty speaking, restlessness, numbness, weakness, seizures, increased sex drive, reverse ejaculation, impotence, missed or early menstrual periods, increased salivation, anemia, reduced levels of certain white blood cells, muscle twitches, blood in the urine, reduced urine flow, increased urinary frequency, and increased appetite. Trazodone may cause elevations in levels of body enzymes, which are used to measure liver function.

Drug Interactions

- Trazodone should not be taken with a monoamine oxidase inhibitor (MAOI) antidepressant. Separate doses of trazodone from an MAOI by 2 weeks.
- Mixing selective serotonin reuptake inhibitors (SSRIs) or other drugs related to serotonin with trazodone may result in symptoms of serotonin syndrome, including irritability, muscle tightness, shivering, jerking, involuntary movements of the arms and legs, and changes in consciousness. Trazodone should not be combined with tryptophan.
- Risk of gastrointestinal bleeding is increased if trazodone is combined with aspirin or nonsteroidal anti-inflammatory drugs (NSAIDs).
- Trazodone may increase the effects of sedatives, alcohol, and other drugs that depress the nervous system.

- Trazodone may cause a small reduction in blood pressure. Your dosage of high-blood-pressure medication may need to be reduced slightly when you start taking trazodone.
- Azole antifungal medications such as itraconazole and ketoconazole, delavirdine, phenothiazine sedatives, and protease inhibitors such as ritonavir, indinavir, and saquinavir slow the clearance of trazodone, increasing the chance of trazodone side effects such as nausea, low blood pressure, and fainting.
- Carbamazepine can reduce the amount of trazodone in the blood, decreasing the effectiveness of the drug, and trazodone may increase levels of carbamazepine.
- Trazodone may increase digoxin or phenytoin blood levels and the risk of side effects.
- Trazodone may interfere with the effectiveness of warfarin (an anticoagulant).

Food Interactions

Take trazodone with food to increase effectiveness and reduce the risk of upset stomach, dizziness, and lightheadedness.

Usual Dose

Adult: 150 mg a day in divided doses with food, to start. This dose may be increased by 50 mg a day every 3–4 days, to a maximum of 400 mg a day. Severely depressed people may be prescribed as much as 600 mg a day. Trazodone can cause drowsiness, which may require the administration of the major portion of the daily dose near bedtime.

Child: not recommended.

Overdosage

Drowsiness and vomiting are the most frequent symptoms of trazodone overdose. Others include very severe side effects, especially those affecting mood and heart function. Fever may be present at first, but as time passes body temperature will drop below normal. Victims must be taken to a hospital emergency room immediately. If you seek treatment, ALWAYS bring the prescription bottle or container.

Special Information

Be careful when driving or performing any task that requires concentration. Avoid alcohol or other depressant drugs while taking trazodone.

Contact your doctor if you develop any side effect, especially blood in the urine, dizziness, or lightheadedness. Trazodone may cause dry mouth, irregular heartbeat, nausea, vomiting, or breathing difficulties.

If you forget a dose, take it as soon as possible. If it is within 4 hours of your next dose, skip the dose you forgot and go back to your regular schedule. Do not take a double dose.

Special Populations

Pregnancy/Breast-feeding: Trazodone may damage the fetus and generally should not be taken by women who are or might be pregnant. Trazodone should be taken during pregnancy only if your doctor determines that the potential benefit outweighs the risks.

Trazodone passes into breast milk. Nursing mothers who must take it should consider using infant formula.

Seniors: Seniors may be more sensitive to trazodone's effects and should start with lower doses.

Generic Name

Treprostinil (tree-PROSS-tin-ill)

Brand Names

Remodulin Tyvaso

Type of Drug

Vasodilator.

Prescribed For

Pulmonary arterial hypertension (PAH).

General Information

Treprostinil injection was introduced 3 years before the inhalation and requires self-inserting a catheter under the skin and using an infusion pump. These requirements expose the patient to important risks, including blood infection. Both forms work identically by dilating pulmonary arteries, and arteries throughout the body, making it easier to move blood through them and for PAH patients to function. However treprostinil's action is short lived and noticeably wears off by the time the next dose is due. Many people plan their treprostinil doses around planned activities to give them maximum flexibility. Treprostinil can be added to bosentan or sildenafil, 2 oral vasodilators often prescribed for PAH.

PAH is high pressure in the arteries that carry blood from your heart to your lungs, where red blood cells pick up oxygen to carry throughout your body. People with PAH do not move enough blood through the lungs because the pulmonary arteries have become hard and stiff. Also, the heart must work harder to pump blood through the arteries because they are not as flexible as they should be. As a result, people with PAH tire easily and can have trouble breathing during normal physical activities such as climbing stairs or walking. Other symptoms of PAH include generally feeling tired, chest pain, and rapid heartbeat. Physical activity gradually becomes more limited as the condition worsens. There is no cure for PAH, but early diagnosis and treatment makes it easier to control.

Cautions and Warnings

Do not take treprostinil if you are **allergic** or **sensitive** to any of its ingredients.

The safety and effectiveness of treprostinil is not known in people with significant lung disease such as **asthma** or **chronic obstructive pulmonary disease**.

This drug can cause low blood pressure in some people.

People with **liver or kidney disease** may be less able to tolerate the medicine because they cannot eliminate it as efficiently from their bodies. Dosage adjustments may be required.

Treprostinil can increase bleeding risk.

Possible Side Effects

- ▼ Most common: cough, headache, nausea, dizziness, flushing, throat irritation or pain, and diarrhea.
- ▼ Common: fainting.
- ▼ Less common: nosebleeds, vomiting blood, and wheezing.
- ▼ Rare: pneumonia. Contact your doctor if you experience anything unusual while taking any medication.

Additional side effects reported with treprostinil injection are rash; jaw pain; swelling in the feet, ankles, or legs; and low blood pressure.

Drug Interactions

- Diuretic drugs, drugs for high blood pressure, and vasodilator drugs taken for other purposes increase the risk of low blood pressure when treprostinil is added.

- Gemfibrozil, glitazone antidiabetes drugs, montelukast, trimethoprim, and the dietary supplement quercetin increase treprostinil blood levels by interfering with its breakdown in the liver. Dose reduction is required while you are taking these medicines to avoid drug side effects.
- Rifampin can reduce blood levels of treprostinil by stimulating its breakdown in the liver. You may have to take more treprostinil if you are also taking rifampin to continue to get the benefit of this medicine.
- Treprostinil increases bleeding by affecting platelets in much the same way as aspirin, clopidogrel, prasugrel, and some other medicines. Your anticoagulant dose should be checked and may need adjustment if you are taking warfarin or another blood thinner.

Food Interactions

Treprostinil should be inhaled while there is nothing in your mouth that might interfere with breathing in the complete dose.

Usual Dose

Remodulin

Adult: Liver function and body weight are considerations when calculating your starting dose. Dose is modified according to your response to the medicine.

Child: not recommended.

Tyvaso

Adult: 3 inhalations 4 times a day, 4 hours apart, to start. Dose is adjusted according to individual tolerance. The ideal maintenance dose is 9 inhalations 4 times a day. Side effects may limit the maximum you can take.

Child: not recommended.

Overdosage

Overdose symptoms can be expected to include facial flushing, headache, low blood pressure, nausea, vomiting, and diarrhea. Contact your doctor or a local poison control center for information. If you seek treatment, ALWAYS bring the prescription bottle or container.

Special Information

Treprostinil inhalation must be taken with the system that comes with the product. It is specially made to give you the correct dose of only the medicine with which it is packaged. Be sure to clean it completely after the last treatment session of the day. Consider having a backup system available in case yours stops working, to avoid interruptions in your treatment.

Do not mix any other inhalation medicine with treprostinil or use the inhalation system for another medicine.

Treprostinil is irritating. Do not swallow it. If gets on your skin or in your eyes, wash it off immediately.

Each treprostinil ampule contains enough medicine for a single day's treatment to use when you set up the machine each morning. Throw away any leftover medicine at the end of the day.

Each treatment session takes about 2 minutes. You must take this medicine exactly as directed. If you forget a dose, take it as soon as you can. If your treatment session is interrupted for any reason, finish it as soon as possible. Do not take a double dose of treprostinil, and do not take more than your doctor has prescribed at any time.

Make sure your doctor knows all the medicines you are taking and that you report taking treprostinil to any other doctors who might prescribe additional medicines.

Special Populations

Pregnancy/Breast-feeding: There is limited information on the effects of this drug in pregnant animals and none in pregnant women. Treprostinil should be taken during pregnancy only if your doctor determines that the potential benefit outweighs the risks.

It is not known if treprostinil passes into breast milk. Nursing mothers who take it should use infant formula.

Seniors: Seniors may be more sensitive to treprostinil because of the increased chance of heart, kidney, or liver disease in older adults.

Generic Name

Tretinoin (TRET-in-oh-in) G

Brand Names

Atralin	Renova
Avita	Retin-A
Refissa	Retin-A Micro

Combination Products
Generic Ingredients: Fluocinolone Acetonide + Hydroquinone + Tretinoin
Tri-Luma

Generic Ingredients: Mequinol + Tretinoin
Solage

The information in this profile also applies to the following drugs:

Generic Ingredients: Tazarotene
Avage Tazorac

Type of Drug

Antiacne; skin irritant and anti-wrinkling agent; and antineoplastic.

Prescribed For

Acne and other skin conditions, skin cancer, acute promyelocytic leukemia (APL), wrinkling, and liver spots caused by chronic sun exposure.

General Information

Tretinoin, also known as retinoic acid or vitamin A acid, works against acne by decreasing the cohesiveness of skin cells, causing the skin to peel. Tazarotene, a retinoid related to vitamin A, is converted to its active form after it is applied to the skin. These drugs are usually not effective in treating severe acne. They are best suited for mild to moderate acne.

Medical research shows that regular application of tretinoin cream to aging skin prevents wrinkling and may even reverse the wrinkling process for some people. Tretinoin causes a temporary "plumping" of the skin when it is applied, peeling the outer layer. This gives the appearance of improved skin and reduced wrinkling. Some tretinoin—about 5%—is absorbed through the skin. When used to treat APL, a blood cancer, tretinoin causes the leukemia cells to mature and reduces the spread of APL cells; the exact way it works is not known.

Cautions and Warnings

Do not use these drugs if you are **allergic** or **sensitive** to any of their ingredients.

Women who are **pregnant** should not use these drugs due to the high risk of birth defects.

These drugs may increase the skin cancer–causing effects of ultraviolet light. If you apply this drug to your skin, you should allow a "rest period" between uses of these drugs and other skin irritants or peeling agents. You must also limit sun exposure to treated areas and avoid sunlamps. If you cannot avoid sun exposure, use sunscreen and protective covering.

Do not apply these drugs close to your eyes, the sides of the nose, or to mucous membrane tissue.

People with APL are at high risk for severe side effects. About 25% of people with APL treated with tretinoin develop a group of symptoms called retinoic acid–APL syndrome. These symptoms include fever, breathing difficulties, weight gain, and fluid in the lungs. Low blood pressure and loss of heart function may also occur.

Forty percent of people who take oral tretinoin develop a rapid increase in white-blood-cell count, which is associated with greater risk of life-threatening complications. Sixty percent of people taking tretinoin develop high blood-cholesterol or triglyceride levels.

Retinoids such as tretinoin have been associated with pseudotumor cerebri (increased pressure in the brain), especially in **children**. Early signs of this problem include swelling in the eyes, headache, nausea, vomiting, and visual difficulties.

Possible Side Effects

Capsules

▼ Most common: headache, fever, weakness, and fatigue. These generally go away with time.

▼ Common: skin changes, dry skin and membranes, bone pain and inflammation, itching, sweating, visual disturbances and other eye problems, hair loss, earache or a feeling of fullness in the ears, not feeling well, shivering, bleeding, infection, swelling in the arms or legs, pain, chest discomfort, weight gain, breathing difficulties, pneumonia, wheezing, abdominal pain, diarrhea, constipation, upset stomach, abnormal heart rhythms, blood-pressure changes, vein irritation, dizziness, tingling in the hands or feet, sleeplessness, depression, confusion, and bleeding in the brain.

▼ Less common: muscle aches, pain in the side, skin irritation, facial swelling, loss of color, lymph system problems, asthma, swollen larynx, gas, swollen liver, hepatitis, ulcer, heart failure, heart attack, heart inflammation, kidney problems (such as kidney failure, painful urination, and frequent urination), enlarged prostate, agitation, hallucination, an

Possible Side Effects *(continued)*

unusual walk, convulsions, coma, depression, paralysis of the face, and a variety of nervous system problems.

▼ Rare: hearing loss. Contact your doctor if you experience anything unusual while taking any medication.

Skin Products

▼ Most common: burning, stinging, tingling, itching, swelling, peeling, or blistering of the skin; formation of crusts on the skin near the application site; and temporary skin discoloration and greater sun sensitivity. All side effects disappear after the drug has been stopped.

▼ Common: skin irritation.

▼ Less common: dry skin, crusting, and rash.

Drug Interactions

Capsules

- Combining tretinoin with ketoconazole and other drugs that affect systems in the liver causes a substantial increase in tretinoin blood levels.

Skin Products

- Other skin irritants will cause excessive sensitivity, irritation, and side effects. Among the substances that cause this interaction are medications that contain sulfur in topical form, benzoyl peroxide, resorcinol, or salicylic acid; abrasive soaps or skin cleansers; cosmetics, creams, or ointments with a severe drying effect; and products with a high alcohol, astringent, spice, or lime content.
- Tretinoin increases the absorption of minoxidil through the skin when they are applied together, leading to lower blood pressure.
- Do not use tretinoin if you are also taking a drug that increases sensitivity to the sun, such as fluoroquinolone antibiotics, tetracyclines, and thiazides.

Food Interactions

Tretinoin capsules are better absorbed when taken with food.

Usual Dose

Capsules: Dosage is individualized for each person. Doses are calculated from height and weight.

Skin Products: Wash the affected area thoroughly, then wait 20–30 minutes and apply a small amount of tretinoin at bedtime.

Overdosage

Ingesting these drugs is like taking vitamin A and can be extremely dangerous for pregnant women, who should not take more vitamin A than is contained in their prenatal vitamins. Children who accidentally swallow tretinoin should be taken to a hospital emergency room. Symptoms include headache, facial flushing, abdominal pain, dizziness, and weakness. These symptoms have resolved without apparent after-effects. If you seek treatment, ALWAYS bring the prescription bottle or container.

Special Information

Your acne may worsen during the first few weeks of treatment because the drug is acting on deeper, hidden lesions. This is beneficial and is not a reason to stop using tretinoin. Results should be seen in 2–3 weeks but may not reach maximum effect for 6 weeks; normal cosmetics can be used during this time.

Keep these drugs away from your eyes, nose, mouth, and mucous membranes. Avoid skin exposure to sunlight or sunlamps.

Applying too much medication will cause skin irritation and peeling but will not increase its effectiveness. Use your fingertip, a gauze pad, or a cotton swab when applying tretinoin to acne lesions to reduce the chances of applying too much medication.

You may feel warmth and slight stinging when you apply these drugs. If you develop a burning sensation, peeling, redness, or are uncomfortable, stop using them for a short time.

Avoid using depilatories or waxing, or any product that might irritate the skin, while using topical tretinoin.

Extreme weather or wind may cause severe irritation of skin treated with tretinoin.

If you forget a dose of tretinoin, do not apply the forgotten dose. Skip it and continue with your regular schedule. Do not apply a double dose.

Special Populations

Pregnancy/Breast-feeding: At very high doses, these drugs cause birth defects in animals. A pregnant woman taking tretinoin capsules is likely to deliver a severely deformed infant. Women who need to take tretinoin capsules should be tested for pregnancy before treatment is started. Use 2 reliable forms of contraception while you are taking tretinoin and for 1 month after treatment has ended. When applied to the skin, tretinoin is rapidly broken down. The topical form of these drugs should not be taken during pregnancy.

It is not known if these drugs pass into breast milk. Nursing mothers who must take them should use infant formula.

Seniors: Seniors may use this product without special precaution.

TriCor *see **Fenofibrate,** page 489*

Type of Drug

Tricyclic Antidepressants

Brand Names

Generic Ingredients: Amitriptyline Hydrochloride G

Generic Ingredients: Amoxapine G

Generic Ingredients: Clomipramine Hydrochloride G
Anafranil

Generic Ingredients: Desipramine Hydrochloride G
Norpramin

Generic Ingredients: Doxepin Hydrochloride G
Silenor

Generic Ingredients: Imipramine G
Tofranil
Tofranil-PM

Generic Ingredients: Nortriptyline Hydrochloride G
Aventyl
Pamelor

Generic Ingredients: Protriptyline G
Vivactil

Generic Ingredients: Trimipramine Maleate G
Surmontil

Combination Products
Generic Ingredients: Amitriptyline Hydrochloride + Chlordiazepoxide G
Limbitrol
Limbitrol DS

Generic Ingredients: Amitriptyline Hydrochloride + Perphenazine G

Prescribed For

Depression, with or without symptoms of anxiety, agitation, or sleep disturbance; neurotic or psychotic depressive disorder, or depression or anxiety associated with disease or alcoholism (not to be taken with alcohol); temporary therapy for urine incontinence in children age 6 and over (imipramine only). Clomipramine is prescribed only for obsessive-compulsive disorder. These medications may also be used for chronic pain due to migraine, tension headache, diabetic neuropathy, tic douloureux, cancer, herpes lesions, and arthritis; pathologic laughing or weeping caused by brain disease; bulimia; sleep apnea; peptic ulcer disease; cocaine withdrawal; panic disorder; eating disorder; premenstrual depression; and skin problems.

General Information

Tricyclic antidepressants block the passage of stimulant chemicals—norepinephrine and/or serotonin—in and out of nerve endings, producing a sedative effect. They also counteract the effects of the neurohormone acetylcholine. Antidepressants work by causing long-term changes in the way nerve endings function. Tricyclic antidepressants can elevate mood, increase physical activity and mental alertness, and improve appetite and sleep patterns after 2–4 weeks of use.

Tricyclic antidepressants have been used in treating nighttime bed-wetting but do not produce long-lasting results. The combination of amitriptyline and perphenazine, a sedative, is used to treat anxiety, agitation, and depression associated with chronic physical or psychiatric disease. The combination of amitriptyline and chlordiazepoxide, an antianxiety drug, is used to treat anxiety and depression. Protriptyline may be especially useful for very withdrawn or lethargic depressed people due to its activating properties. Tricyclic antidepressants are broken down in the liver.

Cautions and Warnings

Do not take tricyclic antidepressants if you are **allergic** or **sensitive** to any of their ingredients or to sulfites.

Antidepressants have been associated with an increased risk of suicide and suicidal thinking, especially in **teenagers** and **young adults**. Younger people who start taking an antidepressant should be observed closely for worsening of their depression, suicidality, or unusual changes in behavior. The risk of suicide is about the same in people age 25–64 and reduced in people age 65 and over. Suicide is always a risk in severely depressed people, who should only be allowed to have minimal quantities of medication in their possession.

Amoxapine may cause very high fever, muscle rigidity, changes in mental state, irregular pulse or blood pressure, sweating, abnormal heart rhythms, and rapid heartbeat. This group of symptoms is associated with neuroleptic malignant syndrome (NMS), which may be fatal. If these symptoms develop, stop taking your medication at once and contact your doctor. Clomipramine may also cause very high fever, especially when used with other drugs; this may also be a sign of NMS.

Amoxapine may increase the risk of potentially irreversible involuntary muscle movements associated with tardive dyskinesia (symptoms include lip smacking or puckering, puffing of the cheeks, rapid or wormlike tongue movements, uncontrolled chewing motions, and uncontrolled arm and leg movements). This condition is more common among the elderly, especially women.

These drugs should not be used if you are recovering from a **heart attack**.

Rapid heartbeat and fainting when rising from a sitting or lying position are problems associated with protriptyline.

These drugs should be taken with caution if you have a history of **epilepsy or other convulsive disorders**, **seizure** (which may be a special problem with clomipramine), **difficulty urinating**, **glaucoma**, **heart disease**, **kidney or liver disease**, or **hyperthyroidism**. Doxepin should not be taken by those with **glaucoma** or **difficulty urinating**.

Antidepressants may aggravate the condition of people who are **schizophrenic** or **paranoid** and may cause people with **bipolar (manic-depressive) disorder** to switch phase. These reactions are also possible when changing or stopping antidepressants.

Tricyclic antidepressants should not be combined with monoamine oxidase inhibitor (MAOI) antidepressants except under close medical supervision.

Possible Side Effects

▼ Most common: sedation and anticholinergic effects, including blurred vision; disorientation; confusion; hallucinations; muscle spasm or tremors; seizures or convulsions; dry mouth;

Possible Side Effects *(continued)*

constipation, especially in older adults; difficulty urinating; worsening glaucoma; and sensitivity to bright light.

- ▼ Less common: blood-pressure changes, abnormal heart rate, heart attack, anxiety, restlessness, excitement, numbness and tingling in the extremities, poor coordination, rash, itching, fluid retention, fever, allergy, changes in blood composition, nausea, vomiting, appetite loss, upset stomach, diarrhea, enlargement of the breasts in men and women, changes in sex drive, and blood-sugar changes.
- ▼ Rare: Rare side effects can occur in almost any part of the body. Contact your doctor if you experience anything unusual while taking any medication.

Drug Interactions

- Combining a tricyclic antidepressant with an MAOI antidepressant may cause high fever, convulsions, and death. Do not take an MAOI until at least 2 weeks after amitriptyline has been discontinued. People who must take both an MAOI and a tricyclic antidepressant require close medical observation.
- Selective serotonin reuptake inhibitors (SSRIs) may increase blood levels of tricyclic antidepressants. Allow up to 5 weeks between switching from fluoxetine to a tricyclic antidepressant.
- Tricyclic antidepressants may increase levels of clonidine, causing dangerously high blood pressure. This combination should be avoided.
- Tricyclics increase the effects of anticholinergic drugs, possibly causing severe constipation.
- Barbiturates, charcoal, and rifamycins may decrease the effectiveness of a tricyclic antidepressant.
- Bupropion, cimetidine, famotidine, haloperidol, nizatidine, ranitidine, and valproic acid may increase the effects of tricyclic antidepressants.
- Combining tricyclic antidepressants and carbamazepine may cause decreases in antidepressant blood levels while increasing carbamazepine levels.
- The blood-thinning effects of dicumarol may be increased by tricyclic antidepressants.
- Combining a tricyclic antidepressant and methylphenidate or a phenothiazine drug may cause severe side effects.

- Tricyclics decrease the blood-pressure-lowering effects of guanethidine.
- These medications may inhibit the effects of levodopa + carbidopa.
- Tricyclic antidepressants may increase the effects of quinolones, such as grepafloxacin and sparfloxacin, increasing the risk of dangerous heart rhythm disorders.
- Smoking may increase the effects of a tricyclic antidepressant.

Food Interactions

You may take a tricyclic antidepressant with food if it upsets your stomach.

Usual Dose

Amitriptyline

Adult: 40–100 mg a day, increased to 150 mg a day if necessary. Hospitalized patients may take up to 300 mg a day if needed. Dosages for conditions other than depression range from 10–300 mg a day.

Child (age 12 and over): 10 mg 3 times a day and 20 mg at bedtime.

Child (under age 12): 0.5–2 mg per lb. per day.

Senior: Lower dosages are recommended, generally 30–50 mg a day.

Amoxapine

Adult and Child (age 17 and over): 100–400 mg a day. Hospitalized patients may need up to 600 mg a day.

Child (under age 17): not recommended.

Senior: Lower dosages are recommended. People over age 60 usually take 100–300 mg a day.

Clomipramine

Adult: 25–250 mg a day.

Child (age 10 and over): 25–200 mg or 1.4 mg per lb. of body weight a day, whichever is less.

Child (under age 10): not recommended.

This drug may be taken at bedtime to minimize daytime sedation.

Desipramine

Adult: 100–200 mg a day. More severely ill patients may need dosages up to 300 mg a day. People taking higher dosages should have regular heart examinations to check for side effects.

Child (age 12 and over) and Senior: Lower dosages are recommended, usually 25–100 mg a day. Doses above 150 mg a day are not recommended for these age groups.

Child (under age 12): not recommended.

Doxepin

Adult and Child (age 12 and over): Start with 25–75 mg a day, then increase as needed to a maximum daily dose of 150 mg a day for mild to moderate disease and 300 mg a day for more severe anxiety or depression. For insomnia: 6 mg once a day (Silenor).

Imipramine

Adult: 100–300 mg a day in divided doses.

Child (age 6 and over): 30–100 mg a day for depression in adolescents; 25 mg a day, given 1 hour before bedtime for nighttime bed-wetting. If bed-wetting does not cease within a week, daily dosage is typically increased to 50–75 mg depending on age—more than 75 mg a day increases side effects without increasing effectiveness. Doses are often taken in mid-afternoon and at bedtime. The dosage should be gradually reduced to help prevent bed-wetting from recurring.

Senior: starting dose—30–40 mg a day; maintenance dose—usually less than 100 mg a day.

Nortriptyline

Adult: 25 mg 3–4 times a day, increased to 150 mg a day if necessary.

Child (age 13 and over) and Senior: Lower dosages are recommended, generally 30–50 mg a day.

Child (under age 13): not recommended.

Protriptyline

Adult: 15–60 mg a day in 3–4 divided doses. Protriptyline must not be taken as a single bedtime dose because of its stimulant effect.

Child (age 13 and over) and Senior: Lower dosages are recommended, usually up to 20 mg a day. Seniors taking more than 20 mg a day should have regular heart examinations.

Child (under age 13): not recommended.

Trimipramine

Adult: 100–300 mg a day in divided doses.

Child (age 13 and over) and Senior: starting dose—50 mg a day; maintenance dose—up to 100 mg a day.

Child (under age 13): not recommended.

Overdosage

Symptoms include confusion, inability to concentrate, hallucinations, drowsiness, lowered body temperature, abnormal heart rate, heart failure, enlarged pupils, convulsions, severely lowered blood pressure, stupor, and coma. Overdose victims should be taken to a hospital emergency room immediately. If you seek treatment, ALWAYS bring the prescription bottle or container.

Special Information

Avoid alcohol and other depressants while taking any tricyclic antidepressant. Do not stop taking your medication without your doctor's knowledge. Abruptly stopping a tricyclic antidepressant may cause nausea, headache, and feelings of ill health.

Tricyclic antidepressants may cause drowsiness, dizziness, and blurred vision. Be careful when driving or doing any task that requires concentration.

The following symptoms may occur early in treatment or when the drug dosage is adjusted up or down: anxiety, agitation, panic attacks, sleeplessness, irritability, restlessness, hostility, aggressiveness, acting impulsively, a manic reaction, deepening of depression, other unusual changes in behavior, and suicidal thinking. Report anything unusual to your doctor at once.

Contact your doctor immediately if you develop seizures, breathing difficulties or rapid breathing, fever and sweating, blood-pressure changes, muscle stiffness, loss of bladder control, or unusual tiredness or weakness.

Dry mouth may lead to an increase in dental cavities and gum bleeding and disease. Maintain good dental hygiene while taking a tricyclic antidepressant.

Discontinue therapy for as long as possible prior to elective surgery.

If your symptoms are unchanged after 6–8 weeks of treatment with an antidepressant, contact your doctor.

These medications may cause sensitivity to the sun. Be sure to wear protective clothing or sunblock if you are exposed to the sun, and avoid prolonged exposure.

If you forget a dose, skip it and go back to your regular schedule. Do not take a double dose.

Special Populations

Pregnancy/Breast-feeding: Tricyclic antidepressants cross into the fetal circulation. Birth defects, including heart, breathing, and urinary problems, have been reported when women took a tricyclic antidepressant during the first 3 months of pregnancy. A tricyclic antidepressant should be taken during pregnancy only if your doctor determines that the potential benefit outweighs the risks.

Small amounts of these drugs pass into breast milk. Nursing mothers who must take a tricyclic antidepressant should use infant formula.

Seniors: Seniors are more sensitive to the effects of these drugs, especially abnormal heart rhythms and other cardiac side effects, and often require a reduced dosage.

Trilipix *see **Fenofibrate,** page 489*

Type of Drug

Triptan-Type Antimigraine Drugs

(TRIP-tan)

Brand Names

Generic Ingredients: Almotriptan
Axert

Generic Ingredients: Eletriptan
Relpax

Generic Ingredients: Frovatriptan
Frova

Generic Ingredients: Naratriptan G
Amerge

Generic Ingredients: Rizatriptan
Maxalt
Maxalt-MLT

Generic Ingredients: Sumatriptan G
Alsuma
Imitrex
Sumavel

Generic Ingredients: Zolmitriptan
Zomig
Zomig ZMT

Combination Products
Generic Ingredients: Sumatriptan + Naproxen
Treximet

Prescribed For

Migraine headache; sumatriptan injection can be used for cluster headaches.

General Information

Triptan-type drugs are used to alleviate symptoms of migraine, which involve severe headaches as well as nausea, vomiting, and increased sensitivity to light and sound. These drugs work by interfering with one type of serotonin receptor in the brain and do not affect other serotonin receptors. This action constricts (narrows) blood vessels in the brain, which are usually dilated (widened) during a migraine attack. While these drugs can alleviate symptoms of migraine, they do not prevent attacks.

Triptan-type drugs are only recommended after analgesics (pain relievers)—such as acetaminophen, aspirin, and other nonsteroidal anti-inflammatory drugs (NSAIDs)—have failed to relieve symptoms. If you experience serious, incapacitating migraines more often than twice a month, your doctor may recommend taking other medications on a regular basis to reduce the number and severity of attacks. Triptan-type drugs generally start to relieve migraine symptoms in about 1 hour; rizatriptan works fastest. They are broken down partially in the liver.

Recent information indicates that these medications may be more effective when taken with an NSAID. Sumatriptan has been combined with an NSAID to make it more convenient to take the 2 medicines together. For more information on Nonsteroidal Anti-inflammatory Drugs (NSAIDs), see page 863.

Cautions and Warnings

Do not take triptans if you are **allergic** or **sensitive** to any of their ingredients. People allergic to sulfa drugs may also be allergic to almotriptan. Stop taking the drug and contact your doctor at once if you develop shortness of breath; wheezing; heart palpitations; swelling of the eyelids, face, or lips; rash; lumps; hives; severe tightness in the chest or throat; or sudden abdominal pain.

You should not take triptan-type drugs if you have uncontrolled **high blood pressure**, **peripheral vascular disease**, or **heart disease**, including angina, uncontrolled high blood pressure, or a history of heart attack, stroke, or mini-stroke. It is strongly recommended that triptan-type drugs not be taken by people who are at risk for heart disease, as indicated by high blood pressure,

arteriosclerosis (hardening of the arteries), **high blood cholesterol**, **smoking**, **obesity**, **diabetes**, and a **family history of heart disease**. If you have any of these risk factors, your doctor must evaluate your heart disease risk before prescribing one of these drugs. People who take triptan-type drugs regularly or who develop risk factors for heart disease should be reevaluated by their doctors. Rarely, serious cardiac problems have occurred after taking one of these drugs.

Strokes and some fatalities have occurred in people taking a triptan-type drug, though these events may have happened because a stroke-related headache was treated with a triptan rather than as a symptom of stroke. People with migraine are more likely to have a stroke or bleeding in the brain. Sumatriptan has been associated with seizures.

Do not take triptans if you suffer from **hemiplegic or basilar migraines**. These drugs are only effective for migraine pain (sumatriptan injection may be used for cluster headaches).

People with severe **liver disease** should not use eletriptan, naratriptan, or sumatriptan. People with mild to moderate liver disease should use any triptan with caution. Rizatriptan and sumatriptan must be used with caution by people with severe **kidney disease**.

People have experienced chest, neck, or jaw tightness and pain after taking 1 of these drugs, but these sensations are rarely associated with heart problems.

Do not take these drugs if your headache is different from your usual migraine pain in any way. A change in the characteristics of your headache may signal a much more serious problem. Contact your doctor at once.

People taking Treximet should contact their doctor at once if they develop any of the following: flu-like symptoms; stomach pain or a sudden or severe abdominal pain; vomiting blood; black, tarry stool; itching, skin rash, or blisters with fever; yellowing of the skin or whites of the eyes; swelling of the arms and legs, hands, feet, face, lips, or tongue; unusual weight gain; or feeling more tired or weaker than usual.

People with **phenylketonuria** should be aware that rizatriptan and zolmitriptan disintegrating tablets contain phenylalanine.

These drugs can collect in the colored part of the eye and cause eye disorders if taken over a long period. Have your eyes checked regularly.

Possible Side Effects

Side effects are usually mild or moderate, do not last long, and may increase with dosage. Some reported side effects (nausea, vomiting, dizziness, fainting, a feeling of ill health, drowsiness, and sedation) are also migraine symptoms.

Rare side effects can affect the heart and blood vessels, nervous system, skin, stomach and intestines, urinary and reproductive systems, blood, muscles, bones, eyes, ears, nose, throat, and other parts of the body. Contact your doctor if you experience anything unusual while taking any medication.

Almotriptan

▼ Most common: nausea, tiredness, tingling in the hands or feet, dry mouth, and headache.

Eletriptan

▼ Most common: weakness, dizziness, sleepiness, and nausea.

▼ Less common: chest, neck, jaw, or throat tightness; dry mouth; upset stomach; flushing; tingling in the hands or feet; abdominal pain or discomfort; and difficulty swallowing.

Frovatriptan

▼ Most common: dizziness, tiredness, and headache.

▼ Less common: tingling in the hands or feet, dry mouth, upset stomach, flushing, skeletal pain, and hot or cold sensations.

Naratriptan

▼ Most common: weakness; nausea; tingling in the hands or feet; dizziness; fatigue; drowsiness; pain or pressure in the neck, throat, or jaw; and generalized pain.

Rizatriptan

▼ Most common: dizziness, tiredness, fatigue, and nausea.

▼ Less common: tingling in the hands or feet; headache; pain or pressure in the neck, throat, chest, or jaw; generalized pain; and dry mouth.

Sumatriptan

▼ Most common: tingling and nasal discomfort (nasal spray).

▼ Less common: unusual sensations of warmth or cold; flushing; heart palpitations; pain, pressure, or tightness in the

Possible Side Effects *(continued)*

jaw, throat, or neck; heaviness, tightness, and pressure in the chest; eye problems; and weakness. At high dosages, agitation, eye irritation, and painful urination may occur.

Zolmitriptan

▼ Most common: dizziness, weakness, sleepiness, tightness in the jaw or neck, tingling, a warm or burning sensation, tiredness, nausea, and fainting.

▼ Less common: diminished sensitivity to stimulation, heart palpitations, chest pain or pressure, sweating, and muscle aches.

Drug Interactions

- Do not take triptans within 24 hours of taking an ergot-based drug (such as dihydroergotamine).
- Do not take more than 1 triptan-type drug within 24 hours of another brand of these drugs.
- Triptans should not be used with a selective serotonin reuptake inhibitor (SSRI) antidepressant, such as fluoxetine, fluvoxamine, paroxetine, or sertraline, or a serotonin-norepinephrine reuptake inhibitor (SNRI) such as duloxetine unless medically necessary. Combining these drugs can lead to serotonin syndrome, a potentially fatal condition. Symptoms include weakness, overly sensitive reflexes, poor coordination, agitation, hallucinations, coma, rapid heartbeat, unstable blood pressure, fever, nausea, vomiting, and diarrhea.
- Monoamine oxidase inhibitor (MAOI) antidepressants can increase blood levels of almotriptan, rizatriptan, sumatriptan, and zolmitriptan, and the risk of their side effects. Do not combine these drugs or take these triptans within 2 weeks of stopping your MAOI medicine.
- Do not use eletriptan within at least 3 days of taking clarithromycin, itraconazole, ketoconazole, nefazodone, nelfinavir, and ritonavir. Almotriptan should be used with caution with these medications.
- Contraceptives increase frovatriptan blood levels and the risk of side effects.
- Cimetidine significantly increases blood levels of zolmitriptan.
- Propranolol may significantly increase eletriptan, frovatriptan, and rizatriptan blood levels.

- If you take Treximet, do not add another pain reliever or fever reducer without first asking your doctor. Because an NSAID is already part of your treatment, adding aspirin or another NSAID increases your risk of stomach damage and bleeding.

Food Interactions

These drugs can be taken without regard to food or meals. Avoid large quantities of grapefruit and starfruit products while you are taking these medicines because they can increase blood levels of the triptan drugs.

Usual Dose

Unless otherwise noted, you may take another dose 2 hours after your first if symptoms improve but then return. If you do not feel better after taking a triptan, call your doctor. Do not take another dose, as you may have a different kind of headache.

Almotriptan

Adult and Child (age 12 and over): 6.25–12.5 mg up to a maximum of 25 mg a day. The safety of treating more than 4 migraines a month has not been established.

Child (under age 12): not recommended.

Eletriptan

Adult: 20–40 mg up to a maximum of 80 mg a day. The safety of treating more than 3 migraines a month has not been established.

Child: not recommended.

Frovatriptan

Adult: 2.5 mg up to a maximum of three 2.5-mg tablets a day. The safety of treating more than 4 migraines a month has not been established.

Child: not recommended.

Naratriptan

Adult: 1–2.5 mg; you may take another dose 4 hours after the first if symptoms return after improvement; up to a maximum 5 mg a day. The safety of treating more than 4 migraines a month has not been established.

Child and Senior: not recommended.

Rizatriptan

Adult

Tablets: 5–10 mg up to a maximum of 30 mg a day. People also taking propranolol should take no more than 5 mg of rizatriptan at a time, up to 15 mg a day. The safety of treating more than 4 migraine headaches a month has not been established.

Disintegrating Tablets: 5–10 mg any time during the attack with or without fluid. Do not take the tablet out of its protective packaging until just before you swallow it. Make sure your hands are dry and place the tablet on your tongue, where it will dissolve and be swallowed with your saliva.

Child: not recommended.

Sumatriptan

The safety of treating more than 4 migraine headaches a month has not been established

Injection

Adult: 6 mg as a subcutaneous injection up to 12 mg a day.

Child: less than 66 lbs.—3 mg; more than 66 lbs.—6 mg.

Nasal Spray

Adult and Child: 1–2 sprays of the 5-mg nasal spray or 1 spray of the 20-mg spray into 1 nostril only (if administering a 10-mg dose, spray 5 mg into each nostril). Do not take more than 40 mg (8 sprays of the 5-mg or 2 sprays of the 20-mg) a day.

Tablets

Adult and Child (age 12 and over): 25–100 mg up to 200 mg a day. People with liver disease should take the lowest effective dosage.

Child (under age 12): 50 mg.

Senior: not recommended.

Sumatriptan + Naproxen

Adult: 1 tablet (85/500 mg) up to 2 tablets a day. Do not treat more than 4 migraines in a month. Do not split, crush, or chew these tablets.

Child and Senior: not recommended.

Zolmitriptan

Adult

Tablets: 1–5 mg up to a maximum of 10 mg a day. People with liver disease should take the lowest effective dosage. The safety of treating more than 3 migraine headaches a month has not been established.

Nasal Spray: one 5-mg dose into 1 nostril. Do not use more than 10 mg (2 sprays) in a 24-hour period. The safety of treating more than 4 migraine headaches in a month has not been established.

Child: not recommended.

Overdosage

Overdose can be expected to cause sedation, convulsions, tremors, swelling, redness in the arms or legs, physical inactivity, slowed breathing, bluish discoloration of the lips or skin under the fingernails, weakness, dilated pupils, paralysis, increased blood pressure, lightheadedness, neck tension, or poor coordination. Take the victim to a hospital emergency room. If you seek treatment, ALWAYS bring the prescription bottle or container.

Special Information

These drugs may make you tired or dizzy. Be careful when driving or performing any task that requires concentration.

These drugs can increase your sensitivity to the sun. Use sunscreen and wear protective clothing.

These drugs are meant only to treat migraine or cluster headaches. They do not work for all types of headache or pain.

You may enhance the effect of triptan-type drugs if you lie down in a quiet, dark room.

Avoid alcohol because it can worsen your headaches.

Contact your doctor if the usual dosage does not relieve 3 consecutive headaches or if your headaches become more frequent or worse.

Special Populations

Pregnancy/Breast-feeding: Animal studies have shown possible toxic effects on the fetus. A triptan-type antimigraine drug should be taken during pregnancy only if your doctor determines that the potential benefit outweighs the risks.

Sumatriptan and eletriptan pass into breast milk. Animal studies show that some other triptan-type drugs may pass into breast milk. Nursing mothers who must take any of these drugs should use infant formula.

Seniors: Migraines occur rarely in seniors so triptans have not been well studied in older adults. Because their liver or kidney function may be decreased, seniors should not take naratriptan or sumatriptan. Almotriptan should be used at the lowest effective dose. Frovatriptan blood levels may be increased in seniors.

Generic Name

Ustekinumab (oos-teh-KIN-u-mab)

Brand Names

Stelara

Type of Drug

Interleukin antagonist.

Prescribed For

Moderate to severe plaque psoriasis.

General Information

Plaque psoriasis is an immune system disorder that results in the rapid overproduction of skin cells characterized by thick patches of inflamed, red skin, often covered with silvery scales. Ustekinumab is a monoclonal antibody that binds with 2 proteins that are key contributors to the overproduction of skin cells. It is slowly absorbed from the injection site, reaching maximum blood concentration in about 2 weeks. Larger doses allow maximum concentration in 1 week. It is intended for people with moderate to severe psoriasis that covers large areas or many different areas of the body, who may benefit from injections, pills, or phototherapy (ultraviolet light with or without pills).

Cautions and Warnings

Do not take this drug if you are **allergic** or **sensitive** to any of its ingredients.

Ustekinumab can interfere with your body's ability to fight infection. It should not be used while you have any **serious infection**. Some specific infections of concern are tuberculosis, salmonella, and mycobacterium, as well as any live-virus vaccination, including BCG vaccine.

Ustekinumab may increase the risk of cancer.

A rare condition known as reversible posterior leukoencephalopathy syndrome (RPLS) occurred in 1 person receiving this medicine. Symptoms include headache, confusion, seizures, and blindness.

The safety of using ustekinumab for more than 2 years is not known.

Possible Side Effects

- ▼ Common: stuffy nose and respiratory infections.
- ▼ Less common: headache, fatigue, diarrhea, back pain, dizziness, throat pain, itching, redness and swelling after the injection, muscle aches, and depression.
- ▼ Rare: RPLS, injection-site infection, pain, bleeding, bruising, irritation, serious infection, and malignancies. Contact your doctor if you experience anything unusual while taking any medication.

Drug Interactions

- Live-virus vaccines should not be used while you are taking this medicine. Your body will not be able respond appropriately.
- Mixing phototherapy for psoriasis or drugs that suppress the immune system with ustekinumab may further suppress your immune system, exposing you to the risk of serious infection.
- Ustekinumab can affect levels of liver enzymes involved in drug breakdown in the blood. If you take cyclosporine, warfarin, or another medicine that affects liver function, your doctor should consider drug monitoring.

Usual Dose

Adult (220 lbs. and over): 90 mg by subcutaneous injection to start and again 1 week later, and then once every 12 weeks.

Adult (under 220 lbs.): 45 mg by subcutaneous injection to start and again 1 week later, and then once every 12 weeks.

Child: not recommended.

Overdosage

Doses up to 2.25 mg per lb. of body weight have been used in clinical studies with no noticeable additional side effects. In the event of an overdose, your doctor will watch you for possible overdose effects.

Special Information

Tell your doctor if you have a tuberculosis or other infection or develop any signs of infection while you are being treated with ustekinumab, including fever; chills; sweats; muscle aches; cough; difficulty breathing; weight loss; spitting up blood; diarrhea; stomach pain; warm, red, and painful skin or sores; burning when you urinate; and extreme tiredness—or if you get infections that keep coming back.

Contact your doctor if you develop headache, confusion, seizures, or vision problems.

A health care professional will give you each injection and check your skin each time.

Ustekinumab injection is colorless to light yellow and may contain a few small translucent or white particles. It should not be used if it is discolored, cloudy, or if other particles are present. The injection does not contain preservatives. Discard any unused product remaining in the vial and/or syringe after each injection.

Special Populations

Pregnancy/Breast-feeding: In animal studies, ustekinumab did not cause birth defects. There is no information about the effect of this medicine on pregnant women. It should be used during pregnancy only if your doctor determines that the potential benefit outweighs the risks.

Ustekinumab is a biological product and will likely pass into breast milk. Nursing mothers who must use this drug should use infant formula.

Seniors: Seniors included in clinical studies had the same reactions and responses as younger adults, though too few were included to establish any meaningful differences.

Generic Name

Valproic Acid (val-PROE-ik) G

Brand Names

Depakene
Stavzor

Generic Ingredients: Divalproex Sodium

Depakote
Depakote ER
Depakote Sprinkle

Type of Drug

Anticonvulsant and antimanic.

Prescribed For

Complex partial seizures and simple and complex absence seizures, prevention of migraine, and mania associated with bipolar disorder; may also be prescribed for borderline personality disorder.

General Information

Valproic acid is chemically unrelated to other drugs used in the treatment of seizure disorders. It may work by increasing levels of gamma-aminobutyric acid (GABA) and improving its effects in the brain. Valproic acid also has a stabilizing effect on cell membranes within the brain, which may account for some of the drug's other effects. It is broken down in the liver. The information in this profile applies to both forms of the drug: valproic acid (Depakene and Stavzor) and its related compound, divalproex sodium (Depakote). Divalproex sodium is made up of equal quantities of valproic acid and sodium valproate.

Cautions and Warnings

Do not take valproic acid if you are **allergic** or **sensitive** to any of its ingredients. Serious drug reactions involving multiple parts of the body have rarely been reported in people who have recently started taking valproic acid.

Use this drug with caution if you have a history of **liver problems**. Liver failure, sometimes resulting in death, has occurred in people taking valproic acid. **Children** under age 2 are at increased risk for liver failure associated with valproic acid, especially if they are also taking other anticonvulsants or have congenital disorders of metabolism, severe seizure disorders, mental retardation, or organic brain disease. After age 2, the risk of a fatal liver reaction decreases sharply. Ammonia in the bloodstream, another factor that worsens liver disease, may also occur with valproic acid. Your doctor should check your liver function before beginning valproic acid treatment and periodically thereafter.

Valproic acid should not be taken by those with known **urea cycle disorders** (a genetic disorder resulting in high levels of ammonia in the bloodstream).

Children and adults taking valproic acid have rarely developed cases of life-threatening pancreatitis (inflammation of the pancreas). Abdominal pain, nausea, vomiting, or appetite loss can be signs of pancreatitis and require immediate medical attention.

Valproic acid can affect platelet function, leading to bruising, bleeding, or changes in blood-clotting function.

Valproic acid may interfere with some urine tests of thyroid function.

Possible Side Effects

Side effects worsen as dosage increases.

▼ Most common: nausea, vomiting, diarrhea, abdominal pain, dizziness, indigestion, sedation or sleepiness, weakness, weight gain, emotional upset, depression, and changes in blood components.

▼ Less common: constipation, increased or decreased appetite, hair loss, change in menstrual periods, headache, loss of eye-muscle control, drooping eyelids, double vision, spots before the eyes, ringing in the ears, loss of muscle control or coordination, and tremors.

Drug Interactions

- Valproic acid may increase the depressive effects of alcohol, sleeping pills, antianxiety drugs, sedatives, phenobarbital, primidone, and other depressant drugs.
- Meropenem, cholestyramine, phenobarbital, primidone, and rifampin may reduce the amount of valproic acid in the blood.
- Dosages of barbiturates, carbamazepine, ethosuximide, lamotrigine, and phenytoin may need to be adjusted when you begin taking valproic acid.
- Aspirin, chlorpromazine, and felbamate may increase the risk of valproic acid side effects by increasing the amount of valproic acid in the blood.
- Mixing topiramate with valproic acid has led to high blood-ammonia levels with or without central-nervous-system symptoms, including sudden changes in mental status with tiredness or vomiting. In most cases, symptoms reverse when either drug is stopped.
- Valproic acid may increase the blood concentration and side effects of tricyclic antidepressants such as amitriptyline and nortriptyline.
- Valproic acid may affect warfarin, an oral anticoagulant (blood thinning) drug; your anticoagulant dose may need to be adjusted.
- Valproic acid may increase blood levels of zidovudine (also known as AZT).

Food Interactions

Food slows the absorption of valproic acid slightly, but you may take it with food if it upsets your stomach. The syrup form can be mixed with food to improve its taste.

Depakote Sprinkle can be taken whole or mixed with 1 tsp. of pudding, applesauce, or other soft food. Swallow the mixture promptly—do not chew.

Usual Dose

Adult: 5–7 mg per lb. a day to a maximum of 27 mg per lb. a day, or 500–1000 mg a day for migraine prevention.

Child (age 10 and over): 5–7 mg per lb. a day to a maximum of 27 mg per lb. a day.

Child (under age 10): not recommended.

Overdosage

Overdose may result in restlessness, hallucinations, flapping of the hands, coma, and death. Contact your local poison control center or take the victim to a hospital emergency room immediately. If you seek treatment, ALWAYS bring the prescription bottle or container.

Special Information

This medication may cause drowsiness. Be careful while driving or performing any task that requires concentration.

Contact your doctor at once if you develop nausea, vomiting, abdominal pain, or loss of appetite.

Do not chew or crush the capsules or tablets.

Do not switch brands of valproic acid without your doctor's knowledge. In at least 1 case, seizures resulted when a person was switched to a new product after 3 seizure-free years on another brand of valproic acid.

Valproic acid can cause mouth, gum, and throat irritation or bleeding, and increased risk of mouth infections. Maintain good dental hygiene while taking this drug. Dental work should be delayed if your blood counts are low.

People with a seizure disorder should carry special identification indicating their condition and any drugs being taken.

If you take valproic acid once a day and forget a dose, take it as soon as possible. If you do not remember until the next day, skip the dose you forgot and continue with your regular schedule. If you take valproic acid 2 or more times a day and forget a dose, take it as soon as possible if you remember within 6 hours of your regular time. Take the remaining daily dosage at evenly spaced intervals. Go back to your regular schedule the next day. Never take a double dose.

Special Populations

Pregnancy/Breast-feeding: Taking valproic acid during the first 3 months of pregnancy may increase the risk of birth defects, when many women are unaware of their pregnancy. Valproic acid should be taken during pregnancy only if your doctor determines that the potential benefit outweighs the risks.

Valproic acid passes into breast milk and may affect a nursing infant. Nursing mothers who must take this drug should use use infant formula.

Seniors: Seniors are more likely to experience side effects due to reduced kidney or liver function and may require lower dosage.

Valtrex *see **Acyclovir,** page 26*

Generic Name

Varenicline (var-EN-ih-clean)

Brand Names

Chantix

Type of Drug

Nicotinic acid receptor antagonist.

Prescribed For

Smoking cessation.

General Information

Varenicline binds to some of the same receptors that nicotine binds to in the nervous system. This binding satisfies the receptor's need for stimulation at a lower level than nicotine while preventing nicotine from binding to the receptor. The receptor blocked by varenicline is linked to another part of the central nervous system thought to be the basis for the feelings of reward associated with smoking. Preliminary studies indicate varenicline may also be beneficial in alcoholism, which involves the same brain receptors as nicotine addiction. It is eliminated unchanged from the body through the kidney in about 24 hours.

Cautions and Warnings

Do not take varenicline if you are **allergic** or **sensitive** to any of its ingredients. Allergic reactions may include severe rash or swelling of the face, lips, larynx (throat), and tongue, which may interfere with breathing. If this happens, go to a hospital at once. Contact your doctor if you develop a sore throat, mouth sores, abnormal heartbeat, sudden difficulty breathing, chest pain, persistent rash, or loss of taste perception.

People taking varenicline have committed or tried to commit suicide and also experienced suicidal thoughts and aggressive and erratic behavior. Some people experiencing these effects had no prior history of mental illness. Report any behavioral changes to your doctor.

People with **kidney disease** should use this drug with caution and may require a lower dose. It can be removed by dialysis.

People with heart disease who use varenicline have an increased risk of a cardiovascular event, including **heart attack**. However, this risk is small compared to the benefits of quitting smoking. Call your doctor if you have difficulty breathing, chest pain, or leg pain when walking. These may be signs of heart disease.

This drug may make you drowsy. Take care while driving or doing anything that requires concentration while you are taking varenicline.

Possible Side Effects

Side effects may increase with increased dosage.

- ▼ Most common: nausea—usually mild or moderate and lasting only a short time, but sometimes lasting for months—vomiting, sleeplessness, abnormal dreaming, constipation, and gas.
- ▼ Common: headache, abdominal pain, upset stomach, dry mouth, sleep disorders, loss of taste, tiredness or lethargy, not feeling well, weakness, and upper-respiratory conditions.
- ▼ Less common: increased or decreased appetite, gastroesophageal reflux disease, runny nose, difficulty breathing, rash, and itching.

Drug Interactions

- Taking supplemental nicotine (such as nicotine gum or patches) with varenicline can lead to more nausea, headache, vomiting, dizziness, upset stomach, and fatigue than with nicotine supplements alone.

- Cimetidine may increase blood levels of varenicline.
- Smoking cessation can change the way some drugs are broken down in the body. Insulin, warfarin, and theophylline doses may have to be altered.

Food Interactions

Varenicline should be taken after meals with a full glass of water.

Usual Dose

Adult: 0.5 mg a day for the first 3 days of treatment, then 0.5 mg morning and night for 4 days, then 1 mg morning and night for a total of 12–24 weeks. Stop smoking after 1 week of treatment or between 8 and 35 days after you have started taking varenicline. People with severe kidney disease may require no more than 0.5 mg twice a day.

Child: not recommended.

Overdosage

There have been only 2 confirmed reports of overdosage with this drug. Symptoms would be expected to be similar to its side effects. Contact your local poison control center or a hospital emergency room for more information. If you seek treatment, ALWAYS bring the prescription bottle or container.

Special Information

Continue trying to quit smoking after the first week of your treatment program, even if you slip up. It may take some time for you to feel comfortable not smoking or for you to stop. An additional 12 weeks of treatment at the full dose is recommended for people who have successfully stopped smoking with varenicline.

If you forget a dose, take it as soon as you remember. If it is almost time for the next dose, skip the one you forgot and continue with your regular schedule. Do not take a double dose.

Special Populations

Pregnancy/Breast-feeding: Animal studies of varenicline have not shown damage to a developing fetus. However, low birth weights and other effects developed in animals given very high doses of the drug. Varenicline should be taken during pregnancy only if your doctor determines that the potential benefit outweighs the risks.

It is not known if this drug passes into breast milk. Nursing mothers who must take this drug should use infant formula.

Seniors: Seniors may require a lower varenicline dosage because of the possibility of age-related reduced kidney function.

Generic Name

Venlafaxine (ven-luh-FAX-ene) G

Brand Names

Effexor
Effexor XR

The information in this profile also applies to the following drugs:

Generic Ingredients: Desvenlafaxine
Pristiq

Generic Ingredients: Duloxetine
Cymbalta

Generic Ingredients: Milnacipran
Savell

Type of Drug

Antidepressant.

Prescribed For

Venlafaxine is prescribed for major depressive disorder, generalized anxiety disorder, and social anxiety disorder. It is also used to treat premenstrual dysphoric disorder, hot flashes, and post-traumatic stress disorder. Desvenlafaxine is prescribed for major depressive disorder. Duloxetine is prescribed for major depressive disorder, generalized anxiety disorder, fibromyalgia, chronic musculoskeletal pain, including low back pain and osteoarthritis, and the management of pain related to diabetes. It may also be used to treat stress urinary incontinence. Milnacipran is prescribed for fibromyalgia.

General Information

Chemically different from other antidepressants, these drugs work by inhibiting the ability of nerve endings in the brain to absorb serotonin, norepinephrine and, to a lesser extent, dopamine. They are known as serotonin-norepinephrine reuptake inhibitors (SNRIs). Venlafaxine passes out of the body primarily via the urine. Duloxetine is broken down in the liver. Milnacipran is mostly released unchanged through the kidneys. The rest is broken down in the liver. It may take several weeks for these drugs to take effect.

Cautions and Warnings

Do not take venlafaxine or duloxetine if you are **allergic** or **sensitive** to any of their ingredients.

Antidepressants can increase the risk of suicidal thinking and behavior in **children** and **teenagers**. Although venlafaxine is not approved for use in children and teenagers, it is sometimes prescribed for this age group. People taking these drugs should be observed for possible worsening of **depression**, suicidal feelings, or unusual behavior changes when treatment is first started and whenever the drug dosage is changed. Symptoms can also occur when people suddenly stop their medicine or quickly lower their daily dose of these medicines.

The first sign of **bipolar disorder** may be a depressive episode. Your doctor should determine if you are at risk for bipolar disorder before prescribing one of these drugs. Antidepressants alone are not used to treat bipolar disorder and may set off a manic episode.

Rarely, people taking antidepressants develop a group of symptoms called serotonin syndrome, consisting of 1 or more of the following symptoms: excitement, a mild manic reaction, restlessness, loss of consciousness, confusion, disorientation, anxiety, agitation, muscle weakness, muscle spasms, tremors, involuntary muscle movements on one side of the body, shivering, dilated pupils, sweating, vomiting, and rapid heartbeat. Serotonin syndrome requires immediate medical treatment.

These medicines can raise blood pressure. Venlafaxine can also increase cholesterol levels. If this happens, your dosage of venlafaxine may need to be reduced. Venlafaxine has not been fully studied in people with recent heart attack or unstable heart disease, although a small study revealed no unusual changes in their electrocardiograms (ECGs). There was no ECG change in a study of people taking duloxetine.

People with uncontrolled **narrow-angle glaucoma** should use these medications with caution and should not use duloxetine. People with a diagnosis of **mania** or **hypomania** (elevated mood, increased activity, decreased need for sleep, grandiosity, racing thoughts) should be cautious when taking these medicines. Report any mood changes to your doctor at once.

People (including children) taking 1 of these medicines often experience weight loss. In studies, children treated with venlafaxine also grew less than those treated with placebo (sugar pill). The difference was greater for those under age 12 than for teens.

People with a **seizure disorder** should take these drugs with caution.

People taking one of these medicines may experience unusual bleeding or very low blood sodium. Sodium levels usually return to normal when you stop taking the medicine, but medical treatment is often necessary.

People with severe **kidney or liver disease** may require reduced dosages of these medications and should not take duloxetine. Liver failure has occurred with duloxetine. You should stop taking duloxetine if you develop symptoms of liver damage, including yellowing of the skin or whites of the eyes.

People taking duloxetine are more likely to develop serious skin reactions. Call your doctor at once if you develop blisters, peeling skin, rash or mouth/throat sores.

Possible Side Effects

Desvenlafaxine

The chance of side effects increases with drug dose.

- ▼ Most common: dizziness, nausea, dry mouth, diarrhea, appetite loss, constipation, headache, sleeplessness or sleepiness, sweating excessively, and sexual side effects in men.
- ▼ Common: vomiting, fatigue, appetite loss, tremors, anxiety, and erectile dysfunction in men.
- ▼ Less common: heart palpitations, rapid heartbeat, blood-pressure increase, chills, nervousness, jittery feelings, irritability, unusual dreams, weakness, weight loss, tingling in the hands or feet, loss of focus, difficult urination, yawning, blurred vision, ringing or buzzing in the ears, taste changes, dilation of the pupils, abnormal or loss of the ability to reach orgasm, and loss of sex drive.

Duloxetine

- ▼ Most common: nausea, dry mouth, constipation, loss of appetite, headache, dizziness, fatigue, and sleeplessness.
- ▼ Common: vomiting, diarrhea, loose stools, weakness, tiredness, sweating, anorexia, upset stomach, and viral infection of the nose, throat, sinuses, ears, Eustachian tubes, trachea, larynx, or bronchial tubes.

Possible Side Effects *(continued)*

- ▼ Less common: tremors, flushing, fever, blurred vision, anxiety, reduced sex drive, abnormal orgasm, muscle cramps or pain, tremors, weight loss, frequent daytime urination, ringing or buzzing in the ears when treatment is stopped, poor sleep quality, difficulty walking, anger and aggression, vaginal bleeding, seizures, uncontrollable leg movements, muscle spasms, erectile dysfunction, and delayed or other ejaculation problems (including ejaculation failure).
- ▼ Rare: Rare side effects can affect almost any part of the body. Contact your doctor if you experience anything unusual while taking any medication.

Milnacipran

- ▼ Most common: nausea, constipation, headache, dizziness, and sleeplessness.
- ▼ Common: rapid heartbeat, vomiting, dry mouth, upper-respiratory infection, migraines, and sweating excessively.
- ▼ Less common: heart palpitations, blurred vision, abdominal pain, chest pain, chills, chest discomfort, blood-pressure increase, appetite loss, tingling in the hands or feet, tremors, reduced sensitivity to touch and other senses, tension headache, anxiety, difficulty breathing, itching, rash, and skin flushing. Men treated with this drug can also experience painful urination, reduced urine flow, difficulty urinating, urinary retention, erection difficulty, failure to ejaculate, reduced sex drive, and pain in the testicles or scrotum.
- ▼ Rare: weight loss, night sweats, high blood cholesterol, hepatitis, and kidney failure. Rare side effects can develop in almost any part of the body. Contact your doctor if you experience anything unusual while taking any medication.

Venlafaxine

Side effects increase with dosage.

- ▼ Most common: blurred vision, tiredness, dry mouth, headache, sweating, dizziness, sleeplessness, nervousness, tremors, weakness, nausea, constipation, diarrhea, appetite loss, vomiting, impotence, and abnormal ejaculation.
- ▼ Less common: changes in sense of taste, ringing in the ears, cough, sore throat, dilated pupils, excessive sweating, high blood pressure, rapid heartbeat, anxiety, reduced

Possible Side Effects *(continued)*

sex drive, agitation, chills, yawning, extreme skin reactions, unusual bleeding, and inability to experience orgasm.

▼ Rare: Rare side effects can occur in almost any part of the body. Contact your doctor if you experience anything unusual while taking any medication.

Drug Interactions

- Taking an SNRI within 2 weeks of taking a monoamine oxidase inhibitor (MAOI) antidepressant may cause severe and sometimes fatal reactions, including high fever, muscle rigidity or spasm, mental changes, and fluctuations in pulse, temperature, or breathing rate. People stopping 1 of these drugs should wait at least 5 days before starting an MAOI.
- These medications should not be combined with other drugs that affect serotonin, due to the risk of serotonin syndrome (see "Cautions and Warnings"). Some of these drugs include other antidepressants, cyclobenzaprine, linezolid, lithium, metoclopramide, tramadol, triptan antimigraine drugs, and tryptophan.
- Mixing these drugs with warfarin, aspirin, NSAIDs, and other anticoagulants increases the risk of serious bleeding.

Desvenlafaxine/Venlafaxine

- Ketoconazole increases blood concentrations of desvenlafaxine and venlafaxine. Other azole antifungal medications may react similarly.
- Desvenlafaxine reduces levels of midazolam.
- Cimetidine can increase levels of venlafaxine in the blood. They should be combined with caution in the elderly and those with reduced liver function.
- Clozapine levels may be increased if taken with venlafaxine, with the potential for increased side effects, including seizures.
- Cyproheptadine decreases the effects of venlafaxine. The combination should be avoided.
- Venlafaxine increases the effects of dextromethorphan.
- Venlafaxine increases blood levels of haloperidol significantly. Haloperidol dosage should be adjusted when given with venlafaxine.
- Venlafaxine reduces levels of indinavir.

- Venlafaxine reduces the blood-pressure-lowering effect of metoprolol. Use caution when mixing these drugs.
- Both propafenone and venlafaxine levels are increased if they are given together. Dosages should be adjusted as necessary.
- The risk of serotonin syndrome is increased if venlafexine is combined with bupropion, fenfluramine, methylene blue, methylphenidate, nefazodone, or rasagiline.

Duloxetine

- The combination of duloxetine and thioridazine should be avoided.
- Duloxetine should not be taken by heavy alcohol users, due to an increased risk of liver damage.
- Cimetidine, ciprofloxacin, fluoxetine, fluvoxamine, paroxetine, quinidine, and terbinafine may increase duloxetine concentrations in the blood. Dosage adjustments may be necessary if duloxetine is combined with any of these.
- Duloxetine may increase concentrations of amphetamine, beta blockers (such as carvedilol, metoprolol, and propranolol), dextroamphetamine, flecainide, phentermine, propafenone, and theophylline. Monitoring and dosage adjustments may be necessary.

Milnacipran

- Milnacipran should not be taken by heavy alcohol users, due to an increased risk of liver damage.
- People switching from clomipramine to milnacipran are more likely to experience euphoria (feeling "high") or dizziness when rising from a sitting or lying position.
- Milnacipran may inhibit the blood-pressure-lowering effects of clonidine.
- Milnacipran may increase the effects of digoxin leading to very low blood pressure and rapid heartbeat. They should not be given together.

Food Interactions

Take each dose of venlafaxine with food. Duloxetine can be taken without regard to food or meals.

Usual Dose

Desvenlafaxine

Adult

Depression: 20–30 mg twice a day to start; maximum dose is 120 mg a day.

Diabetic Pain: 60 mg once a day.

Fibromyalgia and Muscle, Joint, and Back Pain: 30–60 mg a day.

Child: not recommended.

Duloxetine

Adult: 30–60 mg once a day. Dosages up to 120 mg a day in 1 or 2 doses have also been used. Swallow the tablets whole. Do not chew or crush duloxetine tablets or sprinkle them on your food.

Child: not recommended.

Milnacipran

Adult: 50–100 mg twice a day.

Child: not recommended.

Venlafaxine

Adult: 75–225 mg a day, divided into 2–3 doses. Some people may benefit from doses up to 375 mg a day. People with severe kidney or liver disease should receive ½ the usual daily dose. Those with moderate kidney disease may need their daily dosage reduced by only 25%.

Child: not recommended.

Overdosage

Symptoms of venlafaxine overdose may include tiredness, mild convulsions, and cardiac effects. Deaths from milnacipran overdose have been reported. Overdose symptoms include increased blood pressure, halted breathing, heart attack, changes in level of consciousness from sleepiness to coma, confusion, dizziness, and rises in liver enzyme levels. There is limited experience with duloxetine overdose. No cases of fatal duloxetine overdose have been reported, but 4 nonfatal cases have occurred in which people took between 300 and 1400 mg. Overdose victims should be taken to a hospital emergency room. If you seek treatment, ALWAYS bring the prescription bottle or container.

Special Information

Contact your doctor if you develop rash, hives, or any other allergic-type reaction or serious skin reaction.

Contact your doctor if you experience thoughts about suicide or dying; new or worsening depression or anxiety; feelings of panic, restlessness, or agitation; new or worsening irritability, aggressiveness, anger, or violence; an extreme increase in activity and talking (mania) or other unusual changes in behavior or mood; or trouble sleeping.

SNRIs may make you tired; be careful when driving or performing any task that requires concentration. Alcohol should be avoided when taking these drugs.

If you forget a dose, take it as soon as you remember. If it is almost time for your next dose, skip the dose you forgot and continue with your regular schedule. Do not take a double dose.

Do not suddenly stop taking these drugs. Dosage should be gradually reduced over a 2-week period. People stopping these medications may experience agitation, anxiety, confusion, dizziness, emotional disturbances, headache, feeling manic, sleep difficulties, irritability, lethargy, seizures, sensory disturbances (a feeling of electric shock sensations), and ringing in the ears. These effects generally clear up on their own, but some have been reported to be severe and may require further attention from your doctor.

Contact your doctor if you have possible symptoms of low blood-sodium levels, including headache, difficulty concentrating, memory loss, confusion, weakness, and unsteadiness, which can lead to falls. More severe sodium loss and/or sudden sodium loss can lead to hallucinations, fainting, seizures, coma, stopping breathing, and death.

Special Populations

Pregnancy/Breast-feeding: Animal studies of these drugs suggest they may cause problems for a developing fetus. Newborn babies exposed to drugs like duloxetine and venlafaxine late in the third trimester of pregnancy have developed complications requiring prolonged hospitalization, respiratory support, and tube feeding. An SNRI should be taken during pregnancy only if your doctor determines that the potential benefit outweighs the risks.

Desvenlafaxine, duloxetine, and venlafaxine pass into breast milk. It is not known if milnacipran passes into breast milk. Nursing mothers who must take an SNRI should use infant formula.

Seniors: Seniors may be more sensitive to side effects of these drugs because of expected loss of kidney function with advancing age.

Ventolin HFA *see **Albuterol,** page 51*

Brand Names

Veregen

Generic Ingredients

Sinecatechins

Type of Drug

Botanical wart remover.

Prescribed For

External genital and perianal warts.

General Information

This drug is a botanical ointment that is a partially purified fraction of green tea leaves. It is 85–95% catechins and the rest consists of caffeine, theobromine, and undefined botanical ingredients found in green tea leaves. The exact way that sinecatechins ointment works is not known. It is an antioxidant but the importance of that action is not known. In clinical studies of this product, it improved wart clearance by about 20% over that produced by a placebo ointment. It is not known how often warts treated with sinecatechins recur after treatment is completed. If new warts develop during treatment, they should also be treated with the ointment. The effect of this product on spreading genital or perianal warts is not known.

Cautions and Warnings

Do not use sinecatechins ointment if you are **allergic** or **sensitive** to any of its ingredients. Stop using it if you develop an allergic reaction.

This medication has not been studied for use beyond 16 weeks in a row or for more than 1 treatment.

Do not apply this product inside the vagina, anus, or to the eye or inside the mouth. It may be applied only to the skin.

Avoid using this product on an open wound or abraded skin.

Sinecatechins ointment has not been proven safe or effective in people whose immune system is not fully functional.

Avoid sun or ultraviolet light exposure to skin on which the ointment has been applied.

Possible Side Effects

- ▼ Most common: redness; raised blistery rash; skin erosion or ulceration; hardening of the skin to which the ointment is applied; swelling, itching, burning, pain, and discomfort at the site of application.
- ▼ Common: skin peeling.
- ▼ Less common: lymph node swelling, liquid discharge from the skin, bleeding, tightening of the foreskin (in uncircumcised men), allergic reaction, scarring, irritation, and rash.
- ▼ Rare: severe pain and inflammation, irritation of the urinary tract, infection around the area of the anus, skin color changes, dryness, eczema, loss of feeling, and other side effects can also occur. Contact your doctor if you experience anything unusual while taking any medication.

Drug Interactions

- Do not apply any other topical medication or skin product to the treatment area while using sinecatechins ointment.

Usual Dose

Adult: Apply 3 times a day to all warts as directed by your doctor. Do not bandage or wrap the area. Continue using the ointment until all warts have cleared, up to 16 weeks.

Child: not recommended.

Overdosage

There have been no reports of sinecatechins overdose. In the event of an accidental overdose, contact your local poison control center for more information. If you seek treatment, ALWAYS bring the ointment container with you to the hospital emergency room.

Special Information

Wash your hands before and after applying the ointment. You must also wash and dry the skin before you apply the ointment; report severe skin reactions to your doctor. Should the reaction be very severe, you can remove the ointment by washing it off with mild soap and water.

Avoid sexual contact while the ointment is on the skin. If you choose to have sexual contact, wash the ointment off beforehand. Sinecatechins ointment can weaken condoms and diaphragms.

Women using tampons should insert the tampon before applying the ointment to avoid accidentally transmitting the ointment to inside the vagina.

Uncircumcised men treating warts under their foreskin should pull back the foreskin and cleanse the area every day before applying the ointment directly to the warts.

Sinecatechins ointment can stain your clothing and bedding.

Special Populations

Pregnancy/Breast-feeding: This medication did affect some pregnant rabbits but was generally free of birth defects in animal studies. There is no information on how this drug affects pregnant women. Sinecatechins ointment should be used during pregnancy only if your doctor determines that the potential benefit outweighs the risks.

It is not known if sinecatechins ointment passes into breast milk. Nursing mothers who must use it should use infant formula.

Seniors: Only a small number of seniors have used this ointment. It is not known if there are any differences between seniors and younger adults.

VESIcare *see **Overactive Bladder Drugs,** page 884*

Viagra *see **Erectile Dysfunction Drugs,** page 453*

Generic Name

Vigabatrin (vie-GA-ba-trin)

Brand Names

Sabril

Type of Drug

Antiepileptic.

Prescribed For

Vigabatrin is added to other medicines for infantile spasms, epilepsy, complex partial seizures, and secondary generalized seizures when those drugs do not work alone.

General Information

Vigabatrin inhibits an enzyme that is responsible for breaking down the neurotransmitter gamma-aminobutyric acid (GABA), increasing GABA levels. GABA slows central-nervous-system function and works against seizures. It is the first treatment to be approved specifically for infantile spasms, a rare kind of seizure disorder, and has been used as an antiepileptic agent in special situations in which other medicines have not proven effective. Infantile spasms are a severe seizure disorder that usually appears when the baby is 4–8 months old. Infantile spasms can be devastating because of the large number of hard-to-control seizures the child can experience every day.

Cautions and Warnings

Do not take this drug if you are **allergic** or **sensitive** to any of its ingredients.

Vigabatrin carries a risk of blindness. It appears to irreversibly damage parts of the retinal nerve. This damage can occur even with small doses, but the degree of risk increases with daily dose. People who are **partially blind** or have another problem with their sight may be at risk for further damage to their eyesight.

Like other medicines for seizure disorders, vigabatrin dose must be slowly reduced over 2–4 weeks. You risk seizures if you stop taking it without gradual reduction. **Absence seizures** can worsen while taking vigabatrin.

People with a history of **psychosis**, **depression**, or **behavioral problems** can experience worsening of their condition.

Most of this drug is eliminated through the kidneys. People with **reduced kidney function** may require lower doses of vigabatrin.

Possible Side Effects

- ▼ Most common: tiredness and hyperactivity (children).
- ▼ Common: weight gain.
- ▼ Less common: abdominal pain, constipation, vomiting, nausea, headache, dizziness, fainting, nervousness, depression, memory disturbances, double vision and other visual changes, aggression, personality changes, loss of coordination while performing normal movements, weakness, adult hyperactivity, confusion, sleeplessness, and loss of the ability to concentrate.

Possible Side Effects *(continued)*

▼ Rare: anxiety, emotional instability, irritability, tremors, upset stomach, increased appetite, changes in gait or walk, and speech changes. Contact your doctor if you experience anything unusual while taking any medication.

Drug Interactions

- Vigabatrin causes an increase in the breakdown of other seizure-control medicines, including carbamazepine, fosphenytoin, and phenytoin. Dose adjustment may be required.
- Vigabatrin can cause small decreases in phenobarbital blood levels.
- Alcohol and other nervous system depressants can worsen the drowsiness and dizziness associated with vigabatrin.

Food Interactions

This drug can be taken without regard to food or meals. Vigabatrin powder must be dissolved in a small amount of water, fruit juice, infant formula, or milk before you take it. Let the powder completely dissolve and drink all of the liquid right away.

Usual Dose

Adult and Child (age 3 and over): 1–3 g a day in 1 or 2 doses; no more than 6 g a day.

Child (age 1 month–2 years): 25–75 mg per lb. of body weight every day, given in 1 or 2 doses.

Overdosage

Usual overdose symptoms are drowsiness, dizziness, fainting, headache, psychotic reactions, unusual behavior, trouble breathing, slow heartbeat, low blood pressure, agitation, irritability, confusion, difficulty talking, and coma. Overdose victims must be taken to a hospital emergency room. If you seek treatment, ALWAYS bring the prescription bottle or container.

Special Information

See your eye doctor every 6 months while taking vigabatrin.

Contact your doctor immediately if your eyesight changes or you have trouble seeing, or if you experience a personality change.

This drug can make you drowsy. Be very careful driving or doing complex or dangerous tasks while you are taking it.

Do not suddenly stop taking vigabatrin. Dosage should be gradually reduced, particularly in infants and children.

If you forget to take a dose of vigabatrin, take it as soon as you remember. If it is almost time for your next dose, skip the forgotten dose and continue with your regular schedule. Do not take a double dose of this medicine. Contact your doctor if you often forget this medication.

Special Populations

Pregnancy/Breast-feeding: Animal studies show vigabatrin can damage the developing fetus. It should be taken during pregnancy only if your doctor determines that the potential benefit outweighs the risks.

Nursing mothers must use infant formula while taking this medicine because of the risk of blindness and other drug side effects.

Seniors: Seniors may require less medication because of reduced kidney function.

Vigamox *see **Fluoroquinolone Anti-infectives,** page 512*

Generic Name

Vilazodone (vil-AZ-oh-doan)

Brand Names

Viibryd

Type of Drug

Antidepressant.

Prescribed For

Major depression.

General Information

Vilazodone is the first of a new class of antidepressants called indolalkylamines. It is a serotonin reuptake inhibitor (SSRI) but, unlike traditional SSRI medicines, it also stimulates 1 of the key serotonin receptors. Vilazodone is recommended for people who do not do well with other antidepressants, though early studies compared it favorably to other SSRI antidepressants. Because of its dual mechanism, vilazodone may work faster than traditional SSRIs, but it takes at least 2 weeks to reach maximum effect. It is broken down by enzymes produced in the liver.

Cautions and Warnings

Do not use vilazodone if you are **allergic** or **sensitive** to any of its ingredients.

Do not mix this medicine with a monoamine oxidase inhibitor (MAOI) drug or within 2 weeks of having stopped an MAOI because of a serious and possibly fatal interaction. Potential symptoms include tremor, muscle twitching, sweating, nausea, vomiting, flushing, dizziness, elevated body temperature, and symptoms similar to neuroleptic malignant syndrome: seizures, rigidity, and mental status changes that include extreme agitation progressing to delirium and coma.

Rarely, people taking SSRIs develop a group of symptoms called serotonin syndrome, consisting of 1 or more of the following symptoms: excitement, a mild manic reaction, restlessness, loss of consciousness, confusion, disorientation, anxiety, agitation, muscle weakness, muscle spasms, tremors, involuntary muscle movements on one side of the body, shivering, dilated pupils, sweating, vomiting, and rapid heartbeat. Serotonin syndrome requires immediate medical treatment.

Low blood sodium has occurred in people taking SSRI medicines though this has not occurred with vilazodone. People taking a diuretic, those who are **dehydrated**, and **seniors** can be at greater risk of developing low blood sodium with SSRIs.

Antidepressants have been associated with an increased risk of suicide, especially in teenagers. Suicide is always a risk in severely depressed people, who should only be allowed to have minimal quantities of medication in their possession.

Do not use vilazodone if you are recovering from a **heart attack**. People with a history of **heart disease** should not use vilazodone, because it may cause abnormal heart rhythms.

Vilazodone has not been studied in people with **seizure disorders** and should be used with caution if you have this condition.

Vilazodone is not approved for bipolar disorder and should be taken for this purpose only if it has been prescribed by a qualified psychiatrist.

Rarely, priapism (a persistent, painful erection) has occurred with vilazodone. If this happens, stop taking the drug and contact your doctor. One-third of these cases may require surgery or may lead to a permanent inability to achieve erection.

Possible Side Effects

- ▼ Common: diarrhea, nausea, dry mouth, dizziness.
- ▼ Less common: fatigue, feeling jittery, vomiting, upset stomach, gas, stomach pain, tiredness, tingling in the hands or feet, tremors, sleeplessness, unusual dreams, reduced sex drive, restlessness, difficulty achieving orgasm or erection, heart palpitations, joint pain, and increased appetite.
- ▼ Rare: Other side effects appear in fewer than 1 in 1000 people. They can affect your heart, eyes, nervous system, mood, and skin. Contact your doctor if you experience anything unusual while taking any medication.

Drug Interactions

- Mixing vilazodone with an MAOI antidepressant can result in a severe, possibly fatal interaction (see "Cautions and Warnings"). Separate doses of vilazodone and an MAOI by 2 weeks.
- Mixing vilazodone with medications that affect serotonin may result in symptoms of serotonin syndrome (see "Cautions and Warnings"). Some of these drugs include buspirone, other SSRIs, serotonin-norepinephrine reuptake inhibitors (SNRIs), tramadol, triptan antimigraine medications, and tryptophan. Do not mix tryptophan with vilazodone.
- Vilazodone may affect other drugs that act on the nervous system, including alcohol, sedatives, and stimulants.
- Aprepitant, atazanavir, clarithromycin, delavirdine, diltiazem, erythromycin, fluconazole, indinavir, itraconazole, ketoconazole, nefazodone, nelfinavir, ritonavir, saquinavir, telithromycin, verapamil, and voriconazole slow the clearance of vilazodone, increasing the chance of vilazodone side effects. Your doctor may cut your maximum dose of vilazodone in ½ if you are also taking one of these medicines.
- Vilazodone may raise the amount of amodiaquine, cerivastatin, paclitaxel, repaglinide, sorafenib, and torsemide by interfering with their breakdown in the body.

- SSRI medicines can increase bleeding risk. Avoid aspirin, warfarin, and other blood-thinning medicines while taking vilazodone.
- Vilazodone may cause a small reduction in blood pressure. Your dosage of high-blood-pressure medication may need to be reduced slightly when you start taking vilazodone.
- Carbamazepine, corticosteroids, efavirenz, modafinil, nevirapine, oxcarbazepine, phenobarbital, phenytoin, pioglitazone, rifabutin, rifampin, St. John's wort, and troglitazone can speed the breakdown of vilazodone, reducing its effectiveness.

Food Interactions

Take vilazodone with food to maximize the amount of drug absorbed and reduce the risk of upset stomach, dizziness, and lightheadedness. Avoid grapefruit juice because it can slow the clearance of vilazodone from the body.

Usual Dose

Adult: 10 mg once a day for 7 days, then 20 mg once a day for another 7 days, and then an increase to 40 mg once a day.

Child: not recommended.

Overdosage

Vilazodone overdose is likely to make you lethargic or restless, have hallucinations, or become disoriented. Other overdose effects include those associated with serotonin syndrome (see "Cautions and Warnings"). Victims should be taken to a hospital emergency room. If you seek treatment, ALWAYS bring the prescription bottle or container with you.

Special Information

Be careful when driving or performing any task that requires concentration. Avoid alcohol or other depressant drugs while taking vilazodone.

Contact your doctor if you develop any side effect, especially blood in the urine, dizziness, or lightheadedness. Vilazodone may cause dry mouth, irregular heartbeat, nausea, vomiting, or breathing difficulties.

If you forget a dose, take it as soon as possible. If it is within 4 hours of your next dose, skip the dose you forgot and go back to your regular schedule. Do not take a double dose.

Do not stop taking vilazodone unless advised to do so by your doctor. Dosage should be gradually reduced instead of abruptly stopped. Adverse events of abrupt discontinuation of vilazodone include the following: sadness, moodiness, irritability, agitation, dizziness, tingling or electric shock sensations, anxiety, confusion, headache, lethargy, sleeplessness, ringing or buzzing in the ears, and seizures. These reactions generally pass but serious symptoms can occur.

Special Populations

Pregnancy/Breast-feeding: Vilazodone's effect on the developing fetus is not known. Animal studies are not conclusive. Infants born to mothers who take an SSRI-type antidepressant during their pregnancy may need prolonged hospital care due to difficulty breathing or feeding, seizures, temperature instability, vomiting, low blood sugar, abnormal muscle tone, overactive reflexes, tremors, jitteriness, irritability, and constant crying. Vilazodone should be taken during pregnancy only if your doctor determines that the potential benefit outweighs the risks.

Vilazodone passes into breast milk. Nursing mothers who must take it should use infant formula.

Seniors: Seniors may take vilazodone without special precautions, though older adults may be more sensitive to drug side effects.

Vivelle *see **Estrogens,** page 466*

Voltaren *see **Nonsteroidal Anti-inflammatory Drug (NSAID) Eye Drops,** page 860*

Generic Name

Vorinostat (vah-RIN-oh-stat) G

Brand Names

Zolinza

Type of Drug

HDAC inhibitor.

Prescribed For

T-cell lymphoma of the skin.

General Information

Vorinostat is prescribed for people whose lymphoma has persisted, progressed, or recurred on or after 2 systemic treatments for T-cell lymphoma of the skin, which affects fewer than 200,000 Americans. Vorinostat works by inhibiting HDAC enzymes produced in large amounts by certain cancers. In clinical studies of the drug, 25–30% of people taking it responded to treatment. HDAC inhibitors are emerging as a new class of anticancer agents for the treatment of solid and blood cancers.

Cautions and Warnings

Do not take vorinostat if you are **allergic** or **sensitive** to any of its ingredients.

Vorinostat can cause blood clots to form in the lungs or some veins. Anemia and low blood-platelet count may be caused by this drug. Contact your doctor if you develop symptoms of a blood clot (see "Special Information"). Gastrointestinal bleeding can occur with vorinostat. Nausea, vomiting, and diarrhea that are serious enough to require treatment can also occur.

Vorinostat can cause high blood sugar.

Vorinostat can affect your heart, so your doctor will periodically monitor your heart function.

This drug is broken down in the liver and people with **liver disease** must be treated with caution. It has not been studied in people with **kidney disease**.

Possible Side Effects

About 10% of people taking vorinostat must have their drug dose modified due to a drug side effect.

▼ Most common: diarrhea, fatigue, nausea, low blood-platelet count, appetite loss, weight loss, muscle spasms, hair loss, dry mouth, taste changes, kidney damage, chills, vomiting, constipation, dizziness, anemia, leg swelling, headache, and itching.

Possible Side Effects *(continued)*

▼ Common: cough, fever, and upper-respiratory infections.

▼ Rare: Rare side effects can occur in almost any part of the body. Contact your doctor if you experience anything unusual while taking any medication.

Drug Interactions

- Mixing this drug with warfarin and similar blood-thinning drugs can lead to excessive bleeding.
- Mixing vorinostat with valproic acid can increase the risk of bleeding.

Food Interactions

Take vorinostat with food.

Usual Dose

Adult: 400 mg once a day. Dosage may be reduced to 300 mg once a day for 5 days in a row every week if you have trouble tolerating this drug.

Child: Consult your doctor.

Overdosage

Little is known about vorinostat overdose. Overdose victims should be taken to a hospital emergency room. If you seek treatment, ALWAYS bring the prescription bottle or container.

Special Information

Contact your doctor if you develop any of the following symptoms: cough, blood in the sputum, sudden difficulty breathing, rib pain when you take a breath, chest pain, rapid breathing, rapid heart rate, wheezing, clammy skin, bluish skin discoloration, pain in the pelvis area, leg pain, swelling in the legs, a lump (possibly painful) that appears on or near a vein, low blood pressure, dizziness or fainting, sweating, or anxiety. These can be signs that a blood clot formed in a lung or vein.

Drink 2 quarts of liquid every day to avoid becoming dehydrated while taking vorinostat.

If you forget your daily dose of vorinostat, take it as soon as you remember. If it is almost time to take your next dose, skip the forgotten dose and take your next daily dose at the regular time. Do not take a double dose.

Special Populations

Pregnancy/Breast-feeding: Vorinostat can harm a developing fetus. This drug should be taken during pregnancy only if your doctor determines that the potential benefit outweighs the risks.

It is not known if vorinostat passes into breast milk. Nursing mothers who must take it should use infant formula.

Seniors: Seniors may be more sensitive to the side effects of vorinostat, although no dose adjustment is necessary.

Vytorin *see **Ezetimibe,** page 480*

Vyvanse *see **Adderall,** page 38*

Generic Name

Warfarin (WOR-far-in) G

Brand Names

Coumadin Jantoven

Type of Drug

Oral anticoagulant (blood thinner).

Prescribed For

Blood clots or coagulation; also prescribed for reducing the risk of small-cell carcinoma of the lung, recurrent heart attack or stroke, and transient ischemic attack (TIA).

General Information

Warfarin prevents the formation of blood clots or coagulation by suppressing the body's production of vitamin-K-dependent factors essential to the coagulation process. If you are taking warfarin, you must take it exactly as prescribed. Notify your doctor at the earliest sign of unusual bleeding or bruising; blood in your urine or stool; or black, tarry stools. Warfarin may be affected by many other drugs, and these interactions may be dangerous (see "Drug Interactions"). One-third of people respond to warfarin in unexpected ways that can be explained by genetic differences. Lab tests are available to help doctors determine the best dose of warfarin for individual patients. Warfarin may also be extremely dangerous if not used properly. Periodic blood-clotting tests are necessary for proper control of warfarin therapy.

Cautions and Warnings

Do not take warfarin if you are **allergic** or **sensitive** to any of its ingredients.

Warfarin must be taken with care if you have any **blood-clotting disease.** Use of warfarin may be dangerous and should be discussed with your doctor if you have past or planned **eye or nervous system surgery**; **protein C deficiency**—a hereditary condition; **liver inflammation or disease**; **kidney disease**; any **infection** being treated with an antibiotic; active **tuberculosis**; severe or prolonged **dietary deficiencies**; **stomach ulcer or bleeding**; **bleeding from the genital or urinary areas**; **high blood pressure**; severe **diabetes**; **vein irritation**; **disease of the large bowel**, such as **diverticulitis** or **ulcerative colitis**; and subacute bacterial **endocarditis.**

Anticoagulant therapy may increase the release of micro plaques into the bloodstream. These micro plaques may block very small blood vessels, leading to purple toe syndrome (a condition that occurs when pressure exerted by normal walking leads to bleeding into the skin of your toes). This usually goes away when anticoagulant treatment is stopped, but it may be a sign of a more serious problem present in another part of your body.

Women taking anticoagulants may be at risk of ovarian bleeding when they ovulate.

People taking warfarin must be extremely careful to avoid cuts, bruises, or other injuries that may cause internal or external bleeding.

Possible Side Effects

▼ Most common: bleeding, which may occur with usual dosages and even when the results of blood tests used to monitor anticoagulant therapy are normal. If you bleed abnormally while you are taking anticoagulants, contact your doctor immediately. This includes abnormally heavy menstruation or vaginal bleeding between periods.

Possible Side Effects *(continued)*

▼ Less common: abdominal cramps, nausea, vomiting, diarrhea, fever, anemia, adverse effects on blood components, hepatitis, jaundice (symptoms include yellowing of the skin or whites of the eyes), itching, rash, hair loss, sore throat or mouth, red or orange urine, painful or persistent erection, and purple toe syndrome.

Drug Interactions

Anticoagulants may have more drug interactions than any other kind of medication. Your doctor and pharmacist should keep records of all drugs you take in order to anticipate possible interactions. It is essential that your doctor and pharmacist know about every medication you are taking, including over-the-counter drugs containing aspirin and herbal medicine.

- Drugs that may increase the effect of warfarin include the following: acetaminophen; aminoglycoside antibiotics; amiodarone; androgen; aspirin and other salicylate drugs; beta blockers; cephalosporin antibiotics; chloral hydrate; chloramphenicol; chlorpropamide; cimetidine; corticosteroids; cyclophosphamide; dextrothyroxine; diflunisal; disulfiram; erythromycin; fluconazole; gemfibrozil; glucagon; hydantoin antiseizure drugs—blood levels of the hydantoins may also be increased in this interaction; ifosfamide, an influenza virus vaccine; isoniazid; ketoconazole; leflunomide; loop diuretics; lovastatin; metronidazole; miconazole; mineral oil; moricizine; nalidixic acid; nonsteroidal anti-inflammatory drugs (NSAIDs); omeprazole; orlistat; oxandrolone; penicillin; phenylbutazone; propafenone; quinidine; quinine; quinolone antibacterials; sulfa drugs; sulfinpyrazone; tamoxifen; tetracycline antibiotics; thiamine; thyroid hormones; and vitamin E.
- Some drugs decrease the effect of warfarin and the interaction may be just as dangerous. Some examples are alcohol, aminoglutethimide, ascorbic acid (vitamin C), barbiturates, carbamazepine, chlorthalidone, cholestyramine, contraceptive drugs, dicloxacillin, estrogen, ethchlorvynol, etretinate, glutethimide, griseofulvin, meprobamate, nafcillin, rifampin, spironolactone, sucralfate, thiazide-type diuretics, trazodone, and vitamin K.

- Warfarin should not be combined with any anticoagulant supplements, including chamomile, garlic, ginkgo biloba, and ginseng.

Food Interactions

Warfarin is best taken on an empty stomach because food slows the rate at which it is absorbed by the blood. Vitamin K counteracts the effects of warfarin. Avoid eating large quantities of vitamin-K-rich foods, such as spinach and other green, leafy vegetables. Any change in dietary habits or alcohol intake may affect warfarin's action.

Usual Dose

Adult: 2–10 mg on the first day, 2–15 mg or more a day thereafter; dosage must be individualized.

Overdosage

The primary overdose symptom is bleeding. Bleeding may make itself known by the appearance of blood in the urine or stool, an unusual number of black-and-blue marks, oozing of blood from minor cuts, or bleeding from the gums after brushing the teeth. If bleeding does not stop within 10–15 minutes, contact your doctor. Your doctor may tell you to skip a dose of warfarin or go to a hospital or doctor's office for blood evaluations, or may give you a prescription for vitamin K, which antagonizes the effect of warfarin. This last approach has some dangers because it may complicate subsequent anticoagulant therapy. If you seek treatment, ALWAYS bring the prescription bottle or container.

Special Information

Do not change warfarin brands without your doctor's knowledge. Different brands may not be equivalent.

Do not stop taking warfarin unless directed to do so by your doctor.

Do not stop or start ANY other medication without your doctor's or pharmacist's knowledge. Avoid alcohol, aspirin and other salicylates, and drastic changes in your diet, because all of these may affect your response.

Contact your doctor if you develop unusual bleeding or bruising, red or black tarry stool, or red or dark-brown urine.

Warfarin may turn your urine a red or orange color. This is different from blood in the urine—which causes urine to appear red or brownish in color—and generally happens only if your urine has less acid in it than normal.

If you forget a dose, take it as soon as you remember, then continue with your regular schedule. If you do not remember until the next day, skip the missed dose and continue with your regular schedule. Do not take a double dose. Contact your doctor if you miss a dose.

Special Populations

Pregnancy/Breast-feeding: Warfarin is not considered safe for use during pregnancy. It passes into the fetal circulation and causes bleeding, brain and other abnormalities, and stillbirth in 30% of fetuses. In some pregnant women, the benefit of taking warfarin may outweigh its risks, but the drug should not be used during the first 3 months of pregnancy. Pregnant women who need an anticoagulant are often given heparin because it does not cross into the fetal bloodstream.

Warfarin passes into breast milk in an inactive form. Full-term babies are not affected by warfarin. The effect on premature babies is not known. Nursing mothers who must take warfarin should consider using infant formula.

Seniors: Seniors may be more sensitive to the effects of warfarin and obtain maximum benefit with smaller dosages.

Xalatan *see **Prostaglandin Agonists,** page 953*

Type of Drug

Xanthine Bronchodilators (ZAN-thene)

Brand Names

Generic Ingredient: Aminophylline G

Generic Ingredients: Dyphylline
Lufyllin

Generic Ingredients: Oxtriphylline
Choledyl SA

Generic Ingredients: Theophylline G

Elixophyllin
Theo-24
Theo-X
Theochron
Theolair
Uniphyl

Prescribed For

Asthma and bronchospasm associated with emphysema, bronchitis, and other diseases; also prescribed for essential tremors and chronic obstructive pulmonary disease.

General Information

Xanthine bronchodilators are a mainstay of therapy for bronchial asthma and similar diseases. Although the dosage of each of these drugs is different, they all work by relaxing bronchial muscles and helping to reverse spasms. The exact way in which they work is not known.

Some xanthine bronchodilators are sustained-release products that act throughout the day. These minimize potential side effects by avoiding the peaks and valleys associated with immediate-release xanthine drugs. They also allow you to reduce the total number of daily doses.

Initial treatment with a xanthine bronchodilator requires your doctor to take blood samples to assess how much of the drug is in your blood. Dosage adjustments may be required based on these blood tests and on your response to the therapy. Because the liver does not eliminate dyphylline, it is not subject to many of the drug interactions or limitations placed on the other xanthine bronchodilators.

Cautions and Warnings

Do not use a xanthine bronchodilator if you are **allergic** or **sensitive** to any of its ingredients.

If you have a **stomach ulcer**, **congestive heart failure**, **heart disease**, **liver disease**, **low blood-oxygen levels**, or **high blood pressure**, or are an **alcoholic**, you should use this drug with caution.

People with **seizure disorders** should not take a xanthine bronchodilator unless they are receiving appropriate anticonvulsant medicines.

Theophylline may cause or worsen pre-existing **abnormal heart rhythm**. Any change in heart rate or rhythm warrants your doctor's immediate attention.

Status asthmaticus, a medical condition in which the breathing passages are almost completely closed, does not respond to oral bronchodilators. People who experience this condition must be taken to a hospital emergency room at once for treatment.

Serious side effects, including convulsions and serious arrhythmias, may be among the initial signs of drug toxicity and could be fatal. Periodic monitoring of blood levels by your physician is mandatory if you are taking one of these drugs. Do not change your dose without consulting your doctor.

Dosage of dyphylline must be altered in the presence of **kidney failure**.

Xanthine bronchodilators should be used with caution in **children**, who may develop toxic blood levels more easily than adults.

Possible Side Effects

Side effects are directly related to the amount of drug in your blood. As long as you stay in the proper range—below 20 mcg per mL of blood—you should experience few, if any, problems.

- ▼ Most common: nausea; vomiting; stomach pain; diarrhea; headache; irritability; restlessness; difficulty sleeping; rectal irritation or bleeding, especially with suppositories; and rapid breathing.
- ▼ Less common: excitability, heartburn, high blood sugar, muscle twitching or spasms, heart palpitations, seizures, brain damage, or death. These effects are more likely when drug levels reach 35 mcg per mL or more.
- ▼ Rare: vomiting blood, regurgitating stomach contents while lying down, fever, headache, rash, hair loss, and dehydration. Contact your doctor if you experience anything unusual while taking any medication.

Drug Interactions

- Taking 2 xanthine bronchodilators together may increase side effects.
- Xanthine bronchodilators are often given in combination with a stimulant drug such as ephedrine. Such combinations can cause excessive stimulation and should be used only as your doctor specifically directs.
- Reports have indicated that combining allopurinol, beta blockers, calcium channel blockers, cimetidine—and, rarely, ranitidine—clarithromycin, contraceptive drugs, corticosteroids, disulfiram, ephedrine, erythromycin, flu vaccine,

interferon, mexiletine, quinolone antibacterials, thiabendazole, or zafirlukast with a xanthine bronchodilator may increase blood levels of the xanthine bronchodilator. Higher blood levels mean the possibility of more side effects. Tetracycline and alcohol may also increase the risk for xanthine bronchodilator side effects.

- The following drugs may decrease theophylline levels: aminoglutethimide, barbiturates, charcoal, ketoconazole, phenytoin and other hydantoin anticonvulsants, rifampin, sulfinpyrazone, and sympathomimetic drugs. The hydantoin level may also be reduced.
- Smoking cigarettes or marijuana makes xanthine bronchodilators less effective by increasing the rate at which your liver breaks them down. This does not apply to dyphylline.
- Drugs that may either increase or decrease xanthine bronchodilator levels include carbamazepine, furosemide and other loop diuretics, and isoniazid. People combining a xanthine bronchodilator with one of these drugs must be evaluated individually. Consult your doctor when combining xanthine bronchodilators with any of these drugs.
- People with an overactive thyroid clear xanthine bronchodilators faster and may require a larger dose. People with an underactive thyroid have the opposite reaction. Correcting thyroid function through medical or surgical treatment will normalize your response to a xanthine bronchodilator.
- A xanthine bronchodilator may counteract the sedative effect of diazepam and other benzodiazepines.
- Xanthine bronchodilators may interfere with or interact with a number of different drugs used during anesthesia. Your doctor may temporarily alter your bronchodilator dose or change drugs to avoid this problem.
- Blood-lithium levels may be lowered by xanthine bronchodilators.
- Probenecid may increase the effects of dyphylline by interfering with its removal from the body through the kidneys.
- Xanthine bronchodilators may counteract the sedative effects of propofol and zafirlukast.

Food Interactions

To obtain a consistent effect from your medication, take it at the same time each day on an empty stomach, at least 1 hour before or 2 hours after meals.

Theophylline is eliminated from the body faster if your diet is high in protein and low in carbohydrates. Eating char-grilled beef also aids theophylline elimination. Conversely, the rate at which your body eliminates theophylline is reduced by a high-carbohydrate, low-protein diet. You may take some food with a liquid or immediate-release xanthine bronchodilator if it upsets your stomach. Dyphylline is not affected in this way.

Caffeine—a xanthine derivative—may add to the side effects of the xanthine bronchodilators, except dyphylline. Avoid large amounts of caffeine-containing products, such as coffee, tea, cola, cocoa, and chocolate, while taking one of these drugs.

Usual Dose

Aminophylline

Adult and Child (age 16 and over): 100–200 mg every 6 hours. Sustained-release—200–500 mg a day in 1–3 doses.

Child (under age 16): 50–100 mg every 6 hours, or 1–2.5 mg per lb. of body weight every 6 hours.

Dyphylline

Adult: up to 7 mg per lb. of body weight every 6 hours. Dosage is reduced when kidney failure is present.

Child: not recommended.

Oxtriphylline

Adult and Child (age 10 and over): about 2 mg per lb. of body weight every 6 hours. Sustained-release—400–600 mg every 12 hours.

Child (age 1–9): 2.8 mg per lb. of body weight every 6 hours.

Theophylline

Adult: up to 6 mg per lb. of body weight a day, in divided doses at 6- or 8-hour intervals, to a maximum daily dose of 900 mg. Sustained-release—same dosage, but taken 1–3 times a day.

Child (age 12–16): up to 8.1 mg per lb. of body weight a day.

Child (age 9–11): up to 9 mg per lb. of body weight a day.

Child (age 1–8): up to 10.8 mg per lb. of body weight a day.

Infant (under 52 weeks): Your doctor will calculate total daily dosage in mg by a formula that factors in age and weight. Under 6 months, give ⅓ the total daily dosage every 8 hours; age 26 weeks–1 year, give ¼ the total daily dosage every 6 hours.

Premature Infant (age 25 days and over): 0.68 mg per lb. of body weight every 12 hours.

Premature Infant (age 1–24 days): 0.45 mg per lb. of body weight every 12 hours.

Dosage of xanthine bronchodilators is often calculated on the basis of theophylline equivalents and must be tailored to your specific condition. The best dose is the lowest that will control your symptoms. Children break down xanthine bronchodilators faster than adults and usually require more drug per lb. of body weight.

Overdosage

The first symptoms of overdose are loss of appetite, nausea, vomiting, nervousness, difficulty sleeping, headache, and restlessness. These symptoms are followed by rapid or abnormal heart rhythm, unusual behavior, extreme thirst, delirium, convulsions, very high temperature, and collapse. These serious toxic symptoms are rarely experienced after overdose by mouth, which generally produces loss of appetite, nausea, vomiting, and stimulation. The overdose victim should be taken to a hospital emergency room immediately. If you seek treatment, ALWAYS bring the prescription bottle or container.

Special Information

Do not chew or crush coated or sustained-release capsules or tablets. Doing so could result in the immediate release of large amounts of the drug, possibly causing serious side effects.

To ensure consistent effectiveness, take your medication at the same time and in the same way, with or without food, every day.

Contact your doctor if you develop nausea, vomiting, heartburn, sleeplessness, jitteriness, restlessness, headache, rash, severe stomach pain, convulsions, or a rapid or irregular heartbeat. Acute drug toxicity may descend abruptly, with little or no warning; serious side effects such as convulsions, life-threatening arrhythmias, and death may result. Periodic monitoring by your physician is mandatory if you are taking a xanthine bronchodilator.

Do not change xanthine bronchodilator brands without notifying your doctor or pharmacist. Different brands of the same bronchodilator may not be identical in their effect on your body.

If you forget to take a dose of your xanthine bronchodilator, take it as soon as you remember. If it is almost time for your next dose, skip the dose you forgot and continue with your regular schedule. Do not take a double dose.

Special Populations

Pregnancy/Breast-feeding: Xanthine bronchodilators pass into the fetal circulation. They do not cause birth defects, but they may produce dangerous drug levels in a newborn's bloodstream. Babies born to women who take one of these drugs may be nervous, jittery, and irritable, and may gag or vomit when fed. Pregnant women who must use a xanthine bronchodilator to control asthma or other conditions should take one only if their doctor determines that the potential benefit outweighs the risks.

These drugs pass into breast milk and may cause a nursing infant to be nervous and irritable or to have difficulty sleeping. Nursing mothers who must use one of these drugs should use infant formula.

Seniors: Seniors, especially men age 55 and over, may take longer to clear the xanthine bronchodilators from their bodies. Seniors with heart failure or other cardiac conditions, chronic lung disease, a viral infection with fever, or reduced liver function may require a lower dosage of this medication to account for the clearance effect.

Xopenex *see **Albuterol,** page 51*

Yaz *see **Contraceptives,** page 316*

Zetia *see **Ezetimibe,** page 480*

Generic Name

Zonisamide (zoh-NIS-uh-mide) G

Brand Names

Zonegran

Type of Drug

Anticonvulsant.

Prescribed For

Partial seizures.

General Information

The exact way that this drug works is unknown, but studies suggest it may affect sodium and calcium flow in and out of nerve cells.

Cautions and Warnings

Do not take zonisamide if you are **allergic** or **sensitive** to any of its ingredients or to sulfa drugs.

People taking this drug are more likely to have suicidal thoughts or attempt suicide.

Some people taking zonisamide are at a greater risk of developing a dangerous imbalance in body electrolytes (sodium, potassium, chloride, and bicarbonate) known as metabolic acidosis. When this happens, the blood becomes too acidic, causing symptoms of chest pain, heart palpitations, headache, severe anxiety, difficulty seeing, nausea, vomiting, abdominal pain, appetite and weight changes, muscle weakness, and bone pain. Deep, rapid breathing can help to alleviate symptoms, but this condition must be treated in a hospital. Your doctor will check your blood-electrolyte levels before treatment.

Unexplained skin rash may be a sign of a severe reaction that can be fatal. Contact your doctor immediately if you experience this side effect.

Zonisamide has been associated with serious blood conditions.

Zonisamide has been associated with central-nervous-system side effects, including depression, psychosis, sleepiness, psychomotor slowing, and difficulty concentrating.

People with severe **kidney disease** may accumulate ⅓ more zonisamide in their blood than others. Lower dosages may be required. Kidney stones are more likely to develop in people taking zonisamide.

Zonisamide should be used with caution by those with **liver disease**.

People taking zonisamide may be at increased risk of having heatstroke, especially **children**.

People who suddenly stop taking zonisamide may experience increased seizures. Anticonvulsant drugs should be reduced gradually.

Possible Side Effects

- ▼ Most common: sleepiness, appetite loss, dizziness, headache, nausea, agitation, and irritability.
- ▼ Common: anxiety, poor muscle coordination, confusion, depression, difficulty concentrating, memory problems, sleeplessness, abdominal pain, and double vision.
- ▼ Less common: kidney stones, mental slowing, tiredness, unusual eye movements, tingling in the hands or feet, psychotic behavior, constipation, diarrhea, upset stomach, verbal difficulty, taste changes, dry mouth, easy bruising, flu-like symptoms, rash, runny nose, and weight loss.
- ▼ Rare: Rare side effects can occur in almost any part of the body. Contact your doctor if you experience anything unusual while taking any medication.

Drug Interactions

- Some drugs may reduce the amount of zonisamide in the blood by stimulating enzymes that break it down in the liver. They include carbamazepine, phenobarbital, phenytoin, and valproate.
- Acetazolamide, dichlorphenamide, and topiramate may increase the amount of zonisamide in the blood, increasing the risk of side effects, including kidney stone formation.
- Zonisamide should be used with caution with drugs that depress the central nervous system, such as alcohol and narcotic analgesics.

Food Interactions

Zonisamide can be taken without regard to food or meals. Avoid drinking grapefruit juice with zonisamide because it can interfere with enzymes that break down the drug.

Usual Dose

Adult and Child (age 16 and over): 100–400 mg a day. Most people taking zonisamide do well with doses in the 100–200-mg range. Higher doses may offer some additional benefit, but they are also associated with an increase in drug side effects.

Child (under age 16): not recommended.

Overdosage

Overdose symptoms primarily affect the central nervous system, including very low heart rate, coma, low blood pressure, and difficulty breathing. Take the victim to a hospital emergency room. If you seek treatment, ALWAYS bring the prescription bottle or container.

Special Information

Contact your doctor at once if you develop an unexplained skin rash. This may be a sign of a severe reaction.

Sudden back pain, abdominal pain, and blood in the urine may be signs of a kidney stone. Drink plenty of water every day to avoid this problem. Contact your doctor if you experience any of these side effects.

Fever, sore throat, ulcers, and easy bruising can be signs of a blood problem related to zonisamide. Contact your doctor if any of these symptoms develop.

Zonisamide may make you drowsy. Be careful while driving or performing any tasks that require coordination and alertness.

If you forget a dose of zonisamide, take it as soon as you remember. If it is almost time for your next dose, skip the dose you forgot and continue with your regular schedule. Do not take a double dose.

Special Populations

Pregnancy/Breast-feeding: Animal studies of zonisamide have shown it can cause birth defects. Seizure disorder itself has been associated with increased risk of birth defects. Zonisamide should be taken during pregnancy only if your doctor determines that the potential benefit outweighs the risks.

It is not known if zonisamide passes into breast milk. Nursing mothers taking zonisamide should use infant formula.

Seniors: Seniors may require a lower dose of zonisamide due to normal reductions in kidney or liver function.

Zyprexa *see* ***Olanzapine,*** *page 961*

Twenty Questions to Ask Your Doctor and Pharmacist About Your Prescription

Many pharmacies now routinely hand out prescription drug "fact sheets" when a medication is first prescribed. If your pharmacist does not provide you with one, ask him or her for a copy.

1. What is the name of this medication?
2. What results may be expected from taking it?
3. How long should I wait before reporting if this medication does not help me?
4. How does the medication work?
5. What is the exact dosage of the medication?
6. What time of day should I take it?
7. Do alcoholic beverages have an effect on this medication?
8. Do I have to take special precautions with this medication in combination with other prescription medications I am taking?
9. Do I have to take special precautions with this medication in combination with over-the-counter or herbal medications?
10. Does food have any effect on this medication?
11. Are there any special instructions I should have about how to use this medication?
12. How long should I continue taking this medication?

13. Is my prescription renewable?

14. For how long a period may my prescription be renewed?

15. Which side effects should I report, and which ones may I disregard?

16. May I save any unused part of this medication for future use?

17. How should I store this medication?

18. How long may I keep this medication without it losing its strength?

19. What should I do if I miss a dose of this medication?

20. Does this medication come in a less expensive, generic form?

Safe Drug Use

- Store your medications in a sealed, light-resistant container to maintain maximum potency, and be sure to follow any special storage instructions listed on your prescription bottle or container, such as "refrigerate," "do not freeze," "protect from light," or "keep in a cool place." Protect all medications from excessive humidity; do not keep them in your bathroom medicine cabinet.
- Make sure each doctor you see knows about all the medications you use regularly, including prescription, over-the-counter (OTC), and herbal medications.
- Keep a record of any bad reaction you have had to a medication.
- Fill each prescription you are given. If you do not fill a prescription, make sure your doctor knows you are not taking the medication.
- Try to fill your prescriptions at the same pharmacy each time. Your pharmacist will keep a record of all your prescription and OTC medications. This listing, called a "Patient Drug Profile," is used to check for potential problems. You may want to keep your own drug profile and take it to your pharmacist for review whenever a new medication is added.
- Do not take extra medication without consulting your doctor or pharmacist.
- Read all the information that comes with your prescription before taking your medication for the first time. Many, but not all, prescription drugs come with a Patient Information Sheet approved by the U.S. Food and Drug Administration (FDA).
- Follow the label instructions exactly. If you have any questions, call your doctor or pharmacist.
- Report any unusual symptoms that develop after taking any medication.
- Always read and check the prescription label before taking a dose of your medication, especially if you are taking multiple medications. Do not trust your memory.

- Be sure the label stays on the container until the medication is used or destroyed.
- Keep the label facing up when pouring liquid medication from the bottle so that it is not obscured by spilled medicine.
- For liquid medication, do not forget to shake the bottle, unless directed otherwise.
- Do not share your medication with anyone. Your prescription was written for you and only you. Do not use a prescription medication unless it has been specifically prescribed for you.
- If you move to another city, ask your pharmacist to forward your prescription records to your new pharmacy. Carry important medical facts about yourself in your wallet. Such things as drug allergies, chronic diseases (e.g., diabetes), and special requirements may be very useful. Whenever you travel, carry your prescription in its original container.

Safe Use of Eye Drops

To administer eye drops, lie down or tilt your head back. Hold the dropper above your eye, gently squeeze your lower lid to form a small pouch, and release the drop or drops of medication inside your lower lid while looking up. Release the lower lid, keeping your eye open. Do not blink for 40 seconds. Press gently on the bridge of your nose at the inside corner of your eye for 1 minute to help circulate the drug in your eye. To avoid infection, do not touch the dropper tip to your finger, eyelid, or any other surface. Wait at least 5 minutes before using another eye drop or eye ointment.

Safety Tips for Self-injectables

Syringe Storage, Disposal, and Safety

- Store your syringes and needles where others do not have access to them. Some medicines come in pre-filled syringes. Store them according to label directions.
- Do not reuse needles or syringes.
- After you have finished using a syringe and needle, cut the needle off and dispose of the needle and syringe in a puncture-resistant, non-see-through container used only for

this purpose. Containers specifically designed for needle and syringe disposal can be obtained from a pharmacy.

- Most needles have a device built in so that you may safely cut the needle off. If you do not have one of these devices, you can break the needle off by covering the needle with its protective sheath and working it back and forth until it breaks. Broken needles should be discarded in your disposal device or plastic container.
- Keep containers in areas that are child- and animal-proof.
- When the container is full, seal it securely and throw the entire container away with your regular garbage. Do not throw loose syringes into the garbage.
- Do not put containers filled with used syringes in your recycling bin.
- Do not throw loose needles or lancets into the recycling bin or trash.
- Do not put needles and syringes in soda cans or bottles, glass containers, or milk cartons.
- Do not flush needles or lancets down the toilet.

Choosing an Injection Site

Choose an area for injection where the skin is loose and soft, away from joints, nerves, and bones. Try to avoid the panty or belt line at the waist and the seat portion of your buttocks, as daily activity may irritate these areas.

Good places to use for subcutaneous (under the skin) injection include:

- Arms (outer and upper back portion)
- Abdomen (except around navel and waistline)
- Buttocks (upper outer area)
- Thighs (front and sides except at groin and knee)

Rotating Injection Sites

Change the site where you inject your medicine each time. This helps prevent reactions at the injection site. It also gives the site time to heal from the last injection. Keep a record of where and when you last gave yourself an injection to make sure you do not use the same site too often. If your regular injection areas become tender, talk to your doctor about other possible injection sites.

Self-injection and Administering Injections to Another Person

- Before you begin, gather your needle and syringe, medicine, alcohol swabs, and cotton balls or gauze pad. Be sure you also have your needle disposal container nearby.
- Do not use an injection solution if it has particles floating in it.
- Certain injection mixtures should not be shaken. Refer to your product patient information for specific instruction.
- Wash your hands.
- Choose an area for injection. Use a different site each day. Do not use any area in which you feel lumps, bumps, firm knots, or pain. Do not use any area in which the skin is discolored, depressed, scabbed, or has broken open.
- You may use an alcohol swab to clean the skin at the injection site. Let the area air dry. Discard the wipe. Uncap the needle.
- Slowly draw the exact amount of drug prescribed into the syringe, being careful to avoid air bubbles in the solution to be injected.
- Pinch up the skin to prevent injecting the drug into a muscle.
- Hold the syringe like a pencil or dart and insert the needle at a 45° angle to the skin.
- Pull back slightly on the plunger to make sure you have not entered a vein. If blood enters the syringe, remove it and throw it away.
- If no blood enters the syringe, slowly depress the syringe plunger until the contents have been completely injected.
- Hold another alcohol swab on the injection site. Remove the needle from the skin. Gently massage the injection site with a dry cotton ball or gauze pad.
- You may ice the area before and after injection to reduce pain and inflammation.
- If injecting into the leg, extend your leg out to reduce the chance of injecting into a muscle.
- Your doctor, nurse, or pharmacist can help you master this procedure.

Complications of Self-injection

- You may notice bruising around the injection. This is due to the piercing of tiny blood vessels and is generally not a problem.

- Sometimes harmless but unsightly lumpy areas develop a injection sites. This is due to an increase in fatty tissue at the site of injection, especially when injecting daily insulin. Avoid injecting into these fatty lumps.
- Visible depressions in the skin may develop due to a loss of fat tissue at the injection site.
- To avoid infection at injection sites, always wash your hands before you begin the procedure, do not touch the bare needle before the actual injection, and do not reuse or share needles with another person.
- Call your doctor if an injection site becomes infected. Signs of infection include redness, pain, swelling, and possible oozing. You may apply a nonprescription antibiotic cream or ointment to that area, but your doctor should be aware of this complication.

Infusion Therapy

When a patient's condition cannot be effectively treated using oral medication, infusion therapy is often the next choice of treatment. Most infusion therapy is administered by the intravenous (IV) route and is increasingly carried out at home or in an outpatient setting. This is a safe and effective alternative to inpatient care for many diseases and treatments. It may be preferable to a hospital stay and can offer a convenient and effective approach to long-term therapy. Implanted or portable infusion pumps are especially useful in the management of chronic conditions such as diabetes.

Each IV medicine has a unique delivery rate, and the way in which it is administered is selected based on this rate. Some IV drugs are designed for rapid delivery over a few minutes to obtain the best effect and are administered by rapid injection straight into a vein using a syringe. Other drugs are most effective when delivered slowly, either intermittently at specific times or continuously throughout the day in an IV solution.

IV medications are most often given through a catheter inserted into a peripheral vein (any vein not inside the chest or abdomen) but may also be administered through an implanted vascular access port, or through a central line where a catheter is inserted into one of the large veins close to the heart.

Guidelines for giving IV medications must be followed to avoid serious complications from the drug injection. To avoid medication rrors, health care practitioners should always follow the 5 "rights" of medication administration—the right patient, the right drug, the right dose, the right time, and the right route—before administering any medication. If you are receiving an IV medicine, you should also check that the person administering it is following these five "rights." Additionally, some IV medications can cause severe tissue damage if they infiltrate into tissue surrounding the IV site. This can happen if the vein is damaged during insertion or if a vein scars or ruptures. This is particularly likely in elderly people with fragile veins or in those who have had a device incorrectly inserted or in place for too long.

Alert your health care professional immediately if you have any unusual feelings or discomfort during or after the administration of your medication. The following are possible complications of IV therapy:

- Infection
- Movement of the IV fluid into tissue surrounding the IV port (IV infiltration)
- Serious tissue damage when drugs are injected into infiltrated IV sites
- Blood clot formation inside a vein (thrombosis), which may cause swelling or discoloration of the skin
- Injection of air
- Serious drug reactions such as very low blood pressure, heart arrhythmias, and cardiac arrest
- Allergic reaction to the medication
- Pain at the IV site

Preparing for Self-administration

- Wash your hands thoroughly with soap before you start.
- Gather together all of the materials you will need, including the medicine, syringes, needles, and tubing.
- Cleanse the area you will be working on with soap or an alcohol-based hand sanitizer. Alcohol swabs may be used to clean the injection site. This is the most important single step in protecting against infection.
- Wash your hands again for 2 minutes with soap or an alcohol-based hand sanitizer before administering the medicine.

Medicine and Money

- Make sure you tell your doctor everything about your health problem. More information allows your doctor to provide the most effective treatment.
- Do not hesitate to discuss the cost of medical care with your doctor or pharmacist.
- Generic drugs are usually less expensive than brand-name drugs, whether you pay for them out-of-pocket or have a co-pay with your insurance company. A drug often becomes available generically when its patent has expired, typically 20 years after the patent was granted.
- If you suffer from a chronic condition, you will probably save money by buying in larger quantities.
- Prescription prices vary from pharmacy to pharmacy; it may be worthwhile to comparison shop for the more expensive medications. Internet pharmacies may also have low-cost prescription drugs available, although you must allow additional time for delivery. Many pharmacies will match Internet prices, if requested.
- Some insurance companies offer discounted quantities of prescription drugs through a mail-order pharmacy program. Most mail-order programs will fill a three-month supply of medication and only charge the co-pay for a two-month supply. Again, extra time must be factored in for delivery.

The Top 200 Prescription Drugs in the United States

RANKED BY NUMBER OF PRESCRIPTIONS DISPENSED FROM JANUARY TO DECEMBER 2010

(Note: Generic drugs by different manufacturers and different formulations of the same drug have been combined.)

1. Hydrocodone + acetaminophen
2. Lisinopril
3. Simvastatin
4. Levothyroxine
5. Amoxicillin
6. Amlodipine
7. Azithromycin
8. Alprazolam
9. Hydrochlorothiazide
10. Omeprazole
11. Metformin
12. Lipitor
13. Furosemide
14. Metoprolol
15. Atenolol
16. Sertraline
17. Zolpidem
18. Oxycodone + acetaminophen
19. Citalopram
20. Gabapentin
21. Ibuprofen
22. Nexium
23. Prednisone
24. Tramadol
25. Plavix
26. Singulair
27. Lisinopril + hydrochlorothiazide
28. Fluoxetine
29. Lorazepam
30. Warfarin
31. Clonazepam
32. Lexapro
33. Fluticasone
34. Cyclobenzaprine
35. Cephalexin
36. Sulfamethoxazole + trimethoprim
37. Crestor
38. Fexofenadine
39. Amoxicillin + potassium clavulanate
40. Ciprofloxacin
41. Pravastatin
42. Trazodone
43. Lovastatin
44. Triamterene + hydrochlorothiazide
45. Carvedilol
46. Advair
47. Alendronate
48. Ranitidine
49. Meloxicam
50. Diazepam

51. Diovan
52. Naproxen
53. Propoxyphene-N + acetaminophen*
54. Fluconazole
55. Methylprednisolone
56. Doxycycline
57. Paroxetine
58. Oxycodone
59. Clonidine
60. Amitriptyline
61. Allopurinol
62. Enalapril
63. Carisoprodol
64. Acetaminophen + codeine
65. Klor-Con
66. Pantoprazole
67. Actos
68. Potassium chloride
69. Temazepam
70. Seroquel
71. Promethazine
72. Glimepiride
73. Albuterol
74. Tamsulosin
75. Folic acid
76. Levaquin
77. Spironolactone
78. Lantus
79. Nasonex
80. Viagra
81. Amphetamine salt
82. Lyrica
83. Celebrex
84. Triamcinolone
85. Digoxin
86. Lamotrigine
87. Cefdinir
88. Diltiazem
89. Benazepril
90. Topiramate
91. Isosorbide
92. Concerta
93. Ramipril
94. Spiriva
95. Risperidone
96. Premarin
97. Glyburide
98. Penicillin
99. Zetia
100. Lansoprazole
101. Clindamycin
102. Bupropion
103. Metronidazole
104. Vytorin
105. Glipizide
106. Divalproex sodium
107. Abilify
108. Tri-Sprintec*
109. Loestrin 24 Fe
110. Losartan potassium
111. Vyvanse
112. Cialis
113. Suboxone
114. Phentermine
115. Mirtazapine
116. Hydroxyzine
117. Estradiol
118. Aricept
119. Valacyclovir
120. Benicar
121. Diclofenac
122. Januvia
123. Nitrofurantoin
124. Verapamil
125. Lunesta
126. Niaspan
127. Venlafaxine
128. Xalatan

*No longer available.

129. Mupirocin
130. Buspirone
131. Gemfibrozil
132. Ondansetron
133. Famotidine
134. Sumatriptan
135. Promethazine + codeine
136. Propranolol
137. Terazosin
138. Polyethylene glycol
139. Meclizine
140. Acyclovir
141. Fentanyl
142. Methotrexate
143. Finasteride
144. NuvaRing
145. Ocella*
146. Ferrous sulfate
147. Benzonatate
148. Lovaza
149. Yaz
150. Methadone
151. Cheratussin AC
152. Tizanidine
153. Quinapril
154. NovoLog
155. Butalbital + acetaminophen + caffeine
156. Metoclopramide
157. Clotrimazole + betamethasone
158. Doxazosin
159. Methocarbamol*
160. Budeprion
161. Combivent
162. Namenda
163. Detrol
164. Ortho Tri-Cyclen Lo
165. Clobetasol
166. Sprintec*
167. Nifedipine
168. Aspirin
169. Fenofibrate
170. Levetiracetam
171. Nitroglycerin
172. Chlorhexidine gluconate
173. Baclofen
174. Aciphex
175. Losartan + hydrochlorothiazide
176. Endocet
177. Dicyclomine
178. Avapro
179. Clarithromycin
180. Bisoprolol + hydrochlorothiazide
181. Bystolic
182. Glyburide + metformin
183. Adderall
184. Symbicort
185. Zyprexa
186. Nabumetone
187. Boniva
188. Hydroxychloroquine
189. Benztropine
190. Ropinirole
191. Minocycline
192. TriNessa
193. Phenazopyridine
194. Pristiq
195. Lidoderm
196. Phenytoin
197. Ketoconazole
198. Humalog
199. Vigamox
200. Prednisolone

*No longer available.

Index of Generic and Brand-Name Drugs

How to Find Your Medication in *The Pill Book*

- *The Pill Book* lists most medications in alphabetic order by generic name because a medication may have many brand names but has only 1 generic name. Most generic medications produce the same therapeutic effects as their brand-name equivalents but are much less expensive. Drugs that are available generically are indicated by the [G] symbol.
- When a medication has 2 or more active ingredients, it is listed by the most widely known brand name. In some cases, pill profiles are listed by drug type (e.g., Sulfonylurea Antidiabetes Drugs).
- *The Pill Book* includes the names of the top 100 brand-name drugs (cross-referenced to their generic name) in alphabetic order with the pill profiles.
- Most over-the-counter (OTC) medications are not included in *The Pill Book*. For complete information on OTC medications, refer to *The Pill Book Guide to Over-the-Counter Medications*.
- All brand and generic names are listed in the Index. Brand names are indicated by **boldface**.
- Sugar-free and alcohol-free brand-name drugs are indicated by the [S] and [A] symbols in the beginning of each pill profile.

ABOUT THE EDITOR

Educated at Columbia University, Dr. Harold Silverman has been a hospital pharmacist, industry consultant, author, and educator for more than 40 years. Dr. Silverman's professional goal has always been to help people better understand why medicines are prescribed and how to get the most from them.

In addition to *The Pill Book,* Dr. Silverman has also authored *The Women's Drug Store, The Pill Book Guide to Safe Drug Use, The Consumer's Guide to Poison Protection,* and *Travel Healthy.* He is also a co-author of *The Vitamin Book: A No-Nonsense Consumer Guide* and *The Med-File Drug Interactions System.*

Dr. Silverman has contributed more than 70 articles, research papers, and textbook chapters to the professional literature, including *The Merck Manual of Medical Information, Home Edition.* He has taught pharmacology and clinical pharmacy at several universities and has won numerous awards for his work. Dr. Silverman resides in the Washington, D.C. area with his wife Judith Brown and their son Joshua.